CURRENT
Diagnosis & Treatment
Cardiology

FOURTH EDITION

Edited by

Michael H. Crawford, MD
Professor of Medicine
Lucy Stern Chair in Cardiology
Chief of Clinical Cardiology
University of California, San Francisco

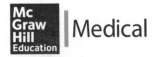

Mc Graw Hill Education | Medical

New York   Chicago   San Francisco   Athens   London   Madrid   Mexico City
Milan   New Delhi   Singapore   Sydney   Toronto

2 3 4 5 6 7 8 9 0   DOC/DOC   18 17 16 15 14

ISBN 978-0-07-180127-0
MHID 0-07-180127-8
ISSN 1079-1051

Notice

Medicine is an ever-changing science. As new research and clinical experience broaden our knowledge, changes in treatment and drug therapy are required. The authors and the publisher of this work have checked with sources believed to be reliable in their efforts to provide information that is complete and generally in accord with the standards accepted at the time of publication. However, in view of the possibility of human error or changes in medical sciences, neither the authors nor the publisher nor any other party who has been involved in the preparation or publication of this work warrants that the information contained herein is in every respect accurate or complete, and they disclaim all responsibility for any errors or omissions or for the results obtained from use of the information contained in this work. Readers are encouraged to confirm the information contained herein with other sources. For example and in particular, readers are advised to check the product information sheet included in the package of each drug they plan to administer to be certain that the information contained in this work is accurate and that changes have not been made in the recommended dose or in the contraindications for administration. This recommendation is of particular importance in connection with new or infrequently used drugs.

This book was set in Minion Pro by Cenveo® Publisher Services.
The editors were Christine Diedrich and Harriet Lebowitz.
The production supervisor was Catherine Saggese.
The cover designer was Thomas DePierro.
Project management was provided by Sapna Rastogi, Cenveo Publisher Services.
RR Donnelley was printer and binder.

This book is printed on acid-free paper.

International Edition ISBN 978-1-25-909532-0 ; MHID 1-25-909532-0.
Copyright © 2014. Exclusive rights by McGraw-Hill Education, for manufacture and export. This book cannot be re-exported from the country to which it is consigned by McGraw-Hill Education. The International Edition is not available in North America.

Contents

30. Pulmonary Hypertension 396

Christopher F. Barnett, MD, MPH & Teresa De Marco, MD

31. Congenital Heart Disease in Adults 416

Ian S. Harris, MD & Elyse Foster, MD

Section VI. Systemic Disease & the Heart

32. Cardiac Tumors 459

Bill P.C. Hsieh, MD & Rita F. Redberg, MD, MSc

33. Cardiovascular Disease in Pregnancy 474

Kirsten Tolstrup, MD

34. Endocrinology & the Heart 494

Eveline Oestreicher Stock, MD

Authors

Amr E. Abbas, MD
Co-Director, Echocardiography Laboratory
Beaumont Hospital
Royal Oak, MI
Aortic Stenosis

Mohamad Alkhouli, MD
Cardiology Fellow
Temple University Hospital
Philadelphia, PA
Lipid Disorders

Karthik Ananthasubramaniam, MD
Associate Professor of Medicine, Wayne State University
Director, Nuclear Cardiology and Echocardiography
    Laboratory
Program Director, Advanced Cardiac Imaging Fellowship
Senior Staff Physician, Division of Cardiology, Department
    of Internal Medicine
Henry Ford Hospital
Detroit, MI
Hypertrophic Cardiomyopathies

Richard W. Asinger, MD
Professor of Medicine, University of Minnesota
Director, Cardiac Rehabilitation Laboratory
Hennepin County Medical Center
Minneapolis, MN
Long-Term Anticoagulation for Cardiac Conditions

Nitish Badhwar, MD
Associate Professor of Medicine
Stone-Chamberlain Chair in Cardiology Associate Chief,
    Cardiac Electrophysiology
University of California
San Francisco, CA
Ventricular Tachycardia

Christopher F. Barnett, MD, MPH
Assistant Professor of Medicine
Division of Cardiology
University of California, San Francisco
San Francisco General Hospital
San Francisco, CA
Pulmonary Hypertension

Andrew J. Boyle, MBBS, PhD
Associate Professor of Medicine
Division of Cardiology
University of California
San Francisco, CA
Acute Myocardial Infarction

Kang-Yuh Chyn, MD, PhD
Assistant Professor of Medicine
University of California, Los Angeles
Staff Cardiologist Cedars-Sinai Medical Center
Los Angeles, CA
Unstable Angina/Non-ST Evaluation Myocardial Infarction

Michael H. Crawford, MD
Professor of Medicine
Lucie Stern Chair in Cardiology
Chief of Clinical Cardiology
University of California
San Francisco, CA
*Approach to Cardiac Disease Diagnosis, Chronic Ischemic
    Heart Disease, Preoperative Evaluation, Syncope,
    Aortic Regurgitation, Mitral Regurgitation, Tricuspid
    and Pulmonic Valve Disease, Infective Endocarditis,
    Myocarditis*

Andrew E. Darby, MD
Assistant Professor of Medicine
University of Virginia
Charlottesville, VA
Sudden Cardiac Death

John P. DiMarco, MD, PhD
Professor of Medicine, University of Virginia
Cardiovascular Division
University of Virginia Health System
Charlottesville, VA
Sudden Cardiac Death

John A. Elefteriades, MD
William W.L. Glenn Professor of Surgery
Director, Aortic Institute at Yale-New Haven
Yale University School
New Haven, CN
Thoracic Aortic Aneurysms & Dissections

Antonio B. Fernandez, MD
Director, Cardiac Intensive Care Unit
Hartford Hospital
Hartford, CT
The Athlete's Heart

Elyse Foster, MD
Director, Adult Non-invasive Cardiology
Arexe Valensky Chair of Cardiology
Professor of Medicine
University of California
San Francisco, CA
Congenital Heart Disease in Adults

Nora F. Goldschlager, MD
Professor of Clinical Medicine
University of California
Chief, Clinical Cardiology, San Francisco General Hospital
Director, CCU, ECG Lab and Pacemaker Clinic, San
    Francisco General Hospital
San Francisco, CA
Conduction Disorders & Cardiac Pacing

James A. Goldstein, MD
Director of Research and Education
Department of Cardiovascular Medicine
Beaumont Health System
Royal Oak, MI
Restrictive Cardiomyopathies

Saurabh Gupta, MD
Director, Cardiac Catheterization Laboratories
Co-Director, Complex Heart Valve Service
Knight Cardiovascular Institute
Oregon Health and Science University
Portland, Oregon
Antiplatelet Therapy

Ian S. Harris, MD
Assistant Professor of Medicine
Director, Adult Congenital Cardiology Program
Division of Cardiology
University of California School of Medicine
San Francisco, CA
Congenital Heart Disease in Adults

Brian D. Hoit, MD
Professor of Medicine and Physiology and Biophysics
Case Western Reserve University
Director of Echocardiography, Case Medical Center
University Hospitals of Cleveland
Cleveland, OH
Tricuspid and Pulmonic Valve Disease

Richard H. Hongo, MD
Assistant Director, Electrophysiology Program
California Pacific Medical Center
San Francisco, CA
Conduction Disorders & Cardiac Pacing

Bill Pei Chin Hsieh, MD
Advanced Cardiac Imaging Fellow
Cedars Sinai Medical Center
Los Angeles, CA
Attending Cardiologist
Long Life Cardiac Center
Alhambra, CA
Cardiac Tumors

Massimo Imazio, MD
Chief of the Myopericardial and Heart Failure Clinic
Cardiology Department, Maria Vittoria Hospital
Torino, Italy
Pericardial Disease

Harish Jarrett, MBChB
Internal Medicine Resident
Temple University Hospital
Philadelphia, PA
Lipid Disorders

Liviu Klein, MD, MS
Assistant Professor of Medicine
University of California, San Francisco
Associate Director,
Mechanical Circulatory Support & Heart Failure Device
    Program
Heart Failure with Reduced Ejection Fraction

Peter R. Kowey, MD
Professor of Medicine
Jefferson Medical College
Chief, Division of Cardiovascular Diseases
Lankenau Hospital
Philadelphia, PA
Supraventricular Tachycardias

D. Elizabeth Le, MD
Staff Physician, Portland VA Medical Center
Clinical Associate Professor of Medicine
Knight Cardiovascular Institute
Oregon Health and Science University
Portland, OR
Mitral Stenosis

Byron K. Lee MD, MAS
Associate Professor of Medicine
Director of the Electrophysiology Laboratories and Clinics
Division of Cardiology
University of California
San Francisco, CA
Supraventricular Tachycardias

Steven J. Lester, MD
Associate Professor of Medicine
Mayo Medical School
Consultant in Cardiology
Mayo Clinic, Arizona
Aortic Stenosis

Ashvarya Mangla, MD
Chief Resident, Internal Medicine
Weiss Memorial Hospital
University of Illinois at Chicago
Chicago, IL
Antiplatelet Therapy

Teresa De Marco, MD
Professor, Clinical Medicine and Surgery
R.H. and Jane G. Logan Endowed Chair in Cardiology
Director, Heart Failure and Pulmonary Hypertension
Medical Director, Heart Transplantation
University of California
San Francisco, CA
Pulmonary Hypertension

Edward McNulty, MD
Clinical Assistant Professor of Medicine
University of California, San Francisco
Assistant Physician-in-Chief, Cardiovascular & Thoracic
    Services
Kaiser San Francisco Medical Center
San Francisco, CA
Cardiogenic Shock

Rajni K. Rao, MD
Cardiology Clinic Practice Chief
Assistant Professor of Medicine
University of California
San Francisco, CA
Pulmonary Embolic Disease

Rita F. Redberg, MD, MSc
Editor, JAMA Internal Medicine
Professor of Medicine
UCSF Division of Cardiology
San Francisco, CA
Cardiac Tumors

Carlos A. Roldan, MD
Professor of Medicine
University of New Mexico School of Medicine
Director, Echocardiography Laboratory
New Mexico VA Health Care Center
Albuquerque, New Mexico
Connective Tissue Diseases & the Heart

Sandeep A. Saha, MBBS
Cardiology Fellow
Rush University Medical Center
Chicago, IL
Pulmonary Embolic Disease

Melvin M. Scheinman, MD
Professor of Medicine Emeritus
Schorenstein Chair in Cardiology
University of California
San Francisco, CA
Atrial Fibrillation

Prediman K. Shah, MD
Shapell and Webb Professor and Director, Atherosclerosis
    Prevention and Treatment Center
Director, Oppenheimer Atherosclerosis Research Center
Cedars Sinai Heart Institute, Los Angeles.
Professor of Medicine, University of California
Los Angeles, CA
Unstable Angina/Non-ST Evaluation Myocardial Infarction

Sanjiv Shah, MD
Associate Professor of Medicine
Director, Heart Failure with Preserved Ejection Fraction
    Program
Division of Cardiology, Department of Medicine
Northwestern University Feinberg School of Medicine
Chicago, IL
Heart Failure with Preserved Ejection Fraction

Sara Sirna, MD
Professor of Medicine
Division of Cardiology
Temple University School of Medicine
Philadelphia, PA
Lipid Disorders

Eveline Oestreicher Stock, MD
Instructor in Medicine
University of California
San Francisco, CA
Endocrinology & the Heart

Paul D. Thompson, MD
Chief of Cardiology
Hartford Hospital
Hartford, CT
The Athlete's Heart

Kirsten Tolstrup, MD
Associate Professor, UNM School of Medicine
Medical Director, Heart Station and Echolab, UNMH
Division of Cardiology
Albuquerque, New Mexico
Cardiovascular Disease in Pregnancy

Wanpen Vongpatanasin, MD
Professor of Medicine
Director, Hypertension Section,
Cardiology Division
University of Texas Southwestern Medical Center
Dallas, TX
Systemic Hypertension

Preface

Current Diagnosis & Treatment: Cardiology is designed to be a concise discussion of the essential knowledge needed to diagnose and manage cardiovascular diseases. *Current Diagnosis & Treatment: Cardiology* cannot be considered a condensed textbook because detailed pathophysiologic discussions are omitted; there are no chapters on diagnostic techniques; and rare or obscure entities are not included. Also, it is not a cardiac therapeutics text because diagnostic techniques, prevention strategies, and prognosis are fully discussed.

INTENDED AUDIENCE

Current Diagnosis & Treatment: Cardiology is designed to be a quick reference source in the clinic or on the ward for the experienced physician. Cardiology fellows will find that it is an excellent review for Board examinations. Also, students and residents will find it useful to review the essentials of specific conditions and to check the current references included in each section for further study. Nurses, technicians, and other health care workers who provide care for cardiology patients will find *Current Diagnosis & Treatment: Cardiology* a useful resource for all aspects of heart disease care.

COVERAGE

The 37 chapters in *Current Diagnosis & Treatment: Cardiology* cover the major disease entities and therapeutic challenges in cardiology. Also, there are chapters on major management issues in cardiology, such as pregnancy and heart disease, the use of anticoagulants in heart disease, and the perioperative evaluation of heart disease patients. Each section is written by experts in the particular area, but has been extensively edited to ensure a consistent approach throughout the book and the kind of readability found in single-author texts.

Since the third edition the book has been reorganized into six sections: Prevention of Cardiovascular Disease, Ischemic Heart Disease, Arrhythmias, Valvular Disease, Cardiomyopathy & Heart Failure, and Systemic Diseases & the Heart. Also, a new chapter on Antiplatelet Therapy has been added. My hope is that the book is found useful and improves patient care. Also, I hope it is an educational tool that improves knowledge of cardiac diseases. Finally, I hope it stimulates clinical research in areas where our knowledge is incomplete.

Michael H. Crawford, MD

Lipid Disorders

Mohamad Alkhouli, MD

Harish Jarrett, MBChB

Sara Sirna, MD

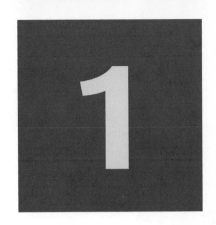

ESSENTIALS OF DIAGNOSIS

- ▶ Elevated plasma levels of low-density lipoprotein cholesterol, non–high-density lipoprotein cholesterol, lipoprotein(a), and apolipoprotein (apo) B-100.
- ▶ Reduced plasma levels of high-density lipoprotein and apo A-I.
- ▶ Elevated plasma levels of triglycerides.
- ▶ Skin xanthomas.

▶ General Considerations

Multiple epidemiologic studies have demonstrated the relationship between cardiovascular mortality and elevated plasma cholesterol levels. Lipid-lowering therapy, particularly with hydroxymethylglutaryl-coenzyme A (HMG-CoA) reductase inhibitors (statins), has demonstrated survival benefit in both primary prevention (patients without evidence of atherosclerotic cardiovascular disease [ASCVD]) and secondary prevention (patients with evidence of ASCVD). As a result, screening, risk stratifying, and treating dyslipidemia have become integral parts of preventive cardiovascular medicine.

A. Lipoproteins and Apolipoproteins

Cholesterol, cholesteryl esters, and triglycerides are the major lipids found in plasma. Cholesterol is an integral component of the cell membrane. It also serves a role in steroid hormone and bile acid synthesis. Triglycerides consist of fatty acid chains and phospholipids. Fatty acid chains are a primary source of energy in humans; phospholipids are key elements of all cell membranes. Cholesterol and triglycerides are insoluble in water and are transported in plasma by lipoproteins, classified as high-density lipoprotein (HDL) cholesterol, low-density lipoprotein (LDL) cholesterol, very-low-density lipoprotein (VLDL) cholesterol, intermediate-density lipoprotein (IDL) cholesterol, and chylomicrons. Lipoproteins consist of a lipid core and a water-soluble phospholipid outer layer that carry apolipoproteins, which are specific proteins that serve as coenzymes or receptor ligands or act as regulators of lipoprotein metabolism. Apolipoprotein (apo) A-I is present in HDL and promotes cholesterol efflux from tissues. Apo B, present as either apo B-100 (VLDL, IDL, LDL) or apo B-48 (chylomicron), serves as the LDL receptor ligand. Apo C-I, apo C-II, and apo C-III participate in triglyceride metabolism, and apo E is present on chylomicrons.

Lipoprotein(a) [Lp(a)] highly correlates with cardiovascular disease (CVD) and consists of an LDL particle and a specific apolipoprotein A. The structure of Lp(a) is similar to plasminogen and is thought to increase thrombogenesis. It is known to predict early atherosclerotic risk independent of other risk factors. Figure 1–1 illustrates the classes of lipoproteins and their characteristics.

B. Metabolism

Transportation of dietary lipids to peripheral tissues and the liver is known as the *exogenous metabolic pathway.* Here, triglycerides are hydrolyzed by pancreatic lipases and are emulsified by bile acids, leading to micelle formation. Micelle uptake occurs in the intestinal brush border where fatty acids are re-esterified and packaged together with apo B-48, phospholipids, and cholesterol to form chylomicrons. Chylomicrons then reach the portal circulation where they are hydrolyzed to release fatty acids by lipoprotein lipase (LPL). LPL activity is regulated through apo C-II, which activates LPL, and apo C-III, which inhibits LPL. The free fatty acids are used by muscle or stored as fat in an insulin-regulated process. As the particles get smaller, the cholesterol and apolipoproteins are transferred to HDL, creating a chylomicron remnant that is then taken up by the liver for degradation in an apo E–mediated process.

The *endogenous metabolic pathway* refers to transport of hepatic lipoproteins to peripheral tissues via LDL. It

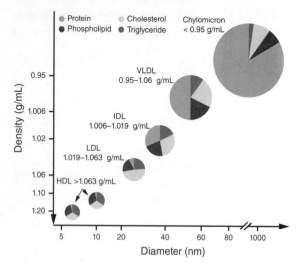

▲ Figure 1–1. Lipoprotein characteristics. HDL, high-density lipoproteins; IDL, intermediate-density lipoproteins; LDL, low-density lipoproteins; VLDL, very-low-density lipoproteins.

ensures a steady supply of substrate given that food supply varies. Here VLDL, a triglyceride-rich lipoprotein, serves a similar role to the chylomicron in the exogenous pathway. VLDL is derived from esterified long-chain fatty acids in the liver. Its triglyceride component is also hydrolyzed by LPL. VLDL acquires apolipoproteins (B-100, C-I, C-II, C-III, and E) from HDL and also exchanges triglycerides for cholesteryl esters in a process mediated by cholesteryl ester transfer protein (CETP). This mechanism allows cholesterol transfer from HDL to VLDL, allowing reverse cholesterol transport. Following hydrolysis, up to 40% of the resulting VLDL remnant, known as IDL, is taken up by the liver in an apo E–mediated transfer, and the remainder is converted to LDL by hepatic lipase. LDL particles mostly contain cholesteryl esters together with apo B-100 and are the main carriers of cholesterol. LDL is internalized through apo B-100, which binds to LDL receptors present on the cell surface. Cells are also capable of synthesizing cholesterol through an enzymatic process that involves HMG-CoA reductase. Figure 1–2 illustrates the endogenous and exogenous lipid metabolism pathways.

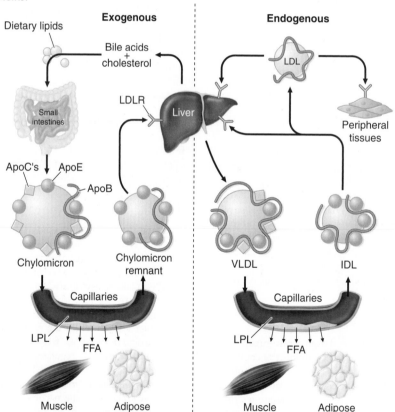

▲ Figure 1–2. Endogenous and exogenous pathways of lipid metabolism. FFA, free fatty acids; IDL, intermediate-density lipoproteins; LDL, low-density lipoproteins; LDLR, low-density lipoprotein receptor; LPL, lipoprotein lipase; VLDL, very-low-density lipoproteins. (Reproduced with permission from Longo DL, et al. *Harrison's Principles of Internal Medicine,* 18th ed. New York: McGraw-Hill; 2012.)

There is an inverse relationship between HDL levels and atherosclerotic coronary artery disease (CAD). HDL is responsible for reverse cholesterol transport. It inhibits lipoprotein oxidation and maintains endothelial integrity. Synthesized mostly in the liver but also in the intestine, the nascent HDL molecule consists of apo A-I, phospholipids, and cholesterol. HDL acquires cholesterol in an apo A-I–mediated process, which is then esterified by lecithin-cholesterol acyltransferase (LCAT) within the HDL particle forming mature HDL-containing cholesteryl esters, which can be taken up by the liver. Cholesterol and triglycerides can also be transferred from HDL to VLDL and chylomicrons via CETP, a process that allows HDL to transport cholesterol between cells, VLDL and chylomicrons, and the liver.

C. Atherosclerosis

Dyslipidemia is a major predisposing factor in the development of atherosclerosis and ASCVD. Elevated plasma LDL concentrations can directly and indirectly contribute to atherogenesis. Oxidized LDL accumulates in subintimal macrophages through active scavenger receptor–mediated uptake that leads to cellular dysfunction, apoptosis, and necrosis. Unlike the LDL receptor–mediated endocytosis, this process is not regulated by cholesterol content. These macrophages are termed foam cells and form subintimal fatty streaks. This culminates in the release of proinflammatory and prothrombotic molecules, which causes endothelial injury. Oxidized LDL can also directly cause endothelial injury through interaction with the cell surface. Endothelial injury results in platelet aggregation and smooth muscle proliferation, which initiates atherosclerotic plaque formation. HDL serves a protective role in atherogenesis. Its antiatherogenic effects are exerted through maintenance of endothelial function, apo A-I–mediated reverse transport of macrophage cholesterol, antioxidant effects, and antithrombotic effects.

▶ Clinical Findings

Patients with dyslipidemia are asymptomatic with the exception of those who present with acute pancreatitis in the setting of severe hypertriglyceridemia. The clinical findings depend on the cause of dyslipidemia.

The most severe forms of hyperlipidemia are caused by genetic disorders of lipoprotein metabolism such as familial hypercholesterolemia (FH). FH is an autosomal dominant disease with defects in the gene for the LDL receptor. The mutant gene prevents the LDL receptor from removing LDLs from the blood. LDL cholesterol levels are typically in excess of 300 mg/dL. Common manifestations include fatty skin deposits called xanthomas over parts of the hands, elbows, knees, and ankles and around the corner of the eye (xanthelasmas). It frequently presents as premature CAD with chest pain (angina) or acute myocardial infarction. Other common primary causes of dyslipidemia are familial combined hyperlipidemia (both high LDL and triglyceride levels) and pure hypertriglyceridemia (very high triglyceride levels).

Table 1–1 summarizes the most common primary causes of dyslipidemia.

A. Secondary Causes of Dyslipidemia

Dyslipidemia develops in many patients as a result of an underlying metabolic abnormality rather than a primary dyslipidemia. Metabolic syndrome is characterized by abdominal obesity, hypertension, insulin resistance ($\pm$ glucose intolerance), prothrombotic state, elevated triglycerides, small LDL particles, and low HDL levels.

Obesity affects over one-third of adults in the United States and represents a significant secondary cause of dyslipidemia due to caloric excess mostly derived from saturated fat and sugar. Decreased insulin sensitivity and increased carbohydrate intake cause an increase in triglyceride formation, which then enters the circulation in the form of VLDL. HDL levels are decreased in obesity. Similarly, patients with type 2 diabetes mellitus are dyslipidemic due to insulin resistance and subsequent insulin excess. This causes an increase in free fatty acid formation in the periphery and in the liver that translates to an increase in VLDL production and hypertriglyceridemia. Lipoprotein catabolism is downregulated due to decreased LPL activity, resulting in further increases in plasma VLDL.

Hypothyroidism commonly results in dyslipidemia due to a decrease in hepatic LDL receptor activity and consequent delayed clearance of LDL. The severity of the dyslipidemia directly correlates with the degree of hypothyroidism, and correction reverses the dyslipidemia.

Liver disease can affect plasma lipid concentrations. Hepatitis is associated with increased VLDL production, and not surprisingly, severe disease and liver failure result in low plasma lipoprotein levels as synthetic function progressively decreases. Cholestatic liver disease results in significant hypercholesterolemia through the accumulation of lipoprotein-X, the deposition of which leads to the appearance of xanthomata in the skin.

Chronic kidney disease is associated with elevation in VLDL as a result of decreased lipolysis and clearance. Nephrotic syndrome results in marked hypercholesterolemia as a result of increased hepatic production of LDL and decreased clearance of VLDL, induced due to low plasma oncotic pressure.

Other secondary causes to consider include cigarette smoking, which decreases plasma HDL concentration. Commonly used drugs such as thiazide diuretics, β-blockers, and estrogen compounds can affect plasma lipid concentrations. Antiretroviral agents, particularly protease inhibitors, are associated with a lipodystrophy syndrome. Antipsychotics are also potential causative agents that are associated with weight gain and insulin resistance.

Table 1–1. Primary Gene Defects

Genetic Disorder	Protein (gene) Defect	Lipoproteins Elevated	Clinical Findings	Genetic Transmission	Estimated Incidence
Lipoprotein lipase deficiency	LPL	Chylomicrons	Eruptive xanthomas, hepato-splenomegaly, pancreatitis	AR	1 in 1,000,000
Familial apolipoprotein C-II deficiency	Ape-CII	Chylomicrons	Eruptive xanthomas, hepato-splenomegaly, pancreatitis	AR	< 1 in 1,000,000
Apo A-V deficiency	ApeA-V	Chylomicrons, VLDL	Eruptive xanthomas, hepato-splenomegaly, pancreatitis	AD	< 1 in 1,000,000
GP1HBP1 deficiency	GP1HBP1	Chylomicrons	Eruptive xanthomas, pancreatitis	AD	< 1 in 1,000,000
Familial hepatic lipase deficiency	Hepatic lipase	VLDL remnants	Pancreatitis, CHD	AR	< 1 in 1,000,000
Familial dysbetalipo-proteinemia	ApoE	Chylomicrons, VLDL remnants	Palmar and tuboeruptive xanthomas, CHD, PVD	AR, AD	1 in 10,000
Familial hypercholesterolemia	LDL receptor	LDL	Tendon xantnomas, CHD	AD	1 in 500
Familial defective apo B-l00	ApoB-100	LDL	Tendon xantnomas, CHD	AD	< 1 in 1000
Autosomal dominant hypercholesterolemia	PCSK9	LDL	Tendon xantnomas, CHD	AD	< 1 in 1,000,000
Autosomal recessive hypercholesterolemia	LDLRAP	LDL	Tendon xantnomas, CHD	AR	< 1 in 1,000,000
Silosterolemia	ABCG5 or ABCG8	LDL	Tendon xanthomas, CHD	AR	< 1 in 1,000,000

AD, autosomal dominant; AR, autosomal recessive; ARH, autosomal recessive hypercholesterolemia; CHD, coronary heart disease; LDL, low-density lipoprotein; LPL, lipoprotein lipase; PVD, peripheral vascular disease; VLDL, very-low-density lipoprotein.
Adapted with permission from Longo DL, et al. *Harrison's Principles of Internal Medicine,* 18th ed. New York: McGraw-Hill; 2012.

▶ **Diagnosis**

The National Cholesterol Education Program, Adult Treatment Panel (NCEP-ATP) III recommends screening for lipid disorders with a fasting lipid profile every 5 years for adults over 20 years old. The US Preventive Services Task Force (USPSTF) advocates for routine screening of men and women above 35 and 45 years old, respectively. The USPSTF also recommends screening at earlier age if risk factors for coronary heart disease (CHD) are present. When lipid abnormalities are discovered, a thorough history should be performed, assessing for symptomatic CVD, as well as attempts to identify potential secondary causes of dyslipidemia. A thorough family history should be obtained, and risk factors such as sedentary lifestyle, obesity, poor diet, and cigarette smoking should be addressed. Physical examination may reveal xanthomas and xanthelasmas, which may aid in the diagnosis of a primary dyslipidemia. Basic metabolic panel, creatinine, and thyroid and liver function tests should be obtained to exclude any secondary causes of hyperlipidemia.

Grundy SM, et al. Diagnosis and management of the metabolic syndrome: an American Heart Association/National Heart, Lung, and Blood Institute Scientific Statement. *Circulation.* 2005;112(17):2735–52. [PMID: 16157765]

▶ **Treatment**

A. LDL Goals

The degree of cardiovascular risk is the major determinant in the decision to commence drug therapy. Current NCEP-ATP-III guidelines incorporate the Framingham 10-year absolute cardiovascular risk rates in identifying target LDL goals for patients with hyperlipidemia. The major risk factors (exclusive of LDL cholesterol) that modify LDL goals are cigarette smoking, hypertension (blood pressure > 140/90 mm Hg

Table 1–2. LDL Treatment Goals

Risk Category	LDL Goal (mg/dL)	LDL Level at Which to Initiate Therapeutic Lifestyle Changes (mg/dL)	LDL Level at Which to Consider Drug Therapy (mg/dL)
CHD or CHD risk equivalent (10-year risk > 20%)	< 100 < 70 (optional)	> 100	> 130
2 risk factors (10-year risk < 20%)	< 130	> 130	10-year risk 10–20% > 130 10-year risk < 10% > 160
0–1 risk factor	< 160	> 160	> 190

CHD, coronary heart disease; LDL, low-density lipoprotein.
Adapted from the Third Report of the Expert Panel on Detection, Evaluation, and Treatment of High Blood Cholesterol in Adults (Adult Treatment Panel III) 2004.

or on antihypertensive medication), low HDL cholesterol (< 40 mg/dL), family history of premature CHD (CHD in male first-degree relative < 55 years; CHD in female first-degree relative < 65 years), and age (men > 45 years; women > 55 years). HDL cholesterol > 60 mg/dL counts as a "negative" risk factor; its presence removes one risk factor from the total count. The presence of peripheral arterial disease, abdominal aortic aneurysm, symptomatic carotid artery disease, or diabetes is considered CHD equivalents. Patients are classified as low, intermediate, and high risk based on the number of their risk factors. The treatment goal and the threshold to initiate drug therapy differ between the three risk groups as illustrated in Table 1–2. Some authorities recommend an LDL goal of ≤ 70 mg/dL for very-high-risk patients (eg, a diabetic patient with recent myocardial infarction), a strategy that has been adapted by most cardiologists.

The major limitation of the Framingham model is that this approach only measures a 10-year and not a lifetime risk of developing CAD. In addition, two major risk factors, diabetes and family history, are not included in the Framingham risk calculation. Therefore, it should be noted that the Framingham risk score may underestimate one's actual risk.

It should be emphasized that treating LDL to optimal target reduces the risk of coronary events but does not eliminate it completely. Patients with LDL at goal who are at very high risk may benefit from further testing to define their "residual risk" of coronary events. Levels of HDL, high-sensitivity C-reactive protein, and Lp(a); particle sizes/numbers; calcium scoring; and vascular intima imaging are useful tools in assessing this residual risk.

It may be reasonable to test serum Lp(a) in those with premature CAD, with a strong family history of premature CAD, or with recurrent disease despite statin treatment. Treatment consists of niacin, 1–3 g mostly in the long-acting form, and aspirin.

B. HDL Goals

Low HDL is an independent risk factor for increased CVD and mortality, although a causal relationship has not been established. High HDL levels convey reduced coronary risk and are associated with a longevity syndrome. Low HDL levels can be caused by genetic mutations, as is the case with familial hypoalphalipoproteinemia, familial HDL deficiency, and Tangier disease. Acquired and often reversible causes include obesity, sedentary lifestyle, cigarette smoking, metabolic syndrome, hypertriglyceridemia, and certain drugs (β-blockers and steroids). These risk factors should be aggressively targeted. As of today, the studies have been inconclusive regarding increasing HDL with pharmacologic intervention and reducing the risk of CHD. In addition, NCEP-ATP-III guidelines highlight that LDL and non-HDL goals should be reached first before HDL goals are addressed.

C. Hypertriglyceridemia and Non-HDL Goals

Hypertriglyceridemia is common and is often associated with obesity, physical inactivity, high-carbohydrate diet, alcohol consumption, and cigarette smoking. Other conditions such as diabetes, metabolic syndrome, and renal disease, as well as drugs (particularly estrogens and protease inhibitors), are also contributory. Patients with hypertriglyceridemia are at increased risk of developing ASCVD. As with low HDL levels, it is unclear whether a causal relationship exists. Current NCEP-ATP-III treatment guidelines recommend reducing serum triglyceride levels in addition to lowering LDL values. Therapeutic lifestyle change should be the major treatment goal given the constellation of risk factors that contribute to the hypertriglyceridemic state.

In addition to aerobic exercise, dietary management should focus on carbohydrate reduction as well as restricting foods that have a high glycemic index. No dietary fat restriction is required, but the correct type of fat consumption should always be emphasized. Patients with extremely high triglyceride levels (> 1000 mg/dL) are at risk of developing acute pancreatitis due to high levels of circulating chylomicrons. In this subgroup of patients, all types of dietary fat should be restricted to reduce this risk. Fibrates, nicotinic

Table 1–3. Triglyceride Treatment Goals

Category	Triglyceride Levels (mg/dL)	Intervention
Optimal	< 150	None
Borderline	150–199	Therapeutic lifestyle change (including weight reduction and aerobic exercise)
High	200–499	Therapeutic lifestyle change. Achieve primary LDL goal. Achieve secondary non-HDL goal. Consider pharmacologic therapy
Very high	> 500	Pharmacologic therapy to decrease triglyceride levels. Once < 500 mg/dL, address LDL goal

HDL, high-density lipoprotein; LDL, low-density lipoprotein.
Adapted the Third Report of the Expert Panel on Detection, Evaluation, and Treatment of High Blood Cholesterol in Adults (Adult Treatment Panel III) 2004.

acid, and fish oils are pharmacologic agents that can reduce triglyceride levels and are discussed separately. Table 1–3 categorizes triglyceride levels and summarizes NCEP-ATP-III guidelines for treating hypertriglyceridemia.

Non-HDL cholesterol is calculated by subtracting HDL from total cholesterol (TC – HDL). This fraction includes all apo B–containing (and therefore atherogenic) lipoprotein particles: LDL, Lp(a), IDL, and VLDL. This measure is useful in the setting of a raised triglyceride level (200–499 mg/dL). The goal non-HDL level is 30 mg/dL higher than the goal LDL level.

National Cholesterol Education Program (NCEP) Expert Panel on Detection, Evaluation, and Treatment of High Blood Cholesterol in Adults (Adult Treatment Panel III). Third Report of the National Cholesterol Education Program (NCEP) Expert Panel on Detection, Evaluation, and Treatment of High Blood Cholesterol in Adults (Adult Treatment Panel III) final report. *Circulation.* 2002;106(25):3143–421. [PMID: 12485966]

D. Nonpharmacologic Treatment

Despite the significant advances in medical treatment, CAD remains the leading cause of death worldwide. This is likely due to the increasing rates of obesity, diabetes, and metabolic syndrome. Therefore, any successful strategy to reduce CHD risk should emphasize weight loss, regular exercise, and a heart-healthy diet.

Dietary fats can be categorized into cholesterol, saturated fatty acids (SFAs), monounsaturated fatty acids (MUFAs),

polyunsaturated fatty acids (PUFAs), and trans-fatty acids. SFAs are mostly derived from animal products that raise both total and LDL cholesterol levels and are strongly associated with increased CVD. Trans-fatty acids result from commercial hydrogenation of PUFAs and decrease HDL levels and elevate LDL levels. Conversely, MUFAs and PUFAs have favorable effects on the lipid profile and may also delay atherosclerosis by limiting oxidization of LDL.

The American Heart Association–advocated diet, previously known as the "Step 1 Diet," recommends that in addition to calorie restriction, there should be a shift in focus to the type of dietary fat consumed. Total fat should comprise no more than 30% (with 7% or less saturated fat) of daily caloric intake, and total cholesterol intake should be less than 300 mg/day.

Another highly successful dietary intervention is the modified Mediterranean diet (MMD). Rich in whole grains, beans, fish, and olive oil, the MMD has shown high adherence rates and a sustainable reduction of coronary events. Thus, diet and exercise remain the foundation of any successful lipid management program.

Kris-Etherton P, et al. AHA science advisory: Lyon Diet Heart Study. Benefits of a Mediterranean-style, National Cholesterol Education Program/American Heart Association Step I Dietary Pattern on Cardiovascular Disease. *Circulation.* 2001;103:1823–5. [PMID: 11282918]
Mozaffarian D, et al. Effects on coronary heart disease of increasing polyunsaturated fat in place of saturated fat: a systematic review and meta-analysis of randomized controlled trials. *PLoS Med.* 2010;7:e1000252. [PMID: 20351774]

E. Pharmacologic Treatment

Most patients with dyslipidemia will require targeted pharmacologic therapy to address their dyslipidemia. Statins are considered the cornerstone in treating dyslipidemia. Other drugs, however, are beneficial as an adjunctive or sole therapy in certain populations.

1. HMG-CoA reductase inhibitors (statins)—Statins (simvastatin, atorvastatin, pravastatin, rosuvastatin, fluvastatin, and lovastatin) are the most commonly used drugs in treating dyslipidemia. They are competitive inhibitors of HMG-CoA reductase, which is required for cholesterol biosynthesis. The decrease in intrahepatic cholesterol levels through this mechanism leads to an increase in LDL receptor expression and increased clearance of plasma LDL and decreased hepatic synthesis of VLDL and LDL. In addition, there is a modest increase in HDL levels. There is a synergistic effect when used in combination with either a cholesterol absorption inhibitor or a bile acid sequestrant, which can be helpful in optimizing LDL levels. They also appear to exert LDL independent anti-inflammatory effects on the endothelium and atherosclerotic plaques. For the most part, statins are well tolerated. Commonly reported side effects include myalgia, myositis reversible transaminitis, and rarely rhabdomyolysis.

Given their efficacy, potency, and tolerability, statins have been the focus of several large-scale prospective randomized studies over the last three decades, which have demonstrated relative cardiovascular risk reduction in primary prevention when compared to placebo. Secondary prevention has also been assessed in major trials (A-to-Z, PROVE-IT, TNT, IDEAL, and SEARCH) and formed the basis of the NCEP-ATP-III (2004) guidelines.

Ray KK, et al. Statins and all-cause mortality in high-risk primary prevention: a meta-analysis of 11 randomized controlled trials involving 65,229 participants. *Arch Intern Med.* 2010;170(12): 1024–31. [PMID: 20585067]

2. Cholesterol absorption inhibitors—Ezetimibe binds to and inhibits the protein Niemann-Pick C1-like 1 (NPC1L1) and inhibits the intestinal absorption of cholesterol. The net effect is a decrease in cholesterol reaching the liver and a subsequent increase in hepatocyte LDL receptor expression, thereby decreasing plasma LDL with no effect on HDL or triglyceride levels. Ezetimibe, the first drug in this class, decreases plasma cholesterol by 15–20% and has a synergistic effect when used in combination with a statin. Major side effects are rare, even when used together with a statin, but liver function should be monitored.

3. Fibric acid derivatives (fibrates)—The major effects of the fibrate class of drugs (gemfibrozil and fenofibrate) are to reduce serum triglyceride levels and raise HDL levels. This effect is mediated by activation of nuclear peroxisome proliferator-activated receptor alpha (PPARα), which results in increased LPL activity and increased VLDL clearance. The elevation of HDL levels is mediated through PPARα-mediated synthesis of apo A-I and apo A-II. Gemfibrozil is indicated in secondary prevention of ASCVD in the setting of hypertriglyceridemia, low HDL, and normal LDL based on the Veterans Administration HDL Intervention Trial (VA-HIT). Common side effects include cholelithiasis, myalgias, and elevated transaminase levels. Combination therapy with statins is effective in treating elevated LDL as well as hypertriglyceridemia; however, fibrates, especially gemfibrozil, can decrease statin elimination and increase the risk of significant myositis and rhabdomyolysis.

4. Bile acid sequestrants (resins)—Bile acid sequestrants interrupt the enterohepatic circulation through binding bile acids and preventing reuptake in the ileum. This results in a decrease in total body and intrahepatic cholesterol, leading to subsequent increase in LDL (apo B and apo E) receptor expression. The LDL receptors (apo B and apo E) then bind LDL cholesterol from the plasma, leading to further decrease in LDL levels. Resins are more effective when used together with a statin. Resins can increase VLDL levels and are therefore restricted to patients with relatively normal triglyceride levels.

Bile acid sequestrants are not absorbed from the gastrointestinal tract, and this reflects their side-effect profile. Bloating and constipation are common and dose dependent, which affects compliance. Bile acid sequestrants can also bind to and impair the absorption of other drugs such as digoxin, warfarin, β-blockers, thiazide diuretics, and fat-soluble vitamins. This effect can be minimized by administering other drugs 1 hour before or 4 hours after the bile acid sequestrant, but this can also affect compliance.

The available bile acid sequestrants, cholestyramine, colestipol, and colesevelam, are not systemically absorbed and thus can be used safely in pregnant patients, patients who are lactating, and children.

5. Nicotinic acid (niacin)—The predominant effect of niacin is to substantially increase HDL levels and decrease triglyceride levels. The mechanism by which niacin increases HDL levels remains unclear. Its effects on plasma triglyceride levels are mediated through enhanced LPL activity as well as inhibition of free fatty acid release from peripheral fat. The main obstacle with niacin therapy has been its tolerability. Common side effects include elevated transaminases, hyperglycemia, gastritis, and flushing. Taking aspirin 30 minutes prior to each dose may reduce flushing. Close monitoring of liver function is warranted due to the risk of niacin-induced hepatitis, which warrants discontinuation of therapy. An escalating dosing schedule can improve tolerability and compliance. Niacin has been shown to be effective in combination with a statin.

The AIM-HIGH Investigators. Niacin in patients with low HDL cholesterol levels receiving intensive statin therapy. *N Engl J Med.* 2011;365:2255–67. [PMID: 22085343]

6. Omega-3 fatty acids (fish oils)—Omega-3 polyunsaturated fatty acids are used in the treatment of hypertriglyceridemia. Eicosapentaenoic acid (EPA) and docosahexaenoic acid (DHA) are the active compounds and are available over the counter and by prescription. They act through an uncertain mechanism to lower triglyceride levels at doses of 3-4 g/day. Fish oils are well tolerated at these doses but can prolong the bleeding time. Studies have shown morbidity and mortality benefit in secondary prevention with ingestion of 1 g of fish oil daily. Future studies are addressing the effects of fish oil on primary prevention. Consuming one to two servings of oily fish per week has been shown to reduce the risk of CVD in adult patients.

F. Treatment in Specific Patient Populations

1. Familial hyperlipidemia—Those who inherit only one copy of the defective gene (familial heterozygous hyperlipidemia) may respond well to high-dose statin therapy and diet and lifestyle modification. Those with severe forms of the disease may require apheresis, an extracorporeal therapy that removes LDL and returns the remainder of the blood to the patient.

2. Diabetics—The insulin-resistant state observed in type 2 diabetes mellitus is associated with hypertriglyceridemia as a result of increased circulating free fatty acids and decreased lipolysis. An increase in VLDL, IDL, and LDL is observed in addition to a decrease in HDL levels. Aggressive LDL reduction confers significant improvements in all-cause mortality in patients with type 2 diabetes mellitus as evidenced by the results from the CARE trial, the Heart Protection Study, and the CARDS study. Thus, type 2 diabetes mellitus is considered a CAD risk equivalent, and the NCEP-ATP-III treatment guidelines reflect these findings with an LDL target of less than 100 mg/dL (2.6 mmol/L) and an optimal target of less than 70 mg/dL (1.8 mmol/L).

3. Stroke—Although an established risk factor for CVD, the link between dyslipidemia and cerebrovascular disease and stroke (cerebrovascular accident [CVA]) remains less clear. Regardless, statin therapy has been shown to be beneficial in both primary and secondary prevention. The HPS, CARE, and ASCOT-LLA trials all demonstrated CVA reduction with statin therapy, even in patients with cholesterol levels in the "normal" range. In addition, the SPARCL trial demonstrated that atorvastatin 80 mg daily reduced recurrent ischemic CVA in patients with a prior history of stroke or transient ischemic attack (TIA). It appears that the non–cholesterol-lowering benefits of statin therapy play a significant role in CVA reduction. This may explain why other lipid-lowering therapies have not shown CVA risk reduction benefits.

4. Hypothyroidism—Hypothyroidism is commonly associated with hyperlipidemia due to decreased LDL receptor activity and with hypertriglyceridemia due to decreased LPL activity. Patients with dyslipidemia should have their thyroid function assessed. If hypothyroidism is diagnosed, treatment with thyroid replacement therapy will result in improvement in the lipid profile.

▶ Prognosis

Hyperlipidemia remains a strong and treatable risk factor for atherosclerotic vascular disease. Major trials have demonstrated the enormous benefit of statin therapy in reducing LDL cholesterol and preventing cardiac events. Potential new therapies targeted toward reducing LDL levels are currently an area of active research. Monoclonal antibody targeted at proprotein convertase subtilisin/kexin 9 (PCKS9), a protease that degrades LDL receptors, has shown very promising results in early phase II trials. This new antibody, yet to be approved by the US Food and Drug Administration, resulted in a 60% additional reduction in LDL in patients already on maximum statin therapy. Another novel agent, mipomersen, achieves LDL reduction by binding to apo B RNA and inhibiting apo B synthesis.

Effective treatment for elevated triglyceride levels has improved the prognosis for patients with hypertriglyceridemia. Therapies that increase HDL levels are also being studied. Torcetrapib, anacetrapib, evacetrapib, and dalcetrapib are CETP inhibitors that raise HDL levels. Investigation with torcetrapib was halted due to an increase in adverse cardiovascular events, but the other agents are currently being studied with promising results. However, there is currently no treatment for low HDL levels, which has been demonstrated to reduce mortality.

Roth EM, et al. Atorvastatin with or without an antibody to PCSK9 in primary hypercholesterolemia. *N Engl J Med.* 2012; 367(20):1891–900. [PMID: 23113833]

Systemic Hypertension

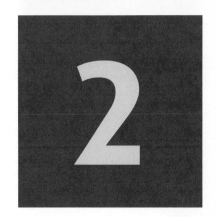

Wanpen Vongpatanasin, MD

ESSENTIALS OF DIAGNOSIS

▶ Prehypertension: systolic pressure of 120–139 mm Hg or diastolic pressure of 80–89 mm Hg.

▶ Stage 1 hypertension: systolic pressure of 140–159 mm Hg or diastolic pressure of 90–99 mm Hg.

▶ Stage 2 hypertension: systolic pressure of at least 160 mm Hg or diastolic pressure of at least 100 mm Hg.

▶ General Considerations

Hypertension is a major public health problem in the United States and many countries worldwide. Prevalence of hypertension in the United States remains unchanged in the past decade at 30%, while prevalence of resistant hypertension (failure to achieve blood pressure [BP] control despite three or more medications) has almost doubled in recent years from 16% to 28%. When the risk is calculated over lifetime, the burden of hypertension in middle-aged men and women is enormous. Eight to nine out of 10 normotensive women or men over the age of 55 are expected to develop hypertension in the next 20 years. Thus, complete understanding of basic pathophysiologic mechanisms and treatment strategies is one crucial step in improving hypertension control.

▶ Pathophysiology & Etiology

Pathophysiology of primary hypertension is complex and heterogeneous. At least one or more of the mechanisms involved in BP regulation, such as vascular, neural, renal, and hormonal mechanisms, contribute to development of primary hypertension. Accordingly, therapy often requires more than one antihypertensive agent or approach to tackle hypertension in the majority of patients.

Systemic vascular resistance and cardiac output are two major determinants of BP. Thus, augmented peripheral vasoconstriction at the level of resistance vessels may lead to hypertension in the presence of normal cardiac output. More recently, large arterial stiffness has been shown to contribute to elevated systolic BP. In many epidemiologic studies, systolic BP increases with age both in men and women. However, after the fifth decade of life, systolic BP continues to increase while diastolic BP starts to fall, causing the pulse pressure to widen. Normally, elasticity of aorta helps absorb pressure during systole, and the elastic recoil of the aorta helps maintain BP during diastole. The loss of aortic elasticity causes BP to rise excessively during systole and decrease markedly during diastole. Furthermore, the aortic pulse wave travels at much faster speed in the stiff artery, and the reflected wave from the peripheral sites further amplifies the systolic BP in the central aorta. Although diastolic BP is traditionally thought to be the most important predictor of cardiovascular risk, it is an important risk factor only for the younger population. For hypertensive patients above the age of 60, systolic BP and pulse pressures are much more important in predicting long-term cardiovascular outcomes.

Neural control of BP also plays an important role in development of hypertension. Overactivity of the sympathetic nervous system has been identified in patients with uncomplicated essential hypertension, and many conditions predispose to hypertension such as obesity, renal failure, and obstructive sleep apnea. Sympathetic overactivity contributes to hypertension by stimulating increase in cardiac output while producing peripheral vasoconstriction. Activation of β_1-adrenergic receptor by norepinephrine released from the sympathetic nerve terminals further increases BP by increasing renin release, causing renal sodium retention. The major hormones that contribute to hypertension include the renin-angiotensin-aldosterone system (RAAS), which will be discussed later in the section on secondary causes of hypertension. Although RAAS triggers hypertension by promoting renal sodium absorption, a large body of evidence from animal experiments suggests that its direct action on the vascular system and the central nervous system further augments hypertension.

► Clinical Findings

A. BP Measurement

Proper BP measurement is essential in the diagnosis and treatment of hypertension. BP monitoring should be done both at home and in the clinic.

1. Clinic BP—In the clinical setting, BP measurement should be performed after patients are sitting quietly for at least 5 minutes with the arm supported at the heart level. The bladder of the cuff should encircle > 80% of the arm, and the width should be about 40% of the arm length. Medical personnel who perform the measurement should avoid talking to the patients during BP measurement because mental stimulation may inadvertently increase BP up to 10–15 mm Hg. Cuff should be inflated 20 mm Hg above systolic BP before deflation, and a minimum of two readings should be obtained at an interval of at least 1 minute. If BP differs by more than 5 mm Hg between the two readings, an additional one or two readings should be taken. During the initial visit, BP should be taken from both arms to exclude subtle stenosis in the subclavian or brachial artery, which could lead to underestimation of actual BP and undertreatment of hypertension. In patients with early onset of hypertension prior to the age of 40, BP should also be obtained from at least one leg to screen for aortic coarctation. In elderly patients and patients with diabetes mellitus or other conditions that predispose to autonomic failure such as Parkinson disease, BP should also be taken after 3 minutes of standing to exclude presence of orthostatic hypotension.

2. Home and ambulatory BP monitoring—Home BP measurement should be encouraged in all hypertensive patients to guide treatment because 20–40% of hypertensive subjects have elevated clinic BP with normal BP outside the doctor's office. This phenomenon, known as the *white-coat effect* (WCE), is more common in older patients, particularly in women with isolated systolic hypertension or diabetes. Accordingly, when home and clinic BP readings provide contradictory results, ambulatory BP monitoring should be considered to verify adequacy of BP control.

It is important to recognize that WCE is not the same as white-coat hypertension (WCH), because the latter is only limited to elevated office BP with normal awake ambulatory BP *without* any antihypertensive treatment. WCH is not associated with increased cardiovascular risks when compared to the population with normal BP both at home and in the clinic. In contrast, hypertensive patients with WCE during drug treatment experience increased cardiovascular events compared to untreated normotensive controls, but at the same risk observed in patients who achieve BP control both in the clinic and out of office with treatment (ie, treated normalized hypertension).

More recently, another subset of hypertensive patients with clinic BP under 140/90 mm Hg but who have elevated out-of-office BP has been recognized. This condition, termed *masked hypertension*, has been identified in 20–45%

of patients with hypertension. Interestingly, patients with masked hypertension experience increased cardiovascular complications similar to patients with sustained hypertension. Whether treatment of masked hypertension will improve cardiovascular outcomes remains unknown.

Franklin SS, et al. Significance of white-coat hypertension in older persons with isolated systolic hypertension: a meta-analysis using the International Database on Ambulatory Blood Pressure Monitoring in Relation to Cardiovascular Outcomes population. *Hypertension*. 2012;59(3):564–71. [PMID: 22252396]

B. Symptoms & Signs

Hypertension is well known as a silent killer because the majority of patients remain asymptomatic until development of target organ damage. However, some patients may have symptoms that could be related to a secondary cause of hypertension. Snoring and daytime somnolence may signify presence of obstructive sleep apnea, whereas episodes of palpitation and paroxysmal hypertension may suggest pheochromocytoma. Presence of muscle weakness, polyuria, and polydipsia might be related to hypokalemia from primary aldosteronism or hypercortisolism. Other symptoms of target organ damage and other coronary risk factors should be assessed because they help to define BP threshold for treatment of hypertension. History taking should also include the onset of hypertension and prior antihypertensive treatment as well as history of side effects from previous medications. The concomitant use of other prescription or nonprescription drugs, such as herbal products, nonsteroidal anti-inflammatory drugs, or decongestant use, which can directly increase BP or interfere with efficacy of antihypertensive medications, should be obtained. In young premenopausal women, method of contraception should be documented because certain antihypertensive medications, such as angiotensin-converting enzyme inhibitors or angiotensin receptor blockers, are teratogenic or fetotoxic. Furthermore, oral contraceptives could cause hypertension in a small number of patients, although the absolute risk is lower than 0.1% with low-dose estrogen preparation. Detailed family history with specific attention to both hypertension and stroke should be obtained because early stroke could be a presenting feature in certain genetic forms of hypertension.

High sodium intake is also a major contributor for uncontrolled hypertension, and detailed dietary assessment should be obtained in patients who fail to achieve BP goals despite multiple medications. Nonadherence to medications is the major cause of apparently resistant hypertension and should be considered in patients on a complex multidrug regimen. Questions related to adherence should not be asked in the manner that sounds judgmental or critical to the patients; otherwise, accurate assessment may not be obtained. Instead of asking, "Do you take medications regularly as the doctors prescribe?", asking patients if they feel that taking multiple medications is difficult or if they have forgotten to take medications in the past 7 days is more likely to uncover a history of nonadherence.

C. Physical Examination

Physical examination should focus on signs of target organ damage such as presence of volume overload, laterally displaced apical impulses, S_3 and/or S_4 gallops, and hypertensive retinopathy. Particular attention should be paid to physical signs that may indicate underlying secondary hypertension. Abdominal bruit may indicate presence of renal artery stenosis. Truncal obesity, dorsocervical fat pads, hirsutism, and abdominal striae may represent cortisol excess. BP gradient between arms and legs and femoral-radial pulse delay may signify coarctation of aorta.

D. Diagnostic Studies

For patients with mild uncomplicated hypertension, serum electrolytes, urinalysis, and complete blood cell count should be obtained during the initial visit to assess renal function and exclude subtle target organ damage. Electrocardiogram should be obtained to screen for left ventricular hypertrophy and presence of conduction system disturbances, which may prohibit the use of β-blockers or nondihydropyridine calcium channel blockers. Echocardiography should be limited to patients with symptoms and signs of congestive heart failure or patients with syncope to exclude presence of dynamic left ventricular outflow tract obstruction, which has been identified in a subset of hypertensive patients with concentric left ventricular hypertrophy. Fasting lipid panel and plasma glucose should also be obtained to assess overall cardiovascular risks. Microalbuminuria should be tested in diabetic patients and patients with severe hypertension.

▶ Differential Diagnosis

In the majority of patients with hypertension, specific etiology cannot be identified, and patients are often labeled as having essential or primary hypertension. However, in approximately 5% of unselected patients with hypertension and 10–20% of all resistant hypertensive cases, causes of hypertension are identifiable and/or potentially reversible. Screening for secondary causes of hypertension is not indicated in every patient with hypertension. Indications for additional workup are as follows:

- Abrupt onset after the age of 55 or before the age of 30
- Accelerated or malignant hypertension with grade 3–4 retinopathy
- Previously, but not presently, controlled
- Poorly controlled hypertension on three or more drugs
- Recurrent flash pulmonary edema
- Hypertension with unexplained renal insufficiency
- Suspected clinical features of secondary causes such as hypokalemia, renal bruits, and truncal obesity

Common secondary causes of resistant hypertension include obstructive sleep apnea, primary aldosteronism, renal parenchymal diseases, and renal artery stenosis. Pheochromocytoma and other endocrine disorders are much less common causes of resistant hypertension.

A. Obstructive Sleep Apnea

Obstructive sleep apnea (OSA) is a well-established independent risk factor for development of hypertension. Because the majority of the population in the United States is overweight or obese, OSA is now a common condition, affecting 10–20% of the population in the United States. Prevalence of OSA in drug-resistant hypertension is much greater, as high as 83% in some studies. Activation of the sympathetic nervous system via activation of chemoreceptor via repetitive hypoxia and hypercapnia is thought to play an important role in the pathogenesis of hypertension. Patients with a history of loud snoring, insomnia, and/or daytime fatigue should undergo polysomnography. Treatment with continuous positive airway pressure (CPAP) has been shown to reduce BP in hypertensive patients with OSA. However, long-term compliance is very poor; less than 50% of patients still continue to use CPAP after 6 months. Therefore, target BP is rarely achieved with CPAP alone, and further adjustment of antihypertensive medications is often needed to reach target goals.

B. Primary Aldosteronism

Aldosterone excess, either from idiopathic bilateral adrenal hyperplasia or aldosterone-producing adenoma, is a common cause of resistant hypertension. Primary aldosteronism (PA) has been identified in 5–10% of unselected patients with hypertension in the primary care setting and up to 20% of patients with resistant hypertension referred to a hypertension clinic or a tertiary care center. Aldosterone induces hypertension not only by increasing renal sodium retention, but also by activation of the sympathetic nervous system. Patients with hyperaldosteronism experienced higher cardiovascular event rates than those with essential hypertension, which is out of proportion to the degree of BP elevation. This is likely to be related to direct cardiovascular toxicity of aldosterone. To screen for PA, plasma renin activity (PRA) or levels and serum aldosterone levels should be obtained. However, the screening test should be performed after discontinuation of thiazide diuretics, direct renin inhibitors, angiotensin-converting enzyme inhibitors (ACEIs), and angiotensin receptor blockers (ARBs) for 2–3 weeks and discontinuation of aldosterone antagonists for at least 6 weeks. During the workup period, patients need to be on other antihypertensive agents such as α-blockers or calcium channel blockers. If needed, addition of β-blockers or central sympatholytic drugs may be added, but this may potentially reduce PRA. Patients who are found to have suppressed renin levels or activity in the presence of elevated serum aldosterone levels of 15 ng/dL or greater should undergo a salt loading test or be referred to hypertension specialists. Patients who have insuppressible aldosterone levels after salt loading should undergo adrenal vein sampling because imaging of adrenal glands is not reliable in separating patients with idiopathic hyperplasia from those with aldosterone-producing adenoma. Treatment includes surgical resection of tumor for patients with aldosterone-producing adenoma, which can cure hypertension in 20–60% of patients, depending on duration of hypertension and presence of target organ complications. Mineralocorticoid receptor antagonists (spironolactone or eplerenone) should be used in patients with bilateral hyperplasia or patients with unilateral adenoma in whom surgical risks are prohibitive.

C. Renal Parenchymal Disease

Renal parenchymal disease could be a cause or a consequence of hypertension. Hypertension is very common in chronic kidney disease (CKD) but is much more difficult to control. Despite requirement for larger numbers of antihypertensive medications, the hypertension control rate in the United States in CKD patients is less than 30% compared with 50% in non-CKD patients. Hypertension related to renal parenchymal disease has traditionally been viewed as being largely volume dependent, due to the failing kidney's inability to excrete salt and water. However, increased systemic vascular resistance from overactivation of the sympathetic nervous system has also been identified in the majority of patients.

D. Renovascular Hypertension

Renovascular hypertension is another common cause of secondary hypertension, accounting for 5–7% of hypertension in patients over the age of 60. Atherosclerosis is the major form of renal artery pathology in the elderly, as fibromuscular dysplasia is seen predominantly in young adults. Screening for renovascular hypertension should be considered in patients with (1) onset of hypertension at < 30 years of age or abrupt onset of hypertension after 55 years of age; (2) accelerated or malignant hypertension; (3) unexplained atrophic kidney or size discrepancy of more than 1.5 cm between each kidney; (4) sudden, unexplained pulmonary edema; (5) unexplained renal dysfunction, including individuals starting renal replacement therapy; and (6) development of new azotemia or worsening renal function after administration of an ACEI or ARB. Imaging of renal arteries with computed tomography (CT) angiography or magnetic resonance angiography should also be obtained in patients with suspected renal artery stenosis. Unfortunately, no currently available invasive or noninvasive studies are sufficiently sensitive or specific in assessing functional significance of a given stenotic lesion or in predicting BP pressure control after revascularization. Renal artery revascularization leads to significant and sustained reduction in BP in patients with fibromuscular dysplasia, but effects on BP control in patients with atherosclerotic renal artery stenosis are much less consistent. Therefore, revascularization should be considered in most patients with fibromuscular dysplasia and selected patients with atherosclerotic renal artery stenosis plus one or more of the following features: (1) bilateral disease or stenosis of the unilateral functioning kidney; (2) rapid decline in renal function; (3) resistant hypertension despite three or more antihypertensive medications; or (4) recurrent pulmonary edema.

E. Pheochromocytoma

Although a screening test for pheochromocytoma is often done in patients with labile hypertension or resistant hypertension, it accounts for < 1% of patients with unselected hypertension. Patients may present with paroxysmal hypertension, palpitation from sinus tachycardia or supraventricular arrhythmia, and panic/anxiety sensation from catecholamine excess. Myocardial infarction, congestive heart failure, and Takotsubo-like cardiomyopathy may be the presenting symptoms, along with hypertension in some patients. Diagnosis requires demonstration of elevated plasma/urinary metanephrines (metanephrine and/or normetanephrine) above 3–4 times the upper limit of normal without other identifiable causes. Patients with paraganglioma or extra-adrenal tumor may have isolated elevation in plasma dopamine, and thus, a plasma catecholamines panel (epinephrine, norepinephrine, and dopamine) should be obtained in patients with suspected pheochromocytoma in the absence of adrenal mass. Borderline elevation in plasma metanephrines or catecholamines is common in hypertensive patients with underlying conditions that cause sympathetic overactivity such as OSA, congestive heart failure, or CKD. These levels may return to normal after correction of the underlying problems. A clonidine suppression test should be obtained in patients with persistent but borderline (less than twofold) elevation in plasma metanephrines or catecholamines to confirm diagnosis. CT or magnetic resonance imaging (MRI) of the abdomen should be used to localize tumor after biochemical confirmation. Metaiodobenzylguanidine scan should be used when CT or MRI fails to reveal tumor.

▶ Treatment

A. Lifestyle Modification

Lifestyle modifications include sodium restriction to less than 1.5–2 g/day. The major source of sodium consumed in the United States comes from processed food including bread and rolls, pasta, cured meat, and snacks. Table salt contributes to only 20% of total sodium consumed. Avoiding table salt alone will not be an effective strategy in limiting sodium intake, and educating patients to read nutritional label is a key to success. A diet rich in fruits and vegetables also reduces BP independent of sodium content.

B. Pharmacologic Intervention

Antihypertensive treatment should be initiated in patients with stage 1 uncomplicated hypertension who fail a trial of lifestyle modification alone. Pharmacologic intervention should be offered promptly without any delay for patients with stage 2 hypertension or those with stage 1 hypertension in the presence of target organ complication, diabetes mellitus, renal failure, or high cardiovascular risks in conjunction with lifestyle modification. The list of antihypertensive drugs available in the United States is shown in Table 2–1.

1. Diuretics—Thiazide diuretics are considered to be the first-line drug therapy for hypertension according to the Seventh Report of the Joint National Committee on Prevention, Detection, Evaluation, and Treatment of High Blood Pressure guidelines due to their efficacy in reducing BP and low cost. Thiazide diuretics promote natriuresis by inhibiting sodium chloride cotransport at the distal convoluted tubule. Among thiazide diuretics, chlorthalidone has the longest half-life of between 40 and 60 hours compared to 8–15 hours for hydrochlorothiazide. Head-to-head comparison studies showed that chlorthalidone is at least two times more potent than hydrochlorothiazide in reducing BP. Thiazide diuretics are known to cause a number of metabolic side effects such as hypokalemia, elevated uric acid, increased fasting triglyceride, and, most importantly, increased risk of diabetes mellitus. Thiazide-induced dysglycemia or insulin resistance is mediated both by hypokalemia and potassium-independent mechanisms, which can be minimized by concomitant administration of the mineralocorticoid receptor antagonist spironolactone and, to a lesser extent, by ACEIs or ARBs.

Loop diuretics promote diuresis by inhibiting $Na^+/K^+/Cl^-$ cotransport at the thick ascending limb of Henle's loop. Although loop diuretics are more potent as diuretic agents than thiazide diuretics, the short half-life limits their efficacy in reducing BP. Furosemide has a half-life of only 1.5–2.5 hours and should be given every 6 hours to have sustained effects on BP; hence the name "Lasix." Thus, it is not recommended for treatment of hypertensive patients with normal renal function. However, it is useful for patients with fluid retention from congestive heart failure, renal failure, or nephrotic syndrome. Among loop diuretics, furosemide has the least predictable absorption, whereas torsemide has the longest half-life.

Mineralocorticoid receptor (MR) antagonists, such as spironolactone and eplerenone, are known to reduce BP by inhibiting MR-dependent activation of the epithelial sodium channel in the cortical collecting duct. Furthermore, inhibition of the sympathetic nervous system and improvement in vascular endothelial function are thought to contribute to the BP-lowering effects of this class of drugs. MR antagonists are effective in lowering BP when either used alone or as add-on therapy for resistant hypertension despite use of three or more drugs. On a milligram-to-milligram basis, eplerenone is less potent than spironolactone in reducing BP in both patients with primary hypertension and PA, and thus, at least a twofold higher dose is often required to achieve BP control. However, spironolactone carries antiandrogenic side effects, including gynecomastia and testicular atrophy, and long-term use at the dose of more than 25 mg/day should be avoided in men. In these patients, the use of eplerenone, which has more than 100-fold lower affinity to androgen receptors than MRs, is preferable. Hyperkalemia is the main side effect of both agents, and serum potassium should be closely monitored in patients with CKD, diabetic patients with hyporeninemic hypoaldosteronism, or those on concomitant treatment with ACEIs, ARBs, or nonsteroidal anti-inflammatory agents. MR antagonists have been shown to reduce mortality in patients with systolic heart failure even with mild symptoms, and they should be considered in treatment of hypertension in patients with impaired ventricular function.

In addition to MR antagonists, direct inhibitors of the epithelial sodium channels (ENaCs), such as amiloride and triamterene, are also effective in lowering BP in patients with low renin essential hypertension. They are particularly useful in patients with gain-in-function mutation in the ENaC, causing excessive renal sodium absorption and renal K wasting, known as Liddle syndrome. Amiloride is also useful in patients with primary aldosteronism who cannot tolerate MR antagonists. Both amiloride and triamterene are often used in a combination pill formulation with hydrochlorothiazide (see Table 2–1).

2. ACEIs—ACEIs reduce BP by inhibiting conversion of angiotensin (Ang) I to potent vasoconstrictor Ang II. ACEIs also prevent degradation of the vasodilator bradykinin, which further contributes to BP reduction. ACEIs are particularly effective in reducing BP in younger patients and Caucasians and tend to be less effective in the setting of the low renin form of hypertension frequently observed in the elderly and black populations. However, the combination of ACEIs with diuretics eliminates racial and age differences in BP response to ACEIs. In addition to BP reduction, ACEIs reduce mortality in patients with congestive heart failure and improve cardiovascular outcomes in high-risk hypertensive patients without heart failure. ACEIs also slow the decline in renal function in patients with diabetic and nondiabetic kidney disease. Thus, they should be used in hypertensive patients with these comorbid conditions. The main side effects of this class of drugs are cough and angioedema from presumably excessive bradykinin accumulation. Hyperkalemia is another side effect, which may limit its use in some patients with severe CKD or bilateral renal artery stenosis.

3. ARBs—ARBs reduce BP by blocking the vasoconstrictor effects of Ang II on angiotensin receptor subtype 1 (AT1R) in the vascular smooth muscle. This class of drugs has remarkably minimal side effects and is generally well tolerated. It avoids side effects of cough and angioedema associated with ACEIs. In placebo-controlled clinical trials,

Table 2–1. Antihypertensive Drugs Available in the United States

Drug	Dose Range, Total mg/day (doses per day)	Drug	Dose Range, Total mg/day (doses per day)
Diuretics		Quinapril	5–80 (1–2)
Thiazide Diuretics		Ramipril	2.5–20 (1)
Hydrochlorothiazide (HCTZ)	6.25–50 (1)	Trandolapril	1–8 (1)
Chlorthalidone	6.25–25 (1)	**Angiotensin Receptor Blockers**	
Indapamide	1.25–5 (1)	Azilsartan	40–80 (1)
Metolazone	2.5–10 (1)	Candesartan	8–32 (1)
Loop Diuretics		Eprosartan	400–800 (1–2)
Furosemide	20–160 (2)	Irbesartan	150–300 (1–2)
Torsemide	2.5–80 (1–2)	Losartan	25–100 (2)
Bumetanide	0.5–2 (2)	Olmesartan	5–40 (1)
Ethacrynic acid	25–100 (2)	Telmisartan	20–80 (1)
Potassium-sparing diuretics		Valsartan	80–320 (1–2)
Amiloride	5–20 (1)	**Direct Renin Inhibitors**	
Triamterene	25–100 (1)	Aliskiren	75–300 (1)
Spironolactone	12.5–400 (1–2)	**α-Blockers**	
Eplerenone	25–100 (1–2)	Doxazosin	1–16 (1)
β-Blockers		Prazosin	1–40 (2–3)
Acebutolol	200–800 (2)	Terazosin	1–20 (1)
Atenolol	25–100 (1)	Phenoxybenzamine	20–120 (2) for pheochromocytoma
Betaxolol	5–20 (1)	**Central Sympatholytics**	
Bisoprolol	2.5–20 (1)	Clonidine	0.2–1.2 (2–3)
Carteolol	2.5–10 (1)	Clonidine patch	0.1–0.6 (weekly)
Metoprolol	50–450 (2)	Guanabenz	2–32 (2)
Metoprolol XL	50–200 (1–2)	Guanfacine	1–3 (1) (q hs)
Nadolol	20–320 (1)	Methyldopa	250–1000 (2)
Nebivolol	5–20 (1)	Reserpine	0.05–0.25 (1)
Penbutolol	10–80 (1)	**Direct Vasodilators**	
Pindolol	10–60 (2)	Hydralazine	10–200 (2)
Propranolol	40–180 (2)	Minoxidil	2.5–100 (1)
Propranolol LA	60–180 (1–2)	**Fixed-Dose Combinations**	
Timolol	20–60 (2)	Aliskiren/HCTZ	75–300/12.5–25 (1)
β/α-Blockers		Aliskiren/valsartan	150–300/160–320 (1)
Labetalol	200–2400 (2)	Amiloride/HCTZ	5/50 (1)
Carvedilol	6.25–50 (2)	Amlodipine/benazepril	2.5–5/10–20 (1)
Calcium Channel Blockers		Amlodipine/olmesartan	5–10/20–40 (1)
Dihydropyridines		Amlodipine/valsartan	5–10/160–320 (1)
Amlodipine	2.5–10 (1)	Amlodipine/valsartan/HCTZ	5–10/160–320/12.5–25
Felodipine	2.5–20 (1–2)	Atenolol/chlorthalidone	50–100/25 (1)
Isradipine CR	2.5–20 (2)	Azilsartan/chlorthalidone	40–80/25 (1)
Nicardipine SR	30–120 (2)	Benazepril/HCTZ	5–20/6.25–25 (1)
Nifedipine XL	30–120 (1)	Bisoprolol/HCTZ	2.5–10/6.25 (1)
Nisoldipine	10–40 (1–2)	Candesartan/HCTZ	16–32/12.5–25 (1)
Nondihydropyridines		Enalapril/HCTZ	5–10/25 (1–2)
Diltiazem CD	120–540 (1)	Eprosartan/HCTZ	600/12.5–25 (1)
Verapamil HS	120–480 (1)	Fosinopril/HCTZ	10–20/12.5 (1)
Angiotensin-Converting Enzyme Inhibitors		Irbesartan/HCTZ	15–30/12.5–25 (1)
Benazepril	10–80 (1–2)	Losartan/HCTZ	50–100/12.5–25 (1)
Captopril	25–150 (2)	Olmesartan/HCTZ	20–40/12.5 (1)
Enalapril	2.5–40 (2)	Spironolactone/HCTZ	25/25 (0.5–1)
Fosinopril	10–80 (1–2)	Telmisartan/HCTZ	40–80/12.5–25 (1)
Lisinopril	5–80 (1–2)	Trandolapril/verapamil	2–4/180–240 (1)
Moexipril	7.5–30 (1)	Triamterene/HCTZ	37.5/25 (0.5–1)
Perindopril	4–16 (1)	Valsartan/HCTZ	80–160/12.5–25 (1)

ARBs reduced mortality in patients with systolic heart failure who were intolerant to ACEIs and offered renal protection in patients with diabetic nephropathy. Thus, they should be considered as part of regimen in hypertensive patients with these clinical features. The combination of ARBs with maximal doses of ACEIs usually yields minimal additional BP reduction and is generally not helpful in improving cardiovascular mortality. Although combination therapy offers synergistic or additive effect in reducing proteinuria, dual renin-angiotensin system blockade is associated with more renal dysfunction than either class of drugs alone. Therefore, it is not recommended as a strategy to control BP in hypertensive patients and should be reserved only for patients with proteinuria from primary renal disease such as immunoglobulin A nephropathy.

3. Calcium channel blockers (CCBs)

CCBs are divided into two major classes: the dihydropyridine (DHP) and nondihydropyridine (non-DHP) CCBs. DHP CCBs include amlodipine, felodipine, nisoldipine, and nicardipine and cause peripheral vasodilation with minimal effects on the heart rate or myocardial contractility. In contrast, non-DHP CCBs (diltiazem and verapamil) exert negative inotropic and chronotropic effects. Non-DHP CCBs are contraindicated in patients with systolic heart failure because of increased cardiovascular mortality and should be avoided in patients with symptomatic bradyarrhythmias or advanced heart block. DHP CCBs have neutral effect on survival in congestive heart failure and may be considered if BP remains elevated despite ACEIs or ARBs in systolic heart failure. All CCBs increase myocardial blood flow and are antianginal. Meta-analysis of clinical trials showed that CCBs are more effective than ACEIs in preventing stroke beyond BP reduction, but less effective than ACEIs and ARBs in preventing coronary heart disease or heart failure. DHP CCBs preferentially dilate afferent arterioles, causing increase in intraglomerular hypertension and are not as effective as ACEIs or ARBs in preventing decline in renal function in diabetic or nondiabetic kidney diseases. Therefore, they should not be used without RAAS blockade in hypertensive patients with CKD.

4. β-Adrenergic receptor blockers (BBs)

BBs reduce BP by decreasing heart rate and myocardial contractility, leading to decreased cardiac output at least initially via inhibition of β_1-adrenergic receptor (AR). Inhibition of renin release from the juxtaglomerular cells via β_1-AR and reduction of norepinephrine release from sympathetic nerve terminals via inhibition of presynaptic β_2-AR also contribute to BP reduction. BBs are divided into two major classes: selective (β_1-specific) and nonselective (β_1- and β_2-AR blockers), as shown in Table 2-2. Activation of β_2-AR leads to peripheral vasodilation and bronchodilation. Thus, nonselective BBs should not be used in patients with asthma or in the setting of sympathetic overactivity, such as clonidine withdrawal or cocaine intoxication because of unopposed α-AR–mediated vasoconstriction. However,

Table 2–2. Selective Versus Nonselective β-Adrenergic Receptor Blockers

Nonselective (ratio β_1:β_2 selectivity)	Selective (ratio β_1:β_2 selectivity)
Propranolol (1:8)	Atenolol (5-10:1)
Carvedilol (1:4-5)	Acebutolol (2:1)
Labetalol (1:2-3)	Metoprolol (2-4:1)
Nadolol (1:23)	Bisoprolol (14:1)
	Esmolol (76:1)
	Nebivolol (320:1)

selectivity to β_1 versus β_2 is dose-dependent and not an all-or-none phenomenon. At higher doses, even selective BBs such as metoprolol, bisoprolol, atenolol, or esmolol may cause bronchospasm and should be used with caution. Certain BBs exert direct vasodilating effects, which enhance antihypertensive efficacy independent of β-AR blockade. For example, labetalol and carvedilol exert α-AR–blocking properties, whereas nebivolol promotes nitric oxide release and possesses antioxidant properties. Although BBs reduce mortality in patients with systolic heart failure and myocardial infarction, older generation BBs, particularly atenolol, are not as effective as other classes of drugs in preventing stroke or all-cause mortality in hypertensive patients with cardiovascular diseases. Thus, atenolol should not be used as initial therapy in patients with uncomplicated essential hypertension, particularly in patients with low renin hypertension, elderly patients, or African Americans.

5. α-AR blockers

α-AR blockers exert antihypertensive effect by inhibiting postsynaptic α_1-ARs in the vascular smooth muscle. α-AR blockers that selectively inhibit α_1-AR antagonists include prazosin, terazosin, and doxazosin, whereas the nonselective blockers, which inhibit both α_1- and α_2-ARs, include phentolamine and phenoxybenzamine. Side effects of α-blockers are orthostatic hypotension, nasal congestion, and volume expansion. Nonselective α-blockers tend to cause more tachycardia because of inhibition of presynaptic α_2-ARs, which normally exert inhibitory influence on norepinephrine release from sympathetic nerve terminals. α-Blockers should not be used as first-line therapy for hypertension because of increased risk of congestive heart failure. However, they are useful as an adjunctive treatment as the fourth- or fifth-line agent when BP fails to reach target goal. They should be considered as the first line of treatment in the setting of pheochromocytoma and are also useful in patients with hypertension related to cocaine intoxication or conditions associated with sympathetic overactivity such as drug or alcohol withdrawal.

6. Central sympatholytic drugs—Central sympatholytic drugs reduce BP mainly by stimulating presynaptic α_2-ARs in the brainstem centers and sympathetic nerve terminals, thereby inhibiting sympathetic nerve discharge and neuronal release of norepinephrine to the heart and peripheral circulation. Drugs in this class include methyldopa, clonidine, guanfacine, and guanabenz. Moxonidine and rilmenidine are also centrally acting drugs used in England and other European countries but are not available in the United States. α-Methyldopa is converted to α-methylnorepinephrine to activate central α_2-ARs in the brainstem, whereas clonidine, guanfacine, and guanabenz are direct α_2-AR agonists. In contrast, moxonidine and rilmenidine predominantly reduce sympathetic nerve activity and BP by stimulating the imidazoline-1 (I_1) receptor, rather than α_2-AR. Because of several major side effects, including fatigue, sedation, and dry mouth, as well as lack of clear-cut cardiovascular benefit, these drugs should be used as fourth-line drug therapy for hypertension. Central sympatholytic drug use should be avoided in patients who are nonadherent to treatment because of precipitation of withdrawal symptoms upon abrupt drug discontinuation. Their use on an as-needed basis for treatment of episodes of asymptomatic BP surge in patients who are not on regular dosing of central α_2-AR agonists should also be discouraged due to rebound hypertension.

7. Direct renin inhibitors (DRIs)—DRIs block catalytic action of circulating renin, thereby preventing formation of Ang I from angiotensinogen. DRIs also inhibit activity of the proenzyme prorenin, which can also cleave angiotensinogen into Ang I upon binding to the prorenin receptors. Inhibitory action of DRIs on renin and prorenin activity results in decreased production of Ang II and BP. Aliskiren is the only drug approved for clinical use in this class so far. Addition of aliskiren to ARBs reduces proteinuria in hypertensive patients with type 2 diabetes mellitus when compared to placebo. However, addition of aliskiren to ARBs or ACEIs is not more effective in reducing left ventricular (LV) mass in hypertensive patients or improving LV remodeling in patients after myocardial infarction than monotherapy with ARBs or ACEIs alone. Furthermore, a recent clinical trial showed that addition of aliskiren to ACEIs or ARBs in patients with diabetes mellitus and established cardiovascular disease failed to improve cardiovascular outcomes and even increased the risk of nonfatal stroke. Thus, the future role of DRIs in the treatment of hypertension is likely to be limited.

8. Direct vasodilators—Hydralazine and minoxidil are the two main drugs in this class, which reduce BP by dilating resistant arterioles with minimal or no effect on the venous circulation. Hydralazine has short plasma half-life of 90 minutes, but its antihypertensive action lasts much longer than its plasma level. Thus, for the ease of administration, hydralazine should be given twice daily in hypertensive patients rather than three times a day, which is the schedule typically used in patients with heart failure. Side effects of hydralazine include lupus-like syndrome, particularly at the higher doses, reflex tachycardia, nausea, vomiting, and diarrhea. Minoxidil promotes vasodilation by activating adenosine triphosphate–sensitive potassium channels in the vascular smooth muscle. Similar to hydralazine, minoxidil-induced BP reduction is usually accompanied by reflex tachycardia and palpitation, and the addition of BBs is often needed to mitigate these side effects. Peripheral edema and volume expansion frequently occur, requiring concomitant diuretic treatment. Less common side effects include hirsutism and pericardial effusion.

Oral nitrates are nitric oxide donors, which produce venodilating effects at low doses and arterial vasodilating effects at higher doses. Although the benefits of nitrates as antianginal drugs are well validated, very few studies have addressed their efficacy as antihypertensive agents. In one small study, isosorbide mononitrate reduced systolic BP in elderly patients with resistant systolic hypertension without affecting diastolic BP. It is unknown whether these data can be extrapolated to other age groups with combined systolic-diastolic hypertension. Headache is the main side effect, and nitrate tolerance is the main limiting factor for long-term use.

C. Management of Uncomplicated Hypertension

In most patients, the goal BP should be < 140/90 mm Hg. Tight control of systolic BP below 120 mm Hg does not reduce cardiovascular death, but reduces the risk of stroke by 40% in patients with diabetes mellitus. Higher systolic BPs (< 150 mm Hg) may be more appropriate for patients > 80 years of age and patients with class 4 or greater CKD. In patients with mild uncomplicated hypertension, thiazide-type diuretics should be considered in patients who have a tendency to be salt sensitive, such as older patients and black patients. For younger patients, ACEIs, ARBs, and CCBs may be more suitable. The use of BBs, particularly older generation BBs such as atenolol, should be avoided in young patients with active lifestyle due to fatiguing side effects and modest efficacy in improving cardiovascular outcomes. BBs are more suitable for patients with compelling indication such as coronary artery disease or congestive heart failure. Treatment of hypertension is also beneficial in elderly patients even > 80 years old in terms of reducing stroke and cardiovascular mortality. In these patients, chlorthalidone or DHP CCB such as amlodipine should be part of the regimen given the proven benefit in reducing stroke and adverse cardiovascular events, particularly in patients with isolated systolic hypertension.

For patients with BP at least 20/10 mm Hg above the goal, the use of combination therapy is preferred over monotherapy to avoid side effects related to the use of a single agent at the high dose that is often needed to control BP. In patients with high cardiovascular risks, the combination of an ACEI and DHP CCB is superior for reducing adverse cardiovascular outcomes than the combination of an ACEI with thiazide-type diuretics. Thus, the addition of DHP CCBs should be considered in such patients whose BP reduction is not adequate with ACEIs alone.

D. Management of Hypertensive Crisis

Hypertensive crisis is a common condition encountered in the emergency department that can be classified as hypertensive emergency or hypertensive urgency. Hypertensive emergency is defined severe elevation in BP (often > 180/120 mm Hg) in the presence of acute target organ damage involving heart, brain, kidneys, or vascular system. Hypertensive urgency is defined as severe hypertension associated with symptoms, such as headache or chest pain, in the absence of any objective evidence of acute target organ damage. Thus, distinction between hypertensive emergency versus urgency is dependent of clinical presentation rather than severity of hypertension alone.

Once patients are identified to have hypertensive crisis, choice of therapy and rapidity of BP reduction are dependent on clinical presentation. In normotensive subjects, cerebral blood flow is maintained at a constant level despite variation in mean arterial BP between 60 and 120 mm Hg by a process known as *cerebral autoregulation*. At the lower end of this range, cerebral vessels dilate to maintain normal perfusion. Only when the mean BP is lower than 50–60 mm Hg, cerebral perfusion becomes pressure-dependent. Similarly, when BP rises to a higher level, myogenic vasoconstriction of the resistant arterioles prevents excessive increase in blood flow and cerebral edema. Patients with well-controlled hypertension have autoregulatory adjustment at the normal BP range similar to normotensives. However, in patients with severe hypertension, this BP range is shifted to the right between 110 and 180 mm Hg (Figure 2–1). Thus, BP lowering in patients with hypertensive encephalopathy should done cautiously by aiming for reduction by 20–25% in the first few hours but not below 140/90 mm Hg (mean BP around 107 mm Hg) in the first 24 hours. Patients with hypertensive urgency could be treated with oral antihypertensive medications in the emergency department and discharged home with close follow-up for titration of BP medications within a few days. Rapid normalization of BP with oral agents in the doctor's office or emergency department in patients with asymptomatic severe hypertension without any target organ damage may provoke hypoperfusion of the vital organs, such as brain and kidneys, and should be avoided.

In contrast to hypertensive encephalopathy, BP should be reduced to < 120/80 mm Hg as soon as possible in patients with hypertensive emergency in the setting of aortic dissection because delay in BP reduction may cause the dissection plane and false lumen to expand, which may jeopardize blood flow to the vital organs. Patients with acute pulmonary edema and acute coronary syndrome should also have more

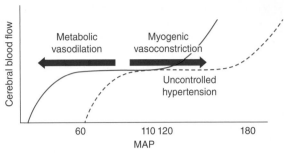

▲ **Figure 2–1.** Relationship between cerebral blood flow (CBF) and mean arterial pressure (MAP) in normotensive subjects (solid line). Normally, CBF is maintained constant at MAP between 60 and 120 mm Hg. However, in patients with uncontrolled hypertension, this relationship is shifted to the right. Therefore, precipitous reduction in BP in these individuals to normal range (MAP < 11 mm Hg in the first 24 hours) may lead to cerebral hypoperfusion.

rapid BP reduction to less than 140/90 mm Hg as soon as possible to decrease LV wall stress, a major determinant of myocardial oxygen demand. Thrombolytic therapy should not be given in patients with ST elevation myocardial infarction until BP is reduced below 180/110 mm Hg to avoid the risk of intracranial hemorrhage. Patients who present with primary intracranial hemorrhage pose a challenge in management because cerebral perfusion pressure is determined both by systemic BP and intracranial pressure. Similarly, for patients with ischemic stroke, rigorous reduction in BP could further compromise the flow to the infarct area and, more importantly, the border zone. More conservative reduction in BP with the goal for BP reduction of approximately 15% within the first hour is generally recommended in these two neurologic emergencies. Treatment of hypertensive emergency in specific clinical settings is summarized in Table 2–3.

Selection of antihypertensive agents in hypertensive emergency also depends on the clinical presentation (Table 2–4). Patients with hypertensive encephalopathy or ischemic stroke should be treated with labetalol, nitroprusside, or nicardipine. Nitroprusside and nitroglycerin should be avoided in patients with intracranial hemorrhage because they may increase intracranial pressure. Phentolamine should be considered in patients with pheochromocytoma or adrenergic crisis such as cocaine intoxication. However, this drug may not be available in many countries, including the United States, on a regular basis. Nicardipine is an alternative therapy for pheochromocytoma. Labetalol, although effective in reversing cocaine-induced increase in BP, should be used with caution in pheochromocytoma because it is still a predominant BB (β-AR to α-AR blockade ratio of 4:1) and

Table 2–3. Treatment of Hypertensive Emergency in Special Populations

Clinical Setting	Rapidity of BP Reduction and Target BP	Antihypertensive Drugs
Hypertensive encephalopathy without stroke	Reduce mean arterial pressure (MAP) by 20–25% over 2–3 hours	Labetalol Nitroprusside Nicardipine
Acute ischemic stroke with indication for thrombolysis and BP > 185/110 mm Hg	Reduce MAP by 15% over 1 hour	Labetalol Nicardipine Nitroprusside
Acute ischemic stroke, not a candidate for thrombolysis, with BP > 220/120 mm Hg	Reduce MAP by 15% over 1 hour	Labetalol Nicardipine Nitroprusside
Intracerebral hemorrhage, with systolic blood pressure (SBP) > 200 mm Hg or MAP > 150 mm Hg	Reduce MAP by 15% over 1 hour. For SBP 150–220 mm Hg, acute lowering of SBP to 140 mm Hg appears safe (*Stroke* 2010;41:2108-29).	Labetalol Nicardipine *(Avoid nitroprusside or nitroglycerin if intracranial pressure is increased.)*
Aortic dissection	Reduce BP to < 120/80 mm Hg immediately	Labetalol Esmolol plus nitroprusside
Acute pulmonary edema	Reduce MAP to 60–100 mm Hg immediately	Nitroglycerin Nitroprusside
Acute coronary syndrome	Reduce MAP to 60–100 mm Hg immediately	Nitroglycerin Labetalol Nicardipine
Adrenergic crisis (pheochromocytoma, clonidine withdrawal, drug or alcohol withdrawal)	Reduce MAP by 20–25% over 2–3 hours	Phentolamine Nicardipine Labetalol
Cocaine overdose	Reduce MAP by 20–25% over 2–3 hours	Phentolamine Labetalol Nicardipine Nitroprusside

may precipitate an unopposed α-AR–mediated vasoconstriction. Nitroprusside is a potent vasodilator but should be used with caution in patients with renal failure given its propensity to cause cyanide toxicity. Nitroglycerin is suitable for use in patients with acute pulmonary edema and acute coronary syndrome because of its antianginal property and ability to relieve pulmonary congestion. Nitrate tolerance may develop quickly with continuous infusion and limit its antihypertensive efficacy. Fenoldopam is a dopamine D_1-like receptor agonist, which reduces BP by promoting peripheral vasodilation. Clevidipine is a newer CCB available in intravenous form with shorter half-life (1 minute) than nicardipine (30–40 minutes). The relatively high cost of these newer agents limits routine use in clinical practice.

E. Management of Resistant Hypertension

Resistant hypertension is defined as failure to achieve BP target goal despite three or more drugs, one of which should be a diuretic. The first simple step in managing resistant hypertension, after excluding WCE, nonadherence to medications, and secondary hypertension, is to determine whether patients are on an appropriate class of diuretics based on renal function. Patients with estimated glomerular filtration rate (eGFR) > 50 mL/min/1.73 m^2 should be treated with thiazide diuretics, particularly chlorthalidone, rather than loop diuretics because of longer half-life and proven efficacy in lowering BP. Patients with an eGFR of 30–40 mL/min/1.73 m^2 or less should be on loop diuretics because the ability of thiazide diuretics to promote diuresis diminishes with impaired renal function. The use of an appropriate drug combination that provides synergistic effect on BP could minimize the number of medications needed to control hypertension. Assessment of hemodynamic variables is also helpful in deciding appropriate drug combination. For example, the use of BBs and a central sympatholytic drug generally yields minimal incremental benefit and is

Table 2–4. Intravenous Antihypertensive Drugs for Hypertensive Emergencies

Drug	Dose	Contraindications and Side Effects
Nitroprusside	Start at 0.25–1.0 mcg/kg/min, increase by 0.5 mcg/kg/min every 5 minutes until goal BP or maximal dose of 10 mcg/kg/min	Renal failure, cyanide toxicity, reflex tachycardia, methemoglobin
Nitroglycerin	Start at 10–20 mcg/min, increase by 5 mcg/min every 5 minutes until goal BP or maximal dose of 200 mcg/min	Headache
Nicardipine	Start at 5 mg/h, increase by 2.5 mg/h every 15–30 minutes until goal BP or maximal dose of 15 mg/h; thereafter decrease to 3 mg/h maintenance	
Clevidipine	Start at 1–2 mg/h, titrate every 90 seconds to 10-minute intervals up to 32 mg/h	Defective lipid metabolism such as pathologic hyper-lipemia or acute pancreatitis
Labetalol	Start at 0.25–0.5 mg/kg at 2–4 mg/min until goal BP, then 5–20 mg/h maintenance	Bradycardia, second- or third-degree atrioventricular (AV) block, bronchospasm, systolic heart failure
Esmolol	0.5–1 mg/kg as bolus; 50–300 mcg/kg/min as continuous infusion plus sodium nitroprusside intravenous gtt; start at 0.25–1.0 mcg/kg/min, increase by 0.5 mcg/kg/min every 5 minutes until goal BP or maximal dose of 10 mcg/kg/min	Bradycardia, second- or third-degree AV block, bronchospasm, systolic heart failure
Phentolamine	1–5 mg, repeat after 5–15 minutes until goal BP is reached; 0.5–1.0 mg/h as continuous infusion	Reflex tachycardia
Fenoldopam	Start at 0.03–0.1 mcg/kg/min, titrated at the increment of 0.05 to 0.1 mcg/kg/min up to 1.6 mcg/kg/min	Increased intraocular pressure, reflex tachycardia

prohibited in patients with bradycardia or heart block. These patients should be treated with vasodilators such as DHP CCBs, ACEIs, ARBs, or hydralazine (Figure 2–2). Patients with elevated resting heart rate are more likely to derive large BP reduction with BBs, diltiazem, or verapamil because elevated heart rate is usually a good indicator for hyperkinetic circulation in hypertensive patients.

Addition of spironolactone should also be considered in patients with resistant hypertension despite adjustment of medications, as mentioned earlier. An increasing body of evidence suggests that low-dose spironolactone between 12.5 and 25 mg/day, which is not likely to produce a major diuretic effect, causes a dramatic fall in BP on average of 25/12 mm Hg, when used as add-on therapy in patients with uncontrolled hypertension. Antihypertensive effect of spironolactone is observed even in patients with essential hypertension without an elevated aldosterone-to-renin ratio. Combination of DHP and non-DHP CCBs appears to have additive effects on peripheral vasodilation and BP, possibly due to binding to different sites of the receptors, and should also be considered in these patients. In contrast, addition of an ARB to ACEI has modest effects on BP, on average of only 5/3 mm Hg. The addition of long-acting nitrates may be considered in patients with isolated systolic hypertension who are refractory to treatment because it has been shown to be beneficial in one small study.

ACCORD Study Group, et al. Effects of intensive blood-pressure control in type 2 diabetes mellitus. *N Engl J Med.* 2010;362: 1575–85. [PMID: 20228401]

Egan BM, et al. Uncontrolled and apparent treatment resistant hypertension in the United States, 1988 to 2008. *Circulation.* 2011;124(9):1046–58. [PMID: 21824920]

HYVET Study Group. Treatment of hypertension in patients 80 years of age or older. *N Engl J Med.* 2008;358(18):1887–98. [PMID: 18378519]

Jamerson K, et al. Benazepril plus amlodipine or hydrochloro-thiazide for hypertension in high-risk patients. *N Engl J Med.* 2008;359:2417–28. [PMID: 19052124]

Krause T, et al. Management of hypertension: summary of NICE guidance. *BMJ.* 2011;343:d4891. [PMID: 21868454]

Mann JF, et al. Renal outcomes with telmisartan, ramipril, or both, in people at high vascular risk (the ONTARGET study): a multicentre, randomised, double-blind, controlled trial. *Lancet.* 2008;372(9638):547–53. [PMID: 18707986]

Raheja P, et al. Spironolactone prevents chlorthalidone-induced sympathetic activation and insulin resistance in hypertensive patients. *Hypertension.* 2012;60(2):319–25. [PMID: 22733474]

▶ Prognosis

Hypertension is a major risk factor for cardiovascular mortality, accounting for 50% of deaths from stroke and 45% from coronary heart disease worldwide. In addition,

Clinical Approach To Refractory Hypertension

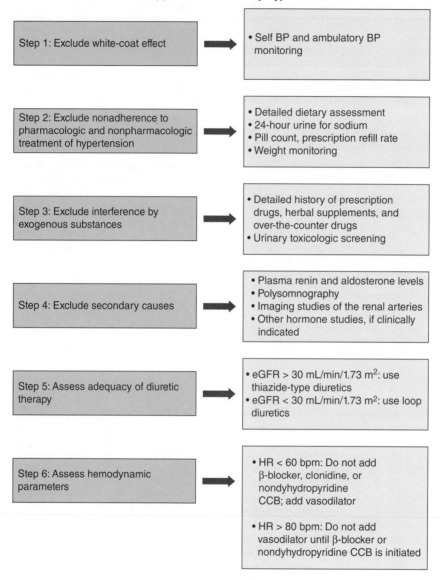

▲ Figure 2–2. Algorithm in management of resistant hypertension. BP, blood pressure; CCB, calcium channel blocker; eGFR, estimated glomerular filtration rate; HR, heart rate.

hypertension is a major risk factor for congestive heart failure, CKD, peripheral arterial disease, and the age-related decline in cognitive function. Presence of either persistent or new-onset LV hypertrophy or renal dysfunction during treatment contributes to poor prognosis. Patients with resistant hypertension experience a 20–25% higher risk of stroke and a 40–50% increase in risk of hospitalization from heart failure than hypertensive patients who achieve BP control with treatment. Thus, prompt evaluation for the underlying causes and intensification of pharmacologic and nonpharmacologic treatment is necessary to prevent target organ complications. Selection of appropriate antihypertensive medications that suit the patient characteristics and risk profile is the key to achieve BP goal. In addition to BP reduction, management of other cardiovascular risk factors is also essential in optimizing overall cardiovascular outcomes in hypertensive patients.

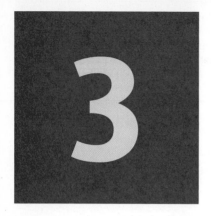

Antiplatelet Therapy

Ashvarya Mangla, MD
Saurabh Gupta, MD

▶ General Considerations

Atherosclerosis is a leading cause of cardiovascular disease. Atherosclerotic plaques can acutely rupture, exposing a necrotic core that sets off the coagulation cascade, ultimately culminating in vascular occlusion. Activation of platelets is the initial event in this cascade and, depending on the vascular bed involved, can cause acute coronary syndromes, ischemic stroke, mesenteric ischemia, or acute limb ischemia. Antiplatelet therapy forms the core of treatment for both acute and chronic atherosclerotic disease. In this chapter, we will discuss antiplatelet therapy in the treatment of cardiovascular disease.

▶ Role of Platelets in Thrombosis

After vascular injury, platelets are bound to exposed collagen and von Willebrand factor (vWF) and activated. Activated platelets then secrete thromboxane A_2 (TXA_2) and adenosine diphosphate (ADP), which leads to platelet aggregation and recruitment of more platelets. The final common pathway of platelet aggregation is mediated by glycoprotein (GP) II_bIII_a receptors that bind to fibrinogen and vWF, leading to platelet plug and clot formation. Antiplatelet agents target different pathways in this cascade (Figure 3–1).

▶ Classification of Antiplatelet Drugs (Figure 3–2)

A. Cyclooxygenase Inhibitors: Aspirin

1. Mechanism of action—Acetylsalicylic acid (ASA, aspirin) in low doses irreversibly inhibits cyclooxygenase-1 (COX-1), which is required for synthesis of TXA_2, a vasoconstrictor required for platelet aggregation. At higher doses, ASA also inhibits COX-2, which is required for prostacyclin production; prostacyclins are inhibitors of platelet aggregation and vasodilators. Thus, for optimal antiplatelet effect, an ASA dose between 75 and 325 mg is recommended. For rapid onset of action, in ASA-naïve patients, a dose of at least 162 mg should be used.

2. Contraindications—ASA is contraindicated in patients with a history of bronchospasm or anaphylactic reaction.

3. Side effects—Dyspepsia, peptic ulcer, erosive gastritis, and upper gastrointestinal bleeding are dose-related side effects. Some patients may develop bronchospasm, urticaria, and rarely anaphylactic reactions. Complex acid–base abnormalities can occur in the setting of aspirin overdose. Some younger patients may have aspirin hypersensitivity with associated nasal polyps, allergic rhinitis, and bronchospasm (Samter's triad). These patients may benefit from aspirin desensitization. Hyporesponsiveness to ASA is defined as the inability of ASA to produce expected inhibitory effects on platelet function. Clinically, this is associated with increased vascular events. Currently, there is no consensus on treatment, although empirically, an ADP receptor antagonist may be added.

4. Uses

A. Acute coronary syndromes—All patients who present with chest pain and electrocardiographic or cardiac biomarker evidence of ST elevation myocardial infarction (STEMI) or non-STEMI (NSTEMI) should be treated with non–enteric-coated aspirin 162–325 mg (preferably crushed and chewed to enable rapid onset of action). Aspirin should be continued indefinitely in all patients who are not allergic at a dose of 75–162 mg/day, once daily. For patients allergic to aspirin, clopidogrel (or another P_2Y_{12} receptor antagonist) is a reasonable alternative.

B. Chronic stable angina—Aspirin 75–162 mg is a standard component of routine management of patients with chronic stable angina and has been demonstrated to reduce morbidity and mortality.

C. Peripheral arterial disease—Patients with symptomatic lower extremity peripheral arterial disease have a high likelihood of disease in other vascular beds and should be treated with aspirin to reduce risk of myocardial infarction (MI), stroke, or vascular death.

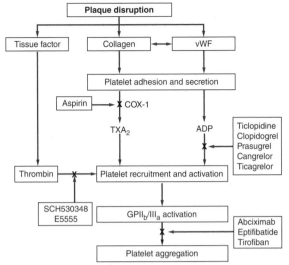

▲ **Figure 3–1.** Site of action of antiplatelet drugs. Aspirin inhibits thromboxane A_2 (TXA_2) synthesis by irreversibly acetylating cyclooxygenase-1 (COX-1). Reduced TXA_2 release attenuates platelet activation and recruitment to the site of vascular injury. Ticlopidine, clopidogrel, and prasugrel irreversibly block P_2Y_{12}, a key adenosine diphosphate (ADP) receptor on the platelet surface; cangrelor and ticagrelor are reversible inhibitors of P_2Y_{12}. Abciximab, eptifibatide, and tirofiban inhibit the final common pathway of platelet aggregation by blocking fibrinogen and von Willebrand factor (vWF) binding to activated glycoprotein (GP) II_b/III_a. SCH530348 and E5555 inhibit thrombin-mediated platelet activation by targeting protease-activated receptor-1 (PAR-1), the major thrombin receptor on human platelets. (Reproduced with permission from Longo DL, et al. *Harrison's Principles of Internal Medicine,* 18th ed. New York: McGraw-Hill; 2012.)

D. **STROKE/TRANSIENT ISCHEMIC ATTACK (TIA)**— Patients with prior ischemic stroke or TIA should receive aspirin 325 mg within the first 48 hours of onset of symptoms. If the patient has received thrombolytic therapy for ischemic stroke, antiplatelet therapy can be started after 24 hours. Therapy should be continued indefinitely at a dose of 75 or 81 mg orally once daily.

E. **PRIMARY PREVENTION**—Currently there is no evidence to support ASA for primary prevention in young patients (males < age 45, women < age 55) or patients over the age of 80 years. Men aged 45–79 years (for reduction of MIs) and women aged 55–79 years (for reduction of ischemic strokes) should take low-dose aspirin for primary prophylaxis if their potential benefit exceeds the risk of GI bleed. Aspirin 75–162 mg/day can be considered in patients with type 1 and type 2 diabetes who have a > 10% 10- year risk of developing coronary artery disease (CAD) based on Framingham risk score.

B. P_2Y_{12} Receptor Blockers

Commercially available products include the irreversible inhibitors ticlopidine, clopidogrel, and prasugrel and the reversible inhibitors cangrelor and ticagrelor.

1. Mechanism of action—These agents inhibit the P_2Y_{12} receptor (required for binding ADP with a resultant increase in platelet aggregation and activation of GP II_bIII_a receptors on platelet surface). Inhibition of these receptors leads to decreased platelet activation and aggregation.

2. Contraindications—Active bleeding and a previous anaphylactic reaction are contraindications to therapy. Prasugrel is contraindicated in patients with a prior history of TIA or stroke and should be used with extreme caution in the elderly (≥ 75 years) or low body weight (< 60 kg) due to increase in the risk of bleeding events. Maintenance doses of aspirin above 100 mg appear to reduce the effectiveness of ticagrelor and should be avoided.

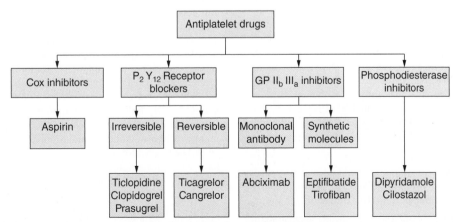

▲ **Figure 3–2.** Classification of antiplatelet drugs based on mechanism of action.

3. Side effects—Bleeding and purpuric lesions rarely occur. Ticlopidine can cause hematologic side effects such as bone marrow suppression, thrombocytopenia, thrombotic thrombocytopenic purpuras, and neutropenia, and regular blood count monitoring is recommended. This drug has largely been supplanted by alternatives with a more favorable risk–benefit ratio. Hematologic side effects are less common with clopidogrel and prasugrel. Skin rashes have also been reported with clopidogrel.

4. Clinically relevant pharmacology— Ticlopidine, clopidogrel, and prasugrel are prodrugs that require metabolism by liver to convert them into active drugs. After a loading dose, platelet inhibition starts in 4–6 hours. Prasugrel is absorbed more completely and has a relatively rapid onset of action. Nonthienopyridines, such as ticagrelor and cangrelor, are absorbed faster, have a more rapid onset, and have a shorter duration of action. In the setting of acute MI-STEMI or NSTEMI, when rapid inhibition of platelets is required, a loading dose of all antiplatelet agents is recommended.

5. Thienopyridine resistance—Some patients treated with adequate doses of clopidogrel still have thrombotic events despite medication compliance. This variability could partially be from genetic polymorphisms in the CYP isoenzymes involved in activation of clopidogrel. The prevalence of polymorphism is as high as 30–50% in certain populations. These genetic polymorphisms do not affect the activity of prasugrel, and it can be an alternative in populations suspected of having genetic predisposition to clopidogrel resistance. In the future, there may be a role for genetic testing prior to initiating clopidogrel.

6. Uses

A. ACUTE CORONARY SYNDROMES—For patients with STEMI, in whom primary percutaneous coronary intervention (PCI) is planned, P_2Y_{12} blockers should be administered as a loading dose, before or at the time of PCI (clopidogrel 300–600 mg, prasugrel 60 mg, or ticagrelor 180 mg). In patients less than 75 years of age who receive fibrinolytic therapy or who do not receive reperfusion therapy, it is reasonable to administer an oral loading dose of clopidogrel 300 mg and continue long-term maintenance therapy (1 year). Prasugrel can be considered once coronary anatomy is known (typically after coronary angiography). Patients with NSTEMI/unstable angina who are selected for early invasive strategy should receive dual antiplatelet therapy including aspirin. The additional agent could be either a P_2Y_{12} or a GP II_bIII_a inhibitor. Dual antiplatelet therapy should be continued for 12 months in patients with an acceptably low risk of bleeding.

B. POST PCI—Patients who undergo PCI should be on dual antiplatelet therapy with aspirin and any of the three P_2Y_{12} inhibitors (clopidogrel, prasugrel, or ticagrelor) for 1 year.

C. ASA ALLERGY—Patients with chronic stable angina, peripheral arterial disease, or a stroke or TIA who are allergic to aspirin can be treated with clopidogrel. Dual antiplatelet therapy with aspirin and P_2Y_{12} receptor antagonists is not indicated in patients without antecedent PCI, and dual antiplatelet therapy with aspirin and clopidogrel is not superior to either agent alone in patients with strokes or TIA.

C. GP II_bIII_a Inhibitors

The monoclonal antibody abciximab and the synthetic compounds eptifibatide and tirofiban are **GP II_bIII_a inhibitors**. Oral GP II_bIII_a receptor antagonists have not been demonstrated to be effective and currently have no role.

1. Mechanism of action—These drugs block the GP II_bIII_a receptors on the platelet surface. These are the most abundant receptors on the platelet surface and are the final common pathway of platelet aggregation and platelet plug formation.

2. Dosage—These agents are typically administered as an intravenous loading dose followed by a continuous infusion. The dose of abciximab does not need to be adjusted for patients with renal disease; however, tirofiban and eptifibatide are renally excreted, and the dose needs to be adjusted in patients with renal disease.

3. Contraindications—Abciximab should not be used in patients in whom PCI is not planned. Tirofiban and eptifibatide are contraindicated in patients with end-stage renal disease.

4. Side effects—Immune-mediated thrombocytopenia and bleeding are the common side effects. Thrombocytopenia is more common with the monoclonal antibody and relatively less common with synthetic agents. For patients being treated with these agents, daily monitoring of blood counts is recommended.

5. Uses: acute coronary syndromes—Patients who present with STEMI and are candidates for primary PCI (with or without stenting) are often treated with a strategy of heparin with a GP II_bIII_a inhibitor at the time of PCI or monotherapy with bivalirudin, in which case GP II_bIII_a inhibitors are reserved for patients with no reflow or with giant thrombus after PCI. In general, there is no role for GP II_bIII_a inhibitors after fibrinolytic therapy (regardless of whether fibrinolysis was successful) due to an increased risk for minor and major bleeding events. Patients with NSTEMI or unstable angina who are selected for early invasive strategy can be treated with GP II_bIII_a inhibitors in addition to aspirin either at the time of presentation or just before PCI. The agents of choice in this setting are eptifibatide and tirofiban. Patients for whom an early conservative strategy is chosen and who continue to have symptoms despite optimal medical therapy can also be considered for GP II_bIII_a inhibitors until the time of PCI.

D. Phosphodiesterase Inhibitors

Dipyridamole and cilostazol are **phosphodiesterase inhibitors.**

1. Mechanism of action—These agents inhibit the enzyme phosphodiesterase, thus increasing the concentration of cyclic adenosine monophosphate (cAMP) in platelets, which in turn inhibits platelet aggregation.

2. Uses

A. **STROKE**—Dipyridamole in combination with aspirin is superior to aspirin alone in secondary prevention of stroke.

B. **PERIPHERAL ARTERIAL DISEASE**—Patients with symptomatic lower extremity peripheral arterial disease and intermittent claudication in the absence of heart failure benefit from addition of cilostazol, with improvement in symptoms and increase in exercise tolerance.

C. **CARDIAC STRESS TESTING**—Due to its vasodilatory properties, dipyridamole is used in chemical stress testing.

▶ Treatment

A. Special Issues with Antiplatelet Therapy

1. Gastrointestinal bleeding—If antiplatelet therapy is indicated in patients with a history of or those at increased risk for gastrointestinal bleeding (advanced age or concomitant warfarin, steroid, or nonsteroidal anti-inflammatory drug use), proton pump inhibitors should be used to prevent recurrence or for prophylaxis. Earlier concerns about diminished efficacy of clopidogrel with the use of proton pump inhibitors have not been validated in randomized clinical trials.

2. Management of patients receiving antiplatelet therapy who require a surgical procedure—Decision to withhold antiplatelet therapy should be individualized for each patient depending on the risk of bleeding and the indication for which the antiplatelet therapy is used. For patients receiving ASA and a P_2Y_{12} receptor antagonist for a bare metal stent (BMS) who require urgent surgery within 6 weeks of placement, dual therapy should be continued in the perioperative period. For patients who are receiving ASA and clopidogrel for a drug-eluting stent (DES) and require urgent surgery within 12 months of placement, therapy should be continued in the perioperative period. Whenever possible, elective surgery in patients receiving ASA and clopidogrel secondary to coronary stent implantation should be deferred for at least 6 weeks after BMS placement and at least 12 months after DES placement.

3. Combined antiplatelet and anticoagulant therapy—Patients with CAD who are on anticoagulant therapy for atrial fibrillation or prosthetic heart valve and undergo PCI should be on dual antiplatelet therapy in addition to anticoagulant therapy. After PCI, the maintenance should consist of a combination of low-dose ASA (75–100 mg), warfarin, and clopidogrel (duration determined by the type of stent—1 month after BMS or 1 year after DES implantation). When warfarin is given in conjunction with clopidogrel or low-dose

ASA, the dose-intensity must be carefully monitored. There is some evidence that a similar strategy of dual antiplatelet therapy with dabigatran may be safe with an acceptably low (albeit increased from baseline) bleeding risk, but caution is warranted until more data are available.

B. Special Populations

1. Antiplatelet therapy in atrial arrhythmias—In patients with atrial fibrillation younger than 60 years without heart disease or risk factors for thromboembolism (lone atrial fibrillation), ASA for primary prevention of stroke is probably reasonable, although the effectiveness of this approach is not well established. For patients at low risk for thromboembolism (age 65–74, female sex, CAD), antiplatelet therapy with aspirin 75–325 mg is a reasonable alternative to anticoagulation. Patients who have just one moderate risk factor for thromboembolism (hypertension, age > 75 years, congestive heart failure, ejection fraction < 35%, diabetes mellitus) may be candidates for antiplatelet therapy with ASA 75–325 mg alone if their risk of bleeding from antithrombotic agent is high, because of patient preference, or if there are issues with sustained monitoring of anticoagulation. Patients with atrial fibrillation or atrial flutter who have more than one moderate risk factor and cannot take anticoagulant therapy for reasons other than bleeding may be started on dual antiplatelet therapy with ASA and clopidogrel, although this therapy is inferior to anticoagulant therapy.

2. Coronary artery bypass grafting (CABG)—When possible, ASA should be administered preoperatively to patients in whom CABG is planned; if not initiated preoperatively, it should be started within 6 hours of surgery and continued indefinitely to prevent graft occlusion. For patients who are intolerant or allergic to aspirin, clopidogrel 75 mg orally once daily can be substituted. Patients on dual antiplatelet therapy with aspirin and P_2Y_{12} receptor blockers scheduled to undergo elective CABG should discontinue clopidogrel and ticagrelor at least 5 days and prasugrel at least 7 days prior to surgery. For urgent surgery, these agents should preferably be discontinued at least 24 hours before surgery to reduce the risk of major bleeding. The GP II_bIII_a inhibitors eptifibatide and tirofiban should be discontinued at least 2–4 hours before surgery and abciximab at least 12 hours before surgery.

3. Pregnancy—Antiplatelet agents can be considered in pregnancy or breastfeeding if maternal benefits clearly outweigh potential fetal risks. Low-dose ASA (75–162 mg daily) is likely safe for use during the first trimester of pregnancy; however, it should be avoided during the third trimester and while breastfeeding. Use of agents other than low-dose ASA should only be considered after weighing maternal benefits with potential risks for the newborn. P_2Y_{12} receptor antagonists should be used during pregnancy or breastfeeding only if clearly indicated.

4. Patients with prosthetic heart valves—The addition of daily ASA (75–100 mg) to therapeutic warfarin is recommended for all patients with mechanical heart valves and those patients with biological valves who have risk factors. For patients with an aortic or mitral bioprosthesis and no risk factors, aspirin is indicated at 75–100 mg/day. For patients unable to take warfarin, ASA is indicated in a dose of 75–325 mg/day (or clopidogrel if intolerant or allergic to ASA).

5. PCI—After PCI, ASA should be continued indefinitely at a dose of 75 or 81 mg once daily. Typically a P_2Y_{12} inhibitor is indicated for at least 12 months regardless of the stent type. In select patients after BMS implantation and an increased risk of bleeding, dual antiplatelet therapy maybe continued for 1 month. Options for P_2Y_{12} inhibitors include clopidogrel 75 mg daily, prasugrel 10 mg daily, or ticagrelor 90 mg twice daily.

Angiolillo DJ, et al. Pharmacologic therapy for acute coronary syndromes. In: Fuster V, et al., eds. *Hurst's the Heart*, 13th ed. New York: McGraw-Hill; 2011.

Fraker TD Jr, et al. 2007 Chronic angina focused update of the ACC/AHA 2002 guidelines for the management of patients with chronic stable angina: a report of the American College of Cardiology/American Heart Association Task Force on Practice Guidelines Writing Group to Develop the Focused Update of the 2002 Guidelines for the management of patients with chronic stable angina. *Circulation*. 2007;116:2762–72. [PMID: 17998462]

Jneid H, et al. 2012 ACCF/AHA focused update of the guideline for the management of patients with unstable angina/non–ST-elevation myocardial infarction (updating the 2007 guideline and replacing the 2011 focused update): a report of the American College of Cardiology Foundation/American Heart Association Task Force on Practice Guidelines. *Circulation*. 2012;126:875–910. [PMID: 22800849]

Kushner FG, et al. 2009 focused updates: ACC/AHA guidelines for the management of patients with ST-elevation myocardial infarction (updating the 2004 guideline and 2007 focused update) and ACC/AHA/SCAI guidelines on percutaneous coronary intervention (updating the 2005 guideline and 2007 focused update): a report of the American College of Cardiology Foundation/American Heart Association Task Force on Practice Guidelines. *J Am Coll Cardiol*. 2009;54(23):2205–41. [PMID: 19942100]

Weitz JI. Antiplatelet, anticoagulant, and fibrinolytic drugs. In: Longo DL, et al., eds. *Harrison's Principles of Internal Medicine*, 18th ed. New York: McGraw-Hill; 2012.

Long-Term Anticoagulation for Cardiac Conditions

4

Richard D. Taylor, MD
Richard W. Asinger, MD

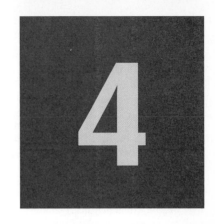

▶ General Considerations

Intracardiac thrombi can form and lead to devastating consequences as a result of obstruction of blood flow and/or peripheral embolization. Long-term anticoagulation is recommended for primary and secondary prevention of thromboembolism in many cardiac conditions, and in selected conditions, it is essential. There are, however, risks associated with the use of anticoagulants, and an understanding of the risks and benefits of anticoagulant therapy for various cardiac conditions is important.

A. Anticoagulants

These agents affect the coagulation protein cascade to reduce thrombosis.

1. Unfractionated heparin—Unfractionated heparin (UFH) binds to antithrombin III, markedly increasing the effect of antithrombin III in neutralizing thrombin. It also inhibits the activation of factors IX and X. The effectiveness of UFH varies greatly from person to person due to its interactions with a number of plasma proteins and the endothelium. Monitoring the effects of full-dose UFH on hemostasis is mandatory. The activated partial thromboplastin time (aPTT) is used to monitor the effects of UFH and is titrated to 1.5–2.0 times greater than control. In certain situations, a higher level of anticoagulation is needed; for example, during coronary interventions where the activated clotting time (ACT) is used to monitor its effect and the dose of UFH is adjusted to keep the ACT 250–300 seconds or greater. When given intravenously, the effects of UFH are immediate. It is usually given as a bolus, followed by a continuous intravenous infusion. It may also be given in therapeutic doses subcutaneously. The effects of UFH will dissipate within 6 hours. Protamine can be given to reverse its effects more quickly. UFH can also be given subcutaneously in smaller doses, which will not affect the aPTT, for primary prevention of deep venous thrombosis.

2. Low-molecular-weight heparin—Low-molecular-weight heparins (LMWHs) are breakdown products of UFH. They have a greater effect on factor X than on thrombin. LMWHs bind less to plasma proteins than UFH, and therefore, the dosing is more predictable. They are more resistant to neutralization by platelet factor 4 than UFH and have less inhibitory effect on platelet function than UFH. LMWHs have a more predictable effect on coagulation than UFH, and laboratory monitoring is usually not necessary, but activated factor Xa levels can be used to monitor their effects. LMWHs are usually administered subcutaneously twice daily. They are not easily reversed by protamine. LMWH can also be given in smaller doses for the primary prevention of deep venous thrombosis.

3. Intravenous thrombin inhibitors—Lepirudin, bivalirudin, and argatroban inhibit thrombin formation and are useful when UFH and LMWH are contraindicated. These agents are administered by bolus followed by a continuous infusion. These agents inactivate both free and fibrin-bound thrombin. They do not bind to plasma proteins and, therefore, have a more predictable pharmacologic response, but their therapeutic window is narrow. The aPTT is used to monitor their effect. The international normalized ratio (INR) is also affected by these agents, making transition to warfarin more difficult. The bleeding risk with the direct thrombin inhibitors may be greater than with UFH. Due to the short half-life of these drugs, bleeding complications can usually be controlled by stopping the infusion. Argatroban is the preferred thrombin inhibitor for patients with renal insufficiency.

4. Fondaparinux—This agent is an analog of pentasaccharides found in UFH and LMWH. It increases the effect of antithrombin and inhibits factor Xa. It has a half-life of 17 hours when given subcutaneously and is given once daily according to the patient's weight: 7.5 mg for 50–100 kg, 5 mg for < 50 kg, and 10 mg for > 100 kg. It should not be used if the creatinine clearance (CrCl) is less than 30 cc/min. It is used for primary prevention of deep vein thrombosis (DVT) and for treatment of DVT and pulmonary embolus.

5. Oral vitamin K antagonists—Coumarins, or vitamin K antagonists, have been the mainstay of oral anticoagulants for more than 50 years. Warfarin is the most commonly used oral anticoagulant. It blocks the conversion of vitamin K to the active moiety, vitamin K epoxide, which is necessary for the synthesis of factors II, VII, IX, and X and proteins C and S. The half-life of warfarin is about 40 hours. It is nearly completely absorbed when given orally and binds to albumin. Its effect on hemostasis is quite variable from person to person and, sometimes, for the same person at different times. Warfarin's effect can be influenced by dietary factors, liver disease, congestive heart failure, hypermetabolic states, and numerous drug interactions. Monitoring the anticoagulant effect of warfarin with a prothrombin time (PT) is mandatory. The PT is now standardized to an international thromboplastin reagent and reported as the INR. Serial INRs are used to monitor warfarin effects and adjust its dose. Warfarin therapy may be started without a loading dose. It usually takes several days for the target INR to be achieved. During initiation of therapy, there may be a brief paradoxical hypercoagulable state due to the inhibition of proteins C and S (anticoagulant factors) before the inhibition of the coagulant factors. For this reason, UFH or LMWH may be used as a bridge until a therapeutic INR is achieved. During initiation of warfarin therapy, the INR should be checked frequently until a stable dose is found that achieves the target INR. Subsequently, the INR should be monitored at least once a month and more frequently if the dose needs to be adjusted. Monitoring can be done by an individual care provider or through an anticoagulation clinic, which tends to be more organized and efficient. Point-of-care monitoring of INR is now available and can be done at home. If warfarin needs to be stopped, the INR will normalize in about 3–4 days. If its anticoagulant effect needs to be reversed more quickly, vitamin K can be administered orally (preferred), subcutaneously or intravenously. The INR will usually correct in 1–2 days if vitamin K is given. If it is necessary to reverse the effects of warfarin more quickly, fresh frozen plasma or prothrombin complex concentrate can be given.

6. New oral anticoagulants—Recently, several new oral anticoagulants have been developed that, in distinction to warfarin, target only a single enzyme in the coagulation cascade. These have targeted thrombin and activated factor Xa. They can be given in a fixed dose that does not require routine monitoring.

A. DIRECT THROMBIN INHIBITORS—These inhibit free thrombin and also thrombin bound to fibrin. Two of these inhibitors, ximelagatran and dabigatran, have been evaluated in phase III clinical trials of nonvalvular atrial fibrillation patients comparing the drug with dose-adjusted warfarin for stroke and systemic embolus as well as bleeding complications. Ximelagatran was associated with liver enzyme elevation and

is no longer used. Dabigatran has been evaluated in a phase III clinical trial in two doses. At 150 mg orally twice a day (bid), dabigatran was superior to warfarin in stroke prevention with a similar incidence of major bleeds. At 110 mg orally bid, dabigatran had a similar incidence of stroke with fewer major bleeds compared to dose-adjusted warfarin. It is excreted primarily through the kidneys and is recommended at 150 mg bid for those with CrCl > 30 cc/min. Based on pharmacodynamics data, a reduced dose of 75 mg bid has been approved by the U.S. Food and Drug Administration for those with CrCl of 15–30 cc/min, although there is no clinical evidence of efficacy. It is not recommended for those with a CrCl < 15 cc/min. The higher dose of 150 mg bid was associated with increased bleeds in those over 75 years of age, and the 110 mg bid dose is recommended in those of age 80 or older by Health Canada. The dose should also be reduced to 110 mg bid for those who weigh < 60 kg. Dabigatran is not metabolized by the cytochrome P450 system, but P-glycoprotein inhibitors can increase its concentration. The European Society of Cardiology (ESC) recommends the lower dose of 110 mg bid for those on verapamil and does not recommended it for those taking dronedarone. Potent P-glycoprotein inhibitors, including St. John's wort, rifampin, carbamazepine, and phenytoin, reduce dabigatran concentration, and it should not be given in combination with these agents. Measurement of the anticoagulant effect is not readily available clinically, although the aPTT is affected. No specific therapy reverses its effect, although hemodialysis will reduce its concentration. In accidental overdose, activated charcoal may be used to absorb it from the stomach. The use of prothrombin complex concentrate and/or activated factor VII maybe helpful in cases of uncontrolled bleeding, but there are no clinical data establishing the efficacy of this approach.

B. FACTOR XA INHIBITORS—A number of factor Xa inhibitors have been or are being developed. Two have been reported in randomized, phase III clinical trials of the incidence of stroke and major bleeds in patients with nonvalvular atrial fibrillation comparing the new anticoagulant with dose-adjusted warfarin (target INR 2.0–3.0). Both rivaroxaban and apixaban are highly selective, reversible, direct factor Xa inhibitors.

Rivaroxaban is a once-a-day drug that is excreted primarily through the kidneys. It is not recommended in patients with a CrCl < 15 cc/min, and there are few data on its efficacy in those with CrCl of 15–30 cc/min. Although drug and diet interactions are minimal, it is metabolized in the liver through cytochrome P450 (CYP)–dependent and –independent mechanisms. It is not recommended for those receiving inhibitors of both CYP3A4 and P-glycoprotein, including azole antimycotics and human immunodeficiency virus (HIV) protease inhibitors. The anticoagulant effect of this drug is not easily measured clinically, although its effect is reflected in the INR. No specific agent is available to reverse its effect. Accidental overdose may be treated with activated charcoal to absorb the drug from the stomach.

Hemodialysis is not effective in reducing its concentration because it is highly protein bound. Its anticoagulant effect can be reversed in vitro with prothrombin complex concentrate, but this has not been demonstrated clinically.

Apixaban is a twice-a-day drug that is metabolized in the liver by CYP3A4-dependent and -independent mechanisms, and about one-quarter is excreted in the urine. It is not recommended for patients with a CrCl < 15 cc/min or in those receiving HIV protease inhibitors. Also there is no easy way to monitor the anticoagulant effect of apixaban clinically, and there is no specific reversal agent. Accidental overdose may benefit from activated charcoal to absorb the drug from the stomach. The use of prothrombin complex concentrate and/or factor VIIa may be helpful for uncontrolled bleeding, but clinical evidence for the efficacy of this approach is limited.

Two other factor Xa inhibitors are in development. Edoxaban is currently being evaluated in a large phase III clinical trial of nonvalvular atrial fibrillation compared with dose-adjusted warfarin. Another factor Xa inhibitor, betrixaban, is also being developed.

B. Risks of Anticoagulant Therapy

Bleeding is the most common serious adverse effect seen with the use of anticoagulant agents. Bleeding complications are more likely to occur in patients who are: of age >65 years; have a history of previous stroke, gastrointestinal tract bleeding, recent myocardial infarction, anemia, renal insufficiency, serious concurrent illness or diabetes; drink alcohol excessively; take antiplatelet agents including aspirin (Table 4–1). Intracranial hemorrhage (ICH) is perhaps the most feared complication of anticoagulant therapy. In the absence of anticoagulation, ICH usually presents suddenly, with rapid progression to the maximal neurologic deficit. ICH that occurs while a patient is receiving anticoagulant therapy, however, can be much more devastating, with continued bleeding and progressive neurologic deterioration. In such situations, reversal of the anticoagulant effect is necessary as soon as possible. Of the anticoagulants available, the incidence of ICH in patients with nonvalvular atrial fibrillation is highest in those prescribed warfarin. For those taking dabigatran or factor Xa inhibitors, the incidence of ICH is significantly less, only one-third the incidence seen with dose-adjusted warfarin. The anticoagulant effect of these newer agents, however, cannot be easily measured clinically, and more problematic is the fact that they have no specific antidote.

Thrombocytopenia can complicate the use of UFH and LMWH in two ways. A dose-dependent lowering of the platelet count is usually not serious and does not necessarily require stopping these agents. The second type of thrombocytopenia is termed "heparin-induced thrombocytopenia" (HIT). It is immune-mediated and can be life-threatening due to arterial and venous thrombus formation. An antibody to heparin interacts with a heparin–platelet factor 4 complex on the platelet surface, resulting in platelet destruction. HIT

Table 4–1. Risk Factors for Bleeding Complications with Anticoagulants

Age > 65 years
History of hemorrhagic stroke
History of stroke
History of gastrointestinal bleeding
INR 4.0
Prosthetic heart valve
Recent myocardial infarction
Anemia
Renal insufficiency
Diabetes
High risk for trauma
Concurrent illness
Multiple medications
Unreliable taking of medications
Unreliable medical follow-up
Antiplatelet use including aspirin
Excessive alcohol intake

INR, international normalized ratio.

usually starts at least 4 days after heparin initiation unless there has been previous heparin exposure. It is not dose-dependent, and there is usually at least a 50% reduction in the platelet count. The diagnosis of HIT can be confirmed with an immunoassay for the antibody–heparin–platelet factor 4 complex. HIT is much less common with LMWH than with UFH, occurring about one-tenth as frequently. The treatment for HIT is immediate discontinuation of all heparin, even low doses used to maintain intravenous access. A direct thrombin inhibitor, such as lepirudin, bivalirudin, or argatroban, should be substituted.

Additional rare complications seen with UFH and LMWH include hyperkalemia (due to hyperaldosteronism), osteoporosis, skin necrosis, and alopecia.

Adverse effects seen with warfarin include skin necrosis and teratogenic effects. Skin necrosis due to warfarin is a rare complication seen within the first few days of treatment. It is most likely to occur in patients with protein C and S deficiencies. Because of its teratogenic effects, warfarin should be used cautiously during pregnancy (if at all), especially in the first trimester and specifically between the 6th and 12th weeks of gestation.

De Caterina R, et al. New oral anticoagulants in atrial fibrillation and acute coronary syndromes: ESC Working Group on Thrombosis-Task force on Anticoagulants in Heart Disease position paper. *J Am Coll Cardiol.* 2012;59:1413–25. [PMID: 22497820]

Furie KL, et al. Oral antithrombotic agents for the prevention of stroke in nonvalvular atrial fibrillation: a science advisory for healthcare professionals from the American Heart Association and American Stroke Association. *Stroke.* 2012;43:3442–53. [PMID: 22858728]

Hirsh J, et al. American Heart Association/American College of Cardiology Foundation guide to warfarin therapy. *J Am Coll Cardiol.* 2003;41(9):1633–52. [PMID: 12742309]
Levine MN, et al. Hemorrhagic complications of anticoagulant treatment. *Chest.* 2001;119(1 Suppl):108S–121S. [PMID: 11157645]

▶ Pathophysiology & Etiology

A. Pathogenesis of Intravascular Thrombi

In the nineteenth century, Virchow theorized that stasis of intracavitary blood, endocardial injury, and a hypercoagulable state were necessary for the formation of intracardiac thrombi. In the normally functioning heart, stasis and thrombosis do not occur, but a high incidence of thrombosis is noted in cardiac chambers that are enlarged or have low flow. Left atrial thrombi can develop in persons with atrial fibrillation and left ventricular thrombi in those with acute myocardial infarction, left ventricular aneurysm, and dilated cardiomyopathy. In these clinical settings, there is generalized or localized low flow in the left atrium and left ventricle, respectively.

Acute ST segment elevation myocardial infarction (STEMI) causes stasis of intracavitary blood (secondary to dysfunction of part of the left ventricle) in the setting of a hypercoagulable state, and left ventricular thrombi are common, particularly if reperfusion therapy is not given or is ineffective. Left ventricular thrombi most commonly develop at the apex of the left ventricle 2–7 days after anterior infarction; they rarely develop with inferior STEMI or non–ST segment elevation myocardial infarction (NSTEMI). Because the left anterior descending coronary artery usually supplies the apex, apical stasis may occur with anterior infarction. Severe apical wall motion abnormalities (ie, akinesia and dyskinesia) precede thrombus formation. Endocardial injury in acute infarction also contributes to thrombosis.

Endocardial abnormalities may be present in other clinical settings such as atrial fibrillation, in which elevated von Willebrand factor is noted in the left atrium. The introduction of a foreign material, such as a prosthetic valve, can provide a nidus for thrombus formation. An inflammatory process that involves the myocardium, secondary to myocarditis or noninfectious endocarditis, may be responsible for thrombus formation, particularly when there is a coexistent hypercoagulable state. Reduced ventricular function may contribute to thrombosis with myocarditis. Eosinophils presumably cause the endothelial injury with Löffler endocarditis that leads to thrombus formation.

The final prerequisite for intracardiac thrombosis is a hypercoagulable state. Activation of the coagulation system can be found in conditions associated with intracardiac thrombi, including acute myocardial infarction and atrial fibrillation. Rare cases of intracardiac thrombi have been reported even with normal wall motion and presumably normal blood flow because of a hypercoagulable state such as factor V Leiden mutation, prothrombin gene mutation, antithrombin deficiency, protein C and S deficiencies, homocysteine deficiency, and antiphospholipid antibody syndrome. Platelets may also play an active role in the formation of intracardiac thrombi and are activated in such clinical situations as acute myocardial infarction and atrial fibrillation.

Although all three of Virchow's prerequisites are operative in specific settings, most clinical data indicate a complex interaction exists, with stasis being the most frequent (or perhaps the most easily demonstrated) factor leading to intracardiac thrombosis.

B. Embolization of Thrombi

The major risk associated with intracardiac thrombi is end organ ischemia/infarction due to embolization. Factors that result in embolization of intracardiac thrombi are poorly understood, but restoration of mechanical function to an area of the heart that was previously noncontractile may result in embolization. Left ventricular thrombi usually form within the first week of an anterior myocardial infarction. However, embolization due to these thrombi usually occurs 5–21 days following infarction, a time at which left ventricular function may be improved, eliminating stasis and expelling the thrombus. Improved myocardial function at the margins of a thrombus could theoretically dislodge the thrombus or change the shape of a thrombus from mural to protruding and lead to embolization.

Recovery of the mechanical function of the left atrium following conversion from atrial flutter or fibrillation has also been implicated in development and embolization of left atrial thrombi. Following conversion of atrial fibrillation to sinus rhythm, the left atrium and/or appendage may be stunned, creating a low-flow state that leads to thrombus formation followed by embolization as its function recovers. Endogenous or pharmacologic thrombolysis could also result in disruption of thrombi and embolization. Embolization is more likely for certain intracardiac thrombi, especially protruding or mobile thrombi. Embolization may also be more likely when larger thrombi are present. Although all the factors that lead to embolization are not known, it is known that embolization is likely to recur in patients who have had previous embolization. Peripheral embolization of intracardiac thrombi can be to the brain, extremities, bowel, spleen, and kidneys. The most frequent site recognized clinically is to the brain, resulting in stroke.

The differentiation of thrombotic from embolic stroke is not always possible, although it is estimated that 15% of all ischemic strokes are cardioembolic. Patients with atrial fibrillation, prosthetic heart valves, or left ventricular mural thrombi are more likely to have cardioembolic events, whereas patients with known carotid artery disease are more likely to have a thrombotic stroke or an artery-to-artery embolus.

Patients who suffer a cardioembolic stroke are at risk for recurrent stroke. Antithrombotic therapy can lower the risk of recurrent stroke, but a serious and potentially life-threatening complication of cardioembolic stroke is intracerebral bleeding secondary to transformation of an ischemic to a hemorrhagic stroke. Computed tomography (CT) scanning should be performed in patients with a cerebral embolus to identify hemorrhage or if there are features indicating a high risk of hemorrhagic transformation. The Cerebral Embolism Study Group recommends that patients with cardiogenic cerebral emboli receive anticoagulation if they are not hypertensive and there is no evidence of intracerebral hemorrhage on CT scan at 24–48 hours. A delay of 7 days might be prudent in those with large cerebral infarction to lower the risk of hemorrhagic transformation.

▶ Diagnostic Studies

An intracardiac source of embolization is often suspected clinically, and a number of diagnostic tests can be used to identify intracardiac thrombi.

Echocardiography is a readily available and reasonably accurate, noninvasive technique for detecting intracardiac thrombi. Transthoracic echocardiography (TTE) is sensitive and specific for detecting left ventricular thrombi (Figures 4–1 and 4–2). Transesophageal echocardiography (TEE) is required to reliably detect left atrial thrombi (Figure 4–3) and atherothrombotic material in the ascending, transverse, and descending thoracic aorta (Figure 4–4). Intravenous echo contrast may help in the correct identification of cardiac masses, especially thrombi (see Figure 4–1).

Serial echocardiography greatly enhanced knowledge of the natural history of intracardiac thrombosis associated with acute myocardial infarction in part because the precise onset of the pathophysiologic thrombotic process can be accurately defined. Doppler studies of blood flow within the left ventricle of patients in whom thrombosis develops have shown that apical patterns of low flow precede thrombus formation. Because high-risk factors (anterior infarction and severe apical wall motion abnormality) are present and can be detected prior to thrombus development, it is possible to initiate prophylactic treatment with anticoagulants and decrease the development of thrombus and subsequent systemic emboli.

Spontaneous echo contrast ("smoke") detected in a cardiac chamber represents low-flow and early rouleaux formation and is frequently associated with thrombus or subsequent development of thrombus. Patients with spontaneous echo contrast or low-flow velocities in the left atrium have a high incidence of left atrial thrombi and thromboembolism.

High-speed contrast CT and magnetic resonance imaging (MRI) can also detect intracardiac thrombus, especially in the left ventricle. These techniques require specialized equipment not always available and are expensive. Delayed enhancement cardiac MRI is, however, highly sensitive and specific in detection of left ventricular thrombi and can be use if TTE including echo contrast is poor quality or indeterminate for left ventricular thrombus or the clinical circumstances dictate.

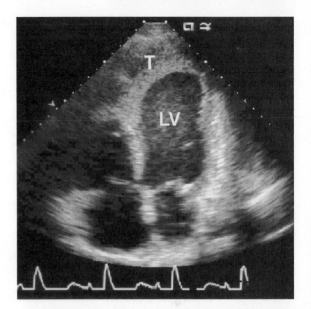

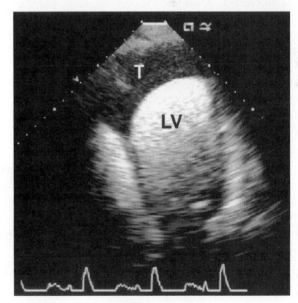

▲ **Figure 4–1.** Mural thrombus (T) in the left ventricle (LV) of a patient with a left ventricular aneurysm following anterior myocardial infarction. Top panel is an apical four-chamber echocardiogram with second harmonic imaging. The thrombus is well imaged, but delineation of the underlying wall motion abnormality is difficult to appreciate. Bottom panel is the same view with a lipid-based echo contrast agent; note the clearer definition of the thrombus and aneurysm.

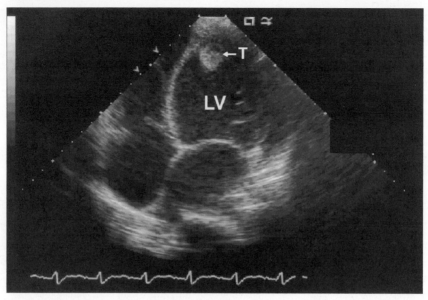

▲ **Figure 4–2.** Apical four-chamber, two-dimensional echocardiogram of a patient with dilated cardiomyopathy showing a protruding thrombus (T) at the apex of the left ventricle (LV).

Although intracardiac thrombi are the most common cardiac cause of peripheral embolization, there are other causes, including valvular vegetations due to infectious or noninfectious endocarditis, calcific emboli due to degenerative aortic and mitral valve disease, tumor emboli from left-sided myxoma, and atheroemboli from friable or mobile plaque in the aorta or great vessels (see Figure 4–4). In addition, embolic events can occur due to paradoxical emboli that originate in the venous system and transverse an intracardiac communication (most commonly a patent foramen ovale) (Figure 4–5). These conditions are readily identified by TTE or TEE, or both.

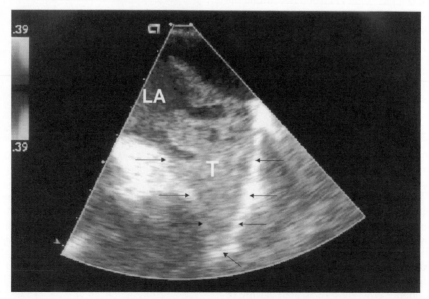

▲ **Figure 4–3.** Transesophageal echocardiogram demonstrating the left atrium (LA) with a large thrombus (T) filling the left atrial appendage. *Arrows* outline the left atrial appendage.

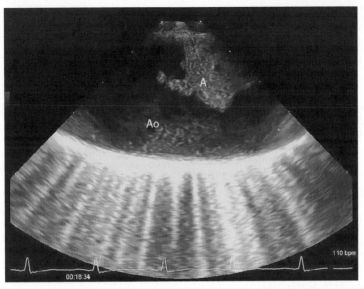

▲ **Figure 4–4.** Transesophageal echocardiogram demonstrating a large atheroma (A) in the transverse thoracic aorta (Ao).

Kirkpatrick JN, et al. Differential diagnosis of cardiac masses using contrast echocardiographic perfusion imaging. *J Am Coll Cardiol.* 2004;43(8):1412–9. [PMID: 15093876]

Mollet NR, et al. Visualization of ventricular thrombi with contrast-enhanced magnetic resonance imaging in patients with ischemic heart disease. *Circulation.* 2002;106(23):2873–6. [PMID: 12460863]

Srichai MB, et al. Clinical, imaging, and pathological characteristics of left ventricular thrombus: a comparison of contrast-enhanced magnetic resonance imaging, transthoracic echocardiography, and transesophageal echocardiography with surgical or pathological validation. *Am Heart J.* 2006;152(1):75–84. [PMID: 16824834]

Thambidorai SK, et al; ACUTE Investigators. Utility of transesophageal echocardiography in identification of thrombogenic milieu in patients with atrial fibrillation (an ACUTE ancillary study). *Am J Cardiol.* 2005;96(7):935–41. [PMID: 16188520]

Weinsaft JW, et al. Detection of left ventricular thrombus by delayed-enhancement cardiovascular magnetic resonance prevalence and markers in patients with systolic dysfunction. *J Am Coll Cardiol.* 2008;52(2):148–57.[PMID: 18598895]

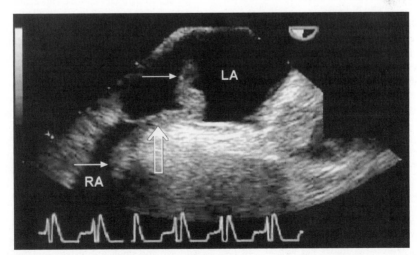

▲ **Figure 4–5.** Transesophageal echocardiogram demonstrating a systemic venous thrombus, which has embolized to the heart and lodged in a patent foramen ovale. LA, left atrium; RA, right atrium. *Arrows* indicate the thrombus; the *open arrow* indicates the patent foramen ovale.

▶ Treatment of Cardiac Conditions Requiring Anticoagulation

Short- and long-term anticoagulation are integral parts of the treatment of many cardiovascular conditions, including acute coronary syndromes, stroke, peripheral arterial disease, and venous thromboembolic disease. These conditions are discussed in other chapters. Long-term anticoagulation will be discussed in this chapter for the following conditions: atrial fibrillation, native valvular heart disease, prosthetic heart valves, left ventricular thrombus with acute myocardial infarction, remote myocardial infarction, left ventricular aneurysm, dilated cardiomyopathy, atherosclerotic sources of emboli, paradoxical emboli associated with a patent foramen ovale, and intracardiac devices.

Guidelines have been written by a number of organizations, including the American Heart Association (AHA), American College of Cardiology (ACC), American College of Chest Physicians (ACCP), and ESC for the management of anticoagulation in a number of conditions. These guidelines vary in their content and format; however, their recommendations are mostly in agreement.

A. Atrial Fibrillation

Atrial fibrillation can result in atrial thrombus formation (most often seen in the left atrial appendage [see Figure 4–3]), which can subsequently result in embolization (most often recognized clinically to the brain resulting in ischemic stroke). The incidence of stroke in patients with atrial fibrillation not related to rheumatic mitral valve disease is 4–5% per year, 4–5 times greater than in similar patients who do not have atrial fibrillation. The incidence of stroke with atrial fibrillation is age related. For those age 50–59 years, the incidence is about 1.5% per year, but this increases to > 10% per year for those 80 years of age and older.

AHA/ACC/ESC has recommended classifying atrial fibrillation as (1) first episode, (2) paroxysmal, (3) persistent, and (4) permanent. Acute atrial fibrillation is that which occurs for the first time. Chronic atrial fibrillation can be paroxysmal, persistent, or permanent. In paroxysmal atrial fibrillation, episodes spontaneously convert to normal sinus rhythm usually within 7 days. In persistent atrial fibrillation, episodes last longer than 7 days and/or conversion to normal sinus rhythm requires cardioversion, either chemical or electrical. In permanent atrial fibrillation, normal sinus rhythm can no longer be restored, and/or the patient and physician no longer attempt to restore or maintain normal sinus rhythm. The risk of stroke is considered the same for all three categories of chronic atrial fibrillation.

Atrial flutter is much less common than atrial fibrillation; however, these two arrhythmias are often seen in the same individual. Patients with atrial flutter are also at risk for thromboembolism, and therefore, the two arrhythmias are treated the same in terms of anticoagulation.

1. Chronic atrial fibrillation (nonvalvular)—The efficacy of long-term therapy with oral anticoagulants (warfarin) for primary and secondary prevention of stroke in patients with nonvalvular atrial fibrillation has been clearly shown in randomized, placebo controlled trials.

The risks of anticoagulant therapy in this particular patient population are considerable. ICH increases significantly with age greater than 75 years and INRs greater than 4.0.

Randomized studies have also evaluated the effects of aspirin in reducing the incidence of stroke in patients with nonvalvular atrial fibrillation. These studies showed little benefit of aspirin, much less than with dose-adjusted warfarin. The combination of aspirin and fixed, low-dose warfarin has been compared with dose-adjusted warfarin and was not as effective in lowering the incidence of stroke. Aspirin plus clopidogrel was more efficacious than aspirin alone for stroke prevention in nonvalvular atrial fibrillation patients, but inferior to dose-adjusted warfarin despite a similar risk of bleeds.

Anticoagulant therapy in atrial fibrillation reduces the incidence of stroke by > 60%. The usually accepted target INR for the prevention of stroke with warfarin is 2.0–3.0, and the time patients are within this range (time in target range) is predictive of the efficacy of anticoagulation—the best results are when patients are in this range > 65% of the time. Its efficacy is diminished if the INR is less than 2.0, and INRs greater than 4.0 are associated with a higher risk of bleeding, including ICH. In view of the higher risk of anticoagulation in the very elderly, the target INR is at times lowered to 2.0–2.5. The newer oral anticoagulants are more effective in maintaining continuous effective anticoagulation.

In patients with atrial fibrillation and coronary artery disease, antiplatelet drugs may be added to warfarin in certain situations. The ACCP guidelines suggest that patients with stable coronary disease (no acute coronary syndrome in the last year) and atrial fibrillation (requiring anticoagulant therapy) should receive warfarin without antiplatelet agents. For atrial fibrillation patients with an acute coronary syndrome, who are not treated with coronary stent(s), anticoagulant therapy with warfarin and a single antiplatelet agent for 1 year is advised. Atrial fibrillation patients at high risk for thromboembolism, in particular those with previous thromboembolism or an acute coronary syndrome, who do not receive a stent should be treated with warfarin and dual antiplatelet agents (aspirin and clopidogrel) for 12 months. After that time, warfarin alone is advised, just as for patients with atrial fibrillation and stable coronary disease. For atrial fibrillation patients requiring anticoagulant therapy who develop an acute coronary syndrome treated with stent(s), the ACCP guidelines advise warfarin and dual antiplatelet therapy for 1 month for bare metal stents and 3–6 months for drug-eluting stents. After these time periods, warfarin and single antiplatelet therapy (frequently clopidogrel) is advised for the remainder of the first year, followed by warfarin alone, just as for atrial fibrillation and stable coronary artery disease. Patients who require long-term anticoagulation with warfarin are preferably treated with a bare metal stent, rather than a drug-eluting stent if possible, to lower the time of exposure to triple therapy and its risk of bleeding complications. Guideline recommendations for the combination of warfarin and antiplatelet agent(s) vary considerably.

2. Balancing the risk of stroke and anticoagulation in patients with nonvalvular atrial fibrillation

In choosing long-term anticoagulation for patients with nonvalvular atrial fibrillation, the balance between risks and benefits should be considered. The Stroke Prevention in Atrial Fibrillation (SPAF) investigators, the Atrial Fibrillation Investigators, the AHA/ACC/ECS, and the ACCP have determined risk factors for stroke in patients with atrial fibrillation. Assessment of patients for these risk factors is helpful in determining antithrombotic therapy. CHADS2 is a modified stroke risk classification that integrates the above schemes (Table 4–2, left column). Congestive heart failure (C), hypertension (H), age greater than 75 years (A), and diabetes (D) are each assigned 1 point. Patients with previous stroke (S) are assigned 2 points. The CHADS2 risk score assists in determining the approach to antithrombotic treatment (Table 4–3, left column). Lowest risk patients have a score of 0 and do not require warfarin. Intermediate-risk patients have a score of 1 and may be treated with anticoagulant or aspirin when the net clinical benefit is considered (stroke risk reduction with anticoagulant versus risk of major bleeding with anticoagulant). High-risk patients have a score of 2 or greater and derive the most benefit from anticoagulants. Patients with atrial fibrillation who have had a previous stroke should receive anticoagulation therapy unless there is a contraindication.

Recently, an alternative risk stratification scheme has been proposed to take into account the importance of age, gender, and coexisting vascular disease. This risk assessment scheme is CHA2DS2-Vasc (see Table 4–3, right column). This acronym is defined similar to CHADS2 with Vasc defined as vascular disease (peripheral or coronary artery disease or atheroma on TEE) and a sex category. Hypertension is defined as a systolic blood pressure greater than 160 mm Hg on treatment. A potential advantage of this scheme is that those with low scores (CHA2DS2-Vasc = 0 or 1) have a very low incidence of stroke if not anticoagulated and may be treated with no antithrombotic or low-dose aspirin. A decision to treat with oral anticoagulants can be based on CHADS2 risk factors complimented by CHA2DS2-Vasc. Patients who have a CHADS2 score of 1 can be reevaluated with CHA2DS2-Vasc. If their CHA2DS2-Vasc score is 1, they are considered intermediate risk and can be treated with either aspirin or dose-adjusted warfarin. If they have a CHA2DS2-Vasc score of 2 or greater, therapeutic anticoagulation should be recommended. Importantly, neither CHADS2 nor CHA2DS2-Vasc has high predictive value, and both serve to guide rather than mandate antithrombotic therapy.

The risk of stroke is similar for patients with chronic paroxysmal, persistent, and permanent atrial fibrillation.

Risk stratification has also been developed for bleeding on anticoagulant therapy with warfarin. Several schemas (HEMOR2RAGE, HAS-BLED, RIETE, and ATRIA) were derived from nonvalvular atrial fibrillation patients. The definitions of clinical risk factors and of major bleeding

Table 4–3. Anticoagulation for Chronic Nonvalvular Atrial Fibrillation by CHADS2 and CHA2DS2-Vasc Risk

CHADS2		CHA2DS2-Vasc	
Score	TE Rate/Year	Score	TE Rate/Year
0	1.9	0	0.2
1	2.8	1	0.6
2	4.0	2	2.2
3	5.9	3	3.2
4	8.5	4	4.8
5	12.5	5	7.2
6	18.5	6	9.7
		7	11.1
		8	11.0
		9	12.2

TE, thromboembolism.

Table 4–2. CHADS2 and CHA2DS2-Vasc Risk Assessment for Anticoagulation in Nonvalvular Atrial Fibrillation

CHADS2		CHA2DS2-Vasc	
CHF	1	CHF	1
Hypertension	1	Hypertension	1
Age > 75	1	Age	
Diabetes	1	65-74	1
Stroke or TIA	2	> 75	2
		Diabetes	1
		Stroke or TIA	2
		Vascular disease	1
		Sex	
		Female	1

CHF, congestive heart failure; TIA, transient ischemic attack.

Table 4-4. Bleeding Risk in Chronic Nonvalvular Atrial Fibrillation by the HAS-BLED Score

HAS-BLED	Points
Hypertension (uncontrolled)	1
Renal disease (Cr > 2.6 mg/dL)	1
Liver disease (bilirubin 2× normal)	1
Stroke history	1
Prior major bleeding	1
Labile INR	1
Age ≥ 65	1
Medications (NSAIDs)	1
Alcohol usage	1

Cr, creatinine; INR, international normalized ratio; NSAIDs, nonsteroidal anti-inflammatory drugs.

vary for these schemas, and none has become the standard. However, the HAS-BLED score has the virtue of simplicity (Table 4-4). Just as for stroke risk standard schemas, the predictive value for hemorrhage with these schemas is not high. Disturbingly, many of the clinical risks for stroke are the same as those for bleeding on warfarin, leading to a clinical conundrum regarding therapeutic anticoagulation. The clinical result of a cardioembolic stroke can be devastating, and this frequently justifies acceptance of the bleeding risk for many patients.

Recently, three new anticoagulants have been developed and compared with warfarin for stroke prevention in nonvalvular atrial fibrillation (Figure 4-6). In contrast to warfarin, which targets all vitamin K–dependent coagulation factors, these agents specifically target just one component of the coagulation cascade with more predictable effects.

Dabigatran is a direct thrombin inhibitor. Dabigatran reaches the colon and may be associated with lower gastrointestinal bleeding, but whether those with previous lower gastrointestinal bleeds are more likely to bleed has not been shown. Dabigatran has, on meta-analysis of studies that included patients with nonvalvular atrial fibrillation and other conditions requiring long-term anticoagulation, been reported to have an increased incidence of acute coronary syndromes in comparison with dose-adjusted warfarin. The increase is not high, however, and may be offset by stroke protection. The anticoagulant effect of dabigatran cannot be precisely determined by routine laboratory tests, although its effects are reflected in the aPTT. There is no specific agent to reverse its anticoagulant effect, but accidental overdose may be treated with activated charcoal to absorb the drug from the stomach. Hemodialysis is effective in reducing its concentration and protein complex concentrate may also be given.

Rivaroxaban is a factor Xa inhibitor and in a dose of 20 mg daily was superior to warfarin for stroke prevention with similar rate of major bleeds in a study of very-high-risk (average CHADS2 score of 3.46) nonvalvular atrial fibrillation patients. Drug and diet interactions are, in general, minimal. It is metabolized in the liver through CYP-dependent and -independent mechanisms and is not recommended for those receiving inhibitors of both CYP3A4 and P-glycoprotein, including azole antimycotics and HIV protease inhibitors. The anticoagulant effect of this drug is not easily measured clinically, and no specific agent is available to reverse its effect. Accidental overdose may be treated with activated charcoal to absorb the drug from the stomach. Hemodialysis is not effective in reducing its concentration because it is highly protein bound. Its anticoagulant effect can be reversed in vitro with prothrombin complex concentrate, but this has not been demonstrated clinically.

Apixaban is also a factor Xa inhibitor and, in a dose of 5 mg bid, was superior to warfarin for prevention of stroke with fewer bleeds. Apixaban is metabolized in the liver via CYP3A4-dependent and -independent mechanisms, and about one-quarter is excreted in the urine. It is not recommended for patients with impaired renal function defined as a CrCl < 15 cc/min or in those receiving HIV protease inhibitors. There is no easy way to monitor the anticoagulant effect of apixaban clinically, and there is no specific reversal agent. Accidental overdose may benefit from activated charcoal to absorb the drug from the stomach. The use of prothrombin complex concentrate and/or factor VIIa may be helpful in uncontrolled bleeding, but there is no clinical evidence of efficacy.

Potential disadvantages of these agents are that their anticoagulation effect cannot be easily measured or reversed if hemorrhage occurs. Other potential limitations are that these agents have only been studied in patients who are "warfarin eligible," and extrapolation to "non–warfarin eligible" patients cannot be advised. In addition, risk factors for major bleeds with these agents have not been determined or validated. There are also no guidelines for the combination of these agents with antiplatelet agents.

An attractive strategy for stroke prevention in nonvalvular atrial fibrillation is rhythm control (ie, convert and maintain normal sinus rhythm with the aim of eliminating atrial fibrillation and hence stroke risk). Several studies have compared the outcomes of patients with atrial fibrillation treated with rate versus rhythm control. The incidence of stroke was similar for both strategies. Importantly, most strokes in these studies occurred in patients not taking anticoagulants or those who had subtherapeutic INRs. In some of these studies, patients in the rhythm control strategy could be taken off anticoagulants if they symptomatically remained in normal sinus rhythm for at least 1 month. Patients may not always be accurate when self-reporting the occurrence of atrial fibrillation based on symptoms. Hence, anticoagulation may have been discontinued when atrial fibrillation persisted, exposing these patients to thromboembolic risk.

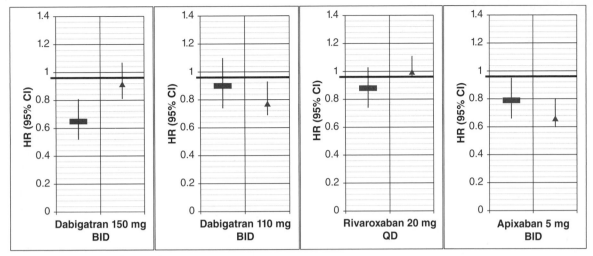

■ = Stroke or systemic embolism

▲ = Major bleeds

HR (95% CI) = Hazard ratios and 95% confidence intervals

▲ **Figure 4-6.** Primary efficacy of stroke or systemic embolism and safety of major bleeding end points for new anticoagulants compared with dose-adjusted warfarin. (Data from De Caterina R, et al. New oral anticoagulants in atrial fibrillation and acute coronary syndromes: ESC Working Group on Thrombosis-Task force on Anticoagulants in Heart Disease position paper. *J Am Coll Cardiol.* 2012;59:1413–25.)

Recommendations regarding discontinuing anticoagulants when a patient is no longer in atrial fibrillation are somewhat vague. (See later discussion of anticoagulation in regard to cardioversion in atrial fibrillation.) The decision to stop warfarin in patients who are no longer in atrial fibrillation should consider risk factors for stroke and anticoagulation.

Catheter ablation is increasingly used in the treatment of highly symptomatic patients primarily with paroxysmal atrial fibrillation. Initial reports of those with long-term success at maintaining sinus rhythm have been encouraging, but whether this lowers the thromboembolic risk and hence indication for anticoagulation has not been determined. This technique should not, at this time, be considered for the purpose of avoiding anticoagulation in patients with nonvalvular atrial fibrillation.

3. Cardioversion of atrial fibrillation—Restoration of sinus rhythm can occur spontaneously or as the result of chemical or electrical cardioversion. Conversion to sinus rhythm can result in systemic emboli through two potential mechanisms. The first is embolization of existing left atrial appendage thrombus, as the mechanical function of the atrium returns following conversion. The second is the development of left atrial appendage thrombus during the postconversion period, when the atrium is mechanically stunned. Embolization of the newly formed thrombus may then occur several days to weeks following conversion, as the mechanical function of the atrium returns. Retrospective

studies have shown up to a 5% incidence of embolic events in patients with atrial fibrillation of unknown duration that were not anticoagulated before cardioversion, compared with less than 1% in those given anticoagulants.

There are two approaches to elective cardioversion to minimize stroke risk: the conventional approach and the TEE-guided approach (Figure 4–7). A randomized study showed that these two approaches were equal in terms of stroke risk. In the conventional approach, patients with atrial fibrillation of unknown or greater than 48 hours duration are treated with warfarin to achieve an INR of 2.0–3.0 or one of the new oral anticoagulants for at least 3 weeks before and at least 4 weeks after successful cardioversion. This recommendation applies regardless of stroke risk factors (CHADS2 or CHA2DS2-Vasc scores). Continuation of anticoagulation beyond 4 weeks depends, however, on stroke risk factors and whether there have been previous episodes of atrial fibrillation. In the TEE-guided approach, patients with atrial fibrillation of unknown or greater than 48 hours duration are therapeutically anticoagulated with UFH to maintain an aPTT of 50–70 seconds, warfarin to maintain an INR of 2.0–3.0, or one of the new anticoagulants and then undergo a TEE. If no left atrial or left atrial appendage thrombus is seen, cardioversion is performed. If sinus rhythm is restored, anticoagulation with warfarin or one of the new anticoagulants should be continued for at least 4 weeks or longer, depending on stroke risk factors. If

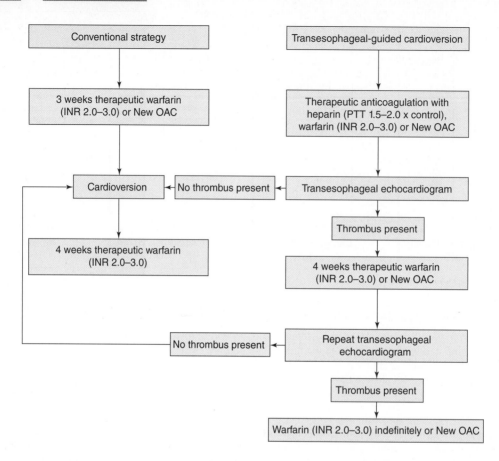

▲ **Figure 4–7.** Anticoagulation strategies for elective cardioversion of atrial fibrillation of unknown duration or lasting longer than 48 hours. INR, international normalized ratio; New OAC, new oral anticoagulant; PTT, partial thromboplastin time.

a left atrial thrombus is seen on TEE, cardioversion should not be performed. These patients should be treated with oral anticoagulant. After 3–4 weeks of therapeutic anticoagulation with warfarin (INR 2.0–3.0) or a newer anticoagulant, TEE can be repeated. If no thrombus is seen, cardioversion can be performed followed by at least another 4 weeks of oral anticoagulant.

For patients with atrial fibrillation of known duration less than 48 hours, according to ACC/AHA/ESC guidelines, anticoagulation is optional prior to and following cardioversion. Whether or not to anticoagulate for the 4 weeks following cardioversion is controversial. The ACCP recommends UFH prior to cardioversion and routine therapeutic anticoagulation for 4 weeks following cardioversion, but the ACC/AHA/ESC recommendations are less directive. These anticoagulation decisions could be based on risk factors and whether there had been previous episodes of atrial fibrillation. For emergency cardioversion (patients with unstable hemodynamics, uncontrolled angina, or congestive heart failure), UFH should be given and the patient treated with oral anticoagulant, either

warfarin or one of the new anticoagulants, for 4 weeks or longer, depending on stroke risk factors.

4. Problems in prescribing anticoagulation for atrial fibrillation—A number of studies have shown that warfarin is not prescribed as often as expected for patients with nonvalvular atrial fibrillation given their hemorrhagic risks, particularly elderly patients. Elderly patients are at high risk for stroke but also at high risk for bleeding complications from warfarin. Often-cited reasons for not prescribing warfarin in those who meet usual criteria for its use include risk of falls, poor compliance, concurrent illnesses, frail state, and history of substance abuse. Applying the results of the placebo-controlled randomized studies to clinical practice is difficult. Patients included in these clinical trials were quite select; in fact, they accounted for less than 10% of those screened. In addition, most studies included very few patients 80 years of age or older. Patients at high risk for bleeding, such as those with recent gastrointestinal tract bleeding, previous ICH, recent stroke, and renal insufficiency, were not included in these studies. It is also important to note that trial protocols required closer monitoring of patients than is usually done in clinical practice. Also, patients included in these studies may be more motivated and compliant than those usually seen in clinical practice. Applying the recommendations derived from these randomized studies requires judgment, and clinicians must consider issues of compliance, risk of trauma and bleeding, and adequacy of follow-up.

The newer anticoagulants offer certain advantages, including the lack of routine monitoring of effect and fewer drug and dietary interactions. The efficacy of these drugs for prevention of stroke was shown to be the same as or better than warfarin (see Figure 4–6), but it is important to remember that these studies were performed in, and hence their results apply to, warfarin-eligible patients; extrapolation to patients not otherwise warfarin candidates cannot be advised.

B. Native Valvular Heart Disease

Thromboembolic complications may occur with a number of valvular conditions. Rheumatic mitral valve disease, particularly when accompanied by atrial fibrillation, has a very high incidence of embolic events. In contrast, patients with mitral valve prolapse and calcific aortic and mitral valve disease (except when atrial fibrillation is also present) are at low risk for embolic events.

1. Rheumatic mitral valve disease—The risk of thromboembolism with mitral stenosis and atrial fibrillation is 18 times greater than matched controls. Patients with rheumatic mitral valve stenosis have at least one chance in five of having a clinically detectable embolic event during their lifetime. Atrial fibrillation is common in patients with rheumatic mitral stenosis, but thromboembolic complications can also occur in patients with rheumatic mitral stenosis who are in sinus rhythm. The ACCP recommends that all patients with rheumatic mitral valve disease and atrial fibrillation or a previous embolic event receive warfarin with a target INR of 2.0–3.0. If an embolic event occurs while a patient is receiving therapeutic anticoagulant therapy, daily aspirin 75–100 mg, dipyridamole 400 mg (in divided doses), or clopidogrel 75 mg should be added. In patients in sinus rhythm with rheumatic mitral stenosis and a left atrial diameter of greater than 5.5 cm by echocardiography, treatment with warfarin with a target INR of 2.0–3.0 had been recommended in the past but currently is not recommended by ACC/AHA guidelines. For patients with rheumatic mitral stenosis undergoing balloon valvuloplasty, warfarin should be given for 3 weeks before and 4 weeks after the procedure.

Balloon valvuloplasty should not be performed on patients with left atrial/appendage thrombus.

Patients with pure rheumatic mitral regurgitation may be at less risk for thromboembolism than those with mitral stenosis because flow through the left atrium is increased due to mitral regurgitation and may lessen the likelihood of thrombus formation. There are no specific recommendations for anticoagulation of patients with rheumatic mitral regurgitation in sinus rhythm. Most patients with rheumatic mitral regurgitation, however, also have some degree of mitral stenosis, and recommendations for anticoagulation for mitral stenosis apply to these patients.

2. Nonrheumatic mitral regurgitation—The routine use of antithrombotic therapy for primary prevention of stroke or systemic embolus in nonrheumatic mitral regurgitation is not recommended. Secondary prevention with warfarin with a target INR of 2.0–3.0 is, however, recommended for those with previous thromboembolism or atrial fibrillation.

3. Mitral valve prolapse—A very small number of patients with mitral valve prolapse experience stroke or transient ischemic attacks despite no other identifiable cause. The mechanism for thromboembolism in mitral prolapse is thought to be fibrinous exudates on the myxomatous valve itself or in the left atrium at the angle formed by the posterior mitral valve leaflet and left atrial wall. No antithrombotic measures are recommended for primary prevention of thromboembolism. Secondary prevention, however, is recommended. The ACCP recommends that patients with mitral valve prolapse who have had documented but unexplained transient ischemic attack or stroke receive long-term treatment with aspirin (50–162 mg daily). For patients with mitral valve prolapse who have had systemic emboli or recurrent transient ischemic attacks despite aspirin therapy, long-term treatment with warfarin, with a target INR of 2.0–3.0, is recommended.

4. Calcific mitral and aortic valve conditions—Calcification of the mitral valve annulus and aortic valve occur commonly in elderly individuals. The incidence of stroke in patients with mitral annular calcification is increased. Embolic events associated with fibrocalcific mitral annular disease occur particularly in those with chronic kidney disease. In addition to thromboembolism, calcified spicules can be dislodged from ulcerated calcific plaques. It may not be possible to differentiate thromboembolism from calcific emboli, although occasionally, calcific emboli may be seen on fundoscopic examination. The ACCP recommends that in the absence of atrial fibrillation, patients with mitral annular calcification complicated by systemic emboli, not documented to be due to calcific emboli, be treated with aspirin 50–100 mg/day. If recurrent thromboembolism is documented on aspirin therapy, dose-adjusted warfarin with a target INR of 2.0–3.0 is recommended. For documented systemic calcific embolism, no specific recommendation is given, although aspirin 50–100 mg daily and statin therapy should be considered. Individuals with calcified aortic valves do not have an increased incidence of strokes compared to controls, although they may be at risk for calcific emboli. Patients with calcification of the aortic valve should not receive warfarin unless they have other indications. For documented calcific embolism, therapy with aspirin 50–100 mg daily and statin therapy should be considered.

5. Endocarditis—The incidence of embolic events in infective endocarditis is quite high. In the preantibiotic era, clinically detected emboli occurred in 70–90% of patients. Currently, the incidence of emboli is 12–40%. In the sulfonamide era, anticoagulant therapy was used to improve penetration of antibiotics into the vegetations. This resulted in a high incidence of cerebral hemorrhage, and the routine use of anticoagulants was abandoned.

Infective endocarditis may occur in patients who have been receiving long-term anticoagulant therapy. If endocarditis develops in a patient with a mechanical prosthetic valve, warfarin should be stopped at the time of initial presentation, until it is clear that invasive procedures will not be required and there are no signs of central nervous system (CNS) involvement. Therapeutic anticoagulation should be restarted when it is clear that the patient does not require interventional procedures or have CNS involvement.

Nonbacterial thrombotic endocarditis (marantic endocarditis) is a condition in which fibrin thrombi are deposited superficially on normal or degenerated cardiac valves. This usually occurs in malignancies, chronic debilitating conditions, and acute fulminant diseases such as septicemia and disseminated intravascular coagulation. The reported incidence of systemic emboli in this condition varies from 14% to 91%. Treatment of nonbacterial thrombotic endocarditis should be directed at the underlying condition. The ACCP recommends UFH for patients with nonbacterial endocarditis with systemic or pulmonary emboli.

C. Prosthetic Heart Valves

Prosthetic heart valves may be either mechanical or bioprosthetic. Mechanical valves require lifelong anticoagulation, whereas bioprosthetic valves usually do not. A mechanical valve prosthesis is more durable than a bioprosthesis, and therefore, it is less likely to require repeat valve surgery. Therefore, it is important to evaluate patients for hemorrhagic risk and likelihood for repeat surgery when choosing the type of prosthetic valve. For older patients, the risk of anticoagulation may be greater than the risk of another operation to replace a bioprosthetic valve. For women of childbearing age, the risks of anticoagulation during pregnancy should be considered in selecting the type of prosthetic heart valve.

1. Mechanical prosthetic heart valves—Mechanical prosthetic heart valves include caged-ball, unileaflet tilting-disk, and bileaflet tilting-disk prosthesis. Caged-ball prosthetic valves are no longer implanted, and patients with these valves are rarely seen. Although flow characteristics vary, all prosthetic valves are foreign material (the sewing ring and the mechanical portions of the prosthesis) placed in the central circulation, providing a potential nidus for thrombus formation. The underlying pathologic process, as well as atrial fibrillation and decreased systolic performance of the left ventricle, are important risk factors for postimplant thromboembolism. The risk of thromboembolism varies for the different types of mechanical prosthetic valves. The lowest risk is for the bileaflet tilting-disk valves and the highest risk is for the caged-ball valves.

The thromboembolic rate of patients with mechanical valves treated with moderate- or high-intensity anticoagulation is similar. However, the hemorrhagic risk is much higher for those receiving high-intensity anticoagulation. Antiplatelet agents may be used in combination with warfarin; the combination has been shown to lower the incidence of thromboembolism, but with an increase in hemorrhagic complications.

Current ACCP recommendations for anticoagulant therapy in patients with a mechanical heart valve are as follows: (1) For patients who have had an aortic valve replacement with a St. Jude or CarboMedics bileaflet valve or a Medtronic Hall unileaflet valve, warfarin with a target INR of 2.0–3.0 should be given. (2) For patients who have had a mitral valve replacement with either a unileaflet or bileaflet valve, warfarin should be given with a target INR of 2.5–3.5. Aspirin in doses of 75–100 mg should be added for patients with high-risk factors for thromboembolism, such as atrial fibrillation, myocardial infarction, low left ventricular ejection fraction, or previous systemic embolism despite warfarin with therapeutic INRs.

The AHA/ACC guidelines differ slightly. They recommend aspirin in addition to warfarin for all patients with mechanical valve prosthesis. In patients with bileaflet tilting-disk valves, warfarin with a target INR of 2.5–3.5 is recommended for the first 3 months after aortic valve replacement. Subsequently, the target INR should be 2.0–3.0. There is less certain evidence for high-risk patients who cannot take aspirin that clopidogrel, 75 mg daily, may be substituted or that warfarin be increased to a target INR of 3.0–4.0.

The ESC recommends warfarin therapy for mechanical valves based on the thrombogenicity of the different types of valves. For low-risk valves (bileaflet tilting-disk), they recommend a target INR of 2.0–3.0. For intermediate-risk valves (unileaflet tilting-disk), they recommend a target INR of 2.5–3.5. For high-risk valves (caged-ball), they recommend a target INR of 3.0–4.0 without other risk factors and 3.5–4.5 if there are other risk factors. They recommend the addition of antiplatelet therapy for concurrent arterial disease, coronary artery stenting, recurrent thromboembolism despite treatment of other risk factors, and optimization of anticoagulation for caged-ball valves. Table 4–5 summarizes anticoagulation recommendations for mechanical prosthetic heart valves.

Anticoagulation with UFH should be started in the postoperative period when adequate hemostasis is achieved and continued until therapy with warfarin is in the therapeutic range for the specific mechanical prosthesis implanted.

An embolic event is the most common adverse consequence seen as a result of thrombosis of a mechanical prosthetic heart valve, but hemodynamic compromise can also occur and be insidious or acutely life-threatening. Thrombi affecting mechanical prosthetic valves can either obstruct or prevent closure of the valve. Fluoroscopic imaging of

Table 4–5. Anticoagulation for Mechanical Prosthetic Valves

Type of Mechanical Prosthetic Valve	Goal of Anticoagulation[1]
Aortic bileaflet tilting disk	INR 2.0–3.0
Aortic unileaflet tilting disk	INR 2.5–3.5
Aortic caged-ball	INR 3.0–4.0
Mitral bileaflet tilting disk	INR 2.5–3.5
Mitral unileaflet tilting disk	INR 2.5–3.5
Mitral caged-ball	INR 3.0–4.0

[1]Add antiplatelet agent for additional risk factors.
INR, international normalized ratio.

prosthetic valve motion can be useful for detecting obstruction by showing reduction in excursion of prosthetic valve leaflet(s). TTE and TEE are the most sensitive and specific diagnostic tests for detecting thrombus complicating a prosthetic valve. According to ACCP guidelines, emergency surgery is reasonable for patients with a thrombosed left-sided prosthetic valve with functional class III–IV symptoms or a large clot burden. Thrombolytic therapy may be considered as first-line therapy for patients with a thrombosed left-sided prosthetic valve and functional class I–II symptoms. Thrombolytic therapy may be considered as first-line therapy in any patient with a left-sided prosthetic valve if emergency surgery is considered to be too high risk or is not available. Thrombolytic therapy is reasonable for a thrombosed right-sided prosthetic heart valve in a patient with functional class III–IV symptoms. UFH is an alternative to thrombolytic therapy in a patient with a thrombosed prosthetic valve with a low clot burden and functional class I–II symptoms. Pannus formation on the sewing ring of the prosthetic valve can cause similar hemodynamic compromise and may be a nidus for thrombus.

2. Bioprosthetic heart valves—Despite the advantages of bioprosthetic valves in terms of central flow and less thrombogenic valve material, thromboembolic complications do occur, particularly in the early postoperative period. The presumed mechanism in this setting is thrombus formation on the sewing ring. A randomized trial of two intensities of anticoagulation following bioprosthetic valve replacement showed similar rates of thromboembolism but fewer hemorrhagic complications for low-intensity anticoagulation.

In the first 3 months following mitral bioprosthetic valve replacement, warfarin is recommended with a target INR of 2.0–3.0. UFH or LMWH should be given postoperatively until the INR is therapeutic for 2 days. Long-term treatment with warfarin is not necessary following bioprosthetic valve replacement in patients who are in sinus rhythm, but long-term therapy with aspirin is recommended. If atrial fibrillation is present, these patients should receive long-term warfarin, as the rate of thromboembolism is high without its use. The AHA/ACC guidelines recommend that patients with a mitral bioprosthesis and risk factors (atrial fibrillation, prior thromboembolic event, left ventricular dysfunction, and a hypercoagulable state) should receive warfarin with a target INR goal of 2.0–3.0. It is also recommended that patients with a bioprosthetic valve receive aspirin in addition to warfarin, if high-risk factors are present.

For the first 3 months following mitral valve repair with an annuloplasty ring, warfarin has been recommended by the ESC and considered reasonable by the ACC/AHA. It is not recommended by the ACCP, provided the patient is in normal sinus rhythm.

For aortic bioprosthetic valves, the ACCP does not recommend long-term warfarin unless high-risk factors are present. Aspirin 50–100 mg should be given during the first 3 months following surgery. Warfarin is not currently recommended for transcatheter aortic bioprosthesis. Instead, aspirin and clopidogrel are recommended for the first 3 months following implant. Table 4–6 summarizes general recommendations for anticoagulants with bioprosthetic valves.

D. Left Ventricular Thrombus

Left ventricular thrombi can complicate myocardial infarction and nonischemic dilated cardiomyopathy. In acute and remote myocardial infarction, the risk factors for ventricular thrombus include anterior myocardial infarction, apical wall motion abnormality, and left ventricular ejection fraction < 40%. No or ineffective reperfusion in acute anterior myocardial infarction is the major risk factor. In dilated cardiomyopathy, left ventricular ejection fraction < 35% is a risk factor for left ventricular thrombus and embolization. Risk factors for embolization of left ventricular thrombus include protrusion into the left ventricle and mobility, a

Table 4–6. Anticoagulation for Bioprosthetic Valves

Postoperative Criteria	Anticoagulation
For first 3 months after surgery	Warfarin INR 2-3
After 3 months	
No atrial fibrillation	Aspirin, 325 mg/day
Aortic + atrial fibrillation	Warfarin, INR 2.0–3.0[1]
Mitral + atrial fibrillation	Warfarin, INR 2.0–3.0[1]

[1]Add antiplatelet agent for additional risk factors.
INR, international normalized ratio.

low left ventricular ejection fraction (< 35%), and within 3 months of acute infarction.

1. Acute myocardial infarction—Postmortem findings of patients with acute myocardial infarction before the reperfusion era indicated a high incidence of left ventricular thrombi, pulmonary and systemic emboli, and coronary artery thrombi. Although embolic events were uncommon, they were frequently devastating since most (> 80%) were to the CNS (87% occur between days 5 and 21 following infarction). The risk of systemic emboli can be decreased with long-term oral anticoagulation. Risk stratification, to identify high- and low-risk groups for the development of thrombus and embolism, can improve the efficacy of anticoagulation following infarction.

Echocardiographic studies have shown thrombus formation to be most common in patients with anterior rather than inferior myocardial infarction. Patients with anterior infarction and akinesia or dyskinesia of the apex are at highest risk. On the basis of clinical and echocardiographic data, there appears to be good rationale to consider long-term (3 months) treatment with oral anticoagulants following anterior infarction in patients who did not receive or achieve effective reperfusion therapy or have decreased left ventricular systolic performance and apical akinesis or dyskinesis. Significantly fewer left ventricular thrombi and embolic events develop in patients receiving therapeutic doses of UFH following acute anterior infarction than in those treated with low-dose or no UFH. Studies of long-term oral anticoagulation following infarction have documented that anticoagulant therapy reduces the incidence of stroke and systemic emboli, although most did not report results based on infarct location.

For patients with anterior STEMI, apical akinesis, or dyskinesis and reduced left ventricular function, who have not received reperfusion therapy, initial anticoagulation with UFH followed by warfarin to maintain an INR of 2.0–3.0 for at least 3 months, in addition to low-dose aspirin (81–162 mg/day) can be recommended. After that time, warfarin could be discontinued if no intracardiac thrombus is detected by echocardiography. Aspirin (325 mg/day) should be continued indefinitely.

Because the incidence of ischemic stroke is low in patients receiving prompt and effective reperfusion therapy, either with thrombolytic or direct percutaneous intervention, it is unclear whether the risk-benefit ratio favors short- or long-term anticoagulation therapy (3 months) to prevent thrombosis and embolization. A reasonable approach is clinical evaluation and echocardiography before the patient is discharged from the hospital. Those with inferior infarction or anterior infarction without akinesia or dyskinesia of the apex and preserved left ventricular systolic performance do not require treatment with warfarin and can be treated with aspirin alone. Patients with left ventricular thrombus on echocardiography are at high risk for thromboembolism, and oral anticoagulation with warfarin is recommended for a period of at least 3 months to maintain an INR of 2.0–3.0. If repeat echocardiography shows resolution of the thrombus at 3 months, oral anticoagulation can be stopped. Aspirin and clopidogrel are usually prescribed for patients who have undergone percutaneous coronary intervention (PCI) for acute STEMI with placement of a stent. For patients who had direct PCI with placement of a bare metal stent and were subsequently shown to have left ventricular thrombus, it is recommended that they receive warfarin in addition to aspirin and clopidogrel for 1 month, then warfarin and single antiplatelet therapy (usually clopidogrel) for the second and third month after infarct. If no thrombus is present after 3 months, warfarin can be stopped and treatment with dual antiplatelet therapy continued for 12 months after infarct. At that time, single antithrombotic therapy should be given and continued indefinitely. If a drug-eluting stent was placed and a left ventricular thrombus was subsequently detected, warfarin, aspirin, and clopidogrel are advised for the first 3–6 months following stent implant. Warfarin can be stopped at that time, and dual platelet therapy should be continued for the remainder of the first year if no left ventricular thrombus can be seen. At that time, a single platelet therapy can be used and continued indefinitely.

2. Remote infarction with thrombus—Antithrombotic management of remote myocardial infarction (> 3 months after the acute event) is controversial. Although traditional studies have not indicated a high risk of embolization, some reports indicate that thrombus detected at least 3 months following infarction still carries a risk for embolism. For patients with remote infarction and left ventricular thrombus seen on echocardiography, treatment with warfarin to maintain an INR of 2.0–3.0 is recommended, particularly if the thrombus is new. A repeat echocardiogram at 3 months can be used to determine whether treatment with warfarin should be continued.

3. Left ventricular aneurysm—Although an uncommon complication of myocardial infarction in the reperfusion era, left ventricular aneurysm provides the necessary substrate for thrombus formation. These aneurysms frequently contain thrombus, but systemic embolization is unusual. It is hypothesized that the low incidence of systemic emboli noted when left ventricular thrombus is flat or "mural" and contained within a discrete aneurysm (see Figure 4–1) relates to a smaller surface area of the clot being exposed to circulating blood. It is unclear whether patients with left ventricular aneurysm warrant long-term anticoagulant therapy for prevention of embolization if flat, mural thrombus is present. However, documented systemic embolization in patients with left ventricular aneurysm and thrombus should prompt therapeutic anticoagulation to maintain an INR of 2.0–3.0 for secondary prevention. Recurrent embolization despite therapeutic anticoagulation in this setting is an indication for left ventricular aneurysmectomy.

4. Dilated cardiomyopathy—Dilated cardiomyopathy may be the end result of many types of heart disease.

Characteristically, generalized four-chamber cardiac enlargement is present with right and left ventricular dysfunction that can cause stasis in any cardiac chamber. These patients have a significant incidence of intracardiac thrombi, particularly in the left ventricle and systemic emboli. In one clinical study, atrial fibrillation was shown to be the only independent predictor for thromboembolism in dilated cardiomyopathy. Another study stressed the importance of severe depression of left ventricular function as a predictor.

The characteristics and the embolic potential of left ventricular thrombi in dilated cardiomyopathy and those in left ventricular aneurysm seem to differ. In dilated cardiomyopathy, left ventricular thrombi may protrude and thus expose a greater surface area to circulating blood (see Figure 4–2). Several studies have indicated that thrombi that protrude into the left ventricular cavity or demonstrate free intracavitary motion are associated with a high risk of embolic events. Thrombi in left ventricular aneurysms are frequently mural and contained within the aneurysm (see Figure 4-1); exposure to circulating blood is minimal because of both their containment and flat shape; patients with these features are at low risk for embolization.

Unlike acute infarction, the natural history of left ventricular thrombus complicating dilated cardiomyopathy is unclear because no clinically apparent event marks the initiation of thrombus development. Studies of intracardiac thrombi complicating dilated cardiomyopathy have, in general, consisted of small numbers of patients, varying definitions of dilated cardiomyopathy, varying proportions of patients with coronary artery disease, and incomplete reporting of anticoagulation status. Aggregate analyses of these clinical and echocardiographic studies indicate that anticoagulation can reduce the thromboembolic rate. Anticoagulation following a thromboembolic event also appears effective as a secondary prevention measure.

Patients with dilated cardiomyopathy are at highest risk for thromboembolic complications if they have atrial fibrillation, severe left ventricular dysfunction, previous thromboembolism, or left ventricular thrombus documented by imaging techniques. For patients with these high-risk characteristics, therapeutic warfarin is recommended to maintain an INR of 2.0–3.0.

For patients with clinical heart failure and reduced left ventricular systolic performance (ejection fraction < 35%), the routine use of therapeutic anticoagulation with warfarin reduces the incidence of stroke but increases the risk of major bleeding, and there is no net clinical benefit. For patients with clinical heart failure and atrial fibrillation, previous thromboembolism, or left ventricular thrombus, therapeutic anticoagulation with warfarin (target INR 2.0–3.0) is recommended.

E. Aortic Atheroma

TEE is often performed in evaluation for a source of cardio-embolism in the setting of stroke or transient ischemic attack and visualizes the ascending, transverse, and descending thoracic aorta. Aortic atheroma detected by this technique (see Figure 4-4) may be a cause of systemic embolus, including stroke. In the Stroke Prevention in Atrial Fibrillation Trial, patients who underwent TEE had a 35% incidence of complex aortic plaque greater than 4 mm thick. The risk of stroke at 1 year in these patients was 12–20%. The risk of stroke in patients with atrial fibrillation without complex aortic plaque was 1.2%. Studies have shown that plaque size greater than 4 mm in thickness and no calcification increase the risk of ischemic events.

Treatment of complex aortic plaque for the primary and secondary prevention of embolic stroke is controversial. While aspirin is generally recommended, warfarin has been reported to be efficacious in some series, particularly for secondary prevention. Patients with complex aortic plaques and embolic events treated with hydroxymethylglutaryl–coenzyme A (HMG-CoA) reductase inhibitors have a significantly lower risk of embolic events than those taking warfarin or aspirin, and HMG-CoA should be given for secondary prevention.

F. Paradoxical Emboli Associated with Patent Foramen Ovale

Intracardiac shunts have the potential to allow for venoarterial or paradoxical emboli (see Figure 4–5). These shunts are usually left to right, but there may also be right-to-left shunting under certain circumstances, such as cough or Valsalva maneuver. Patent foramen ovale is quite common, occurring in up to 15–20% of the population. Asymptomatic patent foramen ovale can be detected on TTE and TEE. The ACCP recommends that asymptomatic patients should not be treated with antithrombotics for primary prevention of systemic embolus. Patients with patent foramen ovale with right-to-left shunt and unexplained systematic embolism or transient ischemic attack should receive antiplatelet therapy for secondary prevention. If they also have venous thrombosis or pulmonary embolism, they will require long-term anticoagulation with warfarin to maintain an INR of 2.0–3.0. If there are recurrent events while on antiplatelet therapy, warfarin should be considered. Recurrent systemic embolus on anticoagulant therapy should prompt consideration for foramen ovale closure (either surgically or percutaneously).

G. Pacemakers, Implantable Cardioverter-Defibrillators, and Other Intracardiac Devices

Anticoagulant therapy is not usually considered for patients with pacemakers and implantable cardioverter-defibrillators (ICDs). However, a number of thromboembolic complications can occur. The intravascular and intracardiac leads used in these devices are foreign bodies that can act as a nidus for thrombus formation. On rare occasions, swelling of the arm on the side of implantation may develop. Ultrasound or venography may indicate obstruction of the subclavian vein. The treatment for subclavian vein thrombosis is UFH followed by oral anticoagulation. The duration of treatment with anticoagulants varies but is usually for at least 3 months. For extreme swelling and pain of the effected extremity, interventional procedures to restore flow in the subclavian vein should be considered. Thrombolytic therapy cannot be used in the immediate post-pacemaker implant period because of the risk of bleeding into the pacemaker pocket.

TEE performed for unrelated indications has demonstrated a high incidence of thrombi on pacing and ICD leads. Often these thrombi are highly mobile. Differentiation from infective endocarditis is mandatory, since the clinical approach and treatment will be affected. The risk for embolization to the pulmonary artery or systemically if there is a patent foramen ovale is unknown. There are no guidelines for treating these thrombi with anticoagulation or for removal of the device. If embolic events have occurred or there are other high-risk factors for thromboembolism, it seems reasonable to initially treat with oral anticoagulants. Follow-up TEE seems reasonable after at least 3 months of therapeutic anticoagulation to determine whether the thrombus has resolved. There is little evidence or experience to guide the duration of treatment.

Technologic advances are leading to the implantation of additional intracardiac devices. Since these devices are foreign bodies, they can act as a nidus for thrombus formation. Percutaneous closure devices for atrial septal defects are available. Current anticoagulation recommendations are for aspirin and clopidogrel for 3 months following the procedure. Warfarin is not recommended. Devices for percutaneous occlusion of the left atrial appendage are currently being investigated for use in nonvalvular atrial fibrillation. Although anticoagulation is required for this procedure, the strategy behind these devices is to avoid long-term anticoagulation. These devices are not yet clinically available.

De Caterina R, et al. New oral anticoagulants in atrial fibrillation and acute coronary syndromes: ESC Working Group on Thrombosis-Task force on Anticoagulants in Heart Disease position paper. *J Am Coll Cardiol.* 2012;59:1413–25. [PMID: 22497820]

Friberg L, et al. Evaluation of risk stratification schemes for ischaemic stroke and bleeding in 182 678 patients with atrial fibrillation: the Swedish Atrial Fibrillation cohort study. *Eur Heart J.* 2012;33(12):1500–10. [PMID: 22246443]

Guyatt GH, et al. Antithrombotic therapy and prevention of thrombosis, 9th ed: American College of Chest Physicians evidence-based clinical practice guidelines. *Chest.* 2012;141 (Suppl):7s–47s. [PMID: 22315257]

Homma S, et al. Warfarin and aspirin in patients with heart failure and sinus rhythm. *N Engl J Med.* 2012;366:1859–69. [PMID: 22551105]

Klein AL, et al; Assessment of Cardioversion Using Transesophageal Echocardiography Investigators. Use of transesophageal echocardiography to guide cardioversion in patients with atrial fibrillation. *N Engl J Med.* 2001;344(19):1411–20. [PMID: 11346805]

Korkeila PJ, et al. Transesophageal echocardiography in the diagnosis of thrombosis associated with permanent transvenous pacemaker electrodes. *Pacing Clin Electrophysiol.* 2006; 29(11):1245–50. [PMID: 17100678]

Lindsay MP, et al. Canadian best practice recommendations for stroke care (update 2010). On behalf of the Canadian Stroke Strategy Best Practices and Standards Writing Group. Ottawa, Ontario, Canada: Canadian Stroke Network; 2010.

Singer DE, et al. Antithrombotic therapy in atrial fibrillation: the Seventh ACCP Conference on Antithrombotic and Thrombolytic Therapy. *Chest.* 2004;126(3 Suppl):429S–56S. [PMID: 15383480]

Uchino K, et al. Dabigatran association with higher risk of acute coronary events–meta-analysis of noninferiority randomized controlled trials. *Arch Intern Med.* 2012;172(5):397–402. [PMID: 22231617]

▶ Special Considerations

A. Pregnancy

Warfarin during pregnancy carries a significant risk for both maternal and fetal complications. Warfarin crosses the placenta and can cause an embryopathy, especially when used between the sixth and twelfth weeks of gestation. Fetal CNS abnormalities may occur with maternal warfarin use in any trimester. UFH and LMWH do not cross the placenta, and therefore, their use in pregnancy may be safer for the fetus. However, both are expensive, difficult to administer, and associated with risks of bleeding, osteoporosis, and HIT (much less likely with LMWH). Low-dose aspirin (< 150 mg/day) is considered safe in the second and third trimesters. Warfarin, UFH, and LMWH can safely be administered to the nursing mother because they do not have an anticoagulant effect in breastfed infants.

When a patient who is receiving long-term warfarin therapy is planning a pregnancy, risks for the fetus should be considered. One approach would be to perform frequent pregnancy tests and substitute UFH or LMWH for warfarin when the patient becomes pregnant. The second approach is to replace warfarin with UFH or LMWH before conception is attempted.

The most common cardiac condition requiring anticoagulation during pregnancy is mechanical prosthetic heart valves. Three different approaches for anticoagulation during pregnancy were evaluated in a review of a number of prospective and retrospective studies (none were randomized): (1) warfarin throughout the pregnancy until close to delivery; (2) warfarin throughout pregnancy except replaced by UFH from the sixth through twelfth weeks; warfarin can then be restarted and used throughout the remainder of pregnancy; and (3) UFH throughout the pregnancy.

The lowest risk for prosthetic valve thrombosis or systemic embolization was warfarin throughout pregnancy, but this strategy was associated with embryopathy in 6.4% of newborns. It appears that warfarin may place the fetus at more risk and the mother at less risk. It is difficult to know whether the higher incidence of thrombotic complications noted with UFH was due to inadequate dosing. There are very few data on the efficacy of LMWH in preventing thrombotic complications during pregnancy. There are medicolegal concerns with the use of warfarin during pregnancy, although it is commonly used in Europe.

The ACCP recommends that women with prosthetic heart valves who are pregnant and routinely require long-term anticoagulants receive adjusted-dose LMWH twice a day throughout pregnancy with doses adjusted to keep the 4-hour postinjection anti-Xa level at approximately 1.0 to 1.2 units/mL or according to weight. An alternative regimen is for UFH throughout pregnancy in doses adjusted to keep the aPTT at least twice control or to attain an anti-Xa level of 0.35–0.70 units/mL. Calcium supplement, 1.2 g/day, is recommended because of the effect of UFH on bone density. Another alternative regimen is to use UFH or LMWH initiated before the sixth week of gestation and continued through the twelfth week. Between the 12th and 36th weeks, adjusted-dose warfarin or LMWH can be given, followed by UFH from the 36th week until delivery. Low-dose aspirin can be added if there are additional high-risk factors. Anticoagulation may be interrupted briefly for delivery and resumed postpartum using UFH or LMWH as a bridge to therapeutic anticoagulation with warfarin.

Women of childbearing age who need to have a prosthetic heart valve should consider their desire to become pregnant when making a decision about the type of valve to be implanted. A bioprosthetic valve or native valve repair that does not require lifelong anticoagulation would be safer in terms of anticoagulation and pregnancy risks.

B. Interruption of Anticoagulation for Surgery and Invasive Procedures

At times, anticoagulant therapy needs to be interrupted because of surgery or other invasive procedures and certain endoscopic procedures. The anticoagulant effects of warfarin persist for several days. Toward the end of this period, there may be inadequate protection from thromboembolism, and this may require short-term anticoagulation with UFH or LMWH. The anticoagulant effects of the newer anticoagulants dissipate more quickly.

Elective and planned surgery and procedures allow for a systematic approach to dealing with anticoagulation issues. Urgent or emergent procedures or surgeries require a different approach to lessen the risk of bleeding and thromboembolic complications.

The risk of bleeding for different procedures and surgeries varies and determines the need for the interruption of anticoagulation therapy. Procedures with a low risk for bleeding include arthrocentesis, cataract surgery, coronary angiography, outpatient dental surgery, and endoscopy without biopsy or intervention. These procedures can be performed without interruption of anticoagulation or only a brief interruption to achieve an INR just below the therapeutic range. Procedures with a high bleeding risk include

open heart surgery, abdominal vascular surgery, intracranial and spinal procedures, major cancer surgeries, and urologic procedures. These procedures require interruption of anticoagulation until a return to normal or near-normal INR measurements.

The risk of thromboembolism when warfarin or any of the new anticoagulants is discontinued varies for different cardiac conditions. In each year after the discontinuation of anticoagulant, the risk of thrombotic complications is as follows: 1% for lone atrial fibrillation and 5% for nonvalvular atrial fibrillation (low risk); 12% for high-risk atrial fibrillation and 10–12% for St. Jude prosthetic aortic valve (intermediate risk); 22% for a mitral mechanical prosthetic valve and up to 91% for multiple mechanical prosthetic valves (high risk). The recommended approach for periprocedural anticoagulation for low-risk patients is to stop anticoagulant 4 days before and administer UFH or LMWH after the procedure until therapeutic oral anticoagulation is achieved (Table 4–7). For intermediate-risk patients, the recommended approach is to stop anticoagulant 4 days before the procedure and start full-dose UFH or LMWH 2 days before the procedure. UFH can be stopped 4 hours prior to the procedure. LMWH should be stopped 24 hours prior to the procedure. After the procedure, UFH or LMWH is recommended along with oral anticoagulant; once therapeutic anticoagulation with an oral agent is achieved, UFH or LMWH should be discontinued. For high-risk patients, anticoagulant should be stopped 4 days prior to the procedure with either UFH (target aPTT of two times control) or LMWH started when the INR is < 2.0. UFH can be stopped 4 hours prior to the procedure and LMWH 24 hours prior to

Table 4–7. Interruption of Anticoagulation for Surgery or Invasive Procedures

Condition	Recommendation
Atrial fibrillation and aortic bileaflet prosthesis without high-risk features[1]	Stop warfarin 4 days before procedure Restart after the procedure as soon as it is safe
All other mechanical valve prostheses[2]	Stop warfarin 3-4 days before the procedure Start unfractionated heparin when INR = 2.0 Stop unfractionated heparin 4-6 hours before procedure Restart unfractionated heparin and warfarin after the procedure as soon as it is safe

[1]High-risk features include atrial fibrillation, previous thromboembolism, hypercoagulable state, and left ventricular dysfunction.
[2]Mitral bileaflet prosthesis, aortic and mitral unileaflet prosthesis, and aortic and mitral ball-cage prosthesis.
INR, international normalized ratio

the procedure. Anticoagulation with UFH or LMWH should be resumed as soon as possible after surgery as a bridge to resumption of long-term oral anticoagulation. The risk for bleeding varies for different procedures. For procedures with a low risk for bleeding on warfarin, an INR of 1.5 may be acceptable. Dental procedures generally do not require stopping warfarin.

The ACC/AHA have established guidelines for bridging anticoagulant therapy in patients with mechanical prosthetic valves. For patients who are at low risk for thrombosis (bileaflet tilting-disk prosthetic aortic valves and no additional risk factors for thromboembolism), warfarin should be stopped 48–72 hours before the procedure to allow the INR to fall below 1.5. Warfarin should be restarted 24 hours after the procedure. Bridging with UFH or LMWH is not necessary. For patients who are at high risk for thrombosis (mechanical aortic valve with risk factors for thromboembolism or any mechanical mitral valve prosthesis), warfarin should be stopped more than 72 hours before the procedure; therapeutic doses of intravenous UFH should be started when the INR falls below 2.0 (usually 48 hours before the procedure); UFH is stopped 4–6 hours before the procedure. UFH and warfarin are restarted as soon after the procedure as possible, and UFH is stopped when the INR is therapeutic.

Emergency surgery and procedures require a different approach. For those on warfarin, immediate reversal with fresh frozen plasma or prothrombin concentrate complex (does not require a large volume load) is recommended; anticoagulants can be restarted when the bleeding risk is acceptably low. The use of vitamin K for those on warfarin is discouraged because it may cause a hypercoagulable state.

The newer oral anticoagulants approved only for patients with nonvalvular atrial fibrillation may also need to be held prior to invasive procedures. Management for elective invasive procedures should be based on the pharmacokinetics and renal function. Dabigatran, rivaroxaban, and apixaban should be discontinued 1–2 days before the procedure for those with CrCl > 50 cc/min. For those with CrCl of 30–50 cc/min, it should be discontinued 3–5 days before the procedure. Resumption of these agents following surgery should only be after hemostasis has been achieved noting that their onset of action is only 2–3 hours. Acute reversal of these agents for emergency surgery is problematic because the anticoagulant effect cannot be easily determined clinically and there is no specific antidote. Activated charcoal can be given to decrease absorption of these agents if they had been recently been ingested. Dabigatran can be dialyzed off and prothrombin concentrate complex and activated factor VII given, but the clinical efficacy of this approach unclear. For rivaroxaban, there is in vitro evidence that prothrombin concentrate complex can reverse its anticoagulant effect, but the clinical efficacy of this approach is unclear. This approach may also be used for those on apixaban.

Bates SM, et al. Venous thromboembolism, thrombophilia, antithrombotic therapy, and pregnancy: American College of Chest Physicians Evidence-Based Clinical Practice Guidelines (8th Edition). *Chest.* 2008;133(6 Suppl):844S–6S. [PMID: 18574280]

Kovacs MJ, et al. Single-arm study of bridging therapy with low-molecular-weight heparin for patients at risk of arterial embolism who require temporary interruption of warfarin. *Circulation.* 2004;110(12):1658–63. [PMID: 15364803]

Vahanian A, et al. Guidelines on the management of valvular heart disease: The Task Force on the Management of Valvular Heart Disease of the European Society of Cardiology. Task Force on the Management of Valvular Hearth Disease of the European Society of Cardiology, ESC Committee for Practice Guidelines. *Eur Heart J.* 2007;28(2):230–68. [PMID: 17259184]

Approach to Cardiac Disease Diagnosis

5

Michael H. Crawford, MD

▶ General Considerations

The patient's history is a critical feature in the evaluation of suspected or overt heart disease. It includes information about the present illness, past illnesses, and the patient's family. From this information, a chronology of the patient's disease process should be constructed. Determining what information in the history is useful requires a detailed knowledge of the pathophysiology of cardiac disease. The effort spent on listening to the patient is time well invested because the cause of cardiac disease is often discernible from the history.

A. Common Symptoms

1. Chest pain—Chest pain is one of the cardinal symptoms (Table 5–1) of ischemic heart disease, but it can also occur with other forms of heart disease. The five characteristics of ischemic chest pain, or angina pectoris, are as follows:

- Anginal pain usually has a substernal location but may extend to the left or right chest, the shoulders, the neck, jaw, arms, epigastrium, and, occasionally, the upper back.
- The pain is deep, visceral, and intense; it makes the patient pay attention but is not excruciating. Many patients describe it as a pressure-like sensation or a tightness.
- The duration of the pain is minutes, not seconds.
- The pain tends to be precipitated by exercise or emotional stress.
- The pain is relieved by resting or taking sublingual nitroglycerin.

2. Dyspnea—A frequent complaint of patients with a variety of cardiac diseases, dyspnea is ordinarily one of four types. The most common is exertional dyspnea, which usually means that the underlying condition is mild because it requires the increased demand of exertion to precipitate symptoms. The next most common is paroxysmal nocturnal dyspnea, characterized by the patient awakening after being asleep or

recumbent for an hour or more. This symptom is caused by the redistribution of body fluids from the lower extremities into the vascular space and back to the heart, resulting in volume overload; it suggests a more severe condition. Third is orthopnea, a dyspnea that occurs immediately on assuming the recumbent position. The mild increase in venous return (caused by lying down) before any fluid is mobilized from interstitial spaces in the lower extremities is responsible for the symptom, which suggests even more severe disease. Finally, dyspnea at rest suggests severe cardiac disease.

Dyspnea is not specific for heart disease, however. Exertional dyspnea, for example, can be due to pulmonary disease, anemia, or deconditioning. Orthopnea is a frequent complaint in patients with chronic obstructive pulmonary disease and postnasal drip. A history of "two-pillow orthopnea" is of little value unless the reason for the use of two pillows is discerned. Resting dyspnea is also a sign of pulmonary disease. Paroxysmal nocturnal dyspnea is perhaps the most specific for cardiac disease because few other conditions cause this symptom.

3. Syncope and presyncope—Lightheadedness, dizziness, presyncope, and syncope are important indications of a reduction in cerebral blood flow. These symptoms are nonspecific and can be due to primary central nervous system disease, metabolic conditions, dehydration, or inner-ear problems. Because bradyarrhythmias and tachyarrhythmias are important cardiac causes, a history of palpitations preceding the event is significant.

4. Transient central nervous system deficits—Deficits such as transient ischemic attacks (TIAs) suggest emboli from the heart or great vessels or, rarely, from the venous circulation through an intracardiac shunt. A TIA should prompt the search for cardiovascular disease. Any sudden loss of blood flow to a limb also suggests a cardioembolic event.

5. Fluid retention—These symptoms are not specific for heart disease but may be due to reduced cardiac function. Typical symptoms are peripheral edema, bloating, weight

Table 5-1. Common Symptoms of Potential Cardiac Origin

Chest pain or pressure
Dyspnea on exertion
Paroxysmal nocturnal dyspnea
Orthopnea
Syncope or near syncope
Transient neurologic defects
Edema
Palpitation
Cough

gain, and abdominal pain from an enlarged liver or spleen. Decreased appetite, diarrhea, jaundice, and nausea and vomiting can also occur from gut and hepatic dysfunction due to fluid engorgement.

6. Palpitation—Normal resting cardiac activity usually cannot be appreciated by the individual. Awareness of heart activity is often referred to by patients as palpitation. Among patients, there is no standard definition for the type of sensation represented by palpitation, so the physician must explore the sensation further with the patient. It is frequently useful to have the patient tap the perceived heartbeat out by hand. Commonly, unusually forceful heart activity at a normal rate (60–100 bpm) is perceived as palpitation. More forceful contractions are usually the result of endogenous catecholamine excretion that does not elevate the heart rate out of the normal range. A common cause of this phenomenon is anxiety. Another common sensation is that of the heart stopping transiently or of the occurrence of isolated forceful beats or both. This sensation is usually caused by premature ventricular contractions, and the patient either feels the compensatory pause or the resultant more forceful subsequent beat or both. Occasionally, the individual feels the ectopic beat and refers to this phenomenon as "skipped" beats. The least common sensation reported by individuals, but the one most linked to the term "palpitation" is rapid heart rate that may be regular or irregular and is usually supraventricular in origin.

7. Cough—Although cough is usually associated with pulmonary disease processes, cardiac conditions that lead to pulmonary abnormalities may be the root cause of the cough. A cardiac cough is usually dry or nonproductive. Pulmonary fluid engorgement from conditions such as heart failure may present as cough. Pulmonary hypertension from any cause can result in cough. Finally, angiotensin-converting enzyme inhibitors, which are frequently used in cardiac conditions, can cause cough.

B. History

1. The present illness—This is a chronology of the events leading up to the patient's current complaints. Usually physicians start with the chief complaint and explore the patient's symptoms. It is especially important to determine the frequency, intensity, severity, and duration of all symptoms; their precipitating causes; what relieves them; and what aggravates them. Although information about previous related diseases and opinions from other physicians are often valuable, it is essential to explore the basis of any prior diagnosis and ask the patient about objective testing and the results of such testing. A history of prior treatment is often revealing because medications or surgery may indicate the nature of the original problem. A list should be made of all the patient's current medications, detailing the dosages, the frequency of administration, whether they are helping the patient, and any side effects.

2. Antecedent conditions—Several systemic diseases may have cardiac involvement. It is therefore useful to search for a history of rheumatic fever, which may manifest as Sydenham chorea, joint pain and swelling, or merely frequent sore throats. Other important diseases that affect the heart include metastatic cancer, thyroid disorders, diabetes mellitus, and inflammatory diseases such as rheumatoid arthritis and systemic lupus erythematosus. Certain events during childhood are suggestive of congenital or acquired heart disease; these include a history of cyanosis, reduced exercise tolerance, or long periods of restricted activities or school absence. Exposure to toxins, infectious agents, and other noxious substances may also be relevant.

3. Atherosclerotic risk factors—Atherosclerotic cardiovascular disease is the most common form of heart disease in industrialized nations. The presenting symptoms of this ubiquitous disorder may be unimpressive and minimal, or as impressive as sudden death. It is therefore important to determine from the history whether any risk factors for this disease are present. The most important are a family history of atherosclerotic disease, especially at a young age; diabetes mellitus; lipid disorders such as a high cholesterol level; hypertension; and smoking. Less important factors include a lack of exercise, high stress levels, the type A personality, and truncal obesity.

4. Family history—A family history is important for determining the risk for not only atherosclerotic cardiovascular disease but also for many other cardiac diseases. Congenital heart disease, for example, is more common in the offspring of parents with this condition, and a history of the disorder in the antecedent family or siblings is significant. Other genetic diseases, such as neuromuscular disorders or connective tissue disorders (eg, Marfan syndrome), can affect the heart. Acquired diseases, such as rheumatic valve disease, can cluster in families because of the spread of the streptococcal infection among family members. The lack of a history of hypertension in the family might prompt a more intensive search for a secondary cause. A history of atherosclerotic disease sequelae, such as limb loss, strokes, and heart attacks, may provide a clue to the aggressiveness of an atherosclerotic tendency in a particular family group.

▶ Physical Findings

A. Physical Examination

The physical examination is less important than the history in patients with ischemic heart disease, but it is of critical value in patients with congenital and valvular heart disease. In the latter two categories, the physician can often make specific anatomic and etiologic diagnoses based on the physical examination. Certain abnormal murmurs and heart sounds are specific for structural abnormalities of the heart. The physical examination is also important for confirming the diagnosis and establishing the severity of heart failure, and it is the only way to diagnose systemic hypertension because this diagnosis is based on elevated blood pressure recordings.

1. Blood pressure—Proper measurement of the **systemic arterial pressure** by cuff sphygmomanometry is one of the keystones of the cardiovascular physical examination. It is recommended that the brachial artery be palpated and the diaphragm of the stethoscope be placed over it, rather than merely sticking the stethoscope in the antecubital fossa. Current methodologic standards dictate that the onset and disappearance of the Korotkoff sounds define the systolic and diastolic pressures, respectively. Although this is the best approach in most cases, there are exceptions. For example, in patients in whom the diastolic pressure drops to near zero, the point of muffling of the sounds is usually recorded as the diastolic pressure. Because the diagnosis of systemic hypertension involves repeated measures under the same conditions, the operator should record the arm used and the position of the patient to allow reproducible measurements to be made on serial visits.

Orthostatic changes in blood pressure are a very important physical finding, especially in patients complaining of transient central nervous system symptoms, weakness, or unstable gait. The technique involves having the patient assume the upright position for at least 90 seconds before taking the pressure to be sure that the maximum orthostatic effect is measured. Although measuring the pressure in other extremities may be of value in certain vascular diseases, it provides little information in a routine examination beyond palpating pulses in all the extremities. Keep in mind, in general, that the pulse pressure (the difference between systolic and diastolic blood pressures) is a crude measure of left ventricular stroke volume. A widened pulse pressure suggests that the stroke volume is large; a narrowed pressure, that the stroke volume is small.

2. Peripheral pulses—When examining the peripheral pulses, the physician is really conducting three examinations. The first is an examination of the cardiac rate and rhythm, the second is an assessment of the characteristics of the pulse as a reflection of cardiac activity, and the third is an assessment of the adequacy of the arterial conduit being examined. The pulse rate and rhythm are usually determined in a convenient peripheral artery, such as the radial. If a pulse is irregular, it is better to auscultate the heart; some cardiac contractions during rhythm disturbances do not generate a stroke volume sufficient to cause a palpable peripheral pulse. In many ways, the heart rate reflects the health of the circulatory system. A rapid pulse suggests increased catecholamine levels, which may be due to cardiac disease, such as heart failure; a slow pulse represents an excess of vagal tone, which may be due to disease or athletic training.

To assess the characteristics of the cardiac contraction through the pulse, it is usually best to select an artery close to the heart, such as the carotid. Bounding high-amplitude carotid pulses suggest an increase in stroke volume and should be accompanied by a wide pulse pressure on the blood pressure measurement. A weak carotid pulse suggests a reduced stroke volume. Usually the strength of the pulse is graded on a scale of 1 to 4, where 2 is a normal pulse amplitude, 3 or 4 is a hyperdynamic pulse, and 1 is a weak pulse. A low-amplitude, slow-rising pulse, which may be associated with a palpable vibration (thrill), suggests aortic stenosis. A bifid pulse (beating twice in systole) can be a sign of hypertrophic obstructive cardiomyopathy, severe aortic regurgitation, or the combination of moderately severe aortic stenosis and regurgitation. A dicrotic pulse (an exaggerated, early, diastolic wave) is found in severe heart failure. Pulsus alternans (alternate strong and weak pulses) is also a sign of severe heart failure. When evaluating the adequacy of the arterial conduits, all palpable pulses can be assessed and graded on a scale of 0 to 4, where 4 is a fully normal conduit, and anything below that is reduced, including 0—which indicates an absent pulse. The major pulses routinely palpated on physical examination are the radial, brachial, carotid, femoral, dorsalis pedis, and posterior tibial. In special situations, the abdominal aorta and the ulnar, subclavian, popliteal, axillary, temporal, and intercostal arteries are palpated. In assessing the abdominal aorta, it is important to make note of the width of the aorta because an increase suggests an abdominal aortic aneurysm. It is particularly important to palpate the abdominal aorta in older individuals because abdominal aortic aneurysms are more prevalent in those older than 70. An audible bruit is a clue to significantly obstructed large arteries. During a routine examination, bruits are sought with the stethoscope head placed over the carotids, abdominal aorta, and femorals at the groin. Other arteries may be auscultated under special circumstances, such as suspected renal artery stenosis (flank bruit).

3. Jugular venous pulse—Assessment of the jugular venous pulse can provide information about the central venous pressure and right-heart function. Examination of the right internal jugular vein is ideal for assessing central venous pressure because it is attached directly to the superior vena cava without intervening valves. The patient is positioned into the semiupright posture that permits visualization of the top of the right internal jugular venous blood column. The height of this column of blood, vertically from the sternal angle, is added to 5 cm of blood (the presumed distance to the center of the right atrium from the sternal angle) to obtain an estimate of central venous pressure in centimeters of blood. This can be converted to millimeters of mercury (mm Hg) with the formula:

$$mm\ Hg = cm\ blood \times 0.736.$$

Examining the characteristics of the right internal jugular pulse is valuable for assessing right-heart function and rhythm disturbances. The normal jugular venous pulse has two distinct waves: a and v; the former coincides with atrial contraction and the latter with late ventricular systole. An absent a wave and an irregular pulse suggest atrial fibrillation. A large and early v wave suggests tricuspid regurgitation. The dips after the a and v waves are the x and y descents; the former coincide with atrial relaxation and the latter with early ventricular filling. In tricuspid stenosis, the y descent is prolonged. Other applications of the jugular pulse examination are discussed in the chapters dealing with specific disorders.

4. Lungs—Evaluation of the lungs is an important part of the physical examination: Diseases of the lung can affect the heart, just as diseases of the heart can affect the lungs. The major finding of importance is rales at the pulmonary bases, indicating alveolar fluid collection. Although this is a significant finding in patients with congestive heart failure, it is not always possible to distinguish rales caused by heart failure from those caused by pulmonary disease. The presence of pleural fluid, although useful in the diagnosis of heart failure, can be due to other causes. Heart failure most commonly causes a right pleural effusion; it can cause effusions on both sides but is least likely to cause isolated left pleural effusion. The specific constellation of dullness at the left base with bronchial breath sounds suggests an increase in heart size from pericardial effusion (Ewart sign) or another cause of cardiac enlargement; it is thought to be due to compression by the heart of a left lower lobe bronchus.

When right-heart failure develops or venous return is restricted from entering the heart, venous pressure in the abdomen increases, leading to hepatosplenomegaly and eventually ascites. None of these physical findings is specific for heart disease; they do, however, help establish the diagnosis. Heart failure also leads to generalized fluid retention, usually manifested as lower extremity edema or, in severe heart failure, anasarca.

5. Cardiac auscultation—Heart sounds are caused by the acceleration and deceleration of blood and the subsequent vibration of the cardiac structures during the phases of the cardiac cycle. To hear cardiac sounds, use a stethoscope with a bell and a tight diaphragm. Low-frequency sounds are associated with ventricular filling and are heard best with the bell. Medium-frequency sounds are associated with valve

opening and closing; they are heard best with the diaphragm. Cardiac murmurs are due to turbulent blood flow, are usually high-to-medium frequency, and are heard best with the diaphragm. Low-frequency atrioventricular valve inflow murmurs, such as that produced by mitral stenosis, are best heard with the bell, however. Auscultation should take place in areas that correspond to the location of the heart and great vessels. Such placement will, of course, need to be modified for patients with unusual body habitus or an unusual cardiac position. When no cardiac sounds can be heard over the precordium, they can often be heard in either the subxiphoid area or the right supraclavicular area.

Auscultation in various positions is recommended because low-frequency filling sounds are best heard with the patient in the left lateral decubitus position, and high-frequency murmurs, such as that of aortic regurgitation, are best heard with the patient sitting.

A. HEART SOUNDS—The **first heart sound** is coincident with mitral and tricuspid valve closure and has two components in up to 40% of normal individuals. There is little change in the intensity of this sound with respiration or position. The major determinant of the intensity of the first heart sound is the electrocardiographic (ECG) PR interval, which determines the time delay between atrial and ventricular contraction and thus the position of the mitral valve when ventricular systole begins. With a short PR interval, the mitral valve is widely open when systole begins, and its closure increases the intensity of the first sound, as compared to a long PR-interval beat when the valve partially closes prior to the onset of ventricular systole. Certain disease states, such as mitral stenosis, also can increase the intensity of the first sound.

The **second heart sound** is coincident with closure of the aortic and pulmonic valves. Normally, this sound is single in expiration and split during inspiration, permitting the aortic and pulmonic components to be distinguished. The inspiratory split is due to a delay in the occurrence of the pulmonic component because of a decrease in pulmonary vascular resistance, which prolongs pulmonary flow beyond the end of right ventricular systole. Variations in this normal splitting of the second heart sound are useful in determining certain disease states. For example, in atrial septal defect, the second sound is usually split throughout the respiratory cycle because of the constant increase in pulmonary flow. In patients with left bundle branch block, a delay occurs in the aortic component of the second heart sound, which results in reversed respiratory splitting; single with inspiration, split with expiration.

A **third heart sound** occurs during early rapid filling of the left ventricle; it can be produced by any condition that causes left ventricular volume overload or dilatation. It can therefore be heard in such disparate conditions as congestive heart failure and normal pregnancy. A **fourth heart sound** is due to a vigorous atrial contraction into a stiffened left ventricle and can be heard in left ventricular hypertrophy of any cause or in diseases that reduce compliance of the left ventricle, such as myocardial infarction.

Although third and fourth heart sounds can occasionally occur in normal individuals, all other extra sounds are signs of cardiac disease. Early ejection sounds are due to abnormalities of the semilunar valves, from restriction of their motion, thickening, or both (eg, a bicuspid aortic valve, pulmonic or aortic stenosis). A midsystolic click is often due to mitral valve prolapse and is caused by sudden tensing in midsystole of the redundant prolapsing segment of the mitral leaflet. The opening of a thickened atrioventricular valve leaflet, as in mitral stenosis, will cause a loud opening sound (snap) in early diastole. A lower frequency (more of a knock) sound at the time of rapid filling may be an indication of constrictive pericarditis. These early diastolic sounds must be distinguished from a third heart sound.

B. MURMURS—**Systolic murmurs** are very common and do not always imply cardiac disease. They are usually rated on a scale of 1 to 6, where grade 1 is barely audible, grade 4 is associated with palpable vibrations (thrill), grade 5 can be heard with the edge of the stethoscope, and grade 6 can be heard without a stethoscope. Most murmurs fall in the 1–3 range, and murmurs in the 4–6 range are almost always due to pathologic conditions; severe disease can exist with grades 1–3 or no cardiac murmurs, however. The most common systolic murmur is the crescendo/decrescendo murmur that increases in intensity as blood flows early in systole and diminishes in intensity through the second half of systole. This murmur can be due to vigorous flow in a normal heart or to obstructions in flow, as occurs with aortic stenosis, pulmonic stenosis, or hypertrophic cardiomyopathy. The so-called innocent flow murmurs are usually grades 1–2 and occur very early in systole; they may have a vibratory quality and are usually less apparent when the patient is in the sitting position (when venous return is less). If an ejection sound is heard, there is usually some abnormality of the semilunar valves. Although louder murmurs may be due to pathologic cardiac conditions, this is not always so. Distinguishing benign from pathologic systolic flow murmurs is one of the major challenges of clinical cardiology. Benign flow murmurs can be heard in 80% of children; the incidence declines with age, but may be prominent during pregnancy or in adults who are thin or physically well trained. The murmur is usually benign in a patient with a soft flow murmur that diminishes in intensity in the sitting position and neither a history of cardiovascular disease nor other cardiac findings.

The **holosystolic,** or **pansystolic,** murmur is almost always associated with cardiac pathology. The most common cause of this murmur is atrioventricular valve regurgitation, but it can also be observed in conditions such as ventricular septal defect, in which an abnormal communication exists between two chambers of markedly different systolic pressures. Although it is relatively easy to determine that these murmurs represent an abnormality, it is more of a challenge to determine their origins. Keep in mind that such conditions as mitral regurgitation, which usually produce holosystolic murmurs, may produce crescendo/decrescendo murmurs, adding to the difficulty in differentiating benign from pathologic systolic flow murmurs.

Diastolic murmurs are always abnormal and are usually graded on a 1 to 4 scale. The most frequently heard diastolic murmur is the high-frequency decrescendo early diastolic murmur of aortic regurgitation. This is usually heard best at the upper left sternal border or in the aortic area (upper right sternal border) and may radiate to the lower left sternal border and the apex. This murmur is usually very high frequency and may be difficult to hear. Although the murmur of pulmonic regurgitation may sound like that of aortic regurgitation when pulmonary artery pressures are high, if structural disease of the valve is present with normal pulmonary pressures, the murmur usually has a midrange frequency and begins with a slight delay after the pulmonic second heart sound. Pulmonic regurgitation is usually best heard in the pulmonic area (left second intercostal space parasternally). Mitral stenosis produces a low-frequency rumbling diastolic murmur that is decrescendo in early diastole, but may become crescendo up to the first heart sound with moderately severe mitral stenosis and sinus rhythm. The murmur is best heard at the apex in the left lateral decubitus position with the bell of the stethoscope. Similar findings are heard in tricuspid stenosis, but the murmur is loudest at the lower left sternal border.

A **continuous murmur** implies a connection between a high- and a low-pressure chamber throughout the cardiac cycle, such as occurs with a fistula between the aorta and the pulmonary artery. If the connection is a patent ductus arteriosus, the murmur is heard best under the left clavicle; it has a machine-like quality. Continuous murmurs must be distinguished from the combination of systolic and diastolic murmurs in patients with combined lesions (eg, aortic stenosis and regurgitation).

Traditionally, the origin of heart murmurs was based on five factors: (1) their timing in the cardiac cycle, (2) where on the chest they were heard, (3) their characteristics, (4) their intensity, and (5) their duration. Unfortunately, this traditional classification system is unreliable in predicting the underlying pathology. A more accurate method, **dynamic auscultation,** changes the intensity, duration, and characteristics of the murmur by bedside maneuvers that alter hemodynamics.

The simplest of these maneuvers is observation of any changes in murmur intensity with normal respiration because all right-sided cardiac murmurs should increase in intensity with normal inspiration. Although some exceptions exist, the method is very reliable for detecting such murmurs. Inspiration is associated with reductions in intrathoracic pressure that increase venous return from the abdomen and the head, leading to an increased flow through the right heart chambers. The consequent increase in pressure increases the intensity of right-sided murmurs. These changes are best observed in the sitting position, where venous return is smallest, and changes in intrathoracic pressure can produce their greatest effect on venous return. In a patient in the supine position, when venous return is near maximum, there may be little change observed with respiration. The ejection sound caused by pulmonic stenosis does not routinely increase in intensity with inspiration. The increased blood in the right heart accentuates atrial contraction, which increases late diastolic pressure in the right ventricle, partially opening the stenotic pulmonary valve and thus diminishing the opening sound of this valve with the subsequent systole.

Changes in position are an important part of normal auscultation; they can also be of great value in determining the origin of cardiac murmurs (Table 5–2). Murmurs dependent on venous return, such as innocent flow murmurs, are softer or absent in upright positions; others, such as the murmur associated with hypertrophic obstructive cardiomyopathy, are accentuated by reduced left ventricular volume associated with the upright position. In physically capable individuals, a rapid squat from the standing position is often diagnostically valuable because it suddenly increases venous return and left ventricular volume and accentuates flow murmurs but diminishes the murmur of hypertrophic obstructive cardiomyopathy. The stand-squat maneuver is also useful for altering the timing of the midsystolic click caused by mitral valve prolapse during systole. When the ventricle is small during standing, the prolapse occurs earlier in systole, moving the midsystolic click to early systole. During squatting, the ventricle dilates and the prolapse is delayed in systole, resulting in a late midsystolic click.

The **Valsalva maneuver** is also frequently used. The patient bears down and expires against a closed glottis, increasing intrathoracic pressure and markedly reducing venous return to the heart. Although almost all cardiac murmurs decrease in intensity during this maneuver, there are two exceptions: (1) The murmur of hypertrophic obstructive cardiomyopathy may become louder because of the diminished left ventricular volume. (2) The murmur associated with mitral regurgitation from mitral valve prolapse may become longer and louder because of the earlier occurrence of prolapse during systole. When the maneuver is very vigorous and prolonged, even these two murmurs may eventually diminish in intensity. Therefore, the Valsalva maneuver should be held for only about 10 seconds, so as not to cause prolonged diminution of the cerebral and coronary blood flow.

Isometric hand grip exercises have been used to increase arterial and left ventricular pressure. These maneuvers increase the flow gradient for mitral regurgitation, ventricular septal defect, and aortic regurgitation; the murmurs should then increase in intensity. Increasing arterial and left ventricular pressure increases left ventricular volume, thereby decreasing the murmur of hypertrophic obstructive cardiomyopathy. If the patient is unable to perform isometric exercises, **transient arterial occlusion** of both upper extremities with sphygmomanometers can achieve the same increases in left-sided pressure.

Noting the changes in murmur intensity in the heart beat following a premature ventricular contraction, and comparing these to a beat that does not, can be extremely useful. The premature ventricular contraction interrupts the cardiac cycle, and during the subsequent compensatory pause, an extra-long diastole occurs, leading to increased left ventricular filling. Therefore, murmurs caused by the flow of blood out of the left ventricle (eg, aortic stenosis) increase in intensity. There is usually no change in the intensity of the murmur of typical mitral regurgitation because blood pressure falls during the long pause and increases the gradient between the left ventricle and the aorta, allowing more forward flow. This results in the same amount of mitral regurgitant flow as on a normal beat with a higher aortic

Table 5–2. Differentiation of Systolic Murmurs Based on Changes in Their Intensity from Physiologic Maneuvers

Maneuver	Origin of Murmur					
	Flow	TR	AS	MR/VSD	MVP	HOCM
Inspiration	– or ↑	↑	–	–	–	–
Stand	↓	–	–	–	↑	↑
Squat	↑	–	–	–	↓	↓
Valsalva	↓	↓	↓	↓	↑	↑
Handgrip/TAO	↓	–	–	↑	↑	↓
Post-PVC	↑	–	↑	–	–	↑

AS, aortic stenosis; Flow, innocent flow murmur; HOCM, hypertrophic obstructive cardiomyopathy; MR, mitral regurgitation; MVP, mitral valve prolapse; PVC, premature ventricular contraction; TAO, transient arterial occlusion; TR, tricuspid regurgitation; VSD, ventricular septal defect; ↑ or ↓, change in intensity of murmur; –, no consistent change pressure and less forward flow. The increased volume during the long pause goes out of the aorta rather than back into the left atrium. Unfortunately, there is no reliable way of inducing a premature ventricular contraction in most patients; it is fortuitous when a physician is present for one. Atrial fibrillation with markedly varying cycle lengths produces the same phenomenon and can be very helpful in determining the origin of murmurs.

Brennan JM, et al. A comparison by medicine residents of physical examination versus hand-carried ultrasound for estimation of right atrial pressure. *Am J Cardiol.* 2007;99(11):1614–6. [PMID: 17531592]

Kobal SL, et al. Comparison of effectiveness of hand-carried ultrasound to bedside cardiovascular physical examination. *Am J Cardiol.* 2005;96:1002–6. [PMID: 16188532]

Marcus GM, et al. Usefulness of the third heart sound in predicting an elevated level of B-type natriuretic peptide. *Am J Cardiol.* 2004;93(10):1312–3. [PMID: 15135714]

B. Diagnostic Studies

1. Electrocardiography—Electrocardiography is perhaps the least expensive of all cardiac diagnostic tests, providing considerable value for the money. Modern ECG-reading computers do an excellent job of measuring the various intervals between waveforms and calculating the heart rate and the left ventricular axis. These programs fall considerably short, however, when it comes to diagnosing complex ECG patterns and rhythm disturbances, and the test results must be read by a physician skilled at ECG interpretation.

Analysis of cardiac rhythm is perhaps the ECG's most widely used feature; it is used to clarify the mechanism of an irregular heart rhythm detected on physical examination or that of an extremely rapid or slow rhythm. The ECG is also used to monitor cardiac rate and rhythm; ambulatory ECG monitoring devices allow assessment of cardiac rate and rhythm on an ambulatory basis. ECG radio telemetry is also often used on hospital wards and between ambulances and emergency departments to assess and monitor rhythm disturbances. There are two types of ambulatory ECG recorders: continuous recorders that record all heart beats over 1 to 7 days and intermittent recorders that can be attached to the patient or implanted subcutaneously for weeks or months and then activated to provide brief recordings of infrequent events. In addition to analysis of cardiac rhythm, ambulatory ECG recordings can be used to detect ST-wave transients indicative of myocardial ischemia and certain electrophysiologic parameters of diagnostic and prognostic value. The most common use of ambulatory ECG monitoring is the evaluation of symptoms such as syncope, near-syncope, or palpitation for which there is no obvious cause and cardiac rhythm disturbances are suspected.

The ECG is an important tool for rapidly assessing **metabolic and toxic disorders** of the heart. Characteristic changes in the ST-T waves indicate imbalances of potassium and calcium. Drugs such as tricyclic antidepressants have characteristic effects on the QT and QRS intervals at toxic levels. Such observations on the ECG can be life-saving in emergency situations with comatose patients or cardiac arrest victims.

Chamber enlargement can be assessed through the characteristic changes of left or right ventricular and atrial enlargement. Occasionally, isolated signs of left atrial enlargement on the ECG may be the only diagnostic clue to mitral stenosis. Evidence of chamber enlargement on the ECG usually signifies an advanced stage of disease with a poorer prognosis than that of patients with the same disease but no discernible enlargement.

The ECG is an important tool in managing suspected **acute coronary syndromes.** In patients with chest pain that is compatible with myocardial ischemia, the characteristic ST-T–wave elevations that do not resolve with nitroglycerin (and are unlikely to be the result of an old infarction) become the basis for thrombolytic therapy or a primary percutaneous intervention. Rapid resolution of the ECG changes of myocardial infarction after reperfusion therapy has prognostic value and identifies patients with reperfused coronary arteries.

Evidence of **conduction abnormalities** may help explain the mechanism of bradyarrhythmias and the likelihood of the need for a pacemaker. Conduction abnormalities may also aid in determining the cause of heart disease. For example, right bundle branch block and left anterior fascicular block are often seen in Chagas cardiomyopathy, and left-axis deviation occurs in patients with a primum atrial septal defect.

2. Echocardiography—Another frequently ordered cardiac diagnostic test, echocardiography is based on the use of ultrasound directed at the heart to create images of cardiac anatomy and display them in real time on a monitor screen. Two-dimensional echocardiography is usually accomplished by placing an ultrasound transducer in various positions on the anterior chest and obtaining cross-sectional images of the heart and great vessels in a variety of standard planes. In general, two-dimensional echocardiography is excellent for detecting any anatomic abnormality of the heart and great vessels. In addition, because the heart is seen in real time, this modality can assess the function of cardiac chambers and valves throughout the cardiac cycle.

Transesophageal echocardiography (TEE) involves the placement of smaller ultrasound probes on a gastroscopic device for placement in the esophagus behind the heart; it produces much higher resolution images of posterior cardiac structures. Transesophageal echocardiography has made it possible to detect left atrial thrombi, small mitral valve vegetations, and thoracic aortic dissection with a high degree of accuracy. Recent advances in image processing of multiplanar images have permitted real-time three-dimensional echocardiography. In its current state of development, it is most useful for evaluating valve structure for planning surgical repair.

The older analog echocardiographic display referred to as M-mode, motion-mode, or time-motion mode, is currently used for its high axial and temporal resolution. It is superior to two-dimensional echocardiography for measuring the size of structures in its axial direction, and its 1/1000-second sampling rate allows for the resolution of complex cardiac motion patterns. Its many disadvantages, including poor lateral resolution and the inability to distinguish whole heart motion from the motion of individual cardiac structures, have relegated it to a supporting role.

Doppler ultrasound can be combined with two-dimensional imaging to investigate blood flow in the heart and great vessels. It is based on determining the change in frequency (caused by the movement of blood in the given structure) of the reflected ultrasound compared with the transmitted ultrasound, and converting this difference into flow velocity. Color-flow Doppler echocardiography is most frequently used. In this technique, frequency shifts in each pixel of a selected area of the two-dimensional image are measured and converted into a color, depending on the direction of flow, the velocity, and the presence or absence of turbulence. When these color images are superimposed on the two-dimensional echocardiographic image, a moving color image of blood flow in the heart is created in real time. This is extremely useful for detecting regurgitant blood flow across cardiac valves and any abnormal communications in the heart.

Tissue Doppler imaging is similar to color-flow Doppler except that myocardial tissue movement velocity is interrogated. This allows for the quantitation of the rate of tissue contraction and relaxation, which is a measure of myocardial performance that can be applied to systole and diastole. Regional differences in myocardial performance can be assessed and used to guide biventricular pacemaker resynchronization therapy.

Because color-flow imaging cannot resolve very high velocities, another Doppler mode must be used to quantitate the exact velocity and estimate the pressure gradient of the flow when high velocities are suspected. Continuous wave Doppler, which almost continuously sends and receives ultrasound along a beam that can be aligned through the heart, is extremely accurate at resolving very high velocities such as those encountered with valvular aortic stenosis. The disadvantage of this technique is that the source of the high velocity within the beam cannot always be determined but must be assumed, based on the anatomy through which the beam passes. When there is ambiguity about the source of the high velocity, pulsed wave Doppler is more useful. This technique is range-gated such that specific areas along the beam (sample volumes) can be investigated. One or more sample volumes can be examined and determinations made concerning the exact location of areas of high-velocity flow.

Two-dimensional echocardiographic imaging of dynamic left ventricular cross-sectional anatomy and the superimposition of a Doppler color-flow map provide more information than the traditional left ventricular cine-angiogram can.

Ventricular wall motion can be interrogated in multiple planes, and left ventricular wall thickening during systole (an important measure of myocardial viability) can be assessed. In addition to demonstrating segmental wall motion abnormalities, echocardiography can estimate left ventricular volumes and ejection fraction. In addition, valvular regurgitation can be assessed at all four valves with the accuracy of the estimated severity equivalent to contrast angiography.

Doppler echocardiography has now largely replaced cardiac catheterization for deriving hemodynamics to estimate the severity of valve stenosis. Recorded Doppler velocities across a valve can be converted to pressure gradients by use of the simplified Bernoulli equation (pressure gradient = $4 \times velocity^2$). Cardiac output can be measured by Doppler from the velocity recorded at cardiac anatomic sites of known size visualized on the two-dimensional echocardiographic image. Cardiac output and pressure gradient data can be used to calculate the stenotic valve area with remarkable accuracy. A complete echocardiographic examination including two-dimensional and M-mode anatomic and functional visualization, and color, pulsed, and continuous wave Doppler examination of blood flow provides a considerable amount of information about cardiac structure and function. A full discussion of the usefulness of this technique is beyond the scope of this chapter, but individual uses of echocardiography will be discussed in later chapters.

Unfortunately, echocardiography is not without its technical difficulties and pitfalls. Like any noninvasive technique, it is not 100% accurate. Furthermore, it is impossible to obtain high-quality images or Doppler signals in as many as 5% of patients—especially those with emphysema, chest wall deformities, and obesity. Although TEE has made the examination of such patients easier, it does not solve all the problems of echocardiography. Despite these limitations, the technique is so powerful that it has moved out of the noninvasive laboratory and is now frequently being used in the operating room, the clinic, the emergency department, and even the cardiac catheterization laboratory, to help guide procedures without the use of fluoroscopy. New hand-held echocardiographic machines may soon rival the cardiac physical examination at the bedside.

3. Nuclear cardiac imaging—Nuclear cardiac imaging involves the injection of tracer amounts of radioactive elements attached to larger molecules or to the patient's own blood cells. The tracer-labeled blood is concentrated in certain areas of the heart, and a gamma ray detection camera is used to collect the radioactive emissions and form an image of the deployment of the tracer in the particular area. The single-crystal gamma camera produces planar images of the heart, depending on the relationship of the camera to the body. Multiple-head gamma cameras, which rotate around the patient, can produce single-photon emission computed tomography (SPECT) images, displaying the cardiac anatomy in slices, each about 1-cm thick. Positron emission tomography (PET) scanning requires special isotopes and imaging equipment, but positrons are less susceptible to attenuation by the chest wall and can detect cellular metabolism as well as perfusion. The presence of metabolism in a malfunctioning or poorly perfused wall suggests myocardial viability.

A. MYOCARDIAL PERFUSION IMAGING—The most common tracers used for imaging regional myocardial blood-flow distribution are thallium-201 and the technetium-99m–based agents, such as sestamibi. Thallium-201, a potassium analog that is efficiently extracted from the bloodstream by viable myocardial cells, is concentrated in the myocardium in areas of adequate blood flow and living myocardial cells. Thallium perfusion images show defects (a lower tracer concentration) in areas where blood flow is relatively reduced and in areas of damaged myocardial cells. If the damage is from frank necrosis or scar tissue formation, very little thallium will be taken up; ischemic cells may take up thallium more slowly or incompletely, producing relative defects in the image.

Myocardial perfusion problems are separated from nonviable myocardium by the fact that thallium eventually washes out of the myocardial cells and back into the circulation. If a defect detected on initial thallium imaging disappears over a period of 3–24 hours, the area is presumably viable. A persistent defect suggests a myocardial scar. In addition to detecting viable myocardium and assessing the extent of new and old myocardial infarctions, thallium-201 imaging can also be used to detect myocardial ischemia during stress testing (see later section on stress testing) as well as marked enlargement of the heart or dysfunction. The major problem with thallium imaging is photon attenuation because of chest wall structures, which can give an artifactual appearance of defects in the myocardium.

The technetium-99m–based agents take advantage of the shorter half-life of technetium (6 hours; the half-life of thallium-201 is 73 hours); this allows for use of a larger dose, which results in higher energy emissions and higher quality images. Technetium-99m's higher energy emissions scatter less and are attenuated less by chest wall structures, reducing the number of artifacts. Because sestamibi undergoes considerably less washout after the initial myocardial uptake than thallium does, the evaluation of perfusion versus tissue damage requires two separate injections.

In addition to detecting perfusion deficits, myocardial imaging with the SPECT system allows for a three-dimensional reconstruction of the heart, which can be displayed in any projection on a monitor screen. Such images can be formed at intervals during the cardiac cycle to create an image of the beating heart, which can be used to detect wall motion abnormalities and derive left ventricular volumes and ejection fraction. Matching wall motion abnormalities with perfusion defects provides additional confirmation that the perfusion defects visualized are true and not artifacts of photon attenuation. Also, extensive perfusion defects and wall motion abnormalities should be accompanied by decreases in ejection fraction.

B. POSITRON EMISSION TOMOGRAPHY—Positron emission tomography (PET) is a technique using tracers that simultaneously emit two high-energy photons. A circular array of detectors around the patient can detect these simultaneous events and accurately identify their origin in the heart. This results in improved spatial resolution compared with SPECT. It also allows for correction of tissue photon attenuation, resulting in the ability to accurately quantify radioactivity in the heart. PET can be used to assess myocardial perfusion and myocardial metabolic activity separately by using different tracers coupled to different molecules. Most of the tracers developed for clinical use require a cyclotron for their generation; the cyclotron must be in close proximity to the PET imager because of the short half-life of the agents. Agents in clinical use include oxygen-15 (half-life 2 minutes), nitrogen-13 (half-life 10 minutes), carbon-11 (half-life 20 minutes), and fluorene-18 (half-life 110 minutes). These tracers can be coupled to many physiologically active molecules for assessing various functions of the myocardium. Because rubidium-82, with a half-life of 75 seconds, does not require a cyclotron and can be generated on site, it is frequently used with PET scanning, especially for perfusion images. Ammonia containing nitrogen-13 and water containing oxygen-15 are also used as perfusion agents. C-11–labeled fatty acids and ^{18}F-fluorodeoxyglucose are common metabolic tracers used to assess myocardial viability, and acetate containing carbon-11 is often used to assess oxidative metabolism.

The main clinical uses of PET scanning involve the evaluation of coronary artery disease. It is used in perfusion studies at rest and during pharmacologic stress (exercise studies are less feasible). In addition to a qualitative assessment of perfusion defects, PET allows for a calculation of absolute regional myocardial blood flow or blood-flow reserve. PET also assesses myocardial viability, using the metabolic tracers to detect metabolically active myocardium in areas of reduced perfusion. The presence of viability implies that returning perfusion to these areas would result in improved function of the ischemic myocardium. Although many authorities consider PET scanning the gold standard for determining myocardial viability, it has not been found to be 100% accurate. Thallium reuptake techniques and echocardiographic and magnetic resonance imaging of delayed myocardial enhancement have proved equally valuable for detecting myocardial viability in clinical studies.

C. RADIONUCLIDE ANGIOGRAPHY—Radionuclide angiography is based on visualizing radioactive tracers in the cavities of the heart over time. Radionuclide angiography is usually done with a single gamma camera in a single plane, and only one view of the heart is obtained. The most common technique is to record the amount of radioactivity received by the gamma camera over time. Although volume estimates by radionuclide angiography are not as accurate as those obtained by other methods, the ejection fraction is quite accurate. Wall motion can be assessed in the one plane imaged, but the technique is not as sensitive as other imaging modalities for detecting wall motion abnormalities. Although still used by some to follow ejection fraction serially, it has largely been replaced by echocardiography.

4. Other cardiac imaging

A. CHEST RADIOGRAPHY—Chest radiography is used infrequently now for evaluating cardiac structural abnormalities because of the superiority of echocardiography in this regard. The chest radiograph, however, is a rapid, inexpensive way to assess pulmonary anatomy and is very useful for evaluating pulmonary venous congestion and hypoperfusion or hyperperfusion. In addition, abnormalities of the thoracic skeleton are found in certain cardiac disorders and radiographic corroboration may help with the diagnosis. Detection of intracardiac calcium deposits by the radiograph or fluoroscopy is of some value in finding coronary artery, valvular, or pericardial disease.

B. COMPUTED TOMOGRAPHIC SCANNING—Computed tomography (CT) has been applied to cardiac imaging by using ECG gating to account for the motion of the heart. The major application of this technology has been the detection of small amounts of coronary artery calcium as an indicator of atherosclerosis in the coronary arterial tree. With the development of multidetector CT and using intravenous contrast agents, noninvasive coronary angiography is possible and has a very high negative predictive value for detecting significant coronary artery lesions. Hybrid PET or nuclear SPECT plus CT scanners are now available and can provide anatomic, perfusion, and viability data. CT scanning is also very useful for detecting thoracic aorta disease, such as dissection and pericardial disease.

C. MAGNETIC RESONANCE IMAGING—Magnetic resonance imaging (MRI) has considerable potential as a technique for evaluating cardiovascular disease. It is excellent for detecting aortic dissection and pericardial thickening and assessing left ventricular volume and mass. Newer computer analysis techniques have solved the problem of myocardial motion and can be used to detect flow in the heart, much as color-flow Doppler is used. In addition, regional molecular disturbances can be created that place stripes of a different density in either the myocardium or the blood; these can then be followed through the cardiac cycle to determine structural deformation (eg, of the left ventricular wall) or the movement of the blood.

Gadolinium-based contrast agents can be injected intravenously to enhance MRI. In delayed images taken after contrast injection (approximately 10 minutes), hyperenhancement of the myocardium suggests irreversible scar formation. This determination can identify nonviable myocardium in patients

Table 5–3. Indications for Stress Testing

Evaluation of exertional chest pain
Assess significance of known coronary artery disease
Risk stratification of ischemic heart disease
Determine exercise capacity
Evaluate other exercise symptoms

with coronary artery disease. The major limitation of cardiac MRI is the length of the studies, their cost, and the relative nonavailability of magnetic resonance systems in acute patient care areas compared with CT.

5. Stress testing—Stress testing in various forms is most frequently applied in cases of suspected or overt ischemic heart disease (Table 5–3). Because ischemia represents an imbalance between myocardial oxygen supply and demand, exercise or pharmacologic stress increases myocardial oxygen demand and reveals an inadequate oxygen supply (hypoperfusion) in diseased coronary arteries. Stress testing can thus induce detectable ischemia in patients with no evidence of ischemia at rest. It is also used to determine cardiac reserve in patients with valvular and myocardial disease. Deterioration of left ventricular performance during exercise or other stresses suggests a diminution in cardiac reserve that would have therapeutic and prognostic implications. Although most stress test studies use some technique (Table 5–4) for directly assessing the myocardium, it is important not to forget the symptoms of angina pectoris or extreme dyspnea: Light-headedness or syncope can be equally important in evaluating patients. Physical findings such as the development of pulmonary rales, ventricular gallops, murmurs, peripheral cyanosis, hypotension, excessive increases in heart rate, or inappropriate decreases in heart rate also have diagnostic and prognostic value. It is therefore important that a symptom assessment and physical examination always be done before, during, and after stress testing.

Electrocardiographic monitoring is the most common cardiac evaluation technique used during stress testing; it should be part of every stress test in order to assess heart rate and detect any arrhythmias. In patients with normal resting ECGs, diagnostic ST depression of myocardial ischemia has a fairly high sensitivity and specificity for detecting coronary artery disease in symptomatic patients if adequate stress is achieved (peak heart rate at least 85% of the patient's

Table 5–4. Methods of Detecting Myocardial Ischemia during Stress Testing

Electrocardiography
Echocardiography
Myocardial perfusion imaging
Positron emission tomography
Magnetic resonance imaging

maximum predicted rate, based on age and sex). Exercise ECG testing is an excellent low-cost screening procedure for patients with chest pain consistent with coronary artery disease, normal resting ECGs, and the ability to exercise to maximal levels.

A **myocardial imaging** technique is usually added to the exercise evaluation in patients whose ECGs are abnormal or, for some reason, less accurate. It is also used for determining the location and extent of myocardial ischemia in patients with known coronary artery disease. Imaging techniques, in general, enhance the sensitivity and specificity of the tests but are still not perfect, with false-positives and false-negatives occurring 5–10% of the time.

Which adjunctive myocardial imaging technology to choose depends on the quality of the tests, their availability and cost, and the services provided by the laboratory. If these are all equal, the decision should be based on patient characteristics. For example, echocardiography might be appropriate when ischemia is suspected of developing during exercise and is profound enough to depress segmental left ventricular performance and worsen mitral regurgitation. On the other hand, perfusion scanning might be the best test to determine which coronary artery is producing the symptoms in a patient with known three-vessel coronary artery disease and recurrent angina after revascularization.

Choosing the appropriate form of stress is also important (Table 5–5). Exercise, the preferred stress for increasing myocardial oxygen demand, also simulates the patient's normal daily activities and is therefore highly relevant clinically. There are essentially only two reasons for not choosing exercise stress, however: the patient's inability to exercise adequately because of physical or psychological limitations; or the chosen test cannot be performed readily with exercise (eg, PET scanning). In these situations, pharmacologic stress is appropriate.

6. Cardiac catheterization—Cardiac catheterization is now mainly used for the assessment of coronary artery anatomy by coronary angiography. In fact, the cardiac catheterization laboratory has become more of a therapeutic than a diagnostic arena. Once significant coronary artery disease is identified, a variety of catheter-based interventions can be used to alleviate the obstruction to blood flow in the coronary arteries. At one time, hemodynamic measurements (pressure, flow, oxygen consumption) were necessary to accurately diagnose and quantitate the severity of valvular heart disease and intracardiac shunts. Currently, Doppler echocardiography has taken over this role almost completely, except in the few instances when Doppler studies are inadequate or believed to be inaccurate. Catheter-based hemodynamic assessments are still useful for differentiating cardiac constriction from restriction, despite advances in Doppler echocardiography. Currently, the catheterization laboratory is also more often used as a treatment arena for valvular and congenital heart disease. Certain stenotic valvular and arterial lesions can be treated successfully with catheter-delivered balloon expansion, the deployment of stents, or stent-mounted bioprosthetic valves. Congenital and acquired shunts can also be closed by catheter-delivered devices.

Myocardial biopsy is necessary to treat patients with heart transplants and is occasionally used to diagnose selected cases of suspected acute myocarditis. For this purpose, a biotome is usually placed in the right heart, and several small pieces of myocardium are removed. Although this technique is relatively safe, myocardial perforation occasionally results.

7. Electrophysiologic testing—Electrophysiologic testing uses catheter-delivered electrodes in the heart to induce rhythm disorders and detect their structural basis. Certain arrhythmia foci and structural abnormalities that facilitate rhythm disturbances can be treated by catheter-delivered radiofrequency energy (ablation) or by the placement of various electronic devices that monitor rhythm disturbances and treat them accordingly through either pacing or internally delivered defibrillation shocks. Electrophysiologic testing and treatment now dominate the management of arrhythmias; the test is more accurate than the surface ECG for diagnosing many arrhythmias and detecting their substrate, and catheter ablation and electronic devices have been more successful than pharmacologic approaches at treating arrhythmias.

8. Test selection—In the current era of escalating healthcare costs, ordering multiple tests is rarely justifiable, and the physician must pick the one test that will best define the patient's problem. Unfortunately, cardiology offers multiple competing technologies that often address the same issues, but in a different way. The following five principles should be followed when considering which test to order:

- What information is desired? If the test is not reasonably likely to provide the type of information needed to help the patient's problem, it should not be done, no matter how inexpensive and easy it is to obtain. At one time, for example, routine preoperative ECGs were done prior to major noncardiac surgery to detect which patients might be at risk for cardiac events in the perioperative period. Once it was determined that the resting ECG was not good at this, the practice was discontinued, despite its low cost and ready availability.

Table 5–5. Types of Stress Tests

Exercise
Treadmill
Bicycle
Pharmacologic
Adenosine
Dipyridamole
Dobutamine
Isoproterenol
Other
Pacing

- What is the cost of the test? If two tests can provide the same information and one is much more expensive than the other, the less expensive test should be ordered. For example, to determine whether a patient's remote history of prolonged chest pain was a myocardial infarction, the physician has a choice of an ECG or one of several imaging tests, such as echocardiography, resting thallium-201 scintigraphy, and the like. Because the ECG is the least expensive test, it should be performed for this purpose in most situations.

- Is the test available? Sometimes the best test for the patient is not available in the given facility. If it is available at a nearby facility and the patient can go there without undue cost, the test should be obtained. If expensive travel is required, the costs and benefits of that test versus local alternatives need to be carefully considered.

- What is the level of expertise of the laboratory and the physicians who interpret the tests? For many of the high-technology imaging tests, the level of expertise considerably affects the value of the test. Myocardial perfusion imaging is a classic example of this. Some laboratories are superlative in producing tests of diagnostic accuracy. In others, the number of false-positive and false-negative results is so high that the tests are rendered almost worthless. Therefore, even though a given test may be available and inexpensive and could theoretically provide essential information, if the quality of the laboratory is not good, an alternative test should be sought.

- What quality of service is provided by the laboratory? Patients are customers, and they need to be satisfied. If a laboratory makes patients wait a long time, if it is tardy in getting the results to the physicians, or if great delays occur in accomplishing the test, choose an alternative laboratory (assuming, of course, that alternatives are available). Poor service cannot be tolerated.

Many other situations and considerations affect the choice of tests. For example, a 50-year-old man with incapacitating angina might have a high likelihood of having single-vessel disease that would be amenable to catheter-based revascularization. It might be prudent to take this patient directly to coronary arteriography with an eye toward diagnosing and treating the patient's disease in one setting for maximum cost-effectiveness. This approach, however, presents the risk of ordering an expensive catheterization rather than a less expensive noninvasive test if the patient does not have significant coronary disease. Physicians are frequently solicited to use the latest emerging technologies, which often have not been proved better than the standard techniques. It is generally unwise to begin using these usually more expensive methods until clinical trials have established their efficacy and cost-effectiveness.

Asch FM, et al. Lack of sensitivity of the electrocardiogram for detection of old myocardial infarction: a cardiac magnetic resonance imaging study. *Am Heart J.* 2006;152(4):742–8. [PMID: 16996851]

Beanlands RS, et al; PARR-2 Investigators. F-18-fluorodeoxyglucose positron emission tomography imaging-assisted management of patients with severe left ventricular dysfunction and suspected coronary disease; a randomized, controlled trial (PARR-2). *J Am Coll Cardiol.* 2007;50(20):2002–12. [PMID: 17996568]

Budoff MJ, et al; American Heart Association Committee on Cardiovascular Imaging and Intervention; American Heart Association Council on Cardiovascular Radiology and Intervention; American Heart Association Committee on Cardiac Imaging, Council on Clinical Cardiology. Assessment of coronary artery disease by cardiac computed tomography: a scientific statement from the American Heart Association Committee on Cardiovascular Imaging and Intervention, Council on Cardiovascular Radiology and Intervention, and Committee on Cardiac Imaging, Council on Clinical Cardiology. *Circulation.* 2006;114(16):1761–91. [PMID: 17015792]

Douglas PS, et al. ACCF/ASE/AHA/ASNC/HFSA/HRS/SCAI/SCCM/SCCT/SCMR 2011 appropriate use criteria for echocardiography. *J Am Coll Cardiol.* 2011;57(9):1126–66. [PMID: 21349406]

Gibbons RJ, et al; American College of Cardiology/American Heart Association Task Force on Practice Guidelines (Committee to Update the 1997 Exercise Testing Guidelines). ACC/AHA 2002 guideline update for exercise testing: summary article: a report of the American College of Cardiology/American Heart Association Task Force on the Practice Guidelines (Committee to Update the 1997 Exercise Testing Guidelines). *Circulation.* 2002;106(14):1883–92. [PMID: 12356646]

Hendel RC, et al. ACCF/ASNC/ACR/AHA/ASE/SCCT/SCMR/SNM 2009 appropriate use criteria for cardiac radionuclide imaging. *J Am Coll Cardiol.* 2009;53(23):2201–29. [PMID: 19497454]

Lucas FL, et al. Temporal trends in the utilization of diagnostic testing and treatments for cardiovascular disease in the United States, 1993-2001. *Circulation.* 2006;113:374–9. [PMID: 16432068]

Patel MR, et al. ACCF/SCAI/AATS/AHA/ASE/ASNC/HFSA/HRS/SCCM/SCCT/SCMR/STS 2012 appropriate use criteria for diagnostic catheterization. *J Thorac Cardiovasc Surg.* 2012;144:39–71. [PMID: 22710040]

Sampson UK, et al. Diagnostic accuracy of rubidium-82 myocardial perfusion imaging with hybrid positron emission tomography/computed tomography in the detection of coronary artery disease. *J Am Coll Cardiol.* 2007;49(10):1052–8. [PMID: 17349884]

Sanz J, et al. Detection of healed myocardial infarction with multidetector-row computed tomography and comparison with cardiac magnetic resonance delayed hyperenhancement. *Am J Cardiol.* 2006;98(2):149–55. [PMID: 16828583]

Taylor AJ, et al. ACCF/SCCT/ACR/AHA/ASE/ASNC/NASCI/SCAI/SCMR 2010 appropriate use criteria for cardiac computed tomography. *J Am Coll Cardiol.* 2010;56:1864–94. [PMID: 21087721]

Chronic Ischemic Heart Disease

6

Michael H. Crawford, MD

ESSENTIALS OF DIAGNOSIS

- ▶ Typical exertional angina pectoris or its equivalents.
- ▶ Objective evidence of myocardial ischemia by electrocardiography, myocardial imaging, or myocardial perfusion scanning.
- ▶ Likely occlusive coronary artery disease because of history and objective evidence of prior myocardial infarction.
- ▶ Known coronary artery disease shown by coronary angiography.

▶ General Considerations

For clinical purposes, patients with chronic ischemic heart disease fall into two general categories: those with symptoms related to the disease, and those who are asymptomatic. Although the latter are probably more common than the former, physicians typically see symptomatic patients more frequently. The issue of asymptomatic patients becomes important clinically when physicians are faced with estimating the risk to a particular patient who is undergoing some stressful intervention, such as major noncardiac surgery. Another issue is the patient with known coronary artery disease who is currently asymptomatic. Such individuals, especially if they have objective evidence of myocardial ischemia, are known to have a higher incidence of future cardiovascular morbidity and mortality. There is, understandably, a strong temptation to treat such patients, despite the fact that it is difficult to make an asymptomatic patient feel better, and some of the treatment modalities have their own risks. In such cases, strong evidence that longevity will be positively influenced by the treatment must be present in order for its benefits to outweigh its risks.

▶ Pathophysiology & Etiology

In the industrialized nations, most patients with chronic ischemic heart disease have coronary atherosclerosis. Consequently, it is easy to become complacent and ignore the fact that other diseases can cause lesions in the coronary arteries (Table 6–1). In young people, coronary artery anomalies should be kept in mind; in older individuals, systemic vasculitides are not uncommon. Today, collagen vascular diseases are the most common vasculitides leading to coronary artery disease, but in the past, infections such as syphilis were a common cause of coronary vasculitis. Diseases of the ascending aorta, such as aortic dissection, can lead to coronary ostial occlusion. Coronary artery emboli may occur as a result of infectious endocarditis or of atrial fibrillation with left atrial thrombus formation. Infiltrative diseases of the heart, such as tumor metastases, may also compromise coronary flow. It is therefore essential to keep in mind diagnostic possibilities other than atherosclerosis when managing chronic ischemic heart disease.

Myocardial ischemia is the result of an imbalance between myocardial oxygen supply and demand. Coronary atherosclerosis and other diseases reduce the supply of oxygenated blood by obstructing the coronary arteries. Although the obstructions may not be enough to produce myocardial ischemia at rest, increases in myocardial oxygen demand during activities can precipitate myocardial ischemia. This is the basis for using stress testing to detect ischemic heart disease. Transient increases in the degree of coronary artery obstruction may develop as a result of platelet and thrombus formation or through increased coronary vasomotor tone. Although it is rare in the United States, pure coronary vasospasm in the absence of atherosclerosis can occur and cause myocardial ischemia and even infarction. In addition, in the presence of other cardiac diseases, especially those that cause a pressure load on the left ventricle, myocardial oxygen demand may outstrip the ability of normal coronary

Table 6–1. Nonatherosclerotic Causes of Epicardial Coronary Artery Obstruction

Fixed	Congenital anomalies
	Myocardial bridges
	Vasculitides
	Aortic dissection
	Granulomas
	Tumors
	Scarring from trauma, radiation
Transient	Vasospasm
	Embolus
	Thrombus in situ

Table 6–2. Risk Factors for Coronary Heart Disease

Major independent risk factors
Advancing age
Tobacco smoking
Diabetes mellitus
Elevated total and low-density lipoprotein (LDL) cholesterol
Low high-density lipoprotein cholesterol
Hypertension
Conditional risk factors
Elevated serum homocysteine
Elevated serum lipoprotein(a)
Elevated serum triglycerides
Inflammatory markers (eg, C-reactive protein)
Prothrombic factors (eg, fibrinogen)
Small, dense LDL particles
Predisposing risk factors
Abdominal obesity
Ethnic characteristics
Family history of premature coronary heart disease
Metabolic syndrome
Obesity
Physical inactivity
Psychosocial factors

arteries to provide oxygenated blood, resulting in myocardial ischemia or infarction. A good example would be the patient with severe aortic stenosis, considerable left ventricular hypertrophy, and severely elevated left ventricular pressures who tries to exercise. The manifestations of chronic ischemic heart disease have their basis in a complex pathophysiology of multiple factors that affect myocardial oxygen supply and demand.

▶ Clinical Findings

A. Risk Factors

Coronary atherosclerosis is more likely to occur in patients with certain risk factors for this disease (Table 6–2). These include advanced age, male gender or the postmenopausal state in females, a family history of coronary atherosclerosis, diabetes mellitus, systemic hypertension, high serum cholesterol and other associated lipoprotein abnormalities, and tobacco smoking. Additional minor risk factors include a sedentary lifestyle, obesity, high psychological stress levels, and such phenotypic characteristics as earlobe creases, auricular hirsutism, and a mesomorphic body type. The presence of other systemic diseases—hypothyroidism, pseudoxanthoma elasticum, and acromegaly, for example—can accelerate a propensity to coronary atherosclerosis. In the case of nonatherosclerotic coronary artery disease, evidence of such systemic vasculitides as lupus erythematosus, rheumatoid arthritis, and polyarthritis nodosa should be sought. Although none of these risk factors is in itself diagnostic of coronary artery disease, the more of them that are present, the greater the likelihood of the diagnosis.

Vasan RS, et al. Relative importance of borderline and elevated levels of coronary heart disease risk factors. *Ann Intern Med.* 2005;142(6):393–402. [PMID: 15767617]
Yusuf S, et al. Effect of potentially modifiable risk factors associated with myocardial infarction in 52 countries (the INTERHEART study): case-controlled study. *Lancet.* 2004;364(9438):937–52. [PMID: 15364185]

B. Symptoms & Signs

The major symptom of chronic ischemic heart disease is angina pectoris, with a clinical diagnosis based on five features:

- The character of the pain is a deep visceral pressure or squeezing sensation, rather than sharp or stabbing or pinprick-like pain.

- The pain almost always has some substernal component, although some patients complain of pain only on the right or left side of the chest, upper back, or epigastrium.

- The pain may radiate from the thorax to the jaw, neck, or arm. Arm pain in angina pectoris typically involves the ulnar surface of the left arm. Occasionally, the radiated pain may be more noticeable to the patient than the origin of the pain, resulting in complaints of only jaw or arm pain. These considerations have led some physicians to suggest that any pain between the umbilicus and the eyebrows should be considered angina pectoris until proven otherwise.

- Angina is usually precipitated by exertion, emotional upset, or other events that obviously increase myocardial oxygen demand, such as rapid tachyarrhythmias or extreme elevations in blood pressure.

- Angina pectoris is transient, lasting between 2 and 30 minutes. It is relieved by cessation of the precipitating event, such as exercise, or by the administration of treatment, such as sublingual nitroglycerin. Chest pain that lasts longer than 30 minutes is more consistent with myocardial infarction; pain of less than 2 minutes is unlikely to be due to myocardial ischemia.

For reasons that are unclear, some patients with chronic ischemic heart disease do not manifest typical symptoms of angina pectoris but have other symptoms that are brought on by the same precipitating factors and are relieved in the same way as angina. Because myocardial ischemia can lead to transient left ventricular dysfunction, resulting in increased left ventricular end-diastolic pressure and consequent pulmonary capillary pressure, the sensation of dyspnea can occur during episodes of myocardial supply-and-demand imbalance. Dyspnea may be the patient's only symptom during myocardial ischemia, or it may overshadow the chest pain in the patient's mind. Therefore, dyspnea out of proportion to the degree of exercise or activity can be considered an angina equivalent. Severe myocardial ischemia may lead to ventricular tachyarrhythmias manifesting as palpitations or even frank syncope. Severe episodes of myocardial ischemia may also lead to transient pulmonary edema, especially if the papillary muscles are involved in the ischemic myocardium and moderately severe mitral regurgitation is produced. The most dramatic result of myocardial ischemia is sudden cardiac death.

Patients with chronic myocardial ischemia can also have symptoms caused by the effects of repeated episodes of ischemia or infarction. Thus, patients may have manifestations of chronic cardiac rhythm disorders, especially ventricular arrhythmias, or chronic congestive heart failure. Patients may have symptoms related to atherosclerosis of other vascular systems. Patients with vascular disease in other organs are more likely to have coronary atherosclerosis. Those with prior cerebral vascular accidents or symptoms of peripheral vascular disease may be so disabled by these diseases that their ability to either perceive angina or generate enough myocardial oxygen demand to produce angina may be severely limited.

C. Physical Examination

The physical examination is often not helpful in the diagnosis of chronic ischemic heart disease. This is because many patients with chronic ischemic heart disease have no physical findings related to the disease, or if they do, the findings are not specific for coronary artery disease. For example, a fourth heart sound can be detected in patients with chronic ischemic heart disease, especially if they have had a prior myocardial infarction; however, fourth heart sounds are very common in hypertensive heart disease, valvular heart disease, and primary myocardial disease. Palpation of a systolic precordial bulge can occur in patients with prior myocardial infarction, but this sign is not specific and can occur in patients with left ventricular enlargement from any cause. Other signs can also be found in cases of chronic ischemic heart disease, such as those associated with congestive heart failure or mitral regurgitation. Again, these are nonspecific and can be caused by other disease processes. Because coronary atherosclerosis is the most common heart disease in industrialized nations, any physical findings suggestive of

heart disease should raise the suspicion of chronic ischemic heart disease.

D. Laboratory Findings

A complete blood count is useful to detect anemia, which will aggravate angina. Thyroid function tests are also important since hyperthyroidism can aggravate angina and hypothyroidism can lead to atherosclerosis. High-sensitivity C-reactive protein (CRP) has been used to detect the increased inflammation of active atherosclerosis. Values greater than 3 mg/L predict coronary events, but the additive value over standard risk factors is unclear. Mortality can be predicted by brain natriuretic peptide (BNP) or troponin levels in patients with coronary artery disease. Presumably, patients with high CRP, BNP, or troponin levels should be treated more aggressively to reduce risk factors.

E. Diagnostic Studies

1. Stress tests—Because angina pectoris or other manifestations of myocardial ischemia often occur during the patient's normal activities, it would be ideal to detect evidence of ischemia at that time. This can be done with ambulatory electrocardiography (ECG). Under unusual circumstances, a patient may have spontaneous angina or ischemia in a medical facility, where it is possible to perform an echocardiogram to assess wall motion abnormalities indicative of ischemia or to inject a radionuclide agent and immediately image the myocardium for perfusion defects. Detection of myocardial ischemia during a patient's normal activities, however, does not have as high a diagnostic yield as exercise stress testing does.

Of the various forms of exercise stress that can be used, the most popular is treadmill exercise, for several reasons: It involves walking, a familiar activity that often provokes symptoms. Because of the gravitational effects of being upright, walking requires higher levels or myocardial oxygen demand than do many other forms of exercise. In addition, walking can be performed on an inexpensive treadmill device, which makes evaluating the patient easy and cost-effective. Bicycling is an alternative form of exercise that is preferred by exercise physiologists because it is easier to quantitate the amount of work the person is performing on a bicycle than on a treadmill. Unfortunately, bicycle exercise does not require as high a level of myocardial oxygen demand as does treadmill walking. Thus, a patient may become fatigued on the bicycle before myocardial ischemia is induced, resulting in lower diagnostic yields. On the other hand, bicycle exercise can be performed in the supine position, which facilitates some myocardial ischemia detection methods such as echocardiography. In patients with peripheral vascular disease or lower limb amputations, arm and upper trunk rowing or cranking exercises can be substituted for leg exercise. Arm exercise has a particularly low diagnostic yield because exercising with the small muscle mass of the arms does not increase myocardial oxygen demand by much. Rowing exercises that involve the arms and the trunk muscles produce higher levels of myocardial oxygen demand that can equal those achieved with bicycle exercise—but not quite the levels seen with treadmill exercise. For these reasons, patients who cannot perform leg exercises are usually evaluated using pharmacologic stress testing.

There are two basic kinds of pharmacologic stress tests. One uses drugs, such as the synthetic catecholamine dobutamine, that mimic exercise; the other uses vasodilator drugs, such as dipyridamole and adenosine, that, by producing profound vasodilatation, increase heart rate and stroke volume, thereby raising myocardial oxygen demand. In addition, vasodilators may dilate normal coronary arteries more than diseased coronary arteries, augmenting any differences in regional perfusion of the myocardium, which can be detected by perfusion scanning. In general, vasodilator stress is preferred for myocardial perfusion imaging, and synthetic catecholamine stress is preferred for wall motion imaging.

2. Electrocardiography—ECG is the most frequently used method for detecting myocardial ischemia because of its ready availability, low cost, and ease of application. The usual criterion for diagnosing ischemia is horizontal or down-sloping ST segment depression, achieving at least 0.1 mV at 80 ms beyond the J point (junction of the QRS and the ST segment). This criterion provides the highest values of sensitivity and specificity. Sensitivity can be increased by using 0.5 mV, but at the expense of lower specificity; similarly, using 0.2 mV increases the specificity of the test at the expense of lower sensitivity. Furthermore, accuracy is highest when ECG changes are in the lateral precordial leads (V_4, V_5, V_6) instead of the inferior leads (II, III, aVF). In the usual middle-aged, predominantly male population of patients with chest pain syndromes, who have normal resting ECGs and can achieve more than 85% of their maximal predicted age-based heart rate during treadmill exercise, the preceding ECG criteria have a sensitivity and specificity of approximately 85%. If the resting ECG is abnormal, if the patient does not achieve 85% of maximum predicted heart rate, or if the patient is a woman, the sensitivity and specificity are lower and range from 70% to 80%. In an asymptomatic population with a low pretest likelihood of disease, sensitivity and specificity fall below 70%.

3. Myocardial perfusion scanning—This method detects differences in regional myocardial perfusion rather than ischemia per se; however, there is a high correlation between abnormal regional perfusion scans and the presence of significant coronary artery occlusive lesions. Thus, when coronary arteriography is used as the gold standard, the sensitivity and specificity of stress myocardial perfusion scanning in the typical middle-aged, predominantly male population with symptoms are approximately 85–95%. Testing an asymptomatic or predominantly female population would result in lower values. Failure to achieve more than 85% of the maximal predicted heart rate during exercise also results in lower diagnostic accuracy. Although treadmill exercise is the preferred stress modality for myocardial perfusion imaging, pharmacologically induced stress with dipyridamole or adenosine produces nearly as good results and is an acceptable alternative in the patient who cannot exercise. **Positron emission tomography** with vasodilator stress also can be used to detect regional perfusion differences indicative of coronary artery disease.

4. Assessing wall motion abnormalities—Reduced myocardial oxygen supply results in diminishment and, if severe enough, failure of myocardial contraction. Using methods to visualize the left ventricular wall, a reduction in inward endocardial movement and systolic myocardial thickening is observed with ischemia. **Echocardiography** is an ideal detection system for wall motion abnormalities because it can examine the left ventricle from several imaging planes, maximizing the ability to detect subtle changes in wall motion. When images are suboptimal (< 5% of cases), intravenous contrast agents can be given to fill the left ventricular cavity and improve endocardial definition. The results with either exercise or pharmacologic stress are comparable to those of myocardial perfusion imaging and superior to the ECG stress test detection of ischemia. The preferred pharmacologic detection method with wall motion imaging is dobutamine because it directly stimulates the myocardium to increase contractility, as well as raising heart rate and blood pressure, all of which increase myocardial oxygen demand. In some laboratories, if the heart rate increase is not comparable to that usually achieved with exercise testing, atropine is added to further increase myocardial oxygen demand. **Magnetic resonance imaging (MRI)** can also be used to assess left ventricular wall motion during pharmacologic stress testing, but there is relatively little experience with this technique.

5. Evaluating global left ventricular performance—Myocardial ischemia, if profound enough, results in a reduction in global left ventricular performance, which can be detected by either a decrease in left ventricular ejection fraction or a failure for it to increase during exercise. Therefore, techniques such as **radionuclide angiography** and single-photon emission computed tomography (SPECT) left ventricular reconstruction have been used to detect changes in global left ventricular function. Because fairly profound ischemia is required to depress global left ventricular function, this method has not been as sensitive as other techniques. Furthermore, myocardial disease can lead to an abnormal exercise ejection fraction response, which lowers the specificity of the test. In addition, age and female gender blunt the ejection fraction response to exercise, making the test less reliable in the elderly and in women. As a result, there is currently little enthusiasm for the use of global left ventricular function tests alone for detecting ischemic heart disease.

6. Evaluating coronary anatomy

A. CORONARY ANGIOGRAPHY—Coronary angiography is the standard for evaluating the anatomy of the coronary artery tree. It is best at evaluating the large epicardial coronary vessels that are most frequently diseased in coronary atherosclerosis. Experimental studies suggest that lesions that reduce the lumen of the coronary artery by 70% or more in area (50% in diameter) significantly limit flow, especially during periods of increased myocardial oxygen demand. If such lesions are detected, they are considered compatible with symptoms or other signs of myocardial ischemia. This assessment is known to be imprecise for several reasons, however. First, the actual cross-sectional area of the coronary artery at the point of an atherosclerotic lesion must be estimated from two-dimensional diameter measurements in several planes. When compared with autopsy findings, stenosis severity is usually found to have been underestimated by the coronary angiography. Second, the technique does not take into consideration that lesions in series in a coronary artery may incrementally reduce the flow to distal beds by more than is accounted for by any single lesion. Thus, a series of apparently insignificant lesions may actually reduce myocardial blood flow significantly. Third, the cross-sectional area is not actually measured routinely. It is instead referenced to a supposed normal segment of artery in terms of a percentage of stenosis or percentage of reduction in the normal luminal diameter or cross-sectional area. The problem with this type of estimate is that it is often difficult to determine what a normal segment of artery is, especially in patients with diffuse coronary atherosclerosis.

Quantitative coronary angiogram measurements are an improvement over this visual inspection technique, but they are not commonly used except in research projects. Epicardial coronary artery anatomy is a static representation at the time of the study. It does not take into consideration potential changes in coronary vasomotor tone that may occur under certain circumstances and further reduce coronary blood flow. In addition, coronary angiography does not adequately evaluate disease in the intramyocardial blood vessels; this may be important in some patients, especially insulin-dependent diabetics. In patients with pure vasospastic angina, the coronary arteries are usually normal or minimally diseased. To establish increased vasomotion as the cause of the angina, provocative tests have been used to induce coronary vasospasm in the cardiac catheterization laboratory. The most popular of these is an **ergonovine infusion,** which is reputed to produce focal vasospasm only in naturally susceptible arteries and not in normal coronary arteries, which usually exhibit only a uniform reduction in vessel diameter. Ergonovine infusion has some risks, however, in that the resultant coronary vasospasm may be difficult to alleviate and can be quite profound. In addition, not all patients with vasospastic angina may respond to this agent. Thus, its use has diminished in favor of ECG monitoring during the patient's normal daily activities.

B. OTHER TECHNIQUES—ECG or imaging evidence of old myocardial infarction is often presumed to indicate that severe coronary artery stenoses are present in the involved vessel. Myocardial infarction, however, can occur as a result of thrombus on top of a minor plaque that has ruptured and occasionally from intense vasospasm or coronary emboli from the left heart. In these cases, coronary angiography would not detect significant (narrowing of > 50% of the diameter) coronary lesions despite the evidence of an old myocardial infarction. Coronary artery imaging is therefore necessary because estimating the degree of stenosis from the presence of infarction is not accurate. The presence of inducible myocardial ischemia almost always correlates with significant coronary artery lesions. Under the right clinical circumstances, coronary angiography can often be avoided if noninvasive stress testing produces myocardial ischemia. Coronary angiography could then be reserved for patients who have not responded to medical therapy and were being considered for revascularization, where visualizing the coronary anatomy is necessary.

Other imaging techniques have also had some success. Echocardiography, especially transesophageal, can often visualize the first few centimeters of the major epicardial coronary arteries, and MRI has also shown promise. At present, neither of these noninvasive imaging techniques has reached the degree of accuracy needed to replace contrast coronary angiography; however, technical improvements may change this in the future.

Cardiac computed tomography (CT) use is expanding. Noncontrast techniques can rapidly detect calcified coronary artery plaque. The amount of plaque can be quantitated, usually as the Agatston score, which is predictive of future coronary events in an incremental fashion beyond traditional risk factors. The major use of CT coronary calcium score may be to further stratify the risk of an event in intermediate-risk patients where the intensity of risk factor reduction could be altered accordingly. Contrast CT angiography can evaluate the lumen of the coronary arteries and is a useful alternative to stress testing for low to intermediate pretest risk of coronary artery disease patients. More recently, hybrid CT and either SPECT or positron emission tomography scanners are being used to visualize coronary lesions and assess their physiologic significance at one setting. Since most patients with a positive CT scan for either coronary calcium or lesions eventually get a stress test, this combination makes sense.

F. Choosing a Diagnostic Approach

Normally, noninvasive testing is performed first in the evaluation of suspected coronary atherosclerosis in symptomatic patients with an intermediate pretest likelihood of disease. There are several reasons for this: There is less risk with stress testing than with invasive coronary angiography, and cardiac CT has almost no risks. Mortality rates for stress testing average 1 per 10,000 patients, compared with 1 per

1000 for coronary angiography. The physiologic demonstration of myocardial ischemia and its extent forms the basis for the therapeutic approach irrespective of coronary anatomy. Mildly symptomatic patients who show small areas of ischemia at intense exercise levels have an excellent prognosis and are usually treated medically. Knowledge of the coronary anatomy is not necessary to make this therapeutic decision. In general, therefore, a noninvasive technique should be used to detect myocardial ischemia and its extent before considering coronary angiography, which is both riskier and more costly. Asymptomatic patients with a low to intermediate pretest likelihood of coronary artery disease may be better served by a noninvasive coronary artery imaging technique, such as cardiac CT; symptomatic patients may be better served by undergoing the combination of cardiac CT and stress perfusion imaging.

Profound symptoms that occur with minimal exertion are almost certainly due to severe diffuse coronary atherosclerosis or left main obstruction, and it is prudent to proceed directly with coronary angiography. Patients with severe unstable angina should undergo coronary angiography because of the potential increased risk posed by stress testing. If this approach is not appropriate in a particular clinical setting, the clinician might medicate the patient and perform careful stress testing after demonstrating a lack of symptoms on medical therapy. Patients with angina or evidence of ischemia in the early period after myocardial infarction are categorized as having unstable angina and should be taken directly to coronary angiography. The postinfarction patient who is not having recurrent ischemia, however, can usually be evaluated by stress testing and then a decision can be made about the advisability of coronary angiography. If the clinical situation is such that it is likely that stress testing will be inaccurate or uninterpretable, CT or invasive coronary angiography should be performed. Left bundle branch block on the ECG, for example, not only renders the ECG useless for detecting myocardial ischemia but may also affect the results of myocardial perfusion imaging and wall motion studies. Noninvasive techniques have poor diagnostic accuracy in morbidly obese female patients who are unable to exercise. In general, patients whose medical conditions preclude accurate stress testing are candidates for direct coronary angiography.

Which type of noninvasive stress testing to select is based on several factors. The most important of these is the type of information desired; second, certain characteristics of the patient, which may make one test more applicable than another; and third, the pretest likelihood of disease. For example, cardiac CT may be most useful in low-risk patients; stress imaging in intermediate-risk patients; and invasive angiography in high-risk patients. Stress perfusion scanning is more likely than echocardiographic imaging to provide adequate technical quality in obese individuals or those with chronic obstructive pulmonary disease. Cost is also an important consideration, and the ECG stress test is the least expensive. In most patients with a low-to-medium clinical

pretest likelihood of disease, using the ECG stress test makes sense, especially because good exercise performance with a negative ECG response for ischemia indicates an excellent prognosis even if coronary artery disease is present. In the patient who is highly likely to have coronary artery disease, however, it is useful to not only confirm the presence of the disease but to document its extent. For this purpose, myocardial imaging techniques are better at determining the extent of coronary artery disease than is the ECG. It is also believed that myocardial perfusion scanning is somewhat better at identifying the coronary arteries involved in the production of ischemia than are techniques for detecting wall motion abnormalities.

Budoff MJ, et al; American Heart Association Committee on Cardiovascular Imaging and Intervention; American Heart Association Council on Cardiovascular Radiology and Intervention; American Heart Association Committee on Cardiac Imaging, Council on Clinical Cardiology. Assessment of coronary artery disease by cardiac computed tomography: a scientific statement from the American Heart Association Committee on Cardiovascular Imaging and Intervention, Council on Cardiovascular Radiology and Intervention, and Committee on Cardiac Imaging, Council on Clinical Cardiology. *Circulation.* 2006;114(16):1761–91. [PMID: 17015792]

Karamitsos TD, et al. Ischemic heart disease: comprehensive evaluation by cardiovascular magnetic resonance. *Am Heart J.* 2011;162(1):16–30. [PMID: 21742086]

▶ Treatment

A. General Approach

Because myocardial ischemia is produced by an imbalance between myocardial oxygen supply and demand, in general, treatment consists of increasing supply or reducing demand—or both. Heart rate is a major determinant of myocardial oxygen demand, and attention to its control is imperative. Any treatment that accelerates heart rate is generally not going to be efficacious in preventing myocardial ischemia. Therefore, care must be taken with potent vasodilator drugs, such as hydralazine, which may lower blood pressure and induce reflex tachycardia. Furthermore, because most coronary blood flow occurs during diastole, the longer the diastole, the greater the coronary blood flow; and the faster the heart rate, the shorter the diastole.

Blood pressure is another important factor: Increases in blood pressure raise myocardial oxygen demand by elevating left ventricular wall tension, and blood pressure is the driving pressure for coronary perfusion. A critical blood pressure is required that does not excessively increase demand, yet keeps coronary perfusion pressure across stenotic lesions optimal. Unfortunately, determining what this level of blood pressure should be in any given patient is difficult, and a trial-and-error approach is often needed to achieve the right balance. Consequently, it is prudent to reduce blood pressure when it is very high, and it may be important to allow it to increase when it is very low. It is not uncommon to encounter patients whose myocardial ischemia has been so vigorously treated with a combination of pharmacologic agents that their blood pressure is too low to be compatible with adequate coronary perfusion. In such patients, withholding some of their medications may actually improve their symptoms. Although myocardial contractility and left ventricular volume also contribute to myocardial oxygen demand, they are less important than heart rate and blood pressure. Myocardial contractility usually parallels heart rate. Attention should be paid to reducing left ventricular volume in anyone with a dilated heart, but not at the expense of excessive hypotension or tachycardia because these factors are more important than volume for determining myocardial oxygen demand.

It is important to eliminate any aggravating factors that could increase myocardial oxygen demand or reduce coronary artery flow (Table 6–3). Hypertension and tachyarrhythmias are obvious factors that need to be controlled. Thyrotoxicosis leads to tachycardia and increases in myocardial oxygen demand. Anemia is a common problem that increases myocardial oxygen demand because of reflex tachycardia; it reduces oxygen supply by decreasing the oxygen-carrying capacity of the blood. Similarly, hypoxia from pulmonary disease reduces oxygen delivery to the heart. Heart failure increases angina because it often results in left ventricular dilatation, which increases wall stress, and in excess catecholamine tone, which increases contractility and produces tachycardia.

The long-term outlook for patients with coronary atherosclerosis must be addressed by reducing their risk factors for the disease. Once a patient is known to have atherosclerosis, risk factor reduction should be fairly vigorous: If diet has not reduced serum cholesterol, strong consideration should be given to pharmacologic therapy because it has been shown to reduce cardiac events. Patients should be encouraged to exercise, lose weight, quit smoking, and try to reduce stress levels. Daily low-dose aspirin is important for preventing coronary

Table 6–3. Factors That Can Aggravate Myocardial Ischemia

Increased myocardial oxygen demand	Tachycardia Hypertension Thyrotoxicosis Heart failure Valvular heart disease Catecholamine analogues (eg, bronchodilators, tricyclic antidepressants, cocaine)
Reduced myocardial oxygen supply	Anemia Hypoxia Carbon monoxide poisoning Hypotension Tachycardia

thrombosis. The use of megadoses of vitamin E, β-carotene, and vitamin C should be discouraged in the patient with known coronary atherosclerosis because clinical trials have not demonstrated efficacy and some have shown harm.

B. Pharmacologic Therapy

1. Nitrates—Nitrates, which work on both sides of the supply-and-demand equation, are the oldest drugs used to treat angina pectoris (Table 6–4). These agents are now available in several formulations to fit the patient's lifestyle and disease characteristics. Almost all patients with known coronary atherosclerosis should carry rapid-acting nitroglycerin to abort acute attacks of angina pectoris. Nitrates work principally by providing more nitrous oxide to the vascular endothelium and the arterial smooth muscle, resulting in vasodilation. This tends to ameliorate any increased coronary vasomotor tone and dilate coronary obstructions. As long as blood pressure does not fall excessively, nitrates increase coronary blood flow. Nitrates also cause venodilation, reducing preload and decreasing left ventricular end-diastolic volume. The reduced left ventricular volume decreases wall tension and myocardial oxygen demand.

Sublingual nitroglycerin takes 30–60 seconds to dissolve completely and begin to produce beneficial effects, which can last up to 30 minutes. Although most commonly used to abort acute attacks of angina, the drug can be used prophylactically if the patient can anticipate its need 30 minutes prior to a precipitating event. Prophylactic therapy is best accomplished, however, with longer-acting nitrate preparations. Isosorbide dinitrate and mononitrate are available in oral formulations; each produces beneficial effects for several hours. Large doses of these agents must be taken orally to overcome nitrate reductases in the liver. Liver metabolism of the nitrates can also be avoided with cutaneous application. Nitroglycerin is available as a topical ointment that can be applied as a dressing; it is also available as a ready-made, self-adhesive patch that delivers accurate continuous dosing of the drug through a membrane. Although the paste and the patches produce similar effects, the patches are more convenient for patients to use.

Sublingual nitroglycerin tablets are extremely small and difficult for patients with arthritis to manipulate. A buccal preparation of nitroglycerin is available, which comes in a larger, more easily manipulable tablet that can be chewed and allowed to dissolve in the mouth, rather than being swallowed. This achieves nitrate effectiveness within 2–5 minutes and lasts about 30 minutes, as do the sublingual tablets. An oral nitroglycerin spray, which may be easier to manipulate and more convenient for some patients, is also available.

The major difficulty with all long-acting nitroglycerin preparations is the development of tolerance to their effects. The exact reason for tolerance development is not clearly understood, but it may involve liver enzyme induction or a lack of arterial responsiveness because of local adaptive factors. Regardless of the mechanism, however, round-the-clock

Table 6–4. Common Oral Antianginal Drugs

Drug	Usual Dose	Comments; Adverse Effects
Nitrates		
Nitroglycerin	0.4–0.6 mg sublingual	Aborts acute attacks; headaches, hypotension
Nitroglycerin	1–3 mg buccal	Larger tablet for handicapped patients
Nitroglycerin	0.4 mg spray	More convenient than pills
Nitroglycerin	0.5–2 in of 2% ointment	Prophylactic therapy; tolerance a problem
Nitroglycerin	0.1–0.6 mg/h patches	Prophylactic therapy; tolerance a problem
Isosorbide dinitrate	10–60 mg three times daily	Need 8 h off every 24 h to avoid tolerance
Isosorbide mononitrate	20 mg twice daily	Take 7 h apart

Drug	Daily Dosage (mg)	Comments; Adverse Effects
β-Blockers		
Propranolol	160–320	Central nervous system side effects—fatigue, impotence—common
Nadolol	80–240	Long half-life, noncardioselective
Timolol	10–45	Noncardioselective
Metoprolol	100–400	Cardioselective
Atenolol	50–200	Cardioselective
Acebutolol	400–1200	Cardioselective, some intrinsic sympathomimetic activity
Betaxolol	5–40	Cardioselective, long half-life
Bisoprolol	5–20	Cardioselective
Pindolol	5–40	Marked intrinsic sympathomimetic activity
Calcium Channel Blockers, Heart Rate Lowering		
Diltiazem	120–360	Heart rate lowering; atrioventricular (AV) block, heart failure, edema
Verapamil	120–480	Heart rate lowering; AV block, heart failure, constipation
Dihydropyridine Calcium Channel Blockers		
Amlodipine	5–10	Least myocardial depression
Nifedipine	30–60	Hypotension, tachycardia
Nicardipine	60–120	Potent coronary vasodilator
Felodipine	5–20	High vascular selectivity
Isradipine	2.5–10	Potent coronary vasodilator
Nisoldipine	10–40	Similar to nifedipine
Sodium Current Inhibitor		
Ranolazine	1000–2000 mg	May increase QT interval on ECG

nitrate administration will lead to progressively increasing tolerance to the drug after 24–48 hours. Because of this, nitroglycerin is usually taken over the 16-hour period each day that corresponds to the time period during which most of the ischemic episodes would be expected to occur. For most patients, this means not taking nitrate preparations before bed and allowing the ensuing 8 hours for the effects to wear off and responsiveness to the drug to be regained. This timing would have to be adjusted for patients with nocturnal angina. The difficulty with the 8-hour overnight hiatus in therapy, however, is that the patient has little protection during the critical early morning wakening period—when ischemic events are more likely to occur. Patients should therefore take the nitrate preparation as soon as they arise in the morning. For this reason, the nitroglycerin patches have a small amount of paste on the outside of the membrane that delivers a bolus of drug through the skin, which quickly elevates the patient's blood level of the drug. It is important that the patient be careful not to wipe this paste off the patch before applying it.

Nitrates, which are effective in preventing the development of angina as well as aborting acute attacks, are helpful in both patients with fixed coronary artery occlusions and those with vasospastic angina. Their potency, compared with other agents, is limited, however, and patients with severe angina often must turn to other agents. In such patients, nitrates can be excellent adjunctive therapy.

2. β-Blockers—β-Adrenergic blocking agents are highly effective in the prophylactic therapy of angina pectoris. They have been shown to reduce or eliminate angina attacks and prolong exercise endurance time in double-blind, placebo-controlled studies. They can be used around the clock because no tachyphylaxis to their effects has been found. β-Blockers mainly work by lowering myocardial oxygen demand through decreasing heart rate, blood pressure, and myocardial contractility. As mentioned earlier, however, they also increase myocardial oxygen supply by increasing the duration of diastole through heart rate reduction. Currently, several β-blocker preparations are available, with one or more features that may make them more—or less—attractive for a particular patient.

Among these features is the agent's pharmacologic half-life, which ranges from 4 to 18 hours. Various delivery systems have been developed to slow down the delivery of short-acting agents and prolong the duration of drug activity through sustained release or long-acting formulations. Note that the pharmacodynamic half-life of β-adrenergic blockers is often longer than their pharmacologic half-life, and drug effects can be detected for days after discontinuation of prolonged β-blocker therapy.

Ideally, β-blockers should be titrated against the heart rate response to exercise because blunting of the exercise heart rate response is the hallmark of their efficacy. Adverse effects of β-blockers include excessive bradycardia, heart block, and hypotension. Nonselective β-blockers can cause bronchospasm, but it occurs less often with the β_1-selective

agents. Blocking β_2-peripheral vasodilatory actions may aggravate claudication in patients with severe peripheral vascular disease. β-Adrenergic stimulation is also important for the gluconeogenic response to hyperglycemia in severely insulin-dependent diabetic patients. Although β-blockers may impair this response, the major problem with their use in insulin-dependent diabetic patients is that the warning signals of hypoglycemia (sweating, tachycardia, piloerection) may be blocked. Because of their negative inotropic properties, β-blockers may also precipitate heart failure in patients with markedly reduced left ventricular performance or acute heart failure.

Other side effects of β-blockers are less predictably related to their anti-β-adrenergic effects. Adverse central nervous system effects are especially troublesome and include fatigue, mental slowness, and impotence. These side effects are somewhat less common with agents that are less lipophilic, such as atenolol and nadolol. Unfortunately, it is these side effects that make many patients unable to tolerate β-blockers.

3. Calcium channel antagonists—Calcium channel antagonists theoretically work on both sides of the supply-and-demand equation. By blocking calcium access to smooth muscle cells, they produce peripheral vasodilatation and are effective antihypertensive agents. In the myocardium, they block sinus node and atrioventricular node function and reduce the inotropic state. They dilate the coronary arteries and increase myocardial blood flow. The calcium channel blockers available today produce a variable spectrum of these basic pharmacologic effects. The biggest group is the dihydropyridine calcium channel blockers, which are potent arterial dilators and thereby cause reflex sympathetic activation, which overshadows their negative chronotropic and inotropic effects.

A second major group of calcium channel blockers are those that lower the heart rate. The two most commonly used drugs in this class are diltiazem and verapamil. Because these drugs have less peripheral vasodilatory action in individuals with normal blood pressure, they produce little reflex tachycardia. The average daily heart rate is usually reduced with these agents because their inherent negative chronotropic effects are not overridden; negative inotropic effects are also more common with these agents. Hypertensive and normotensive individuals seem to have a different vascular responsiveness to the rate-lowering calcium channel blockers. Interestingly, in hypertensive individuals, rate-lowering calcium channel blockers lower the blood pressure as well as the dihydropyridine agents. Diltiazem is more widely used because of its low side-effect profile. Verapamil, which is an excellent treatment for patients with supraventricular arrhythmias, has potent effects on the arteriovenous (AV) node; this can cause excessive bradycardia and heart block in patients with angina pectoris. Verapamil is also more likely than diltiazem to precipitate heart failure, and it often produces troublesome constipation, especially in elderly individuals. All the calcium channel blockers can produce peripheral edema. This is due not to their negative inotropic effects but rather to an imbalance between the efferent and afferent peripheral arteriolar tone, which increases capillary hydrostatic pressure. Other adverse effects of these drugs are idiosyncratic and include gastrointestinal and dermatologic effects.

Calcium channel blockers are titrated to the patient's symptoms because there is no physiologic marker of their effect, in contrast to the heart rate response to exercise with β-blockers. This makes choosing the appropriate dosage difficult, and many clinicians increase the dose until some side effect occurs and then they reduce it. The most common side effects are related to the pharmacologic effects of the drugs. With the dihydropyridines, vasodilatory side effects, such as orthostatic hypotension, flushing, and headache, occur. Hypotension is less common with the heart rate–lowering calcium channel blockers, and their side effects are more related to cardiac effects, such as excessive bradycardia. These drugs are very useful because they are excellent for preventing angina pectoris, lowering high blood pressure, and, in the case of the heart rate–lowering agents, controlling supraventricular arrhythmias.

4. Ranolazine—Ranolazine partially inhibits fatty acid oxidation and increases glucose oxidation, which generates more adenosine triphosphate for each molecule of oxygen consumed. This shift in substrate selection may reduce myocardial oxygen demand without altering hemodynamics. Since all other antianginal agents reduce heart rate and blood pressure, this gives ranolazine an advantage. Studies have shown that ranolazine provides additive benefits to standard treatment described earlier and is useful as monotherapy. It has few adverse effects, but experience with this agent is limited.

5. Combination therapy—Although monotherapy is desirable for patient convenience and cost considerations, many patients, especially those with severe inoperable coronary artery disease, require more than one antianginal agent to control their symptoms. Because all antianginal agents have a synergistic effect in preventing angina, the initial choices should be for agents with complementary pharmacologic effects. For example, nitrates can be added to β-blocker therapy: Nitrates have an effect on dilating coronary arteries and increasing coronary blood flow, and their peripheral effects may increase reflex sympathetic tone and counteract some of the negative inotropic and chronotropic effects of the β-blockers. This has proved to be a highly effective combination. Similarly, combining a β-blocker with dihydropyridine drugs, when the β-blockers suppress the reflex tachycardia produced by the dihydropyridine, has also proved to be highly effective. Combinations of the heart rate–lowering calcium channel blockers and nitrates have also proved efficacious. Extremely refractory patients may respond to the combination of a dihydropyridine calcium channel blocker and a heart rate–lowering calcium channel blocker.

Combining a dihydropyridine calcium channel blocker and nitrates makes little sense, however, because of the high likelihood of producing potent vasodilatory side effects. This combination may excessively lower blood pressure to the point that coronary perfusion pressure is compromised and the patient's angina actually worsens. In fact, in as many as 10% of patients with moderately severe angina, both the nitrates and the dihydropyridine calcium channel blockers alone have been reported to aggravate angina. Although few corroborative data exist, this percentage is certainly higher with the combination of the two agents.

The most difficult cases often involve triple therapy, with a calcium channel blocker, a β-blocker, and a nitrate. Although there are few objective data on the benefits of this approach, it has proven efficacious in selected patients. The major problem with triple therapy is that side effects, such as hypotension, are increased, which often limits therapy. Ranolazine has no hemodynamic effects and can be used for those patients refractory to their current regimen but with heart rate or blood pressure levels as low as is tolerable. It has been successfully combined with atenolol, amlodipine, and diltiazem.

6. Adjunctive therapy—All patients with coronary artery disease should take aspirin (81–325 mg/day), and selected high-risk patients should also take clopidogrel. These drugs reduce platelet aggregation and retard the growth of atherothrombosis. Also important is correction of dyslipidemia, smoking cessation, exercise, weight loss, control of hypertension, and management of stress. In patients with known coronary artery disease, it is important to decrease low-density lipoprotein (LDL) cholesterol and perhaps increase high-density lipoprotein (HDL) cholesterol to published targets (< 100 mg/dL and > 40 mg/dL, respectively). Angiotensin-converting enzyme (ACE) inhibitors may have a protective effect in patients with coronary artery disease, especially postmyocardial infarction. β-Blockers are also indicated for postmyocardial infarction, but their use in chronic coronary artery disease without infarct or angina is controversial. However, both β-blockers and ACE inhibitors would be preferred agents for blood pressure control in patients with chronic coronary artery disease.

C. Revascularization

1. Catheter-based methods—The standard percutaneous coronary intervention (PCI) is balloon dilatation with placement of a metal stent. Such treatment is limited to the larger epicardial arteries and can be complicated by various types of acute vessel injury, which can result in myocardial infarction unless surgical revascularization is immediately performed. Smaller arteries may be amenable to plain old balloon angioplasty (POBA), and large arteries with complicated lesions may be candidates for other forms of PCI. PCI requires intense antiplatelet therapy, usually with aspirin and clopidogrel, to prevent stent thrombosis. After the stent has been covered with endothelium, this risk is much less.

In the absence of acute complications, initial success rates for significantly dilating the coronary artery are greater than 85%, and the technique can be of tremendous benefit to patients—without their undergoing the risk of cardiac surgery. The principal disadvantage to PCI is restenosis, which occurs in about one-third of patients treated with a bare metal stent during the first 6 months. Drug-eluting stents have reduced restenosis to 10% or less but have been associated with a small incidence of late thrombosis. Although many agents are under intense investigation, there is currently no systemic pharmacologic approach to preventing restenosis.

PCI is ideal for symptomatic patients with one or two discrete lesions in one or two arteries. In patients with more complex lesions or those with three or more vessels involved, bypass surgery is preferable for several reasons. First, the restenosis risk is the same for each lesion treated by PCI, so that if enough vessels are worked on the risk of restenosis in one of them will approach 100%. Second, the ability to completely revascularize patients with multivessel disease is less with PCI compared with bypass surgery. Finally, some clinical trials have shown that diabetic patients have better outcomes after bypass surgery relative to PCI.

2. Coronary artery bypass graft surgery—Controlled clinical trials have shown that coronary artery bypass graft (CABG) surgery can successfully alleviate angina symptoms in up to 80% of patients. These results compare very favorably with pharmacologic therapy and catheter-based techniques and can be accomplished in selected patients with less than 2% operative mortality rates. Although the initial cost of surgery is high, studies have shown it can be competitive with repeated angioplasty and lifelong pharmacologic therapy in selected patients.

The standard surgical approach is to use the saphenous veins, which are sewn to the ascending aorta and then, distal to the obstruction, in the coronary artery, effectively bypassing the obstruction with blood from the aorta. Although single end-to-side saphenous-vein-to-coronary-artery grafts are preferred, occasionally surgeons will do side-to-side anastomoses in one coronary artery (or more) and then terminate the graft in an end-to-side anastomosis in the final coronary artery. There is some evidence that although these skip grafts are easier and quicker to place than multiple single saphenous grafts, they may not last as long. The major problems with saphenous vein grafts are recurrent atherosclerosis in the grafts, which is often quite bulky and friable, and ostial stenosis, probably from cicatrization at the anastomotic sites. Although these problems can be approached with PCI and other interventional devices, the success rate of catheter-delivered devices to open obstructed saphenous vein grafts is not as high as that seen with native coronary artery obstructions, and many patients require repeat saphenous vein grafting after an average of about

8 years. It is believed that meticulous attention to a low-fat diet, cessation of smoking, and the ingestion of one aspirin a day (80–160 mg) will retard the development of saphenous vein atherosclerosis; some patients do well for 20 years or more after CABG.

There is now considerable evidence that arterial conduits make better bypass graft materials. The difficulty is finding large enough arteries that are not essential to other parts of the body. The most popular arteries used today are the internal thoracic arteries. Their attachment to the subclavian artery is left intact, and the distal end is used as an end-to-side anastomosis into a single coronary artery. If a patient requires more than two grafts, some surgeons, rather than using a saphenous vein, have used the radial artery or abdominal vessels, such as the gastroepiploic. There are less data on these alternative conduits, but theoretically, they would have the same advantages as the internal thoracic arteries in terms of graft longevity. Efforts at preventing bypass graft failure are worthwhile because the risk of repeat surgery is usually higher than that of the initial surgery. There are several reasons for this, including the fact that the patient is older, the scar tissue from the first operation makes the second one more difficult, and finally, any progression of atherosclerosis in the coronary arteries makes finding good-quality insertion sites for the graft more difficult.

D. Selection of Therapy

Pharmacologic therapy is indicated when other conditions may be aggravating angina pectoris and can be successfully treated. For example, in the patient with coexistent hypertension and angina, it is often prudent to treat the hypertension and lower blood pressure to acceptable levels before pursuing revascularization for angina because lowering the blood pressure will often eliminate the angina. For this purpose, it is wise to use antihypertensive medications that are also antianginal (eg, β-blockers, calcium channel blockers) rather than other agents with no antianginal effects (eg, ACE inhibitors, centrally acting agents). The presence of heart failure can also produce or aggravate angina, and this should be treated. Care must be taken in choosing antianginal drugs that do not aggravate heart failure. For this reason, nitrates are frequently used in heart failure and angina because these drugs may actually benefit both conditions. Rate-lowering calcium channel blockers should be avoided if the left ventricular ejection fraction is below 35%, unless it is clear that the heart failure is episodic and is being produced by ischemia. In this situation, however, revascularization may be a more effective strategy. β-Blockers can be effective, but they must be started at low doses and uptitrated carefully. Although β-blockers are now part of standard therapy for heart failure, there is little data on their use in patients with angina and reduced left ventricular performance. Finally, the presence of ventricular or supraventricular tachyarrhythmias may aggravate angina. Rhythm disorders also afford an opportunity for using dual-purpose drugs. The heart rate–lowering calcium channel blockers may effectively control supraventricular arrhythmias and also benefit angina. β-Blockers can often be effective treatment for ventricular arrhythmias in patients with coronary artery disease and should be tried before other, more potent antiarrhythmics or devices are contemplated. Keep in mind that digoxin blood levels may be increased by concomitant treatment with calcium channel blockers. In addition, the combination of digoxin and either heart rate–lowering calcium channel blockers or β-blockers may cause synergistic effects on the atrioventricular node and lead to excessive bradycardia or heart block.

The major indication for revascularization of chronic ischemic heart disease is the failure of medications to control the patient's symptoms. Drug-refractory angina pectoris is the major indication for revascularization. Note that myocardial ischemia should be established as the source of the patient's symptoms before embarking on revascularization, since symptoms may actually be due to gastroesophageal reflux. Consequently, some form of stress testing that verifies the relationship between demonstrable ischemia and symptoms is advisable before performing any revascularization procedure.

In some other instances—patient preference, for example—revascularization therapy might be considered before even trying pharmacologic therapy. Some patients do not like the prospect of lifelong drug therapy and would rather have open arteries. Although this is a valid reason to perform revascularization, the clinician must be careful that his or her own enthusiasm for revascularization as treatment does not pressure the patient into such a decision. Other candidates for direct revascularization are patients with high-risk occupations who cannot return to these occupations unless they are completely revascularized (eg, airline pilots).

Revascularization is preferred to medical therapy in managing certain types of coronary anatomy that are known (through clinical trials) to have a longer survival if treated with CABG rather than medically. Such lesions include left main obstructions of more than 50%, three-vessel disease, and two-vessel disease in which one of the vessels is the left anterior descending artery. Currently, left main stenoses are not effectively treated with catheter-based techniques, but two- and three-vessel coronary disease could potentially be treated by PCI. Clinical trials have shown equivalent long-term outcomes between PCI and CABG in patients with multivessel disease.

CABG is also recommended for patients with two- or three-vessel coronary artery disease and resultant heart failure from reduced left ventricular performance, especially if viable myocardium can be demonstrated. Because the tests for viable myocardium are not perfect, however, many clinicians believe that all these patients should be revascularized in the hope that some myocardial function will return. This seems a prudent approach, given that donor hearts for cardiac transplantation are difficult to obtain—and many patients with heart failure and coronary artery disease improve following bypass surgery.

Surgery is also recommended when the patient has a concomitant disease that requires surgical therapy, such as significant valvular heart disease, heart failure in the presence of a large left ventricular aneurysm, or mechanical complications of myocardial infarction, such as a ventricular septal defect. In the presence of hemodynamic indications for repairing these problems, any significant coronary artery disease that is found should be corrected with bypass surgery at the same time.

The risk of bypass surgery in a given individual must also be considered because several factors can increase the risk significantly and might make catheter-based techniques or medical therapy more desirable. Age is always a risk factor for any major surgery, and CABG is no exception. Also, female gender tends to increase the risk of CABG, possibly because women are, on average, smaller and have smaller arteries than men. Some data indicate that if size is the only factor considered, gender disappears as a risk predictor with CABG. Other medical conditions that may complicate the perioperative period (eg, chronic kidney disease, obesity, lung disease, diabetes) also raise the risks of surgery. Another factor (discussed earlier) is whether this is a repeat bypass operation. The technical difficulties are especially troublesome when a prior internal thoracic artery graft has been placed because this artery lies right behind the sternum and can be easily compromised when reopening the chest.

The choice between catheter-based techniques and CABG surgery is based on several considerations: Is it technically feasible to perform either technique with a good anticipated result? What does the patient wish to do? The patient may have a strong preference for one technique over the other. Again, the clinician must be careful not to unduly influence the patient in this regard, lest it give the appearance of a conflict of interest. Consideration must also be given to factors that increase the risk of surgery. The most difficult decision involves the patient who is suitable for either surgery or a catheter-based technique. The few controlled, randomized clinical trials that have been done on such patients have shown equivalent clinical results with PCI and surgery in terms of mortality and symptom relief. Note that this is accomplished by PCI at the cost of repeated procedures in many patients. Despite the necessity for these repeated procedures, the overall cost of bypass surgery is higher over the short term. Unfortunately, the trials do not outline clear guidelines for choosing PCI or CABG in the patient who is a good candidate for either treatment; this continues to be a decision to be made by the clinician and the patient on a case-by-case basis. The availability of minimally invasive surgery has pushed the balance between CABG and PCI a little toward CABG, but not all patients are suitable for a minimally invasive approach.

Bhatt DL, et al; CHARISMA Investigators. Clopidogrel and aspirin versus aspirin alone for the prevention of atherothrombotic events. *N Engl J Med.* 2006;354(16):1706–17. [PMID: 16531616]

Boden WE, et al; COURAGE Trial Research Group. Optimal medical therapy with or without PCI for stable coronary disease. *N Engl J Med.* 2007;356(15):1503–16. [PMID: 17387127]

Chaitman BR, et al. Anti-ischemic effects and long-term survival during ranolazine monotherapy in patients with chronic severe angina. *J Am Coll Cardiol.* 2004;43(8):1375–82. [PMID: 15093870]

Chaitman BR, et al; Combination Assessment of Ranolazine in Stable Angina (CARISA) Investigators. Effects of ranolazine with atenolol, amlodipine, or diltiazem on exercise tolerance and angina frequency in patients with severe chronic angina: a randomized controlled trial. *JAMA.* 2004;291(3):309–16. [PMID: 14734593]

Fihn SD, et al. 2012 ACCF/AHA/ACP/AATS/PCNA/SCAI/STS guideline for the diagnosis and management of patients with stable ischemic heart disease. *J Am Coll Cardiol.* 2012;60(24): e44–164. [PMID: 23182125]

Levine GN, et al. 2011 ACCF/AHA/SCAI guideline for percutaneous coronary intervention. *J Am Coll Cardiol.* 2011;58(24): e44–122. [PMID: 22070834]

▶ Prognosis

There are two major determinants of prognosis in patients with chronic ischemic heart disease. The first is the clinical status of the patient, which can be semiquantitated by the Canadian Cardiovascular Society's angina functional class system. In this system, class I is asymptomatic, II is angina with heavy exertion, III is angina with mild-to-moderate exertion, and IV comprises patients who cannot perform their daily activities without getting angina or who are actually experiencing angina decubitus. The higher the Canadian class, the worse is the prognosis. Clinical status can also be determined by exercise testing. If patients can exercise more than 9 minutes or into stage IV of the modified Bruce protocol, their prognosis is excellent. However, the presence of either angina or significant ischemic ST depression on the exercise test indicates a poorer prognosis. In addition, when using perfusion scanning, the more extensive the perfusion abnormalities with exercise, the worse is the prognosis. Left ventricular dysfunction with exercise, as evidenced by a decrease or a failure to increase the ejection fraction on left ventricular imaging, or by significant lung uptake of thallium during stress perfusion imaging, also connotes a worse prognosis. Perhaps the most powerful predictor for future mortality is the resting left ventricular ejection fraction; values of less than 50% are associated with an exponential increase in mortality.

A second prognostic system is based solely on coronary anatomy. The more vessels involved, and the more severely they are involved, the worse the prognosis. This observation has formed the anatomic basis for revascularization in patients with coronary artery disease. Although this approach has some appeal, it has never been proven that revascularization in asymptomatic patients improves their prognosis. Even in patients with left main and severe three-vessel disease, proof is lacking that prophylactic revascularization is of any value if the patients are asymptomatic. Theoretical considerations suggest that ischemia—even in the absence of angina—that can be demonstrated by stress testing or ambulatory ECG recordings would support a decision to revascularize based on anatomy and the presence of ischemia. Although this seems like a much stronger case for revascularization in an asymptomatic patient, such treatment has not been proven efficacious in clinical trials.

The simplicity of the coronary anatomy approach to prognosis has resulted in considerable clinical data on the longevity of patients with chronic ischemic heart disease. Patients with one-vessel coronary artery disease have about a 3% per year mortality rate; this rate is less if the vessel is the right or circumflex coronary artery and somewhat more if it is the left anterior descending artery. Patients with two-vessel disease have a 5% or 6% mortality rate per year; in patients with three-vessel disease, this increases to 6–8% a year. Patients with left main disease, with or without other coronary occlusions, have about an 8–12% yearly mortality rate. Similar data do not exist for the clinical classification of patients because of the complexities of determining risk by this approach. A positive treadmill exercise test, at a low workload, for either angina or ischemic ST changes connotes a yearly mortality rate of 5%. This is less if the patient exercised a long time and had good left ventricular function and no previous myocardial infarction. It is worse if the patient exercised only a very short time on the treadmill and had evidence of left ventricular dysfunction or a prior myocardial infarction. How much modern pharmacologic and revascularization therapy can influence these prognostic figures is unclear at present.

Vidal-Perez R, et al. Determinants of cardiovascular mortality in a cohort of primary care patients with chronic ischemic heart disease. BARBANZA Ischemic Heart Disease (BARIHD) study. *Int J Cardiol.* 2012 Feb 2. [Epub ahead of print] [PMID: 22305776]

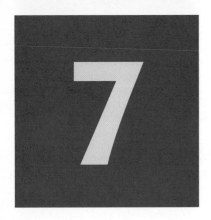

Unstable Angina/Non-ST Elevation Myocardial Infarction

Kuang-YuhChyu, MD, PhD

Prediman K. Shah, MD

▶ General Considerations

A. Background

Unstable angina and non-ST elevation myocardial infarction (USA/NSTEMI) are a part of the wide spectrum of clinical manifestations of atherosclerotic coronary artery disease (Table 7–1). Compared with ST elevation myocardial infarction (STEMI), the incidence of USA/NSTEMI has been increasing. According to the National Registry of Myocardial Infarction (NRMI) database, from 1994 to 1999, the prevalence of STEMI decreased from 36.4% to 27.1% with concomitant rise of NSTEMI from 45% to 63%. Similar trends were also observed in a population study from 1999 to 2008. Despite this, the age-adjusted mortality for NSTEMI patients has been gradually declining, likely due to advancement in the treatment for acute coronary syndrome.

B. Pathophysiology

Angina pectoris is the symptomatic equivalent of transient myocardial ischemia, which results from a temporary imbalance in the myocardial oxygen demand and supply. Most episodes of myocardial ischemia are generally believed to result from an absolute reduction in regional myocardial blood flow below basal levels, with the subendocardium carrying a greater burden of flow deficit relative to the epicardium, whether triggered by a primary reduction in coronary blood flow or an increase in oxygen demand. USA/NSTEMI shares a more or less common pathophysiologic substrate with STEMI, which is usually due to ruptured or unstable atherosclerotic plaques with overlying thrombus formation, leading to reduced coronary blood flow. The differences in clinical presentation result largely from the differences in the magnitude of coronary occlusion, the duration of the occlusion, the modifying influence of local and systemic blood flow, and the adequacy of coronary collaterals.

▶ Clinical Findings

A. Symptoms

USA/NSTEMI is a clinical syndrome characterized by symptoms of ischemia, which may include classic retrosternal chest pain or such pain surrogates as a burning sensation, feeling of indigestion, or dyspnea (Table 7–2). Anginal symptoms may also be felt primarily or as radiation in the neck, jaw, teeth, arms, back, or epigastrium. The pain of unstable angina typically lasts 15–30 minutes; it can last longer in some patients. In some patients, particularly the elderly, dyspnea, fatigue, diaphoresis, light-headedness, a feeling of indigestion and the desire to burp or defecate, or nausea and emesis may accompany other symptoms or may be the only symptoms. It has been estimated that about 43.6% of patients with USA/NSTEMI presented without chest pain. The clinical presentation of unstable angina can take any one of several forms.

There may be an onset of ischemic symptoms in a patient who had been previously free of angina, with or without a history of coronary artery disease. If symptoms are effort-induced, they are often rapidly progressive, with more frequent, easily provoked, and prolonged episodes. Rest pain may follow a period of crescendo effort angina or may exist from the beginning.

Symptoms may intensify or change in a patient with antecedent angina. Pain may be provoked by less effort and be more frequent and prolonged than before. The response to nitrates may decrease and their consumption increase. The appearance of new pain at rest or with minimal exertion is particularly ominous. On the other hand, recurrent long-standing ischemic symptoms at rest do not necessarily constitute an acute ischemic syndrome. Ischemic symptoms may recur shortly after (usually within 4 weeks) an acute myocardial infarction (MI), coronary artery bypass surgery, or catheter-based coronary artery intervention. In some

Table 7–1. Clinical Spectrum of Atherosclerotic Coronary Artery Disease

Subclinical symptoms or asymptomatic
Stable angina
Acute coronary syndromes
   Unstable angina
   Acute myocardial infarction
   Acute pulmonary edema
Sudden death

patients, an acute unstable coronary syndrome may manifest as acute pulmonary edema or sudden cardiac death.

B. Physical Examination

No physical finding is specific for USA/NSTEMI, and when the patient is free of pain, the examination may be entirely normal. During episodes of ischemia, a dyskinetic left ventricular apical impulse, a third or fourth heart sound, or a transient murmur of ischemic mitral regurgitation may be detected. Similarly, during episodes of prolonged or severe ischemia, there may be transient evidence of left ventricular failure, such as pulmonary congestion or edema, diaphoresis, or hypotension. Arrhythmias and conduction disturbances may occur during episodes of myocardial ischemia.

The findings from physical examination, especially as they relate to signs of heart failure, provide important prognostic information. An analysis of data from four randomized clinical trials (GUSTO IIb, PURSUIT, and PARAGON A and B) revealed that Killip classification, a commonly used classification based on physical examination of patients at presentation of STEMI, is a strong independent predictor for short- and long-term mortality, with

Table 7–2. Clinical Presentation of Unstable Angina

New onset of ischemic symptoms
   At rest only
   During exertion only
   At rest and exertion
Intensification of previous ischemic symptoms
   Increased frequency, severity, duration
   Change in pattern (eg, symptoms at rest)
Recurrence of ischemic symptoms within 4-6 weeks after an acute myocardial infarction
Other
   Recurrence of ischemia within 4-6 weeks following bypass surgery or coronary revascularization
   Recurrent acute pulmonary edema
   Prinzmetal (variant) angina

higher Killip class associated with higher mortality rate. This has also been recently confirmed using data from the Canadian Acute Coronary Syndrome Registries.

C. Diagnostic Studies

USA/NSTEMI is a common reason for admission to the hospital, and the diagnosis, in general, rests entirely on clinical grounds. In a patient with typical effort-induced chest discomfort that is new or rapidly progressive, the diagnosis is relatively straightforward, particularly (but not necessarily) when there are associated electrocardiogram (ECG) changes. Often, however, the symptoms are less clear-cut. The pain may be atypical in terms of its location, radiation, character, and intensity, or the patient may have had a single, prolonged episode of pain, which may or may not have resolved by the time of presentation. The physician should strongly suspect unstable angina, particularly when coronary artery disease or its risk factors are present. When in doubt, it is safer to err on the side of caution and consider the diagnosis to be unstable angina until proven otherwise. Even though dynamic ST-T changes on the ECG make the diagnosis more certain, between 5% and 10% of patients with a compelling clinical history (especially middle-aged women) have no critical coronary stenosis on coronary angiography. In rare instances, especially in women, spontaneous coronary artery dissection, unrelated to coronary atherosclerosis, may be the basis for an acute coronary syndrome. In general, the more profound the ECG changes, the greater the likelihood of an ischemic origin for the pain and the worse the prognosis.

1. ECG and Holter monitoring—ECG abnormalities are common in patients with USA/NSTEMI. In view of the episodic nature of ischemia, however, the changes may not be present if the ECG is recorded during an ischemia-free period or the ischemia involves the myocardial territories (eg, the circumflex coronary artery territory) that are not well represented on the standard 12-lead ECG. Therefore, it is not surprising that 40–50% of patients admitted with a clinical diagnosis of unstable angina have no ECG abnormalities on initial presentation. The ECG abnormalities tend to be in the form of transient ST segment depression or elevation and, less frequently, T-wave inversion, flattening, peaking, or pseudo-normalization (ie, the T wave becomes transiently upright from a baseline state of inversion or vice versa). It must be emphasized, however, that a normal or unremarkable ECG should never be used to disregard the diagnosis of unstable angina in a patient with a compelling clinical history and an appropriate risk-factor profile.

Continuous ambulatory ECG recording reveals a much higher prevalence of transient ST-T wave abnormalities, of which 70–80% are not accompanied by symptoms (silent ischemia). These episodes, which may be associated with transient ventricular dysfunction and reduced myocardial perfusion, are much more prevalent in patients with ST-T changes on their admission tracings (up to 80%) than in persons without such changes. Frequent and severe ECG changes on ECG monitoring, in general, indicate an increased risk of adverse clinical outcome.

2. Angiography—More than 90–95% of patients with a clinical syndrome of unstable angina have angiographically detectable atherosclerotic coronary artery disease of varying severity and extent. The prevalence of single-, two-, and three-vessel disease is roughly equal, especially in patients older than 55 and those with a past history of stable angina. In relatively younger patients and in those with no prior history of stable angina, the frequency of single-vessel disease is relatively higher (50–60%). Left main coronary disease is found in 10–15% of patients with unstable angina. A subset of patients (5–10%) with angiographically normal or near normal coronary arteries may have noncardiac symptoms masquerading as unstable angina, the clinical syndrome X (ischemic symptoms with angiographically normal arteries and possible microvascular dysfunction), or the rare primary vasospastic syndrome of Prinzmetal (variant) angina. It should be recognized, however, that most patients (even those with Prinzmetal angina) tend to have a significant atherosclerotic lesion on which the spasm is superimposed. In general, the extent (number of vessels involved, location of lesions) and severity (the percentage of diameter narrowing, the minimal luminal diameter, or the length of the lesion) of coronary artery disease and the prevalence of collateral circulation, as judged by traditional angiographic criteria, do not differ between patients with unstable angina and those with stable coronary artery disease. The morphologic features of the culprit lesions do tend to differ, however. The culprit lesion in patients with unstable angina tends to be more eccentric and irregular, with overhanging margins and filling defects or lucencies. These findings (on autopsy or in vivo angioscopy) represent a fissured plaque, with or without a superimposed thrombus. Such unstable features in the culprit lesion are detected more frequently when angiography is performed early in the clinical course.

3. Noninvasive tests—Any form of provocative testing (exercise or pharmacologic stress) is clearly contraindicated in the acute phase of the disease because of the inherent risk of provoking a serious complication. Several studies of patients who had been pain-free and clinically stable for more than 3–5 days, however, have shown that such testing, using ECG, scintigraphic, or echocardiographic evaluation, may be safe. Provocative testing is used primarily to stratify patients into low- and high-risk subsets. Aggressive diagnostic and therapeutic interventions can then be selectively applied to the high-risk patients; the low-risk patients are treated more conservatively. In general, these studies have shown that patients who have good exercise duration and

ventricular function, without significant inducible ischemia or ECG changes on admission, are at a very low risk and can be managed conservatively. On the other hand, patients with ECG changes on admission, a history of prior MI, evidence of inducible ischemia, and ventricular dysfunction tend to be at a higher risk for adverse cardiac events and therefore in greater need of further and more invasive evaluation.

4. Biomarkers—Blood levels of specific myocardial biomarkers such as cardiac troponins are, by definition, not elevated in unstable angina; if they are elevated without evolution of Q waves, the diagnosis is generally an NSTEMI. This distinction is somewhat arbitrary, however. Patients with negative biomarkers within 6 hours of symptom onset need to have them remeasured within 8–12 hours.

Elevated levels of circulating biomarkers, such as high-sensitivity C-reactive protein, fibrinogen, brain natriuretic peptide, and glucose, have been reported in patients presenting with USA/NSTEMI. The presence of such markers may be useful in risk stratification for clinical outcomes; however, their roles in diagnosing USA/NSTEMI and determining whether treatment strategies based on these biomarkers would alter clinical outcomes have not been established.

Canto AJ, et al. Differences in symptom presentation and hospital mortality according to type of acute myocardial infarction. *Am Heart J.* 2012;163:572–9. [PMID: 22520522]

Khot UN, et al. Prognostic importance of physical examination for heart failure in non-ST-elevation acute coronary syndromes: the enduring value of Killip classification. *JAMA.* 2003;290(16): 2174–81. [PMID: 14570953]

Movahed MR, et al. Mortality trends for non-ST-segment elevation myocardial infarction (NSTEMI) in the United States from 1988 to 2004. *Clin Cardiol.* 2011;34:689–92. [PMID: 22095658]

Rogers WJ, et al. Temporal trends in the treatment of over 1.5 million patients with myocardial infarction in the US from 1990 through 1999: the National Registry of Myocardial Infarction 1, 2 and 3. *J Am Coll Cardiol.* 200036(7):2056–63. [PMID: 11127441]

Segev A, et al. Prognostic significance of admission heart failure in patients with non-ST-elevation acute coronary syndromes (from the Canadian Acute Coronary Syndrome Registries). *Am J Cardiol.* 2006 Aug 15;98(4):470–3. [PMID: 16893699]

Shah PK. Pathophysiology of plaque rupture and the concept of plaque stabilization. *Cardiol Clin.* 2003;21(3):303–14. [PMID: 14621447]

Yeh RW, et al. Population trends in the incidence and outcomes of acute myocardial infarction. *N Engl J Med.* 2010;362:2155–65. [PMID: 20558366]

▶ Differential Diagnosis

Conditions that simulate or masquerade as unstable angina include acute MI, acute aortic dissection, acute pericarditis, pulmonary embolism, esophageal spasm, hiatal hernia, and chest wall pain. Careful attention to the history, risk factors, and objective findings of ischemia (transient ST-T changes and mild elevations of troponins in particular) remain the cornerstones for the diagnosis.

A. Acute Myocardial Infarction

Although MI often produces more prolonged pain, the clinical presentation can be indistinguishable from that of unstable angina. As stated earlier, this distinction should be considered somewhat arbitrary because abnormal myocardial technetium-99m pyrophosphate uptake, mild creatine kinase elevations detected on very frequent blood sampling, and increases in troponin T and I levels (released from necrotic myocytes) are observed in some patients with otherwise classic symptoms of unstable angina.

B. Acute Aortic Dissection

The pain of aortic dissection is usually prolonged and severe. It frequently begins in or radiates to the back and tends to be relatively unrelenting and often tearing in nature; transient ST-T changes are rare. An abnormal chest radiograph showing a widened mediastinum, accompanied by asymmetry in arterial pulses and blood pressure, can provide clues to the diagnosis of aortic dissection, which can be verified by bedside echocardiography (transesophageal, with or without transthoracic echocardiography), magnetic resonance imaging (MRI), computed tomography (CT) scanning, or aortography.

C. Acute Pericarditis

Acute pericarditis may be difficult to differentiate from unstable angina. A history of a febrile or respiratory illness suggests the former. The pain of pericarditis is classically pleuritic in nature and worsens with breathing, coughing, deglutition, truncal movement, and supine posture. A pericardial friction rub is diagnostic, but is often evanescent, and frequent auscultation may be needed. Prolonged, diffuse ST elevation that is not accompanied by reciprocal ST depression or myocardial necrosis is typical of pericarditis. Leukocytosis and an elevated erythrocyte sedimentation rate are common in pericarditis but not in unstable angina. Echocardiography may detect pericardial effusion in patients with pericarditis; diffuse ventricular hypokinesis may imply associated myocarditis. Regional dysfunction, especially if transient, is more likely to reflect myocardial ischemia.

D. Acute Pulmonary Embolism

Chest pain in acute pulmonary embolism is also pleuritic in nature and almost always accompanied by dyspnea. Arterial hypoxemia is common, and the ECG may show sinus tachycardia with a rightward axis shift. Precordial ST-T wave abnormalities may simulate patterns of anterior myocardial ischemia or infarction. A high index of suspicion, combined with a noninvasive assessment of pulmonary ventilation-perfusion mismatch, evidence of lower extremity deep venous thrombosis, CT angiography, and possibly pulmonary angiography, is necessary to exclude the diagnosis.

E. Gastrointestinal Causes of Pain

Various gastrointestinal pathologies can mimic unstable angina. These include esophageal spasm, peptic ulcer, hiatal hernia, cholecystitis, and acute pancreatitis. A history compatible with those conditions, the response to specific therapy, and appropriate biochemical tests and imaging procedures should help clarify the situation. It should be noted that these abdominal conditions may produce ECG changes that simulate acute myocardial ischemia.

F. Other Causes of Chest Pain

Many patients present with noncardiac chest pain that mimics unstable angina, and sometimes no specific diagnosis can be reached. The pain may be musculoskeletal, or there may be nonspecific changes on the ECG that increase the diagnostic confusion. In these patients, a definite diagnosis often cannot be reached despite careful clinical observation. When the pain has abated and the patient is stable, a provocative test for myocardial ischemia may help rule out ischemic heart disease. Although coronary angiography may provide evidence of atherosclerotic coronary artery disease, anatomic evidence does not necessarily prove an ischemic cause for the symptoms. In some patients, acute myocarditis may also produce chest pain syndromes simulating unstable angina and acute MI. Recreational drug use (cocaine and methamphetamine) may also produce clinical syndromes of chest pain, sometimes related to drug-induced acute coronary syndrome precipitated by the vasoconstrictor and prothrombotic effects of these drugs.

▶ Treatment

In treating unstable angina, the initial objective is to stratify patients for their short-term morbidity and mortality risks based on their clinical presentations. After risk stratification, management objectives include eliminating episodes of ischemia and preventing acute MI and death.

A. Initial Management

During this early in-hospital phase, therapy is primarily aimed at stabilizing the patient by stabilizing the culprit coronary lesion and thus preventing a recurrence of myocardial ischemia at rest and progression to MI.

1. General measures—Patients whose history is compatible with a diagnosis of unstable angina should be promptly hospitalized in an intensive or intermediate care unit. General supportive care includes bed rest with continuous monitoring of cardiac rate and rhythm and frequent evaluation of vital signs; relief of anxiety with appropriate reassurance and, if necessary, anxiolytic medication; and treatment of associated precipitating or aggravating factors such as hypoxia, hypertension, dysrhythmias, heart failure, acute blood loss, or thyrotoxicosis. A 12-lead ECG should be repeated if it is initially unrevealing or if any significant change has occurred in symptoms or clinical stability. Serial cardiac biomarker evaluation should be performed as a part of an NSTEMI rule-out protocol and to evaluate the extent of myocardial damage and used for outcome risk stratification.

2. Outcome risk stratification—The Global Registry of Acute Coronary Events (GRACE) and Thrombolysis in Myocardial Infarction (TIMI) risk scores are the two commonly used risk scores to predict short-term risk of events and are helpful for clinical decision making. GRACE score is calculated based on the sum of the scores assigned to clinical parameters such as age, heart rate, systolic blood pressure, serum creatinine, Killip classification, presence of cardiac arrest, ST segment deviation, and elevation of cardiac enzymes. The score predicts outcome events reasonably well both in test and validation cohorts, predicting greater than 3% in-hospital death with a score higher than 140. Calculation of GRACE score is somewhat complex, but an online version of the GRACE risk score calculator is available at www.outcomes.org/grace. The TIMI score contains less clinical variables with 1 point assigned to each variable; hence, it is easier for clinical usage and performs relatively well in predicting outcome. However, the TIMI score lacks several key factors compared to the GRACE score, and thus is not as accurate in predicting outcomes as the GRACE score. The TIMI calculator is available at www.timi.org.

3. Anti-ischemic medications

A. Nitrates—Nitrates are generally considered one of the cornerstones of therapy (Table 7–3); however, their use is largely based on clinical experience, not on randomized clinical trials. Nitrates relieve and prevent ischemia by improving subendocardial blood flow in the ischemic zone through their vasodilator actions, predominantly on the large epicardial vessels, including the stenotic segments and the coronary collaterals. Nitrates directly stimulate cyclic guanosine monophosphate (GMP) production, achieving vasodilatory effect in the vascular smooth muscle without requiring an intact or functional endothelium; hence, their effects are generally well preserved in atherosclerosis. Reduction of left ventricular preload and afterload by peripheral vasodilator actions may contribute to the reduction of myocardial ischemia. Although nitrates may reduce the number of both symptomatic and asymptomatic episodes of myocardial ischemia in unstable angina, no effect has yet been demonstrated on the incidence of progression to MI or death.

In the very acute phase, it is preferable to use intravenous nitroglycerin to ensure adequate bioavailability, a rapid onset and cessation of action, and easy titration of doses. Oral, sublingual, transdermal, and transmucosal preparations are better suited for subacute and chronic use. To minimize the chances of abrupt hypotension, nitroglycerin infusion should be started at 10 mcg/min and the infusion rate titrated according to symptoms and blood pressure. The goal is to use the lowest dose that will relieve ischemic symptoms without incurring side effects. The side effects of nitrates include hypotension, reflex tachycardia associated with hypotension; occasional profound bradycardia, presumably related to vagal stimulation; headaches; and facial flushing. Rare side effects include methemoglobinemia, alcohol intoxication, and an increase in intraocular and intracranial pressure. Because the magnitude of reduced arterial pressure that a patient can tolerate without developing signs of organ hypoperfusion varies, it is difficult to define an absolute cut-off point. A reasonable approach in normotensive patients without heart failure is to maintain the arterial systolic blood pressure no lower than 100–110 mm Hg; in hypertensive patients, reduction below 120–130 mm Hg may be unwise.

Continuous and prolonged administration of intravenous nitroglycerin for more than 24 hours may lead to the attenuation of both its peripheral and coronary dilator actions. This effect is due to the development of tolerance in some patients. At the present time, however, there is no easy and practical way to avoid or overcome this problem other than escalating the dose to maintain reduction in measurable end points (eg, the arterial blood pressure).

With the increasing use of phosphodiesterase-5 inhibitors (such as sildenafil) for erectile dysfunction among patients with coronary artery disease or the recreational use of such medication, it is important to obtain a history of whether the patient has taken such medication 24 hours prior to presentation of USA/NSTEMI. Nitrate-mediated vasodilation in the presence of phosphodiesterase-5 inhibition can lead to prolonged hypotension or even death.

Table 7–3. Effects of Medical Therapy in USA/NSTEMI

Therapy	Recurrent Ischemia	Progression to Acute Myocardial Infarction	Mortality
Nitrates	↓↓	?	?
Calcium channel blockers	↓↓	?[1]	?[1]
β-Blockers	↓↓	↓?	↓?
Aspirin/clopidogrel	↓?	↓↓	↓↓
UFH/LMWH	↓↓	↓↓↓	↓↓↓

↓, reduction in frequency; ?, benefit not clearly established; LMWH, low-molecular-weight heparin; UFH, unfractionated heparin.
[1]Increased risk with nifedipine and decreased risk with diltiazem in non-Q wave infarction in two studies.

B. β-BLOCKERS—The evidence for use of β-blockers in USA/NSTEMI extrapolates mostly from studies in STEMI or stable angina patients. Use of β-blockers has been shown to reduce the frequency of both symptomatic and asymptomatic ischemic episodes in stable as well as unstable angina. These protective effects are generally attributed to their negative chronotropic and inotropic effects, which reduce the imbalance of myocardial oxygen demand and supply. Their ability to reduce the risk of infarct development is less clear, but they do decrease reinfarction and mortality rates in postinfarction patients. The mechanism of their protective effect against reinfarction remains unexplained, although it has been speculated that they reduce the risk of plaque rupture by reducing mechanical stress on the vulnerable plaque. It is also unclear whether β-blockers offer any additional benefit in unstable angina patients who are already receiving nitrates and antiplatelet-anticoagulant therapy.

β-blockers administered orally, not intravenously, can be started early (within 24 hours after admission) in the absence of contraindications such as congestive heart failure, hemodynamic instability, heart block, or active reactive airway disease. The choice of β-blockers depends on pharmacokinetic consideration as well as physician familiarity; however, β-blockers without intrinsic sympathomimetic activity, such as propranolol, atenolol, or metoprolol, are preferred.

C. CALCIUM CHANNEL BLOCKERS—Calcium channel blockers are also frequently used in managing ischemic heart disease. Their beneficial effects in myocardial ischemia are generally attributed to their ability to improve myocardial blood flow by reducing coronary vascular tone and dilation of large epicardial vessels and coronary stenoses through an endothelium-independent action. They also reduce myocardial workload through their negative chronotropic (diltiazem and verapamil) and inotropic and peripheral vasodilator effects. Because exaggerated vasoconstriction may play a role in unstable angina, calcium channel blockers have been used in its management. In general, although calcium channel blockers have been shown to reduce the frequency of ischemic episodes in unstable angina, their protective effect against the development of acute MI has not been definitively demonstrated. In fact, the use of such calcium channel blockers as nifedipine tends to increase the risk of ischemic complications in unstable angina. Such adverse effects may well be due to reflex tachycardia or coronary steal caused by the arteriole-dilating actions of dihydropyridine calcium channel blockers. The protective effects of the heart rate-slowing calcium channel blocker diltiazem have been reported in patients with a non-Q wave MI and preserved ventricular function. As in the case of β-blockers, the additive benefits of calcium channel blockers in patients with unstable angina who are receiving nitrates and antithrombotic therapy have not been defined, and their use should also be considered an adjunct to such drugs.

4. Antiplatelet therapy—Platelet activation and aggregation leading to coronary thrombosis is the hallmark feature underlying the pathophysiology of acute coronary syndrome. Hence, inhibition of platelet activation via pharmacologic blockade of signaling pathways such as cyclooxygenase-1 or P_2Y_{12} receptor plays a central role in managing acute coronary syndrome.

A. ASPIRIN—Aspirin irreversibly inhibits cyclooxygenase-1 and reduces thromboxane A_2 production; hence, it reduces platelet aggregation by this pathway. It has been shown to reduce the risk of developing MI by about 50% in at least four randomized trials. The protective effect of aspirin in unstable angina has been comparable, in the dosage range of 75–1200 mg/day. Because of the potential for gastrointestinal side effects, low doses of aspirin (75–81 mg/day) are preferable for daily maintenance. A higher loading dose of 160–325 mg on the first day is recommended in order to initiate the antiplatelet effect more rapidly.

B. P_2Y_{12} RECEPTOR INHIBITORS—Adenosine diphosphate (ADP) is one of the inducers of platelet activation by binding to a G-protein–coupled P_2Y_{12} receptor with subsequent activation of GP II_bIII_a receptor and stabilization of platelet aggregation. Currently available P_2Y_{12} receptor inhibitors include ticlopidine, clopidogrel, prasugrel, and ticagrelor.

(1) Ticlopidine—Ticlopidine was the first P_2Y_{12} receptor inhibitor that was approved for use for secondary prevention of stroke and MI and for prevention of stent closure after percutaneous coronary intervention (PCI). Ticlopidine is a prodrug and requires biotransformation to active metabolite in liver. Its use can cause rare, but life-threatening side effects including thrombotic thrombocytopenic purpura or neutropenia; hence, its use has been replaced by other P_2Y_{12} receptor inhibitors.

(2) Clopidogrel—Clopidogrel is also a prodrug requiring hepatic metabolism to form active metabolite to irreversibly inhibit P_2Y_{12} receptor. Extrapolation based on the CURE trial suggested that the combination of aspirin and clopidogrel appears to modestly reduce the combined incidence of cardiovascular death, MI, or stroke in USA/NSTEMI patients who are not undergoing revascularization procedures. However, this small additional benefit is at the expense of increased major or minor bleeding and cost.

The majority of clinical trials (CREDO, PCI-CURE, CLARITY, and COMMIT) testing the efficacy of aspirin and clopidogrel focus on high-risk acute coronary syndrome patients undergoing PCI. Based on these trials, current guidelines recommend treatment with aspirin and clopidogrel for 12 months for acute coronary syndrome patients undergoing PCI. The suggested loading and daily maintenance dose for clopidogrel are 300 mg and 75 mg, respectively. A higher loading dose (600 mg) and higher daily maintenance dose (150 mg) of clopidogrel for the first 7 days, using a dose of 75 mg/day thereafter,

Table 8–1. ESC/ACC Definition of Myocardial Infarction

Criteria for acute MI

The term acute myocardial infarction (MI) should be used when there is evidence of *myocardial necrosis* in a clinical setting consistent with *acute myocardial ischemia*. Under these conditions *any one of the following* criteria meets the diagnosis for MI:

1. Typical rise and fall of biochemical markers of myocardial necrosis (preferably cardiac troponin) with at least one of the following:
   a. Ischemic symptoms
   b. Development of pathologic Q waves on the ECG
   c. ECG changes indicative of ischemia (ST segment – T-wave changes)
   d. Imaging evidence of new loss of viable myocardium or new regional wall motion abnormality.
   e. Identification of an intracoronary thrombus by angiography or autopsy
2. Cardiac death with symptoms suggestive of myocardial ischemia and presumed new ischemic ECG changes or new LBBB
3. Percutaneous coronary intervention (PCI)–related MI is arbitrarily defined by elevation of cTn in patients with normal baseline values or a rise of cTn values > 20% if the baseline values are elevated and are stable or falling. In addition, either (i) symptoms suggestive of myocardial ischemia or (ii) new ischemic ECG changes or (iii) angiographic findings consistent with a procedural complication or (iv) imaging demonstration of new loss of viable myocardium or new regional wall motion abnormality are required
4. Stent thrombosis associated with MI when detected by coronary angiography or autopsy in the setting of myocardial ischemia and with a rise and/or fall of cardiac biomarkers
5. Coronary artery bypass grafting (CABG)–related MI is arbitrarily defined by elevation of cardiac biomarkers in patients with normal baseline values. In addition, either (i) new pathologic Q waves or new LBBB, or (ii) angiographic documented new graft or new native coronary artery occlusion, or (iii) imaging evidence of new loss of viable myocardium or new regional wall motion abnormality

Criteria for prior MI

Any one of the following criteria satisfies the diagnosis for prior MI:

1. Development of new pathologic Q waves on serial ECGs. The patient may or may not remember previous symptoms. No other nonischemic cause
2. Imaging evidence of a region of loss of viable myocardium that is thinned and fails to contract, in the absence of a nonischemic cause
3. Pathologic findings of a healed or healing MI

cTn, cardiac troponin; ESC/ACC, European Society of Cardiology/American College of Cardiology; CK-MB, myocardial muscle kinase isoenzyme; ECG, electrocardiogram; LBBB, left bundle branch block; MI, myocardial infarction.

Adapted, with permission, from Thygesen K, et al. Third universal definition of myocardial infarction. *J Am Coll Cardiol.* 2012;60(16): 1581–98.

acute infarction. In these cases, vasoconstriction secondary to endothelial dysfunction and a propensity to thrombosis are of sufficient magnitude and duration to cause thrombus formation. Oxygen consumption and possibly direct myocyte toxicity also increase with cocaine use. In addition,

thrombosis in situ can apparently cause infarction among women who take estrogens (especially if they smoke). An increasingly recognized differential diagnosis of acute MI is stress cardiomyopathy (also known as apical ballooning syndrome or takotsubo cardiomyopathy). This entity can present with a variety of symptoms and ECG changes, including ST elevation, and there is akinesis of the anterior and inferior walls and apex of the left ventricle in the absence of coronary artery disease. It is often accompanied by severe emotional stress. The diagnosis is one of exclusion, after angiography demonstrates patent coronary arteries. The treatment is supportive and the prognosis is good: recovery of ventricular function is the norm.

In addition to blockage of coronary arteries (reduced "supply"), acute MI may be seen when myocardial oxygen requirements are elevated (increased "demand"). This often occurs when other medical illnesses coexist with ischemic heart disease. Pulmonary embolism, pneumonia, arrhythmia, septic shock, severe anemia, or great emotional distress can increase myocardial oxygen demand, reduce coronary perfusion pressure, or evoke paradoxical coronary artery responses and lead to MI. However, these tend to be smaller infarctions with no ECG ST elevation that are diagnosed by elevated biomarkers.

Libby P, et al. Inflammation and atherosclerosis. *Circulation.* 2002;105(9):1135–43. [PMID: 11877368]

Roger VL, et al. Heart Disease and stroke statistics—2012 update. A report from the American Heart Association. *Circulation.* 2012;125:e12–e230. [PMID: 22179539]

Wittstein IS, et al. Neurohumoral features of myocardial stunning due to sudden emotional stress. *N Engl J Med.* 2005;352(6):539–48. [PMID: 15703419]

▶ Clinical Findings

A. Symptoms & Signs

Chest discomfort is the most common symptom; it is usually described as "pressure," "dull," "squeezing," or "aching," although it may be described differently because of individual variability, differences in articulation or verbal abilities, or concomitant disease processes. The discomfort is usually in the center of the chest and commonly radiates to the left arm or the neck. However, it may also radiate to the right arm, epigastrium, jaw, teeth, or back. The nature of the pain may lead patients to place a hand or fist over the sternum (Levine sign). These clinical signs and symptoms were originally defined in groups of males. It is now clear that women often have more atypical symptoms.

Associated symptoms may include dyspnea, nausea (particularly in inferior infarction), palpitations, and a sense of impending doom.

Patients, especially those with diabetes or hypertension, may have atypical presentations; for example, a diabetic person may have abdominal pain that mimics the discomfort commonly associated with gallstones. In elderly patients, heart failure is often the presenting symptom. Up to 42% of women and 30% of men present with MI without chest pain. The diagnosis of MI should be considered in patients in whom symptoms are atypical yet compatible with ischemia (paroxysms of dyspnea, for example) or in those with atypical chest discomfort. Patients can also have discomfort that is sharper or that radiates to the back. These patients can have pericarditis alone, pericarditis induced by infarction, or a dissecting aortic aneurysm—with or without concomitant infarction.

B. Physical Examination

The physical examination is a critical and underappreciated part of the initial assessment of patients with suspected acute MI. Findings may vary tremendously, from markedly abnormal, with signs of severe congestive heart failure (CHF), to totally normal.

On general inspection, most patients with a large MI appear pale or sweaty and may be agitated or restless. Heart rate should be measured for arrhythmia, heart block, or sinus tachycardia. This is crucial before administration of β-blockers. Assessment of blood pressure is important because severe hypertension (which may be due to the pain) is a contraindication to fibrinolytic treatment and must be treated emergently. Conversely, hypotension in the setting of acute MI may be due to cardiogenic shock, which alters treatment strategy. Fibrinolytic treatments are not effective in cardiogenic shock, and the patient should be considered for an urgent intra-aortic balloon pump (IABP) and primary percutaneous coronary intervention (PCI).

The jugular venous pulse should be carefully examined. Its elevation in the setting of inferior MI without left heart failure suggests right ventricular MI. Detection of right ventricular MI is vital because it portends a much worse prognosis than isolated inferior MI, and the management strategy is different than isolated inferior MI. Whereas elevated jugular venous pulse in left ventricular MI with left ventricular failure may respond to diuresis, right ventricular MI may require intravenous fluid therapy to maintain left ventricular filling.

Cardiac auscultation should be specifically targeted to complications of MI (see later discussion in this chapter) and detection of important comorbidities. Acute MI may result in ischemic mitral regurgitation with a soft S_1 and a pansystolic murmur. Acquired ventricular septal defect (VSD) may also result in a pansystolic murmur, but it is usually loud and high-pitched and has a normal S_1 and usually occurs later (see later Complications of Myocardial Infarction section). Both ischemic mitral regurgitation and acquired VSD may result in heart failure. The presence of a pericardial friction rub may indicate established infarction that has happened days earlier. Heart failure due to large infarctions may result in a third heart sound. Signs of left heart failure, such as

rales and pulmonary hypertension, should also be sought. Important comorbidities, such as concomitant severe aortic stenosis, should also be documented because they may change the initial reperfusion strategy from fibrinolysis or PCI to cardiac surgery with coronary artery bypass graft (CABG) and aortic valve replacement simultaneously.

Alternative diagnoses may also be suggested by clinical examination. The presence of atrial fibrillation or prosthetic valve may suggest that thromboembolism to the coronary artery is the cause of the coronary occlusion. Furthermore, a brief assessment of pulse equality and blood pressure in both arms should be performed. Inequalities in perfusion between arms may indicate aortic dissection, causing compromised blood flow in the branch vessels of the aortic arch. Aortic dissection may also be responsible for occlusion of the ostium of the coronary artery causing the acute MI. This is a surgical emergency and should not be treated with anticoagulation or fibrinolysis. Therefore, a focused clinical examination is an essential part of the initial patient assessment and can be invaluable in guiding therapy.

C. Diagnostic Studies

1. Electrocardiography—The most rapid and helpful test in assessing patients with suspected acute MI is the 12-lead ECG. It should be performed as soon as possible, preferably within 10 minutes, after the patient's arrival in the emergency department or clinician's office, since the presence or absence of ST elevation determines the preferred management strategy. For a diagnosis of ST elevation MI (STEMI), ST elevation must be present in at least two contiguous leads. For anterior MI, the precordial (V) leads demonstrate ST elevation (Figure 8–1), and if there is lateral wall involvement, I and aVL may also show ST elevation. In inferior MI, leads II, III, and aVF are affected.

In addition to standard ECG leads, right ventricular leads should be recorded in all patients with inferior MI. Inferior MI is usually caused by occlusion of the right coronary artery, which may also cause right ventricular infarction. Differentiating right ventricular infarction from left ventricular infarction is imperative because the management is different.

In posterior MI, usually due to circumflex artery occlusion, the only changes seen on a standard ECG may be reciprocal ST depression and R waves (reciprocal of Q waves) in the anterior leads. This ECG pattern should prompt the use of posterior ECG leads V_{7-9}, which may show ST elevation. Even in the absence of ST elevation in posterior leads, true posterior infarction pattern on ECG in the presence of symptoms suggestive of MI should be treated like STEMI.

Non-ST elevation MI (NSTEMI) has a variable presentation on ECG. There may be no ECG changes, or patients may have ST depression, T-wave flattening, or T-wave inversion. Preexisting abnormalities like T-wave inversion may also "pseudo-normalize" in NSTEMI, making it even more

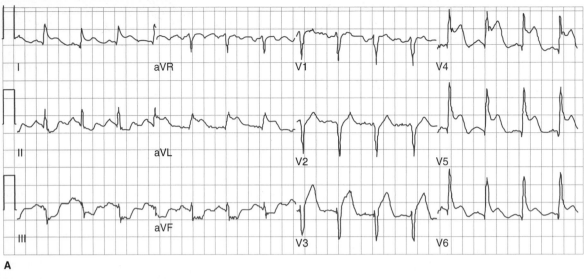

A

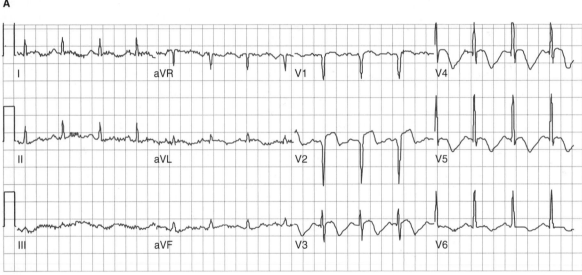

B

▲ **Figure 8–1.** Electrocardiogram (ECG) changes in anterolateral ST elevation myocardial infarction (STEMI). **A:** Initial ECG on presentation shows ST segment elevation in the precordial leads, as well as I and aVL, indicative of acute anterolateral STEMI due to proximal left anterior descending (LAD) coronary artery occlusion. Note the reciprocal ST depression in the inferior leads. **B:** Following reperfusion, subsequent ECG 48 hours later demonstrates resolution of both the anterolateral ST elevation and the reciprocal changes. Note the Q wave in V_2 and the development of T-wave inversion.

difficult to diagnose on ECG. Because determining whether ECG changes are new or old may be difficult, serial ECGs are necessary to diagnose dynamic changes. In patients with symptoms suggestive of MI and no evidence of ST elevation on ECG, the diagnosis of acute coronary syndrome is made. This encompasses unstable angina pectoris and NSTEMI. The distinction between these two entities is made on the presence or absence of elevated biomarkers of MI.

2. Cardiac biomarkers—The diagnosis of infarction requires increases in molecular markers of myocardial injury (Figure 8–2). Myoglobin release from injured myocardium occurs quite early and is very sensitive for detecting infarction. Unfortunately, it is not very specific because minor skeletal muscle trauma also releases myoglobin. Myoglobin is cleared renally, so even minor decreases in glomerular filtration rate lead to elevation. The other early markers advocated

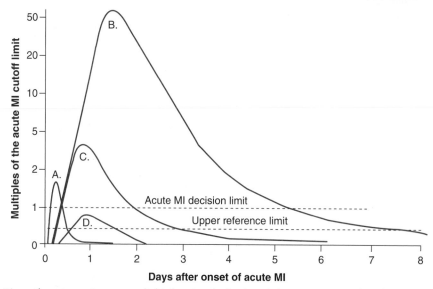

▲ **Figure 8–2.** Biomarkers in acute myocardial infarction (MI). Plot of the appearance of cardiac markers in blood versus time after onset of symptoms. Peak A, early release of myoglobin or CK-MB isoforms after acute MI. Peak B, cardiac troponin after acute MI. Peak C, CK-MB after acute MI. Peak D, cardiac troponin after unstable angina. Data are plotted on a relative scale, where 1.0 is set at the acute MI cutoff concentration. (Reprinted, with permission, from Wu AH, et al. *Clin Chem.* 1999;45:1104.)

by some are isoforms of creatine kinase (CK). This marker has comparable early sensitivity and specificity to myoglobin. The marker of choice in past years was the MB isoenzyme of creatine kinase (CK-MB). A typical rising-and-falling pattern of CK and CK-MB (in the proper clinical setting) was sufficient for the diagnosis of acute infarction. In the typical pattern of CK release after infarction, the enzyme marker level exceeds the upper bound of the reference range within 6–12 hours after the onset of infarction. Peak levels occur by 18–24 hours and generally return to baseline within no more than 48 hours. However, elevations can occur due to release of the enzyme from skeletal muscle. The lack of a rising-and-falling pattern should raise the suspicion that the release is from skeletal muscle, which is usually due to a chronic skeletal muscle myopathy. Elevations of CK in patients with hypothyroidism (where clearance of CK is slowed) and those with renal failure (where clearance is normal because CK is not cleared renally) are caused, in part, by myopathy.

Cardiac troponins I and T are proteins found in cardiac muscle cells and released into the circulation from damaged cardiac myocytes during acute MI. Troponin levels (either I or T) are significantly more sensitive and specific for myocardial damage than CK. Troponin becomes detectable in serum between 4 hours and 6 hours after onset of an acute MI, peaks and then falls to lower levels, and remains elevated at these low levels for 5–7 days (see Figure 8–2). Thus, the late or retrospective diagnosis of acute MI can be made with this marker, making the use of lactate dehydrogenase isoenzymes superfluous. Therefore, because of its sensitivity and

specificity for cardiac muscle damage as well as its early rise and continued low-level detectability, troponin is the preferred biomarker for diagnosis of acute MI. Furthermore, it has been shown to correlate with prognosis even in the absence of CK or CK-MB elevation. Newer high-sensitivity troponin markers are in development, and these have the potential to detect myocardial necrosis at lower levels and more rapidly.

Coronary recanalization, whether spontaneous or induced pharmacologically or mechanically, alters the timing of all markers' appearance in the circulation. Because it increases the rapidity with which the marker is washed out from the heart, leading to rapid increases in plasma, the diagnosis of infarction can be made much earlier—generally within 2 hours of coronary recanalization. Although patency can be approximated from the marker rise, distinguishing between thrombolysis in myocardial infarction (TIMI) II and TIMI III flow is not highly accurate. It should also be understood that peak elevations are accentuated, which must be taken into account if the clinician wants to use peak values as a surrogate for infarct size.

3. Imaging—In the emergency setting, most diagnoses of acute MI are made on history, physical examination, and ECG. However, when the history is atypical and the ECG is equivocal or uninterpretable, performance of a rapid bedside echocardiogram may demonstrate a new regional wall motion abnormality with preserved wall thickness, suggestive of acute MI. In most cases of STEMI, however, echocardiography is not warranted because it delays reperfusion therapy.

Echocardiography is also helpful in diagnosing complications of MI, such as VSD, papillary muscle rupture or free wall rupture, and tamponade.

In NSTEMI that is diagnosed on elevated plasma levels of cardiac biomarkers, nuclear scintigraphy or echocardiography may help determine the region of the heart affected by the MI, but these are not standard diagnostic tools.

Canto JG, et al. Association of age and sex with myocardial infarction symptom presentation and in-hospital mortality. *JAMA.* 2012;307:813–22. [PMID: 22357832]

Hassan AKM, et al. Usefulness of peak troponin-T to predict infarct size and long-term outcome in patients with first acute myocardial infarction after primary percutaneous coronary intervention. *Am J Cardiol.* 2009;103:779–84. [PMID: 19268731]

Menown IB, et al. Early diagnosis of right ventricular or posterior infarction associated with inferior wall left ventricular acute myocardial infarction. *Am J Cardiol.* 2000;85(8):934–8. [PMID: 10760329]

Thygesen K, et al. Third universal definition of myocardial infarction. *J Am Coll Cardiol.* 2012;60(16):1581–98. [PMID: 22958960]

▶ Treatment

The goals of treatment in acute MI are stabilization of the patient and salvage of as much myocardium as possible. A number of general measures should be performed in all patients. In patients with ST elevation—who are at highest risk for complications and have ongoing cardiomyocyte necrosis—immediate reperfusion of the infarct artery should be attempted. The management of acute MI is summarized in Table 8–2.

Early recognition of symptoms of myocardial ischemia may lead to faster treatment and salvage of myocardium. Therefore, it is recommended that patients at risk for MI be educated about the symptoms suggestive of acute MI and call for emergency help immediately if they have these symptoms.

A. Prehospital Management

Aspirin, 162–325 mg, should be given immediately. Continuous cardiac monitoring, oxygen, and sublingual nitroglycerin should be administered to all patients with suspected acute MI. Communities usually have organized protocols for ambulance personnel regarding (1) whether or not they should obtain a 12-lead ECG, (2) whether there are designated hospitals that receive patients in whom an acute MI is suspected, or (3) whether the patient should be taken to the nearest emergency department. In some regions of the world, fibrinolytic treatment is initiated in the ambulance, based on a 12-lead ECG.

B. Emergency Department Therapy

On arrival, all patients with suspected acute MI should have a 12-lead ECG performed immediately. If aspirin has not

Table 8–2. Overview of Management of Acute Myocardial Infarction

Prehospital management
Aspirin
Call 911
Continuous cardiac monitoring
Consider prehospital 12-lead ECG
Emergency department treatment
Intravenous access
Continuous cardiac monitoring
12-lead ECG
Aspirin
Oxygen
Nitroglycerin
Morphine
Heparin
β-Blocker
Reperfusion strategies
Primary PCI vs fibrinolysis for STEMI
Antiplatelet therapy for NSTEMI, possibly followed by elective PCI
In-hospital management
Initial bedrest
Continuous cardiac monitoring
Oxygen for hypoxemia
Nitroglycerin for ongoing pain
ACE inhibitor, β-blocker, aspirin, thienopyridine, statin
Postdischarge
Prognostic indicators
Cardiac rehabilitation
Aggressive secondary prevention with smoking cessation, therapeutic lifestyle changes, and medications

ACE, angiotensin-converting enzyme; ECG, electrocardiogram; NSTEMI, non-ST elevation myocardial infarction; PCI, percutaneous coronary intervention; STEMI, ST elevation myocardial infarction.

been given, then 162–325 mg of aspirin should be administered immediately. All patients with suspected MI should have continuous cardiac ECG monitoring, and intravenous access (two separate intravenous lines) should be gained in all patients. Sublingual nitroglycerin and intravenous morphine should be administered if patients have active chest pain. Oxygen saturations should be monitored noninvasively, rather than by arterial blood gas measurement. Supplemental oxygen, 2–4 L/min, should be given to all patients, particularly if they are hypoxemic. A portable chest radiograph should be ordered but should not delay reperfusion, unless a diagnosis of aortic dissection is strongly considered. Echocardiography may be considered if the diagnosis of MI remains in doubt (eg, equivocal history, uninterpretable ECG). Oral β-blockers should be administered to all patients with acute MI, unless there is a contraindication, such as hypotension, bradycardia, or asthma. This has been shown to improve outcomes and limit the size of infarction. Intravenous β-blockers could be considered when there is hypertension or tachyarrhythmia, for example (Table 8–3). However, they should be avoided in

Table 8–3. Standard Doses of Commonly Used Agents in Patients with Acute Myocardial Infarction

Agents	Dosage	Comments
Antiarrhythmics		
Lidocaine	Initial bolus of 1 mg/kg and 2 mg/min infusion; additional bolus doses to 3 mg/kg may be necessary	For symptomatic arrhythmias and sustained ventricular tachycardia and ventricular fibrillation, not arrest
Procainamide	20 mg/min–1 g, then 2–4 mg/min drip	May cause hypotension, QRS or QT lengthening, or toxicity
Magnesium	1–2 g over 1–2 min or infusion of 8 g over 24 h	Observe for changes in heart rate, blood pressure
Amiodarone	15 mg/min × 10 min, then 1 mg/min × 6 h and 0.5 mg/min × 24 h	For refractory ventricular tachycardia, ventricular fibrillation and arrest
β-Blockers		
Esmolol	250 mcg/kg IV loading dose, then 25–50 mcg/kg/min to maximum dose of 300 mcg/kg/min	Very short half-life
Metoprolol	5 mg every 5 min IV × 3 then 25–50 mg every 12 h orally	Long duration of action; may exacerbate heart failure
Propranolol	0.1 mg/kg over 5 min IV, followed by 20–40 mg every 6 h orally	Long duration of action; may exacerbate heart failure
Calcium channel blockers		
Diltiazem	20–25 mg IV test dose, then 10–15 mg/h as needed; 90–120 mg three times daily orally	May exacerbate heart failure
Inotropes and pressors		
Amrinone	Initial bolus of 0.75 mg/kg, then 5–10 mg/kg/min	May exacerbate ischemia
Dobutamine	Begin at 2.5 mcg/kg/min and titrate to effect	Increases in heart rate > 10% may exacerbate ischemia
Dopamine	Start at 2 mcg/kg/min, titrate to effect	May exacerbate pulmonary congestion and ischemia
Norepinephrine	Start at 2 mcg/min, titrate to effect	Temporizing treatment only
Vasodilators		
Nitroglycerin	Begin at 10 mcg/min IV, titrate to effect	Avoid reducing blood pressure by > 10% if normotensive, > 30% if hypertensive
Nitroprusside	Begin at 0.1 mcg/kg/min, titrate to effect	Mean dose 50–80 mcg/kg/min
Nesiritide	2 mcg/kg bolus followed by 0.01 mcg/kg/min infusion, can increase by 0.005 to maximum infusion 0.03 mcg/kg/min	Hold diuretics and other vasodilators. Keep systolic blood pressure > 100 mm Hg
Anticoagulants		
Unfractionated heparin	5000-unit bolus followed by 1000 units/h adjusted by aPTT	Less efficacious than LMWH
Enoxaparin	1 mg/kg SQ every 12 h, can give immediate 30-mg bolus intravenously if necessary	Hard to reverse effects; avoid in patients with renal failure
Dalteparin	120 international units/kg every 12 h	Avoid in patients with renal failure
Abciximab	0.25 mg/kg followed by 0.125 mcg/kg/min × 12 h, maximum time–24 h	Care necessary if renal failure; thrombocytopenia greater with repeated use
Eptifibatide	180 mcg/kg bolus × 2 (30 min later) followed by 2 mcg/kg/min for as long as 96 h for ACS, 24 h post PCI	Care necessary if renal failure

(continued)

Table 8-3. Standard Doses of Commonly Used Agents in Patients with Acute Myocardial Infarction (*Continued*)

Agents	Dosage	Comments
Tirofiban	0.4 mcg/kg/min × 30 min followed by 0.1 mcg/kg/min for up to 108 h for ACS, 12-19 h for PCI	Care necessary if renal failure
Clopidogrel	600 mg loading dose, then 75 mg/day × at least 1 month, preferably for 12 months	TTP possible
Prasugrel	60 mg loading dose, then 10 mg daily for 12 months	Contraindicated if prior stroke or TIA, weight < 60 kg, or age > 75 years
Ticagrelor	Ticagrelor 180-mg loading dose then 90 mg twice daily for 12 months	May cause bradycardia or shortness of breath

ACS, acute coronary syndromes; aPTT, activated partial thromboplastin time; IV, intravenous; LMWH, low-molecular-weight heparin; PCI, percutaneous coronary intervention; SQ, subcutaneous; TIA, transient ischemic attack; TTP, thrombotic thrombocytopenic purpura.

patients with signs of heart failure, in those with contraindications to β-blockers, and in those at high risk for cardiogenic shock (age > 70 years, heart rate > 110/min or < 60/min, systolic blood pressure < 120 mm Hg, or prolonged time since the onset of symptoms).

An anticoagulant should be administered to all patients with acute MI, unless a contraindication exists. In patients with ST elevation who receive fibrinolytics, 48 hours of anticoagulant should be administered. Acceptable choices for anticoagulants include unfractionated heparin (UFH), low-molecular-weight heparin (LMWH), and fondaparinux. For patients with ST elevation undergoing primary PCI, acceptable choices for anticoagulants include UFH, LMWH, and bivalirudin. UFH is preferred to LMWH in most institutions for primary PCI because it has a short half-life, it can be turned off rapidly if there is a complication during invasive therapy, and it can be monitored during procedures with a bedside activated clotting time test. In contrast, LMWHs have a long half-life, and there is no bedside test of their anticoagulant efficiency.

C. Reperfusion Therapy

1. Patients with STEMI—All patients with STEMI who seek medical care within the first 12 hours after symptom onset should be considered for urgent reperfusion of the infarct-related artery, but the earlier therapy is begun, the greater the benefit. In addition, those patients who seek medical care within 12–24 hours of symptom onset may be considered for reperfusion, particularly if chest pain is ongoing or heart failure or shock has developed, but the benefit of reperfusion therapies after more than 12 hours is less well established. The definitive therapies for reperfusion in STEMI are fibrinolysis or PCI. Both of these strategies improve patency of the infarct-related artery, reduce infarct size, and lower mortality rates. Therefore, one or the other method should be performed as quickly as possible. The goal of reperfusion therapies in the United States is a door-to-needle

time of 30 minutes (for fibrinolysis) and a door-to-balloon inflation time of less than 90 minutes (for PCI). PCI has been shown to be superior to fibrinolysis when it is performed without significant delay by experienced clinicians in experienced centers (Figure 8–3). However, significant delays in performing PCI reduce its benefit over fibrinolytic therapy. There are special cases where primary PCI is always preferred over fibrinolysis: cardiogenic shock, severe CHF or pulmonary edema (Killip class III), or if there are contraindications to fibrinolysis (Table 8–4). These patients may require insertion of an IABP and may benefit from mechanical reperfusion with primary PCI. The different management of patients with these high-risk clinical features underscores the need for careful clinical examination of all patients with chest pain.

Recent data suggest that all patients with STEMI, whether they undergo primary PCI or fibrinolytic therapy, benefit from early administration of a thienopyridine in addition to aspirin. Acceptable alternatives include clopidogrel, prasugrel (only if undergoing primary PCI), or ticagrelor. However, thienopyridines may cause an increase in bleeding complications if the patient undergoes CABG surgery.

2. Patients with NSTEMI—These patients should not be treated with fibrinolytics. The definitive management of NSTEMI involves anticoagulation, platelet inhibition, and consideration for an early invasive strategy (ie, routine coronary angiography with or without PCI during the index hospitalization).

For detailed discussion of NSTEMI, see Chapter 7.

D. In-Hospital Management

All patients with acute MI should be admitted for continuous cardiac monitoring. Patients should have bed rest for the first 12–24 hours following MI and reperfusion, but in the absence of ongoing ischemia, they should be mobilized after this time. All patients should receive the appropriate

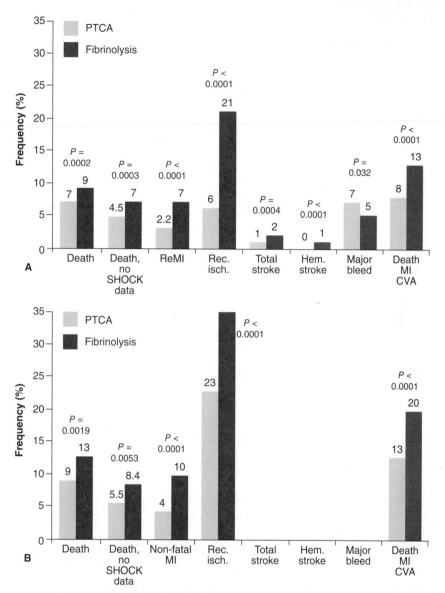

▲ **Figure 8–3.** Percutaneous coronary intervention (PCI) versus fibrinolysis for ST elevation myocardial infarction (STEMI). Short-term (4–6 weeks; **A**) and long-term (**B**) outcomes for various end points shown are plotted for STEMI patients randomized to PCI or fibrinolysis for reperfusion in 23 trials (n = 7739). Primary angioplasty for acute STEMI improves both short- and long-term outcomes. CVA, cerebrovascular accident; Hem. stroke, hemorrhagic stroke; Rec. isch., recurrent ischemia; ReMI, recurrent myocardial infarction. (Modified, with permission, from Keeley EC, et al. *The Lancet.* 2003;361:13 and Antman EM, et al. *J Am Coll Cardiol.* 2004;44:671.)

cardiac diet, adhering to the National Cholesterol Education Program (NCEP) Adult Treatment Panel III (ATP III) dietary guidelines, as well as education regarding the necessary dietary changes they should make after discharge.

Within the first 24 hours of presentation, the long-term medical management of patients with both STEMI and

NSTEMI should be commenced. Angiotensin-converting enzyme (ACE) inhibitors should be given on day 1, if the patient's blood pressure allows, particularly in those with anterior MI or impaired left ventricular function. ACE inhibitors reduce left ventricular remodeling and heart failure and should be continued long-term. β-Blockade should have

Table 8–4. Contraindications for Fibrinolysis Use in STEMI

Absolute contraindications
  Any prior ICH
  Known structural cerebral vascular lesion (eg, AVM)
  Known malignant intracranial neoplasm (primary or metastatic)
  Ischemic stroke within previous 3 months
  Suspected aortic dissection
  Active bleeding or bleeding diathesis (excluding menses)
  Significant closed head or facial trauma within 3 months
  Severe uncontrolled hypertension (SBP > 180 mm Hg and/or DBP
    > 110 mm Hg)

Relative contraindications
  History of prior ischemic stroke greater than 3 months, dementia, or
    known intracranial pathology not covered in contraindications
  Traumatic or prolonged (> 10 minutes) CPR or major surgery in
    previous 3 weeks
  Recent internal bleeding (within 4 weeks)
  Noncompressible vascular punctures
  For streptokinase/anistreplase: prior exposure (> 5 days ago) or
    prior allergic reaction to these agents
  Pregnancy
  Active peptic ulcer
  Current use of anticoagulants: the higher the INR, the higher the
    risk of bleeding

AVM, arteriovenous malformation; CPR, cardiopulmonary resuscitation; DBP, diastolic blood pressure; ICH, intracranial hemorrhage; INR, international normalized ratio; SBP, systolic blood pressure; STEMI, ST elevation myocardial infarction.

already been started in the emergency department and should be continued orally in all patients, unless there are absolute contraindications, and should also be continued long-term. Aspirin, 162–325 mg daily, should be administered initially, then 81 mg daily for life. Thienopyridines (clopidogrel, prasugrel, or ticagrelor) should be continued for 12 months. Hydroxymethylglutaryl-coenzyme A (HMG-CoA) reductase inhibitors (statin therapy) should be given soon after MI and should be continued at high dose long-term.

During hospitalization, all patients should be educated about adhering to therapeutic lifestyle changes, including dietary and lifestyle measures, smoking cessation, and medication compliance. Patients should be referred to a cardiac rehabilitation program to consolidate these messages and develop an appropriate exercise regimen. This has been shown to reduce mortality after MI.

E. Primary PCI Versus Fibrinolysis

The goal of reperfusion is to rapidly restore blood flow to the myocardium to prevent ongoing ischemic cell death. Therefore, whichever means can achieve reperfusion most quickly should be used. Primary PCI results in improved patency rates of the infarct-related artery, as well as improved TIMI flow grade, compared with fibrinolysis. In general, the patency rate with primary PCI is 90% or higher, whereas with thrombolysis, the rate is about 65% and recurrent events are more common. With modern advances, coronary stenting has further improved long-term outcomes over balloon angioplasty alone. PCI has therefore been widely accepted as the treatment of choice for STEMI in centers that can perform primary PCI rapidly and effectively (Figure 8–4). However, very early after the onset of

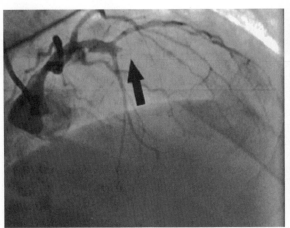
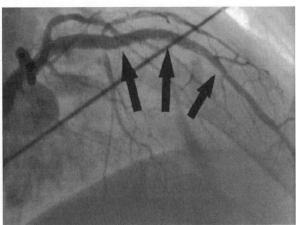

A   B

▲ **Figure 8–4.** Primary percutaneous coronary intervention (PCI) for acute myocardial infarction (MI). **A:** Initial angiography of a patient presenting with acute anterior ST elevation myocardial infarction (STEMI) shows an occluded left anterior descending (LAD) coronary artery (*arrow*). **B:** Following angioplasty and stenting, patency of the LAD is restored.

symptoms, when the thrombus in the infarct-related artery is still soft, fibrinolysis may recanalize the artery as quickly as, if not more so than, primary PCI. This is true in the first hour and possibly the first 3 hours after symptom onset. Therefore, fibrinolysis is an acceptable treatment in these early time points. However, after 3 hours, primary PCI has a clear benefit over fibrinolysis and should be considered the preferred therapy. It bears restating that primary PCI should only be performed in centers skilled in the treatment of STEMI that can achieve rapid reperfusion, with a goal door-to-balloon inflation time of 90 minutes.

In deciding whether elderly patients with acute STEMI should undergo PCI or fibrinolytic therapy, the risks and benefits must be weighed carefully. Elderly patients with STEMI are at high risk for increased morbidity and mortality with thrombolytic agents. Indeed, some studies suggest that these agents have no benefit in this group. On the other hand, PCI is clearly beneficial. However, if PCI cannot be accomplished, individual decisions concerning the risk (which is substantial, especially in regard to intracranial bleeding) and the potential benefits must be balanced. Given the high (20–30%) mortality rate from STEMI in the elderly, some increased risk may be reasonable.

F. Fibrinolytic Agents

There are a number of fibrinolytic agents that have been successfully used in acute MI. Table 8–5 shows the currently approved agents for use in the United States. A brief discussion of each is warranted before deciding on the most appropriate agent. Plasmin, the key ingredient in the fibrinolytic system, degrades fibrin, fibrinogen, prothrombin, and a variety of other factors in the clotting and complement systems. This effect inhibits clot formation and can lead to bleeding. Patients with acute MI and ST segment elevation have little evidence of spontaneous or intrinsic fibrinolysis, despite the intense thrombotic stimulus present. This may be due in part to increased levels of circulating plasminogen activator inhibitor (PAI-1) in plasma or PAI-1 that is elaborated locally from platelets. The pharmacologic administration of fibrinolytic agents (see Table 8–5) to such patients seems reasonable. Plasminogen activators can be administered intravenously or directly into the coronary artery. Although more rapid patency occurs with local administration and lower doses can be used, given the need for early treatment, plasminogen activators are generally administered intravenously.

In addition to invoking fibrinolysis and inhibiting clotting by degrading clotting factors, all plasminogen activators enhance clot formation. These effects seem greater with nonspecific plasminogen activators such as streptokinase and urokinase and could partly explain why fibrin-specific activators such as t-PA open arteries more rapidly. The enhancement of coagulation by plasminogen activators suggests an important role for the concomitant use of antithrombotic agents.

Table 8–5. Fibrinolytic Agents

Agent	Dosage	Adjunctive Treatments
Streptokinase	1,500,000 units over 1 h	Aspirin, ± heparin
Tissue plasminogen activator		
Standard	15 mg bolus, then 50 mg over 30 min and 35 mg over next 60 min	Aspirin, heparin essential
Patients weighing less than 65 kg	1.25 mg/kg over 3 h, 10% of dose as initial bolus	
Urokinase	3,000,000 units over 1 h	Aspirin, ± heparin
Reteplase	10 mg initial bolus, second 10-mg bolus after 30 min	Aspirin, heparin essential
Tenecteplase	< 60 kg: 30-mg bolus	Aspirin, heparin essential
	60–70 kg: 35-mg bolus	
	71–80 kg: 40-mg bolus	
	81–90 kg: 45-mg bolus	
	> 90 kg: 50-mg bolus	

All fibrinolytic agents increase the risk of bleeding, and therefore, patients at high risk for life-threatening bleeding should not be given fibrinolysis (see Table 8–4).

1. Streptokinase—Streptokinase is derived from streptococcal bacteria and activates plasminogen indirectly, forming an activator complex with a slightly longer half-life than streptokinase alone (23 minutes versus 18 minutes after a bolus). Because it activates both circulating plasminogen and plasminogen bound to fibrin, both local and systemic effects occur; that is, circulating fibrinogen degrades substantially (fibrinogenolysis, as well as fibrinolysis, occurs).

Because antibodies to the streptococci exist in many patients, allergic reactions can occur; anaphylaxis is rare, however, and the use of corticosteroids to avoid allergic reactions is no longer recommended. When streptokinase is administered intravenously, a large dose is necessary to overcome antibody resistance. Because a dose of 250,000 units will suffice in 90% of patients, the recommended dose of 1.5 million units over a 1-hour period is generally more than adequate to overcome resistance. Patients who are known to have had a severe streptococcal infection or to have been treated with streptokinase within the preceding 5 or 6 months (or longer) should not receive the agent.

Rapid administration of streptokinase, even at the recommended dose, can cause a substantial reduction in blood pressure. Although this might be considered a potential benefit of the agent, it may also be detrimental. The rate of the infusion should therefore be reduced in response to significant hypotension, and the blood pressure should be monitored closely. Because streptokinase is more procoagulant than other thrombolytic agents, it should not be surprising that patients benefit to a greater extent from the concomitant use of potent antithrombins such as hirudin. However, in combination with glycoprotein (GP) II_bIII_a inhibitors, streptokinase seems to be associated with markedly increased bleeding rates.

2. Urokinase—Urokinase is a direct activator of plasminogen. It has a shorter half-life than streptokinase (14 ± 6 minutes) and is not antigenic. Its effects on both circulating and bound-to-fibrin plasminogen are similar to those from streptokinase. It is therefore difficult to understand why intravenous doses of urokinase (2.0 million units as bolus or 3 million units over 90 minutes) seem to induce coronary artery patency more rapidly than does streptokinase. There is substantial synergism between urokinase and t-PA.

3. Tissue plasminogen activator—The initial human t-PA was made by recombinant DNA technology. The half-life in plasma was short (4 minutes) as a bolus but longer (46 minutes) with prolonged infusions. Despite the short half-life, lytic activity persisted for many hours after clearance of the activator. Although t-PAs are considered "fibrin-specific," no activator is totally fibrin-specific, and fibrin specificity is lost at higher doses. At clinical doses, however, less fibrinogen degradation took place than with nonspecific activators. t-PA clearly opened coronary arteries more rapidly than nonspecific activators, and this is likely why its use improved mortality rates. Bleeding was not less, and there was a slight increase in the number of intracranial bleeds, which was in part due to the need for dosage adjustment for lighter-weight patients.

The original regimen for the use of t-PA was 100 mg over 3 hours: 10 mg as a bolus, followed by 50 mg over the first hour and 40 mg over the next 2 hours. Patients who weighed less than 65 kg received 1.25 mg/kg over 3 hours with 10% of the total dose given as a bolus. An alternative front-loaded regimen was found to be more effective and included an initial bolus of 15 mg, followed by 50 mg over 30 minutes and 35 mg over the next 60 minutes. Doses higher than 100 mg are associated with a higher incidence of intracranial bleeding.

4. Reteplase—Reteplase, a mutant form of t-PA, lacks several of the structural areas of the parent molecule (the finger domain, kringle 1, and the epidermal growth factor domain). It is less fibrin-specific (causes more systemic degradation of fibrinogen) than the parent molecule and has a longer half-life. Accordingly, it is used as a double bolus of 10 units initially followed by a second bolus 30 minutes later, and this requires no adjustment for patient weight. Although not

shown to be superior to t-PA, many clinicians have elected to use reteplase because of the convenience of the double bolus administration.

5. Tenecteplase—Tenecteplase is also a mutant form of t-PA. It has substitutions in the kringle 1 and protease domains to increase its half-life, increase its fibrin specificity, and reduce its sensitivity to its native inhibitor (PAI-1). Although not shown to be superior to t-PA, tenecteplase is generally being used in preference to the parent molecule because of the convenience of a single bolus dose.

Regardless of the fibrinolytic agent used, all patients should receive aspirin and heparin (either UFH or LMWH) to counteract the procoagulant effect of the fibrinolytic agent.

Intravenous heparin, used with plasminogen activators, improves the rapidity with which patency is induced; it is essential for maintaining coronary patency, especially with t-PA–type agents. Its use is less necessary after treatment with streptokinase, probably because of the anticoagulant effects of fibrinogen depletion and degradation products.

The standard dose of UFH is usually a bolus of 5000 units, followed by a 1000-unit-per-hour infusion until the partial thromboplastin time can be used to titrate a dose between 1.5 and 2 times the normal range. It has become clear that optimal titration of UFH is problematic and that if the activated partial thromboplastin time is either too high or too low, some benefit is lost. For this reason, the use of LMWH has been recommended. With the exception of patients with renal failure, a dose of 1 mg/kg of enoxaparin and 120 unit/kg of dalteparin provide consistent reduction in anti-Xa levels and thus consistent anticoagulation. This is probably the reason that recent studies suggest LMWH is more effective for the treatment of patients with acute MI. In addition, because LMWH inhibits Xa activity predominantly, there is some suggestion that discontinuing it may be less problematic than is the case for UFH, which has fewer effects on Xa and more direct effects (when combined with antithrombin 3) on thrombin itself. The ability to use LMWH intravenously in the catheterization laboratory has not been a problem in regions where this strategy has been embraced.

G. Adverse Effects of Fibrinolytic Therapy

The most serious complication of treatment with thrombolytic agents is bleeding, particularly intracranial hemorrhage; however, catheter-based interventions substantially reduce this complication. The mechanism of bleeding with thrombolytic agents is unclear but has been related to the efficacy of the agent; the concomitant use of antithrombotic agents, such as heparin and aspirin; and the degree of hemostatic perturbation induced by the plasminogen activators. In most studies, the incidence of stroke and intracranial bleeding has been slightly higher with t-PA–type activators. This may be in keeping with the greater efficacy and rapidity of their effects. Although most bleeding occurs early during treatment, bleeding can occur 24–48 hours later, and vigilance even after the first few hours is important.

Intracranial bleeding is by far the most dangerous bleeding complication because it is often fatal. For most plasminogen activators, the incidence of intracranial hemorrhage is less than 1%, but it may be as high as 2–3% in elderly patients. Risk factors for intracranial bleeding include a history of cerebrovascular disease, hypertension, and age. These factors must be taken into account when determining whether a thrombolytic agent has an appropriate benefit-to-risk relationship. Changes in mental status require an immediate evaluation—clinical and computed tomography or magnetic resonance imaging. If bleeding is strongly suspected, heparin should be discontinued or neutralized with protamine.

There also is a substantial incidence of nonhemorrhagic, probably thrombotic, stroke that may be partly due to dissolution of thrombus within the heart, followed by migration. The exact mechanisms of this phenomenon are unclear. In some studies, the excess of strokes with t-PA has been found to be related to this phenomenon, and in other studies, it has been due to an apparent increase in intracranial bleeding.

Bleeding outside the brain can occur in any organ bed and should be prevented whenever possible. The puncture of noncompressible arterial or venous vessels is relatively contraindicated in all cardiovascular patients: those with unstable angina one day may be candidates for thrombolytic treatment on the next. Blood gas determinations should therefore be avoided if possible and oximeters used instead in cardiovascular patients. It should be understood that central lines placed in cardiovascular patients pose a substantial risk should there be a subsequent need for a lytic agent. Foley catheters and endotracheal (especially nasotracheal) intubation can also predispose to significant hemorrhage. Bleeding should be watched for assiduously. If severe bleeding occurs while heparin is in use, it should be antagonized with protamine. In general, this and supportive measures are all that can be done. In some studies, there appears to be a slightly higher incidence of extracranial bleeding with nonspecific activators than with t-PA; this finding has not been consistent. In an occasional patient, who begins to bleed shortly after receiving the plasminogen activator, aminocaproic acid, which changes the activation of plasminogen, may be useful. Otherwise, discontinuation of the drug and conservative local measures are all that can be done. If volume repletion is necessary, red blood cells are preferred to whole blood, and cryoprecipitate is preferred to fresh frozen plasma because it does not replenish plasminogen.

Allergic reactions related to the use of streptokinase are unusual but should be identified when they occur. Mild reactions, such as urticaria, can be treated with antihistamines; more severe reactions, such as bronchospasm, may require corticosteroids or epinephrine.

Bleeding after primary PCI can also be substantial, particularly if GP II_bIII_a agents are administered. The use of newer closure devices are touted by some clinicians, but close observation is the key to minimizing bleeding from the catheter site. On occasion, platelet transfusions may be necessary.

Antman EM, et al. 2007 Focused update of the ACC/AHA 2004 guidelines for the management of patients with ST-elevation myocardial infarction. J Am Coll Cardiol. 2008;51:210–47. [PMID: 18191746]

Jneid H, et al. 2012 ACCF/AHA focused update of the guideline for the management of patients with unstable angina/non-ST-elevation myocardial infarction (updating the 2007 guideline and replacing the 2011 focused update): a report of the American College of Cardiology Foundation/American Heart Association Task Force on Practice Guidelines. J Am Coll Cardiol. 2012;60:645–81. [PMID: 22809746]

Kushner FG, et al. 2009 Focused updates: ACC/AHA guidelines for the management of patients with ST-elevation myocardial infarction (updating the 2004 guideline and 2007 focused update) and ACC/AHA/SCAI guidelines on percutaneous coronary intervention (updating the 2005 guideline and 2007 focused update): a report of the American College of Cardiology Foundation/American Heart Association Task Force on Practice Guidelines. J Am Coll Cardiol 2009;54:2205–41. [PMID: 19942100]

Sabatine MS, et al; CLARITY-TIMI 28 Investigators. Addition of clopidogrel to aspirin and fibrinolytic therapy for myocardial infarction with ST-segment elevation. N Engl J Med. 2005;352(12):1179–89. [PMID: 15758000]

Stone GW, et al. Bivalirudin during primary PCI in acute myocardial infarction. N Engl J Med. 2008;358:2218–30. [PMID: 18499566]

Yusuf S, et al; Clopidogrel in Unstable Angina to Prevent Recurrent Events Trial Investigators. Effects of clopidogrel in addition to aspirin in patients with acute coronary syndromes without ST-segment elevation. N Engl J Med. 2001;345(7):494–502. [PMID: 11519503]

▶ Complications of Myocardial Infarction

The complications of acute MI are listed in Table 8–6.

A. Cardiogenic Shock

Cardiogenic shock is characterized by peripheral hypoperfusion and hypotension refractory to volume repletion. This occurs secondary to inadequate cardiac output resulting from severe left ventricular dysfunction.

Table 8–6. Complications of Acute Myocardial Infarction

Cardiogenic shock
Congestive heart failure
Ischemic mitral regurgitation
Ventricular septal defect
Free wall rupture
Recurrent ischemia
Pericarditis
Conduction disturbances
Arrhythmias
Mural thrombus
Aneurysm or pseudoaneurysm of the left ventricle
Right ventricular infarction

Goals of therapy for cardiogenic shock include hemodynamic stabilization to ensure adequate oxygenation of perfused tissue and prompt assessment for reversible causes of the cardiogenic shock. If reversible causes are not found, immediate reperfusion, especially with PCI, is indicated (see Chapter 9).

B. Congestive Heart Failure

In general, there is greater urgency in treating patients with CHF during the early phases of acute MI because such patients often have multivessel disease and are at increased risk for recurrent infarction and increased infarct size. A high degree of suspicion and close monitoring are key to anticipating this complication of acute MI.

Echocardiography has been the technique of choice in evaluating such patients from a perspective of both valvular and myocardial function. Swan-Ganz pulmonary artery catheterization can also be used to aid diagnosis and to assess ongoing management. Management strategies depend on the clinical history of the patient. Patients with new-onset acute CHF are typically euvolemic and benefit from nitrate therapy for ischemia. These patients in general should not receive diuretics initially because diuretic therapy often complicates the clinical course with the development of hypotension. In addition, reduced respiratory effort, reduced heart rate, and normalization of oxygen saturation are central to early clinical management.

Nitroglycerin is often the best agent to use for ischemia in patients with CHF. In some instances, the hemodynamic profile provided by nitroprusside may be desirable. However, nitroprusside may exacerbate ischemia by inducing a coronary steal phenomenon; in this setting, nitroprusside would be a second-line therapy.

Continuous positive airway pressure can reduce the work of breathing in patients with pulmonary edema and should be considered early in these patients.

Intravenous ACE inhibitor therapy should not be used in this setting. Hypotension is a complicating factor because it reduces coronary perfusion and may lead to further ischemia. Low-dose dobutamine, starting at 2.5 mcg/kg/min, can be used to achieve hemodynamic benefit. Also, phosphodiesterase inhibitors can be considered, although their vasodilating effects may limit their inotropic benefit in patients with significant hypotension.

The use of Swan-Ganz catheterization monitoring is controversial, and no randomized controlled data support their use as a first-line recommendation in the management of CHF with acute MI. However, Swan-Ganz monitoring can be beneficial in verifying diagnosis, and its use in the early phases of management may allow rapid titration of parenteral therapy.

Once hemodynamic stabilization has been achieved, which is generally within the first 6–12 hours, initiation of oral agents is appropriate. Drugs of choice in this setting are ACE inhibitors, which improve cardiac performance, have beneficial effects on ventricular remodeling, and have been demonstrated not only to reduce morbidity but also to reduce mortality rates in patients with CHF. Oral β-blocker therapy should also be initiated early in the treatment of these patients; however, this should be done in a stepwise fashion in relation to ACE inhibitor therapy to avoid hypotensive effects.

Aldosterone blockade with spironolactone or eplerenone should be given to patients with left ventricular impairment (left ventricular ejection fraction < 40%) or clinical heart failure or both following MI. Aldosterone blockade should be started, in addition to ACE inhibitors, in patients who do not have significant renal impairment or hyperkalemia. The serum potassium level should be monitored closely, since both eplerenone and spironolactone can cause hyperkalemia.

C. Acute Mitral Valve Regurgitation

The development of acute severe mitral valve regurgitation occurs in approximately 1% of patients with acute MI and contributes to 5% of deaths. Acute mitral regurgitation occurs as a result of papillary muscle rupture most commonly involving the posterior medial papillary muscle because its singular blood vessel supply is derived from the posterior descending coronary artery. In contrast, the anterior lateral papillary muscle much less commonly ruptures because it has a dual blood supply derived from the left anterior descending and circumflex coronary arteries. Rupture of the papillary muscle may be complete or partial with the development of a flail mitral valve leaflet. Pulmonary edema usually ensues rapidly and occurs within 2–7 days after inferior infarction. The intensity of associated murmur varies depending on the extent of unobstructed flow back into the left atrium. If severe regurgitation is present, no murmur may be audible. As a result, a high degree of suspicion is needed to promptly diagnose acute mitral regurgitation. Two-dimensional echocardiography can be used to demonstrate the partial or completely ruptured papillary muscle head and the flail segment of the mitral valve. Typically, hyperdynamic left ventricular function is demonstrated, and its occurrence in severe CHF should prompt the diagnosis. The treatment of choice is to stabilize the patient hemodynamically with the use of intravenous vasodilators and possibly intra-aortic balloon counterpulsation. The basis of a successful outcome, however, is prompt emergency surgery. The operative mortality rate in this setting can be up to 10%, but this affords most opportunity for survival. Mitral valve repair with reimplantation of the severed papillary muscle is the preferred technique as an alternative to mitral valve replacement. The mortality rate is unacceptably high in the absence of prompt surgery.

Ischemic mitral regurgitation without papillary muscle rupture occurs in up to 50% of patients with acute inferior wall MI. In those patients in whom severe CHF symptoms develop, hemodynamic compensation needs to be undertaken and could include the use of IABP for adequate afterload reduction. Treatment of ischemia in this setting may include reperfusion therapy with PCI, intravenous vasodilator therapy, and mechanical support. Once the acute phase of the infarction is past, resolution of the severe mitral regurgitation may occur, which then avoids the need for surgery.

D. Acute Ventricular Septal Rupture

Rupture of the ventricular septum has been reported to occur in up to 3% of acute MIs and contributes to about 5% of deaths. Typically, half of VSDs occur in anterior wall MIs, often in patients with their first infarction, with peak incidence occurring 3–7 days after initial infarction. Findings associated with VSD can be confused with acute mitral regurgitation because both can result in hypotension, severe heart failure, and prominent murmur. However, the diagnosis of VSD should be suspected clinically when a new pansystolic murmur is noted. Generally, the murmur is most prominent along the left sternal border and may have an associated thrill. Prompt surgical intervention is recommended, which, if successful, can reduce the mortality rate from nearly 100% to below 50%.

Although percutaneous repair of postinfarction VSDs in the catheterization laboratory using septal occluding devices has been reported, surgical repair remains the gold standard.

E. Cardiac Rupture

Rupture of the free wall of the left ventricle occurs in approximately 1–3% of patients with acute infarction and accounts for up to 15% of peri-infarction deaths. Free wall rupture may occur as early as within the first 48 hours of infarction. Fifty percent of ruptures occur within the first 5 days of infarction and 90% within the first 2 weeks. Rupture may be due to expansion of the peri-infarct zone, with thinning of the infarcted wall occurring in response to increased stress. The paradoxical motion of the infarcted segment at the margin of the infarcted zone may also contribute stress, resulting in muscle rupture. Patients may complain of recurrence of chest pain, and an ECG may show persistent ST elevation with Q waves. Prompt intervention at that time may include echocardiography with pericardiocentesis, IABP placement, and urgent cardiac catheterization with anticipation of immediate surgery. Unfortunately, all too often signs of cardiac rupture are not present until acute hemodynamic decompensation occurs with cardiac arrest due to electromechanical dissociation. The rate of cardiac rupture following MI is decreasing due to early reperfusion therapy. However, the mortality rate remains extremely high. Successful treatment of cardiac rupture requires the clinician to have a high index of suspicion and undertake immediate intervention if there is to be any possibility of preventing death.

F. Recurrent Ischemia

Episodes of chest pain recur in up to 60% of patients after infarction. When chest discomfort recurs early (within 24 hours of MI), the discomfort usually reflects the process of completing the infarction. Chest discomfort may reflect the effects of ongoing ischemia or recurrent infarction. In this situation, prompt reassessment and treatment are critical. Patients with hemodynamic compromise in association with new ECG changes in the distribution other than that of the infarct-related artery are at significant risk and require prompt attention, often including coronary angiography with catheter-based intervention.

In patients who were treated initially with reperfusion therapy and have recurrent chest pain, prompt evaluation is needed to assess the adequacy of anticoagulation and the possibility of reocclusion of the culprit coronary artery. Adequacy of adjunctive therapy in the setting of recurrent chest pain is necessary, and often adjustments in drug doses are required. Occasionally short-term use of intravenous nitroglycerin and intravenous β-blockers is required to quiet the ischemic episode. In this setting, GP II_bIII_a inhibitors should be considered if no contraindications are present. In patients who have had coronary angiography and PCI, correlation between angiographic findings and the 12-lead ECG should be made. Acute stent thrombosis will usually be seen on the ECG as recurrence of ST elevation. This requires emergent repeat catheterization. Conversely, patients with diffuse coronary artery disease may have ischemia due to narrowing in the nonculprit coronary arteries, precipitated by stress or tachycardia, for example. The treatment of this is anticoagulation, GP II_bIII_a inhibitors, and β-blockers.

In patients with NSTEMI, recurrent chest pain is a marker of significant risk for reinfarction, especially if transient ST segment and T-wave changes are noted or if persistent ST segment depression is associated with the initial presentation. Prompt coronary angiography and PCI are often required in this setting.

G. Pericarditis

Pericarditis is common in patients with acute MI, particularly in the course of transmural infarctions. In general, the larger the area of infarction, the more likely pericarditis will develop. Pericarditis may be clinically silent or may be associated with a pericardial rub, pleuritic chest pain, or pericardial effusion as suggested by chest radiograph or two-dimensional echocardiography. The associated chest discomfort, classically described as being relieved by sitting up, may also be associated with a description of shortness of breath and epigastric discomfort with inflammation of the contiguous diaphragm. Pericardial rubs are most commonly heard when the patient is seated with held inspiration. Late pericardial inflammation occurring 2 weeks to 3 months after MI is termed "Dressler syndrome" and most likely reflects an autoimmune mechanism. Dressler syndrome is often associated with large serosanguinous pleural and pericardial effusions, and tamponade develops in persons who die of this syndrome. The treatment of choice for Dressler syndrome is aspirin, or colchicine, and in some instances, corticosteroids may be necessary. The use of corticosteroids, however, is not generally advocated because of the high frequency of relapse when corticosteroid therapy is discontinued. Echocardiographic assessment is appropriate as a follow-up tool in these patients to determine the extent of effusion if present and to exclude tamponade or the possibility of partial myocardial rupture. Nonsteroidal anti-inflammatory drugs (NSAIDs) should be avoided in patients with ischemic heart disease, particularly those with evidence of acute infarction. Agents such as indomethacin inhibit new collagen deposition and, therefore, may impair the healing process necessary for stabilization of the infarcted region. This may, in a small number of patients, contribute to the development of myocardial rupture. When used in cases refractory to aspirin, NSAIDs should be used for the shortest time possible and tapered as rapidly as possible. In addition, recent data have linked the use of NSAIDs and cyclooxygenase-2 (COX-2) inhibitors to increased rates of cardiac events. Therefore, the use of NSAIDs and COX-2 inhibitors should be minimized or discouraged. Heparin use early in acute MI should not be stopped if pericarditis is present. However, the presence of Dressler syndrome is a contraindication to heparin use, because of its high incidence of hemorrhage into the pericardial fluid with resulting tamponade.

H. Conduction Disturbances

The presence of a conduction disturbance is associated with increased in-hospital and long-term mortality rates. The prognostic significance and management of these disturbances may vary with the location of the infarction, the type of conduction disturbance, associated clinical findings, and the extent of hemodynamic compromise. Patients whose conduction disturbances result in bradycardias and produce hemodynamic compromise generally require transvenous pacing. Bradycardias, especially those associated with inferior infarction, can often be treated with atropine. Recurrent episodes, however, warrant insertion of a pacemaker. Often ventricular pacing to provide a back-up rate is all that is required. A need for improved hemodynamics may be a reason to consider atrioventricular (AV) sequential pacing.

1. Anterior STEMI—The highest risk conduction disturbances occur in these patients. Abnormalities are present early after the onset of infarction and are usually the result of extensive infarction producing pump failure; treatment with a pacemaker may not improve the prognosis. Conduction disturbances in this circumstance are generally right bundle branch block (RBBB), with or without concomitant fascicular block. RBBB without fascicular block may have the same incidence of progression to complete heart block (20–40%)

as does an RBBB with fascicular block. Patients with RBBB and a fascicular block with anterior MI should be considered for placement of temporary transvenous pacing and be observed for evidence of progression to complete heart block, warranting permanent transvenous pacing.

Left bundle branch block (LBBB) is most often a chronic manifestation of hypertension and myocardial dysfunction rather than an acute abnormality. In a setting of acute MI, however, it is often difficult to determine whether the LBBB is new. Recommendations have been to use pacemakers for patients with LBBB known to be new; this approach has also been advocated for patients with RBBB. Given the present availability of external pacemakers, these issues appear to be less critical.

In the absence of the signs and symptoms of hemodynamic instability or evidence of the progression to heart block, it is reasonable to observe patients with RBBBs or LBBBs and to use external pacing if conduction disturbances develop. Once such a disturbance develops, a transvenous pacemaker is indicated, and it is likely that AV sequential devices would be of benefit.

2. Inferior MI—Conduction disturbances with acute inferior MI are often less critical, but they do suggest a poorer prognosis. The conduction disturbances that commonly occur represent involvement of the AV node and usually include first-degree AV block, Mobitz I (Wenckebach) or Mobitz II second-degree AV block with narrow QRS complexes, and complete heart block with a junctional rhythm. Conduction disturbances are more common in patients with right ventricular infarction. If hemodynamic stability is maintained, patients with these conduction disturbances do not require pacemakers, and they often respond to the administration of atropine (0.5 mg intravenously). If hemodynamic compromise occurs in association with either Wenckebach block or a junctional rhythm, however, or if any arrhythmia requires treatment with more than one dose of atropine, a transvenous pacemaker is warranted. Large initial or total doses of atropine can lead to tachycardia with exacerbation of ischemia and, at times, ventricular tachycardia (VT) or ventricular fibrillation (VF). For patients with right ventricular infarction and hemodynamic compromise associated with the loss of atrial kick, an AV sequential pacemaker is recommended. In general, hemodynamically significant conduction disturbances occur in patients with inferior infarction early during the evolution of infarction; late conduction disturbances are usually well tolerated. Some of these conduction disturbances respond to an intravenous infusion of 250 mg of aminophylline.

3. Mobitz II second-degree AV block—Mobitz II second-degree AV block and complete heart block with a wide QRS complex are both absolute indications for transvenous pacemaker insertion. Such disturbances can occur from electrolyte abnormalities or conduction system disease, but they are most often associated with hemodynamic abnormalities caused by bradycardia. The use of temporary AV sequential pacing may benefit patients who have hemodynamic abnormalities; these patients are also likely to require permanent pacing (see the section, Prognosis, Risk Stratification, & Management).

I. Other Arrhythmias

1. Sinus tachycardia—Sinus tachycardia occurs in up to 25% of patients with acute MI. It is a marker of physiologic stress (pain, anxiety, hypovolemia) and often indicates the presence of CHF. In some patients, such as those with right ventricular infarction, it may represent relative or absolute volume depletion. In general, although tachycardia increases myocardial oxygen consumption and can exacerbate ischemia, it should not be treated as a discrete entity. The proper approach is to treat the underlying physiologic drive. It may be unwise to block a tachycardia that is compensating for the increased cardiac work required, for example, by sepsis. Accordingly, β-blockers should only be used once it is clear that no underlying abnormality is inducing the tachycardia or that the underlying abnormality (eg, hyperthyroidism) is amenable to such treatment. Making this determination may require hemodynamic monitoring.

2. Supraventricular tachycardia—Paroxysmal supraventricular tachycardia (PSVT), atrial flutter, and atrial fibrillation can all occur with acute MI. Atrial fibrillation is by far the most common arrhythmia and is often associated with the presence of high atrial filling pressures. The presence of supraventricular tachycardia should lead to consideration of CHF as a cause. A complete differential diagnosis, including conditions such as hyperthyroidism, pulmonary embolism, pericarditis, and drug-induced arrhythmias, is appropriate. Paroxysmal supraventricular tachycardia should be treated immediately because of the high likelihood in this setting that the tachycardia will induce ischemia. Adenosine in bolus doses of 6–12 mg intravenously is the initial approach of choice and often terminates the tachycardia. If it does not, cardioversion should be considered prior to other treatment, unless the PSVT terminates and restarts recurrently. Prolonged pharmacologic management before cardioversion may complicate the procedure, and the delay may induce toxicity if the heart rate is rapid, even in the absence of overt hemodynamic compromise. For recurrent or once-terminated PSVT (depending on the mechanisms of the tachycardia; see Chapter 11), small doses of digitalis, diltiazem, verapamil, or a class I antiarrhythmic agent are reasonable choices for maintenance, as long as the indications and contraindications for each of these agents are kept in mind.

Atrial flutter and atrial fibrillation are generally markers of CHF. Frequently the diagnosis of flutter or fibrillation is made after administration of adenosine; once diagnosed, control of the ventricular response is critical. This can generally be accomplished with digitalis, verapamil, or diltiazem in conventional doses (see Chapter 12) once the CHF is treated. Intravenous diltiazem is effective in an emergency situation, usually with an initial test dose of 20–25 mg. If the response

is favorable, a titrated dose of 10–15 mg/h should be used. Intravenous diltiazem should be used cautiously in patients with acute MI and CHF. Cardioversion is indicated if a rapid ventricular response persists; the ventricular rate is difficult to control; or there are signs of hypotension, CHF, or recurrent ischemia. In general, PSVT and atrial flutter require 100 J as the initial shock energy; atrial fibrillation requires 200 J.

Arrhythmias that recur after transient reversion in response to pharmacologic maneuvers or cardioversion require additional treatment. Treatment of the underlying initiating stimulus is critical. β-Blockers can also be used to control the ventricular response acutely or for maintenance.

3. Ventricular arrhythmias—The incidence of postinfarct malignant ventricular arrhythmias in patients with acute MI appears to be diminishing, perhaps because of the use of reperfusion therapy. It also is conceivable that interventions such as intravenous β-blockers have also contributed to this decline. Because of the diminishing incidence of VT and fibrillation in patients with acute infarction, as well as an unfavorable benefit-risk ratio, the use of prophylactic lidocaine is not recommended. Although prophylactic lidocaine reduces the incidence of VF, it is associated in many series with an increase in cardiac death, possibly because it abolishes ventricular escape rhythms in patients who may also be prone to bradycardia. Because warning arrhythmias, once considered progenitors of VF, do not appear to be highly predictive, it is recommended that only symptomatic arrhythmias and VT be indications for treatment.

VT with hemodynamic compromise, angina, or pulmonary edema, and VF should be treated with immediate electric shock. Sustained monomorphic VT without hemodynamic compromise, angina, or pulmonary edema can be treated with amiodarone. Amiodarone should be administered as an initial bolus of 150 mg over 10 minutes. If arrhythmias persist, additional boluses of 150 mg every 10–15 minutes can be given; however, the total dose should never exceed 2.2 g in 24 hours. Hypotension and CHF can be induced during the acute administration of amiodarone as a result of its negative inotropic effects. If amiodarone does not relieve the symptoms or the arrhythmias, patients can be treated with intravenous procainamide. The initial loading dose is 1 g, at no more than 50 mg/min, followed by a 2–6 mg/min drip. The infusion rate should be reduced if hypotension occurs; this effect is due to procainamide's α-adrenergic effects. If successful, the drug is continued until the patient is hemodynamically stable; it can then be tapered after initiation of treatment with secondary-prevention agents and an assessment made in terms of long-term risk stratification. On rare occasions, a pacemaker may need to be placed in the right ventricle to compete with or overdrive-suppress malignant ventricular arrhythmias. This is usually reserved for rhythms refractory to pharmacologic therapy and can, on occasion, be life-saving. The ventricular pacemaker is generally set at 90–110 bpm, or whatever rate is necessary to suppress the ventricular arrhythmias.

Accelerated idioventricular rhythm occurs in up to 40% of patients and can in some instances be a marker of reperfusion. This rhythm is generally thought to be benign and is usually not treated.

J. Mural Thrombi

Patients with acute MI are at risk for the development of endocardial thrombi for a variety of reasons. Left ventricular thrombus develops in up to 40% of patients with anterior wall infarction but uncommonly in inferior infarcts. Large areas of dyskinesis with poor flow are prone to develop clots. Because there may be a return in contractility in the borders of the infarcted zone during the remodeling process, it could paradoxically be that clots develop more readily in patients with larger infarctions, but those with somewhat smaller infarctions tend to have them result in emboli more frequently. It has been recommended that all patients with an anterior wall MI be considered for anticoagulation during hospitalization and for 3–6 months thereafter. If anticoagulation is not used routinely, echocardiographic evaluation for the presence of mural thrombi is recommended. Because short-term anticoagulation until the ventricle is remodeled might well be adequate for most patients, the value of long-term (3 months or more) anticoagulation is unclear. In the absence of contraindications, it is probably worthwhile to use heparin during hospitalization and subsequently to use warfarin for 3 months for patients with anterior infarction. Because it has not been established whether low doses of warfarin are as effective as larger doses in inhibiting left ventricular mural thrombi, only a full dose (international normalized ratio [INR] 2.0–2.5) is recommended. Anticoagulation may be valuable for some patients for other reasons, such as atrial fibrillation. Patients with inferior or non-Q wave infarctions do not require routine anticoagulation following MI but should receive warfarin if mural thrombi are detected by echocardiography. Some clinicians use echocardiographic criteria to select patients who should be treated; others would treat any thrombus detected.

In the current era of routine aspirin and clopidogrel use after MI, there are few data on which patients should receive warfarin. It is prudent to fully anticoagulate patients with established mural thrombi, and those with other reasons for warfarin therapy, such as atrial fibrillation or aspirin allergy. Other cases, including anterior MI, should be judged individually with the risk of thromboembolism from mural thrombus balanced against the risk of bleeding from warfarin.

Mural thrombi can form in the atrium as well as in the ventricle. Atrial fibrillation is common in patients with CHF; in the setting of atrial fibrillation, stagnation of blood in the atrial appendage leads to a high incidence of clots. This condition can be established only with transesophageal echocardiography, but it may explain the high incidence of emboli in patients with paroxysmal atrial fibrillation. Accordingly, patients with atrial fibrillation should receive anticoagulation, not only because of their

increased incidence of thrombus but because it appears that emboli can be prevented in this group with reasonably modest doses of anticoagulants (goal INR 2.0–2.5). Anticoagulation is discussed in depth in Chapter 4.

Patients with CHF and acute MI are at increased risk for pulmonary emboli because of deep venous thrombosis in the calf and thigh. This may be prevented by the use of warfarin. An argument can be made to consider the use of warfarin in any patient with acute infarction who has had no contraindications for several months. Because aspirin was withheld in some studies, it is unclear whether it offers similar benefits, which would allow it to be substituted for warfarin. In the current era of aspirin plus thienopyridine following MI, warfarin should be considered for MI with extensive wall motion abnormality, including anterior MI, and any MI with established mural thrombus on echocardiography. However, it is probably not necessary in other patients.

K. Aneurysm and Pseudo-Aneurysms

Large areas of infarction tend to thin and bulge paradoxically. These large dyskinetic areas eventually form discrete aneurysms with defined borders. In general, treatment involves the same principles as those for patients with heart failure: vasodilatation and adequate control of filling pressures to reduce pulmonary congestion. Often patients with large dyskinetic areas will have a component of heart failure.

Occasionally, while aneurysms are forming, a myocardial rupture will occur. A small amount of rupture can become tamponaded by the pericardium, leading to what is known as a pseudo-aneurysm. Pseudo-aneurysms, which tend to have narrow necks and are not lined with endocardium, function like aneurysms in that they fill with blood during ejection, reducing systolic performance. In addition to reducing stroke volume and leading to increases in ventricular volume as a compensatory response with concomitant increases in pulmonary congestion, pseudo-aneurysms are prone to rupture. The larger the pseudo-aneurysm, the greater is the possibility of rupture. Accordingly, the diagnosis of pseudo-aneurysm usually leads to relatively prompt surgery. Although pseudo-aneurysms can occur with both anterior and inferior MIs, true aneurysms are unusual in the inferior-posterior distribution. A large aneurysmal dilatation is therefore more apt to be a pseudo-aneurysm in an inferior-posterior location.

L. Right Ventricular Infarction

Right ventricular involvement in acute inferior wall MI is common. Hemodynamically significant right ventricular dysfunction, however, is uncommon, occurring in relatively few patients with right ventricular infarction. Substantial right ventricular infarction contributing to hemodynamic compromise occurs in up to 20% of patients with inferior and posterior infarction. These patients often clinically demonstrate hypotension and elevated jugular venous pressure but clear lung fields in the setting of acute inferior wall infarction. ST segment elevation in right-sided leads (V_3R or V_4R) and right ventricular wall motion abnormalities on echocardiography help confirm the diagnosis of right ventricular involvement. With right ventricular infarction, the right ventricle becomes noncontractile, and cardiac output is maintained by increased excursion of the septum into the right ventricle and by elevated right-sided filling pressures. The incidence of high-grade AV block is also increased in patients with right ventricular infarction.

If reperfusion is not possible, the stunned right ventricle tends to resolve its dysfunction. Support entails intravenous fluid administration if left ventricular filling pressures are reduced, and occasionally the use of positive inotropic therapy or AV sequential pacing, or both, is required. Early treatment with intravenous diuretics may lead to hypotension and confound patient presentation; therefore, focused clinical examination on presentation is paramount. Patients who display the development of shock despite supportive treatment may benefit from catheter-based intervention (angioplasty and stenting) of the occluded right coronary artery. The balance between the extent of right ventricular and left ventricular dysfunction, however, determines long-term outcome.

Crenshaw BS, et al. Risk factors, angiographic patterns, and outcomes in patients with ventricular septal defect complicating acute myocardial infarction. GUSTO-I (Global Utilization of Streptokinase and TPA for Occluded Coronary Arteries) Trial Investigators. *Circulation.* 2000;101(1):27–32. [PMID: 10618300]

Figueras J, et al. Changes in hospital mortality rates in 425 patients with acute ST-elevation myocardial infarction and cardiac rupture over a 30-year period. *Circulation.* 2008;118:2783–9. [PMID: 19064683]

Hochman JS, et al. Early revascularization in acute myocardial infarction complicated by cardiogenic shock. SHOCK Investigators. Should We Emergently Revascularize Occluded Coronaries for Cardiogenic Shock. *N Engl J Med.* 1999;341(9): 625–32. [PMID: 10460813]

Welch PJ, et al. Management of ventricular arrhythmias: a trial-based approach. *J Am Coll Cardiol.* 1999;34(3):621–30. [PMID: 10483940]

▶ Prognosis, Risk Stratification, & Management

A. Risk Predictors

1. Infarct size—Infarct size is an important determinant of long-term risk: the larger the infarction, the poorer is the long-term prognosis. This association is easy to demonstrate in patients with first infarctions. In patients with multiple infarctions, the cumulative amount of damage is predictive. Measures that estimate cumulative infarct size (eg, ejection fraction, sestamibi scanning) provide important prognostic information. Nonetheless, the presence of an adverse prognosis does not, in and of itself, mandate a more aggressive therapeutic approach. However,

ACE inhibitors and β-blockers are important adjunctive therapies.

2. Infarct type—Patients with NSTEMI are more prone to recurrent episodes of chest discomfort and infarction than are patients with STEMI. Patients with STEMI have an adverse short-term prognosis and should be considered for immediate reperfusion therapy; they often manifest arrhythmias that, especially in association with a low left ventricular ejection fraction, are an important marker of an adverse prognosis. Often these are the patients who have CHF during hospitalization for acute infarction. Their prognosis is worse than that of patients without heart failure, even if the left ventricular ejection fraction appears reasonably well preserved.

3. Malignant arrhythmias—Many patients who suffer malignant arrhythmias during evolution of the infarction are also at increased risk. The one exception appears to be patients with primary VF (ie, VF with no complication of infarction).

B. Risk Assessment

Advanced age (> 65 years), prior MI, anterior location of infarction, postinfarction angina, NSTEMI, mechanical complications of infarction, CHF, and the presence of diabetes all suggest higher risk for reinfarction or death in the 6 months following infarction. These patients require aggressive risk stratification prior to hospital discharge after infarction.

1. Myocardial ischemia—Patients with recurrent ischemia during hospitalization are generally considered unstable because of the adverse prognosis associated with recurrent angina following MI. For patients with multiple episodes of recurrent chest discomfort, or ischemia in a distribution distant from the current infarction, cardiac catheterization is recommended to permit consideration of PCI.

In patients without complications, who are not receiving reperfusion therapy, ECG treadmill stress tests provide additional prognostic information. Thallium or sestamibi scintigraphy adds to the sensitivity and specificity of this analysis. Nuclear or echocardiographic imaging can be used in patients whose ECGs cannot be interpreted because of drug effects, resting ST-T wave changes, or conduction disturbances. Patients who are unable to exercise may benefit from pharmacologic stress tests, such as dobutamine echocardiography or dipyridamole or adenosine nuclear stress imaging. The inability to exercise is in itself a marker of poor prognosis.

Patients who have received thrombolytics or PCI and have not had recurrent episodes of chest discomfort constitute a very low-risk group for which the ability of any stress testing method to predict events is significantly reduced. Generally, however, patients who have been treated with thrombolytic agents and have evidence of ischemia undergo invasive investigation with cardiac catheterization.

The evidence that the prognosis of patients with NSTEMI is adequately determined by stress testing is controversial and in part depends on the nature of the stress procedure, perhaps including whether patients exercise vigorously enough. There is some suggestion that because most stress tests during acute hospitalization tend to be submaximal, a maximal stress test 6–8 weeks after the infarction is most appropriate for thorough risk stratification.

2. Ventricular function—Patients with complications of infarction or any findings of CHF should have a noninvasive evaluation of ventricular function during their acute hospitalization. Assuming the absence of intercurrent events, one evaluation of ventricular function generally suffices.

In the absence of such an assessment, a stress echocardiogram can provide information concerning both ischemia and ventricular performance. Advocates believe that the combination of these parameters is important; detractors argue that the evaluation of ischemia is less complete than can be accomplished with radionuclide scintigraphy.

The evaluation of some patients with poor ventricular function may also require determining the presence of viable but dysfunctional myocardium (stunned or hibernating regions). Sophisticated metabolic studies using positron emission tomography seem to have the most promise for delineating the regions apt to improve with revascularization; however, they are not widely available for routine use. The response of dysfunctional regions may also be evaluated with dobutamine echocardiography (improved function is thought to be predictive of viable myocardium) or delayed thallium imaging (delayed uptake suggests viability). The absence of late gadolinium uptake by injured myocardium on magnetic resonance imaging also suggests viability.

3. Arrhythmias—Patients who have VT or recurrent episodes of VF after the first day require further evaluation. Evaluation is mandatory for patients who have recurrent arrhythmias without easily remediable causes, especially sustained VT, which generally requires invasive electrophysiologic studies. Although treadmill- and ambulatory ECG-guided therapies are equivalent in some studies, the use of invasive electrophysiologic studies to select and titrate antiarrhythmic agents or choose a mechanical device provides one approach. Recent data suggest that if the ejection fraction is < 35% and VT is present that implantable cardioverter-defibrillators (ICDs) save lives.

At present, it is unclear how to manage less severe arrhythmias, which may include frequent ectopy or nonsustained VT. Signal-averaged ECG can be used in such patients; although a negative study is reassuring, the sensitivity of the procedure for detecting risk is inadequate. Recent data suggest that prophylactic ICDs in the 6 weeks following MI for ejection fraction < 35% do not reduce mortality. Therefore, depressed ejection fraction alone, in the absence of life-threatening arrhythmias, following MI is not an indication for ICD therapy. Patients should have optimal medical therapy, and left ventricular ejection fraction should be reassessed after 6 weeks.

Patients who have had bradycardias often require pacemakers. Long-term pacemakers improve the prognosis for patients in whom complete heart block has developed via a mechanism involving bundle branch block. Some clinicians advocate pacing for patients who had transient complete heart block without the development of bundle branch blocks (those with inferior MI and narrow QRS complexes), but supportive data are not conclusive. There also is controversy concerning the use of pacemakers in patients with conduction disturbance such as RBBB and anterior fascicular block, who may (or may not) have had transient Mobitz II second-degree AV block; the benefits of pacing have yet to be established.

C. Risk Management

Patients with recurrent ischemia, severe ventricular arrhythmias, reduced ejection fraction (< 40%), or evidence of severe ischemia during stress testing require cardiac catheterization. Although, in general, treatment is guided by anatomic considerations and their relationship to a long-term prognosis, the ability to predict—from the anatomy—which vessels are apt to be involved in subsequent events is poor. Furthermore, it is unclear that mechanical interventions will reduce the incidence of infarction or death except in well-defined subsets of patients (eg, those with left main disease, proximal three-vessel disease, and a reduced ejection fraction).

1. Risk factor modification—Central to the patient's in-hospital treatment is the identification of factors that increase the risk for progression of coronary artery disease. These include the traditional risk factors for atherosclerosis: hypertension, diabetes, smoking, cholesterol abnormalities, family history, and a sedentary lifestyle. Attempts to modify the diet, stop smoking, and increase exercise should begin once the patient has left the intensive care unit. Although such efforts will vary with each patient, a structured program with active follow-up of patients to ensure some level of success may be helpful.

Recent statin therapy trials support aggressive reduction in cholesterol for the stabilization, and possibly regression, of atherosclerosis. Therefore, a very aggressive approach toward the reduction of low-density lipoprotein (LDL) cholesterol and increases in high-density lipoprotein is justified early (within the first 24–48 hours) in postinfarction management. All post-MI patients should receive a statin and aim to achieve an LDL of < 70 mg/dL.

2. Secondary prevention—β-Blockers should be given to all patients who have had acute STEMIs and NSTEMIs, with or without reperfusion therapy. Patients with CHF tend to benefit most with gradual titration of dose.

Although secondary-prevention trials with aspirin have not indicated statistically significant benefits, most studies do show a trend toward improvement, and meta-analysis supports the concept that aspirin improves prognosis after acute infarction. Whether this benefit is synergistic with the effects of β-blockers is unclear. Nonetheless, it appears reasonable for patients to start taking low doses of aspirin (81–325 mg/day) after acute MI and to continue aspirin long-term. Patients treated with primary PCI should be treated with aspirin.

Long-term treatment with ACE inhibitors is recommended for patients at risk for ventricular remodeling and the sequelae associated with that process. In general, this includes patients with left ventricular ejection fractions of < 45%. Given the results of recent trials, even patients with a low normal ejection fraction after infarction should be considered for ACE inhibitor treatment, particularly with an anterior MI.

3. Rehabilitation—Studies of exercise rehabilitation have been confounded by the fact that individuals who participate in such programs generally have favorable risk factor and psychological profiles that lessen their risk of recurrent events. It has been argued that the improved prognosis of such patients is related to these initial characteristics—and not to the effects of exercise training. Nonetheless, exercise training clearly improves peripheral muscle efficiency, and intense long-term physical training (5 days a week for at least 9 months) has been shown to reduce the development of cardiac ischemia. Therefore, exercise rehabilitation programs are recommended whenever possible for postinfarction patients.

The amount of exercise prescribed must obviously be based on the patient's heart rate and blood pressure. These should be monitored as the patients start to walk during the convalescent phase in the hospital, and marked increases (eg, blood pressure > 140/90 mm Hg) should be avoided. The patient's rehabilitation activity schedule should be reduced if this level of hypertension occurs. This may also indicate the need for treatment with β-blockers or ACE inhibitors to reduce the labile hypertensive response. In any event, the response of blood pressure and heart rate to exercise must be monitored. Phase II of the program begins at hospital dismissal and generally continues for 8–12 weeks. Objectives should include further patient education, risk factor modification, and gradual resumption of normal work and recreational activities.

4. Psychological factors—It is now clear that as many as 20–25% of patients with acute MI meet formal clinical criteria for depression. It also appears that this is an adverse prognostic feature and that such patients have increased morbidity and mortality rates. Although there is some argument that this is so because these patients have more severe disease, this hypothesis has not been supported by recent studies. It may well be that whatever leads to depression is negatively synergistic with underlying coronary artery disease, as suggested by the increase in catecholamines in such patients. Regardless of the mechanism, however, careful consideration of the presence or absence of depression in patients is recommended. Psychological consultation should be sought for patients in whom depression is suspected, and treatment should be initiated to improve both the quality of the individual's life and—to the extent that there is an interaction with ischemic heart disease—the prognosis. Because tricyclic antidepressants initially liberate catecholamines and may thereby induce adverse effects, drug treatment has previously been thought to be problematic in cardiovascular patients. On the other hand, these agents have membrane-stabilizing effects that may reduce the propensity to arrhythmias, and it is believed that the potential for risk has been exaggerated. Newer agents that antagonize serotonin as their primary mode of action may be safer, but cognitive therapy has also been shown to be effective.

Ades PA. Cardiac rehabilitation and secondary prevention of coronary heart disease. *N Engl J Med.* 2001;345(12):892–902. [PMID: 11565523]

Antman EM, et al. The TIMI risk score for unstable angina/non-ST elevation MI: a method for prognostication and therapeutic decision making. *JAMA.* 2000;284(7):835–42. [PMID: 10938172]

Hohnloser SH, et al; DINAMIT Investigators. Prophylactic use of an implantable cardioverter-defibrillator after acute myocardial infarction. *N Engl J Med.* 2004;351(24):2481–8.

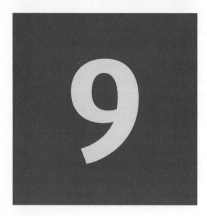

Cardiogenic Shock

Edward McNulty, MD

ESSENTIALS OF DIAGNOSIS

- ► Tissue hypoperfusion: depressed mental status, cool extremities, decreased urinary output.
- ► Hypotension: systolic blood pressure < 90 mm Hg.
- ► Reduced cardiac output: cardiac index < 2.2 L/min/m².
- ► Adequate intravascular volume: pulmonary artery wedge pressure > 15 mm Hg.

► General Considerations

Cardiogenic shock is an extremely morbid condition. Despite recent advances in treatment, nearly 50% of patients with cardiogenic shock still do not survive to hospital discharge. Cardiogenic shock develops as a result of the failure of the heart in its function as a pump, resulting in inadequate cardiac output. This failure is most commonly caused by extensive myocardial damage from an acute myocardial infarction (MI), but other mechanical complications of an acute MI, valve lesions, arrhythmias, and cardiomyopathies can also lead to cardiogenic shock.

► Definition

Cardiogenic shock is defined by both the clinical signs of a reduced cardiac output and associated hemodynamic findings. Clinical signs of reduced cardiac output include cool extremities, weak distal pulses, altered mental status, and diminished urinary output (> 30 mL/h). Hemodynamic findings in cardiogenic shock include a reduced cardiac output without evidence of hypovolemia. One commonly used set of hemodynamic criteria are as follows: (1) a systolic blood pressure of < 90 mm Hg for at least 30 minutes (or the need for medications or devices to maintain a systolic blood pressure ≥ 90 mm Hg), (2) a pulmonary capillary wedge pressure (PCWP) of > 15 mm Hg (which excludes hypovolemia), and (3) a cardiac index < 2.2 L/min/m².

► Etiology

Acute MI accounts for most cases of cardiogenic shock. Acute MI results in cardiogenic shock in 5–10% of patients presenting for emergency care; however, it is likely that cardiogenic shock develops in many more patients following an acute MI, but they do not survive to receive medical attention. Cardiogenic shock may occur in a patient with a massive first infarction, or it may occur with a smaller infarction in a patient with a weakened heart from prior MIs. "Mechanical" complications of an acute MI can also cause shock, and these include ventricular septal defect (VSD), acute mitral regurgitation as a result of papillary muscle rupture, and myocardial free wall rupture with tamponade. Right ventricular infarction in the absence of significant left ventricular infarction or dysfunction can lead to shock. Refractory tachyarrhythmias or bradyarrhythmias, usually in the setting of preexisting left ventricular dysfunction, are occasionally a cause of shock and can occur with either ventricular or supraventricular arrhythmias. Cardiogenic shock may occur in patients with end-stage cardiomyopathies (ischemic, valvular, hypertrophic, restrictive, or idiopathic in origin). Cardiogenic shock may also be the presenting manifestation of acute myocarditis (infectious, toxic, rheumatologic, or idiopathic). A more recently recognized entity is **stress cardiomyopathy** (also known as apical ballooning syndrome or takotsubo cardiomyopathy) in which severe heart failure and sometimes cardiogenic shock result from extreme emotional distress. Finally, certain endocrine abnormalities may cause severe cardiac dysfunction and cardiogenic shock (Table 9–1).

Babaev A, et al. Trends in management and outcomes of patients with acute myocardial infarction complicated by cardiogenic shock. *JAMA.* 2005;294(4):448–54. [PMID: 16046651]
Hochman JS, et al. Cardiogenic shock complicating acute myocardial infarction–etiologies, management and outcome: a report from the SHOCK Trial Registry. Should We Emergently Revascularize Occluded Coronaries for Cardiogenic Shock?

J Am Coll Cardiol. 2000;36(3 Suppl A):1063–70. [PMID: 10985706]

Sharkey SW, et al. Acute and reversible cardiomyopathy provoked by stress in women from the United States. *Circulation.* 2005;111(4):472–9. [PMID: 15687136]

▶ Pathogenesis

The principle feature of shock is hypotension with evidence of end-organ hypoperfusion. In cardiogenic shock, this occurs as a consequence of inadequate cardiac function. The usual response to low cardiac output is sympathetic stimulation to increase cardiac performance and maintain vascular tone. This results in tachycardia and increased myocardial contractility (β-adrenergic–mediated effects) and peripheral vasoconstriction (an α-adrenergic–mediated effect). The classic patient with cardiogenic shock has evidence of peripheral vasoconstriction (cool, moist skin) and tachycardia. Corresponding typical hemodynamics are a reduced cardiac output and increased systemic vascular resistance (SVR), defined as:

$$\text{SVR (in dynes} \times \text{s/cm}^5) = (\text{mean arterial pressure} - \text{right atrial pressure})/(\text{cardiac output})$$

Recent evidence suggests that many patients with cardiogenic shock do not have these typical hemodynamics and instead have a lower SVR much like patients in septic shock. In fact, it has been postulated that a systemic inflammatory response–like syndrome with a low SVR may be encountered in up to 25% of patients in cardiogenic shock. Furthermore, patients with severe septic shock often have depressed myocardial function, and patients with cardiogenic shock can have a component of hypovolemia. Thus, there can be considerable overlap in pathophysiologies.

A. Cardiogenic Shock after Acute MI

If at least 40% of the left ventricular myocardial muscle mass is lost, either acutely or as a result of prior damage, cardiogenic shock can result from pump failure (ie, there is not sufficient left ventricular muscle mass to maintain forward cardiac output). This usually occurs as a consequence of an MI. The initial event in an acute MI is obstruction of a coronary artery, commonly termed the "infarct-related artery." The acute obstruction decreases oxygen supply to a portion of the heart, resulting in myocardial ischemia and infarction, which in turn leads to diminished myocardial contractility. The ensuing drop in cardiac output and blood pressure leads to decreased perfusion pressures in other coronary beds. (Coronary perfusion becomes compromised when the aortic diastolic pressure falls below 50–55 mm Hg.) This results in further ischemia, especially if stenoses are present in these non–infarct-related vessels, and additional deterioration in left ventricular function occurs. Indeed, most patients with shock after acute MI have extensive coronary disease, and mortality correlates with the extent of coronary disease (Figure 9–1).

The process of ischemia and infarction leading to myocardial dysfunction leading to further ischemia, and so on, has been appropriately termed "a vicious cycle." Evidence for this vicious cycle is found in autopsy studies that show infarct extension at the edges of an infarct in addition to discrete, remote infarctions throughout the ventricle. This also explains the finding that cardiogenic shock can occur immediately, provided sufficient myocardium is dysfunctional, or occur hours after the initial infarct as a consequence of this vicious cycle. Tissue hypoperfusion also leads to accumulation of lactic acid. Acidemia is detrimental to left ventricular contractility, and this is another example of a vicious cycle contributing to the pathophysiology of cardiogenic shock.

B. Mechanical Complications of Acute MI

The pathophysiology of cardiogenic shock due to mechanical complications of acute MI is somewhat different. The three main mechanical problems are (1) acute mitral regurgitation as a consequence of papillary muscle rupture, (2) VSD, and (3) myocardial free wall rupture leading to cardiac tamponade. These mechanical problems all occur in a bimodal distribution, with some occurring earlier in the presentation and others occurring later, and are a consequence of weakened, necrotic myocardium.

The papillary muscles anchor the mitral valve apparatus to the left ventricle. Proper papillary muscle function is vital in ensuring that the two mitral valve leaflets close

Table 9–1. Causes of Cardiogenic Shock

I. Acute myocardial infarction (MI)
   A. Pump failure
   B. Mechanical complications of acute MI
      1. Acute mitral regurgitation
      2. Ventricular septal defect
      3. Free wall rupture/tamponade
   C. Right ventricular MI
II. End-stage, severe cardiomyopathies secondary to
   A. Valvular disease
   B. Chronic ischemic disease
   C. Restrictive/infiltrative
   D. Idiopathic
III. Acute myocarditis: viral/infectious, toxic
IV. Stress cardiomyopathy
V. ndocrine disease (eg, hypothyroidism, pheochromocytoma)
   A. Bradyarrhythmias
   B. Tachyarrhythmias
VI. Secondary to medications
VII. Posttraumatic

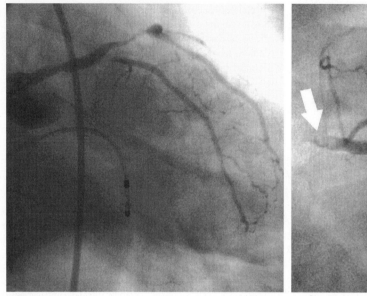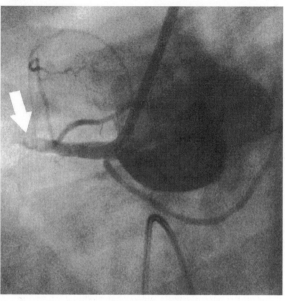

A   B

▲ **Figure 9–1.** Coronary angiogram of patient with an acute myocardial infarction and cardiogenic shock. Severe disease in left coronary system (**A**) and acute occlusion with thrombus in the right coronary artery (**B**).

completely to prevent leakage or regurgitation of blood backward into the left atrium. Papillary muscle rupture is a term used somewhat erroneously; rupture and avulsion of the entire papillary muscle usually result in such severe regurgitation that it is rapidly fatal. If only a portion of the papillary muscle ruptures, then severe mitral regurgitation ensues, leading to pulmonary edema and a reduced forward cardiac output. This accounts for up to 7% of patients with cardiogenic shock after an acute MI. The sympathetic nervous system response to cardiac failure results in increased SVR (afterload) and a further increase in the regurgitant fraction, another example of a vicious cycle contributing to cardiogenic shock.

Rupture of the myocardial free wall results in bleeding into the relatively nondistendible pericardial space and leads rapidly to pericardial tamponade and cardiovascular collapse. Often this is immediately fatal, but occasionally, patients survive and cardiogenic shock develops. The incidence of free wall rupture in patients with cardiogenic shock is as high as 3%.

Rupture of the intraventricular septum with the formation of a VSD has an incidence of approximately 0.3% in patients with acute MI and accounts for up to 6% of patients with cardiogenic shock after an acute MI. A large VSD causes significant shunting of blood from the left ventricle to the right ventricle and results in right ventricular volume and pressure overload (Figure 9–2). Shock usually develops as a consequence of reduced forward cardiac output. As with acute mitral regurgitation, the sympathetic nervous system response results in

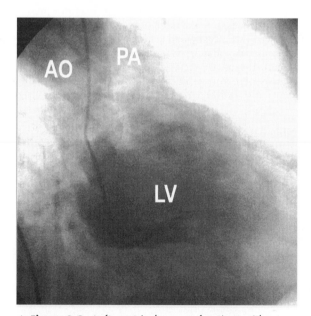

▲ **Figure 9–2.** Left ventriculogram of patient with ventricular septal defect. Note that contrast injected into the left ventricle (LV) opacifies both the aorta (AO) and the pulmonary artery (PA). (The right ventricle is superimposed upon the left in this projection and therefore is not visualized.)

increased afterload, thereby shunting an even larger fraction of the cardiac output across the interventricular septum.

C. Right Ventricular Infarction

Right ventricular infarctions occur in approximately 40% of patients with inferior MIs. Right ventricular infarctions may result in cardiogenic shock without significant left ventricular dysfunction. Failure of the right ventricle leads to diminished right ventricular stroke volume, which results in a decreased volume of blood returning to the left ventricle. This markedly diminished left ventricular preload, even with normal left ventricular contractility, causes a decreased systemic cardiac output. The right ventricle also becomes dilated, which results in displacement of the intraventricular septum to the left. If severe, this can actually impair left ventricular filling, with physiology similar to that seen in cardiac tamponade. Since left ventricular filling pressures are not elevated in pure right ventricular failure, pulmonary congestion will not be evident.

D. Arrhythmias

A variety of arrhythmias can contribute to the development of shock. A sustained arrhythmia, that is, one that does not culminate in ventricular fibrillation and sudden death, is generally a cause of shock only in the already compromised ventricle. Atrial and ventricular tachyarrhythmias can result in diminished time for ventricular filling in diastole as well as the loss of the atrial contribution to ventricular diastolic filling. This results in a diminished preload, which in turn results in a decreased stroke volume. These factors may be enough to result in cardiogenic shock in patients with already impaired left ventricular function or with conditions such as severe aortic stenosis in which the left ventricle is especially sensitive to filling pressures. Bradyarrhythmias reduce cardiac output as a consequence of the slow heart rate. Because total cardiac output is a function of heart rate and stroke volume (cardiac output = stroke volume × heart rate), a markedly decreased heart rate, especially with concomitant left ventricular dysfunction may, result in shock.

E. Other Causes of Cardiogenic Shock

Many forms of heart disease can result in an end-stage dilated cardiomyopathy. These patients may be in such acutely decompensated states that they are in frank cardiogenic shock.

Birnbaum Y. Ventricular septal rupture after acute myocardial infarction. *N Engl J Med.* 2002;347(18):1426–32. [PMID: 12409546]

Bowers TR, et al. Patterns of coronary compromise resulting in acute right ventricular ischemic dysfunction. *Circulation.* 2002;106(9):1104–9. [PMID: 12196336]

Crenshaw BS, et al. Risk factors, angiographic patterns, and outcomes in patients with ventricular septal defect complicating acute myocardial infarction. GUSTO-I (Global Utilization of Streptokinase and TPA for Occluded Arteries) Trial Investigators. *Circulation.* 2000;101(1):27–32. [PMID: 10618300]

Jacobs AK, et al. Cardiogenic shock caused by right ventricular infarction: a report from the SHOCK registry. *J Am Coll Cardiol.* 2003;41(8):1273–9. [PMID: 12706920]

Kohsaka S, et al. Systemic inflammatory response syndrome after acute myocardial infarction complicated by cardiogenic shock. *Arch Intern Med.* 2005;165(14):1643–50. [PMID: 16043684]

Menon V, et al. Outcome and profile of ventricular septal rupture with cardiogenic shock after myocardial infarction: a report from the SHOCK trial registry. Should We Emergently Revascularize Occluded Coronaries in Cardiogenic Shock? *J Am Coll Cardiol.* 2000;36(3 Suppl A):1110–6. [PMID: 10985713]

Slater J, et al. Cardiogenic shock due to cardiac free-wall rupture or tamponade after acute myocardial infarction: a report from the SHOCK trial registry. Should We Emergently Revascularize Occluded Coronaries for Cardiogenic Shock? *J Am Coll Cardiol.* 2000;36(3 Suppl A):1117–22. [PMID: 10985714]

Webb JG, et al. Implications of the timing of onset of cardiogenic shock after acute myocardial infarction: a report from the SHOCK trial registry. Should We Emergently Revascularize Occluded Coronaries in Cardiogenic Shock? *J Am Coll Cardiol.* 2000;36(3 Suppl A):1084–90. [PMID: 10985709]

Wong SC, et al. Angiographic findings and clinical correlates in patients with cardiogenic shock complicating acute myocardial infarction: a report from the SHOCK trial registry. Should We Emergently Revascularize Occluded Coronaries for Cardiogenic Shock? *J Am Coll Cardiol.* 2000;36(3 Suppl A):1077–83. [PMID: 10985708]

▶ Clinical Findings

A. History

The symptoms that precede the development of cardiogenic shock depend on the cause. Patients with acute MIs often have the typical history of acute onset of chest pain, possibly in the setting of known coronary artery disease. Often, however, patients seek medical care days later following unrecognized MIs once cardiogenic shock has developed. In such cases, there is often no history of antecedent chest pain, but instead the insidious onset of dyspnea and weakness culminating in shock. Patients may be obtunded and lethargic as a result of decreased central nervous system perfusion. Mechanical complications of acute MI tend to occur several days to a week following the initial infarction but can occur earlier. They may be heralded by chest pain, but they more commonly present abruptly as acute dyspnea. Patients with arrhythmias may have a history of palpitations, presyncope, syncope, or a sensation of skipped beats. Regardless of the cause, however, by the time shock develops, the patient may be unable to give any useful history.

B. Physical Examination

The physical examination reveals signs consistent with hypoperfusion.

1. Vital signs—Hypotension is present (systolic blood pressure < 90 mm Hg). The heart rate is commonly elevated, and the respiratory rate is generally increased as a result of hypoxia from pulmonary congestion.

2. Neurologic—Patients may be confused, lethargic, or obtunded as a consequence of cerebral hypoperfusion.

3. Pulmonary—Patients may use accessory muscles of respiration and may have paradoxical respirations. The chest examination in most cases shows diffuse rales, often to the apices. Patients with isolated right ventricular infarction will not have pulmonary congestion.

4. Cardiovascular system—Jugular venous pulsations are commonly elevated. Peripheral pulses will be weak. The apical impulse is displaced in patients with dilated cardiomyopathies, and the intensity of heart sounds is diminished, especially in patients with pericardial effusions. A third or fourth heart sound suggesting significant left ventricular dysfunction and/or elevated filling pressures may be present. A mitral regurgitation murmur (holosystolic, usually at the apex) or a VSD murmur (harsh, holosystolic at the sternal border) can help in diagnosing these causes. Patients with a free wall rupture that is partially contained may have a pericardial friction rub. Patients with significant right heart failure may have signs on abdominal examination of liver enlargement with a pulsatile liver in the presence of significant tricuspid regurgitation.

5. Extremities—Peripheral edema may be present. Cyanosis and cool, moist extremities are indicative of diminished tissue perfusion. Profound peripheral vasoconstriction can result in mottling of the skin (livedo reticularis).

C. Laboratory Findings

Patients with recent or acute MIs will have elevations in cardiac-specific enzymes (CPK-MB, troponin). Renal and hepatic hypoperfusion may result in elevations in serum creatinine and in transaminases (alanine transaminase [ALT] and aspartate transaminase [AST]). Coagulation abnormalities may be present in patients with hepatic congestion or hepatic hypoperfusion. An anion gap acidosis may be present, and the serum lactate level may be elevated.

D. Diagnostic Studies

While further diagnostic studies are important in clarifying the diagnosis, it must be emphasized that rapid, definitive therapy should not be delayed once the diagnosis is apparent. In general, patients with cardiogenic shock and suspected acute MI should proceed to cardiac catheterization as quickly as possible.

1. Electrocardiography—The electrocardiogram (ECG) may be helpful in distinguishing between causes of cardiogenic shock. Patients with coronary disease and acute MI may show evidence of both old (Q waves) and new infarctions (ST segment elevation). Right-sided chest leads in patients with inferior MIs can detect the presence of a right ventricular infarction (ST elevation in V_4R). Although ST elevations are often present on the ECGs of patients with cardiogenic shock, patients with non-ST segment elevation MIs represent up to 50% of patients with cardiogenic shock. The ECG also readily aids in the diagnosis of arrhythmias contributing to cardiogenic shock.

2. Chest radiography—The chest radiograph may show an enlarged cardiac silhouette (cardiomegaly) and evidence of pulmonary congestion in patients with severe left ventricular failure. A VSD or severe mitral regurgitation associated with an acute infarction will lead to pulmonary congestion but not necessarily cardiomegaly. Findings of pulmonary congestion may be less prominent—or absent—in the case of predominantly right ventricular failure or in patients with superimposed hypovolemia.

3. Echocardiography—Given that it is noninvasive and able to be performed rapidly at the bedside, echocardiography is extremely useful in the diagnosis of cardiogenic shock. Furthermore, mechanical complications of an acute infarction can be readily diagnosed via echocardiography. Information obtained by echocardiography includes assessment of right and left ventricular size and function, valvular function (stenosis or regurgitation), right and left ventricular filling pressures, and the presence of pericardial fluid with tamponade.

4. Hemodynamic monitoring—Routine use of invasive pulmonary artery catheters in critically ill patients is controversial. However, this procedure is recommended in certain situations and can help in establishing the diagnosis and cause of cardiogenic shock. Catheters are usually placed from a central vein into the right heart and advanced into a pulmonary artery. By occluding flow temporarily in a branch of the pulmonary artery ("wedging" the catheter), an estimate of left atrial pressure can be obtained (the PCWP). The presence of a wedge pressure higher than 15 mm Hg in a patient with acute MI generally, but not always, indicates adequate intravascular volume. Patients with primarily right ventricular failure or significant superimposed hypovolemia may have cardiogenic shock with a normal or reduced PCWP. The presence of a large "v wave" on the PCWP tracing is consistent with significant mitral regurgitation, but may also be seen with a VSD or a very stiff left ventricle. A pulmonary artery catheter also allows calculation of the SVR. Hemodynamic criteria for cardiogenic shock vary and include a cardiac index of less than 2.2 L/min/m². (Cardiac index is preferred to cardiac output as a measure because it normalizes the cardiac output for body size.) It is important to note that some patients with chronic heart failure but not in cardiogenic shock have cardiac outputs in this range and are in fact ambulatory in a "compensated" state. Patients in cardiogenic shock usually have suffered an acute insult and cannot compensate.

5. Oxygen saturation—Invasive measurement of the mixed venous oxygen saturation can be obtained from pulmonary artery catheters and may be helpful in two ways.

First, knowing the mixed venous oxygen saturation allows the arteriovenous difference in oxygen content to be calculated. The arteriovenous difference in oxygen content is inversely proportional to the cardiac output; it increases as more oxygen is extracted from the blood in the setting of low cardiac output. Serial determinations can be useful in monitoring a patient's course and response to therapy. Secondly, oxygen saturations obtained invasively with a pulmonary artery catheter may also be helpful in diagnosing a VSD. The shunting of oxygenated blood from the left ventricle to the right ventricle across the septal defect results in an abnormal "oxygen saturation step-up" when comparing oxygen saturations from the right atrium with those obtained from the right ventricle.

E. Left Heart (Cardiac) Catheterization

Left heart catheterization and invasive coronary angiography should be performed without delay in patients with ST segment elevation MI, since survival and myocardial salvage depend on the time to reperfusion. This also applies to patients in cardiogenic shock with ST segment elevation. In patients with cardiogenic shock without ST-segment elevation but with evidence of MI, cardiac catheterization should be expedited as well. In the cardiac catheterization laboratory, obstructions in coronary arteries or bypass grafts can be detected, appropriate treatments planned (either bypass surgery or percutaneous coronary intervention [PCI]), and an intra-aortic balloon pump (IABP) or left ventricular assist device placed if necessary.

▶ Treatment

Although some general therapeutic considerations are applicable to all patients in cardiogenic shock, treatment is most effective when the cause is identified. In many situations, this identification allows rapid correction of the underlying problem. In fact, survival in most forms of shock requires a quick, accurate diagnosis. The patient is so critically ill that only prompt, directed therapy can reverse the process. The already high mortality rates in cardiogenic shock are even higher in patients for whom treatment is delayed. Therefore, although measures aimed at temporarily stabilizing the patient may provide enough time to start definitive therapy, potentially life-saving treatment can be carried out only when the cause is known (Table 9–2).

A. Acute Myocardial Infarction

In patients with cardiogenic shock caused by a large amount of infarcted or ischemic myocardium, the most effective treatment for decreasing mortality is prompt revascularization, with either PCI or coronary artery bypass grafting (CABG) surgery. A number of pharmacologic and nonpharmacologic measures may be helpful in stabilizing the patient prior to revascularization.

Table 9–2. Management of Cardiogenic Shock

I. Diagnosis[1]
  A. Electrocardiogram
  B. Chest radiography
  C. Laboratory tests (complete blood count, coagulation profile, CK-MB, cardiac troponin, electrolytes + blood urea nitrogen/creatinine, arterial blood gases)
  D. Echocardiography
  E. Pulmonary artery catheterization (if diagnosis is in question, patient receiving inotropes/vasopressors, or patient is not responding to treatment)
  F. Cardiac catheterization
II. Treatment
  A. Oxygen supplementation; intubation, ventilation
  B. Vasopressors/inotropes; consider careful intravenous fluids, arterial line and pulmonary artery catheter insertion to guide management; correct underlying causes of acidemia
  C. Intra-aortic balloon pump, if needed
  D. For suspected acute MI: aspirin, heparin, urgent cardiac catheterization, revascularization (PCI, CABG); fibrinolysis if a delay in PCI is anticipated

[1]Patients with suspected acute MI should proceed directly to cardiac catheterization; this should generally not be delayed to facilitate additional diagnostic tests.
CABG, coronary artery bypass grafting; MI, myocardial infarction; PCI, percutaneous coronary intervention.

1. Ventilation-oxygenation—Because respiratory failure usually accompanies cardiogenic shock, every effort should be made to ensure adequate ventilation and oxygenation. Adequate oxygenation is essential to avoid hypoxia and further deterioration of oxygen delivery to tissues. Patients with cardiogenic shock should receive supplemental oxygen, and many require mechanical ventilation. Hypoventilation can lead to respiratory acidosis, which could exacerbate the metabolic acidosis already caused by tissue hypoperfusion. Acidosis worsens cardiac function and makes the heart less responsive to inotropic agents. A substantial proportion of the cardiac output in patients with cardiogenic shock is devoted to the "work of breathing," so mechanical ventilation is also advantageous in this regard.

2. Fluid resuscitation—Although hypovolemia is not the primary defect in cardiogenic shock, a number of patients may be relatively hypovolemic when shock develops following MI. The causes of decreased intravascular volume include increased hydrostatic pressure and increased permeability of blood vessels as well as patients simply being volume depleted for many hours. The physical examination may not always be helpful in determining the adequacy of the left ventricular filling pressure. In selected patients, invasive monitoring with a pulmonary artery catheter can be helpful in determining the optimal volume status. Some patients with cardiogenic shock will actually have improved hemodynamics with slightly higher than normal filling pressures.

Ventricular compliance is reduced in acute ischemia; the pressure–volume relationship changes such that cardiac output may be optimized at slightly higher filling pressures. In general, a PCWP of 18–22 mm Hg is considered adequate; further increases will lead to pulmonary congestion without a concomitant gain in cardiac output. Fluid administration, when indicated by low or normal PCWP, should be undertaken in 200–300 mL boluses of saline, followed by careful reassessment of hemodynamic parameters, especially cardiac output and PCWP, and generally should not be undertaken in patients with marginal oxygenation or in those not already mechanically ventilated.

3. Inotropic/vasopressor agents—A variety of drugs are available for intravenous administration to increase the contractility of the heart, the heart rate, and peripheral vascular tone. It is important to note that these agents also increase myocardial oxygen demand; improvements in hemodynamics and blood pressure therefore come at a cost, which can be deleterious in patients with ongoing ischemia. Furthermore, β-agonists can precipitate tachyarrhythmias, and α-agonists can lead to dangerous vasoconstriction and ischemia in vital organ beds. When using these agents, attention should be given to the patient as a whole rather than focusing solely on a desired arterial pressure.

A. Digoxin—Although digoxin benefits patients with chronic congestive heart failure, it is of less benefit in cardiogenic shock because of its delayed onset of action and relatively mild potency (compared with other available agents).

B. β-Adrenergic agonists—Dopamine is an endogenous catecholamine with qualitatively different effects at varying doses. At low doses (> 3 mcg/kg/min), it predominantly stimulates dopaminergic receptors that dilate various arterial beds, the most important being the renal vasculature. Although used frequently in low doses to improve renal perfusion, there is scant evidence to support the clinical usefulness of this strategy. Intermediate doses of 3–6 mcg/kg/min cause β_1-receptor stimulation and enhanced myocardial contractility. Further increases in dosage lead to predominant α-receptor stimulation (peripheral vasoconstriction) in addition to continued β_1 stimulation and tachycardia. Dopamine increases cardiac output, and its combination of cardiac stimulation and peripheral vasoconstriction may be beneficial as initial treatment of hypotensive patients in cardiogenic shock.

Dobutamine is a synthetic sympathomimetic agent that differs from dopamine in two important ways: It does not cause renal vasodilatation, and it has a much stronger β_2 (arteriolar vasodilatory) effect. The vasodilatory effect may be deleterious in hypotensive patients because a further drop in blood pressure may occur. On the other hand, many patients with cardiogenic shock experience excessive vasoconstriction with a resultant elevation in afterload (SVR) as a result of either the natural sympathetic discharge or the treatment with inotropic agents, such as dopamine, that also have prominent vasoconstrictor effects. In such patients, the combination of cardiac stimulation and decreased afterload with dobutamine may improve cardiac output without a loss of arterial pressure.

Other agents that are used include isoproterenol and norepinephrine. Isoproterenol is also a synthetic sympathomimetic agent. It has very strong chronotropic and inotropic effects, resulting in a disproportionate increase in oxygen consumption and ischemia. It is therefore not generally recommended for cardiogenic shock except occasionally for patients with bradyarrhythmias. Norepinephrine has even stronger α and β_1 effects than dopamine and may be beneficial when a patient continues to be hypotensive despite large doses of dopamine (> 20 mcg/kg/min). A recent randomized trial suggests that norepinephrine may be superior to dopamine in the treatment of cardiogenic shock.

4. Vasodilators—Vasodilation (especially of the arterioles to reduce SVR) can be effective in increasing cardiac output in patients with heart failure by countering the peripheral vasoconstriction caused by endogenous catecholamines. Although these agents have a role in treating acute, decompensated heart failure, they are rarely used in patients with cardiogenic shock given the risk of worsening hypotension. The IABP (see below) is generally more effective for reducing SVR without the risk of untoward hypotension.

5. Circulatory support devices—Among the mechanical devices developed to assist the left ventricle until more definitive therapy can be undertaken, the IABP has been in use the longest and is the most well studied. The IABP is placed in the descending aorta, usually via the femoral artery. Its inflation and deflation are timed to the cardiac cycle (generally synchronized with the ECG). The balloon inflates in diastole immediately following aortic valve closure. The augmentation of diastolic pressure that occurs when the balloon inflates increases coronary perfusion as well as that of other organs. The balloon deflates at the end of diastole, immediately before left ventricular contraction, abruptly decreasing afterload and thereby enhancing left ventricular ejection. Unlike β-agonists, these benefits come without increases in myocardial demand.

Indications for use of the IABP include cardiogenic shock, especially when caused by ventricular septal rupture and acute mitral regurgitation. In both ventricular septal rupture and mitral regurgitation, the principle benefit is the decrease in afterload that occurs as the balloon deflates; this results in a larger fraction of the left ventricular volume being ejected forward into the aorta rather than into the left atrium (mitral regurgitation) or the right ventricle (ventricular septal rupture). An IABP should be placed as soon as possible in an effort to support these patients until emergency surgery can be performed. The most common side effects of the IABP are local vascular complications, but these have diminished substantially with the smaller caliber devices used currently. Nonrandomized data have shown that patients in cardiogenic shock treated with an IABP fare better than those not treated with an IABP. Recently, a randomized trial (IABP SHOCK II) showed similar outcomes with or without IABP use following revascularization. The IABP is therefore most useful as a temporizing agent, either to keep patients alive until revascularization or until more aggressive support can be initiated in patients who may be transplant candidates.

A number of other circulatory support devices have been developed in recent years with the ability to provide even more circulatory support than the IABP. Devices can be implanted surgically (such as the left ventricular assist device [LVAD]) or percutaneously and are capable of creating flow rates of 3–5 L/min (close to a normal cardiac output). These devices can be used until cardiac transplantation can be facilitated or occasionally to support patients who ultimately recover. Large-scale, randomized data to support their use are lacking as of this time.

6. Revascularization—Revascularization, either by PCI or CABG surgery, decreases mortality in patients in whom cardiogenic shock develops following MI. The multicenter, randomized SHOCK trial (Should We Emergently Revascularize Occluded Coronaries for Cardiogenic Shock) showed a trend toward improved survival at 30 days in patients randomized to early revascularization (either PCI or CABG within 6 hours of enrollment). The survival benefit for early revascularization became significant at 6 months, a benefit that persisted to 6 years. Although the mortality of patients treated with a strategy of early revascularization was still high, the absolute reduction in mortality was substantial (13% at 1 year); stated alternatively, the "number needed to treat" with revascularization was approximately eight to prevent one death at 1 year, which is low and provides strong support for revascularization in these circumstances. Of note, patients 75 years of age and older did not benefit from revascularization at 1 year in the randomized trial but did benefit in the nonrandomized but much larger SHOCK registry. Many experts believe that the SHOCK trial was underpowered to show a mortality difference at 30 days and, based on the 6-month and now 6-year data, American College of Cardiology (ACC)/American Heart Association (AHA) guidelines recommend emergency revascularization for patients (especially those under the age of 75) with cardiogenic shock complicating acute MI.

A. PERCUTANEOUS CORONARY INTERVENTION—Patients undergoing PCI in the SHOCK trial had a similar benefit to those having bypass surgery. Mortality from cardiogenic shock has decreased over the past decade in parallel with increasing use of PCI for these patients. Although retrospective, other studies from large populations have shown that PCI use is associated with lower mortality in patients with cardiogenic shock.

B. CABG SURGERY—Despite the marked absolute reduction in mortality observed among patients treated with bypass surgery in the SHOCK trial, only a small proportion of patients with cardiogenic shock undergo urgent bypass surgery (approximately 3% in the National Registry of Myocardial Infarction 2004 database). Nevertheless, patients with multivessel disease in cardiogenic shock should be evaluated for bypass surgery, and for patients with mechanical complications of MI, surgery offers the best hope for survival at present.

7. Fibrinolytic therapy—Fibrinolytic therapy refers to treating patients with acute ST segment elevation MIs with drugs that have fibrinolytic properties (that dissolve occlusive thrombus within coronary arteries or grafts). Although PCI is superior therapy to fibrinolysis for ST segment elevation MI, fibrinolysis is the recommended therapy if there will be a considerable delay in facilitating PCI. Most trials of fibrinolytic therapy excluded patients with cardiogenic shock. In earlier trials that included patients with cardiogenic shock, there was no benefit to fibrinolytic therapy over placebo. It has been suggested that the low-flow state present in shock may contribute to the limited efficacy of fibrinolytic therapy. In contrast to these older studies, in the SHOCK trial and registry, patients treated medically with fibrinolytic therapy fared better than those medically treated without fibrinolytic therapy. Additional evidence comes from meta-analyses of more recent fibrinolytic trials that revealed improved survival among hypotensive patients treated with fibrinolytics. Fibrinolytic therapy for patients with an acute MI complicated by cardiogenic shock may be useful for patients early in their presentation in whom there will be a delay in timely cardiac catheterization and revascularization.

8. Other medical therapies—Aspirin and heparin are indicated in patients with MIs and cardiogenic shock, provided mechanical complications requiring surgery are not present. β-Blockers are contraindicated in patients in cardiogenic shock. Platelet glycoprotein (GP) II_bIII_a inhibitors block the final pathway of platelet activation and aggregation and are beneficial in patients with acute coronary syndromes. Several clinical trials of GP II_bIII_a inhibitors included patients with cardiogenic shock. Patients in cardiogenic shock treated with the GP II_bIII_a inhibitor eptifibatide had improved survival in the PURSUIT trial, and patients in cardiogenic shock at presentation who undergo PCI and are treated with the GP II_bIII_a inhibitor abciximab have improved survival. These agents are probably most effective when initiated during cardiac catheterization, after the coronary anatomy is defined, but may have a role for patients who must be transferred for cardiac catheterization. For patients who eventually stabilize and in whom hypotension is no longer a concern, most clinicians would recommend other medical therapies benefiting patients with heart failure including angiotensin-converting enzyme inhibitors.

B. Mechanical Complications

Acute mitral regurgitation secondary to papillary muscle dysfunction, myocardial free wall rupture, and VSD are true emergencies. The definitive therapy for these catastrophes is surgical repair, although there are reports of using percutaneously placed devices to successfully repair VSDs. If the patient is to survive, all efforts must be made to get the patient to the operating room as soon as possible after the diagnosis is made. Pharmacologic agents and the IABP (see previous section on circulatory support devices) are useful as temporizing measures.

C. Right Ventricular Infarction

Cardiogenic shock may occur with right ventricular MI and no or only minimal left ventricular dysfunction. Recent data have questioned the long-accepted notion that patients with shock from an isolated right ventricular MI have a better prognosis than those with primarily left ventricular dysfunction. In the SHOCK registry, patients with a right ventricular MI and shock fared similarly to those with primarily left ventricular dysfunction. Hemodynamic data suggesting right ventricular dysfunction out of proportion to left ventricular dysfunction and ST elevation in lead RV_4 on a right-sided ECG are helpful in establishing the diagnosis, and assessment of right ventricular function on echocardiography can confirm the diagnosis. In cases of shock from right ventricular failure, initial treatment is aggressive fluid resuscitation to increase right ventricular preload and output. Significant amounts of fluid (1–2 L or more) may be required to develop an adequate preload for the failing right ventricle. Inotropic agents are usually necessary when the right ventricular failure is so profound that shock continues despite adequate volume administration, and the IABP may be helpful in this situation. Heart block is common in patients with right ventricular MIs. Patients with right ventricular infarction are relatively dependent on right atrial contraction. As a result, single-chamber right ventricular pacing may be inadequate in patients who require pacing, and atrioventricular sequential pacing may be required to improve cardiac output.

D. Arrhythmias

Arrhythmias contributing to cardiogenic shock are readily recognized with ECG monitoring and should be promptly treated. Tachyarrhythmias (ventricular tachycardia and supraventricular tachycardia) should be treated with electrical cardioversion in patients with hemodynamic compromise. Bradyarrhythmias may respond to pharmacologic agents (atropine, isoproterenol) in some circumstances, but external or transvenous pacing may be required.

Antoniucci D, et al. Abciximab therapy improves survival in patients with acute myocardial infarction complicated by early cardiogenic shock undergoing coronary artery stent implantation. *Am J Cardiol.* 2002;90(4):353–7. [PMID: 12161221]

Brodie BR, et al. Comparison of late survival in patients with cardiogenic shock due to right ventricular infarction versus left ventricular pump failure following primary percutaneous coronary intervention for ST-elevation acute myocardial infarction. *Am J Cardiol.* 2007;99(4):431–5. [PMID: 17293178]

De Backer D, et al. Comparison of dopamine and norepinephrine in the treatment of shock. *N Engl J Med.* 2010;362(9):779–89. [PMID: 20200382]

Dzavik V, et al; SHOCK Investigators. Early revascularization is associated with improved survival in elderly patients with acute myocardial infarction complicated by cardiogenic shock: a report from the SHOCK trial registry. *Eur Heart J.* 2003;24(9):828–37. [PMID: 12727150]

Fang J, et al. Trends in acute myocardial infarction complicated by cardiogenic shock, 1979–2003, United States. *Am Heart J.* 2006;152(6):1035–41. [PMID: 17161048]

Hochman JS, et al. Early revascularization and long-term survival in cardiogenic shock complicating acute myocardial infarction. *JAMA.* 2006;295(21):2511–5. [PMID: 16757723]

Martinez MW, et al. Transcatheter closure of ischemic and posttraumatic ventricular septal ruptures. *Catheter Cardiovasc Interv.* 2007;69(3):403–7. [PMID: 17195200]

Thiele H, et al. Intraaortic balloon support for myocardial infarction with cardiogenic shock. *N Engl J Med.* 2012;367(14):1287–96. [PMID: 23281982]

White HD, et al. Comparison of percutaneous coronary intervention and coronary artery bypass grafting after acute myocardial infarction complicated by cardiogenic shock: results from the Should We Emergently Revascularize Occluded Coronaries for Cardiogenic Shock (SHOCK) trial. *Circulation.* 2005;112(13):1992–2001. [PMID: 16186436]

▶ Prognosis

Over the past 25 years, the prognosis of patients with cardiogenic shock has improved from over 80% in-hospital mortality in the late 1970s to under 50% mortality in recent years. Revascularization (primarily PCI) appears to be the major contribution to improved outcomes. Demographic features associated with a better prognosis include younger age and male gender. Delayed time to revascularization predicts a worse outcome. Other clinical predictors of poorer outcome include a lower ejection fraction, extensive coronary disease, a left main or vein graft acute occlusion, higher heart rate, lower systolic blood pressure, and severe mitral regurgitation. Cardiac power (mean arterial pressure × cardiac output) was the strongest hemodynamic predictor of outcome in the SHOCK registry.

Evaluation & Treatment of the Perioperative Patient

10

Sanjiv J. Shah, MD

Michael H. Crawford, MD

The prevalence of cardiovascular disease and the death rate associated with it rise sharply after age 45, an age when the incidence of noncardiac surgeries is also increasing, and approximately one-third of the 25 million surgical procedures done annually are performed in patients with cardiovascular diseases. Cardiac deaths and nonfatal myocardial infarction (MI) occur in about 0.2% of all cases of general anesthesia and surgery (about 500,000 events annually). Cardiac deaths account for approximately 40% of all perioperative mortality, the same proportion as sepsis, although in many cases the cause of death is multisystem organ failure. These figures underestimate the total effect of cardiovascular diseases because another 500,000 persons a year suffer nonfatal MI, unstable angina, or congestive heart failure (CHF) perioperatively, prolonging both their time in the intensive care unit and the total hospital stay.

Although there is great potential to reduce perioperative cardiovascular risk, it is also impractical, unnecessary, and potentially harmful to perform cardiovascular testing in all patients prior to noncardiac surgery. Therefore, it is important to determine perioperative risk, decide whether cardiac testing is appropriate, and provide prophylactic treatment to reduce risk.

▶ Preoperative Risk Assessment

An individual patient's preoperative risk profile depends on three main factors: the patient's age, current medical and functional status, and the type of surgery. Preoperative electrocardiography can detect arrhythmias and prior silent MI, but it rarely changes management. Preoperative echocardiography would probably provide more useful information, but the cost effectiveness of such testing has not been determined.

Table 10–1 lists cardiac risk based on type of noncardiac surgery. In the evaluation of perioperative patients, understanding the nature of the surgery is of prime importance. Is this an emergency surgery? If yes, the clinician should advise to proceed with the surgery and evaluate the patient's cardiac risk postoperatively. On the other hand, if the patient is young, without systemic disease, and undergoing a minor surgery or procedure, the clinician should advise to proceed with surgery without further cardiac workup. However, most patients who require perioperative cardiac consultation are not so straightforward. In these patients, there are various algorithms that can help identify perioperative risk and the need for further cardiac testing.

A. Algorithms

1. Revised Cardiac Risk Index (RCRI)—This algorithm is simple to use, and it helps identify patients who require β-blockers perioperatively. *However, the RCRI may have less accuracy in patients undergoing major vascular surgery.* Use the RCRI as follows:

a. Assign 1 point to each of the following risk factors if present:

- High-risk surgery (intraperitoneal, intrathoracic, suprainguinal vascular)
- Ischemic heart disease (history of MI or current angina, use of sublingual nitroglycerin, recent abnormal stress test, Q waves on electrocardiogram [ECG], or history of coronary revascularization with ongoing chest pain)
- History of heart failure
- History of cerebrovascular disease (stroke, transient ischemic attack)
- Diabetes mellitus requiring insulin
- Preoperative creatinine > 2.0 mg/dL

b. Assign a risk class to determine the major cardiac complication rate to help counsel the patient and also the surgeon:

- Class I: zero risk factors, 0.4%
- Class II: one risk factor, 0.9%
- Class III: two risk factors, 6.6%
- Class IV: three or more risk factors, 11.0%

Table 10–1. Cardiac Risk Stratification for Noncardiac Surgical Procedures

High (reported cardiac risk often > 5%)
    Emergent major operations, particularly in the elderly
    Aortic and other major vascular surgery
    Anticipated prolonged surgical procedures associated with large
      fluid shifts and/or blood loss (eg, liver transplantation)
Intermediate (reported cardiac risk generally < 5%)
    Carotid endarterectomy surgery
    Head and neck surgery
    Intraperitoneal and intrathoracic surgery
    Orthopedic surgery
    Peripheral vascular surgery
    Prostate surgery
Low (reported cardiac risk generally < 1%)
    Endoscopic procedures
    Superficial procedure
    Cataract or other eye surgery
    Breast surgery

    c. Patients who are categorized as having risk class III or IV may require additional cardiac testing for risk stratification and more aggressive perioperative medical management to reduce the risk of complications.

2. American College of Cardiology/American Heart Association (ACC/AHA) guidelines—These guidelines are somewhat cumbersome. In simplified terms, the ACC/AHA guidelines recommend noninvasive cardiac stress testing in patients with two or more of the following risk factors:

- Intermediate clinical predictors: mild angina, prior MI, compensated or prior heart failure, diabetes mellitus, or renal insufficiency

- Poor functional capacity (< 4 metabolic equivalents): cannot walk more than one or two blocks on level ground; cannot do light housework, such as washing dishes or dusting; cannot climb a flight of stairs or walk up a hill

- High-risk surgery: vascular surgery, prolonged procedure, or anticipated large fluid shifts or blood loss

3. Online cardiac risk calculator—With the increased use of mobile computerized devices by physicians, access to interactive surgical databases is possible. This has been used successfully by cardiac surgeons to assess the risk of cardiac surgery by the use of the Society of Thoracic Surgery (STS) database and the Euroscore from the European Society of Cardiology database. These societies collect data from their members about each surgery performed and its outcome. Then they use multiple regression analysis of the clinical variables in the database to compare with a specific patient's same variables entered into a Web-based calculator to determine the risk of a proposed surgery. The beauty of these databases is that they are constantly being updated, so as surgical techniques and medical therapy improve these

advances are reflected in the risk calculation. A similar schema has been proposed and tested for noncardiac surgery by a group of investigators in Canada and has been shown to be superior to the RCRI. It is based on five variables: the type of surgery; the functional status of the patient; serum creatinine; American Society of Anesthesiology class; and age. We predict that such online Web-based approaches will be the dominant approach to preoperative risk stratification for noncardiac surgery in the future.

B. Intermediate-Risk Patients

Although perioperative management of low-risk and high-risk patients is relatively straightforward, the management of patients who fall into the intermediate-risk group is more challenging. Low-risk patients can proceed to surgery without further cardiac evaluation. For high-risk patients, management should include one or more of the following: postpone or cancel surgery until high-risk features improve or resolve, start treatment of the underlying high-risk features, or proceed to invasive testing. In high-risk patients with a high pretest probability of disease, noninvasive tests are not helpful, because a negative result will most likely be a false negative.

Intermediate-risk patients derive the most benefit from perioperative medical management or stress testing, or both.

For most patients in the intermediate-risk category, it is important to obtain imaging with the stress test because ECG alone is unlikely to move the posttest probability beyond the threshold for treatment or no treatment.

1. Exercise versus pharmacologic stress testing—The choice between exercise and pharmacologic stress testing follows the same guidelines as those for routine, nonperioperative stress testing. Exercise testing can provide valuable information on functional capacity, but patients may not be able to reach 85% of maximal predicted heart rate due to deconditioning or β-blocker use. Since β-blockers are important in the perioperative period, withholding them is not ideal.

Dipyridamole or adenosine is preferred in cases where arrhythmia (eg, rapid atrial fibrillation) or frequent premature atrial or ventricular beats are present. These agents are relatively contraindicated in patients with significant bronchospasm, in whom dobutamine is the agent of choice.

2. Type of imaging technique—When choosing either echocardiography or nuclear imaging (the two most commonly available stress imaging modalities), it is most important to determine which modality has better reliability and expertise at the clinician's hospital or clinic. In published studies, both imaging techniques have good negative predictive value (> 90%) but poor positive predictive value (< 25%). Echocardiography with contrast (to assist in endocardial border definition) may be more helpful in obese patients (who may have more attenuation defects on nuclear imaging). Nuclear imaging may be more useful in patients with left bundle branch block and when atrial fibrillation is present. Newer modalities include rubidium positron emission tomography (PET) scanning, which provides better resolution images. However, patients must be cooperative and must be able to hold still for longer periods of time. Cardiac computed tomography provides anatomic assessment of the coronary arteries but does not provide data on ischemic burden and has not been adequately evaluated in the perioperative setting.

C. Understanding Cardiac Complications

Despite the risks during general anesthesia, including myocardial depression, transient hypotension, and tachycardia, very few cardiac events occur during the surgery itself. The incidence of perioperative cardiac complications actually peaks between 2 and 5 days postoperatively. These data imply that factors activated during or following surgery, and not only the surgery itself, are crucial in determining adverse outcomes.

Pneumonitis and microatelectasis produce ventilation-perfusion mismatch, and sedation or analgesia may cause respiratory depression and interfere with coughing, all of which contribute to arterial hypoxemia. Thrombocytosis and a generalized hypercoagulable state, caused by increased fibrinogen and activators from the damaged tissue, favor thrombosis. At the same time, sympathetically mediated increases in heart rate, blood pressure, and contractility increase myocardial oxygen consumption, whereas thrombotic tendencies, anemia, and arterial desaturation impede oxygen delivery to the myocardium. In a patient with underlying coronary artery disease, this situation may lead to myocardial ischemia or infarction. The imbalance may be further exaggerated because antihypertensive or anginal medications are often withheld. By the third or fourth postoperative day, the patient is hypermetabolic, with negative nitrogen and potassium balances. A natriuresis follows, which can produce hypovolemia and further activate the sympathetic nervous system.

All of these factors provide the exact setting in which a perioperative MI may occur. Perioperative MI carries a high mortality and presents atypically (usually without chest pain). Clues such as hypotension, pulmonary edema, altered mental status, and arrhythmia may be the only signs alerting the clinician to the possibility of a perioperative MI. Therefore, those caring for perioperative patients must have a high level of suspicion in order to detect perioperative MI.

Fleisher LA, et al. ACC/AHA 2007 guidelines on perioperative cardiovascular evaluation and care for noncardiac surgery: executive summary: a report of the American College of Cardiology/American Heart Association Task Force on Practice Guidelines (Writing Committee to Revise the 2002 Guidelines on Perioperative Cardiovascular Evaluation for Noncardiac Surgery). *J Am Coll Cardiol.* 2007;50:1707–32. [PMID: 17950159]

Gupta PK, et al. Development and validation of a risk calculator for prediction of cardiac risk after surgery. *Circulation.* 2011;124:381–7. [PMID: 21730309]

▶ Treatment to Reduce Perioperative Risk

Knowledge of how new therapies can reduce cardiac risk has progressed rapidly in recent years. Perioperative medicine now provides "risk management" (through medicine such as β-blocker) in addition to the standard risk prediction. In general, the higher the patient's risk, the greater benefit derived from the use of therapies such as β-blockers and statins. Therefore, healthcare providers should risk stratify patients, and then use this to determine whether or not to treat.

A. β-Blockers

These agents are first-line therapy to reduce perioperative morbidity and mortality in high-risk patients. Current guidelines have advocated β-blockers in almost all intermediate- or high-risk patients undergoing noncardiac surgery. However, two recent studies in vascular surgery patients did not show a benefit, and a meta-analysis of seven randomized controlled trials did not conclusively show a benefit with β-blockers. Another recent retrospective review of 600,000 patients showed that β-blocker benefit was greater in higher risk patients. Therefore, the decision to use β-blockers should be individualized. If the patient is already taking a β-blocker for other reasons (eg, coronary artery disease), β-blockers should be continued in the perioperative setting.

In patients deemed to benefit from β-blockers in the perioperative setting, oral metoprolol is started on the day of the perioperative visit. For patients who were taking β-blockers before the surgery, the dose is titrated to a heart rate of 60 bpm. Postoperatively, metoprolol is started at 5–10 mg intravenously every 4–6 hours as needed to keep the heart rate at 60–70 bpm until the patient can take oral medications. Oral β-blockers are then continued for 30 days postoperatively and indefinitely in patients who were previously taking these medications.

B. Statins

One small randomized controlled trial and several observational studies have found a benefit to statin use, with greater benefit in higher risk patients, especially major vascular surgery patients. Therefore, if there are no contraindications, high-risk patients should be taking a statin prior to major noncardiac surgery. Also, patients already on statins should have them continued because there is evidence that stopping them is associated with a higher perioperative MI rate.

C. Clonidine

There is evidence that clonidine (an α_2-adrenergic agonist) reduces MI and mortality in high-risk vascular surgery patients. Clonidine's transdermal delivery system works well in the perioperative setting, but clonidine is not ideal for outpatient management and carries the risk of rebound hypertension. For these reasons, clonidine should not be used routinely, but can be a good choice for in-hospital control of hypertension in the perioperative patient who cannot take oral medications.

D. Calcium Channel Blockers

Verapamil and diltiazem (centrally acting calcium channel blockers) are second-line therapy for reducing perioperative ischemia or arrhythmia, or both. Use in high-risk patients who have a contraindication to β-blockers.

E. Aspirin

Many patients are taking aspirin for known cardiovascular disease or for its prevention. Aspirin has been shown to mildly increase bleeding risk with surgery, but there are few data on how to manage aspirin perioperatively in patients without coronary stents. A few observational studies have shown increased cardiovascular event rates if aspirin is stopped, but there are not clear guidelines on how to manage aspirin. It seems reasonable to continue low-dose aspirin therapy if a small increase in bleeding risk is acceptable. This is often not the case for cerebral or eye surgery, but perfectly acceptable in orthopedic surgery, for example. If a patient is not on aspirin, it does not make sense to start it before surgery no matter what the indication. If aspirin needs to be stopped, it should be stopped 7–10 days prior to surgery.

F. Deep Venous Thrombosis Prophylaxis

Although not a routine part of perioperative cardiac risk assessment and treatment, it is important to check for appropriate perioperative deep venous thrombosis (DVT) prophylaxis since DVT (with resultant pulmonary embolism) can cause significant cardiac instability and death. Low-molecular-weight heparins are being used increasingly in place of unfractionated heparin and appear to be equivalent or, in some cases, superior.

G. Endocarditis Prophylaxis

Recommendations for management of endocarditis prophylaxis have changed dramatically with the publication of the new AHA guidelines. In general, the new AHA guidelines advocate less use of antibiotic prophylaxis because of the lack of evidence of benefit in humans and the fact that transient bacteremia occurs frequently, and there is no evidence that dental and other procedures increase rates of bacteremia more than activities of daily living alone. The AHA guidelines state that only patients at the highest risk for endocarditis should receive antibiotic prophylaxis. These high-risk patients include those with prosthetic cardiac valve, previous infective endocarditis, unrepaired cyanotic congenital heart disease (including palliative shunts and conduits), completely repaired congenital heart defect with prosthetic material or device during the first 6 months after the procedure, repaired congenital heart defects with residual defects

at site of prosthetic material that prevent endothelialization, and patients who have undergone heart transplantation in whom significant valvular heart disease develops.

Prophylaxis for dental procedures in the aforementioned patients is only recommended if the procedure involves manipulation of gingival tissue, manipulation of periapical region of teeth, or perforation of the oral mucosa.

Endocarditis prophylaxis is no longer recommended for genitourinary or gastrointestinal procedures.

H. Perioperative Medication Management

Management of outpatient medications in the perioperative period is underappreciated but extremely important for ensuring an optimal patient outcome. Many times, essential medications are discontinued and not restarted before the patient is discharged from the hospital, leading to potentially disastrous outcomes. Other times, the conversion of oral to intravenous (and back to oral) dosing of medications causes under- or overtreatment.

1. Anticoagulation management—Nowhere is perioperative medication management more important than in anticoagulation, since use of anticoagulants can cause increased bleeding intra- and postoperatively. Alternatively, too little anticoagulation can lead to severe morbidity (eg, stroke, MI, and stent thrombosis) and even death.

A. ORAL ANTICOAGULANTS—One of the most common reasons for cardiac consultation (besides assessing perioperative risk) is to manage oral anticoagulants (OACs) perioperatively. Although the risks of discontinuing OAC therapy 4 days prior to surgery are low, in the few patients in whom thromboembolism develops, the results (stroke, pulmonary embolism, MI, or death) can be devastating. Therefore, in high-risk patients, bridging with unfractionated or intravenous heparin is important and can reduce perioperative risk of thromboembolism. However, use of heparins can increase bleeding. Therefore, it is important to carefully select patients who will need bridging with heparin. The keys to optimal OAC management are to identify the indication for OAC and assess the patient's risk for thromboembolism. Bridging with heparin is advised in the following situations: atrial fibrillation and rheumatic heart disease; history of thromboembolism; mechanical heart valve; hypercoagulable state; venous or arterial thromboembolism in prior 3 months; or acute intracardiac thrombus visualized on echocardiogram.

Bridging is advised on a case-by-case basis (weighing risks and benefits) in patients with significant (recurrent) cerebrovascular disease, bioprosthetic valve in mitral position, atrial fibrillation with multiple risk factors for cardiac embolism, and history of venous thromboembolism (> 3 months ago). Bridging is not advised in patients with bioprosthetic valve in the aortic position, atrial fibrillation without multiple risk factors for cardiac embolism, or a history of one remote (> 6 months ago) venous thromboembolism.

Warfarin should be stopped 4 days prior to surgery if preoperative international normalized ratio (INR) is 2.0–3.0 (with modification of timing if INR is < 2.0 or > 3.0). Newer OACs may need to be held for longer periods of time. In patients who require bridging with a heparin, there is evidence that low-molecular-weight heparin (eg, enoxaparin) is just as effective and safe (if not more so) than unfractionated heparin. Enoxaparin (1 mg/kg twice daily), if not contraindicated, is started 36 hours after the last dose of warfarin and is discontinued 24 hours prior to surgery. On postoperative day 1, warfarin is restarted at the preoperative outpatient dose. At 24 hours postoperatively, the patient is evaluated and enoxaparin is restarted if hemostasis has been achieved. Once INR is in the therapeutic range, enoxaparin can be discontinued. Consult manufacturer's guidelines for bridging with the newer OACs.

B. Antiplatelet therapy in patients with coronary stents—Controversy exists regarding the optimal management of antiplatelet therapy in patients undergoing noncardiac surgery, especially in patients with drug-eluting stents. It appears that decreased endothelialization of drug-eluting stents predisposes these patients to stent thrombosis for quite some time after stent placement.

In patients who do not have a coronary stent and who are at low risk for perioperative cardiac events, aspirin, clopidogrel, and newer antiplatelet agents should be discontinued 7–10 days prior to noncardiac surgery and resumed when hemostasis is achieved postoperatively.

In patients with coronary stents, especially drug-eluting stents, the risk of stent thrombosis greatly increases when aspirin and other antiplatelet drugs are stopped prematurely. Recent AHA/ACC guidelines state that aspirin and clopidogrel should not be discontinued for at least 1 month after bare metal stent and for at least 12 months after the placement of a drug-eluting stent. With some of the newer drug-eluting stents, discontinuation of dual antiplatelet therapy may be possible at 6 months. If surgery cannot be deferred, aspirin should be continued in the perioperative period, and in extremely high-risk patients, intravenous glycoprotein II_bIII_a inhibitors (which have a shorter half-life than clopidogrel) can be used to try to prevent stent thrombosis (although the increased risk of significant bleeding must also be taken into consideration).

It is now clear that cardiologists must discuss with their patients the need for prolonged dual antiplatelet therapy prior to percutaneous coronary intervention, so that if noncardiac surgery is possible in the near future, drug-eluting stents should be avoided.

2. Antiarrhythmics—These medications should be continued up to the day of surgery and, if necessary, in the immediate postoperative period (in an intravenous form).

Amiodarone is a common oral antiarrhythmic that needs to be converted to an intravenous format in the perioperative period. Since intravenous bolus of amiodarone can cause hypotension, it is more ideal to add up the total daily oral dose of amiodarone and convert that dose to a prolonged or continuous infusion (eg, instead of giving 200 mg intravenously as a bolus once daily, give 0.15 mg/min intravenously continuously over 24 hours, or give the 200 mg intravenously over 4–6 hours).

Digoxin dose should generally be reduced slightly in the perioperative period, especially in elderly patients or those in whom worsening renal function is to be expected.

3. Nonsteroidal anti-inflammatory drugs (NSAIDs)—These medications can predispose elderly and other high-risk patients to perioperative renal failure, especially with perioperative dehydration and hypotension. Therefore, NSAIDs should be discontinued at least 3 days prior to surgery and restarted if necessary upon discharge from the hospital.

I. Prophylactic Coronary Revascularization

For patients who are intermediate or high risk and who eventually undergo coronary angiography, there are three possibilities: no significant coronary artery disease, left main or triple-vessel coronary artery disease, and single- or two-vessel coronary artery disease.

1. No significant coronary artery disease—Noncardiac surgery can proceed without further testing, although perioperative risk reduction with β-blockers and other agents may be important.

2. Left main or triple-vessel coronary artery disease—These patients, who are on the opposite extreme, are very high risk and should undergo prophylactic coronary artery bypass grafting. Alternatively, in institutions with expertise, percutaneous coronary intervention is another possibility.

3. Single- or two-vessel coronary artery disease—In these patients, the decision for prophylactic revascularization is more difficult. However, there are no convincing data that revascularization, especially with surgery, is superior to maximal medical therapy for the prevention of short- and long-term cardiac events. Therefore, in patients found to have single- or two-vessel coronary disease, medical management in the perioperative period, even before high-risk vascular surgery, is just as safe as prophylactic revascularization and does not delay noncardiac surgery. If patients must undergo percutaneous coronary intervention preoperatively, balloon angioplasty alone avoids the necessity to continue dual antiplatelet therapy. If stents are placed, it is extremely important to follow recommendations for perioperative management of dual antiplatelet therapy (see earlier section, Perioperative Medication Management).

Devereaux PJ, et al. How strong is the evidence for the use of perioperative beta blockers in non-cardiac surgery? Systematic review and meta-analysis of randomized controlled trials. *BMJ*. 2005;331(7512):313–21. [PMID: 15996966]

Grines CL, et al; American Heart Association; American College of Cardiology; Society for Cardiovascular Angiography and Interventions; American College of Surgeons; American Dental Association; American College of Physicians. Prevention of premature discontinuation of dual antiplatelet therapy in patients with coronary artery stents: a science advisory from the American Heart Association, American College of Cardiology, Society for Cardiovascular Angiography and Interventions, American College of Surgeons, and American Dental Association, with representation from the American College of Physicians. *Circulation.* 2007;115(6):813–8. [PMID: 17224480]

Lindenauer PK, et al. Lipid-lowering therapy and in-hospital mortality following major noncardiac surgery. *JAMA.* 2004; 291(17):2092–9. [PMID: 15126437]

Lindenauer PK, et al. Perioperative beta-blocker therapy and mortality after major noncardiac vascular surgery. *N Engl J Med.* 2005;353(4):349–61. [PMID: 16049209]

Poldermans D, et al. Pre-operative risk assessment and risk reduction before surgery. *J Am Coll Cardiol.* 2008;51:1913–24. [PMID: 18482658]

Wilson W, et al; American Heart Association Rheumatic Fever, Endocarditis, and Kawasaki Disease Committee; American Heart Association Council on Cardiovascular Disease in the Young; American Heart Association Council on Clinical Cardiology; American Heart Association Council on Cardiovascular Surgery and Anesthesia; Quality of Care and Outcomes Research Interdisciplinary Working Group. Prevention of infective endocarditis: guidelines from the American Heart Association: a guideline from the American Heart Association Rheumatic Fever, Endocarditis, and Kawasaki Disease Committee, Council on Cardiovascular Disease in the Young, and the Council on Clinical Cardiology, Council on Cardiovascular Surgery and Anesthesia, and the Quality of Care and Outcomes Research Interdisciplinary Working Group. *Circulation.* 2007;116(15):1736–54. [PMID: 17446442]

▶ Special Populations

A. Liver Transplantation

Liver failure patients have a unique cardiovascular physiology characterized by high cardiac output and a reduced response to cardiac stress, which some have called cirrhotic cardiomyopathy. Often these patients have low peripheral vascular resistance, bradycardia, left ventricular hypertrophy, and prolonged QTc interval on ECG. Today these patients are older, sicker, and have more comorbidities than before. The most common causes of perioperative death in these patients are arrhythmias, heart failure, and MI. Once the new liver is reperfused, there is an increase in preload, which will exacerbate cardiac stress. In addition, coronary artery disease (CAD) is common in these patients, and those with known CAD have worse outcomes. Thus, these are high-risk patients, and determining who has CAD is important because it may preclude liver transplantation.

Noninvasive stress testing has been less valuable in pre–liver transplant patients. Although preferred by many, dobutamine stress echo (DSE) has lower sensitivity in these patients. Nuclear perfusion testing has lower specificity.

Given the enormous resources needed to transplant these patients successfully, all except the lowest risk patients are assessed by coronary angiography, usually invasively. Coronary computed tomography angiography may be adequate, but there are few data on this technique in these patients. Certainly patients with known CAD, diabetes, age > 50 years, renal dysfunction, and two or more major risk factors are high risk for CAD and should be studied. Some centers study almost all patients. There are no data demonstrating improved outcomes with revascularization of significant coronary artery lesions, but doing so may allow the patient to be transplanted.

Transthoracic echocardiography is important in the evaluation of pre–liver transplant patients. Reduced left ventricular (LV) function may be detected but is not an absolute contraindication for transplant, because it may improve afterward. However, it indicates that aggressive heart failure prophylactic measures should be taken. Some patients have LV outflow tract obstruction, which is also not a contraindication to surgery, but requires special management techniques during the perioperative period. Prolonged QTc on ECG is also not a contraindication to surgery but should motivate a search for treatable causes, so the incidence of ventricular arrhythmias can be reduced. Some centers are employing cardiac magnetic resonance imaging to detect myocardial iron deposits, which indicate a higher risk of heart failure postoperatively but are not an absolute contraindication to surgery.

The most serious cardiovascular abnormality in pre–liver transplant patients is portopulmonary hypertension, which is caused by abnormal pulmonary vasoconstriction and, if not effectively treated, is a contraindication to transplantation. Echocardiographic screening that shows an elevated estimated systolic pulmonary artery pressure or right ventricular dysfunction indicates the need for right heart catheterization. A mean pulmonary artery pressure > 35 mm Hg, a pulmonary vascular resistance > 3 Wood units, and a pulmonary artery wedge pressure < 15 mm Hg contraindicate surgery unless treatment with pulmonary vasodilator drugs is successful in lowering the pulmonary pressure.

B. Aortic Stenosis

In patients with severe or critical aortic stenosis, risks of a perioperative cardiac complication are high. The risk correlates with aortic valve mean gradient, as measured by echocardiography. Even moderate aortic stenosis (mean gradient of > 25 mm Hg) has been associated with an adjusted relative risk of 5.2 for perioperative cardiac complications.

Noninvasive stress testing is unnecessary and potentially dangerous in these patients. If the patient has symptomatic aortic stenosis, postpone the noncardiac surgery until after the patient undergoes coronary angiography, aortic valve replacement, and coronary artery bypass grafting (if the patient is found to have significant CAD). In asymptomatic patients with severe aortic stenosis, preoperative aortic valve replacement (prior to elective noncardiac surgery) is usually the best option because of the very high-risk nature of these patients. If aortic valve replacement is not an option, percutaneous aortic valvuloplasty can be considered as a temporizing measure, because it carries a significant risk of aortic stenosis recurrence. Also, the procedural risks must be weighed against the risk of cancelling surgery or operating with significant aortic stenosis. Percutaneous aortic valve replacement is another option but has not been tested extensively in this situation.

C. Heart Failure

Patients with a history of hospitalization for heart failure, and especially those with current signs and symptoms of heart failure, are at high risk for perioperative cardiac events. In these patients, heart failure should be treated and volume status optimized prior to surgery, since the risks of heart failure outweigh those associated with delaying surgery in most cases. As the number of patients with heart failure increases along with the aging population, more patients who undergo noncardiac surgery will have a history of heart failure. Even though heart failure indicates a greater risk of perioperative cardiac events than CAD, there are few studies on the optimal perioperative treatment of patients with heart failure, especially those with preserved ejection fraction.

D. Pulmonary Hypertension

In patients with significant pulmonary hypertension, the risks of general anesthesia are extraordinarily high. Pulmonary hypertension can be thought of as a fixed obstruction to cardiopulmonary blood flow, and therefore, it prevents the increase in cardiac output necessary in the perioperative state. Therefore, it is very similar to critical aortic or mitral stenosis in this aspect. In these cases, a pulmonary hypertension specialist should be consulted. Elective surgeries should be postponed indefinitely until the patient is treated with pulmonary vasodilators to reduce the perioperative risk. If surgery is absolutely necessary, it is advisable that these patients undergo continuous monitoring with pulmonary artery catheter intraoperatively. Intraoperative inhaled nitric oxide can be used to decrease pulmonary artery pressures.

E. Pacemakers, Defibrillators, & Atrial Fibrillation

There is a small risk that prolonged electrocautery could trigger, reprogram, or inadvertently offset an implantable cardioverter-defibrillator (ICD). Electrocautery may also interfere with pacemaker output, and anesthetic agents may interfere with pacing thresholds. Some manufacturers have recommended that the device be inactivated during surgery. Supraventricular tachycardias, which are fairly common in the postoperative period, may exceed the rate threshold of the ICD and can cause inappropriate shocks to be delivered. ICDs should be interrogated before surgery to assess underlying rhythm and frequency of discharges. In pacemaker-dependent patients, the rate response feature should be tuned off. The ICD defibrillation capacity should be disengaged just prior to surgery and resumed immediately after surgery, and an external defibrillating device with personnel able to handle it should be close to the patient at all times during the period that the ICD is off. Of note, an anteroposterior lead placement of the external pacer paddles away from the device pocket is required in the event of external cardioversion or defibrillation. Preoperative atrial fibrillation is associated with a higher risk of perioperative adverse cardiovascular events, especially stroke. Anticoagulation should be restarted as soon as hemostasis is achieved postoperatively. The most common problem with atrial fibrillation patients is rapid rate after surgery. Optimization of rate control preoperatively should be accomplished if possible.

Christ M, et al. Preoperative and perioperative care for patients with suspected or established aortic stenosis facing noncardiac surgery. *Chest.* 2005;128(4):2944–53. [PMID: 16236971]

Kertai MD, et al. Optimizing the prediction of perioperative mortality in vascular surgery by using a customized probability model. *Arch Intern Med.* 2005;165(8):898–904. [PMID: 15851641]

Raval Z, et al. Cardiovascular risk assessment of the liver transplant candidate. *J Am Coll Cardiol.* 2011;58:223–31. [PMID: 21737011]

Van Diepen S, et al. Mortality and readmission of patients with heart failure, atrial fibrillation, or coronary artery disease undergoing noncardiac surgery: an analysis of 38,047 patients. *Circulation.* 2011;124:289–96. [PMID: 21709059]

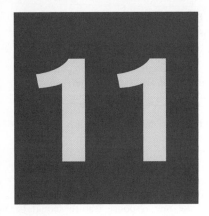

Supraventricular Tachycardias

Byron K. Lee, MD

Peter R. Kowey, MD

ESSENTIALS OF DIAGNOSIS

▶ Heart rate greater than 100 bpm.

▶ Rhythm is supraventricular in origin.

▶ General Considerations

Supraventricular tachycardias (SVTs) are rapid rhythm disturbances originating from the atria or the atrioventricular (AV) node. In the absence of a bundle branch block, there is intact conduction to the ventricles via the right and left bundles leading to a narrow and normal-appearing QRS. Therefore, these arrhythmias are also often called narrow complex tachycardias. Since many of the SVTs are episodic, many clinicians also refer to this group of arrhythmias as paroxysmal SVTs. Radiofrequency ablation has become an important therapeutic option in the management of SVTs because of its ability to cure these arrhythmias safely. Table 11–1 outlines the pharmacologic therapy for SVTs.

▶ Pathophysiology & Etiology

Arrhythmias occur as a result of three main mechanisms: reentry, which is most common; enhanced or abnormal automaticity; and triggered activity.

Reentrant arrhythmias sustain themselves by repetitively following a revolving pathway comprising two limbs, one that takes the impulse away from and one that carries it back to the site of origin. For reentry to exist, an area of slow conduction must occur, and each limb must have a different refractory period (see the discussion on AV nodal reentrant tachycardia). In this situation, pacing (by inducing refractoriness in one limb of the circuit) can typically initiate a reentrant tachycardia. Once established, pacing can also terminate the tachycardia by interfering with impulse propagation in one of the limbs.

The second mechanism, **automaticity,** refers to spontaneous and, often, repetitive firing from a single focus, which may either be ectopic or may originate in the sinus node. It should be noted that automaticity is an intrinsic property of all myocardial cells. This mechanism comprises two subcategories. **Enhanced automaticity** is defined as a focus that fires spontaneously and may originate in the sinus node, subsidiary pacemakers in the atrium including the Eustachian ridge, Bachmann bundle, coronary sinus and AV valves, the AV node, His-Purkinje system, and the ventricles. **Abnormal automaticity** is usually secondary to a disease process causing alterations in ionic flow that produces a lower (ie, more positive) resting diastolic membrane potential. Threshold potential is therefore more easily attained, thereby increasing the probability of a sustained arrhythmia.

The third mechanism, **triggered arrhythmias,** depends on oscillations in the membrane potential that closely follow an action potential. In the absence of a new external electrical stimulus, these oscillations, or **after-depolarizations,** cause new action potentials to develop. Thus, each new action potential results from the previous action potential. These arrhythmias can be produced by early or late after-depolarization, depending on the timing of the first after-depolarization relative to the preceding action potential (the one that spawned the triggered activity). In **early after-depolarizations,** membrane repolarization is incomplete, which allows an action potential to be initiated by a subthreshold stimulus. This type is often associated with electrolyte disturbance and may be the mechanism responsible for arrhythmogenesis related to the prolonged QT syndrome and torsades de pointes caused by quinidine. With **delayed after-depolarization,** membrane repolarization is complete, but an abnormal intracellular calcium load causes spontaneous depolarization. The reason for the high calcium levels is unclear, but it can be related to inhibition of the sodium pump by drugs such as digoxin. In either type of arrhythmia, the process may be repetitive and lead to a sustained tachycardia.

Table 11–1. Antiarrhythmic Drugs for Supraventricular Tachycardias

Agent	Indication	Intravenous Dose	Oral Dose	Adverse Effects	Drug Interactions
Class Ia					
Quinidine	AF, AFL, AVNRT, AVRT	6–10 mg/kg over 20–30 min	200–400 mg q4–6h; q8h with long-acting preparations	Hypotension (especially IV), ventricular proarrhythmia, GI disturbance, thrombocytopenia	↑ Digitalis level ↑ Warfarin effect ↑ Metoprolol, propranolol, propafenone levels
Procainamide	AF, AFL, AVNRT, AVRT	*Bolus:* 15 mg/kg given as 20 mg/min *Infusion:* 2–4 mg/min	50 mg/kg/day q3–4h; twice daily dosage with long-acting preparation	GI disturbance, hypotension, SLE, agranulocytosis, FUO hemolytic anemia, myasthenia gravis aggravation, ventricular proarrhythmia	↑ Procainamide level with cimetidine, quinidine, and amiodarone
Class 1c					
Flecainide	AF, AFL, AT, AVNRT, AVRT	N/A	50–200 mg q12h	Ventricular proarrhythmia, CHF, GI disturbance, CNS (dizziness, tremor, light-headedness)	↑ Digitalis level ↑ Flecainide level with amiodarone, cimetidine, Norpace, propranolol ↓ Flecainide level with smoking
Propafenone	AF, AFL, AVNRT, AVRT	N/A	150–300 mg q8h or 225–425 mg bid (long-acting form)	GI disturbance, CNS (dizziness), metallic taste, CHF, first-degree AVB, IVCD, positive ANA	Synergism with β-blockers
Class II (IV)					
Esmolol	Ventricular rate control for AF, AFL, ST, AT	*Bolus:* 500 mcg/kg over 1–2 min *Infusion:* 50–200 mcg/kg/min	N/A	CHF, AVB, bradycardia, bronchospasm	
Propranolol	Ventricular rate control for AF, AFL, ST, AT	1–5 mg at 1 mg/min	20–320 mg/day q6h, q8h, q12h, or once daily, depending on preparation	CHF, AVB, bradycardia, bronchospasm	
Class III					
Sotalol	AF, AFL, AVNRT, AVRT, AT	N/A	80–160 mg q12h	Dyspnea, fatigue, dizziness, CHF, bradycardia, ventricular proarrhythmia, bronchospasm	Synergism with Ca^{2+} antagonists or β-blockers

(continued)

Table 11-1. Antiarrhythmic Drugs for Supraventricular Tachycardias *(Continued)*

Agent	Indication	Intravenous Dose	Oral Dose	Adverse Effects	Drug Interactions
Amiodarone	AF, AFL, AVNRT, AVRT, AT	*Bolus:* 150 mg over 10 min; *Infusion:* 1 mg/min × 6 h, then 0.5 mg/min	100–400 mg once daily	Pulmonary toxicity, CHF, tremor, bradycardia, ↑ LFTs, corneal deposits, skin discoloration, GI intolerance, hyper-/hypothyroidism	↑ Digoxin levels; ↑ Warfarin effect; ↑ Quinidine, procainamide/NAPA, flecainide; ↑ Phenytoin level
Ibutilide	AF, AFL	1 mg bolus over 10 min; second bolus, if needed, after 10-min wait	N/A	Ventricular proarrhythmia, hypotension, GI disturbance	
Dofetilide	AF, AFL	N/A	125–500 mcg twice daily modified by algorithm	Ventricular proarrhythmia, headache, chest pain, nausea, dizziness	Contraindicated with verapamil, cimetidine, ketoconazole, trimethoprim
Class IV					
Diltiazem	AF, AFL, AVNRT, AVRT, AT, MAT	*Bolus:* 0.25 mg/min over 2 min then 0.35 mg/kg in 15 min if needed; *Infusion:* 5–15 mg/h	90–360 mg/day in 1–4 divided doses, depending on preparation	Hypotension, bradycardia, CHF, AVB	Synergism with β-blockers
Verapamil	AF, AFL, AVNRT, AVRT, AT, MAT	2.5–20 mg over 20 min in divided doses	40–120 mg q8h; 240–360 mg once daily of long-acting preparation	Hypotension, bradycardia, CHF, AVB	Synergism with β-blockers
Class V					
Adenosine	SVT diagnosis, AVNRT, AVRT, AT termination	6 mg IV rapid bolus followed by 12 mg × 2 if needed; half dosage if administered in central line	N/A	Chest tightness, facial flushing, dyspnea, AVB	↑ Activity by dipyridamole; ↓ Activity by theophylline
Digoxin	Ventricular rate control for AF, AFL, AT (generally not very effective in active patients)	Up to 1.0 mg bolus in divided doses followed by 0.125–0.375 mg/day	0.125–0.375 mg/day in single dose	GI disturbance, conduction defects, atrial/ventricular arrhythmias, headache, visual disturbances	*Digoxin level:* amiodarone, quinidine, verapamil, indomethacin, spironolactone, alprazolam, erythromycin, tetracycline; ↓ *Digoxin level:* antacids, cholestyramine, rifampin, neomycin; ↑ Risk of digitalis toxicity with potassium-depleting diuretics

AF, atrial fibrillation; AFL, atrial flutter; ANA, antinuclear antigen; AT, atrial tachycardia; AVB, atrioventricular block; AVNRT, atrioventricular nodal reentrant tachycardia; AVRT, atrioventricular reciprocating tachycardia; CHF, congestive heart failure; CNS, central nervous system; FUO, fever of unknown origin; GI, gastrointestinal; IV, intravenous; IVCD, intraventricular conduction delay; LFT, liver function tests; MAT, multifocal atrial tachycardia; N/A, not applicable; NAPA, N-acetyl procainamide; SLE, systemic lupus erythematosus; ST, sinus tachycardia.

▶ General Diagnostic Approach

A systematic approach to interpreting the 12-lead electrocardiogram (ECG) will allow accurate determination of the type of SVT in most cases (Figure 11–1). The first step is to determine whether the rhythm is regular or irregular. If it is irregular, the rhythm is likely either atrial fibrillation, atrial flutter with variable conduction, or multifocal atrial tachycardia (MAT). The appearance of the P waves or lack of P waves will usually distinguish between these three entities. In atrial fibrillation, there is chaotic atrial activity. In atrial flutter, P waves are seen at rate of 240–320 bpm. In MAT, there are P waves preceding each QRS complex, and there are at least three different P-wave morphologies.

If the SVT is regular, there are several main types of SVT to consider. The SVT could be sinus tachycardia, sinus node reentry, atrial flutter, atrial tachycardia, AV nodal reentrant tachycardia (AVNRT), junctional tachycardia, or atrioventricular reciprocating tachycardia (AVRT). The type of regular SVT can be usually identified by examining four aspects of the 12-lead ECG: onset and termination, heart rate, P wave morphology, and R-P relationship. Sinus tachycardia and junctional tachycardia typically have very gradual onset, whereas the other SVTs usually start and stop more suddenly.

Rate can also be helpful since sinus tachycardia cannot typically go over 220-age bpm and the heart rate in atrial flutter is often a multiple of 300. P-wave morphology can be helpful since retrograde P waves (negative in the inferior leads: II, III, and aVF) favor AVNRT and junctional tachycardia. Finally, R-P relationship refers to the distance from the R wave to the next P wave during tachycardia. If this distance is longer than the P-R interval, the SVT is termed "long R-P," whereas if this distance is short, it is termed "short R-P" (Figure 11–2).

SINUS TACHYCARDIA & SINUS NODE REENTRY

1. Sinus Tachycardia

ESSENTIALS OF DIAGNOSIS

▶ Onset and termination: gradual.

▶ Heart rate: 100 to (220 – age) bpm.

▶ P wave: identical to normal sinus rhythm P wave.

▶ R-P relationship: long.

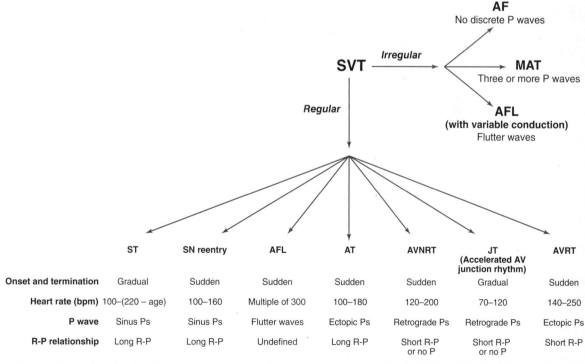

	ST	SN reentry	AFL	AT	AVNRT	JT (Accelerated AV junction rhythm)	AVRT
Onset and termination	Gradual	Sudden	Sudden	Sudden	Sudden	Gradual	Sudden
Heart rate (bpm)	100–(220 – age)	100–160	Multiple of 300	100–180	120–200	70–120	140–250
P wave	Sinus Ps	Sinus Ps	Flutter waves	Ectopic Ps	Retrograde Ps	Retrograde Ps	Ectopic Ps
R-P relationship	Long R-P	Long R-P	Undefined	Long R-P	Short R-P or no P	Short R-P or no P	Short R-P

▲ **Figure 11–1.** Algorithm for distinguishing supraventricular tachycardias. AF, atrial fibrillation; AFL, atrial flutter; AT, atrial tachycardia; AVNRT, atrioventricular nodal reentrant tachycardia; AVRT, atrioventricular reciprocating tachycardia; JT, junctional tachycardia; MAT, multifocal atrial tachycardia; SN, sinus node; ST, sinus tachycardia; SVT, supraventricular tachycardia.

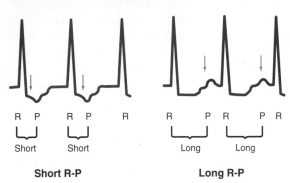

▲ **Figure 11–2.** *Short R-P* refers to a regular supra-ventricular tachycardia (SVT) where the R-P interval is shorter than the P-R interval. *Long R-P* refers to a regular SVT where the R-P interval is longer than the P-R interval.

▶ General Considerations

When the sinus node fires at a rate of more than 100 bpm, the rhythm is, with one exception, considered sinus tachycardia (see later section, Sinus Node Reentry). The onset and termination of sinus tachycardia are invariably gradual. The range for heart rate in sinus tachycardia is 100 to (220 – age) bpm; faster rates usually imply a different cause. Confirming that the tachycardic P waves are identical in morphology and axis to the normal sinus rhythm P waves is essential to the diagnosis. Like normal sinus rhythm, the R-P relationship in sinus tachycardia is typically long R-P, unless the patient has a very long P-R interval, which can usually be seen on the baseline ECG.

Sinus tachycardia is usually a physiologic response, activated when the body requires a higher heart rate to meet metabolic demands or maintain blood pressure. Common causes are exercise, hypotension, hypoxemia, heart failure, sepsis, fever, hyperthyroidism, fluid depletion, and blood loss.

The heart rate achieved is proportional to the intensity of the stimulus, but the rapidity with which the heart rate increases and decreases is a function of how quickly the stimulus is applied and withdrawn.

▶ Treatment

Vagal maneuvers slow the tachycardia gradually but only while being performed; when the vagal stimulus is removed, the heart rate gradually returns to where it started.

Attempting to slow the heart rate pharmacologically can be detrimental because it counteracts the compensatory mechanism provided by the tachycardia. Therefore, management is usually focused on treating the underlying cause of the sinus tachycardia.

2. Sinus Node Reentry

 ESSENTIALS OF DIAGNOSIS

▶ Onset and termination: sudden.
▶ Heart rate: 100–160 bpm.
▶ P wave: identical to normal sinus rhythm P wave
▶ R-P relationship: long.

▶ General Considerations

This uncommon rhythm accounts for less than 5% of SVTs. It uses the sinus node or perinodal tissue as a critical part of the reentrant circuit, producing P waves identical to those seen during normal sinus rhythm. The heart rate usually falls between 100 and 160 bpm. Like sinus tachycardia, the R-P relationship is typically long R-P. Unlike sinus tachycardia, sinus node reentry is initiated by an ectopic beat rather than a physiologic stimulus and possesses the characteristics typical of a reentrant circuit. It therefore begins and ends abruptly and responds to vagal maneuvers and pharmacologic interventions by terminating rather than slowing.

▶ Treatment

The arrhythmia can be terminated quickly with intravenous adenosine, verapamil, or diltiazem, or via carotid massage. Long-term treatment uses β-blockers and calcium channel blockers. The largest reported series of patients treated with catheter ablation described success in all 10 patients. No complications were reported. Other smaller series found similar efficacy.

Sperry RE, et al. Radiofrequency catheter ablation of sinus node reentrant tachycardia. *Pacing Clin Electrophysiol.* 1993;16(11):2202–9. [PMID: 7505935]

ATRIAL FLUTTER

 ESSENTIALS OF DIAGNOSIS

▶ Onset and termination: sudden.
▶ Heart rate: usually a multiple of 300.
▶ P waves: flutter waves at 250–340 bpm.
▶ R-P relationship: undefined due to flutter waves.
▶ Prominent neck vein pulsations of about 300/min.

▶ General Considerations

Atrial flutter is usually associated with organic heart disease and is second in frequency only to atrial fibrillation in post–coronary bypass surgery patients, with an incidence of up to 33%. With a typical atrial rate of 300 bpm (range 250–340 bpm), atrial flutter usually produces a "sawtooth" appearance (F waves). As is the case with atrial fibrillation (see Chapter 12), the ventricular rate depends on conduction through the AV node. Unlike atrial fibrillation, the ventricular impulses are transmitted at some integer fraction of the atrial rate. In rare circumstances, 1:1 conduction may occur. Fixed 2:1, 3:1, or 4:1 block is the usual scenario. However, variable block can also occur, leading to one of the three types of irregular SVTs (see Figure 11–1). If flutter is suspected but F waves are not clearly visible, vagal maneuvers or pharmacologic agents, such as adenosine, can help unmask the flutter waves by enhancing the degree of AV block.

▶ Pathophysiology

Atrial flutter occurs in a variety of forms; the most common is isthmus-dependent counterclockwise atrial flutter; followed by the isthmus-dependent clockwise atrial flutter; and then the atypical, nonisthmus-dependent variety. The counterclockwise flutter is recognized electrocardiographically by negative F waves in leads II, III, and aVF and positive F waves in lead V_1. The single reentrant wavefront proceeds up the interatrial septum, across the roof of the right atrium, down the lateral wall, and across the inferior wall. Clockwise flutter, on the other hand, has positive F waves in leads II, III, and aVF and negative F waves in lead V_1. The reentrant circuit in this case moves in the reverse direction. In both of these types of atrial flutter, the atrial rates range between 250 and 340 bpm.

▶ Clinical Findings

Symptoms attributable to atrial flutter are secondary to the ventricular response in addition to any underlying cardiac diseases. Dizziness, palpitations, angina-type chest pain, dyspnea, weakness, fatigue, and, occasionally, syncope may be the presenting symptoms. In those patients with poor left ventricular function, overt congestive heart failure may ensue.

Clinical evaluation is similar to that described for atrial fibrillation (see Chapter 12), but underlying heart disease is detected more often with atrial flutter than with fibrillation.

▶ Prevention

Several antiarrhythmic agents can prevent recurrences of atrial flutter. It appears that both class Ia and Ic agents are effective. Class III agents, such as sotalol and amiodarone, can also work very well. Dofetilide, a newer class III agent, which blocks the rapid form of the delayed rectifier current, Ik_r, has also been found effective in converting to and maintenance of sinus rhythm. Its administration requires initiation in the hospital and an ECG-monitored setting. Drugs that are contraindicated with its use include verapamil, ketoconazole, cimetidine, trimethoprim, prochlorperazine, megestrol, and hydrochlorothiazide. With regard to safety, dofetilide has an overall proarrhythmic event rate of approximately 0.9%, which is less than the 3.3% seen in patients with congestive heart failure or the 2.5% in patients with previous ventricular tachycardia.

It should be emphasized that an AV nodal blocking agent should be started before initiating a class I drug. If the AV node is unblocked, a type I agent could facilitate conduction of atrial flutter by improving nodal conduction or by slowing the flutter rate and paradoxically increasing the ventricular response.

▶ Treatment

A. Conversion

Once the diagnosis of atrial flutter is made, assessment of the patient's status will dictate whether to perform cardioversion immediately. Immediate cardioversion can be accomplished with synchronized direct-current (DC) cardioversion, rapid atrial pacing to interrupt the macroreentrant circuit, or intravenous infusion of an antiarrhythmic agent. For DC cardioversion, as little as 25 J may be all that is required; however, at least 50 J is recommended to avoid extra shocks, and 100 J will terminate almost all episodes of atrial flutter. The major drawback with DC cardioversion is the need to administer sedation.

Rapid atrial pacing is another method that may terminate the arrhythmia. Pacing is best performed in the right atrium at a rate faster than the flutter rate, which allows the circuit to be entered by the pacing impulse. If the extrinsic pacing rate exceeds the rate that can be sustained through the zone of slow conduction, the flutter wavefront can be interrupted and will no longer be present when the pacing is stopped. If the patient has a pacemaker or implantable cardiac defibrillator with an atrial lead, pace termination can be done painlessly via the device. An alternative method uses a swallowed transesophageal electrode. Because of the interposed tissue, a high current is often necessary to capture and pace the atrium reliably, which may cause significant discomfort to the patient. Of note, overdrive pacing may precipitate atrial fibrillation, which usually terminates spontaneously after several minutes. Should the atrial fibrillation persist, however, control of the ventricular response rate is typically easier when compared with atrial flutter.

Finally, rapid pharmacologic cardioversion can be considered with intravenous agents such as ibutilide. Ibutilide is a unique class III antiarrhythmic agent with a rate of conversion of approximately 60% in patients with atrial flutter of less than 45 days duration. Cardioversion can be expected within 30 minutes of administration. The major complication with this agent is the development of torsades de pointes, which can occur in up to 12.5% of patients, with 1.7% requiring cardioversion for sustained polymorphic ventricular tachycardia. These occur primarily within the first hour after administration. For this reason, patients given ibutilide are typically kept on monitor for several hours after administration. Procainamide is another intravenous agent that can be given to pharmacologically convert atrial flutter.

B. Rate Control

In general, controlling the ventricular rate in atrial flutter is more difficult than in atrial fibrillation. β-Blockers and calcium channel blockers are moderately effective in controlling the rate. Digoxin is less helpful since it only weakly blocks AV node conduction. Intravenous amiodarone, which has some β-blocking effect, has been shown to be at least as efficacious as digoxin.

C. Catheter Ablation and Other Modalities

The reentrant circuit in typical atrial flutter has been successfully mapped and includes an area of slow conduction called the isthmus, which is bound by the tricuspid annulus, the inferior vena cava, and the os of the coronary sinus. Ablation in the isthmus region interrupts the reentrant circuit and has been shown to be highly efficacious (90–100%) in permanently eliminating atrial flutter. In cost-effective analysis, ablation appears to be the preferred approach over cardioversion and pharmacologic prevention. Non–isthmus-dependent atypical atrial flutters can be more difficult to ablate. However, with current three-dimensional mapping systems (electroanatomic and noncontact high resolution), even these types of atrial flutter are being ablated with high success rates.

If attempts to ablate atrial flutter fail, the ventricular rate can be controlled by transcatheter ablation of the AV node or His bundle. With a long-standing, there may be a subsequent improvement in left ventricular function.

D. Stroke Prophylaxis

Atrial flutter is a recognized cause of peripheral embolization and stroke. The current recommendation is to treat patients with atrial flutter just as atrial fibrillation in terms of stroke prophylaxis. Many patients have bouts of atrial fibrillation even after successful atrial flutter ablation. Therefore, rigorous monitoring after atrial flutter ablation is recommended to determine which patients need long-term aspirin or anticoagulant therapy.

Calkins H, et al. Results of catheter ablation of typical atrial flutter. *Am J Cardiol.* 2004;94(4):437–42. [PMID: 15325925]

Feld G, et al. Radiofrequency catheter ablation of type 1 atrial flutter using large-tip 8- or 10-mm electrode catheters and a high-output radiofrequency energy generator: results of a multicenter safety and efficacy study. *J Am Coll Cardiol.* 2004;43(8):1466–72. [PMID: 15093885]

Nakagawa H, et al. Characterization of reentrant circuit in macro-reentrant right atrial tachycardia after surgical repair of congenital heart disease: isolated channels between scars allow "focal" ablation. *Circulation.* 2001;103(5):699–709. [PMID: 11156882]

Tomson TT, et al. Risk of stroke and atrial fibrillation after radiofrequency catheter ablation of typical atrial flutter. *Heart Rhythm.* 2012;9(11):1779–84. [PMID: 22813577]

MULTIFOCAL ATRIAL TACHYCARDIA

 ESSENTIALS OF DIAGNOSIS

▶ Heart rate: up to 150 bpm.
▶ P waves: three or more distinct P waves in a single lead.
▶ Variable P-P, P-R, and R-R intervals.

▶ General Considerations

Multifocal atrial tachycardia (MAT) is an irregular SVT that constitutes less than 1% of all arrhythmias. It is related to pulmonary disease in 60–85% of cases, with chronic obstructive pulmonary disease (COPD) exacerbation being the most common. In addition, MAT is precipitated by respiratory failure, acute decompensated cardiac function, and infection. It has also been reported to be associated with hypokalemia, hypomagnesemia, hyponatremia, pulmonary embolism, cancer, and valvular heart disease, and can also occur in the postoperative setting. It affects children and adults. Distention of the right atrium from elevated pulmonary pressures causes multiple ectopic foci to fire, with ventricular rates not usually exceeding 150 bpm. Whether this rhythm is due to abnormal automaticity or triggered activity is uncertain, but the ability of verapamil to suppress the ectopic atrial activity by virtue of its calcium channel–blocking properties supports the latter assumption.

Three ECG criteria must be met to diagnose MAT (Figure 11–3): (1) the presence of at least three distinct P-wave morphologies recorded in the same lead; (2) the absence of one dominant atrial pacemaker; and (3) varying P-P, P-R, and R-R intervals.

MAT is often misdiagnosed as atrial fibrillation. Although both are irregular, the former has distinct P waves with an intervening isoelectric baseline. At times, MAT may progress to atrial fibrillation.

▶ Treatment

The primary treatment for MAT should be directed at the underlying disease state. Oral and intravenous verapamil and several formulations of intravenous β-blockers have been effective to varying degrees in either slowing the heart rate (without terminating the rhythm) or in converting the arrhythmia to sinus rhythm. Intravenous magnesium and potassium, even in patients with serum levels of these electrolytes within the normal range, convert a significant percentage of these patients to sinus rhythm. Digoxin is not effective in treating this condition. Moreover, treatment with digoxin may precipitate digitalis intoxication. In addition, if the arrhythmia is secondary to delayed after-depolarizations, further aggravation may occur with digitalis because this drug increases delayed

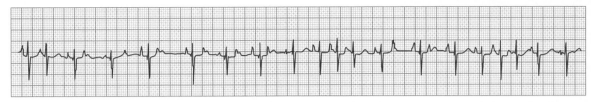

▲ **Figure 11–3.** Multifocal atrial tachycardia. The presence of at least three distinct P-wave morphologies, the absence of one dominant pacemaker focus, and varying P-P, R-R, and PR intervals establish the diagnosis.

after-depolarizations. Medications that cause atrial irritability, such as theophylline and β-agonists, should be withdrawn whenever possible.

Application of radiofrequency energy for both AV node modification and AV node ablation with subsequent implantation of a pacemaker has been reported. The numbers of patients in the studies were very small, and there are no long-term results. Nevertheless, ablation of the AV node has been shown to reduce symptomatic MAT, resulting in improved quality of life, reduced hospital admissions for recurrent symptomatic MAT, and improved left ventricular function.

▶ **Prognosis**

Because of the severity of the precipitating underlying diseases, MAT portends a poor outcome. Mortality during the hospitalization when the arrhythmia is first diagnosed is between 30% and 60%, with death being attributed to the disease state rather than the tachycardia itself. In one study of patients with pulmonary disease who were admitted for acute respiratory failure, the in-hospital mortality rate for those with MAT was 87%, compared with 24% for those in a different rhythm.

Bradley DJ, et al. The clinical course of multifocal atrial tachycardia in infants and children. *J Am Coll Cardiol.* 2001;38(2):401–8. [PMID: 11499730]

Ueng KC, et al. Radiofrequency catheter modification of atrioventricular junction in patients with COPD and medically refractory multifocal atrial tachycardia. *Chest.* 2000;117(1):52–9. [PMID: 10631199]

ATRIAL TACHYCARDIA

 ESSENTIALS OF DIAGNOSIS

▶ Onset and termination: sudden.

▶ Heart rate: 100–180 bpm.

▶ P wave: distinct P waves that differ from sinus P waves.

▶ R-P relationship: long.

▶ **General Considerations**

Atrial tachycardia originates from an ectopic site in the atrium, and therefore, the P waves are usually quite different than the sinus P waves. It has been demonstrated that these arrhythmias arise from well-defined anatomic regions, including the crista terminalis, the tricuspid and mitral annuli, the right and left atrial appendage, and the region within or surrounding the pulmonary veins. In situations where the P wave is identical to the sinus P wave, the SVT is usually designated to be sinus node reentry or sinus tachycardia. The onset of atrial tachycardia is typically sudden; however, there can be some acceleration at the beginning, which is called the "warm-up" phase. Rates can range from 100 to 180 bpm and, rarely, over 200 bpm. The R-P relationship is usually long, unless there is a very long P-R interval, which can sometimes be appreciated on the baseline ECG. The episodes may either be brief and self-terminating or chronic and persistent, eventually leading to a tachycardia-induced cardiomyopathy if left untreated. Short nonsustained bursts of atrial tachycardia can be seen in 2–6% of young healthy adults on Holter evaluations.

In patients with paroxysmal sustained atrial tachycardia, there is a higher likelihood of associated organic heart disease, including coronary artery disease, valvular heart disease, congenital heart disease, and other cardiomyopathies. Frequently, a transient automatic atrial tachycardia will be present, the cause of which can usually be determined from the associated clinical setting. Some of the most frequent causes include acute myocardial infarction (in which case, it is seen in 4–19% of patients), electrolyte disturbances (especially hypokalemia), chronic lung disease or pulmonary infection, acute alcohol ingestion, hypoxia, and use of cardiac stimulants (theophylline, cocaine).

The form that occurs almost exclusively, and not uncommonly, in children is a continuous tachycardia with heart rates of about 175 bpm. Symptoms are severe, and congestive heart failure frequently develops as a result of a tachycardia-induced cardiomyopathy. The arrhythmia may be transient in younger children, but when it persists in older children, it should be considered permanent. Fortunately, if the tachycardia can be terminated, cardiac function returns to normal. When it appears in adults, the continuous variety manifests milder symptoms.

Atrial tachycardias may have an automatic, triggered, or microreentrant mechanism. Although precisely defining the basic mechanism of a particular atrial tachycardia may be difficult, understanding their basic principles may help with choosing therapy.

▶ Treatment

A. Pharmacologic Therapy

Although there are no large-scale trials in the medical treatment of atrial tachycardias, reported data show that β-blockers and calcium channel blockers are at least partially effective, particularly if the underlying mechanism of the tachycardia is abnormal automaticity or triggered activity. Because of their safety profile, these drugs are usually first-line medical therapy.

Other antiarrhythmic drugs may be effective in treating some patients with atrial tachycardias. However, there are no large-scale trials comparing the drugs or even trials comparing drugs to placebo. Therefore, drug therapy is largely empiric, and drug choice is determined more by side-effect profile and risk of proarrhythmia than by suspected efficacy. The use of class Ic antiarrhythmic drugs may be somewhat successful. Flecainide and propafenone are often well tolerated in patients without structural heart disease and thus can be considered a reasonable first-line antiarrhythmic therapy. Quinidine and procainamide are less well tolerated. Class Ib agents are generally not effective for atrial tachycardias; however, there may be a small subset of lidocaine-sensitive atrial tachycardias in which mexiletine may be effective. Sotalol may also be effective, in part because of its inherent β-blocker (class II) properties. It is generally better tolerated than quinidine and may provide rate control during recurrences. Nevertheless, because sotalol also has class III properties, it will prolong the QT interval and may predispose patients to torsades de pointes, similar to quinidine and procainamide. Amiodarone may be effective, especially in resistant tachycardias. In addition, it is the least proarrhythmic and is generally used as first-line drug therapy in patients with depressed left ventricular function. Newer class III drugs, such as dofetilide, may be effective for atrial tachycardias, but there are few data about their use in atrial arrhythmias, except atrial fibrillation and atrial flutter.

B. Ablation

Ablation for atrial tachycardias has been proven safe and effective, with reported success rates between 77% and 100%. It also has been shown to improve patient quality of life scores. Therefore, ablation should be indicated for all symptomatic patients who have persistent symptoms despite medical therapy or intolerable side effects from medicines. Furthermore, patients who are not willing to undergo medical therapy should also be considered. Recently, the use of electromagnetic and noncontact mapping systems has significantly improved ablative therapy by decreasing fluoroscopic

time, mapping time, and number of radiofrequency applications, thereby increasing efficacy.

Heck PM, et al. The challenging face of focal atrial tachycardia in the post AF ablation era. *J Cardiovasc Electrophysiol.* 2011;22(7):832–8. [PMID: 21635611]

Kalman JM, et al. Localization of focal atrial tachycardias–back to the future . . . when (old) electrophysiologic first principles complement sophisticated technology. *J Cardiovasc Electrophysiol.* 2007;18(1):7–8. [PMID: 17240545]

Sanders P, et al. Characterization of focal atrial tachycardia using high-density mapping. *J Am Coll Cardiol.* 2005;46(11):2088–99. [PMID: 16325047]

ATRIOVENTRICULAR NODAL REENTRANT TACHYCARDIA

 ESSENTIALS OF DIAGNOSIS

▶ Onset and termination: sudden.

▶ Heart rate: usually 120–200 bpm but can be faster; neck pulsations correspond to heart rate.

▶ P waves: retrograde P waves; P waves not visible in 90% of cases.

▶ R-P relationship: short, if P waves visible.

▶ General Considerations

Atrioventricular nodal reentrant tachycardia (AVNRT) is more common in women than in men. Heart rates usually fall in the range of 120–200 bpm, although rates up to 250 bpm have been recorded. Palpitations are almost universally reported. A feeling of diuresis, noted with other supraventricular arrhythmias, is significantly more common in AVNRT and has been correlated with elevated right atrial pressures and elevated atrial natriuretic peptide. Neck pulsations are common (Brugada phenomenon) and are secondary to simultaneous contraction of the atria and ventricles against closed mitral and tricuspid valves. Dizziness and lightheadedness can occur, but frank syncope is very unusual. Sudden death has been reported but is extremely rare. Although symptoms may occur at any age, the distribution of when the tachycardia and symptoms commonly start appears to be bimodal. The initial episode may begin during the second decade of life, only to disappear and then reappear during the fourth and fifth decades of life.

▶ Pathophysiology

Conduction from the right atrium to the ventricles is normally over a singular AV nodal pathway, with no route of reentry back into the atrium. In persons with dual AV nodal pathways, an atrial impulse may travel antegrade from the atrium over one limb of the AV node and then back to the atrium over another limb in a retrograde fashion. When only one cycle occurs, a single echo beat in the form of a retrograde P wave may be seen on the ECG. If this echo beat can again penetrate the AV node antegrade, the cycle can perpetuate itself, leading to AVNRT. It is estimated that dual AV nodal pathways exist in up to one-fourth of the population, but only a fraction of these people ever manifest a tachycardia.

If each limb of the circuit conducted impulses equally, echo beats and sustained AVNRT would not occur. An atrial impulse traveling down both limbs at the same speed would cause each limb to be refractory when that impulse reached the bottom of the node, preventing the impulse in each limb from going back up the other. Instead, the limbs have varying conduction speeds and refractory periods. The faster conducting limb, called the β or fast pathway, has a longer refractory period, whereas the reverse is true for the second limb, called the α or slow pathway. A premature atrial or ventricular depolarization is often the trigger of AVNRT. The typical AVNRT circuit occurs with a self-perpetuating impulse that travels down the slow pathway and up the fast pathway.

Conduction up the fast pathway is usually so rapid that retrograde atrial depolarization is simultaneous or almost simultaneous with antegrade ventricular activation. This causes the low-amplitude P wave to become obscured in the much higher amplitude QRS complex. Therefore, the P wave is not visible 50–60% of the time. In 20–30% of cases, the P wave distorts the terminal portion of the QRS causing a pseudo-S wave in the inferior leads and a pseudo-R' in lead V_1, and in approximately 10% of cases, the P wave distorts the QRS complex (Figure 11–4). Since the P wave usually occurs simultaneous to or just after the QRS, the common variety of AVNRT is a short R-P tachycardia.

AVNRT, once initiated, can perpetuate itself without the participation of either the atria or ventricles. Therefore, on rare occasions, the tachycardia can occur with a 2:1 block in either direction, leading to two atrial depolarizations for every ventricular depolarization or two ventricular depolarizations for every atrial depolarization.

▶ Prevention

Prevention of AVNRT is directed at slowing or blocking conduction in either the fast or slow pathway. Typical AV nodal blocking agents such as β-blockers, calcium channel blockers, and digoxin are most effective on the antegrade slow pathway. The more potent class Ia antiarrhythmic drugs may be necessary to inhibit conduction in the retrograde fast pathway. Class Ic drugs and amiodarone and sotalol (class III) affect both pathways.

▶ Treatment

A. Vagal Maneuvers

Vagal maneuvers should be considered, barring any contraindications, before embarking on medical therapy. The Valsalva maneuver and carotid sinus massage can immediately terminate the tachycardia by increasing refractory time in the AV node. In patients over 50 years old, bruits should be ruled out before carotid sinus massage to avoid embolic stroke. Medications may render the arrhythmia more susceptible to termination with vagal maneuvers. Therefore, these can be attempted immediately after each round of drug therapy if the tachycardia persists.

B. Pharmacologic Therapy

Terminating an acute episode of AVNRT in the hospital setting has been made simpler with the availability of intravenous adenosine. Adenosine temporarily stops conduction in the AV node, thereby terminating the reentrant circuit in AVNRT. It is fast acting, typically reaching and acting on the AV node within seconds of administration. With a clinical half-life of 10 seconds, commonly reported sensations such as breathlessness, chest heaviness, and flushing disappear quickly. The routine dosage is 6 mg followed by up to two more boluses of 12 mg. If adenosine is ineffective, intravenous verapamil can be used, but it takes longer to act. Diltiazem, given as intravenous bolus, can also be effective in aborting the tachycardia. Hypotension occurs with about a 10% incidence and is usually rapidly reversed with fluid administration. Although intravenous β-blockers, procainamide, and digoxin are other second-line choices, they can be advantageous in recurrent cases because of their slower clearance from the body.

C. Catheter Ablation

Radiofrequency lesions delivered via an ablation catheter can be directed at either the fast or slow pathway; the latter is preferred since it is associated with a lower risk of complete heart block.

The inferior origin of the slow pathway is variable within the triangle of Koch, but it is usually anterior and superior to (and sometimes within) the os of the coronary sinus. These anatomic landmarks and gross intracardiac electrogram patterns can be used to position the ablation catheter for successful modification of the AV node. The fast pathway is left unaltered and can still be used for transmission of sinus impulses to the ventricles. Long-term freedom from recurrent AVNRT is about 95%, and the risk of complete heart block as a result of inadvertent fast pathway or nodal damage is 0–5%.

A relatively new form of ablation is cryoablation, using a supercooling catheter, which can reversibly or permanently damage endocardial tissue. This novel approach allows for testing the acceptability of a particular ablation site. Should heart block occur prior to irreversible tissue damage, then rewarming can be performed with no untoward effects.

Gupta D, et al. Cryoablation compared with radiofrequency ablation for atrioventricular nodal re-entrant tachycardia: analysis of factors contributing to acute and follow-up outcome. *Europace*. 2006;8(12):1022–6. [PMID: 17101629]

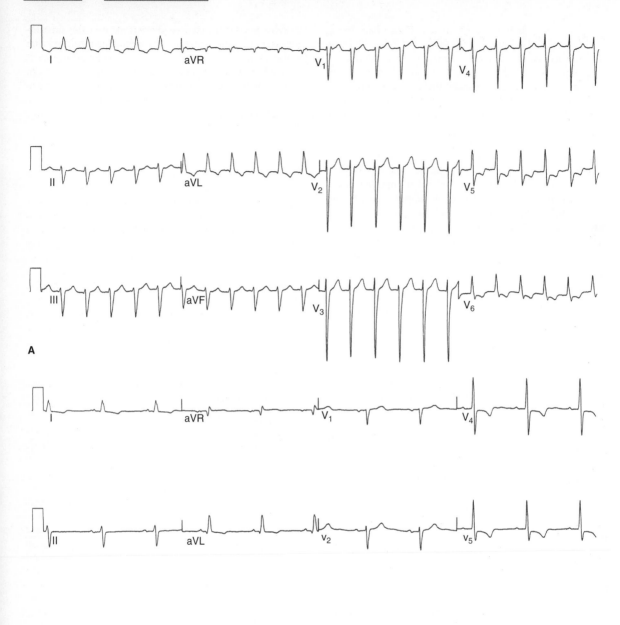

▲ **Figure 11–4. A:** Supraventricular tachycardia without easily identifiable P waves but with pseudo R′ in lead V₁ compatible with atrioventricular nodal reentrant tachycardia. **B:** Postconversion tracing. Note normal QRS in lead V₁ when patient displays normal sinus rhythm.

Rodriguez-Entem FJ, et al. Cryoablation versus radiofrequency ablation for the treatment of atrioventricular nodal reentrant tachycardia: results of a prospective randomized study. *J Interv Card Electrophysiol.* 2013;36:41–5. [PMID: 23080326]

Wu J, et al. Mechanisms underlying atrioventricular nodal conduction and the reentrant circuit of atrioventricular nodal reentrant tachycardia using optical mapping. *J Cardiovasc Electrophysiol.* 2002;13(8):831–4. [PMID: 12212708]

JUNCTIONAL TACHYCARDIA (ACCELERATED AV JUNCTIONAL RHYTHM)

 ESSENTIALS OF DIAGNOSIS

- ▶ Onset and termination: gradual.
- ▶ Heart rate: 70–120 bpm.
- ▶ P waves: retrograde.
- ▶ R-P relationship: short, if P waves visible.

▶ General Considerations

Unlike AVNRT, which presents with recurrent tachycardia episodes of sudden onset, junctional tachycardia, which is sometimes also called nonparoxysmal junctional tachycardia (NPJT), usually starts gradually and sometimes almost imperceptibly. It is easily differentiated from AVNRT by a heart rate between 70 and 120 bpm, gradual onset and termination, and lack of termination with vagal maneuvers. Although heart rates of less than 100 bpm can be seen, it is, nevertheless, a tachycardia because the rates are faster than the 40–60 bpm seen with a junctional escape rhythm.

▶ Clinical Findings

The heart rate at onset is just slightly faster than that of the rhythm preceding it, with gradual acceleration until the final rate is achieved. AV dissociation is common, occurring in 85% of cases caused by digoxin (see following discussion). When the conduction to the atria is intact, retrograde P waves may appear immediately before or after the QRS complex, or they may be obscured within the QRS. Discharge from the AV node is regular, but if antegrade second-degree AV block (almost always the result of digoxin excess), exit block, or atrial capture beats coexist with junctional tachycardia, the rhythm will appear irregular. Enhanced vagal tone or vagolytic agents will either slow down or speed up the arrhythmia, respectively.

Usually seen in the setting of organic heart disease, the cause of this rhythm is almost always identifiable. At one time, digoxin excess accounted for up to 85% of cases of junctional tachycardia. Awareness of the drug's side effects and the availability of other AV nodal blocking agents have diminished the incidence. Nevertheless, in patients being treated with digoxin

for atrial fibrillation, clinicians should suspect this arrhythmia when the ECG demonstrates a regularized ventricular response. Acute inferior infarction accounts for 20% of junctional tachycardias, and this rhythm may be present in up to 10% of all infarcts in this location, with onset usually within the first 24 hours and disappearance in several days. Junctional tachycardia may follow open heart surgery (valve replacement more often than bypass surgery), or it can be caused by myocarditis (especially rheumatic) and, rarely, congenital heart disease. In all cases, the tachycardia resolves along with the acute underlying event or with digoxin withdrawal.

▶ Treatment

Treatment is usually directed at the underlying causative factor. Because the rhythm rarely causes deleterious hemodynamic effects, treatment of the rhythm itself is usually not indicated. If digoxin toxicity is the cause, it should be withdrawn. If digoxin is not the cause, digoxin, β-blockers, or calcium channel blockers can be used to slow down the rate if necessary. Catheter ablation can also be performed, but it carries a risk of complete heart block since the origin of the arrhythmia is near the AV node. However, cryoablation has been used in this setting and may be safer.

Hamdan MH, et al. Role of invasive electrophysiologic testing in the evaluation and management of adult patients with focal junctional tachycardia. *Card Electrophysiol Rev.* 2002;6(4):431–5. [PMID: 12438824]

Law IH, et al. Transcatheter cryothermal ablation of junctional ectopic tachycardia in the normal heart. *Heart Rhythm.* 2006;3(8):903–7. [PMID: 16876738]

ATRIOVENTRICULAR RECIPROCATING TACHYCARDIA

 ESSENTIALS OF DIAGNOSIS

- ▶ Onset and termination: sudden.
- ▶ Heart rate: 140–250 bpm.
- ▶ P wave: ectopic.
- ▶ R-P relationship: short.
- ▶ Delta wave on baseline ECG if bypass tract conducts antegrade.

1. Bypass Tracts & the Wolff-Parkinson-White Syndrome

▶ General Considerations

Congenital bands of tissue that can conduct impulses but lie outside the normal conduction system are called accessory pathways, or bypass tracts. These pathways are responsible for a variety of mechanistically distinct tachycardias by providing preferential conduction between different areas within the heart.

▶ Epidemiology

Accessory pathways are quite prevalent in the general population, with a 2:1 male-to-female predominance. The presence of a bypass tract, however, does not mean that a tachyarrhythmia is a certainty because less than half of persons with documented bypass tracts ever sustain an arrhythmia. The actual number depends on the population studied and varies from 13% in a healthy outpatient population to 80% in the hospital setting.

Approximately 5–10% of patients with documented bypass tracts have concomitant structural heart disease. Ebstein anomaly is the most common, accounting for 25–50% of the anomalies in this group. Of patients with Ebstein anomaly, 8–10% have coexistent bypass tracts, mostly on the right side. The association of right-sided accessory pathways with structural heart disease is strong: 45% of patients with right-sided (and only 5% of those with left-sided) pathways display some type of heart disease.

A familial tendency toward bypass tracts has been seen in some instances, with a fourfold to tenfold increase in incidence among first-degree family members.

▶ Pathophysiology

A. Anatomy

Anatomically, the atria and ventricles are in apposition, separated by an invagination known as the AV groove. Paroxysmal tachycardias mediated by accessory pathways that cross the groove and electrically link the atria and ventricles, when combined with a short P-R interval (< 0.12 seconds), a wide QRS, and secondary repolarization abnormalities, define the Wolff-Parkinson-White syndrome. When this ECG pattern is seen without the tachycardia, it is called Wolff-Parkinson-White pattern or ventricular preexcitation.

Although the most common site of insertion is between the lateral aspect of the left atrium and left ventricular myocardium, pathways can cross the AV groove anywhere in its course (except the region between the aortic and mitral valves) to connect the left or right atrium to its respective ventricle (Figure 11–5). In noting the distribution of accessory pathways, 46–60% are located in the left free wall, 25% within the posteroseptal space, 13–21% in the right free wall, and 2% in the anteroseptal space. Females have right-sided accessory pathways and Asians have right anterior accessory pathways more frequently than other groups, suggesting that pathogenesis of these pathways has a genetic component. Each location produces a distinct ECG pattern (Figure 11–6),

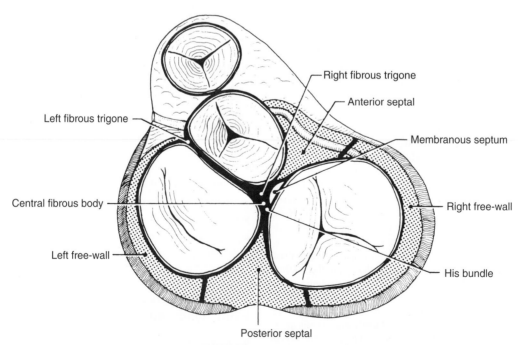

▲ **Figure 11–5.** Cross-sectional diagram of the atrioventricular groove. Atrioventricular bypass tracts may cross the groove anywhere in its course except in the region bounded by the left and right fibrous trigones. (Reprinted, with permission, from Cox JL, et al. *J Thorac Cardiovasc Surg.* 1985;90:490.)

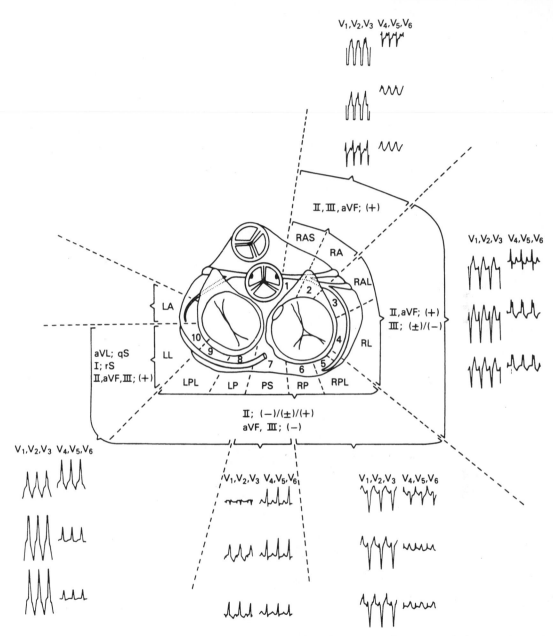

▲ **Figure 11–6.** Single atrioventricular bypass-tract localization based on maximally preexcited electrocardiographic morphology of the QRS. LA/LL, left anterior or left lateral accessory pathways; LPL/LP, left posterolateral or left posterior accessory pathways; PS, posteroseptal accessory pathways; RAL/RL, right anterolateral or right lateral accessory pathways; RAS/RA, right anteroseptal or right anterior accessory pathways; RP/RPL, right posterior or right posterolateral accessory pathways; +, positive delta wave; −, negative delta wave; ±, isoelectric delta wave. (Reprinted, with permission, from Fananapazir L, et al. *Circulation.* 1990;81:578.)

but in the 13% of patients with two or more bypass tracts, the ECG tracing can be confounding and show multiple QRS morphologies.

B. Cardiac Electrical Conduction

Unlike the AV node, whose function is to delay atrial impulses en route to the ventricles, most bypass tracts conduct rapidly and without delay, which accounts for the short P-R interval often seen in sinus rhythm in these patients.

Impulses that reach the ventricles over a bypass tract spread through cell-to-cell conduction within the myocardium, activating the ventricles in series rather than in parallel. This relatively slow process is manifested as a wide QRS complex.

Sinus impulses are not restricted to using the AV node or the bypass tract only to reach the lower chambers. Instead, both may contribute to ventricular activation. This produces a QRS that is initially wide, reflecting conduction over the bypass tract, with the latter portion of the QRS appearing normal and narrow, indicating that the remainder of the ventricle has been depolarized via the normal conduction system (the AV node and His-Purkinje system). The initial slurred upstroke of the QRS, a delta wave, indicates ventricular preexcitation, which can be defined as ventricular depolarization that begins earlier than would be expected by conduction over the AV node alone. The degree of preexcitation and P-R shortening depends on the proportion of ventricular activation occurring over the AV node and the bypass tract. This, in turn, is related to two factors. The first is the conduction velocity of the bypass tract relative to the AV node. The faster the bypass tract can conduct impulses to the ventricles in relation to the AV node, the earlier the ventricle will preexcite, and vice versa. The second factor is the location of the tract, and more specifically, its proximity to the sinus node and AV node. A sinus impulse will encounter a right-sided free-wall bypass tract earlier than it will the AV node, and this favors a short P-R interval with a high degree of ventricular preexcitation (Figure 11–7A). On the other hand, a sinus beat will encounter the AV node early in its course while traveling to a pathway in the lateral left atrium, allowing ventricular activation to occur primarily by the normal conduction system. A narrow, minimally (if at all) preexcited QRS complex with a normal or near-normal P-R interval may be seen (Figure 11–7B). Changes in autonomic tone, by modifying the conduction velocity and refractoriness over both the pathway and the AV node, can produce varying degrees of preexcitation at different times in the same patient (Figure 11–7C).

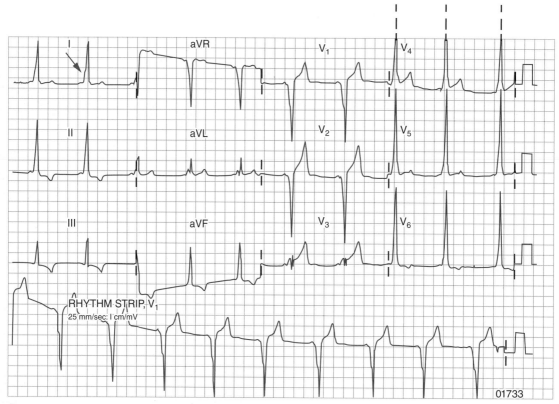

A

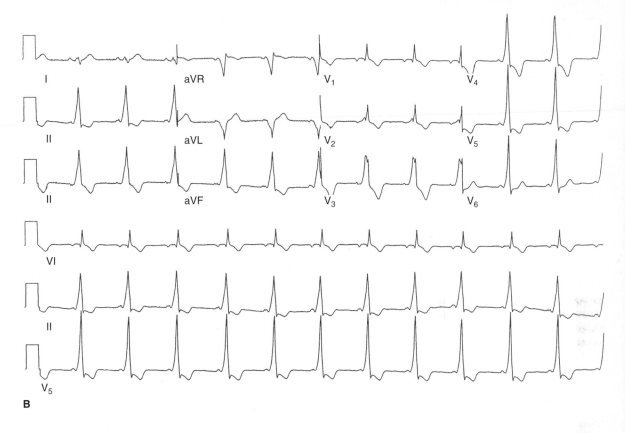

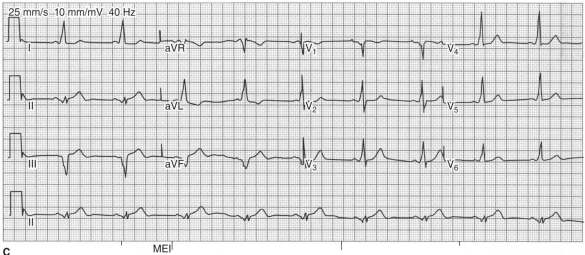

▲ **Figure 11–7.** Ventricular preexcitation over a bypass tract in sinus rhythm. Note the short P-R interval. **A:** Right anterior bypass tract. The delta wave is positive in most leads (*arrow*), and negative in aVR and V₁-V₃. **B:** Left lateral bypass tract. The isoelectric delta wave in V₁ gives the appearance of a normal PR interval. Inspection of the simultaneously recorded rhythm strip leads (*lower three panels*) reveals delta wave onset to be at the end of the P wave in leads II and V₅. **C:** Posterior septal bypass tract. A short time after this tracing was obtained, the patient exhibited minimal to no preexcitation. This was due to fluctuations in autonomic tone causing enhanced conduction through the AV node.

If the delta wave axis of a maximally preexcited beat is discordant from the accompanying preexcited QRS axis, or if more than one preexcited QRS morphology is noted, there may be multiple bypass tracts.

C. Mechanism

1. Atrioventricular reciprocating tachycardia—An inherent property of accessory pathways is their ability to conduct in a retrograde direction more easily than antegrade. The AV node, on the other hand, conducts more efficiently antegrade. For this reason, reentrant rhythms in this setting most commonly use the AV node to go from atrium to ventricle and the bypass tract to return to the atrium. Orthodromic AVRT (antegrade conduction over the AV node) accounts for 70–80% of arrhythmias in patients with AV bypass tracts, with heart rates of 140–250 bpm (Figure 11–8). Antidromic AVRT, in which the atrial impulse is carried to the ventricle over the bypass tract and reenters the atrium via retrograde conduction over the AV node, is rare, occurring in approximately 5–10% of cases. Because conduction to the ventricles during orthodromic AVRT occurs over the normal conduction system, the QRS is narrow, unless bundle branch aberrancy is present. During antidromic AVRT, the QRS is wide and maximally preexcited as a result of the complete lack of AV nodal contribution to ventricular depolarization. When two or more bypass tracts are present, each tract may act as the antegrade or retrograde limb (or both), especially with

involvement of the AV node. There is a higher incidence of ventricular fibrillation in patients with multiple accessory pathways. Additionally, multiple pathways are more common in patients with antidromic SVT and in patients with Ebstein anomaly.

Tachycardia is usually initiated by a premature atrial or ventricular beat. In orthodromic tachycardia, a premature atrial beat conducts down the AV node to depolarize the ventricle, and the bypass tract carries the impulse back to the atrium (Figure 11–9). A ventricular premature beat finding the AV node refractory might initiate an identical tachycardia by first conducting up the bypass tract to the atrium. Antidromic tachycardia initiates in an identical fashion but with a reversed direction of conduction.

Atrial fibrillation accounts for only 19–38% of arrhythmias in the population with accessory pathways, but it is potentially more lethal than the reciprocating tachycardias discussed earlier. It is more common in patients with antegrade conducting accessory pathways and in pathways with a short antegrade refractory period. By virtue of their short refractory periods, bypass tracts (unlike the AV node) have the potential to conduct very rapidly to the ventricles at ventricular rates of 250–350 bpm (Figure 11–10) with the possibility of degeneration to ventricular fibrillation. A reputed marker for sudden death in patients with atrial fibrillation is a shortest preexcited R-R interval of ≤ 250 ms (corresponding to a heart rate of ≥ 240 bpm) between two fully preexcited beats. The finding of a short R-R interval

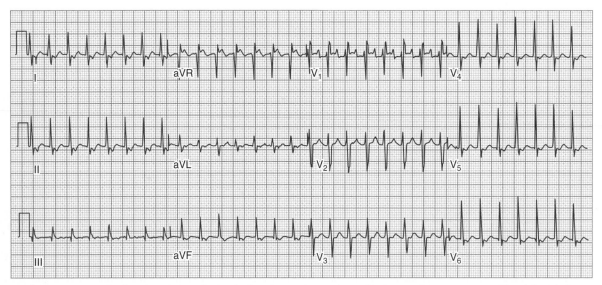

▲ **Figure 11–8.** Orthodromic atrioventricular (AV) reciprocating tachycardia (O-AVRT) in a patient with a left-sided bypass tract. The circuit conducts from atria to ventricles over the AV node and from ventricles to atria retrograde over the bypass tract. This mechanism accounts for the narrow QRS and the retrograde P waves inscribed in the early portion of the T waves. Although the electrocardiogram with atrioventricular nodal reentrant tachycardia (AVNRT) may appear similar, a ventriculoatrial conduction time of more than 100 ms, as measured from QRS onset to P wave onset, greatly favors O-AVRT. The time in this tracing is 110 ms.

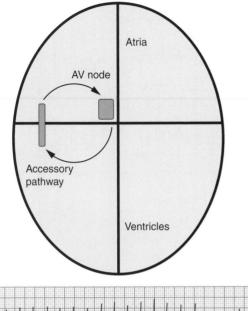

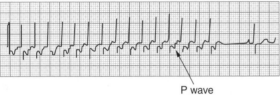

P wave

▲ **Figure 11–9.** The reentry circuit of orthodromic atrioventricular (AV) reciprocating tachycardia (O-AVRT). The atrioventricular (AV) node serves as the antegrade limb of the reentry circuit, and an accessory pathway serves as the retrograde limb. In this case, the accessory pathway is located in the free wall of the right ventricle. The wave of depolarization travels from the AV node to the accessory pathway through the ventricle and from the accessory pathway to the AV node through the atrium. Because the ventricles are depolarized by the normal conduction system, the QRS is narrow unless there is a bundle branch block. Also shown is an ECG example of O-AVRT, at a rate of about 210 bpm. A P wave is present in the left half of the RR cycle (*arrow*) because retrograde conduction through the accessory pathway is more rapid than antegrade conduction through the AV node.

actually has a low positive predictive value, however, because sudden death in this syndrome is still rare.

During atrial fibrillation, the ECG reveals an irregularly irregular rhythm with QRS complexes of varying morphologies, representing conduction to the ventricles via the AV node (normally conducted narrow complexes), the bypass tract (wide, preexcited complexes), and both (fusion beats, harboring elements of both the normally conducted and preexcited beats). In this setting, the bypass tract may be called a

bystander since it is not integral to the tachycardia. Patients with AV bypass tracts have a higher incidence of atrial fibrillation than does the general population, possibly because of the degeneration of reentrant tachycardia or of microreentry within the atrial portion of the bypass tract. It has been shown that ablation of the bypass tract can frequently also eliminate atrial fibrillation.

2. Concealed bypass tracts—Between 15% and 50% of patients with no evidence of preexcitation during sinus rhythm are found to have bypass tracts that conduct only in the retrograde direction. By definition, concealed bypass tracts (their presence cannot be detected by standard ECG) do not display delta waves on the ECG during sinus rhythm, but they can still support an orthodromic AVRT and account for about 30% of orthodromic tachycardias.

Differentiating orthodromic AVRT from AVNRT on the ECG can be difficult. The incidence of both tachycardias being operative at different times in the same person is reported to be between 1.7% and 7%. Therefore, although the presence of a delta wave on the nontachycardiac tracing makes it statistically unlikely that AVNRT was the documented tachycardia, it does not exclude the possibility completely.

Because of the simultaneous atrial and ventricular activation that occurs during AVNRT, the P waves formed as a result of retrograde conduction to the atrium are usually obscured by or merged with the QRS complex. Likewise, because of the short retrograde conduction time via the bypass tract, orthodromic AVRT usually is a short R-P tachycardia, albeit the R-P interval is somewhat longer than with AVNRT (see Figure 11–8). In AVRT, the P waves are usually located within the ST segment and are not obscured or merged with the QRS.

▶ Treatment

A. Vagal Maneuvers

The management of orthodromic AVRT or antidromic AVRT is similar to that of AVNRT. Since the AV node is an integral part of the reentry circuit in AVRT, blocking the AV node terminates the tachycardia. Therefore, vagal maneuvers such as the Valsalva maneuver or carotid sinus massage can be tried first.

B. Pharmacologic Therapy

Intravenous adenosine almost always terminates these tachycardias. Other AV nodal blocking agents such as β-blockers, calcium channel blockers, and digoxin can also be helpful. Just as in AVNRT, vagal maneuvers can be retried after each dose of these longer acting AV nodal blocking agents.

In contrast to orthodromic or antidromic AVRT, patients with atrial fibrillation or atrial flutter and a bystander bypass tract should not be given AV nodal blocking agents. This point is crucial since these types of medicines can precipitate ventricular fibrillation. Blocking the AV node enhances conduction down the bypass tract, making all the

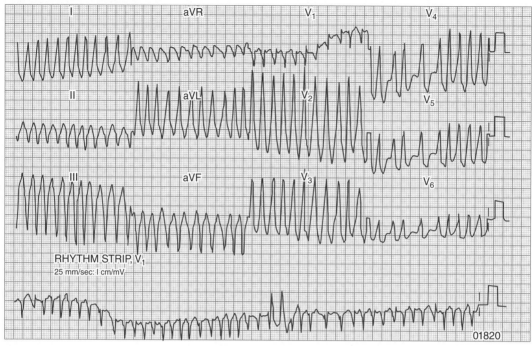

▲ **Figure 11–10.** Atrial fibrillation with antegrade conduction over a left posterolateral bypass tract. Although most beats are fully preexcited, several of the beats in the rhythm strip are narrower, indicating combined conduction over both the bypass tract and the atrioventricular node. Antidromic atrioventricular reciprocating tachycardia (A-AVRT) would have a similar appearance on 12-lead electrocardiogram, but the rhythm irregularity and the varying degrees of preexcitation nullify this possibility. (Reprinted, with permission, from Zipes DP. Specific arrhythmias: diagnosis and treatment. In: Braunwald E, ed. *Heart Disease. A Textbook of Cardiovascular Medicine.* Philadelphia: WB Saunders; 1988.)

complexes wide. Furthermore, the bypass tract can often conduct faster than the AV node, increasing ventricular rates to sometimes over 200 bpm. The aberrant conduction and rapid rate can lead to disorganized ventricular conduction, resulting in ventricular fibrillation. The drug of choice for patients with atrial fibrillation or atrial flutter and a bystander bypass tract is intravenous procainamide or another drug that preferentially blocks the bypass tract. This shunts more conduction through the AV node, which narrows the QRS complexes and often slows down the overall ventricular rate.

Asymptomatic patients showing delta waves on the ECG generally do not require treatment unless they are involved in a high-risk profession such as commercial pilots, police officers, and firefighters. Patients with occasional or rare bouts of minimal or mildly symptomatic palpitations from orthodromic or antidromic AVRT can often be safely treated with such agents as β-blockers or calcium channel blockers to prevent recurrent episodes. However, due to the potential of ventricular fibrillation, these AV node blocking agents should be used with great caution or not at all in

patients who have also demonstrated atrial fibrillation or atrial flutter.

C. Radiofrequency Catheter Ablation Therapy

Patients who experience significant symptoms such as dizziness, presyncope, or syncope should undergo an electrophysiologic study with concomitant radiofrequency ablation. In addition, patients with frequent symptoms who do not respond to or who wish to avoid drug therapy can also undergo ablative therapy. Recent guidelines indicate that ablation can be considered first-line therapy for patients with symptomatic Wolff-Parkinson-White syndrome.

The right internal jugular or femoral vein ablation approach is used for accessory pathways located on the right side of the heart. Left-sided pathways can be approached from the left ventricle with the retrograde technique or transseptally from within the left atrium using the Brockenbrough technique. A steerable catheter is moved around the mitral or tricuspid annulus until the site of shortest impulse transit between the atrium and ventricle is found. This mapping process localizes the bypass tract. Frequently, an impulse can be recorded directly from the bypass tract, further confirming its localization. Once identified, radiofrequency energy delivered to the tract through the mapping catheter permanently destroys the tract and prevents further transmission of electric impulses over it.

Given its curative potential, a high success rate (95% in experienced hands, even with multiple bypass tracts), and a low complication rate, radiofrequency catheter ablation is now a very common treatment for accessory pathways (Table 11–2). As with other supraventricular arrhythmias, new mapping systems have been developed that decrease fluoroscopy and procedure time as well as allowing the operator to return to specific locations if needed.

D. Surgical Ablation Therapy

In rare instances, patients will have multiple pathways or pathways that are inaccessible to an ablation catheter. These patients may undergo surgical division of their tracts.

Table 11–2. Complications of Radiofrequency Ablation of Accessory Pathways[1]

Complication	Incidence (%)
Death	0.08
Nonfatal complications	
Cardiac tamponade	0.5
Atrioventricular block	0.5
Coronary artery spasm	0.2
Mild mitral regurgitation	0.2
Coronary artery thrombosis	0.1
Pericarditis	0.1
Mild aortic regurgitation	0.1
Transient neurologic deficit	0.1
Bacteremia	0.1
Femoral artery complications	
Thrombotic occlusion	0.2
Large hematoma	0.2
Atrioventricular fistula	0.1

[1]The incidence of death is based on unpublished data from the University of Oklahoma, the University of Alabama, the University of Michigan, Duke University, and the University of California, San Francisco. The incidence of nonfatal complications is based on pooled data from seven published studies.

2. Other Bypass Tracts

A variety of bypass tracts other than AV tracts (Kent fibers) also exist. Atriohisian fibers connecting the atrium to the His bundle have been demonstrated. This led to the description of the Lown-Ganong-Levine (LGL) syndrome, which refers to those patients with a short P-R interval, normal QRS, and recurrent SVT. However, current data suggest that LGL syndrome does not truly exist since atriohisian pathways have not been shown to support any type of reentry tachycardia.

Atriofascicular fibers, which are also known as Mahaim fibers, typically run from the lateral right atrium to the right bundle branch. The tract is capable of antegrade conduction only, and therefore, only antidromic AVRT is possible. Because the antegrade reentrant circuit engages the right bundle branch, the tachycardia QRS complex typically has a left bundle branch block pattern. Treatment considerations are the same as for Wolff-Parkinson-White syndrome.

Hsu JC, et al. Differences in accessory pathway location by sex and race. *Heart Rhythm.* 2010;7(1):52–6. [PMID: 19914144]

Kalarus Z, et al. Influence of reciprocating tachycardia on the development of atrial fibrillation in patients with preexcitation syndrome. *Pacing Clin Electrophysiol.* 2007;30(1):85–92. [PMID: 17241320]

Kothari S, et al. Atriofascicular pathways: where to ablate? *Pacing Clin Electrophysiol.* 2006;29(11):1226–33. [PMID: 17100675]

DIFFERENTIATION OF WIDE QRS COMPLEX TACHYCARDIAS

With the exception of the AV node, the refractory period of cardiac tissue for a given beat is directly related to the interval between that beat and the preceding beat; the slower the heart rate, the longer is the recovery period with each beat. Furthermore, because the stability of refractoriness depends on the stability of the heart rate, a beat-to-beat change in refractoriness accompanies variability in the heart rate.

When an early supraventricular beat occurs in the midst of a regular rhythm, the tissues do not have a chance to shorten (or reset) their refractory periods; the result may be aberrant conduction (a transient functional refractoriness, or block) in one of the bundle branches. The shorter the interval between the early beat and the preceding one, the greater is the probability that the early beat will be aberrant (Ashman phenomenon). Ashman phenomenon is also associated with the irregularity and frequent pauses of atrial fibrillation (Figure 11–11). Aberrancy may continue for a variable period before normal conduction resumes.

Aberrant conduction is often seen at the onset of any SVT that uses the AV node for antegrade conduction. (This excludes tachycardias that conduct antegrade over a bypass tract.) The right bundle branch, with its longer refractory period, is more subject to block than is the left, but occasionally the left bundle becomes refractory earlier. Once the tachycardia has been established and refractory periods

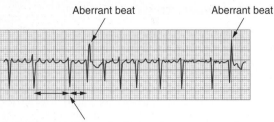

Aberrant beat   Aberrant beat

Long interval before a short interval

▲ **Figure 11–11.** Atrial fibrillation with ventricular aberration from Ashman phenomenon. The long interval before the short interval sets up the aberrant conduction in the ventricle.

stabilized, this normal functional aberrancy may give way to normal conduction, with resumption of a narrow QRS.

Deciding whether a wide-complex tachycardia is supraventricular or ventricular in origin is often difficult. Only when AV dissociation or capture or fusion beats are present can a ventricular rhythm be diagnosed with certainty. The low sensitivities of these findings (20% for AV dissociation) do not provide a firm diagnosis in more than a minority of wide-complex tachycardias, however.

Classic criteria that examine V_1 when a right bundle branch block pattern is present, the QRS width and axis, the presence of positive or negative concordance across the precordium, and various combinations of QRS patterns in different leads may support a diagnosis, but they have been found lacking in diagnostic power because of their low sensitivity, low specificity, or both. A proposed algorithm separates supraventricular from ventricular tachycardia with 99% sensitivity and 97% specificity. However, this algorithm, which is also known as the "Brugada criteria," has had lower sensitivity and specificity in recent studies.

Lau EW, et al. Comparison of two diagnostic algorithms for regular broad complex tachycardia by decision theory analysis. *Pacing Clin Electrophysiol.* 2001;24(7):1118–25. [PMID: 11475829]

OTHER SUPRAVENTRICULAR ARRHYTHMIAS

1. Sinus Node Arrhythmia

 ESSENTIALS OF DIAGNOSIS

▶ Cyclic heart rate variation with respiration.
▶ P-P interval variability ≥ 160 ms or 10%.
▶ P-wave morphology identical to normal sinus rhythm P wave.

▶ General Considerations

A cyclic increase and decrease in heart rate normally accompany inspiration and expiration, respectively, and the irregularity in rhythm (mediated by vagal tone) is often imperceptible. More marked degrees of rate excursion can occur, especially at slower heart rates, but these are not considered to be sinus arrhythmia unless the shortest and longest P-P interval varies by 0.16 seconds or more, or by 10% or more. This respiratory form of sinus arrhythmia is common in younger people. It becomes less prevalent with increasing age and in conditions associated with autonomic dysfunction, such as diabetes mellitus. Enhancement of vagal tone with agents such as digoxin and morphine may also cause sinus arrhythmia.

▶ Treatment

Because of its benign nature, no treatment is required for sinus arrhythmia.

2. Wandering Atrial Pacemaker

 ESSENTIALS OF DIAGNOSIS

▶ Progressive cyclic alteration in P wave morphology.
▶ Heart rate: 60–100 bpm.

▶ General Considerations

The presence of more than one pacemaker within the atria (which may or may not include the sinus node) causes variation in the P-P interval, P-wave morphology, and P-R interval. The heart rate remains within the normal range.

There is controversy over the cause of this rhythm. Some authorities believe that wandering atrial pacemaker and MAT are the same rhythm artificially separated by heart rate and that both are attributable to underlying pulmonary disease. Others believe that it is an exaggerated form of a respiratory sinus arrhythmia, with the uncovering of latent atrial and sinus node pacemakers when the primary sinus node pacemaker cycles to a slow rate with expiration.

The significance ascribed to a wandering atrial pacemaker should probably be interpreted in the setting in which it is seen. In those with lung disease, it may simply be a reflection of that process. In the elderly, it may suggest sinus node disease or sick sinus syndrome, and in the young and athletic heart, it may represent heightened vagal tone.

▶ Treatment

The rhythm itself is usually benign and typically requires no intervention. If the rhythm is secondary, treating the underlying etiology may be warranted.

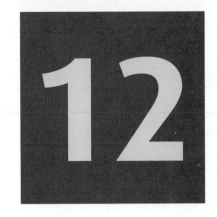

Atrial Fibrillation

Melvin M. Scheinman, MD

ESSENTIALS OF DIAGNOSIS

▶ Irregularly irregular ventricular rhythm.
▶ Absence of P waves on the electrocardiogram.

▶ General Considerations

Atrial fibrillation, the most common sustained clinical arrhythmia, is diagnosed by finding an irregularly irregular ventricular rhythm without discrete P waves (Figure 12–1). The QRS complex is usually narrow, but it may be wide if aberrant conduction or bundle branch block is present. Atrial fibrillation associated with the Wolff-Parkinson-White syndrome may occur with very rapid ventricular rates and may be life-threatening. This arrhythmia is diagnosed by its very rapid irregular rate associated with wide preexcited QRS complexes and requires emergency treatment (see later section, Long-Term Approach).

Approximately 4% of the population over age 60 years has sustained an episode of atrial fibrillation, with a particularly steep increase in prevalence after the seventh decade of life. Risk factors for development of atrial fibrillation include heart failure, hypertensive cardiovascular disease, coronary artery disease, and valvular heart disease. Moreover, both sustained and paroxysmal atrial fibrillation have important implications for the development of a cerebrovascular accident (CVA) or other systemic emboli. It is estimated that 15–20% of CVAs in nonrheumatic patients are due to atrial fibrillation.

▶ Clinical Findings

A. Symptoms & Signs

When called on to manage new-onset atrial fibrillation, it is important to establish the precipitating factors because the type of associated condition determines long-term prognosis.

In some patients, episodes of atrial fibrillation may be initiated by caffeine, alcohol, or marijuana use. Atrial fibrillation may result from acute intercurrent ailments. For example, this arrhythmia may develop in patients with hyperthyroidism or lung disease, or after either cardiac or pulmonary surgery, especially in older patients. Atrial fibrillation is also seen in patients with acute pulmonary embolism, myocarditis, or acute myocardial infarction, particularly when the last condition is complicated by either occlusion of the right coronary artery or heart failure. When atrial fibrillation occurs in these settings, it almost always abates spontaneously if the patient recovers from the underlying problem. Hence, management usually involves administration of drugs to control the heart rate, and long-term antiarrhythmic therapy is generally not needed.

Alternatively, atrial fibrillation may occur in association with structural cardiac disease. Important associated conditions include rheumatic mitral stenosis, hypertension, hypertrophic cardiomyopathy, or chronic heart failure. In contrast to patients with acute intercurrent ailments, those with structural heart disease may expect (even with antiarrhythmic therapy) many recurrences, and chronic atrial fibrillation may supervene.

Lone fibrillation is the term used to describe patients with atrial fibrillation not associated with known cardiac conditions or noncardiac precipitants. The natural history of the atrial fibrillation for those with lone atrial fibrillation is similar to that in patients with structural cardiac disease, in that episodes of atrial fibrillation are likely to recur and, eventually, the arrhythmia may become sustained.

B. Initial Evaluation

The initial evaluation is mainly directed at diagnosing associated conditions (eg, valvular heart disease, hypertension, evidence of heart failure). The cardiac examination during atrial fibrillation will show an irregularly irregular rhythm, variability of the first heart sound, and augmentation of a systolic murmur after long pauses. The initial evaluation

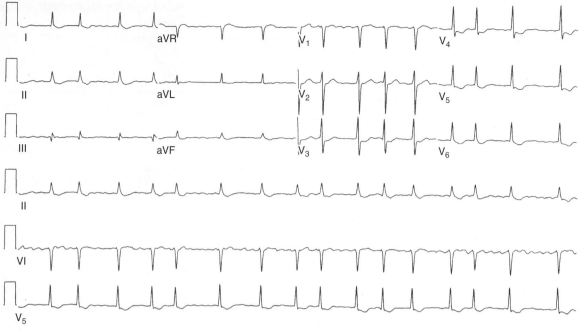

▲ **Figure 12–1.** The 12-lead electrocardiogram shows the typical rapid irregular rhythm seen with atrial fibrillation.

of new-onset atrial fibrillation also includes a detailed history focusing on possible precipitating factors as well as the presence of organic cardiac disease. As such, the initial evaluation includes, at a minimum, a careful physical examination, 12-lead electrocardiogram (ECG), chest radiograph, echocardiogram, and tests of thyroid function. Further testing will depend on various aspects of the history or physical examination. Ambulatory ECG monitoring may be helpful in diagnosing the patient with paroxysmal atrial fibrillation. For example, if atrial fibrillation is usually precipitated by exercise, then an exercise treadmill test is appropriate. In the patient with frequent episodes of paroxysmal atrial fibrillation, a 24- to 48-hour ambulatory ECG recording may discern whether atrial fibrillation was triggered by another arrhythmia, such as a premature atrial complex alone, or whether the fibrillation was preceded by an episode of supraventricular tachycardia. In addition, patients with vagally mediated fibrillation will typically have episodes either after heavy meals or during sleep. These clues may help identify those patients who may respond to specific approaches (see later section, Treatment).

▶ Differential Diagnosis

The ECG diagnosis of atrial fibrillation is usually straightforward and is characterized by an irregularly irregular rhythm with a narrow QRS complex unless there is associated bundle branch block. The chief diagnostic problem relates to patients showing short bursts of irregular atrial tachycardia (which are common on random ambulatory ECG recordings in the elderly). In addition, patients with atrial flutter may have varying atrioventricular (AV) conduction, which may serve to mimic atrial fibrillation. Careful evaluation of all leads looking for the characteristic flutter pattern is important. Less commonly, patients presenting with multifocal atrial tachycardia may mimic the irregularity found in those with atrial fibrillation. Careful analysis in the latter group shows an irregular atrial tachycardia with at least three P-wave morphologies. A very uncommon arrhythmia that may mimic atrial fibrillation is seen in patients with dual AV nodal physiology with dual conduction over the fast and slow AV nodal pathways. For this diagnosis, identify that a single sinus P wave is associated with two QRS complexes. These patients are readily cured with slow pathway ablation.

▶ Treatment

The objectives of therapy include (1) achieving rate control, (2) restoring sinus rhythm (where feasible), and (3) decreasing the risk of CVA. The principles of treatment discussed in this chapter largely follow those promulgated in the recent American College of Cardiology (ACC)/American Heart Association (AHA)/European Society of Cardiology (ESC) guidelines.

European Heart Rhythm Association, et al. ACC/AHA/ESC 2006 guidelines for the management of patients with atrial fibrillation—executive summary: a report of the American College of Cardiology/American Heart Association Task Force on Practice Guidelines and the European Society of Cardiology Committee for Practice Guidelines (Writing Committee to Revise the 2001 Guidelines for the Management of Patients with Atrial Fibrillation). *J Am Coll Cardiol.* 2006;48(4):854–906. [PMID: 16904574]

Wann SL, et al. 2011 ACCF/AHA/HRS focused update on the management of patients with atrial fibrillation (updating the 2006 guideline); a report of the American College of Cardiology/American Heart Association Task Force on Practice Guidelines. *J Am Coll Cardiol.* 2011;57(2):223–42. [PMID: 21177058]

A. Rate Control

If the patient has atrial fibrillation and a rapid rate associated with severe heart failure or cardiogenic shock, emergency direct-current cardioversion is indicated. For patients with atrial fibrillation associated with rapid rate but with stable hemodynamics, attempts to achieve acute rate control are indicated. Drugs to slow the ventricular rate in patients with atrial fibrillation (Table 12–1) include digitalis preparations, calcium channel blockers (verapamil or diltiazem), and β-blockers. If rapid rate control is desired, then calcium channel blockers and β-blockers are far more effective than digitalis. In addition, a common misconception is that digitalis therapy is associated with acute conversion to sinus rhythm, but carefully controlled studies have shown that conversion to sinus rhythm is no more likely with digoxin than with placebo. As emphasized later, digitalis and intravenous calcium channel blocker therapy are contraindicated in patients with Wolff-Parkinson-White syndrome and atrial fibrillation. Intravenous diltiazem has been shown to be safe and effective for patients with atrial fibrillation and a modest degree of heart failure. In patients refractory to these agents, intravenous amiodarone may be effective but requires many hours before rate control is achieved. In patients with a known history of congestive heart failure, use of intravenous β-blockers or calcium channel blockers may aggravate cardiac failure. In this subset, digitalis or intravenous amiodarone would be the preferred agent for rate control.

B. Long-Term Antiarrhythmic Therapy and Elective Cardioversion

For patients who have had a single, initial episode of atrial fibrillation with no significant hemodynamic problems, no specific therapy is required because repeat episodes may not occur for many years. In contrast, patients who manifest frequent recurrences may be candidates for long-term antiarrhythmic therapy with class Ia (quinidine, procainamide, and disopyramide), class Ic (propafenone and flecainide), or class III (sotalol, amiodarone, dronedarone, and dofetilide) agents, all of which are more effective than placebo in maintaining sinus rhythm (Figure 12–2).

C. Antiarrhythmic Drug Therapy for Atrial Fibrillation

For patients with lone atrial fibrillation, use of any of the antiarrhythmic drugs listed is appropriate. In general, the class Ic agents (flecainide or propafenone) are the first choice in terms of efficacy and lowest incidence of side effects. It would be wise, for example, to withhold amiodarone as a first-line drug in view of the potential for adverse effects. Only two drugs have been proved safe for patients with severe congestive heart failure: dofetilide and amiodarone.

For patients with atrial fibrillation associated with coronary artery disease, consider use of sotalol as initial drug therapy. This agent has class III antiarrhythmic effects and is a potent β-blocker. Class Ic drugs should not be used in patients with significant structural cardiac disease or in those

Table 12–1. Intravenous Pharmacologic Agents for Heart Rate Control in Atrial Fibrillation

Drug	Loading Dose	Onset	Maintenance Dose	Major Side Effects
Diltiazem	0.25 mg/kg IV over 2 min	2–7 min	5–15 mg/h infusion	Hypotension, heart block, HF
Esmolol	0.5 mg/kg over 1 min	5 min	0.05–0.2 mg kg^{-1} min^{-1}	Hypotension, heart block, bradycardia, asthma, HF
Metoprolol	2.5–5 mg IV bolus over 2 min; up to 3 doses	5 min	NA	Hypotension, heart block, bradycardia, asthma, HF
Propranolol	0.15 mg/kg IV	5 min	NA	Hypotension, heart block, bradycardia, asthma, HF
Verapamil	0.075–0.15 mg/kg IV over 2 min	3–5 min	NA	Hypotension, heart block, HF
Digoxin	0.25 mg IV each 2 h, up to 1.5 mg	2 h	0.125–0.25 mg daily	Digitalis toxicity, heart block, bradycardia

HF, heart failure; NA, not applicable.
Reprinted, with permission, from Fuster V, et al. *J Am Coll Cardiol.* 2001;38:266i.

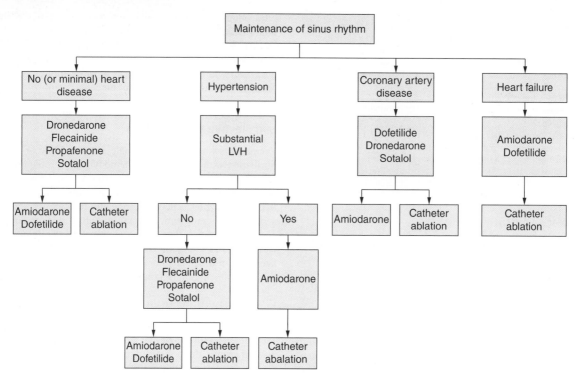

▲ **Figure 12–2.** Therapy to maintain sinus rhythm in patients with recurrent paroxysmal or persistent atrial fibrillation. Drugs are listed alphabetically and not in order of suggested use. The seriousness of heart disease progresses from left to right, and selection of therapy in patients with multiple conditions depends on the most serious condition present. LVH, left ventricular hypertrophy. (Reproduced, with permission, from Wann SL, et al. *J Am Coll Cardiol.* 2011;57[2]:223–42.)

with ischemic heart disease. Sotalol may be safe and effective for patients with hypertension and atrial fibrillation without significant left ventricular hypotrophy. Similarly, class Ic drugs may be used in well-controlled hypertension, but without left ventricular hypertrophy.

In addition, extracardiac factors are very important in the choice of antiarrhythmic drugs. For example, dose adjustments are mandatory for patients with renal insufficiency. This is especially true for sotalol and dofetilide. Dofetilide, for example, requires hospital admission, calculation of the creatinine clearance, and drug titration according to the QT corrected for heart rate as well as renal function. An algorithm for antiarrhythmic drug usage is summarized in Figure 12–2, and drug doses are listed in Table 12–2.

Even with drug therapy, recurrence rates for atrial fibrillation approach 50% per year (as opposed to recurrences with placebo therapy of 75% per year). In addition, these agents may be associated with significant side effects. For class Ia drugs, these include induction of torsades de pointes, especially for those with congestive heart failure. For example, a meta-analysis compared quinidine with placebo

for patients with atrial fibrillation and found that death from all causes was higher in the groups treated with quinidine. In addition, in the Stroke Prevention in Atrial Fibrillation (SPAF) trials, substantial numbers of patients were treated with antiarrhythmic agents; in patients with heart failure, those treated with class I drugs had significantly increased mortality rates compared with those not treated with antiarrhythmic drugs. Great care must be exercised in the use of these agents, balancing the benefits against the potential for adverse effects. General rules include avoidance of all class Ia drugs or sotalol for patients with congestive heart failure and avoidance of class Ic agents for patients with structural heart disease. In addition, sotalol is contraindicated for patients with severe depression of the left ventricular ejection fraction and/or severe left ventricular hypertrophy. Patients with significant sinus node or AV conduction disease may require pacemaker therapy before use of antiarrhythmic drugs because these drugs may further depress sinus node or AV conduction. The only drugs that appear to be both effective and safe for patients with heart failure and atrial fibrillation are amiodarone and dofetilide. Amiodarone is associated

Table 12–2. Typical Doses of Drugs Used to Maintain Sinus Rhythm in Atrial Fibrillation, Listed Alphabetically

Drug	Daily Dosage	Potential Adverse Effects
Amiodarone	100–400 mg	Photosensitivity, pulmonary toxicity, polyneuropathy, GI upset, bradycardia, torsades de pointes (rare), hepatic toxicity, thyroid dysfunction
Disopyramide	400–750 mg	Torsades de pointes, HF, glaucoma, urinary retention, dry mouth
Dofetilide	500–1000 mcg	Torsades de pointes
Dronedarone	400 mg	Contraindicated for those with severe or worsening heart failure or in those with persistent AF and cardiovascular risk factors
Flecainide	200–300 mg	Ventricular tachycardia, congestive HF, increased rate with conversion to atrial flutter
Procainamide	1000–4000 mg	Torsades de pointes, lupus-like syndrome, GI symptoms
Propafenone	450–900 mg	Ventricular tachycardia, congestive HF, increased rate with conversion to atrial flutter
Quinidine	600–1500 mg	Torsades de pointes, GI upset, increased rate with conversion to atrial flutter
Sotalol	240–320 mg	Torsades de pointes, congestive HF, bradycardia, exacerbation of chronic obstructive or bronchospastic lung disease

AV, atrioventricular; GI, gastrointestinal; HF, heart failure.
Modified, with permission, from Fuster V, et al. *J Am Coll Cardiol.* 2001;38:266i.

with a host of both cardiac (eg, severe sinus bradycardia or arrest or AV block) and noncardiac (eg, thyroid abnormalities, pulmonary fibrosis) adverse effects, but low-dose amiodarone (ie, 200 mg/day) appears to be effective and very well tolerated. Dofetilide has a narrow therapeutic window and can cause life-threatening arrhythmias; it can be used in patients with atrial fibrillation and congestive heart failure but requires a 2- to 3-day in-hospital stay for monitoring of the agent. Dronedarone is the newest agent approved for treatment of atrial fibrillation. This drug is a derivative of amiodarone and has most of the physiologic effects of amiodarone. This drug has limited efficacy and should not be used in patients with severe or worsening heart failure or in those with persistent atrial fibrillation and cardiovascular risk factors (see later discussion of CHADS2 score).

D. Chemical Cardioversion

Recent studies have emphasized the use of drugs for acute conversion of atrial fibrillation. It has been shown that intravenous ibutilide and intravenous dofetilide (not available in the United States) are effective for conversion of approximately 50% of patients with recent-onset atrial fibrillation. It should be emphasized that ibutilide should be used only in a monitored environment. The usual dose is 1 mg over 10 minutes, followed by a 10-minute interlude, followed by an additional 1 mg over 10 minutes if necessary. A defibrillator should be readily available, because the incidence of sustained torsades de pointes is 1–2%. Ibutilide should be avoided for patients with severe heart failure bradycardia or a prolonged QT interval.

E. Other Drugs for Chemical Cardioversion

Other drug combinations have also been found effective. For example, it has been found that use of large oral doses of either flecainide (300 mg) or propafenone (600 mg) may terminate up to 80% of episodes of atrial fibrillation within 2 hours (pill-in-the-pocket). This approach should be used only in patients who are pretreated with β-blocking drugs and in the absence of significant cardiac disease or heart failure. It is best to assess first-time use of the "pill-in-the-pocket" approach in a hospital setting.

F. Anticoagulant Therapy

The risk of CVA in patients with nonrheumatic atrial fibrillation is 4–7% per year. Patients at particularly high risk include those over age 75 years or with hypertension, a history of heart failure, increased left atrial size, diabetes, or prior CVA. The risks of CVA are similar in patients with paroxysmal versus chronic atrial fibrillation. Risk of stroke is assessed by noting the CHADS2 score: C (congestive heart failure), H (hypertension), A (age > 75 years), D (diabetes), S (previous stroke). According to current AHA and ACC guidelines, aspirin therapy is acceptable for those with CHADS2 score of 0 or 1, whereas anticoagulants are advised for those with CHADS2 score ≥ 2 who have no contraindications for anticoagulant therapy. More recent risk criteria also include female sex, age over 65, and evidence of coronary or peripheral vascular disease (CHA2DS2-Vasc score). When compared with CHADS2, CHA2DS2-Vasc

Table 12–3. Risk Factor Scoring for Cerebrovascular Accident and Risk of Hemorrhage from Anticoagulant Therapy

	Risk Factor	Score
1. CHADS2	Congestive heart failure	1
	Hypertension	1
	Age > 75	1
	Diabetes	1
	Stroke	2
2. CHA2DS2-Vasc	Congestive heart failure or	1
	EF ≤ 35%	1
	Hypertension	1
	Age > 65	2
	Age > 75	1
	Diabetes	2
	Stroke (TIA or systemic emboli)	1
	Vascular disease (peripheral vascular disease, previous MI)	1
	Sex (female)	
3. HAS-BLED	Hypertension (uncontrolled)	1
	Renal disease (Cr > 2.6 mg/dL)	1
	Liver disease (bilirubin 2× normal)	1
	Stroke history	1
	Prior major bleeding	1
	Labile INR	1
	Age ≥ 65	1
	Medications (NSAIDs)	1
	Alcohol usage	1

Cr, creatinine; EF, ejection fraction; INR, international normalized ratio; MI, myocardial infarction; NSAIDs, nonsteroidal anti-inflammatory drugs; TIA, transient ischemic attack.

performed better in predicting those at high risk or those at very low risk for stroke. Warfarin anticoagulation is recommended for those with a CHA2DS2-Vasc score ≥ 2 (Table 12–3). Numerous studies have documented the remarkable efficacy of warfarin in decreasing the risk of emboli by 45–85% in patients with nonrheumatic atrial fibrillation with a low risk of significant hemorrhage, provided the international normalized ratio (INR) is in the range of 2.0–2.5. However, some patients have a considerable risk of bleeding, which can be estimated by scores such as the HAS-BLED (see Table 12–3). In general, if the HAS-BLED score exceeds the CHADS2 score, the benefits of anticoagulation may be outweighed by the risk of bleeding. Risk associated with bleeding exceeds the possible benefit of anticoagulant therapy in younger patients with lone atrial fibrillation because the risk of emboli is very low in this group.

Several newer anticoagulant drugs (dabigatran, rivaroxaban, and apixaban) have recently been approved for anticoagulant therapy of patients with nonvalvular atrial fibrillation. These drugs have proved to be either equivalent or actually superior in efficacy and safety compared with warfarin. The advantages of the newer agents include obviating the need for INR blood tests and fewer drug–drug or drug–food interactions compared with warfarin. All of the newer agents require careful monitoring of renal function per serial measurement of creatinine clearance (CrCl) because dose adjustment is required in the face of reduced renal function (Table 12–4). In addition, specific inhibitors (in the event of bleeding) are not currently available.

The role of aspirin therapy for patients with atrial fibrillation remains controversial. In one study, 75 mg of aspirin failed to decrease the stroke risk compared with placebo (5.5%/year). In contrast, the SPAF I trials showed that a higher dose of aspirin, 325 mg, appeared to be of benefit in patients under 75 years of age. In a follow-up study (SPAF II), the incidence of stroke was higher with aspirin (4.8%) compared with warfarin (3.6%). The SPAF III trials demonstrated that aspirin (325 mg/day) and fixed low-dose warfarin (1, 2, or 3 mg) were ineffective for stroke prevention. Therefore, the weight of current data favors use of warfarin with an INR of 2.0–3.0 as the best strategy to prevent systemic embolization. Recent studies showed that a newer anticoagulant (apixaban) was more effective than aspirin in those with nonvalvular atrial fibrillation who could not take warfarin.

Table 12–4. Anticoagulant Therapy

Drug	Dose	Side Effects or Precautions
Warfarin	Determined by INR measurement	Many drug-drug or drug-food (ie, green leafy vegetables) interactions
Dabigatran	150 mg bid for CrCl > 30 mL; 75 mg bid for CrCl 15–30; contraindicated for CrCl < 15 mL	(1) When converting patients from warfarin to dabigatran, wait until INR > 2 (2) Gastrointestinal upset (3) Interactions with dronedarone, ketoconazole, etc.
Rivaroxaban	CrCl > 50 mL/min–20 mg/day; CrCl 15–50 mL/min–15 mg/day	Interacts with drugs that inhibit (ie, ketoconazole) or induce CYP3A4 enzymes (rifampin, etc.)

CrCl, creatinine clearance; INR, international normalized ratio.

Olesen JB, et al. Validation of risk stratification schemes for predicting stroke and thromboembolism in patients with atrial fibrillation: nationwide cohort study. *BMJ.* 2011;342:d124. [PMID: 21282258]

G. Direct-Current Cardioversion

Direct-current cardioversion is a very effective technique for restoration of sinus rhythm. Because of the benefits of sinus rhythm in terms of improved cardiac output and decreased risk of embolic phenomena, in general, at least one attempt should be made to restore sinus rhythm. Several precautions are in order. If the patient has a history of recurrent episodes of atrial fibrillation, then he or she should be pretreated with an antiarrhythmic agent because reversion to atrial fibrillation after shock therapy is very high. Use of antiarrhythmic drugs before direct-current shock, however, is inappropriate for the patient with an initial episode of well-tolerated atrial fibrillation. Unless urgent cardioversion is required because of hemodynamic decompensation, severe ischemia, or congestive heart failure, it is imperative to follow one of several options for reducing the risk of systemic embolization:

a. For patients with atrial fibrillation of less than 48 hours in duration, it would appear to be safe to proceed with application of direct-current shock.

b. If atrial fibrillation persists for more than 48 hours, then the risk of embolization increases and anticoagulants are required prior to ablation. One recommended option for patients with atrial fibrillation of more than 48 hours in duration is to perform transesophageal echocardiography (TEE), which is excellent for detecting clots in the left atrium or the left atrial appendage. Evidence from several studies indicates that the finding of either a clot or spontaneous echocardiographic contrast in the left atrium is associated with higher risks of systemic embolization. In the absence of such findings on TEE, systemic emboli are rare. Therefore, patients with recent-onset atrial fibrillation with no evidence of atrial clots or spontaneous contrast by TEE may undergo direct-current cardioversion after initiation of heparin therapy. A recent report from the ACUTE trial showed that patients with atrial fibrillation treated based on TEE-guided therapy versus a group treated with a 3-week course of anticoagulant therapy had similar rates of thromboembolism (< 1%). It must be appreciated that atrial function is depressed (atrial stunning) after cardioversion and that anticoagulant therapy is recommended for at least 1 month after cardioversion. This is true whether the duration of atrial fibrillation was either less than or greater than 48 hours. For patients with clot or dense spontaneous echocardiographic contrast with TEE, full anticoagulant therapy with an INR of 2.0–3.0 is recommended for at least 2–3 weeks before cardioversion.

c. An alternative approach is that patients with atrial fibrillation of greater than 48 hours be fully anticoagulated for at least 3 consecutive weeks before attempting direct-current cardioversion and for about 4 weeks afterward to decrease the risk of an embolism after successful reversion to sinus rhythm. This approach tends to be less efficient than the TEE-guided approach for recent-onset atrial fibrillation, but is an acceptable alternative treatment for atrial fibrillation.

Direct-current external shock is usually performed in a monitored area under supervision of an anesthesiologist. Pads are placed in an anterior-posterior orientation in order to maximize current delivered to the atrium. It is wise to check the arterial oxygen saturation and serum potassium level before cardioversion. Direct-current shocks beginning with at least 150 J biphasic are used in an attempt to achieve sinus rhythm. Multiple shocks of lesser energy are to be avoided. If the patient fails to revert after maximal external shocks (360 J biphasic), then successful cardioversion can almost always be achieved by the use of supplemental doses of ibutilide. Ibutilide has been shown to lower the atrial defibrillation threshold. An attempt at internal cardioversion using small-energy shocks delivered between the coronary sinus and the right atrium is seldom necessary because the previously described treatments are almost always effective.

H. Long-Term Approach

Clinicians should be especially careful to identify patients whose atrial fibrillation might be cured. Examples include patients with hyperthyroidism as well as those in whom other cardiac arrhythmias appear to trigger atrial fibrillation. For example, patients with atrial flutter or paroxysmal supraventricular tachycardia may experience atrial premature impulses during tachycardia that trigger atrial fibrillation. In selected patients, it is possible to apply catheter ablation to cure the underlying supraventricular arrhythmia and, hence, prevent the trigger for atrial fibrillation. Therefore, in the evaluation of patients with atrial fibrillation, initial testing should include obtaining a thyroid-stimulating hormone assay, an echocardiogram, and a 48-hour ambulatory ECG recording for those with paroxysmal atrial fibrillation. In analyses of these recordings, the clinician seeks evidence for triggering arrhythmias. In addition, the clinician looks for vagal triggers of atrial fibrillation, such as sinus bradycardia associated with sleep or heavy meals, that initially may be treated with vagolytic antiarrhythmic agents such as disopyramide. Alternatively, if atrial fibrillation appears only with enhanced sympathetic tone, such as with exercise, a trial of β-blocker therapy is appropriate.

One important special circumstance is that of atrial fibrillation in the patient with Wolff-Parkinson-White syndrome. These patients may have a very rapid irregular rate and wide complex tachycardia owing to conduction over the accessory pathway (Figure 12–3). After recognition of this entity, appropriate immediate therapy includes use of intravenous ibutilide or procainamide or direct-current cardioversion. It is important to remember that intravenous digoxin and calcium channel blockers are contraindicated. In addition, use of lidocaine, β-blockers, or adenosine is not effective and is contraindicated because they delay appropriate therapy. After the rhythm is stabilized, these patients should undergo catheter ablation of the accessory pathway.

The natural history of atrial fibrillation associated with structural cardiac disease or in lone atrial fibrillation patients is spontaneous recurrence of the arrhythmia. Unfortunately, no drug is universally effective, and the decision of how many drugs to try before a judgment is made to terminate antiarrhythmic drugs and focus on rate control depends on how symptomatic the patient is during atrial fibrillation. If the episodes are poorly tolerated, then multiple drug trials or even various ablative procedures may be required (see later section, Nonpharmacologic Treatment of Atrial Fibrillation). On the other hand, if rate control can be readily achieved with drugs, such as digoxin, β-blockers, or calcium antagonists that block AV nodal conduction and the patient has a good symptomatic outcome, then an acceptable alternative is to use drugs that control rate combined with long-term anticoagulant treatment. A large, randomized trial (AFFIRM)

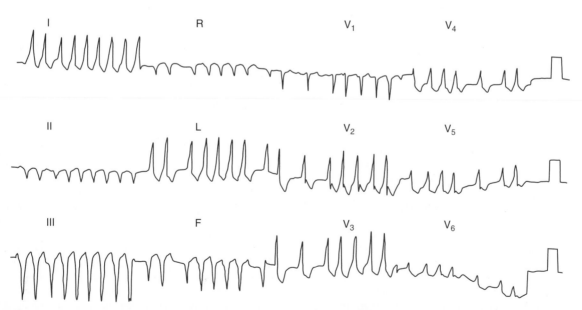

▲ **Figure 12–3.** The 12-lead electrocardiogram shows a rapid irregular rhythm with broad QRS complex. This is pathognomonic of atrial fibrillation in a patient with Wolff-Parkinson-White syndrome. This arrhythmia requires urgent treatment. Acceptable therapy includes use of intravenous ibutilide or procainamide or direct-current shock.

compared the strategy of rate control and anticoagulation versus maintaining sinus rhythm with antiarrhythmic drugs. The AFFIRM trial randomized over 4000 patients with atrial fibrillation to either rate or rhythm control. The patient cohort consisted in large measure of older (mean age 69 years) patients who were not very symptomatic. They found no difference in mortality or quality of life between groups. The rhythm control group had a higher incidence of hospitalizations and episodes of torsades de pointes. In addition, stroke risk was related to presence of no or inadequate anticoagulant treatment. This study showed that for most patients with atrial fibrillation, rate control was equally effective as rhythm control and that long-term anticoagulation therapy is required for both groups.

Wyse DG, et al; Atrial Fibrillation Follow-up Investigation of Rhythm Management (AFFIRM) Investigators. A comparison of rate control and rhythm control in patients with atrial fibrillation. *N Engl J Med.* 2002;347(23):1825–33. [PMID: 12466506]

I. Nonpharmacologic Treatment of Atrial Fibrillation

Because pharmacologic therapy for atrial fibrillation is not ideal, a number of nonpharmacologic treatment modalities have been introduced. Current ACC/AHA/ESC guidelines allow for catheter ablation for treatment of atrial fibrillation after one failed drug trial. Recent studies used wide-area ablative lesions around the pulmonary veins in order to create entrance and exit block from those triggering foci. Other foci may evacuate from the coronary sinus, vein of Marshall, or the superior vena cava and may require ablation as well. In addition, some groups advocate ablation of complex fractionated potentials (CAFÉ) or use of a roof line between the upper right and left superior pulmonary vein or an ablation line from the mitral annulus to the left inferior pulmonary vein (mitral isthmus line). The initial success rate for ablation of paroxysmal atrial fibrillation is 70–90%, but the 5-year success rate is approximately 50%.

Patients with persistent tachycardia may suffer from a tachycardia-induced cardiomyopathy with left ventricular failure superimposed on their native cardiac disease. Hence, in the management of chronic atrial fibrillation, rate control is an important objective that must be achieved either via AV nodal blocking drugs or, failing these, with catheter ablative procedures. Catheter ablation of the AV junction involves insertion of an electrode catheter in the region of the His bundle with application of radiofrequency energy in order to destroy AV conduction. The chief benefit of this technique is achievement of perfect rate control without need for drugs. The drawbacks include the need for permanent pacing and a continued need for anticoagulant therapy.

For most of these patients, especially for those with left ventricular ejection fraction greater than 40%, single chamber pacing appears to be sufficient. In some patients, left ventricular function may deteriorate, and biventricular pacing may be helpful (PAVE trial).

It has been shown that atrial-based pacing systems will decrease the incidence of atrial fibrillation in patients with the tachycardia-bradycardia syndrome. In addition, pacing may allow for safe use of antiarrhythmic drugs. In patients with vagally mediated atrial fibrillation, atrial pacing may be effective in decreasing episodes of atrial fibrillation. Experimental studies have shown that either dual-site atrial pacing (ie, from coronary sinus and right atrium) or pacing from the atrial septum in conjunction with antiarrhythmic therapy may suppress atrial fibrillation, but this technique has not been shown to be clinically useful.

Bhargava M, et al. Impact of type of atrial fibrillation and repeat catheter ablation on long-term freedom from atrial fibrillation: results from a multicenter study. *Heart Rhythm.* 2009;6:1403–12. [PMID: 19716348]

Ouyang F, et al. Long-term results of catheter ablation in paroxysmal atrial fibrillation: lessons from 5-year follow-up. *Circulation.* 2010;122:2368–77. [PMID: 21098450]

Weerasooriya R, et al. Catheter ablation for atrial fibrillation: are results maintained at 5 years of follow-up? *J Am Coll Cardiol.* 2011;57:160–6. [PMID: 21211687]

▶ Prognosis

Atrial fibrillation, particularly associated with rapid rates, carries significant negative prognostic implications for those with associated structural cardiac disease or heart failure. For example, loss of the atrial booster pump function for those with less compliant ventricles (ie, hypertrophic myopathy) may result in hemodynamic collapse. In addition, persistent, rapid rates may induce a tachycardia-mediated cardiomyopathy with similar negative prognostic implications. This is why, depending on the clinical scenario, maintenance of sinus rhythm or rate control is such an important therapeutic concern.

Although anticoagulants and perhaps aspirin can reduce the risk of stroke or other systemic emboli, the risk is never zero, whether the patient has paroxysmal, persistent, or permanent atrial fibrillation. Also, in patients with cardiovascular disease, the presence of atrial fibrillation always increases the risk of major adverse cardiac events. It is not clear whether various treatment approaches substantially alter this adverse prognosis. However, maintenance of sinus rhythm compared to rate control does not seem to improve long-term survival.

Ventricular Tachycardia

Nitish Badhwar, MD

ESSENTIALS OF DIAGNOSIS

- ▶ Nonsustained: three or more consecutive QRS complexes of uniform configuration of ventricular origin at a rate of more than 100 bpm.
- ▶ Sustained: lasts more than 30 seconds; requires intervention for termination.
- ▶ Monomorphic ventricular tachycardia.
- ▶ Polymorphic ventricular tachycardia: beat-to-beat variation in QRS configuration.

The magnitude of ventricular tachycardia (VT), one of the most common health problems encountered in clinical practice, can best be appreciated in terms of its various clinical manifestations, which include ventricular fibrillation (sudden cardiac death [SCD]), syncope or near syncope, and wide QRS tachycardia.

The most serious is its degeneration into ventricular fibrillation, producing cardiac arrest and SCD that accounts for 200,000 deaths a year. The second most serious clinical presentation is syncope. Although the overall prevalence of VT-related syncope is unclear, it is estimated to be frequent because inducible VT (via electrical stimulation) is the most common arrhythmia detected in patients with unexplained syncope. A high prevalence of SCD (> 20% incidence within the ensuing 12 months) is noted in patients with syncope from cardiovascular causes, suggesting that undiagnosed VT may be an underlying cause of sudden death in patients with unexplained syncope. The third most significant clinical manifestation of VT is a wide QRS complex tachycardia that is often hemodynamically well tolerated.

DIAGNOSTIC ISSUES

1. Underdiagnosis

VT as a cause of morbidity and mortality is grossly underdiagnosed, potentially leading to mismanagement. This may be particularly true when the clinical presentation is unexplained syncope because no concomitant electrocardiographic (ECG) documentation is available. In the case of cardiac arrest or SCD, acute myocardial infarction rather than an arrhythmic problem is often assumed to be responsible. Most persons who have suffered sudden death have no evidence of acute myocardial necrosis, even though the episode often occurs in patients with underlying coronary artery disease. Managing the underlying coronary artery disease with no regard to treating the concomitant VT is inadequate.

2. Misdiagnosis

When hemodynamically stable VT is recorded on the surface ECG, it is often misdiagnosed as supraventricular tachycardia (SVT) with aberrant conduction. Any subsequent management is therefore directed toward SVT. Although the exact logic for this line of thinking is unclear, the main reason may be that the hemodynamic stability is associated with the broad QRS rhythm and thus the erroneous belief that the problem cannot be VT.

The clinical presentation of VT depends on many factors, including rate, ventricular function, presence of concomitant coronary artery disease, the presence or absence of cardioactive drugs, and even the patient's posture at the time of onset. Hemodynamic tolerance of VT can, therefore, vary considerably in different situations; at times, it can vary in the same patient, and it is prudent not to exclude the diagnosis of VT on the basis of hemodynamic tolerance alone. It must be understood that approximately 80% of the patients with sustained wide QRS tachycardia have VT. To avoid misdiagnosis, the clinician can either use the established ECG criteria (discussed in the next section) that distinguishes VT from SVT with aberrant conduction or simply assume the presence of VT. The assumption of VT is more often correct; it is also safer because misdiagnosing VT as SVT is a riskier judgment error than vice versa.

3. Diagnostic Approach to the Patient with Wide QRS Complex Tachycardia

The diagnosis of wide QRS complex tachycardia by ECG analysis has always been a challenge for clinicians. The differential diagnosis includes VT, SVT with aberrant conduction, and preexcited tachycardia in patients with Wolff-Parkinson-White (WPW) syndrome. Figure 13–1 depicts, schematically, the reasons for normal and broad QRS complexes. Preexcited tachycardia results from antegrade activation of the ventricle via an accessory pathway in patients with WPW syndrome, which can present with atrial fibrillation, atrial flutter, atrial tachycardia, atrioventricular nodal reentry tachycardia (AVNRT), or antidromic tachycardia (Figure 13–2). Preexcited tachycardia is a rare cause of wide QRS complex tachycardia (5–8% of cases); however, the QRS pattern of preexcited QRS complex can be difficult to distinguish from VT because in both instances

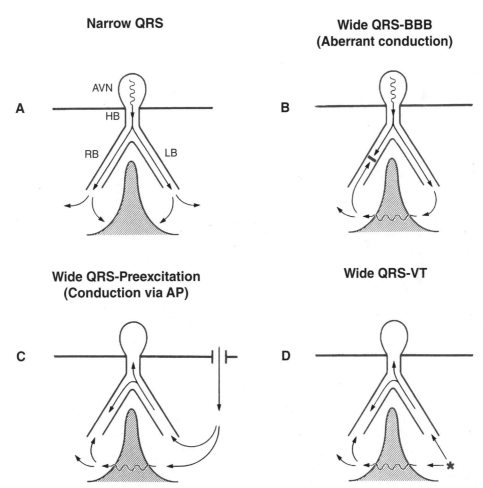

▲ **Figure 13–1.** Mechanism of wide QRS. **A:** Narrow QRS from simultaneous activation of the right and left ventricles. In the three types of wide QRS shown in **B–D,** there is sequential rather than simultaneous activation of the left and right ventricle and a variable amount of muscle-to-muscle conduction. AP, accessory pathway; AVN, atrioventricular node; BBB, bundle branch block; HB, His bundle; LB, left bundle; RB, right bundle. (Reproduced, with permission, from Akhtar M, et al. Electrophysiological spectrum of wide QRS complex tachycardia. In: Zipes DP, et al., eds. *Cardiac Electrophysiology. From Cell to Bedside.* Philadelphia: WB Saunders; 1990.)

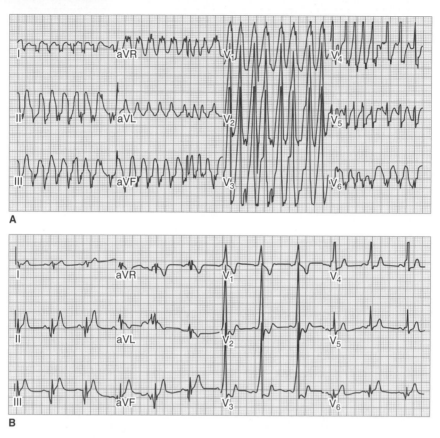

A

B

▲ **Figure 13–2. A**: Preexcited wide complex tachycardia in a patient with Wolff-Parkinson-White (WPW) and atrial fibrillation **B**: Sinus rhythm electrocardiogram showing short PR interval and delta wave consistent with left posterior WPW. (Reproduced, with permission, from Turakhia MP, et al. *Indian Pacing Electrophysiol J.* 2009;9[2]:130–3.)

the QRS starts with muscle-to-muscle conduction. ECG artifact can also mimic wide QRS complex tachycardia and be misdiagnosed as VT, leading to expensive testing and even placement of implantable cardioverter-defibrillator (ICD). Clues to the diagnosis include absence of hemodynamic deterioration, an unstable baseline, association with body movement, and ability to march the normal QRS complexes through the artifact ("notches sign") at sinus R-R interval (Figure 13–3). A number of surface ECG criteria, including the atrioventricular (AV) relationship, the QRS complex

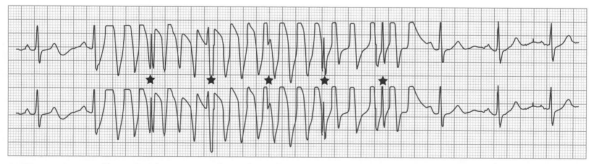

▲ **Figure 13–3.** Artifact mimicking ventricular tachycardia. The QRS complexes are seen as notches that are marching at the regular sinus interval (★). (Reproduced, with permission, from Badhwar N, et al. *J Intensive Care Med.* 2012;27[5]:267–89.)

duration, specific QRS morphology, and the QRS complex axis, have been established to distinguish VT from SVT with aberrant conduction. These criteria are helpful in arriving at an accurate diagnosis if they are used in a systemic fashion.

▶ Atrioventricular Relationship

In SVT, the arrhythmia arises in the atria or AV junction and reaches the ventricles through the AV node and His-Purkinje system. Because the atrial arrhythmia is the primary event, either a 1:1 AV response or a varying degree of AV block occurs, but in either case, the atrial rates equal or exceed ventricular rates. During VT, a retrograde block often leads to either AV dissociation or a varying degree of ventriculoatrial conduction ratios, but the ventricular rates equal or exceed the atrial rate. When AV dissociation can be recognized, it is the most reliable criterion for VT (Figures 13–4 and 13–5). This criterion lacks sensitivity, however, because the P waves can be identified on the surface ECG in only 25% of patients with VT. In patients with slower VT and AV dissociation, intermittent ventricular capture can result in fusion with narrow QRS complexes during wide QRS complex tachycardia. This useful but rarely observed finding is also 100% specific for the diagnosis of VT.

▶ QRS Complex Duration

For the reasons listed earlier, the QRS complex duration is the widest in VT and narrowest in aberrant conduction. To distinguish VT from SVT with aberrant conduction on the basis of QRS duration alone, however, some specific aspects must be considered. In the absence of cardioactive drugs and extensive myocardial fibrosis, aberrancy rarely results in a QRS duration of more than 140 ms with a right bundle branch block (RBBB) pattern (see Figure 13–5) or more than 160 ms with a left bundle branch block (LBBB) configuration. In the presence of intramyocardial conduction delay from drugs (such as class I antiarrhythmic agents) and myocardial fibrosis, the QRS width may also exceed these values in SVT with aberrant conduction. Conversely, on a rare occasion, VT can present as a narrow QRS tachycardia (< 120 ms that is narrower than the conducted QRS complex) when there is near-simultaneous activation of the two ventricles, perhaps from the septum.

▶ Specific QRS Morphology

The prevalence of LBBB versus RBBB morphology among the causes of wide QRS is comparable in both VT and SVT with aberrant conduction; it is therefore of no diagnostic value. The typical RBBB is a triphasic complex best seen in V_1 as rsR′ or rSR′ pattern and in lead I as qRs, qRS pattern. Similarly, a typical LBBB has no initial q wave in lead I and a small r and a rapid S wave in V_1. Because of the myocardial origin of most forms of VT, however, the QRS appearance is not exactly like a typical LBBB or RBBB. Many ECG criteria, therefore, have exploited this difference to separate VT from aberrant conduction. A study that analyzed the morphology of premature ventricular complexes and aberrantly conducted beats of RBBB morphology in V_1 found that the triphasic RsR′ pattern with R′ > R was predominant in aberrant conduction (70%) compared with premature ventricular complexes (6%). Monophasic pattern or R > R′ was seen in the premature ventricular complex beats. The limitation of that study is that origin of the anomalous beats (SVT versus VT) was also based on the ECG (presence or absence of preceding P wave). A retrospective ECG analysis

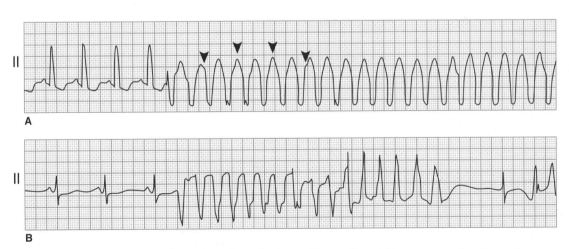

▲ **Figure 13–4. A**: Monomorphic ventricular tachycardia (VT), with a uniform QRS appearance for all complexes. Arrowheads indicate superimposed P waves. **B**: Polymorphic VT, with a beat-to-beat variation in the QRS morphology; QT-interval prolongation follows the termination of the VT episode. (Reproduced, with permission, from Akhtar M. *Circulation.* 1990;82:1561.)

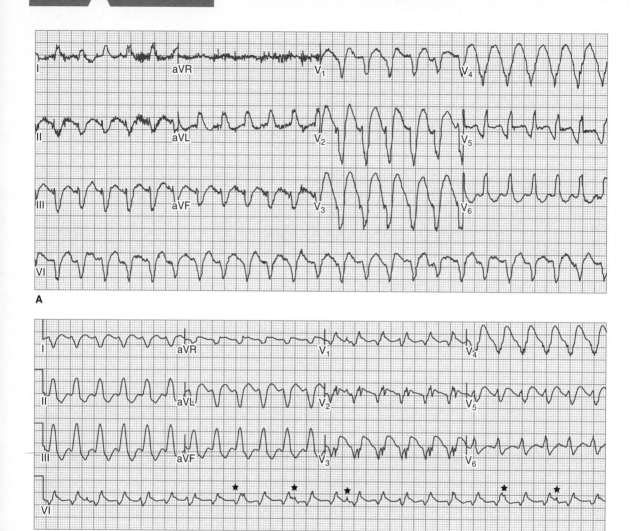

▲ **Figure 13–5.** **A**: Scar-related ventricular tachycardia (VT), with a left bundle branch block left axis morphology in a patient with ischemic cardiomyopathy and previous myocardial infarction. **B**: Right bundle branch block right axis morphology VT in the same patient at the same rate suggesting that both forms of VT have the same circuit (that revolves around the mitral annulus) with different exits causing the difference in morphology. Atrioventricular dissociation is noted in the rhythm strip on V_1 (★) that is 100% specific for VT.

of 70 patients with SVT and 70 patients with VT in whom His bundle recordings were used to determine the site of origin of the wide QRS complex tachycardia found that VT was favored by monophasic or biphasic R waves in V_1 and an R:S ratio less than 1 in V_6 in patients with RBBB morphology and any Q wave in V_6 in patients with LBBB morphology. A study of 150 consecutive wide QRS complex tachycardia cases found that 12-lead QRS morphology during wide QRS complex tachycardia was different from that during preexisting bundle branch block in sinus rhythm, favoring a

diagnosis of VT. The investigators also noted that a positive QRS concordance (positive complexes V_1–V_6) is uncommon in aberrancy, but a negative QRS concordance can occur during aberrant conduction in a small percentage of cases. Another study that evaluated wide QRS complex tachycardia with LBBB morphology in V_1 found that an R wave of > 30 ms, notching in the down stroke of the S wave and an RS (beginning of QRS complex to nadir of S wave) interval > 60 ms in V_1 or V_2, and any Q wave in V_6 favored a diagnosis of VT. In a prospective analysis of wide QRS complex tachycardia (with RBBB and LBBB morphology), the following two criteria for a diagnosis of VT were proposed: (1) absence of R-S in all precordial leads, and (2) R-S interval > 100 ms (measured from the beginning of the QRS complex to the nadir of the S wave) in any precordial lead. Finally, the presence of QR complex in any lead during wide QRS complex tachycardia also favors a diagnosis of VT.

▶ QRS Complex Axis

The axis orientation on a 12-lead ECG ranging from normal (−30° to +90°), left (−31° to −90°), or right (+91° to +180°) has significant overlap across the causes of wide QRS complex tachycardia and is of little diagnostic value. The axis range of −91° to 180°, however, is usually not seen in aberrant conduction. The axis location of this extreme during SVT is, therefore, unlikely unless there was a nonarrhythmic reason for it, such as severe right ventricular hypertrophy or lung disease. Similarly, a combination of right axis with LBBB pattern is almost always seen in patients with VT. A previous history of myocardial infarction (MI) and an axis change of more than 40° between sinus rhythm and wide QRS complex tachycardia may independently favor VT over SVT.

▶ History, Physical Examination, and 12-Lead ECG

A detailed history and physical examination can provide clues to the diagnosis of wide QRS complex tachycardia. A history of MI favors VT as the diagnosis of wide QRS complex tachycardia. The presence of irregular cannon waves and variable intensity of S_1 suggest AV dissociation and are indicative of VT. Carotid massage (performed carefully after ruling out a bruit) that leads to termination of wide QRS complex tachycardia suggests SVT as the mechanism of the arrhythmia (an exception is idiopathic VT arising from the right ventricular outflow tract).

An old ECG in sinus rhythm showing Q waves indicates VT; SVT is the diagnosis if the old ECG shows bundle branch block pattern that matches the 12-lead ECG during wide QRS complex tachycardia; and preexcited tachycardia is inferred from the ECG showing WPW pattern that is similar to wide QRS complex tachycardia ECG pattern. It is essential to obtain a 12-lead ECG during wide QRS complex tachycardia to compare it to the sinus rhythm ECG and look for subtle findings like AV dissociation and narrow beats (fusion and capture) that might not be evident in some leads. Table 13–1 outlines an approach to diagnosing wide QRS complex tachycardia by analyzing the ECG. The first step is to read the ECG with emphasis on rate, regularity (atrial fibrillation with preexcited tachycardia is irregular), axis (extreme northwest axis suggests VT), and morphology in V_1. The next step is looking for AV dissociation (V > A) that is facilitated by marching the sinus P waves at the onset and termination of the wide QRS complex tachycardia if available. Narrow QRS complexes in a wide QRS complex

Table 13–1. Approach to the ECG with Wide QRS Complex Tachycardia

1. **Read the ECG:** rate, rhythm, axis, morphology in V_1 (predominantly upright, RBBB; downward, LBBB)
2. **AV dissociation**
3. **Narrow complex beat:** fusion or capture
4. **Brugada criteria:** RS (measured from beginning of QRS to the nadir of S wave) in precordial leads
   a. Absence of RS in all precordial leads favors VT
   b. RS > 100 ms in any precordial lead favors VT
5. **Morphology criteria:**
   a. RBBB (rsR′): R′ > r in lead V_1 favors SVT. Other morphologies favor VT.
   b. LBBB: Kindwall criteria in leads V_1, V_2 favor VT R > 30 ms, notch in S wave, QRS onset to S > 60 ms Q wave in V_6
   c. Peak R-wave duration in lead II > 50 ms favors VT
   d. Lead aVR criteria that favor VT (any one of the following): Initial R wave, initial r or q wave > 40 ms, notch in initial downstroke of QRS complex, voltage change in initial 40 ms (v_i)/voltage change in terminal 40 ms (v_t) < 1

AV, atrioventricular; ECG, electrocardiogram; LBBB, left bundle branch block; RBBB, right bundle branch block; SVT, supraventricular tachycardia; VT, ventricular tachycardia.

tachycardia (caused by capture and fusion of conducted beats through the AV node-His-Purkinje system) are also 100% specific for VT. The next step is to use the Brugada criteria by evaluating the R-S complexes in precordial leads. Absence of R-S complex in all precordial leads or a R-S greater than 100 ms in one precordial lead favor a diagnosis of VT. The last step is using the morphology criteria to differentiate VT from SVT. Morphology criteria for RBBB and LBBB in leads V_1, V_2, and V_6 have been discussed earlier. The onset of QRS complex to peak of the R wave or nadir of S wave in lead II > 50 ms favors a diagnosis of VT. New criteria based only on analysis of lead avR during tachycardia have been proposed to differentiate SVT from VT. Criteria in avR that favor VT include presence of initial R wave, initial r or q wave > 40 ms, notch in initial downstroke of QRS complex, and voltage change in initial 40 ms (v_i)/voltage change in terminal 40 ms (v_t) < 1. The morphology criteria have certain limitations because idiopathic VT (fascicular VT, outflow tract VT) and bundle branch reentrant VT can have a typical bundle branch block pattern on the ECG and can be misdiagnosed as SVT with aberrancy, whereas some patients with SVT who take antiarrhythmic medications can have atypical bundle branch block pattern on the ECG, leading to a misdiagnosis of VT.

Vereckei A, et al. New algorithm using only lead aVR for differential diagnosis of wide QRS complex tachycardia. *Heart Rhythm.* 2008;5(1):89–98. [PMID: 18180024]

CLASSIFICATIONS OF VENTRICULAR TACHYCARDIA

The spectrum of VT in Table 13–2 lists the two most common varieties encountered in clinical practice and their underlying causes. This classification helps approach the diagnosis in a systematic fashion and directs the physician to specific therapeutic options.

Monomorphic VT is a form of VT in which the QRS complex configuration is uniform from beat to beat in all the surface ECG leads (see Figure 13–4A). In **polymorphic VT,** a beat-to-beat variation occurs in the QRS complex configuration in any of the ECG leads (see Figure 13–4B). These diagnoses may be difficult, however, when a single-surface ECG lead is recorded. As used in the literature, sustained VT is a tachycardia that lasts for 30 seconds or requires intervention for termination. The definition does not imply that a prolonged episode of VT lasting less than 30 seconds has any less clinical significance. Nonsustained VT is a term used to describe any three or more consecutive QRS complexes of ventricular origin with a rate of more than 100 bpm. When describing nonsustained VT, it is important to mention the number of complexes and rate in order to convey a clear picture of the event. In this chapter, VT is considered sustained unless specifically stated otherwise.

VT is most commonly associated with structural heart disease; 15–20% of VT episodes reported in various series is seen in patients without structural heart disease and is referred to as idiopathic VT. This distinction is important because the therapeutic approach to VT is different in patients with structural heart disease compared with patients with idiopathic VT in which case catheter ablation can be curative.

Table 13–2. Classification and Causes of Common Ventricular Tachycardias

Monomorphic ventricular tachycardia
Chronic coronary artery disease
Idiopathic dilated cardiomyopathy
Arrhythmogenic right ventricular cardiomyopathy
No structural heart disease
Right bundle branch block configuration
Left bundle branch block configuration
Repetitive monomorphic ventricular tachycardia
Other forms
Polymorphic ventricular tachycardia
Prolonged QT interval (torsades de pointes)
Congenital
Acquired
Normal QT interval
Acute ischemia
Other

VENTRICULAR TACHYCARDIA ASSOCIATED WITH STRUCTURAL HEART DISEASE

1. Monomorphic Ventricular Tachycardia in Association with Chronic Coronary Artery Disease

This is the most common form encountered in clinical practice as well as the most extensively investigated in clinical and electrophysiology laboratories. The underlying substrate is usually an area of fibrosis that provides an anatomic obstacle around which the reentrant impulse can propagate. The extent and architecture of the scar may determine the propensity to VT in a given situation. For example, a homogeneous scar with no surviving conducting tissue is less likely to cause arrhythmias than is fibrosis interspersed with streaks of healthy myocardium. In some situations, acute myocardial ischemia or infarct can produce the conditions of slow conduction and block necessary for reentry. Although nonreentrant mechanisms (eg, abnormal automaticity, triggered activity) may cause VT in these settings, reentry is the most common mechanism.

As myocardial activation spreads from the reentrant circuit, the resultant QRS morphology is determined by the direction of the activation vector. Because of the myocardial origin of this type of VT, some characteristic features are expected: (1) The initial part of the QRS complex will generally be inscribed slowly because of muscle-to-muscle propagation. (2) The resultant QRS width is often markedly increased because of this intramyocardial conduction delay. (3) Because the impulse is not activating the ventricles via the bundle branches, the QRS pattern is not likely to be typical of either the RBBB or LBBB. (4) When there is no septal scar, VT originating in the left ventricle activates the ipsilateral ventricle, followed by the interventricular septum and then the right ventricle. This causes an atypical RBBB pattern. (5) VT that originates in the right ventricle shows a LBBB pattern. (6) When the tachycardia originates close to a septal scar, it may show an LBBB pattern even if the reentrant circuit resides in the left ventricle. (7) ECG leads can be used to localize the site of origin of VT from the left ventricle as follows: (a) Positive QRS complex in lead avR and negative in lead V_4 suggests apical site of origin and vice versa for basal sites. (b) Positive QRS complexes in leads II, III, and avF suggest anterior site of origin, whereas negative QRS complex in these leads is seen in VT arising from inferior wall. (c) Positive QRS complex in leads I and avL is seen in VT arising from the septum, whereas a negative QRS in these leads suggests origin from the lateral wall. Figure 13–5 shows scar-related VT in a patient with previous history of MI. The VT has one reentrant circuit in the left ventricle with two different morphologies based on different exit sites.

After an initial documentation on the surface ECG, or when VT is suspected by virtue of underlying coronary artery disease and symptoms such as syncope, a further workup is often critical for characterization of VT. Ambulatory monitoring is of limited value because sustained

VT is not commonly seen on a daily basis. In most situations, invasive electrophysiologic studies are indicated for these patients for both diagnostic and therapeutic purposes.

2. Monomorphic Ventricular Tachycardia in Association with Idiopathic Dilated Cardiomyopathy

Monomorphic VT associated with idiopathic dilated cardiomyopathy and valvular disease is indistinguishable from VT in chronic coronary artery disease in approximately 60% of patients. The underlying substrate is most probably fibrosis, providing both the anatomic obstacle and the pathway for reexcitation. Invariably, however, these patients have conduction slowing in the His-Purkinje system as a part of the diffuse myocardial disease process, and the baseline ECG shows evidence of nonspecific intraventricular conduction defect. The resultant tachycardia uses the bundle branches and the bundle of His for sustained reentry. Bundle branch reentry could manifest as either an LBBB or RBBB pattern (Figure 13–6). Because ventricular myocardial activation occurs via the bundle branches, a typical LBBB or RBBB configuration is generally noted. Although the prevalence of bundle branch reentry is particularly high in patients with idiopathic dilated cardiomyopathy, it does occur in dilated cardiomyopathy regardless of the underlying pathology.

Bundle branch reentry is also fairly common in patients with aortic and mitral valve disease. Due to the close anatomic relationship between the proximal His-Purkinje system and annuli of these valves, His-Purkinje system conduction delays can occur in association with valvular disease. Frequently, sustained bundle branch reentry is observed soon after valve surgery, probably related to aggregation of local substrata.

3. Monomorphic Ventricular Tachycardia in Arrhythmogenic Right Ventricular Cardiomyopathy

Arrhythmogenic right ventricular cardiomyopathy is a disease that causes fibrofatty infiltration in the right ventricle

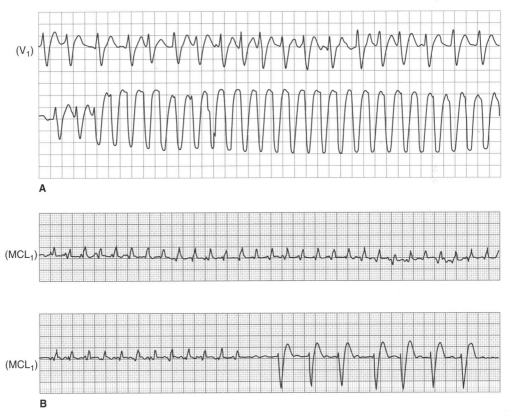

▲ **Figure 13–6.** Bundle branch reentrant ventricular tachycardia with typical left (**A**) and right (**B**) bundle branch morphologies, recorded at different times in a patient with idiopathic dilated cardiomyopathy. Note the underlying intraventricular conduction defect during baseline rhythm, before onset (**A**) and after termination (**B**). (Reproduced, with permission, from Tchou P, et al. *Circulation* 1988;78:246.)

Table 13–3. Idiopathic Ventricular Tachycardia

Monomorphic Ventricular Tachycardia	Polymorphic Ventricular Tachycardia
Outflow Tract VT	Long QT syndrome
RVOT-VT	Brugada syndrome
LVOT-VT	Short coupled torsades
Aortic cusp VT	Short QT syndrome
Fascicular VT	Catecholaminergic polymorphic VT
LAF-VT	Idiopathic VF
LPF-VT	Early repolarization syndrome
Septal VT	
Adrenergic monomorphic VT	
Annular VT	
Mitral annular	
Tricuspid annular	

LAF, left anterior fascicular; LPF, left posterior fascicular; LVOT, left ventricular outflow tract; RVOT, right ventricular outflow tract; VF, ventricular fibrillation; VT, ventricular tachycardia.
Modified, with permission, from Badhwar N, et al. *Curr Probl Cardiol.* 2007;32:7.

with a characteristic ECG morphology of LBBB with inferior axis (Figure 13–9). Lead I has a QS or qR complex in anterior sites and dominant R wave in posterior sites, while avL shows negative complex in septal sites and positive complex in lateral sites. Based on the site of origin, outflow tract VT can be classified as (1) VT that arises from the right ventricular outflow tract, (2) VT that arises from the left ventricular outflow tract, or (3) VT that arises from the aortic cusps (cusp VT). Cusp VT shows earlier precordial transition (< V_2) and a broader R-wave duration in V_1 and V_2. It is important to differentiate right ventricular outflow tract VT from VT associated with arrhythmogenic right ventricular cardiomyopathy that also has an LBBB morphology.

Right ventricular outflow tract VT is more common in women and is usually seen in third to fifth decade of life, whereas left ventricular outflow tract VT is equally distributed between men and women. Symptoms include palpitations, dizziness, atypical chest pain, and syncope. There are three predominant clinical forms of this syndrome: (1) nonsustained repetitive monomorphic VT alternating with periods of sinus rhythm, (2) paroxysmal exercise-induced sustained VT, and (3) frequent premature ventricular complexes that occasionally present as bigeminal rhythm giving rise to tachycardia-induced cardiomyopathy. In some patients, the tachycardia is provoked by exercise and

isoproterenol infusion, suggesting that catecholamines triggered after depolarization may be the underlying mechanism. In most situations, intravenous adenosine will terminate the VT, and triggered activity dependent on cyclic adenosine monophosphate (AMP) may be the mechanism. Immediate termination of right ventricular outflow tract VT can also be achieved with carotid sinus massage, verapamil, and lidocaine. β-Blockers are especially effective for those with exercise-induced outflow tract VT, and a synergistic action is noted with calcium channel blockers. Antiarrhythmic agents, such as procainamide, flecainide, amiodarone, and sotalol, are also effective in these patients. Catheter ablation using radiofrequency energy to cure patients with outflow tract VT is associated with a high success rate due to the focal origin of this form of VT.

3. Annular Ventricular Tachycardia

Mitral annular VT arises from the mitral annulus in the left ventricle and is associated with RBBB morphology. Palpitations are the presenting manifestation in these patients due to repetitive monomorphic VT or frequent monomorphic premature ventricular complexes. The mechanism is thought to be triggered rhythm that terminates with the administration of intravenous adenosine and verapamil. The ECG in mitral annular VT shows a delta wave-like beginning of the QRS complex similar to that seen in patients with left-sided WPW syndrome. Catheter ablation is associated with a high success rate (> 90%), making it a suitable alternative to drug therapy in these patients.

Recently, VT arising from the tricuspid annulus has been described which is associated with LBBB morphology. Tricuspid annulus VT originates more often in the septal region (74%) than in the free wall (26%). The septal VT had an early transition in precordial leads (V_3), narrower QRS complexes, and Qs in lead V_1 with absence of "notching" in the inferior leads, whereas the free wall VT was associated with late precordial transition (> V_3), wider QRS complexes, absence of Q wave in lead V_1, and "notching" in the inferior leads. The success rate for catheter ablation of the free wall VT was 90% compared with 57% in the septal group (since its origin is in close proximity to the normal AV nodal conduction).

Badhwar N, et al. Idiopathic ventricular tachycardia: diagnosis and management. *Curr Probl Cardiol.* 2007;32(1):7–43. [PMID: 17197289]

DIAGNOSTIC STUDIES

Patients with sustained VT that is either documented via ECG or suspected from symptoms such as syncope or presyncope should undergo additional studies, which can confirm the diagnosis of wide QRS tachycardia, determine whether VT is the cause of unexplained symptoms, identify the underlying substrate, and determine the direction of therapy.

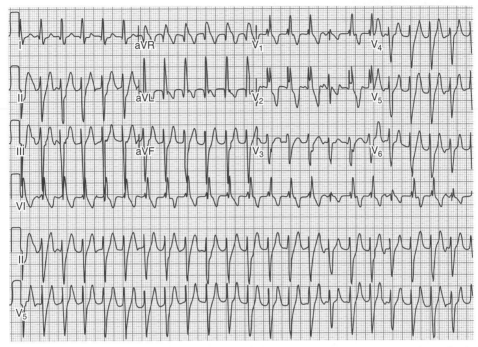

▲ **Figure 13–8.** Twelve-lead electrocardiogram of verapamil-sensitive idiopathic ventricular tachycardia (VT) arising from the left posterior fascicle with a right bundle branch block superior axis morphology. The duration of the QRS complex and the RS interval are narrower than that noted in VT associated with structural heart disease. However, the presence of atrioventricular dissociation and fusion beats (*arrows*) is diagnostic of VT. (Reproduced, with permission, from Badhwar N, et al. *Curr Probl Cardiol.* 2007;32:7.)

In most patients with documented sustained VT, the critical components of the workup include assessment of the nature and extent of any underlying heart disease and an electrophysiologic evaluation. A noninvasive cardiovascular workup includes ambulatory monitoring to detect heart rate variability or a daily fluctuation of arrhythmia; exercise testing to detect coronary artery disease or provoke catecholamine-sensitive VT; and an echocardiographic examination to uncover structural heart disease. Cardiac catheterization is strongly recommended for patients in whom coronary artery disease is suspected. Although a 12-lead ECG is usually adequate to make an accurate diagnosis of VT (versus SVT), the precise nature may not be clear in many patients unless electrophysiologic studies are performed.

When VT is suspected but not documented, its induction in the laboratory is critical to the decision to undertake any therapeutic approach. By inducing or replicating VT in the laboratory, its rate, morphology, origin, hemodynamic tolerance, and response to intravenous drugs can be evaluated.

Catheter ablation using radiofrequency or electrical energy is an effective form of treatment in patients with bundle branch reentry, idiopathic VT, and, in some cases, VT in association with prior MI. Thorough electrophysiologic testing is crucial for a successful outcome in these cases.

Many patients with VT have extensive cardiac pathology, including abnormalities of sinus node function and AV conduction. These abnormalities can be further aggravated with the administration of antiarrhythmic drugs. Electrophysiologic studies can frequently identify the nature and determine both the extent of these abnormalities and the need for additional therapeutic interventions (eg, permanent pacing for bradycardia).

Aside from arrhythmia assessment and cardiac substrate identification, the role of further tests in this population is dictated by the initial findings. When reversible abnormalities, such as myocardial ischemia, are detected, every attempt should be made to correct them. Paying separate attention to arrhythmias is critical because monomorphic VT is unlikely to be controlled without addressing specific VT management.

MANAGEMENT OF MONOMORPHIC VENTRICULAR TACHYCARDIA

Because monomorphic VT is most commonly due to underlying myocardial fibrosis, the pharmacologic treatment outlined here primarily relates to this substrate. The same approach can be used in other situations, but it may not be as applicable.

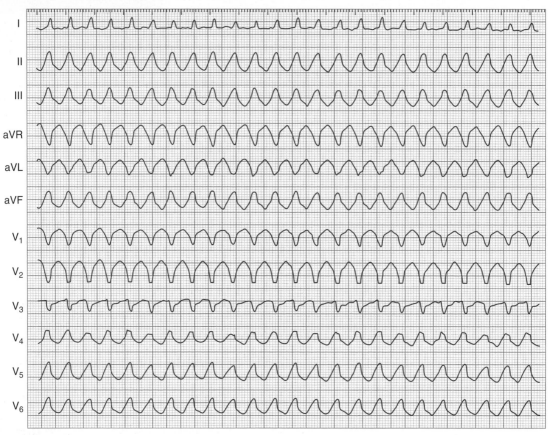

▲ **Figure 13–9.** Twelve-lead electrocardiogram that is typical of ventricular tachycardia (VT) in the absence of structural heart disease, originating in the right ventricular outflow tract. There is left bundle branch block morphology with late transition (V$_4$) in the precordial leads and an inferior axis in the limb leads. Negative QRS complex in lead avL suggest a septal origin. (Reproduced, with permission, from Badhwar N, et al. *Curr Probl Cardiol.* 2007;32:7.)

► Immediate Termination

The method of VT termination in the acute settings depends on the hemodynamic tolerance of the tachycardia. When the patient loses consciousness or has severe hypotension, a synchronized direct-current (DC) cardioversion should be attempted. Sedation prior to cardioversion is advised in patients who are awake. With hemodynamically well-tolerated VT, there is ample time to gather complete information, including a 12-lead ECG, before initiating therapy. Intravenous amiodarone is the drug of choice for treating VT. VT in association with acute MI may respond to lidocaine (2–3 mg/kg). Intravenous procainamide (10–15 mg/kg) at a rate of 50–100 mg/min is also effective, but it can lead to hypotension. Intravenous calcium channel blockers such as verapamil should not be administered unless the supraventricular nature of a sustained wide QRS tachycardia (SVT with aberrant conduction) is certain. The only type of VT

that responds to verapamil is uncommon. When VT is triggered or aggravated by exercise, intravenous β-blockers may be tried as the initial therapy unless there are contraindications to their use. If there is any uncertainty regarding the safety of β-blockers in patients with VT, it is somewhat safer to use agents with a short half-life, such as esmolol.

When pharmacologic intervention fails, overdrive termination can be tried. It does require insertion of a pacing catheter but can be quite useful in patients with frequent recurrent VT. Cardioversion is necessary in many situations, particularly if a prolonged VT episode is undesirable, such as in the setting of ischemic heart disease. It should also be emphasized that careful attention should be paid to other factors contributing to ventricular arrhythmogenesis, such as acidosis, hypoxia, electrolyte abnormalities, and the use of drugs. If such factors are involved, pharmacologic treatment alone may fail to control the VT.

▶ Prevention

Although acute termination of VT is relatively straightforward in most situations, the prevention of recurrences is often a challenge. The empiric use of antiarrhythmic drugs is not encouraged because of potential harm to the patient—as well as their unproven efficacy. Because VT represents a potentially life-threatening arrhythmia, establishing an effective form of therapy is desirable before the patient is discharged, especially for patients with VT-related syncope or cardiac arrest. In most situations, the therapy must be individualized, which requires understanding the type of VT, any underlying heart disease, left ventricular function, and the clinical presentation.

A. Pharmacologic Therapy

For monomorphic VT in association with chronic coronary artery disease or any other type of fibrosis, a variety of therapeutic options are now available. These include antiarrhythmic drugs, VT focal ablative therapy, and ICDs. Among the antiarrhythmic drugs, class I agents (Table 13–4) have moderate efficacy; quinidine and procainamide (class Ia) have been used extensively. In recent years, however, their use has progressively declined because of both excessive patient intolerance and lack of efficacy. Class Ib drugs such as mexiletine are weak antiarrhythmic agents when used alone, but they seem more useful in combination with Ia drugs. Class Ic drugs have moderate efficacy but a significant proarrhythmic potential; they are mainly used in patients with idiopathic VT. Exercise-induced VT generally responds well to β-blockers, and serial exercise stress tests can be used to judge drug efficacy. Because other forms of VT in patients with coronary artery disease may respond to β-blockers, they are frequently used alone or in combination with other antiarrhythmic drugs when the patient can tolerate them. At present, class III agents (eg, amiodarone, sotalol, azimilide) are the most promising antiarrhythmic agents for control of VT and ventricular fibrillation (VF). After a loading dose of 1200–1800 mg/day for 1–2 weeks, amiodarone can be used

in a maintenance dose of 200–400 mg/day. It is associated with long-term side effects that can affect the thyroid, lungs, gastrointestinal tract, eyes, skin, genitourinary system, and central nervous system. Baseline thyroid function test, liver function test, pulmonary function test, and ophthalmologic examination should be done in patients when amiodarone therapy is started, with repeat tests every 6 months. The usual daily dose of sotalol is 120–240 mg/day with monitoring of the ECG for QT prolongation during its administration or with any change in dosage. It should be pointed out that in high-risk patients with coronary artery disease and reduced left ventricular function, none of the antiarrhythmics, including amiodarone, have been shown to decrease mortality compared with placebo. Regardless of the method used, a failure of drug response is usually an indication for nonpharmacologic treatment, which can produce excellent results.

B. Nonpharmacologic Therapy

1. Implantable cardioverter-defibrillators—These devices clearly provide the most effective form of therapy for preventing SCD in patients with VT. The ICD does not prevent VT from occurring, however; it is designed only to terminate the tachycardia or fibrillation. Most episodes of VT can be terminated with overdrive pacing; this form of therapy is usually not perceptible to the patient. There are relatively few contraindications to ICD treatment; these include incessant VT and VF secondary to reversible causes such as antiarrhythmic drugs, electrolyte abnormalities, and acute ischemia. ICDs have demonstrated a remarkable effectiveness in prevention of SCD, with an overall 1-year survival rate of 92% in patients with documented life-threatening ventricular tachyarrhythmias. A meta-analysis of ICD trials showed that the relative risk reduction of sudden death with ICDs in secondary prevention is 50% and that for primary prevention is 37% (see Chapter 15).

2. Surgical ablation—In patients with coronary artery disease and prior MI, the VT often originates close to the infarct, thus providing the opportunity for surgical destruction of the VT site of origin. It should be considered in patients undergoing coronary artery bypass surgery who have a ventricular aneurysm or infarction and mappable VT. In patients with a left ventricular ejection fraction of at least 25%, this type of surgery can be carried out with relatively low risk and a cure rate of approximately 75%. There has been a decline in primary surgical therapy for patients with VT with the advent and widespread use of ICDs.

3. Catheter-based ablation—The development of radiofrequency catheter ablation as a therapeutic option for the treatment of arrhythmias has dramatically altered the approach to the tachycardic patient. Since its introduction in 1986, radiofrequency ablation has provided actual cure for thousands of patients with debilitating symptoms from paroxysmal SVTs and certain VTs. ICDs are the standard

Table 13–4. Antiarrhythmic Drugs

Class	Drug
Ia	Quinidine, procainamide, disopyramide
Ib	Mexiletine, lidocaine
Ic	Flecainide, propafenone, others (Ethmozine)
II	β-Blockers
III	Amiodarone, sotalol, bepridil
IV	Calcium channel blockers

therapy for sustained VT in patients with structural heart disease. In patients who experience recurrent shocks from the ICD, radiofrequency catheter ablation may be used in an attempt to modify or eliminate the VT circuit and thereby reduce the number of shocks a patient may experience. Catheter ablation in this setting is usually palliative with elimination of all VT circuits achieved in 50–60% of patients by the most experienced operators.

It is almost always curative, however, for sustained VT from bundle branch reentry from any cause seen in patients with dilated cardiomyopathy. High success rates (85–100%) make radiofrequency catheter ablation a good alternative to drug therapy in patients with idiopathic VT. Radiofrequency catheter ablation is likely to play a greater role in management of VT in the future due to the development of advanced mapping systems, better catheter design, and incorporation of real-time anatomy using computed tomography scans and magnetic resonance imaging.

Recent consensus guidelines recommend catheter ablation for patients with structural heart disease in each of the following conditions: (1) symptomatic sustained monomorphic VT, including VT terminated by an ICD, that recurs despite antiarrhythmic drug therapy or when antiarrhythmic drugs are not tolerated or not desired; (2) incessant sustained monomorphic VT or VT storm that is not due to a transient reversible cause; (3) patients with frequent premature ventricular contractions, nonsustained VT, or VT that is presumed to cause ventricular dysfunction; (4) bundle branch reentrant or interfascicular VTs; and (5) recurrent sustained polymorphic VT and VF that is refractory to antiarrhythmic therapy when there is a suspected trigger that can be targeted for ablation.

Aliot EM, et al. EHRA/HRS expert consensus on catheter ablation of ventricular arrhythmias. *Europace.* 2009;11:771–817. [PMID: 19443434]

Bardy GH, et al; Sudden Cardiac Death in Heart Failure Trial (SCD-HeFT) Investigators. Amiodarone or an implantable cardioverter-defibrillator for congestive heart failure. *N Engl J Med.* 2005;352(3):225–37. [PMID: 15659722]

Ezekowitz JA, et al. Implantable cardioverter defibrillators in primary and secondary prevention: a systematic review of randomized, controlled trials. *Ann Intern Med.* 2003;138(6): 445–52. [PMID: 12639076]

Goldschlager N, et al. A practical guide for clinicians who treat patients with amiodarone: 2007. *Heart Rhythm.* 2007;4(9): 1250–9. [PMID: 17765636]

Zipes DP, et al. ACC/AHA/ESC 2006 guidelines for management of patients with ventricular arrhythmias and the prevention of sudden cardiac death. *J Am Coll Cardiol.* 2006;48(5):e247–346. [PMID: 16949478]

POLYMORPHIC VENTRICULAR TACHYCARDIA

Recognition of polymorphic VTs and their distinction from the monomorphic variety represent the crucial first step toward appropriate management. These tachycardias tend to be rapid; they generally produce symptoms of hypotension and can readily degenerate into VF. At least two types can be recognized that must be distinguished by the presence or absence of prolonged myocardial recovery.

1. Polymorphic Ventricular Tachycardia in the Setting of Prolonged QT Interval

This condition is often referred to as torsades de pointes. It can be congenital or acquired. Although the precipitating factor can differ between the two varieties, both show a prolonged QT (QTc) interval and slow, prominent, or unusual-looking T waves.

▶ Clinical Findings

Congenital long QT syndrome (LQTS) can occur with deafness (Jervell and Lange-Nielsen syndrome) or without deafness (Romano-Ward syndrome). It is mainly characterized by episodes of torsades de pointes that are often triggered by adrenergic stimulation, which can be brought about by physical exertion or mental or emotional stress. The QT interval prolongation may be subtle and can be unmasked by long pauses or adrenergic stimuli such as exercise. The electrophysiologic mechanism may be early after-depolarization for initiation and reentry for sustenance. The clinical presentation includes episodes of lightheadedness, near syncope, syncope, and, in some cases, cardiac arrest. There are no obvious associated cardiac abnormalities. Characteristic patterns of QT prolongation on the ECG provide a clue to the three most common forms of LQTS (Figure 13–10). It is now clear that congenital LQTS is caused by ion channel defects. LQT_1 and LQT_2 are K^+ channel abnormalities, but LQT_3 is an Na^+ channel mutation. At least eight genetic mutations at different loci have been identified. Congenital LQTS has been proposed as one of the causes of sudden infant death syndrome; however, most of these patients have the first event around 9 to 12 years of age. LQT_1 and LQT_2 account for 80% of the cases. LQT_3 is only seen in 10% of the cases, but it accounts for most of the lethal cases of LQTS. Exercise and sudden auditory stimuli are triggers for LQT_1 and LQT_2, respectively, whereas LQT_3 patients have most of the events during sleep at slower heart rates. Female sex, congenital deafness, baseline QT interval > 500 ms, a prolonged interval from the peak of the T wave to the end of the T wave, and males with LQT_3 are associated with a high risk of sudden death.

Acquired LQTS can be caused by a variety of pharmacologic agents and metabolic factors (a partial list is given in Table 13–5). These patients have a partial defect in the K^+ channel I_{Kr} that becomes a complete defect in the presence of the offending agents. The main ECG abnormality is that of prolonged QT interval and often an unusual appearance of the T wave, frequently referred to as the slow wave (Figure 13–11). The QT interval prolongation may not

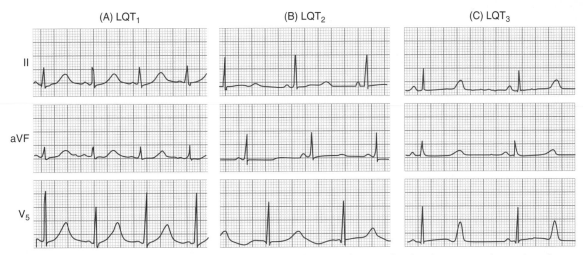

▲ Figure 13–10. Genotype-specific T-wave morphology on electrocardiogram (ECG) in long QT syndrome (LQTS) patients. **A:** ECG in LQT$_1$ showing broad-based T waves. **B:** ECG in LQT$_2$ showing low-amplitude T waves with notches. **C:** ECG in LQT$_3$ showing extended ST segment with relatively narrow peaked T waves. (Reproduced, with permission, from Moss AJ, et al. *Circulation*. 1995;92:2929.)

always be striking at the normal rates but should show a measurable increase after a pause, for example, following a premature beat. Extreme caution must be exercised in such individuals because a recurrence is likely if challenged with the same triggers. The actual list of potentially offending agents may be quite long because many pharmacologic agents have not been tested for such adverse side effects as prolongation of the QT interval, and only the widely known culprits are listed in Table 13–5.

▶ Management

The key to managing torsades de pointes related to acquired prolonged QT interval is recognizing it. Frequently, these patients have underlying monomorphic VT that is being treated with antiarrhythmic agents. The emergence of torsades de pointes in this setting may not be interpreted correctly as a side effect of the medication but as a lack of sufficient control that requires more aggressive but similar

Table 13–5. Causes of Acquired Long QT Syndrome

Antiarrhythmic drugs	**Psychiatry drugs**
Class Ia	Antidepressants (tetra/tricyclic), antipsychotic (phenothiazines, haloperidol, sertindole)
Quinidine (I_{Kr}, I_{To}, and I_{Ks}), disopyramide, procainamide	**Cholinergic antagonists**
Class III	Cisapride (I_{Kr}), organophosphates (insecticides)
Sotalol (I_{Kr}, I_{To}), d-sotalol, amiodarone (I_{Kr}, I_{Ks}), ibutilide, dofetilide (I_{Kr})	**Inotropic drugs**
	Amrinone, milrinone
Antibiotics	**Poisons**
Macrolides (erythromycin [I_{Kr}], clarithromycin, clindamycin), trimethoprim-sulfamethoxazole, pentamidine, imidazoles (ketoconazole)	Arsenic, organophosphates (insecticides, nerve gas)
	Metabolic abnormalities
	Hypokalemia (I_{Kr}), hypomagnesemia, hypocalcemia
Histamine receptor antagonists	**Bradyarrhythmias**
Terfenadine,[1] astemizole[1] (I_{Kr})	Complete atrioventricular block, sick sinus syndrome
Serotonin receptor antagonists	**Starvation**
Ketanserin (I_{Kr}, I_{To})[2]	Anorexia nervosa, "liquid protein" diets, gastroplasty, ileojejunal bypass
Serotonin receptor inhibitors	**Nervous system injury**
Sertindole (I_{Kr}),[2] zimeldine[2]	Subarachnoid hemorrhage, thalamic hematoma, right neck dissection or hematoma, pheochromocytoma
Diuretics	
Indapamide (I_{Ks})	

[1]Withdrawn from the U.S. market.
[2]Not available in the United States.

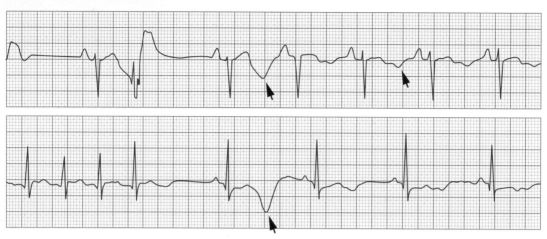

▲ **Figure 13–11.** Prolonged QT interval with slow wave. The T wave has an unusual appearance, and both the QT-interval prolongation and T-wave morphologic abnormality are more pronounced after the pause. The slow wave is indicated by the *arrows*. (Reproduced, with permission, from Jackman WM, et al. *Prog Cardiovasc Dis*. 1988;31:115.)

therapy. When the proper diagnosis is made, the treatment is withdrawal of the offending agent and replacement of electrolytes. Intravenous magnesium has been shown to decrease early after-depolarizations. The prompt replacement of potassium and calcium is also critical. Because hemodynamic stability is necessary to excrete the offending pharmacologic agent, the immediate suppression of torsades de pointes is desirable and can be accomplished with overdrive pacing or using such drugs as isoproterenol or atropine. When it is related to pauses and bradycardia, pacemaker support may be needed.

The mainstay of long-term treatment in congenital LQTS is β-blockade, and up to 5 mg/kg/day of propranolol (or 1 mg/kg/day of nadolol) may be necessary in some situations. Because cardiac slowing can also be arrhythmogenic, permanent pacing is often performed and is the therapy of choice in LQT_3 where β-blockers are contraindicated. Specific drugs that block the culprit ion channels include nicorandil in LQT_1, potassium supplements and spironolactone in LQT_2, and mexiletine in LQT_3. Clearly, drugs that prolong the QT interval must be avoided. Left stellate sympathectomy has been carried out with variable success in difficult cases. In individuals with recurrent syncope or cardiac arrest, ICDs remain a viable option to prevent SCD.

2. Polymorphic Ventricular Tachycardia with a Normal QT Interval

It is not uncommon to see short episodes of polymorphic VT without any QT interval prolongation. Sustained forms of such arrhythmias can lead to VF. The true nature of this

problem can be readily appreciated by observation of the QT interval prior to the tachycardia and, more reliably, following the pause that ensues after termination of VT. If no QT prolongation is noted, the following possibilities must be entertained.

Acute ischemia should be suspected with polymorphic VT in the presence of a normal QT interval. Although the exact prevalence of this type of VT is unknown, it is probably more common than realized. The VT tends to be rapid and has a tendency to degenerate into VF (Figure 13–12). Acute ischemia must be excluded in all patients with polymorphic VT in association with normal QT interval. The acute ischemia might be related to underlying coronary stenosis or coronary artery spasm brought about by a variety of factors. Prompt diagnosis and therapy are critical for preventing VT-related SCD in these patients. The workup includes coronary arteriography and an assessment for coronary artery spasm. The traditional diagnostic criteria—history of chest pain or obvious ST abnormalities—may not be present prior to the episode. A high index of suspicion is likely to lead to a correct diagnosis. This type of VT can seldom be induced in the laboratory, and the electrophysiologic mechanism for it remains unclear. The treatment, in essence, is directed toward eliminating myocardial ischemia; it might include myocardial revascularization or antiischemic drugs such as β-blockers or calcium channel blockers.

Polymorphic VT with normal QT interval can also occur in patients without substrates for myocardial ischemia but with chronic fibrosis or hypertrophy; sometimes, it can occur with no obvious pathology. It is prudent to exclude all the previously mentioned correctable causes before a diagnosis of this idiopathic variety is made. In some cases, the

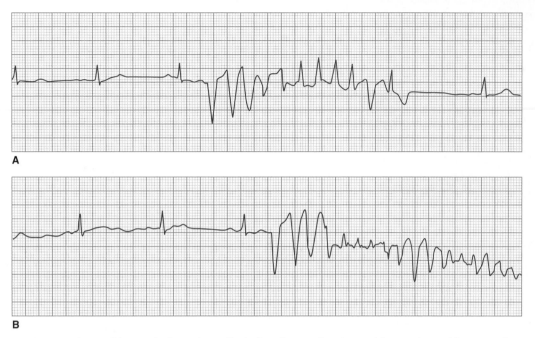

▲ **Figure 13–12.** Polymorphic ventricular tachycardia (VT) and normal QT interval in a patient with severe three-vessel disease. **A:** Several nonsustained polymorphic VT episodes. **B:** Degeneration to ventricular fibrillation, requiring direct-current cardioversion.

polymorphic VT may be inducible, suggesting a reentrant nature. Although such an arrhythmia can occur in patients with healed MI, it is also sometimes seen in patients with hypertrophic and congestive cardiomyopathy. This type of polymorphic VT does not provide a reliable end point for drug testing or VT surgery. Antiarrhythmic drugs, particularly amiodarone, may be useful as are ICDs in preventing SCD in this population.

PROGNOSIS

VT as a warning sign for SCD differs vastly in various clinical situations. The initial presentation and the left ventricular function are, perhaps, the most important determinants. Recurrent cardiac arrest or SCD is more likely in patients who have had a previous similar presentation, and syncope resulting from VT also carries a poor prognosis. On the other hand, SCD in the event of VT recurrence is less likely in patients with hemodynamically well-tolerated VT. Reduced left ventricular function and VT carry a worse prognosis than does either alone.

Chiang CE, et al. The long QT syndromes: genetic basis and clinical implications. *J Am Coll Cardiol.* 2000;36(1):1–12. [PMID: 10898405]

Priori SG, et al. Risk stratification in the long-QT syndrome. *N Engl J Med.* 2003;348(19):1866–74. [PMID: 12736279]

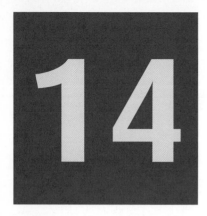

Conduction Disorders & Cardiac Pacing

Richard H. Hongo, MD

Nora F. Goldschlager, MD

ESSENTIALS OF DIAGNOSIS

Sinus node dysfunction ("sick sinus syndrome")

▶ Sinus bradycardia: sinus rate of less than 60 bpm.

▶ Sinoatrial exit block, type I: progressively shorter P-P intervals, followed by failure of occurrence of a P wave.

▶ Sinoatrial exit block, type II: pauses in sinus rhythm that are multiples of basic sinus rate.

▶ Sinus arrest, sinus pauses: failure of occurrence of P waves at expected times.

Atrioventricular (AV) block

▶ First degree: prolonged PR interval more than 200 ms.

▶ Second degree

• Type I: progressive increase in PR interval, followed by failure of atrioventricular (AV) conduction and nonoccurrence of a QRS complex.

• Type II: abrupt failure of AV conduction not preceded by increasing PR intervals.

▶ "2:1 block:" due to lack of consecutive PR intervals; unable to assign either type I or type II block.

▶ "Advanced:" AV conduction ratio ≥ 3:1.

▶ Third degree ("complete"): independent atrial and ventricular rhythms, with failure of AV conduction despite temporal opportunity for it to occur.

▶ General Considerations

The clinical presentation of patients with conduction system disease is determined by two underlying abnormal conditions: the inability to maintain or increase the sinus rate in response to metabolic need, and atrioventricular (AV)

dyssynchrony (inappropriately timed atrial and ventricular depolarization and contraction sequences).

▶ Pathophysiology & Etiology

A. Sinus Node Dysfunction

Sinus node dysfunction ("sick sinus syndrome") is usually due to a degenerative process that involves the sinus node and sinoatrial (SA) area (Table 14–1). Often, the degenerative process and associated fibrosis also involve the approaches to the AV node and the AV node itself, as well as the intraventricular conduction system; as many as 25–30% of patients with sinus node dysfunction have evidence of AV and bundle branch conduction delay or block.

Respiratory sinus arrhythmia, in which the sinus rate increases with inspiration and decreases with expiration, is not an abnormal rhythm and is most commonly seen in young healthy persons. Nonrespiratory sinus arrhythmia, in which phasic changes in sinus rate are not due to respiration, may be accentuated by the use of vagal agents, such as digitalis and morphine, and is more likely to be observed in patients who are older and who have underlying cardiac disease, although the arrhythmia is not itself a marker for structural heart disease; its mechanism is unknown. Ventriculophasic sinus arrhythmia is an unusual rhythm that occurs during advanced second-degree or complete AV block; it is characterized by shorter P-P intervals that enclose QRS complexes and longer P-P intervals that do not enclose QRS complexes. The mechanism is not known with certainty, but may be related to the effects of the mechanical ventricular systole. The ventricular contraction increases the blood supply to the sinus node, thereby transiently increasing its firing rate; the resulting increase in intra-atrial pressure causes subsequent inhibition of the sinus rate. Ventriculophasic sinus arrhythmia is not a pathologic arrhythmia and should not be confused with premature atrial depolarizations or SA block. None of the sinus arrhythmias indicate sinus node dysfunction.

Table 14–1. Causes of Sinus Node Dysfunction

Idiopathic
    Degenerative process
    Normal aging
Acute myocardial ischemia or infarction
    Right or left circumflex coronary artery occlusion
    Jarisch-Bezold reflex
Medications
    β-Blockers
    Rate-sparing calcium channel blockers
     Diltiazem, verapamil
    Digitalis (with high prevailing vagal tone)
    Class I antiarrhythmic agents
    Class III antiarrhythmic agents (amiodarone, dronedarone, sotalol)
    Clonidine

Sinus node dysfunction is present when marked sinus bradycardia, pauses in sinus rhythm (sinus arrest), SA block, or a combination of these exist (Figures 14–1 through Figure 14–5). Some clinically normal individuals who do not have structural heart disease can experience significant sinus bradycardia and prolonged sinus pauses under conditions of high vagal tone such as sleep. In some patients, a trigger, such as vomiting or coughing, can be identified; in other patients, high levels of acetylcholine may be responsible. Vagal stimulation, often from an identifiable trigger (Table 14–2), is commonly responsible for significant sinus bradyarrhythmias occurring in patients in an intensive care setting.

SA block may take the form of progressive delay in transmission of the sinus-generated impulse through the SA node to the atrium, finally resulting in a nonconducted sinus impulse and an absent P wave on the surface electrocardiogram (ECG) (Wenckebach, or type I second-degree exit block; see Figures 14–1 and 14–4), or abrupt failure of transmission of the sinus impulse to the atrium (type II second-degree exit block; see Figure 14–1). In type I second-degree exit block, there is less incremental delay with each successive impulse transmission through the SA nodal tissue (similar to type I AV nodal block); thus, the P-P intervals become progressively shorter until a P wave fails to occur. In type II second-degree exit block, abrupt failure of sinus impulse conduction to the atria can take the form of 2:1, 3:1 (and so on) SA block. Fixed 2:1 SA exit block cannot be distinguished from sinus bradycardia on the surface ECG.

Bradycardia-tachycardia syndrome is characterized by episodes of both bradycardias and supraventricular tachycardias (Figure 14–6). The bradycardia is due to sinus node dysfunction (sinus arrest or SA exit block) with associated junctional or ventricular escape rhythms. The supraventricular tachycardias may be atrial tachycardia, atrial flutter, atrial fibrillation, AV reciprocating tachycardia, or AV nodal

reentry tachycardia (see Chapter 11); more than one type of tachycardia may occur in the same patient. Bradycardia-tachycardia syndrome often represents diffuse conduction system disease, but is not necessarily associated with structural heart disease.

Sinus bradycardia not uncommonly results from medications, particularly β-blockers, the rate-limiting calcium channel-blocking agents verapamil and diltiazem, and some commonly used antiarrhythmic agents such as sotalol, dronedarone, and amiodarone (see Figure 14–2). If these medications are necessary to treat the patient, permanent cardiac pacing is indicated.

The natural history of sinus node dysfunction is one of variable progression to an absence of identifiable sinus activity, with the process taking from 10 to 30 years. The condition itself is not associated with a high risk of arrhythmic death, although the morbidity caused by a sudden onset of bradycardia can be considerable. The ultimate prognosis for the patient with sinus node dysfunction typically depends on the presence and severity of underlying heart disease, rather than on the bradyarrhythmia itself.

B. Atrioventricular Block

Delay or block can occur anywhere along the course of the AV conducting system that is made up of the AV node, His bundle, and Purkinje fibers (left and right bundle branches). Like sinus node dysfunction, AV nodal-His block and bundle branch block (BBB) are often the result of sclerodegenerative processes. These processes can also involve the approaches to the AV node. Acquired AV nodal block is often due to acute ischemia and infarction (especially involving the inferior wall and right ventricle), infection, trauma, and medications (Table 14–3).

The AV node, or junction, is made up of three regions: atrionodal, central compact, and nodal-His. Cells of the atrionodal region have a relatively fast depolarization rate (45–60 bpm) and are responsive to autonomic nervous system input, whereas cells of the nodal-His region have a slower depolarization rate (about 40 bpm) and are generally unresponsive to autonomic influences. The site of origin of a junctional rhythm will therefore determine its rate, responsiveness to vagal and adrenergic input, and consequently the presence and severity of clinical symptoms.

The natural history of patients with AV block depends on whether or not there is an underlying cardiac condition with its own prognosis; however, the site of the block and the resulting rhythm disturbances themselves contribute to prognosis. First-degree AV block has little prognostic import. Persistent second-degree (types I and II), advanced second-degree (two or more consecutive nonconducted P waves), and complete AV block can all be associated with adverse outcomes, including death, unless the arrhythmias are vagally mediated or are due to other reversible causes.

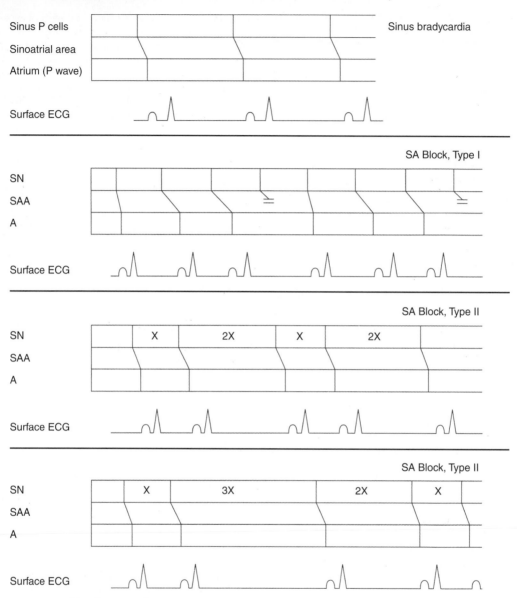

▲ **Figure 14–1.** Ladder diagrams illustrating sinus bradycardia and sinoatrial block, types I and II. ECG, electrocardiogram; SA, sinoatrial; SAA, sinoatrial area; SN, sinoatrial node.

▶ Clinical Findings

A. Symptoms & Signs

The symptoms resulting from conduction disorders reflect cerebral hypoperfusion, low cardiac output at rest or during exercise, and rarely, hemodynamic collapse. Symptoms, which are often subtle, can be episodic or chronic and can change over time. Because a patient often adapts activity levels

to compensate for the impairment in heart rate response, significant symptoms may not be evident unless the patient is closely questioned about specific activities and effort tolerance, or the clinician actually observes the patient during performance of activities of daily living such as walking or during formal treadmill exercise tests.

Syncope is the classic symptom of cerebral hypoperfusion due to bradycardia; however, symptoms of presyncope

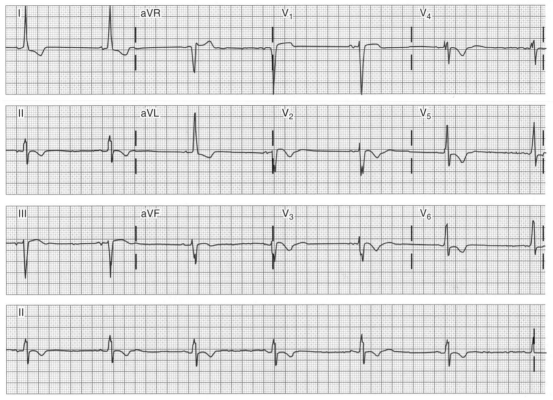

▲ **Figure 14–2.** This 83-year-old woman was being treated for systolic heart failure and was receiving 200 mg/day of amiodarone for episodes of nonsustained ventricular tachycardia. She complained of profound effort fatigue but no symptoms of heart failure. Electrocardiogram reveals an atrial bradycardia at a rate of about 38 bpm. The P waves vary in morphology, suggesting some wandering of the atrial pacemaker. Left axis deviation and a left intraventricular conduction delay with ST- and T-wave abnormalities are present. The atrial bradycardia was presumed to be due to the amiodarone, which was discontinued, resulting in appreciable increase in a stable sinus rhythm, with amelioration of the patient's effort fatigue.

such as dizziness, lightheadedness, and confusion can reflect the same pathophysiology and warrant the same aggressive approach to diagnosis and management. It should be emphasized that patients with cerebral hypoperfusion often have impairment of memory surrounding the presyncopal or syncopal episodes and may therefore be unable to provide an adequate or accurate history surrounding the events; witnesses, if present, can contribute significant information in these cases.

Patients with sinus node dysfunction or AV block, in whom the escape pacemaker is unresponsive to autonomic nervous system input, cannot increase their heart rate in response to increases in oxygen demand. They are, therefore, intolerant of effort and will report symptoms of exercise-related breathlessness, weakness, and fatigue. These symptoms, which can be disabling, are often confused with other conditions such as hypothyroidism, medications, underlying heart disease, deconditioning, or simply older age.

During periods of AV block, the atria and ventricles often depolarize and contract asynchronously or with inappropriate and suboptimal timing between atrial and ventricular contractions. There are variable increases in atrial pressures and volumes depending on the degree to which the AV valves are open or closed at the onset of ventricular systole. The resulting atrial stretch and secretion of atrial natriuretic peptide produce reflex systemic hypotension and cerebral hypoperfusion. In addition, the increases in left atrial and pulmonary venous pressures can cause shortness of breath and pulmonary venous congestion, including frank pulmonary edema. The mistaken diagnosis of refractory left ventricular dysfunction is not infrequently made in this situation.

Patients who have the bradycardia-tachycardia syndrome (see Figure 14–6) have symptoms referable to both the bradycardia and the tachycardia. During tachycardia, the patient can experience uncomfortable palpitations,

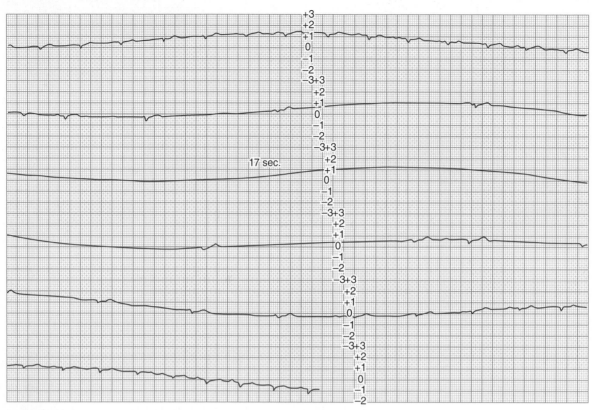

▲ **Figure 14–3.** Continuous modified lead-II ambulatory electrocardiographic recording in a patient with recurrent presyncopal spells. Sinus rhythm is present in the top strip; the second strip shows marked sinus slowing, followed by a 17-second period of sinus arrest without the appearance of a QRS escape rhythm. Sinus rhythm reappears in the fourth strip, gradually increasing its rate until stable rhythm is restored in the bottom strip. The absence of an escape rhythm raises the possibility of diffuse disease of the conduction system and impulse-generating tissue.

breathlessness, chest discomfort, and at times, symptoms of cerebral hypoperfusion from excessively rapid heart rates.

More rarely, bradycardias can lead to a potentially lethal form of polymorphic ventricular tachycardia known as bradycardia- or pause-dependent ventricular tachycardia

(Figure 14–7); this tachycardia is often triggered in the setting of QT interval prolongation brought on by the longer R-R intervals associated with either bradycardia or pauses (torsade de pointes ventricular tachycardia). Symptoms in these patients can include not only palpitations, presyncope, and syncope, but also cardiac arrest.

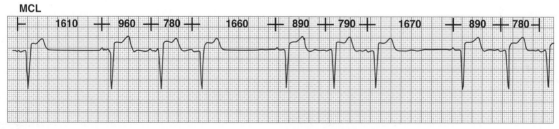

▲ **Figure 14–4.** Progressive decrease in P-wave cycle lengths followed by a pause in P-wave rate, indicating type I second-degree sinoatrial block. The pauses in sinus rate are less than twice the preceding sinus cycle lengths, satisfying the criteria for Wenckebach periodicity. MCL, modified chest lead.

Continuous MCL$_1$ Rhythm Strips

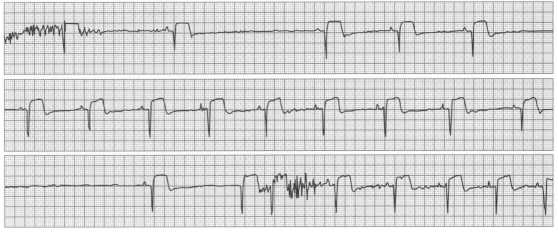

▲ **Figure 14–5.** Irregular pauses in sinus rate, which occur abruptly and are not multiples of a basic sinus-cycle length. Best characterized as sinus pauses rather than sinoatrial block or sinus arrest, this rhythm indicates the existence of sinus node dysfunction. MCL$_1$, modified chest lead.

Table 14–2. Conditions Associated with Vagally Mediated Bradyarrhythmias

Highly conditioned state
Sleep
Vomiting, retching
Suctioning
Nasal intubation
Gastric intubation
Urination
Defecation
Coughing
Swallowing
Central nervous system trauma with high intracranial pressure
Isotonic exercise conditioning

Table 14–3. Causes of Acquired AV Nodal-His Block

Idiopathic
Degenerative process
Ischemic heart disease (inferior wall, septal area, right ventricle)
Calcific aortic and mitral valve disease
AV nodal/His ablative procedures
Medications
    Digitalis, β-blockers, calcium channel blockers (verapamil, diltiazem), sotalol, dronedarone, amiodarone
Infections (including aortic valve endocarditis)
Inflammatory diseases (myocarditis)
Infiltrative diseases
    Amyloidosis, neoplasm, sarcoidosis, hemochromatosis
Neuromuscular diseases
    Myotonic muscular dystrophy, Kearns-Sayre syndrome, Erb dystrophy (limb-girdle muscular dystrophy), peroneal muscular atrophy
Collagen-vascular diseases
Trauma
Aortic valve surgery

AV, atrioventricular.

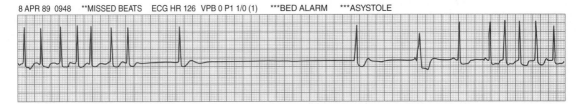

8 APR 89 0948   **MISSED BEATS   ECG HR 126 VPB 0 P1 1/0 (1)   ***BED ALARM   ***ASYSTOLE

▲ **Figure 14–6.** Lead II rhythm strip characteristic of bradycardia-tachycardia syndrome, recorded from a patient with palpitations and intermittent dizzy spells.

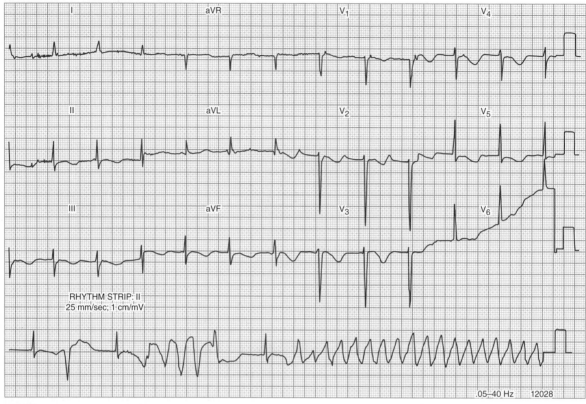

▲ **Figure 14–7.** Pause-dependent ventricular tachycardia causing loss of consciousness in a patient with syncopal and presyncopal spells. Note the markedly prolonged QT interval, which is longer and more bizarre when associated with the longer RR cycle lengths.

B. Physical Examination

The physical examination of the patient with bradycardia reflects the origin of the QRS rhythm and the AV relationship more so than the heart rate per se. Junctional or ventricular escape rhythms resulting from atrial bradycardia or AV block produce AV dyssynchrony. This dyssynchrony results in varying degrees of atrial contribution to ventricular filling, as well as varying stroke outputs and systolic blood pressures. Because AV dyssynchrony causes changes in the positions of the mitral and tricuspid valves relative to their fully closed or open positions, the intensity of the first heart sound will vary, as will the audibility of atrial gallop (S_4) sounds and the intensity of semilunar valve systolic ejection murmurs and AV valve regurgitant murmurs.

Examination of the venous pulse contour in the neck can reveal cannon *a* waves (due to atrial systole occurring against closed AV valves) and prominent *cv* waves (due to ventricular contraction occurring with the AV valves partially or even completely open), and the diagnosis of AV block can occasionally be made by recognizing these findings. Central venous pressure elevation (not to be confused with *a* and

cv waves) is a common physical finding that is independent of the venous pulse contour.

The carotid pulse may vary in volume and upstroke velocity in patients with AV dyssynchrony. Examination of the chest may disclose rales, which reflect increased pulmonary venous pressure and valvular regurgitation rather than systolic or diastolic ventricular dysfunction. The liver may be enlarged and may pulsate because of transmitted *a* and *cv* waves. Peripheral edema may also be present if the AV dyssynchrony is chronic.

These same physical findings can also occur in patients who have sinus rhythm but develop AV dyssynchrony from being paced by a single-chamber ventricular system. In these patients, symptoms of weakness, fatigue, and congestive heart failure, together with physical findings indicating AV dyssynchrony, constitute the "pacemaker syndrome," and this syndrome is treated by upgrading the single-chamber ventricular pacing system to a dual-chamber system in which sensing of the atrial rhythm triggers a paced ventricular response to restore AV synchrony (see later section, Permanent Pacing).

In addition to the findings described earlier, marked bradycardia (< 40 bpm) may result in ventricular dilatation in order to use the Frank-Starling effect to boost stroke volume and increase cardiac output despite the slow heart rate. This dilatation may lead to left ventricular gallop sounds and regurgitant murmurs, which disappear when normal heart rate is returned. Also, the enlarged ventricles may be palpable.

C. Diagnostic Studies

1. Sinus node dysfunction

A. ELECTROCARDIOGRAPHY—The P waves inscribed on the surface ECG represent atrial depolarizations. Sinus node depolarization precedes atrial depolarization and is not seen on the surface ECG. The P waves that result from sinus-generated impulses must be inferred from their morphology and axis.

The sinus P wave has a mean frontal plane axis of +15 to +75° and is upright in leads I, II, and aVF, inverted in lead aVR, and variable in leads III and aVL. In the horizontal plane, the sinus P wave can be inverted in lead V_1 but is upright in leads V_3–V_6. Respiratory variation in the sinus P-wave contour can be seen in the inferior leads and should not be confused with wandering atrial pacemaker, which is unrelated to breathing. Sinus arrhythmia is present when the P-wave morphology is normal and consistent and the P-P intervals vary by more than 160 ms. SA block exists when some impulses generated by the sinus pacemaking cells do not exit the SA node to depolarize the atria; in the absence of atrial depolarization, a P wave will not be inscribed on the surface ECG. High-degree (advanced) SA block, in which most of the sinus impulses fail to exit the SA node to the atrium, is inscribed on the surface ECG as pauses in sinus rhythm. These pauses often cannot be differentiated from sinus arrest caused by failure of impulse generation by the sinus node. If the pauses between sinus P waves are multiples of a basic P wave rate, however, the diagnosis of type II second-degree SA block can be made.

B. ELECTROPHYSIOLOGIC STUDIES—Sinus node function can be evaluated in the electrophysiology laboratory by means of simultaneous surface and intracardiac electrographic recordings made during basal conditions, physiologic and pharmacologic interventions, and atrial pacing. This evaluation can be undertaken in patients with either symptomatic sinus bradycardia or bradycardia-tachycardia syndrome. It can also be used in patients with recurrent syncope of unclear etiology, although the diagnostic yield and predictive value for the condition is limited. Measurements include the intrinsic heart rate, the sinus node recovery time (SNRT), the SA conduction time (SACT), and the response to parasympathetic (vagal) stimulation as assessed by carotid sinus massage.

The intrinsic heart rate (ie, the rate independent of autonomic influences) is the sinus rate during pharmacologic denervation of the sinus node using a β-blocker and atropine. The intrinsic heart rate is sometimes used to distinguish healthy persons from those with sinus node dysfunction.

Sinus node recovery time is the interval between the end of a period of pacing-induced overdrive suppression of sinus node activity and the return of sinus node function, manifested on the surface ECG by the postpacing sinus P-wave interval. The measured SNRT depends on several factors, among them the proximity of the pacing catheter to the sinus node, the SACT, the presence or absence of SA entrance block (in which atrial impulses fail to enter and depolarize the sinus node), and local neurohormonal influences. In normal persons, atrial pacing at rates of 120–130 bpm for 30 seconds or more is followed by a return of sinus node activity at a reproducible interval, with the basic sinus rate generally being achieved within three postpacing beats. The usual SNRT is less than 1.5 seconds, although considerable variation may exist depending on the prevailing autonomic tone. The corrected sinus node recovery time can be calculated by subtracting the basic sinus rate from the sinus node recovery time; a normal value is usually between 350 and 550 ms. In patients with sinus node dysfunction, sinus node recovery times are not reproducible and tend to be longer after more prolonged periods of pacing; return to the basic sinus rate within three postpacing beats is also inconstant and may be followed by additional (secondary) pauses in rate.

SA conduction time reflects the time taken by a premature atrial-pacing stimulus delivered near the sinus node area to traverse the atrial tissue to reach the sinus node and prematurely depolarize it, the time to the formation of the next sinus impulse following the premature depolarization, and the return of the sinus-generated impulse through atrial tissue to the recording electrode. The SA conduction time is often prolonged in patients with clinical evidence of sinus node dysfunction other than sinus bradycardia alone.

Because the electrophysiologic tests of sinus node function are neither specific nor sensitive, they can sometimes show abnormal results in patients without sinus bradycardia and normal results in those with symptomatic sinus node disease. The test results should not, therefore, be relied on in isolation when making clinical decisions regarding either diagnosis or treatment.

Some of the problems of poor sensitivity and specificity can be overcome by recording the sinus node electrogram from an electrode catheter positioned in the vicinity of the sinus node (at the junction of the superior vena cava and the right atrium). The sinus node electrogram, however, cannot be reproducibly recorded in as many as 50% of patients. Sinus node electrography can distinguish between SA exit block and sinus arrest, and studies have shown that most pauses in sinus rhythm are due to SA exit block. Notwithstanding these technologic advances, the diagnosis of sinus node dysfunction generally remains a clinical one.

C. EXERCISE TESTING—Treadmill exercise testing can be of substantial value in assessing chronotropic response ("chronotropic competence") to increases in metabolic needs in patients with sinus bradycardia in whom sinus node dysfunction is suspected. The definition of chronotropic incompetence is not agreed upon, but it is reasonable to designate it as consisting of either an inability to achieve a heart rate exceeding 75% of age-predicted maximum (usually taken as 220 – age), or 100–120 bpm at maximum effort. Irregular (and nonreproducible) increases, and even decreases, in sinus rate during exercise can also occur, but are rare. Similarly rare are abrupt changes in rate occurring during the postexercise recovery period. Chronotropic incompetence can result from medications (see Table 14–1) and should be distinguished from intrinsic sinus node dysfunction.

The Bruce treadmill exercise protocol, which is usually used to diagnose the presence and severity of coronary artery disease, is generally inappropriate for patients with sinus node dysfunction, in whom the goal is to assess heart rate at lower workloads expected to be encountered during average daily activities. Specific protocols, such as the chronotropic assessment exercise protocol (CAEP), have therefore been developed for this purpose. In addition to documenting chronotropic incompetence, treadmill exercise testing can be used to aid in optimal programming of rate-adaptive cardiac pacemakers that are usually required in these patients.

2. Atrioventricular block

A. ELECTROGRAPHY AND ELECTROCARDIOGRAPHY—The advent of intracardiac His bundle electrography has provided important information regarding normal and abnormal AV conduction in humans. The technique involves positioning a multipolar electrode catheter across the tricuspid valve in proximity to the AV nodal-His bundle area to record electrical activity as it passes through these structures. Because of its location, the catheter records electrical activity at the level of the low right atrium, His bundle, and proximal right bundle branch in addition to ventricular electrical activity. The sinus node pacemaker cells normally initiate the cardiac impulse, but they are not registered on either the surface ECG or the His bundle electrogram. The onset of the P wave on the surface ECG signifies the beginning of atrial depolarization; because the intracardiac electrode catheter lies at the level of the low right atrium, the early regions of atrial depolarization will not be detected by it; as the atrial depolarization wavefront passes through the region in which the catheter is located (the low right atrium), a deflection is registered (A). As the impulse traverses the His bundle, another deflection is registered, representing its depolarization (H). The His bundle deflection is followed by a ventricular deflection (V), which is registered at the time the wavefront of ventricular depolarization reaches the electrodes and often follows the onset of inscription of the QRS complex on the surface ECG.

His bundle electrography is useful in indicating the site of AV conduction delay or block. Normally, the conduction time through the AV node is 90–150 ms, and the conduction time through the His-Purkinje system is 35–55 ms. In a patient with a prolonged PR interval, a prolonged AH interval signifies delayed impulse conduction within the AV node, and a prolonged HV time represents delayed impulse conduction within the His bundle or the bundle branches. Conduction delay within the His bundle itself manifests as more than one His deflection ("split" His deflections).

In **first-degree AV block** (a delay in conduction between the atria and the ventricles), all atrial impulses are conducted to the ventricles; it is characterized by a prolonged PR interval that exceeds 200 ms (Figure 14–8). The components of the PR interval are interatrial conduction (10–50 ms), AV nodal conduction (90–150 ms), and intra-His and His-Purkinje conduction (35–55 ms). The conduction delay in first-degree AV block can thus represent prolonged intraatrial, AV nodal, intra-His, or His-Purkinje conduction, and the recordings help clarify the location of the delay.

In patients with a QRS complex that is narrow and normal-appearing, first-degree AV block is AV nodal in more than 85% and is intra-His in less than 15%. In patients with a wide QRS complex, first-degree AV block is AV nodal in less than 25%, infranodal in about 45%, and at more than one site in about 33%.

In **second-degree AV block,** not all atrial impulses are conducted to the ventricles. The ratio of P waves to QRS complexes describes the AV conduction ratio. **Type I (Wenckebach) second-degree AV block** is present when the conduction of atrial impulses to the ventricles is progressively delayed because of AV (generally AV nodal) refractoriness, with eventual failure of conduction of an atrial impulse to the ventricles. The AV conduction ratio in type I second-degree AV block can be 3:2, 4:3, 5:4, and so on; this ratio is also referred to as a **Wenckebach period.** AV conduction ratios in type I second-degree AV block need not be constant, and therefore, the Wenckebach period may not be reproducible. Because type I second-degree AV block usually occurs within the AV node, the PR interval of the first conducted P wave of the Wenckebach period is often prolonged, and because this conduction disturbance does not involve the bundle branches, the QRS complexes are expected to be narrow and normal-appearing unless there is preexisting bundle branch disease.

In a typical, or classic Wenckebach period, the PR intervals progressively lengthen, the R-R intervals progressively shorten, and the R-R interval encompassing the nonconducted P wave is less than twice the preceding R-R interval. Typical Wenckebach periods are usually seen with low AV conduction ratios (3:2, 4:3, and 5:4), but as the AV conduction ratio increases (exceeding 6:5), more and more Wenckebach sequences are atypical and do not follow the rules. If the sinus rate is not constant, for example in vagal bradycardias, sequences that resemble Wenckebach conduction (referred to as "vagotonic block") often occur; they should, however, not be considered type I second-degree

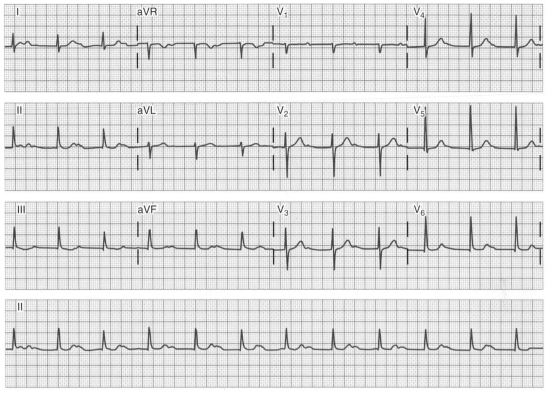

▲ **Figure 14-8.** Sinus rhythm with marked first-degree atrioventricular (AV) block. All P waves are conducted to the ventricles. The PR intervals are about 480 ms. The RP intervals are shorter than the PR intervals, which, in some patients, can cause symptoms due to suboptimally timed AV depolarization-contraction sequences. Despite the length of the PR intervals, this conduction disturbance is generally benign; evolution to second-degree AV block can take years.

AV block, in which the sinus rate must be constant for the diagnosis to be made.

In **type II second-degree AV block,** atrial impulses intermittently fail to be transmitted to the ventricles, but progressive conduction delay prior to the conduction failure does not occur. Because prior conduction delay from the atria is not present, the failure of antegrade conduction is often abrupt and unpredictable and may be advanced. In contrast to type I second-degree AV block, in which the conduction delay is usually in the AV node, the conduction delay in type II second-degree AV block can be within the His bundle or, more commonly, distal to the His bundle in the bundle branches. If the block is within the His bundle, the QRS complexes will be narrow and normal-appearing, or only mildly aberrant, unless preexisting BBB is present. If the block is infra-His, the QRS complexes will show a BBB pattern. In contrast to type I second-degree AV block, the PR interval of the conducted P waves is constant and often (but not always) normal (Figure 14–9).

Second-degree AV block with a 2:1 AV conduction ratio may represent either AV nodal or His-Purkinje block (Figures 14–10 and 14–11). Two consecutive PR intervals are not recorded in 2:1 AV conduction; therefore, the presence or absence of progressive PR prolongation cannot be ascertained, and distinguishing the diagnoses may be difficult. If the PR interval of the conducted P waves is prolonged and the QRS complexes are narrow and normal-appearing, AV nodal block is probably present. If the PR interval of the conducted P waves is normal and the QRS complexes have a BBB pattern, His-Purkinje block is probably present. If the PR interval of the conducted P wave is prolonged and the QRS complexes have a BBB pattern, or if the PR interval of the conducted P wave is normal and the QRS complexes appear normal, it may not be possible to distinguish between the two types, and more than one site of AV block may also be present. Altering the AV conduction ratio by means of carotid sinus massage (to produce sinus and AV nodal slowing) or intravenous atropine (to enhance sinus rate and AV nodal conduction) will often allow identification of the nature of the AV block and thus its location (see Figure 14–9).

In **advanced second-degree AV block** the AV conduction ratio is 3:1 or greater, and atrial impulses are only occasionally conducted to the ventricles. In contrast, in **complete AV block,** no atrial impulses are conducted to the ventricles despite temporal opportunity for this to occur, and the atria and ventricles are depolarized by their respective pacemakers that are independent of each other (Figure 14–12). The atrial rate in complete AV block is almost always faster than the ventricular rate. The QRS rhythm, or the escape rhythm, originates distal to the site of block and may be in the AV junction, His bundle, bundle branches, or distal Purkinje system. The morphology of the QRS complexes and their rate will depend on their site of origin. A narrow QRS complex escape rhythm originates from the AV junction. On the other hand, a wide QRS complex rhythm is not a reliable guide to the origin of the rhythm because rhythms originating in the longitudinally separated predivisional region of the His bundle can have a wide QRS complex.

If the atrial rate is not sinus, the existence of advanced or complete AV block is diagnosed by the presence of a slow ventricular rate with varying intervals between the QRS complexes or by a slow and regular QRS rate (Figure 14–13), respectively. Atrial fibrillation and flutter are commonly associated with advanced AV block and slow QRS rates. The rate of the ventricular rhythm, as well as the QRS-complex morphology, will depend on the site of origin of the rhythm. A regular rhythm in a patient with atrial fibrillation confirms the presence of complete AV block, with a QRS pacemaker

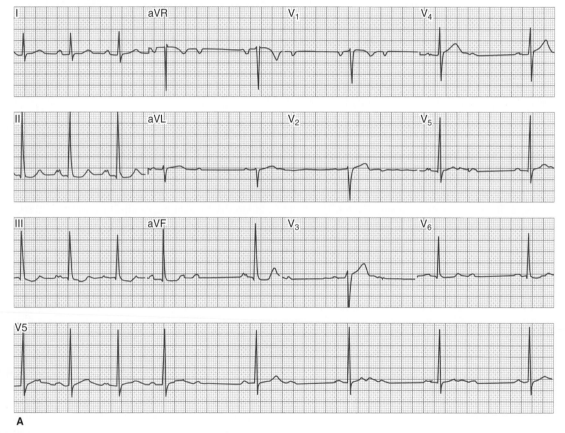

A

▲ **Figure 14–9. A:** This electrocardiogram was recorded in a patient with presyncopal spells who was about to undergo exercise treadmill testing. The atrial rhythm is sinus at a rate of about 68 bpm. The PR intervals of the conducted QRS complexes are all about 240 ms. The QRS complexes are narrow, and nondiagnostic ST- and T-wave abnormalities are present. A 2:1 atrioventricular (AV) conduction develops abruptly during the recording. The prolonged PR intervals of the conducted P waves, as well as the narrow morphology of the QRS complexes (indicating absence of bundle branch system disease), could suggest that the 2:1 AV conduction represents AV nodal block; intra-His block, however, is suggested by the absence of prolongation of the PR intervals prior to the nonconducted P waves. Changing of the AV conduction ratio from 2:1 to 3:2, 5:4, and so on, would help establish the presence of AV nodal block. This could be achieved by atropine or exercise testing, during which adrenergic drive would be expected to facilitate AV conduction. (*continued*)

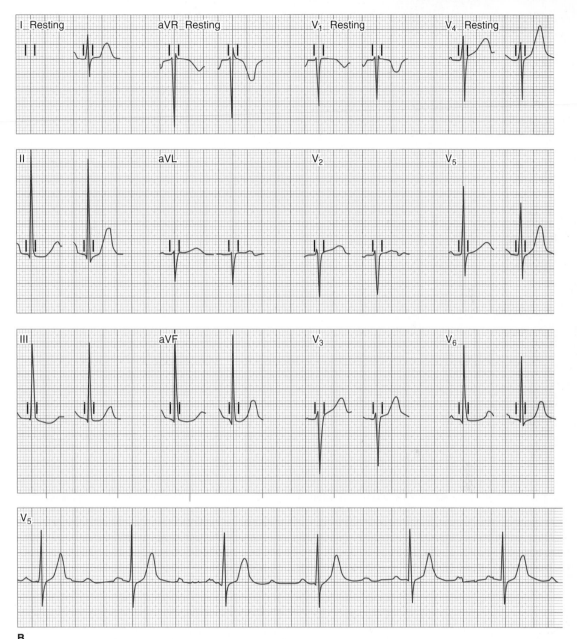

B

▲ **Figure 14–9.** (*Continued*) **B:** The patient achieved stage IV of the Bruce protocol during treadmill testing. The atrial rate was 150 bpm. At peak effort and for the first 2 minutes of the postexercise recovery period, 3:1 atrioventricular (AV) block developed abruptly and was associated with the patient's typical presyncopal symptoms. AV block developing during exercise, although decidedly rare, is always abnormal, and if the QRS complexes are narrow or normal appearing, indicate intra-His block. Permanent cardiac pacing is required.

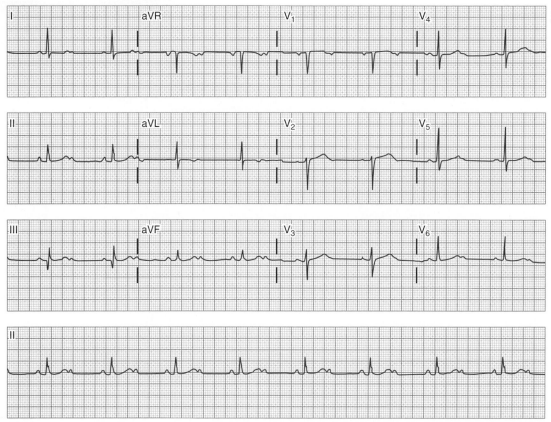

▲ **Figure 14–10.** The atrial rhythm is sinus, and 2:1 atrioventricular (AV) conduction is present. The PR intervals of the conducted beats are normal at about 190 ms. The QRS complexes are narrow and normal appearing. The 2:1 AV conduction could represent either AV nodal or His-Purkinje block. When AV nodal block is present, the PR intervals of the conducted complexes are often prolonged and the QRS complexes narrow and normal appearing, whereas in infra-Hisian block, the PR intervals of the conducted complexes are generally normal and the QRS complexes broad, indicating bundle branch disease. In this tracing, the PR intervals are normal. The site of block cannot be known with certainty from this tracing, and manipulation of the AV conduction ratio by atropine or exercise, which facilitates AV conduction, might be required. AV nodal block generally does not require cardiac pacing. If the block is within the His bundle, both the PR interval and QRS complex width are typically normal (electrophysiologic study may be needed to distinguish from AV nodal block), and permanent cardiac pacing is indicated.

originating below the level of conduction block that is independent of the atrial rhythm.

In **vagotonic block,** a high degree of vagal tone, such as occurs with sympathetic withdrawal during sleep or in highly conditioned athletes, may be associated with slowing of the sinus rate, pauses in sinus rhythm, variable degrees of delay in AV conduction manifested by prolongation of PR intervals (often irregular), and failure of conduction of P waves resembling type I or II second-degree AV block (Table 14–4). It is important to recognize vagotonic block because it often occurs in normal individuals as well as in patients with inferior or right ventricular myocardial infarction, or any other clinical condition in which hypervagotonia is present

(see Table 14–2). It not uncommonly accompanies the use of certain medications, notably β-blocking agents, some antihypertensive drugs, and occasionally, digitalis. It can also be seen during swallowing (deglutition bradycardia), coughing (tussive bradycardia), and yawning. In the critical care setting, vagotonic block (and significant bradycardia) can occur during endotracheal suctioning or esophagogastric intubation, and in patients with elevated intracranial pressure.

B. **Exercise testing**—Unlike the value of exercise testing in sinus node dysfunction for both diagnosis and evaluation of chronotropic competence, exercise testing in patients with AV block is generally not useful. AV node conduction is

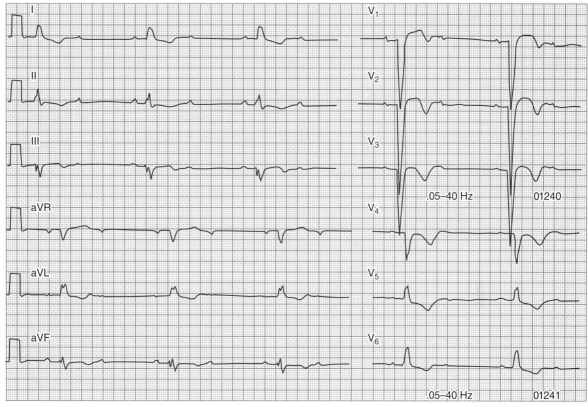

▲ **Figure 14–11.** Second-degree atrioventricular (AV) block, with 2:1 conduction ratio and evidence of bundle branch disease. The first-degree block of the conducted P waves and the left bundle branch block pattern of the conducted QRS complexes make localization of the site of block difficult; the prolonged PR interval suggests AV nodal disease, whereas the wide QRS complexes support infra-Hisian disease; electrophysiologic study may be necessary to decide whether permanent cardiac pacing is required.

enhanced by the vagolysis and increased sympathetic drive that occurs with exercise. Thus, patients with first-degree AV block and type I second-degree AV block are expected to have shorter PR intervals during exercise; in patients with type I second-degree AV block, a longer Wenckebach period can develop (eg, 3:2 at rest becoming 6:5 during exercise). Patients with 2:1 AV conduction, in whom the site of conduction block may be uncertain, can benefit from exercise testing by observing whether the AV conduction ratio increases in a Wenckebach-like manner (eg, to 3:2 or 4:3) or decreases (eg, to 3:1 or 4:1) (see Figure 14–9). In the latter case, the increase in the sinus rate finds the His-Purkinje system refractory, causing the higher degrees of block. This response is always abnormal because it indicates intra- or infra-His block, which will require permanent cardiac pacing.

▶ Treatment

The major reversible causes of conduction system disturbances are high vagal tone and medications. High vagal tone, whether or not it is accompanied by withdrawal of sympathetic tone, can cause or contribute to both atrial and ventricular bradycardia. Vagally mediated bradycardias are usually transient and not accompanied by symptoms of presyncope or frank syncope, and no treatment is needed. If necessary, intravenous atropine can be used to facilitate AV nodal conduction to avoid ventricular bradycardia; however, the atropine-induced increase in atrial rate can lead to a paradoxical slowing of ventricular rate as a result of more rapid stimulation of, and encroachment on, the refractory period of the AV conduction system ("time-dependent" refractoriness). Moreover, the effects of intravenous atropine are short-lived, and its long-term use is accompanied by significant side effects.

In contrast to the majority of vagally mediated bradycardias, "vasovagal" episodes (hypotension with variable degrees of bradycardia or asystole) can be frequent, abrupt, unpredictable, and disabling. These highly symptomatic episodes, also referred to as neurocardiogenic or neurally mediated syncopal syndromes, can require heart rate support with

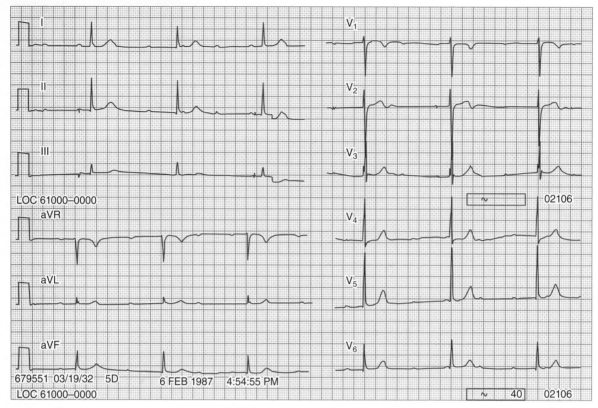

▲ **Figure 14–12.** Complete atrioventricular (AV) block. The atrial and ventricular rhythms are independent of each other. The narrow, normal-appearing QRS complexes suggest that the AV block is within the AV node or the His bundle.

oral theophylline or ephedrine. In some circumstances, they can also require permanent dual-chamber cardiac pacing, using special algorithms to detect an abrupt fall in heart rate and respond with tachypacing until the spontaneous heart rate increases. Intravascular volume support with fluids, support hosiery, and even mineralocorticoids can also be helpful. Because left ventricular baroreceptor stimulation (from vigorous systolic ventricular contraction) and its consequent reflex peripheral vasodilation play a role in this syndrome, drugs having negative inotropic effects (eg, β-blockers, disopyramide) have been used in management, although there is evidence that these agents have limited, if any, efficacy. α-Agonists, such as midodrine, have also been used with some success. In addition, because a central effect is recognized, anticholinergic agents and serotonin reuptake inhibitors have been used with variable success.

Commonly used medications that cause or contribute to bradycardia do so by enhancing vagal tone (eg, digitalis), reducing the facilitation of AV conduction that results from sympathetic tone (eg, β-blockers and antiarrhythmic agents with β-blocking properties such as sotalol and propafenone),

or direct action on SA and AV conduction tissue (eg, verapamil and diltiazem). Simple withdrawal of these medications will reverse the bradycardia, although the process may require several days. If the offending medications are necessary to treat other conditions such as angina pectoris or heart failure and cannot be discontinued, permanent cardiac pacing will be required (Table 14–5).

It is important to exclude AV nodal blocking medications, such as digitalis preparations, β-blockers, and rate-limiting calcium channel blockers, as a cause of, or contributor to, slow ventricular rates in atrial fibrillation and flutter; withdrawal of these drugs or reduction in dosage can result in reversal of the AV block and permanent cardiac pacing may be avoided. If the ventricular rhythm is slow in the absence of these agents, intrinsic AV conduction system disease is likely to be present, and permanent cardiac pacing will usually be indicated. Electrical cardioversion of the atrial arrhythmia should be undertaken with caution, if at all, in patients with slow ventricular rates in the absence of medication; because of diffuse underlying conduction disease, postcardioversion sinus bradycardia or even asystole can occur.

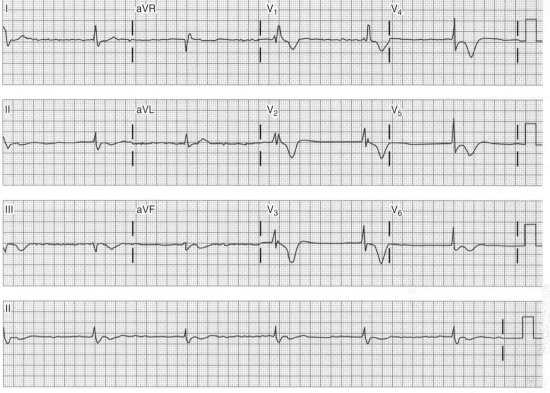

▲ **Figure 14–13.** The atrial rhythm is fibrillation. The QRS rhythm is regular at a rate of about 33 bpm and displays a right bundle branch block pattern. The regularity of the rhythm indicates complete atrioventricular (AV) block, and the rate and morphology suggest a ventricular focus of origin. This rhythm could be due to digitalis toxicity or to the effects of calcium channel or β-blockers; if offending medications cannot be discontinued, permanent cardiac pacing is indicated. This rhythm and rate are also seen in the absence of medications and after radiofrequency ablation of the AV node to treat uncontrolled ventricular rate in patients with atrial fibrillation; permanent cardiac pacing is required.

In bradycardia-tachycardia syndrome, prolonged pauses in sinus rhythm frequently occur following an abrupt termination of the tachycardia. These pauses are often associated with symptoms of cerebral insufficiency, and cardiac pacing is frequently required. Alternatively, elimination of the tachycardia by radiofrequency ablation can potentially avert the need for cardiac pacing; severity of the underlying sinus node dysfunction, however, may still make cardiac pacing necessary even after ablation.

Although cardiac pacing using AAIR or DDDR devices (see later section, Permanent Pacing) may serve to suppress the tachycardias to some degree, treatment with antiarrhythmic agents is usually required. When the tachycardia occurs despite antiarrhythmic drug therapy, control of the ventricular rate also becomes necessary, but AV nodal blocking agents are often only partially effective in achieving this control; moreover, their use can be associated with significant side effects. Radiofrequency AV node ablation, together with dual-chamber cardiac pacing, has thus emerged as a useful and cost-effective technique in the management of this rhythm disturbance. When treating bradycardia-tachycardia syndrome, current pacemakers use a special algorithm to switch from a DDD or DDDR mode of operation to a VVI, VVIR, DDI, or DDIR mode on sensing an atrial tachyarrhythmia, and back again to DDD or DDDR mode when a normal atrial rate is sensed; this helps maintain an even pulse rate whether in or out of tachycardia.

Table 14–4. Diagnostic Clues to Vagally Mediated Atrioventricular Block

Concomitant slowing of sinus rate
Changing PR intervals, often with irregularity of sinus rates
Atypical Wenckebach periods, often with inconstant PP intervals
Inconstant escape rates
Inconstant escape foci
Transient nature of episodes
Reversed or abolished by intravenous atropine or an increase in sympathetic tone

Table 14–5. Common Indications for Permanent Cardiac Pacing

Acquired AV block
Third-degree (complete) and advanced second-degree
    With symptoms (including symptoms resulting from necessary medications)
    With asystole ≥ 3 seconds, rate of escape pacemaker < 40 bpm, or escape rhythm below the AV node in awake patients
    With AF and ventricular pauses ≥ 5 seconds, or after AV node ablation
Second-degree
    Type II
    Type I in patients with symptoms
Acute myocardial infarction
    With persistent second- and third-degree AV block
    With transient advanced second- and third-degree AV block and bundle branch block
Sinus node dysfunction
With symptoms (including symptoms resulting from necessary medications)
With rates < 40 bpm in awake patients
With symptomatic chronotropic incompetence
Carotid sinus hypersensitivity
With recurrent syncope caused by spontaneous carotid sinus stimulation
With hypersensitive cardioinhibitory response (asystole ≥ 3 seconds) during carotid sinus massage
Neurocardiogenic syncope
With symptomatic bradycardia documented spontaneously or during tilt-table testing

AF, atrial fibrillation; AV, atrioventricular.
Based on ACC/AHA/HRS 2008 Guidelines for Device-Based Therapy of Cardiac Rhythm Abnormalities by Epstein AE, et al. *Circulation.* 2008;117:e350–408.

Table 14–6. Common Uses for Temporary Cardiac Pacing

Therapeutic
To provide adequate heart rate in patients with symptomatic bradycardia from sinus node dysfunction or advanced second-degree and complete AV block while awaiting definitive therapy
To terminate some supraventricular and ventricular tachycardias by overdrive suppression or entrainment (eg, atrial flutter, monomorphic ventricular tachycardia)
Prophylactic
To prevent advanced second-degree and complete AV block in some patients with acute myocardial infarction and in some patients after cardiac surgery (eg, aortic valve replacement)
To prevent bradycardia-dependent ventricular tachycardia
Diagnostic
To determine the site of AV block
For evaluation for optimal type of permanent pacing system

AV, atrioventricular.

A. Cardiac Pacing

Temporary or permanent cardiac pacing, in which an electrical stimulus depolarizes cardiac tissue, is indicated when bradycardia causes symptoms of cerebral hypoperfusion or hemodynamic decompensation. Occasionally, patients with bradycardia-dependent ventricular tachycardia require pacing to prevent the pauses in rhythm that lead to the tachyarrhythmia (Tables 14–5 and 14–6; see Figure 14–7). Although emergency pacing can be accomplished temporarily by transcutaneous pacing systems, in all but the most critical situations, stable temporary pacing is best ensured by the transvenous insertion of electrodes into the right atrium, right ventricle, or both. Permanent cardiac pacing is also usually performed through the transvenous route; in some circumstances, however, epicardial placement of electrodes via thoracotomy or a subxiphoid approach is still used.

1. Temporary pacing

A. Transmyocardial pacing—Transmyocardial pacing involves the percutaneous placement of cardiac pacing wires into the ventricular cavity or onto the ventricular wall through a transthoracic needle. The reliability of this technique is poor, and it is a highly invasive procedure with significant potential morbidity. Transmyocardial pacing is performed only in an emergency setting, usually during cardiac arrest, when transvenous pacing cannot be accomplished rapidly or when transcutaneous pacing is unavailable or unsuccessful. The reported incidence of successful capture with transthoracic pacing varies from 5% to 90%; typically, it is 21–40%.

Often, however, because of the clinical circumstances in which this type of pacing is used, electrical capture is not followed by mechanical systole. The major complications of transthoracic pacing include myocardial or coronary artery laceration, pericardial tamponade, pneumothorax, and hepatic or gastric damage. Transthoracic pacing should therefore be reserved for situations of the utmost gravity where no other pacing system is feasible or available. External (transcutaneous) pacing should always be tried first, because it is probably as efficacious (if not more so) and is associated with significantly less morbidity. Transthoracic pacing should never be used in awake or stable patients. The technique is now all but obsolete.

B. Transcutaneous pacing—This method, in which electrical current is delivered to the heart through the skin via large surface electrodes, is usually reserved for standby prophylaxis in patients recognized to be at high risk for bradycardia, for example during inferior and large anterior wall acute myocardial infarctions (Table 14–7), and in some patients with suspected sinus node dysfunction who are undergoing elective cardioversion. Because of its ease of use and relative efficacy, this pacing modality has virtually eliminated the need for transmyocardial pacing in emergency situations.

Table 14–7. Conditions Considered Risks for Advanced Second-Degree or Complete Atrioventricular Block During Acute Myocardial Infarction[1]

Inferior-wall MI, especially if it involves the interventricular septum, posterior wall, and right ventricle, with first-degree AV block; second-degree AV block, type I (usually intra-AV nodal); or second-degree AV block, type II (often intra-His)
Extensive anteroseptal MI, with new bifascicular block with a normal PR interval or with first-degree AV block; second-degree AV block, type II; first-degree AV block with bifascicular block (not known to be old); or alternating bundle branch block

[1]The incidence of AV block during acute myocardial infarction has decreased considerably in the current era of fibrinolytic and direct percutaneous revascularization therapies.

AV, atrioventricular; MI, myocardial infarction.

The transcutaneous pacing system uses two large, low-impedance surface electrodes placed on the anterior and posterior chest walls. A long duration pacing stimulus output of 20–40 ms (not programmable by the operator) and current output of more than 100 milliamperes (mA) (programmable by the operator) are often necessary to overcome the impedance offered by the chest wall, muscle and bone, and intrathoracic structures. The transcutaneous pacemaker paces the ventricle and inhibits its output when it senses spontaneous ventricular electrical activity, thus functioning in VVI (demand) mode (see later section, Permanent Pacing). Because the pacing pulses are 20–40 ms in duration and the current output is large, they create a deflection of high amplitude on the surface ECG recording that should not be confused with QRS complexes. If ventricular depolarization (capture) is occurring, the pacer output pulse will be followed by a QRS complex that is best seen on the pacemaker generator's oscilloscope and strip-chart recording. Significant distortion, or total obscuration, of the paced QRS complex can exist on the bedside rhythm monitor or surface ECG recording. Ventricular capture should always be verified by confirming the presence of a pulse, either through palpation or through visualizing a proper waveform with pulse oximetry or arterial pressure monitoring. Skeletal muscle twitching occurs at a stimulus output of 30 mA, but ventricular capture does not usually occur until 35–80 mA; sedation of the awake patient is usually required to mitigate the painful muscle contractions.

Transcutaneous cardiac pacing can be effective in up to 70% of patients and has its best use in an emergency situation when pacing of short duration is required or as a bridge to permanent cardiac pacemaker implantation. The majority of pacing failures (specifically, failure to capture) occur in patients during the advanced stages of cardiopulmonary arrest. The likelihood of successful transcutaneous pacing in patients with cardiac arrest of more than 15 minutes in duration is approximately 33–45%. Failure to capture can

also occur after prolonged (hours to days) pacing and likely represents increases in impedance; repositioning of the electrodes can restore pacing capability.

C. TEMPORARY TRANSVENOUS PACING—Although transcutaneous pacing offers ease of use, rapid initiation of pacing therapy, and very low complication rates, transvenous pacing is far more stable and better tolerated if pacing is needed for longer than 20–30 minutes. Transvenous pacing is usually performed by placing an electrode catheter in the right ventricle. In rare cases where temporary atrial pacing is also required, catheters can be positioned in the right atrium or in the proximal portion of the coronary sinus.

Venous access can be obtained by several approaches. The internal jugular, subclavian, and femoral veins are all potential sites for introduction of the pacing catheter into the right heart, although the femoral vein is the least desirable due to the potential for pacing lead dislodgement and infection. The median cubital and basilic veins can also be used, but these sites are also associated with a high incidence of lead dislodgement (because of arm motion) and are rarely, if ever, used today.

Prior to obtaining venous access, the existence of a bleeding diathesis or coagulopathy should be excluded or corrected if possible. If this is not possible, the femoral vein should be considered as the initial access site because it is easier to apply pressure and achieve hemostasis in this region if a complication occurs. Other factors, such as the patient's pulmonary status, location of dialysis shunts, previous neck surgery, or radiation therapy should be taken into account when considering the appropriate site for venous access. The presence of a prosthetic tricuspid valve is a contraindication to right ventricular pacing; in this circumstance, left ventricular pacing can be performed by positioning the pacing catheter in the left ventricular veins via the coronary sinus.

There are two main types of transvenous pacing catheters. The flexible balloon-tipped catheter is advanced into the heart in a similar way as a Swan-Ganz catheter, using blood flow to guide it into the right ventricle; it is important to note that during a cardiac arrest, the inflation of the balloon will be useless because of the lack of circulation. The position of the catheter tip within the heart is confirmed either through assessing the electrogram recorded from the pacing catheter tip (negative pole connected to any precordial lead on an ECG machine) or by observing capture of ventricular tissue. Once the catheter tip crosses the tricuspid valve, the balloon should be deflated to allow advancement into the ideal right ventricular apical position. Balloon-tipped pacing catheters can be inserted at the bedside if necessary. The nonfloating, rigid, fixed-curve catheters are easier to manipulate and are more stable once positioned in the right ventricle; because of their rigid design they are typically placed only under fluoroscopic guidance. In general, temporary transvenous pacing lead positioning should be accomplished using fluoroscopy whenever feasible.

Ventricular capture thresholds should be < 2 mA (or < 2 volts [V] with some pulse generators) and ideally < 1 mA (or < 1 V) in stable lead positions and should not change with coughing or deep breathing. Atrial leads are typically less stable, and capture thresholds around 2 mA (or 1–2 V) are acceptable. The presence of myocardial infarction, ischemia, antiarrhythmic drug therapy, hyperkalemia, and other metabolic derangements can increase capture thresholds. Current or voltage output of the pulse generator should be programmed to at least twice capture threshold.

Sensing thresholds can also be affected by myocardial ischemia or infarction, hyperkalemia, and class I antiarrhythmic agents, leading to undersensing ("failure" to sense). Ectopic ventricular depolarizations are often undersensed because of poor intracardiac signal quality. These considerations need to be borne in mind when setting the sensitivity of the pacemaker; inappropriate pacing occurring because of an undersensed QRS complex can initiate ventricular tachyarrhythmias if the pacing stimulus falls on the terminal portion of the QRS complex or T wave.

A daily chest radiograph and paced 12-lead ECG should be obtained and compared with prior studies to check for possible lead migration. Pacing and sensing thresholds should be checked at least daily, with any significant changes being investigated for possible lead migration, lead disconnection from the pulse generator, or change in the patient's clinical status. Pulse generator battery status should be monitored by the appropriate biomedical personnel, and batteries replaced as needed. Temporary leads and access sites should be changed at least every 3 or 4 days to decrease the risk of infection and venous thrombosis.

Although temporary transvenous pacing is relatively low risk, there are potentially serious complications. Complication rates range from 4% to 20% and include pneumothorax, hemothorax, arterial puncture, air embolism, serious bleeding, myocardial perforation, cardiac tamponade, nerve injury, thoracic duct injury, catheter-related arrhythmias, infection, and thromboembolism. The risk of complications is increased if pacing is initiated in emergent situations. To minimize risk, transvenous pacing should be accomplished when the patient is relatively hemodynamically stable. It is important to remember that if the patient has left bundle branch block (LBBB), pacing catheter manipulation in the area of the right bundle branch can result in complete AV block; in these circumstances, transcutaneous pacing should be in place should rate support be required.

2. Permanent pacing—Because of the complexity of pacing system design, an identification code has been developed that describes the function of currently available pacemaker generators. The "mode" code consists of three primary letters. The first letter stands for the chamber in which pacing is occurring: A for atrium, V for ventricle, and D for dual, or both. The second letter stands for the chamber in which sensing of the electrical signal occurs: A, V, D, or O for neither. The third letter refers to the mode of response of

the generator to the sensed signal: I for inhibited output, D for both inhibited and triggered output that is delivered in response to a sensed signal (eg, a paced ventricular complex delivered in response to a sensed P wave), and O for not applicable. Currently available pacing systems incorporate one or two sensors that allow the pacing rate to increase and decrease with changes in metabolic need; sensor-based pacing systems thus adapt the pacing rate to the activities of daily living. Pacing systems with this feature add an R following the three primary letters (eg, AAIR, DDDR), indicating the existence of rate-adaptive capability. Current pacemakers have numerous functions that can be altered noninvasively by a programmer; such units are described as having multifunction programmability (Table 14–8). Several of the newer temporary pulse generators also have such features.

A. MODES OF PACING

(1) Asynchronous pacing (VOO, AOO, DOO)— In the asynchronous mode of pacemaker function, no electrical signals are sensed, and the pulse generator delivers output pulses without regard to any electrical activity occurring

Table 14–8. Some Programmable Functions and Parameters of Cardiac Pacemakers

Standby rate (base rate, lower rate limit): The rate at which the patient is paced unless the spontaneous rhythm is faster

Upper rate limit: The highest rate at which the ventricles are paced 1:1 in response to the atrial rate

AV interval: The interval between the paced or sensed P wave and the delivery of the ventricular pacing stimulus

Atrial refractory period: The time after a sensed P wave or delivered atrial output during which the atrial channel is refractory to electrical signals; the refractory period that follows a paced QRS complex is referred to as the PVARP

Ventricular refractory period: The time after a sensed QRS or delivered ventricular output during which the ventricular channel is refractory to electrical signals

Sensitivity (atrial and ventricular channels): The amplitude of the intrinsic atrial and ventricular depolarizations that are to be sensed

Energy output (atrial and ventricular channels): Volts, current and pulse duration

Modes of function[1]**:** AAI, VVI, AOO, VOO, VDD, DDI, DOO, DDD, OOO

Sensor ("on" or "off"): Rate-adaptive programming either activated or deactivated

Sensor-based parameters: Time to achieve peak pacing rate; time to decline to standby rate; criteria for sensor activation

Mode switch ("on" or "off"): Upon sensing an atrial tachyarrhythmia, a DDD(R)[1] device will automatically switch to DDI(R) or VVI(R) mode of function, and will automatically switch back to DDD(R) mode upon sensing normal atrial rhythm

[1]Pacemaker codes: A, atrium; D, dual; I, inhibited; O, nonapplicable; R, rate-adaptive function; V, ventricle.
AV, atrioventricular; PVARP, postventricular atrial refractory period.

spontaneously within the heart (Figure 14–14). Because the native cardiac rhythm is not sensed, competitive rhythms (paced and native depolarizations) can result. Asynchronous pacemaker generators are no longer manufactured; however, the asynchronous pacing mode can be programmed. Asynchronous pacing also occurs whenever a magnet is placed over an implanted generator in order to evaluate capture function. With a magnet in place, asynchronous pacing and concomitant occurrence of the spontaneous rhythm result in iatrogenic parasystole (Figure 14–15). At the energy output of today's generators (1.5–7.5 V), induction of repetitive ventricular or atrial rhythms is usually not observed, although this possibility exists, especially if myocardial ischemia or electrolyte imbalance is present.

(2) Single-chamber demand pacing [VVI(R), AAI(R)]— Both sensing and pacing circuits are present in these units. When a spontaneous intracardiac signal is sensed, VVI and AAI pulse generators will inhibit their output and no pacemaker

stimulus artifact will appear. Electrical signals sensed by demand pacemaker generators can originate not only from the heart but also from the environment (electrocautery, cellular telephones, electronic article surveillance systems, tasers), from the patient (muscle potentials), or from the pacing system itself (lead fracture or insulation breaks). Such sensed signals may cause inhibition of output, leading to pauses in paced rhythm; this phenomenon is termed "oversensing" (Tables 14–9 and 14–10), a problem that can generally be corrected by noninvasive programming or, in the case of lead fracture or insulation break, by replacement of the lead. Current generator design and programming capability have not only helped to reduce problems of oversensing but have also simplified their correction.

The pacing function of a demand pulse generator cannot be evaluated if the patient's spontaneous rhythm exceeds the programmed standby (base) rate of the generator. Applying a magnet over the pulse generator converts it to an asynchronous

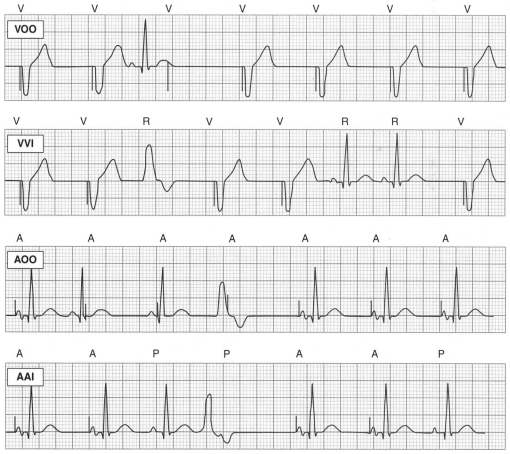

▲ **Figure 14–14.** Schematic illustrations of various pacing modes. (See Permanent Pacing section for explanation of symbols.) A, atrial pacing stimulus; P, spontaneous P wave; R, spontaneous QRS; V, ventricular pacing stimulus. *(continued)*

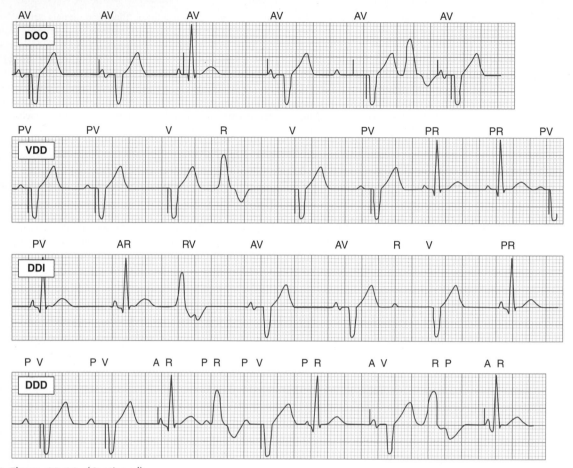

▲ **Figure 14–14.** (*Continued*)

mode of function, and capture (stimulation) of the atria or ventricles by the pacemaker can be confirmed, provided that the pacing stimuli fall outside the refractory period of the cardiac tissue. Conversely, if the patient's rhythm is continually paced, the sensing function of the generator cannot be evaluated. Programming the device to a lower rate may allow the emergence of a spontaneous cardiac rhythm, which should then be sensed, resulting in inhibition of pacemaker output.

Continuous single-chamber ventricular pacing will result in AV dyssynchrony (unless the atrial rhythm is fibrillation). Although the symptoms attributable to bradycardia are alleviated through ventricular rate support from the pacemaker, these may be replaced by symptoms due to AV dyssynchrony, or pacemaker syndrome. Either single-chamber atrial pacing (with intact AV conduction) or dual-chamber pacing is a solution to avoid pacemaker syndrome.

(3) Single-lead P-synchronous pacing (VDD)—These are systems in which electrodes for both the atrium and the ventricle are located on a single lead. The lead is positioned in the right ventricle where the tip electrodes sense and pace the ventricle; atrial electrodes are located on the lead body, at the level of the atrium and only sense, at least at the present time. When the atrial electrodes sense an electrical signal, a ventricular pacing stimulus is delivered after a programmable AV delay that corresponds to the PR interval. If a spontaneous QRS complex occurs, the ventricular output is inhibited. Tracking of the atrial rhythm in a 1:1 relationship allows the ventricular paced rate to change with the sinus rate. The programmed upper rate is the maximum ventricular paced rate that can occur in a 1:1 relationship to atrial activity, and prevents rapid ventricular paced rates should the atrial rate become too fast. If the atrial rate exceeds the programmed upper rate limit, the paced ventricular rate can become irregular because of an electronic Wenckebach protection, can slow to one-half the programmed upper rate limit, or can fall back gradually until 1:1 tracking can resume. This last feature results in disengagement of the tracking function, which causes transient AV dyssynchrony (Figure 14–16).

Without magnet

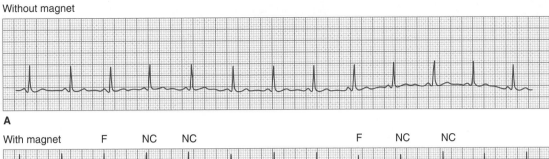

A

With magnet   F   NC   NC   F   NC   NC

B

▲ **Figure 14–15.** A VVI pacing system. **A:** Normal sinus rhythm is present. Sensing function is presumed to be normal because no ventricular pacing artifacts are occurring. **B:** With a magnet in place over the pulse generator, ventricular pacing stimuli are emitted asynchronously, resulting in a rhythm that competes with the sinus rhythm. The large magnitude of the pacing artifacts indicates that the lead configuration is unipolar. The large unipolar stimulus obscures the resulting QRS complex; however, because T waves are present following some of these pacing stimuli, capture is confirmed. Both sensing and pacing functions are normal. F, true fusion complexes, with ventricular depolarization resulting from both sinus and paced impulses. NC, noncapture because of pacing stimuli falling in the refractory period of ventricular muscle; this has been referred to as "functional" noncapture.

Table 14–9. Pacing System Malfunctions and Clues to Their Recognition

Failure to sense (undersensing)
Single-chamber systems
  ECG will show earlier-than-expected appearance of pacing-stimulus artifact
Dual-chamber systems
  Atrial undersensing: Delivery of atrial pacing stimuli despite occurrence of spontaneous P waves; failure to track intrinsic atrial activity at the programmed AV interval
  Ventricular undersensing: Delivery of ventricular pacing stimuli despite occurrence of spontaneous QRS complexes
Oversensing
  ECG will show inappropriate inhibition of atrial or ventricular output stimuli; oversensing in the atrial channel causes earlier-than-expected ventricular pacing stimuli
Failure to capture
Pacing stimuli not followed by atrial or ventricular depolarization (assuming muscle tissue is not refractory)
Failure of output
  Absence of pacing stimulus outputs, with oversensing excluded

AV, atrioventricular; ECG, electrocardiogram.

Table 14–10. Causes of Pacemaker Oversensing

Electromagnetic interference
Power transformers, power lines; welding equipment; household appliances such as razors and garage-door openers (unusual with today's pulse generators), microwave ovens operating at high power; rotating radar detectors; metal-detector gates (older generation designs); transcutaneous nerve stimulators; cardioverting and defibrillating devices (external or implanted internally); diathermy; lithotriptors; electrocautery; electrocoagulation; MRI; ionizing radiation; tasers; cellular telephones if used on the side ipsilateral to the pulse generator (some models); electronic article surveillance monitors
Physiologic intracardiac signals
R-wave sensing (AAI[1] systems), T-wave sensing (VVI systems), P-wave sensing (VVI systems) (unusual)
Physiologic extracardiac signals
Muscle potentials (eg, diaphragm, pectoral)
Signals generated within the pacing system
Leads
Conductor-wire fracture causing a voltage transient; insulation defect
Pulse generator
Afterpotential sensing of late portions of the pacing stimulus itself (unusual); component malfunction

[1]Pacemaker codes: A, atrium; I, inhibited; V, ventricle.
MRI, magnetic resonance imaging.

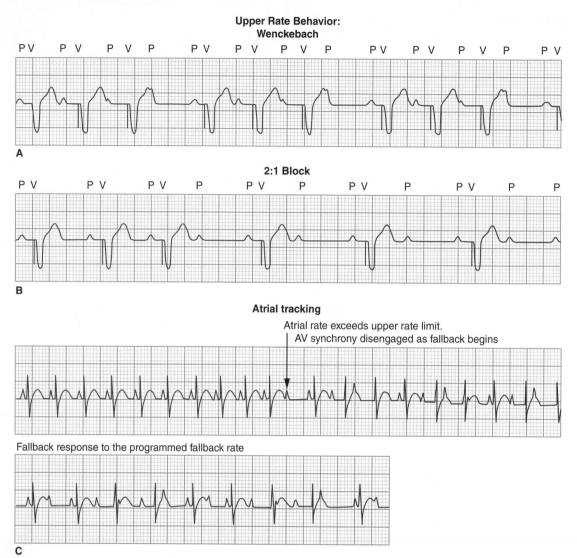

▲ **Figure 14–16.** Schematic illustration of responses from pulse generators at the atrial-driven upper rate limit. The pacemaker will not allow the ventricular paced rate to exceed this programmed upper rate. Atrial rhythms that can exceed the upper rate limit include sinus tachycardia, atrial tachycardia, atrial flutter, and atrial fibrillation. The pacemaker-mediated tachycardia (see text) will also not exceed the programmed upper rate. **A:** Lengthening of the interval between the sensed P wave and the triggered ventricular-paced complex so as not to violate the upper rate limit (Wenckebach): the P wave that is not followed by a paced QRS complex falls in the refractory period of the atrial channel and is not sensed, resulting in absence (nondelivery) of the ventricular stimulus output. **B:** In 2:1 block, alternate P waves fall in the atrial refractory period and are not sensed: they are not followed by a paced ventricular event. **C:** In fallback, the ventricular paced rate gradually slows once the programmed upper rate has been achieved. During the fallback period, tracking of the atrial rate is disengaged, and AV synchrony is no longer present. The ventricular paced rate will again track the atrial rate once the latter falls below the programmed upper rate. The fallback response avoids abrupt decreases in paced ventricular rate. Pacemakers that function in a rate-adaptive mode can have their sensor-based upper rate limit exceed the previously described upper tracking limit.

If no atrial activity is sensed, as occurs in sinus bradycardia, these pulse generators pace the ventricles on demand at the programmed standby rate; atrial pacing does not occur, at least at the present time. Thus, at slow atrial rates, the pacing system behaves as though it were a VVI system, and AV synchrony is lost (see Figure 14–14). Although this pacing system seems ideal for patients with normal sinus rhythm and AV block, atrial bradycardia, which occurs commonly over ensuing years, either spontaneously or as a result of medications, makes the VDD device ultimately suboptimal for most patients.

(4) Dual-chamber pacing [DDD(R)]—These pacing systems are capable of sensing and pacing in both the atrium and the ventricle on demand (see Figure 14–14). They therefore approach the physiology of normal AV conduction. The ability to sense retrograde atrial depolarizations can lead to ventricular stimulus delivery and ventricular pacing in response; if the paced ventricular depolarization travels retrograde to the atrium to depolarize it, the process can become repetitive. This event creates an artificial extra-AV-nodal bypass tract, causing a "pacemaker-mediated tachycardia." Specific algorithms have been designed to terminate these tachycardias and are automatic once they have been programmed.

Dual-chamber devices depend on a stable atrial rhythm for optimum function. Because of their potential for rapid paced ventricular rates, these systems should not be used with atrial arrhythmias such as chronic fibrillation or flutter, multifocal tachycardia, or refractory automatic tachycardia; single-chamber VVI(R) devices should be used instead.

If the atrial tachyarrhythmias are paroxysmal, however, a programmed "mode switch" feature should be programmed on that automatically changes the mode from DDD(R) to either DDI(R) or VVI(R) modes when a rapid atrial rate is detected; this removes the ability to track the atrial rate as long as the atrial tachyarrhythmia persists (Figure 14–17). Studies have established that in patients with bradycardia, compared with ventricular pacing, atrial-based pacing reduces the incidence of atrial fibrillation and may reduce stroke.

Rate-adaptive pacing systems are appropriate for patients with permanent atrial arrhythmias with slow ventricular response and for patients whose sinus node dysfunction prevents rate acceleration, but who would benefit from an increase in paced ventricular or atrial rates, respectively, in response to increases in metabolic demand. Current sensors measure body motion and acceleration, minute ventilation, QT interval, or intracardiac impedance; sensors to measure other parameters (eg, right ventricular dP/dt [rate of rise of pressure within the right ventricle]) are under development. Changes within the sensor's established parameters, designed to reflect physiologic needs, result in changes in paced rates. Sensor-based pacing rate depends on the individual sensor used, however; for example, if an activity sensor is being used, the paced rate can increase in response to body vibrations that are unrelated to actual physical activity, such as

shivering or tremor. This can cause problems in hospitalized patients, especially those in intensive care units. Several manufacturers, therefore, currently incorporate two sensors into their pacemakers to confirm the need for appropriate changes in pacing rate. For example, the activity sensor input can be confirmed by a more physiologic sensor such as minute ventilation, resulting in a more specific and accurate response to the change in pacing rate for the particular change in metabolic need. Recognition of sensor-based pacing and changing pacing rates is necessary to avoid erroneous diagnoses of pacemaker malfunction.

A growing number of studies have reported that right ventricular pacing can be detrimental, especially in patients with left ventricular systolic dysfunction. The left ventricular dyssynchrony caused by pacing from the right ventricle is thought to induce further cardiomyopathy and systolic heart failure due to functional LBBB. Dyssynchrony-induced cardiomyopathy has also been observed in patients with spontaneous LBBB, where abnormal electrical activation can initiate electrical remodeling that leads to myocardial remodeling; this form of cardiomyopathy can be reversed with cardiac resynchronization therapy through biventricular pacing. When there is preexisting cardiomyopathy, biventricular pacing can address the dyssynchrony caused by unavoidable right ventricular pacing.

In patients who do not need continuous ventricular pacing, a new development in dual-chamber pacing design provides various parameters that can be programmed to minimize unnecessary ventricular pacing. The AV delay can be programmed to automatically extend to allow native AV conduction as much as possible. Another programmable solution is managed ventricular pacing (MVP) mode (Medtronic, Inc., Minneapolis, MN) that maintains AAI(R) mode until AV block is detected, at which time it automatically switches to DDD(R) mode; AAI(R) mode is restored when the pacemaker detects resumption of native AV conduction.

The type of pacing system implanted is indicated on an identification card supplied to the patient by the manufacturer; patients should carry these cards with them at all times. It is important to note, however, that such information does not guarantee the operation of a particular mode of function, rate, or any parameter that can be programmed by the patient's pacemaker physician. As pulse-generator design and function increase in complexity, it is best to assume that the pacemaker is performing normally until proved otherwise (there are, of course, malfunctions and "pseudo" malfunctions; these are addressed in the following sections). Similarly, ECGs in paced patients should be considered to reflect normal device function unless they are interpreted otherwise by personnel experienced in pacemaker ECG.

B. UNIPOLAR AND BIPOLAR PACING—Unipolar pacing systems have the cathode (stimulating electrode) in the heart and the anode at the generator. The distance between the

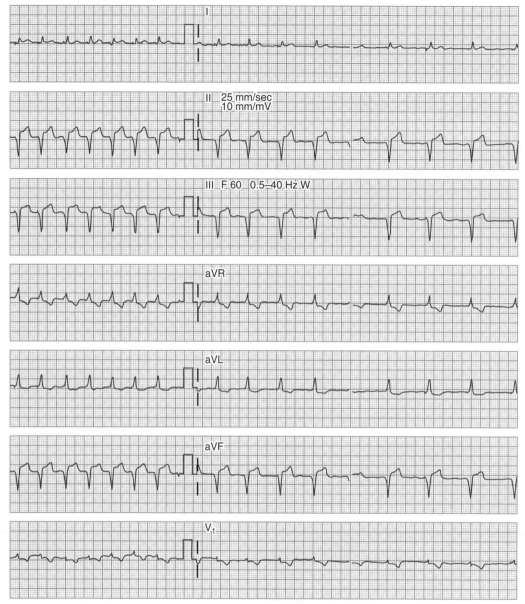

▲ **Figure 14–17.** Depiction of mode-switch operation of a dual-chamber pacemaker. In the initial portion of the rhythm strip, tracking of atrial fibrillation is occurring, resulting in a rapid paced ventricular rate. When the algorithm in the pacemaker recognizes the atrial tachyarrhythmia, automatic change of mode of function to VVIR takes place, terminating the rapid paced ventricular rate. On sensing restoration of a normal atrial rhythm, the device will automatically restore its dual-chamber mode of operation.

cathode and anode in these systems results in the inscription of large pacing artifacts whose direction (pacing-artifact axis) in the frontal plane points toward the anode in analog ECG recorders, but not in digital recorders in which stimulus artifact amplitudes and axes vary due to digital sampling of the pacing stimulus (see below).

Bipolar pacing systems have both lead electrodes within the heart, usually less than 1 cm apart, in either or both atrium and ventricle. Either the distal (tip) electrode or the proximal (ring) electrode of the lead can serve as the cathode. Because of the small interelectrode distance, the pacing artifacts are small and their direction in the frontal

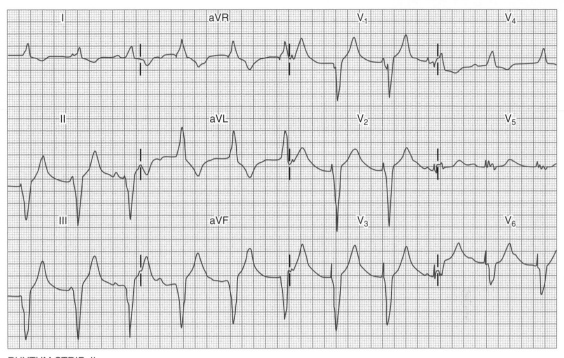

RHYTHM STRIP: II
25 mm/sec; 1 cm/mV

▲ **Figure 14–18.** Bipolar VVI pacing system. All QRS complexes are paced. Note the small magnitude of the pacing artifacts. The simultaneous recordings indicate that in some leads the pacing stimuli are virtually invisible.

plane reflects the direction of current flow (Figure 14–18). It is common for the small pacing artifacts to appear to be absent on ECGs and ECG monitoring strips; even computer-interpreted ECGs may fail to indicate that a pacemaker is present. Identification of paced (as opposed to spontaneous) P waves and QRS complexes must therefore be undertaken; often, magnet application with comparison of paced P and QRS morphologies with the initially recorded complexes is necessary to accomplish this.

In sum, ECGs recorded on digital rather than analog machines can show marked variations in both amplitude and polarity of pacing artifacts. Because the digital equipment samples the pacing stimuli at specific time intervals and then recreates them on paper, the inscribed stimulus artifacts are not seen in real time. In some ECG leads, the pacing stimuli may not be visible at all, raising the questions of spontaneous wide QRS complex rhythms or even failure of generator output. It is important to recognize this recording artifact in patients with pacemakers to avoid an erroneous diagnosis of pacemaker malfunction. It is equally important to document the morphology of paced complexes so that when the pacing stimuli cannot be seen, normal pacemaker function can be assumed until an accurate evaluation can be made.

Some permanent bipolar pacing systems offer lead polarity that can be programmed to unipolar; therefore, the presence of a bipolar lead on chest radiograph does not ensure bipolar lead function, and the ECG appearance of the pacing artifacts may differ from what is expected.

C. ELECTROCARDIOGRAPHIC PATTERNS OF PACED COMPLEXES—These patterns depend on how the myocardium is depolarized. Paced atrial complexes reflect the sequence of atrial activation initiated by the pacing impulse and thus, in part, the site of the pacing electrode(s). Because the atrial electrodes can be located in the atrial appendage or screwed into any portion of atrial tissue, paced P wave contours and axes will vary.

Pacing from the right ventricular apex produces paced QRS complexes that have a LBBB configuration (reflecting right ventricular myocardial depolarization before left ventricular depolarization) and a superior mean frontal plane axis (the apex of the heart is depolarized before the base; Figure 14–19). Paced QRS complexes usually have a duration of 120–180 ms; if they are substantially longer, intrinsic myocardial disease, hyperkalemia, or antiarrhythmic drug therapy (eg, amiodarone) should be suspected.

Pacing from the right ventricular outflow tract also results in QRS complexes that have a LBBB pattern, but the

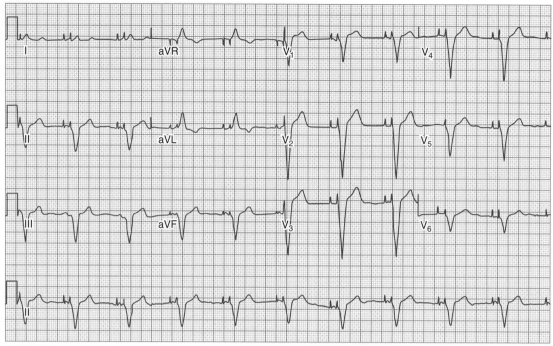

▲ **Figure 14–19.** Atrioventricular pacing with ventricular pacing from the area of the right ventricular apex, yielding superiorly directed paced QRS complexes with a left BBB pattern. The paced P-wave morphology and axis are similarly determined by the location of the pacing lead tip.

mean frontal plane axis is inferiorly directed (the base of the heart is depolarized before the apex). Occasionally, pacing from the interventricular septum can result in paced QRS complexes that show an indeterminate conduction delay pattern; they can even be narrow and relatively normal-appearing. This reflects almost simultaneous activation of both the right and left sides of the interventricular septum.

Pacing from the left ventricular epicardium produces paced QRS complexes having a right BBB pattern, reflecting left ventricular myocardial activation in advance of right ventricular activation. The mean frontal-plane QRS axis will depend on the location of the epicardial electrodes relative to each other (bipolar system) or to the pulse generator serving as anode (unipolar system).

Over the last decade, left ventricular pacing has been accomplished from the coronary veins approached via the coronary sinus. This technique is used along with simultaneous, or near simultaneous, pacing from the right ventricle in patients with advanced heart failure and wide QRS complexes (≥ 120 ms) in order to "resynchronize" ventricular depolarization-contraction. The biventricular-paced QRS complexes can be narrower and more normal-appearing than the patient's spontaneous QRS complexes, reflecting electrical resynchronization and suggesting a beneficial result of this therapy; electrical synchrony, however, does not necessarily correlate with mechanical synchrony, and a persistently wide QRS complex does not predict failure of therapy. The mean frontal plane axis of the paced complexes will vary with the location of the electrodes. Because the timing of the two ventricular leads can now be programmed separately, and either lead can be activated first by up to 80 ms, biventricular paced QRS complexes can be preceded by tightly coupled double-pacing artifacts (Figure 14–20).

Spontaneous QRS complexes occurring in patients with pacemakers often show marked T-wave inversion (Figure 14–21). This phenomenon has been explained as "T-wave memory" or the temporary persistence of abnormal repolarization "learned" by the myocardium during pacing. The ECG abnormality should not be interpreted as acute or chronic myocardial disease (including ischemia and infarction) in the absence of clinical indications.

D. PACEMAKERS AND MAGNETIC RESONANCE IMAGING—
Traditionally, magnetic resonance imaging (MRI) has been contraindicated in patients with pacemakers. This is based on a number of observed deleterious effects that the strong magnetic field can have on a pacemaker and on a handful of reported deaths possibly associated with MRI scanning. Potential effects range from activation of rate-adaptive sensors causing rapid pacing rates to reverting of the pacemaker

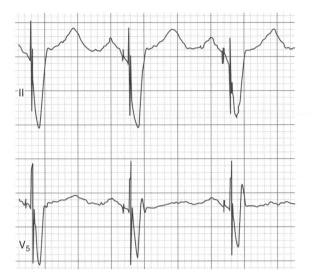

▲ **Figure 14-20.** Lead II and V_5 in patient with a biventricular pacing system, programmed with a VV timing set to LV first by 60 ms. Two distinct ventricular stimulus output artifacts are seen tightly coupled at the onset of the paced QRS complex, following a sensed P wave.

generator to a default mode and settings. There is also concern that the magnetic field can induce movement of current in the pacemaker lead, leading to heating at the lead tip-tissue interface with acute rises in capture threshold; in a pacemaker-dependent patient, critical loss of capture could then ensue.

There are instances where the benefits of MRI scanning (eg, early detection of cancer, imaging of the brain) need to be weighed against the potential risks to the patient with a pacemaker. Protocols have been established by different institutions that allow for non–pacemaker-dependent patients to undergo MRI scanning under close observation after making temporary programming changes that will minimize interaction with the magnetic field. Pacemakers implanted in the last 10 years have advanced electromagnetic interference protection that decreases the likelihood of encountering a problem. Pacemakers and leads that are Food and Drug Administration–approved to be used with MRI have recently become available, and MRI compatibility is projected to eventually become a standard feature of pacemakers in the future. MRI compatibility should be part of the discussion with patients prior to pacemaker implantation, and the choice of pacemaker type should be a factor, especially if there are underlying conditions that will likely require future MRI scans (eg, history of cancer, orthopedic problems, neurologic abnormalities).

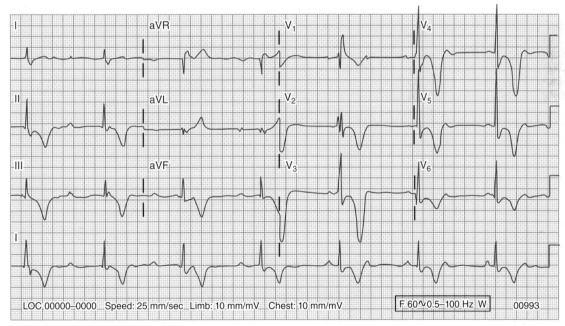

LOC 00000–0000   Speed: 25 mm/sec   Limb: 10 mm/mV   Chest: 10 mm/mV   F 60~0.5–100 Hz W   00993

▲ **Figure 14-21.** Twelve-lead electrocardiogram in patient with a DDD pacing system, temporarily programmed to a rate of 30 bpm to permit emergence of the native rhythm. The intrinsic rhythm is sinus with complete atrioventricular (AV) block and right bundle branch block. Because no pacing artifacts are occurring, sensing function is normal in both atrium and ventricle. The deeply inverted T waves in the inferior and precordial leads represent a nonspecific abnormality commonly observed in patients with pacemakers; they do not represent myocardial injury.

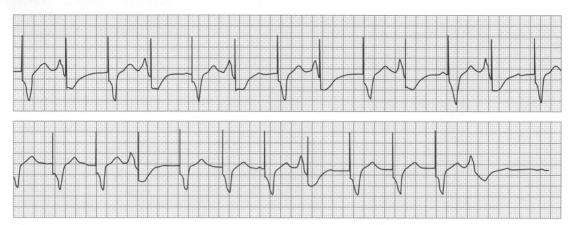

▲ **Figure 14–22.** Failure to sense spontaneous ventricular complexes in a patient with a VVI pacing system. Because the signal quality of depolarization originating in ventricular tissue is often poor, this is not uncommon. Repetitive ventricular beating induced by the stimulus-on-ST complex is, however, rare in stable patients.

B. Pacing System Malfunctions

Pacing system malfunctions fall into four general categories: (1) undersensing, or "failure" to sense; (2) oversensing, or the sensing of unwanted signals; (3) failure to capture and stimulate myocardial tissue; and (4) failure of output. Undersensing of cardiac electrical signals because of poor intrinsic signal quality does not represent sensing failure as such, but rather the inability to detect the suboptimal signal itself; undersensed P waves and QRS complexes are not rare. Premature ventricular complexes (see Table 14–9; Figure 14–22) generate suboptimal signals because they originate from within the myocardium, away from the normal conduction apparatus; they can occur in patients without structural heart disease, during acute myocardial ischemia and infarction, or as a result of drug toxicity and electrolyte imbalance. Undersensed P waves can be caused by changes in atrial volume, ectopic atrial rhythms, or retrograde atrial depolarizations. Undersensing of spontaneous complexes and consequent failure to inhibit output results in the delivery of an earlier-than-expected pacing stimulus, which can, on occasion, induce repetitive rhythms.

Ventricular pacing artifacts can sometimes occur after the onset of spontaneous QRS complexes that have a right BBB configuration, raising concern of undersensing. This happens because of delayed conduction in the right bundle branch: the wavefront of ventricular depolarization does not reach the lead electrode in the right ventricle (especially the apex) in time to inhibit the output of the pacing stimulus. This phenomenon of stimulus delivery within a QRS complex, called "pseudofusion" (as opposed to true fusion), may also be observed in patients with inferior and right ventricular myocardial infarction and is probably due to the conduction delay resulting from ventricular scarring. The same principles apply to patients who have a left ventricular epicardial electrode and either underlying LBBB or ventricular

scarring and to patients who have a right atrial electrode and an intra-atrial conduction delay. Undersensing in these cases is due to intrinsic conduction system disease rather than to a malfunctioning unit. The problem is managed by extending the programmed AV delay (in the case of ventricular pseudofusion), programming a higher sensitivity, or if necessary, increasing the pacing rate to overdrive the native rhythm.

Oversensing refers to sensing of unwanted electrical signals such as T waves, myopotentials, and environmental signals (eg, electrocautery; see Table 14–10). Programming the pulse generator to sense only electrical signals of larger magnitude will often solve the problem. When a programmer is not immediately available, placing a magnet over the pulse generator will temporarily eliminate the oversensing by converting the generator to a nonsensing asynchronous mode. Because competitive rhythms with the magnet in place can induce ventricular tachyarrhythmias, these patients should be in a monitored unit.

Failure to capture exists when pacing stimuli do not depolarize nonrefractory myocardium (Figure 14–23; Table 14–11). This condition may result from poor electrode position; a subthreshold programmed output; output reduction due to battery depletion; or an increase in myocardial stimulation threshold that usually results from acute myocardial infarction, drug toxicity, electrolyte imbalance, cardiopulmonary resuscitation, or fibrosis at the electrode-tissue interface. Pacemaker noncapture can be managed by noninvasive programming of the generator's energy output (voltage and pulse duration), surgical repositioning of the lead, or generator exchange, depending on the underlying problem.

The difference between failure to capture (stimulus artifact is present) and failure of output (lack of stimulus output when such output is expected and indicated) should be recognized. If the pacing stimulus has not been delivered (Table 14–12), capture cannot be ascertained. Applying

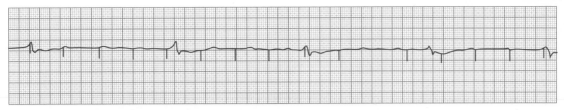

▲ **Figure 14–23.** Failure to capture and sense in a patient following cardiac arrest; a temporary transvenous pacing system had been placed in the right ventricular apex. The QRS complexes are spontaneous and occur at a severely slow rate; they do not follow pacing stimuli.

a magnet will aid in determining the cause for the lack of stimulus output. Asynchronous pacing will result with magnet application if the lack of pacing stimulus output results from inhibition due to oversensing. If there is a true problem with delivery of a stimulus output, no stimulus output and therefore no paced complexes will be seen despite magnet application. The main causes of failure of output are battery depletion and generator component failure. This is to be distinguished from the situation when pulse generator output is occurring normally but the current is not reaching body tissues to depolarize it, due to lead fracture or insulation break, and loose set screw (loss of connection between the lead connector pin and the pacemaker generator). Management of pacemaker failure of output will require replacement of the generator, whereas lead problems usually require lead replacement, and loose set screws are addressed merely by restoring a good connection between the lead connector pin and the generator.

C. Assessment of Pacing System Function

All patients should have a 12-lead ECG, with and without a magnet applied, to allow identification of spontaneous (where present), purely paced, and fusion P waves and QRS complexes, as well as sensing and pacing functions in both atria and ventricles. The (nonprogrammable) pacing rate with a magnet in place is not the same as the programmed rate, and the mode of function with the magnet in place may differ from the programmed mode (eg, a DDD system may have a magnet mode that is VOO, although this is currently a rare event; Figure 14–24). The magnet mode, rate, and AV

interval for each device is manufacturer and model specific, and may vary, with a number of stimuli delivered at one rate and AV interval, followed by another rate and AV interval.

In addition, all patients should have highly penetrated posteroanterior and lateral chest radiographs in order to assess the leads and, when possible, to identify the pacemaker's manufacturer and model number. The number and type (unipolar, bipolar, MRI-compatible) of leads can be ascertained, as well as the positions of the lead tips and pulse generator. Lead tips lying outside the cardiac silhouette suggest the possibility of myocardial perforation. Occasionally, lead insulation degradation, wire fracture, or improper connections between the lead and generator can be seen.

More sophisticated evaluation techniques, such as interrogation of the programmed parameters of the pulse generator, sensing and pacing threshold determination, and

Table 14–11. Causes and Management of Pacemaker Noncapture

Tissue refractoriness: Verify capture during temporal opportunity
Lead dislodgement: Reposition lead, or program lead polarity
Increase in myocardial stimulation threshold: Program higher energy output; treat underlying cause if possible
Lead-insulation break: Repair or replace lead; unipolarize lead
Conductor-wire fracture: Replace lead
Inappropriately low programmed output: Program higher output
Generator end of life: Replace generator

Table 14–12 Causes of Absence of Pacing Stimulus Output and Response to Magnet Application

Cause	Response to Magnet
Normal inhibition by P waves and QRS complexes	Pacing stimuli will be delivered asynchronously
Oversensing	Pacing stimuli will be delivered asynchronously
Lead fracture	Pacing stimuli may not be seen if the break in the wire is complete (current does not reach body tissues); may be seen as multiples of a basing pacing rate, or may be seen intermittently (make-break circuit); may have variable amplitude
Lead–generator disconnection or improper connection	Same as for lead fracture
Battery failure (end of life)	Pacing stimuli at slow rate, no visible pacing stimuli, noncapture, failure to sense
Battery component failure	Variable response

Without Magnet

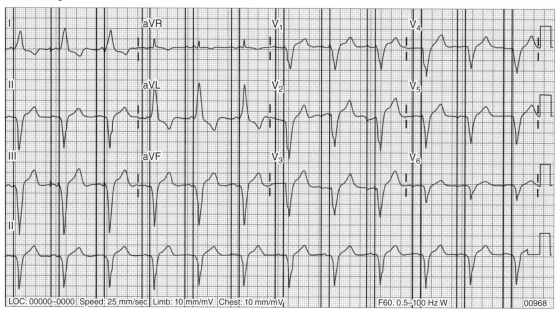

A

With Magnet

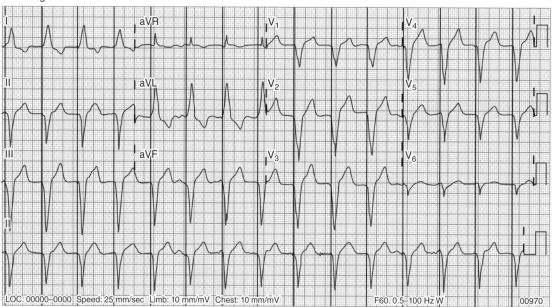

B

▲ **Figure 14-24. A:** Atrioventricular sequential pacing. The large magnitude of the pacing artifacts indicates unipolar pacing in both chambers. Because atrial pacing stimuli are followed by P waves, and ventricular stimuli are followed by QRS complexes, pacing function is normal in both chambers. Sensing function cannot be evaluated because spontaneous P waves and QRS complexes are not occurring. **B:** Twelve-lead electrocardiogram, recorded with magnet in place. The mode of function is VOO (asynchronous ventricular pacing) at the factory-designated rate of about 88 bpm. This is normal function for this particular device.

recording of intracardiac electrograms, can be necessary to detect and then determine the cause of pacemaker malfunction; these evaluations should be performed by a pacemaker specialist.

Epstein AE, et al. ACC/AHA/HRS 2008 guidelines for device-based therapy of cardiac rhythm abnormalities: a report of the ACC/AHA Task Force on Practice Guidelines (Writing Committee to Revise the ACC/AHA/NASPE 2002 guideline update for implantation of cardiac pacemakers and anti-arrhythmia devices). *Circulation*. 2008;117(21):e350–408. [PMID: 18483207]

Gillis AM, et al. HRS/ACCF expert consensus statement on pacemaker device and mode selection. *Heart Rhythm*. 2012;9(8): 1344–65. [PMID: 22858114]

Healey JS, et al. Cardiovascular outcomes with atrial-based pacing compared with ventricular pacing: meta-analysis of randomized trials, using individual patient data. *Circulation*. 2006;114(1):11–7. [PMID: 16801463]

Misiri J, et al. Electromagnetic interference and implanted cardiac devices: the nonmedical environment (part I). *Clin Cardiol*. 2012;35(5):276–80. [PMID: 22539305]

Misiri J, et al. Electromagnetic interference and implanted cardiac devices: the medical environment (part II). *Clin Cardiol*. 2012;35(6):321–8. [PMID: 22539263]

Nazarian S, et al. A prospective evaluation of a protocol for magnetic resonance imaging of patients with implanted cardiac devices. *Ann Intern Med*. 2011;155(7):415–24. [PMID: 21969340]

Wilkoff BL, et al. Dual-chamber pacing or ventricular backup pacing in patients with an implantable defibrillator: the Dual Chamber and VVI Implantable Defibrillator (DAVID) Trial. *JAMA*. 2002;288(24):3115–23. [PMID: 12495391]

Wood MA, et al. Clinical outcomes after ablation and pacing therapy for atrial fibrillation. A meta-analysis. *Circulation*. 2000;101(10):1138–44. [PMID: 10715260]

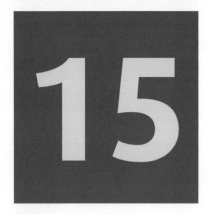

Sudden Cardiac Death

Andrew E. Darby, MD
John P. DiMarco, MD, PhD

▶ Unexpected death occurring within an hour of onset of symptoms.

▶ Primary electrical mechanisms include ventricular fibrillation, ventricular tachycardia, asystole, and pulseless electrical activity.

▶ General Considerations

Each year in the United States, more than 350,000 individuals die suddenly of some form of cardiovascular disease. Because of the many advances made during the past 30 years in clinicians' ability to identify and modify the risk factors associated with sudden death, to resuscitate victims of cardiac arrest, and to prescribe specific antiarrhythmic therapy to prevent recurrences, age-adjusted sudden death mortality rates have declined dramatically. However, the number of elderly individuals in the population has increased, and sudden cardiac arrest remains an important problem.

For general clinical purposes, the term "sudden cardiac death" is usually reserved for those deaths in which the patient had stable cardiac function until the terminal event, with death occurring within a short time (often defined as less than 1 hour) of the onset of symptoms. Some experts prefer the term "instantaneous death," namely, death with immediate collapse without preceding symptoms. Instantaneous death is usually assumed to be due to a primary arrhythmia, but other catastrophic events, such as a massive pulmonary embolism, the rupture of an aortic aneurysm, or a stroke, can also cause instantaneous death. It is also important to note that not all arrhythmic deaths are sudden. For example, a patient who is resuscitated from a cardiac arrest may die days or weeks later from complications of the arrest. This death would be due to an arrhythmia but would not meet the standard time-based definition for instantaneous or sudden death.

Effective evaluation and treatment of patients at risk for cardiac arrest and sudden death require an understanding of the responsible pathophysiologic mechanisms, the strategies proposed for primary prevention, the techniques and results of resuscitation, and the treatment modalities for secondary prevention in survivors of an initial episode.

Roger VL, et al. Heart disease and stroke statistics – 2012 update: a report from the American Heart Association. *Circulation.* 2012;125:e2–220. [PMID: 22179539]

▶ Pathophysiology & Etiology

A number of different electrophysiologic mechanisms may be responsible for sudden cardiac death. When ambulatory electrocardiographic (ECG) recordings from the time of an out-of-hospital cardiac arrest are examined, ventricular fibrillation and rapid ventricular tachycardia are the most commonly documented initial arrhythmias. Bradyarrhythmias, including atrioventricular block, asystole, or electromechanical dissociation, are also observed. The prevalence of these latter arrhythmias is higher in the setting of progressive and advanced underlying heart disease; in the elderly, and in patients whose sudden death is precipitated by an acute catastrophe, such as a pulmonary embolism, an acute myocardial infarction, rupture of a major vessel, or a major neurologic insult. Extrapolation of the mortality rate from data recorded by the Resuscitation Outcomes Consortium suggests that 382,800 people experience out-of-hospital cardiac arrests in the United States each year. Among out-of-hospital cardiac arrests treated by emergency medical personnel, only 23% have an initial rhythm of ventricular tachycardia or ventricular fibrillation or are shockable by an automated external defibrillator. Interestingly, the incidence of cardiac arrest with an initial rhythm of ventricular fibrillation has decreased over time, although the incidence of cardiac arrest with any rhythm has not decreased. The focus of this chapter will be principally those sudden deaths for which an arrhythmia was the primary cause.

A. Coronary Artery Disease

Although sudden death occurs in all forms of heart disease, in the United States and Europe, coronary artery disease is the most common cardiac diagnosis seen in sudden death victims (Table 15–1). Several mechanisms can produce potentially fatal arrhythmias among patients with coronary artery disease, and it is often difficult to define the precise factors that gave rise to a given episode. At one extreme is the patient with a previously normal ventricle who has an acute occlusion of a major epicardial coronary artery in whom ventricular fibrillation then develops during the first minutes of an acute infarction. This patient represents an example of pure ischemic injury without associated prior scar. At the other end of the spectrum is the patient with a history of a single-vessel occlusion and an old myocardial infarction, in whom postinfarction scarring has provided the anatomic substrate for a rapid reentrant ventricular tachycardia that results in hemodynamic collapse and sudden death. Acute ischemia need not be involved as a trigger in the latter situation. In coronary artery disease, the individuals at highest risk for sudden death have both multivessel disease and myocardial scarring from one or more prior infarctions. Even in such individuals, sudden cardiac arrest may be the first clinical manifestation of the disease. As treatment of acute myocardial infarction has become more aggressive during the past 20 years, the nature of the typical scar that results from a myocardial infarction has also changed. Dense scar tissue with aneurysm formation, the classic substrate associated with uniform morphology ventricular tachycardia, is now seen less often. After early pharmacologic or mechanical reperfusion, the current standards of therapy, the infarct zone shows mostly patchy fibrosis, and in such areas, disorganized arrhythmias predominate. In patients with this complex substrate, sudden death is thought to result from a complex interaction between some triggering event, such as ischemia, autonomic nervous system dysfunction, electrolyte imbalance, or drug toxicity, and the unstable electrophysiologic milieu created by prior infarction.

Autopsy and clinical studies have highlighted this complexity. Coronary artery thrombi or plaque rupture may be detected in up to 50% of sudden death victims, but new Q-wave myocardial infarctions will develop in only about 25% of patients resuscitated from an out-of-hospital cardiac arrest. Angiographic studies in cardiac arrest survivors have shown that a high proportion of persons have long, diffusely irregular, and ulcerated coronary lesions similar to those seen in patients with acute coronary syndromes. It has also been demonstrated that therapy directed at ischemia reduces the incidence of sudden death. Aggressive surgical revascularization has been shown to decrease late sudden death mortality. In the Coronary Artery Bypass Graft (CABG-Patch) trial, no survival benefit over control was seen in patients who received an implantable cardioverter-defibrillator (ICD) at the time of their revascularization surgery. Based on this confusing overall picture, it is prudent in any individual with coronary disease to consider ischemia as an important, potentially reversible risk factor for sudden death, even in the absence of clinical angina. In previously asymptomatic individuals, coronary artery disease may still be the cause of sudden death. Significant coronary artery disease may be asymptomatic or unrecognized, and the general population contains a large number of such individuals. Up to 50% of all sudden cardiac deaths due to coronary artery disease may occur in individuals not previously known to have the condition.

Other diseases of the coronary arteries are rare causes of sudden death. An anomalous origin of a coronary artery may give rise to either myocardial scarring with late ventricular tachycardia or to arrhythmias mediated by acute intermittent ischemia. Similar mechanisms affecting patients with coronary artery spasm, embolism, trauma, dissections, or arteritis may cause sudden death.

Table 15–1. Cardiac Conditions Associated with Sudden Death

Diseases of the coronary arteries
  Atherosclerotic
    Acute ischemia or infarction
    Prior myocardial infarction
  Congenital coronary anomalies
  Others
    Spasm
    Arteritis
    Dissection
Diseases of the aorta
  Marfan syndrome
  Aortic aneurysm
Diseases of the myocardium
  Hypertrophic cardiomyopathies
  Dilated cardiomyopathies
  Left ventricular noncompaction
  Valvular heart disease
  Arrhythmogenic right ventricular cardiomyopathy/dysplasia
  Congenital heart disease
  Infiltrative cardiomyopathy (eg, sarcoidosis)
  Primary pulmonary hypertension
  Myocarditis
  Chagas disease
  Neuromuscular disorders with cardiac involvement
Primary electrophysiologic disorders
  Long QT syndrome: acquired and congenital
  Brugada syndrome
  Catecholaminergic polymorphic ventricular tachycardia
  Preexcitation syndromes
  Congenital atrioventricular block
Other
  Drug ingestion
  Commotio cordis
  Electrolyte disorders
  Diet related

B. Hypertrophic Cardiomyopathy

Hypertrophic cardiomyopathy is the most common genetic cardiovascular disorder with an estimated prevalence of 1 in 500. In hypertrophic cardiomyopathy, sudden death tends to occur in young adults who often have had no prior cardiac symptoms. There appears to be an excess of events during vigorous exercise, and hypertrophic cardiomyopathy is the leading cause of sudden death among competitive athletes in the United States. Teenagers or young adults in some kindreds with familial hypertrophic cardiomyopathy have a higher incidence of sudden death than do older members. In other families, sudden death in young adults is uncommon but may occur after heart failure has developed.

Several clinical risk factors for sudden death in patients with hypertrophic cardiomyopathy have been determined. These include a family history of sudden death; recurrent, unexplained syncope; nonsustained ventricular tachycardia during ambulatory monitoring; hypotension during exercise; and severe (> 30 mm) left ventricular hypertrophy. The presence of myocardial scarring on a magnetic resonance scan is a new risk factor that has recently been identified. Hypertrophic cardiomyopathy is a genetic disease primarily affecting the cardiac sarcomere with 60–70% of cases accounted for by sarcomere mutations. Genetic studies of patients with hypertrophic cardiomyopathy have revealed more than 900 mutations in 13 different genes. Some mutations (eg, those in troponin T) may be associated with a high risk of sudden death even in the absence of marked left ventricular hypertrophy. Polymorphic ventricular tachycardia or ventricular fibrillation, rather than monomorphic ventricular tachycardia with a scar-related intramyocardial circuit, is thought to be the initial arrhythmia at the time of cardiac arrest in patients with hypertrophic cardiomyopathy. Due to the severe hypertrophy and conduction system disease seen in patients with hypertrophic cardiomyopathy, sustained ventricular tachycardia due to reentry in the His-Purkinje system may occur and result in hemodynamic collapse with sudden death. Patients with hypertrophic cardiomyopathy are also at risk for sudden death due to atrioventricular block and supraventricular arrhythmias because any change in rhythm that produces significant ischemia in the hypertrophied ventricular wall may degenerate to a fatal arrhythmia.

C. Nonischemic Dilated Cardiomyopathy

Nonischemic dilated cardiomyopathy is the primary cardiac diagnosis in about 10% of patients who have been resuscitated after cardiac arrest. Sudden death accounts for about half of all deaths in patients with this diagnosis. In contrast to the situation in some forms of hypertrophic cardiomyopathy, sudden death tends to occur relatively late in the course of dilated cardiomyopathy, after hemodynamic symptoms have been present for some time. A variety of arrhythmias have been implicated in patients with this condition; both monomorphic and polymorphic ventricular tachycardias are seen in patients with nonischemic dilated cardiomyopathies.

Intraventricular conduction delays may lead to ventricular tachycardia caused by macroreentry in the His-Purkinje system. In patients with this arrhythmia, catheter ablation of one of the bundle branches may be curative. In patients with cardiomyopathies and very advanced heart failure, bradyarrhythmias, rather than tachyarrhythmias, are the initial recorded rhythm in up to 50% of cardiac arrests. Some forms of familial dilated cardiomyopathy (eg, lamin A/C mutation carriers) are associated with markedly increased risks for sudden death, and such patients will often require intervention outside of standard guidelines.

D. Other Cardiac Diseases

In **valvular heart disease,** sudden death can occur in several ways. Sudden death is usually related to exertion in young adults with congenital aortic stenoses. In other forms of valvular heart disease, sudden death is usually a late occurrence seen in patients with advanced heart failure and ventricular hypertrophy. Although symptomatic atrial and ventricular arrhythmias are common in patients with mitral valve prolapse, truly life-threatening arrhythmias are rare, except in the presence of some complicating condition, such as a LQTS, electrolyte imbalance, or drug toxicity. In pulmonary hypertension, sudden death may occur from hemodynamic causes, bradyarrhythmias, or tachyarrhythmias.

Arrhythmogenic right ventricular cardiomyopathy (ARVC) is a regional myopathy with primarily right ventricular involvement. When genetic studies have been performed, mutations in one of the desmosomal proteins are often found. These patients usually have left bundle branch block morphology ventricular tachycardias. Symptoms and signs of right ventricular dysfunction may or may not be present in patients with ARVC and ventricular tachycardia, and the clinical course is highly variable. It has been suggested that ARVC with extensive disease (including left ventricular involvement), one or more affected family members with sudden death, or undiagnosed syncope (when ventricular tachycardia or ventricular fibrillation has not been excluded as the cause of syncope) may indicate an increased risk of sudden death and prompt consideration for a primary prevention ICD.

In most forms of **congenital heart disease,** sudden arrhythmic death in the absence of severe heart failure, ventricular hypertrophy, or hypoxemia is uncommon. However, late ventricular tachycardia that arises from the right ventriculotomy scar or the septal repair may develop in some patients who have undergone a successful surgical repair of Fallot tetralogy.

E. Inherited Arrhythmia Syndromes

The **congenital long QT syndrome** (LQTS) is a family of disorders characterized by prolongation of cardiac repolarization with a prolonged QT interval on the scalar ECG and a tendency to develop polymorphic ventricular tachycardia that may degenerate to ventricular fibrillation. It occurs with an estimated prevalence of 1 in 3000 to 5000 in the general population. The most common types of the LQTS are caused by mutations in genes that encode ion channel proteins. The resultant ion channel dysfunction causes a prolonged repolarization phase of the ventricular action potential. This promotes polymorphic ventricular tachycardia triggered by oscillations in the action potential called early after-depolarizations. Electrolyte imbalance, bradycardia or pauses, sudden sympathetic stimulation, and drug effects all may further prolong repolarization in individuals with these mutations and trigger acute episodes. Factors significantly affecting outcome include QTc duration (ie, increased risk of ventricular arrhythmias with QTc > 500 ms); age-gender interactions (increased event rate in males during childhood and females after onset of adolescence); LQTS genotype (LQT_3 responds less well to β-blocker therapy); and syncope despite treatment with a β-blocker. Interestingly, family history of sudden death does not seem to be a marker of life-threatening cardiac events in LQTS patients. It is important to recognize patients with LQTS because standard antiarrhythmic drugs may worsen their condition and other QT-prolonging agents must be avoided.

A **short QT syndrome** caused by a gain in function mutation in a repolarizing potassium current that is associated with sudden death has also been described. The syndrome is characterized by short QT intervals (< 350 ms) and high incidence of syncope, sudden death, and atrial fibrillation.

The **Brugada syndrome** is another familial condition associated with sudden death. These individuals have an incomplete or complete right bundle branch block on their ECG with ST segment elevation in V_1 and V_2. These patients will manifest spontaneous episodes of polymorphic ventricular tachycardia and ventricular fibrillation, often during sleep. Some patients with Brugada syndrome have a mutation in the sodium channel gene (SCN5A) with a decrease in the inward sodium current during the plateau phase of the action potential. The unusual ECG manifestations are believed to be due to more pronounced ion channel dysfunction in the right ventricular epicardium.

Catecholaminergic polymorphic ventricular tachycardia (CPVT) is a rare syndrome in which bursts of rapid ventricular tachycardia occur during sympathetic stimulation or exercise. This syndrome is genetically heterogenous, with mutations in the genes encoding the cardiac ryanodine receptor type II and calsequestrin. These genetic mutations result in deranged calcium homeostasis with increased intracellular calcium, thereby predisposing to an increased risk of ventricular arrhythmias. β-Blockers are indicated for symptomatic patients. An ICD may be indicated for CPVT patients with syncope or sustained ventricular tachycardia despite treatment with β-blockers.

Advancements in genetic testing have facilitated the diagnosis and risk stratification of patients with inherited arrhythmia syndromes. Most of these diseases are caused by single genetic mutations that are heritable (often in an autosomal dominant fashion). However, the genetic cause has been identified for only a portion of these life-threatening

disorders (up to 75% of LQTS cases; 65% of hypertrophic cardiomyopathy; 50% of ARVC and CPVT; and 25 to 30% of dilated cardiomyopathy and Brugada syndrome). Genome-wide association studies (GWAS) analyze the entire human genome in large cohorts seeking to establish a correlation between common genetic mutations and disease. Specifically, GWAS assess the impact of single nucleotide polymorphisms (SNPs; genetic mutations that are common [> 1%] in the general population) on the susceptibility to arrhythmias. GWAS have identified mutations that affect the QT interval and may modulate the risk of sudden cardiac death in the LQTS. Further research may identify mutations that influence the risk of sudden death in other cardiac conditions as well as the susceptibility to drug-induced QT prolongation and torsade de pointes.

Barsheshet A, et al. Genetics of sudden cardiac death. *Curr Cardiol Rep.* 2011;13:364–76. [PMID: 21789574]

Cerrone M, et al. Genetics of sudden death: focus on inherited channelopathies. *Eur Heart J.* 2011;32:2109–20. [PMID: 21478491]

Milan DJ, et al. Genome-wide association studies in cardiac electrophysiology: recent discoveries and implications for clinical practice. *Heart Rhythm.* 2010;7:1141–8. [PMID: 20423731]

F. Drug-Induced Arrhythmias

Drug toxicity can also result in sudden death. A variety of medications can affect cardiac electrophysiology and lead to fatal arrhythmias. Even when prescribed for atrial fibrillation or supraventricular tachycardia, all antiarrhythmic drugs may be associated with a proarrhythmic response in the ventricle. Other cardiac and noncardiac drugs can also cause arrhythmias. The most common mechanism is I_{Kr} blockade. Multiple factors are often required for drug-induced proarrhythmia. Risk factors include electrolyte disturbances, age, female gender, genetic polymorphisms or mutations, left ventricular hypertrophy, and bradycardia.

Patients with severe electrolyte disturbances and abnormal dietary histories (eg, anorexia nervosa and liquid protein diets) are also susceptible to potentially fatal ventricular arrhythmias even in the absence of significant heart disease.

G. Other Arrhythmias

Several electrophysiologic abnormalities can produce sudden death without associated major structural heart disease. **Supraventricular arrhythmias,** if associated with very rapid ventricular rates, can cause hemodynamic collapse and degenerate to ventricular fibrillation. Atrial fibrillation with rapid conduction over an accessory pathway in a patient with **Wolff-Parkinson-White syndrome** is the supraventricular arrhythmia most frequently associated with sudden death, but other supraventricular arrhythmias have also occasionally been implicated. Although sudden death due to a ventricular preexcitation syndrome is rare, it may be the first clinical manifestation of the condition.

Bradyarrhythmias may also be associated with sudden death. In **congenital complete heart block,** the escape pacemaker may deteriorate over time, with ventricular arrhythmias appearing as the patient's bradycardia becomes more and more inappropriate. Most previously healthy adults in whom a bradycardia develops as a result of sinus node dysfunction or heart block will have some functioning escape pacemaker that can, at least briefly, support vital organs. Therefore, sudden death is uncommon with these arrhythmias in the absence of severe ventricular dysfunction, another complicating disease, electrolyte imbalance, drug toxicity, or a prolonged delay in treatment of the bradycardia.

A recently recognized syndrome of sudden death in young individuals with structurally normal hearts is **commotio cordis.** Ventricular fibrillation develops after the patient receives a sharp blow to the chest, often while engaged in sports. Animal models have shown that a critically timed and placed chest impact during a vulnerable portion of the T wave can initiate ventricular fibrillation. It is assumed that a similar mechanism is responsible for the human syndrome.

Not all ventricular arrhythmias in patients with structurally normal hearts carry a risk for sudden death. Sudden death is very rare in individuals with structurally normal hearts who initially present with a stable **monomorphic ventricular tachycardia.** The two most common forms of sustained monomorphic ventricular tachycardia in patients with structurally normal hearts arise either from the right ventricular outflow tract with a left bundle branch block pattern and an inferior axis or from the inferior septal region with a right bundle branch block and left axis pattern. Both of these forms of ventricular tachycardia are usually hemodynamically well tolerated and rarely result in sudden cardiac death.

▶ Management of Cardiac Arrest: Initial Resuscitation

The introduction of transthoracic defibrillation 50 years ago sparked the development of community-based programs to resuscitate persons who suffered cardiac arrest out of the hospital. The most successful systems involve an educated lay public that can provide basic cardiopulmonary resuscitation (CPR), judicious community placement of automatic external defibrillators (AEDs) for nonprofessional use, and trained responders who can provide advanced life support in the field. The most important factor influencing survival is the time from cardiac arrest to restoration of an organized cardiac rhythm. If an effective rhythm is not restored within 4–8 minutes, survival with well-preserved neurologic function becomes unlikely. Bystander CPR can extend this window for survival by a few minutes.

Because early defibrillation is the key to survival, community programs to speed defibrillation have been widely introduced but with modest results. Initial efforts involved emergency medical technicians trained in both basic and advanced cardiac life support who responded to the emergency call. The success of these programs was limited by the ability of these trained responders to reach the patient within the first critical minutes after the arrest.

Public access to AEDs has been shown to improve survival for out-of-hospital cardiac arrest patients. When an AED is connected to an unconscious individual by electrode pads placed on the chest, a microprocessor within the device analyzes the patient's rhythm. Ventricular fibrillation and rapid ventricular tachycardia are accurately identifiable as "shockable" rhythms, and the AED instructs the rescuer to push a button to deliver a shock. AEDs designed for home use by minimally trained lay family members are now commercially available, and a wearable vest AED that does not require a rescuer for activation has recently been introduced. The greatest success with AED usage has been in public places like casinos, sports venues, and transportation centers where arrest victims are likely to be observed quickly and security personnel trained in AED usage are present. Basic CPR techniques have also evolved, with the current emphasis placed on maintenance of effective chest compression.

A discussion of the techniques for basic and advanced cardiac life support is beyond the scope of this chapter. For patients with ventricular tachycardia or fibrillation, early cardioversion or defibrillation is the key to survival. For patients with asystole or pulseless electrical activity, the prospects for survival remain poor unless some reversible cause can be identified and immediately corrected.

▶ Management of Cardiac Arrest Survivors: In-Hospital Phase

Even in communities that have effective programs for prehospital cardiac care, only a fraction of cardiac arrest patients will survive to hospital admission. The immediate goal for rescuers in the field is restoration of spontaneous circulation. If that can be achieved, preservation of the brain, heart, and other vital organs must be considered. Potential complications of the resuscitation must be identified and treatment instituted. The probable cause, including reversible precipitating events, the nature and severity of any underlying heart disease, and the arrhythmia probably responsible for the episode, should be determined. Finally, therapy can be selected and its potential for success evaluated.

A. Complications of Resuscitation

Only a fraction of cardiac arrest survivors who receive early defibrillation will be alert and oriented with full recovery of function at the time of hospital admission. Most patients will have pulmonary, cardiac, or neurologic complications resulting from the period of arrest or the resuscitation itself. Pulmonary complications are usually due either to aspiration of gastric contents or to mechanical injury to the thoracic cage during closed-chest compressions. The chest wall should be carefully inspected, palpated, and stabilized, if necessary. In extreme cases, bony thoracic fractures may result in a flail chest, or hepatic or splenic lacerations may occur. Chest radiography may be helpful in detecting aspiration, but repeated examinations may be necessary to document the delayed appearance of infiltrates. If a central line has been placed, the chest radiograph is also useful to confirm catheter position and to exclude a pneumothorax. Mechanical ventilation is often required in the early period after admission to allow adequate oxygenation and pulmonary cleansing; this may require the use of muscle relaxants and sedation. Over oxygenation should be avoided.

Early revascularization should be attempted in all cardiac arrest survivors who present with a new ST segment elevation myocardial infarction and should be considered whenever acute ischemia was a likely contributor to the arrest. Some cardiac arrest centers have urged that all cardiac arrest survivors undergo coronary angiography immediately after resuscitation, but this may not be possible in all hospitals. If an acute total coronary occlusion is identified, revascularization is indicated.

Cardiac arrest even without a new coronary occlusion produces a period of global cardiac ischemia, frequently resulting in a period of cardiac stunning, defined as a reversible depression in cardiac systolic function. Inotropic or even mechanical (eg, intra-aortic balloon counterpulsation) support may be necessary to maintain vital organ perfusion during the early phase after resuscitation. Any acute assessment of ventricular function may overestimate the amount of permanent dysfunction, and a low ejection fraction measured in the first several days after arrest may not be an accurate gauge of eventual cardiac function. Arrhythmias are frequently seen during the period immediately after resuscitation. They may be similar to those that originally produced the arrest, or they may be new rhythm disturbances caused by poor hemodynamic function and multiorgan failure. No single therapy will be predictably effective against these arrhythmias, and antiarrhythmic agents, β-adrenergic blockers, positive inotropic agents, and other measures to improve hemodynamic function must be tried. Recent studies using intravenous amiodarone prior to hospital admission have demonstrated improvements in rates of return of spontaneous circulation and survival-to-hospital admission but no clear benefit in survival-to-hospital discharge.

If spontaneous circulation can be restored and the patient is admitted to the hospital, neurologic damage is the major cause of death and long-term disability. Neurologic damage occurs quickly during a cardiac arrest. Unless defibrillation with restoration of spontaneous circulation was almost immediate, patients will be unconscious when admitted to the hospital, and an accurate evaluation of the potential for functional recovery is often difficult in this early stage. Brainstem reflexes may be preserved, but their presence does not necessarily predict a favorable outcome. Generalized or focal seizure activity, decerebrate or decorticate posturing, and involuntary respiratory efforts may make mechanical ventilation difficult. Neuromuscular blocking agents, anticonvulsants, and sedation are often required, further hampering any ability to make an accurate neurologic assessment. Studies have demonstrated

that mild therapeutic hypothermia (32–34°C for 24 hours) significantly improves neurologic recovery in unconscious resuscitated cardiac arrest patients. Advanced life support protocols now call for therapeutic cooling to be started in the field or immediately upon hospital arrival (Figure 15–1). In patients who received therapeutic hypothermia, the prognosis is good if they regain consciousness within 72 hours of arrest. Many will recover completely with minimal or no long-term neurologic impairment. Therapeutic hypothermia does not rule out early revascularization, and both strategies should be employed. If coma persists longer than 72 hours, only a minority of patients survive. Those who do will often have persistent severe motor and cognitive deficits. Somatosensory evoked potential testing, measurement of brain-specific enolases, and electroencephalogram data may help to determine prognosis. Decisions about prolonged artificial support of these latter patients are often difficult and require that a variety of medical, ethical, and social factors be taken into consideration.

Nolan JP, et al. Post-cardiac arrest syndrome: epidemiology, pathophysiology, treatment and prognostication. A scientific statement from the International Liason Committee on Resuscitation; The American Heart Association Emergency Cardiovascular Care Committee; the Council on Cardiovascular Surgery and Anesthesia; the Council on Cardiopulmonary, Perioperative, and Critical Care; the Council on Clinical Cardiology; the Council on Stroke. *Resuscitation*. 2008;79: 350–79. [PMID: 18963350]

Peberdy MA, et al. Part 9: post-cardiac arrest care: 2010 American Heart Association guidelines for cardiopulmonary resuscitation and emergency cardiovascular care. *Circulation*. 2010; 122:S768–86. [PMID: 20956225]

Stub D, et al. Post cardiac arrest syndrome: a review of therapeutic strategies. *Circulation*. 2011;123:1428–35. [PMID: 21464058]

Young GB. Neurologic prognosis after cardiac arrest. *N Engl J Med*. 2009;361:605–11. [PMID: 19657124]

B. Diagnostic Studies

1. Noninvasive evaluation for structural heart disease—

Once the patient has recovered to the point that long-term survival seems likely, efforts should be made to define fully the type and extent of underlying cardiac disease.

A. ELECTROCARDIOGRAPHY—Although the ECG usually provides the first information available, the initial ECG after defibrillation may be misleading. Transient ST segment elevation in leads with prior Q waves is common and does not always signify a new infarction as the primary cause of the arrest. However, patients with a new ST elevation myocardial infarction are candidates for acute mechanical or pharmacologic reperfusion, and it is better to proceed to catheterization whenever doubt exists., More commonly, the ECG after resuscitation will show such evidence of chronic disease, including old Q waves, conduction defects, or hypertrophy. ST segment and T-wave abnormalities appear in virtually all patients following resuscitation and

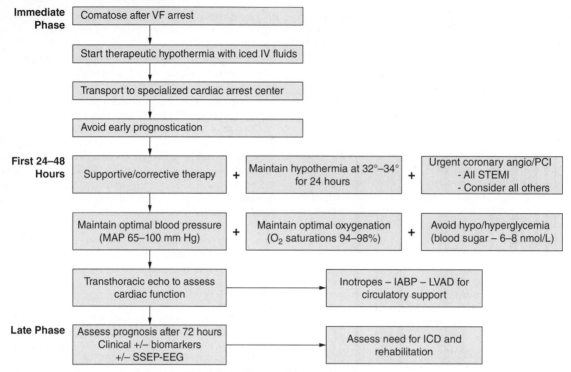

Immediate Phase
- Comatose after VF arrest
- Start therapeutic hypothermia with iced IV fluids
- Transport to specialized cardiac arrest center
- Avoid early prognostication

First 24–48 Hours
- Supportive/corrective therapy + Maintain hypothermia at 32°–34° for 24 hours + Urgent coronary angio/PCI - All STEMI - Consider all others
- Maintain optimal blood pressure (MAP 65–100 mm Hg) + Maintain optimal oxygenation (O₂ saturations 94–98%) + Avoid hypo/hyperglycemia (blood sugar – 6–8 nmol/L)
- Transthoracic echo to assess cardiac function → Inotropes – IABP – LVAD for circulatory support

Late Phase
- Assess prognosis after 72 hours Clinical +/– biomarkers +/– SSEP-EEG → Assess need for ICD and rehabilitation

▲ **Figure 15–1.** Proposed management algorithm for out-of-hospital cardiac arrest victims. IABP, intra-aortic balloon pump; ICD, implantable cardioverter-defibrillator; IV, intravenous; LVAD, left ventricular assist device; MAP, mean arterial pressure; PCI, percutaneous coronary intervention; SSEP-EEG, somatosensory evoked potential–electroencephalography; STEMI, ST elevation myocardial infarction; VF, ventricular fibrillation.

are of limited significance. The ECG may also be useful in the diagnosis of congenital and acquired LQTS, the Brugada syndrome, preexcitation syndromes, cardiomyopathies, and congenital heart disease.

B. Echocardiography—Echocardiography performed in the coronary care unit can provide a noninvasive assessment of cardiac function and anatomy shortly after resuscitation. An early, two-dimensional echocardiogram can provide valuable information about chamber size, wall thickness, valvular abnormalities, coronary artery anomalies, and ventricular function. Since myocardial stunning is common after arrest, improvements in ejection fraction over time occur frequently so serial studies are often helpful.

C. Other noninvasive tests—Other noninvasive tests may also be appropriate in some cases. Magnetic resonance imaging is particularly valuable in patients with congenital heart disease including coronary artery anomalies and ARVC with myocarditis. Positron emission tomography, magnetic resonance imaging, and isotope perfusion scans may be useful for assessing viability in regions of poor ventricular function. Preserved viability may influence decisions concerning the appropriateness of any attempts at revascularization.

2. Invasive evaluation for structural heart disease—Cardiac catheterization provides the most complete assessment of the structure, function, and blood supply of the heart, and it should be performed in virtually all survivors of cardiac arrest. Coronary artery disease is found in about 80% of cardiac arrest patients in the United States and Europe.

The prognosis of a patient who survives a cardiac arrest in the acute phase of a myocardial infarction is determined by the total amount of ventricular damage, the severity of residual ischemia, and the completeness of recovery from any noncardiac complications of the arrest. Treatment of these patients should be similar to that for other acute infarct patients, and special steps to define long-term antiarrhythmic therapy are not required. The role of ischemia in cardiac arrest patients without new Q-wave infarction is controversial. As noted earlier, "high risk" coronary artery lesions are often seen on coronary angiograms in cardiac arrest survivors and at autopsy in those who suffered sudden death. If these lesions are seen in patients with totally normal ventricular function, ischemia from these lesions alone may be responsible for the arrest. Correcting the ischemia through revascularization is the most appropriate—and sometimes the only required—therapy. More commonly, both a potential for acute ischemia and a fixed scar will be present. Transient ischemia may be a trigger for the arrhythmia. Since other triggers may exist, therapy should consider both the ischemia trigger and the underlying substrate.

3. Diagnosis of arrhythmias—A variety of arrhythmias can cause cardiac arrest and sudden death. Supraventricular arrhythmias with rapid ventricular rates and primary bradyarrhythmias are infrequent causes of cardiac arrest. However, it is important to identify patients with these arrhythmias because they will require a different therapeutic approach. Ventricular tachycardia and ventricular fibrillation are the most common causes of out-of-hospital cardiac arrest, and the evaluation and treatment of these arrhythmias will be the focus of the rest of this chapter.

A. NONINVASIVE EVALUATION—The role of noninvasive testing in patients who have suffered cardiac arrest is limited because a history of cardiac arrest has already placed them in a high-risk group. Noninvasive tests, however, are often used to assess the risk for future events in patients with known cardiac disease.

Exercise testing may be useful in some cases of exercise-induced ventricular tachycardia or in some patients with cardiac arrest to determine the presence of inducible ischemia. Abnormal prolongation of the QT interval in patients with LQTS and the appearance of arrhythmias in patients with congenital heart block may also be useful markers of future risk. In most cases, however, exercise testing is used to provide information about the potential for ischemia, rather than to diagnose the mechanism of arrhythmia or to guide therapy.

Ambulatory ECG monitoring is rarely useful in cardiac arrest survivors, but the presence of frequent and complex ventricular premature beats and abnormal heart rate variability are risk factors for sudden death during follow-up in patients with many forms of heart disease. In population studies, frequent or complex ventricular ectopy is associated with an increased risk of both sudden and nonsudden cardiac death. Unfortunately, the prognostic value of ambulatory ECG monitoring data in any individual patient is limited by poor day-to-day reproducibility of the data. The use of antiarrhythmic drug therapy guided by suppression of ventricular ectopic activity has not been shown to improve survival. Other noninvasive tests have been used to risk stratify patients. Tests that assess microvolt T-wave alternans during exercise, late potentials on a signal averaged ECG, heart rate variability, and baroreceptor sensitivity have been proposed, but their value in individual patients is controversial.

B. INVASIVE EVALUATION—Invasive evaluation involves a baseline electrophysiologic study that uses programmed electrical stimulation to initiate and characterize the patient's arrhythmia. As ICDs have become more accepted as the most effective therapy to prevent cardiac arrest, electrophysiologic studies have been relegated to a secondary role. They are now used to help define an arrhythmia mechanism if either an unusual mechanism of arrhythmia or an arrhythmia that

might be susceptible to ablation is suspected. The ability to identify an effective antiarrhythmic drug by serial testing is limited, and the failure rate of drug therapy selected by the technique is unacceptably high. However, electrophysiologic studies may be useful for characterizing the effects of drug therapy on tachycardias. Drug therapy may change the rate of many ventricular tachycardias and can affect defibrillation thresholds. Data obtained from electrophysiologic studies during drug therapy can be used to guide programming of ICDs.

▶ Treatment of Cardiac Arrest Survivors

Treating the cardiac arrest survivor requires a comprehensive strategy that must consider both aggressive and appropriate management of the underlying cardiac disease process as well as specific antiarrhythmic therapy.

A. Antiarrhythmic Drug Therapy

The role of antiarrhythmic drugs in the treatment of cardiac arrest survivors has changed substantially in the last 20 years. This change in strategy has been based on the results of randomized clinical trials for the primary and secondary prevention of sudden death. These trials have shown that therapy with class I antiarrhythmic drugs does not improve, and may worsen, survival when used for primary prevention in patients after myocardial infarction. When used in patients with a history of sustained ventricular tachycardia or ventricular fibrillation, class I drugs are inferior to sotalol and amiodarone. The latter drugs have, in turn, been shown to be less effective for improving survival than is therapy with an ICD.

Antiarrhythmic drugs, however, are still valuable for individual patients. Unstable arrhythmias are common in the immediate period after resuscitation. Intravenous amiodarone and β-blockers are the most effective treatments in this setting. Many patients with an ICD, in the absence of drug therapy, may have frequent episodes of sustained or nonsustained ventricular tachycardia that would trigger ICD therapy. Sotalol, a class III agent with β-adrenergic blocking activity, and amiodarone have been shown in randomized trials to decrease the frequency of ICD therapy. The usual dosage range for sotalol is 80–160 mg twice daily. Sotalol is cleared by the kidneys, and the dose should be adjusted in patients with renal insufficiency. QT interval prolongation that may result in torsades de pointes is the most worrisome complication. d,l-Sotalol is a potent β-adrenergic blocker, and bradycardia may limit therapy. Sotalol also lowers defibrillation thresholds. Amiodarone, if not started intravenously, is usually administered with an oral loading dose of 5–10 g in the first 1–2 weeks of therapy, followed by a daily dose of 200–300 mg. Common adverse reactions during amiodarone therapy include thyroid dysfunction, photosensitivity and skin discoloration, neuromuscular complaints, and abnormal liver function tests. Amiodarone-induced pulmonary toxicity can be life-threatening if unrecognized and occurs in approximately 1–2% of patients in the first year of therapy and in 0.5% of patients per year thereafter. Some patients will not be candidates for or will not desire ICD therapy. In those cases, sotalol or amiodarone would be the drugs of choice. Effective pharmacologic treatment to prevent ischemia and heart failure progression is also critical to long-term management.

B. Revascularization

Revascularization may play an important role in the care of both survivors of cardiac arrest and patients at risk for sudden death. In patients with ischemic heart disease and chronic stable angina, coronary revascularization decreases sudden death rates, with the greatest benefits being observed in patients with multivessel disease and depressed left ventricular function. Among cardiac arrest survivors, revascularization is indicated in patients with evidence of active ischemia or extensive areas of hibernating, dysfunctional but viable, myocardium. If no significant prior scarring is evident, revascularization alone may provide effective therapy for selected patients. In the presence of prior scarring, however, revascularization alone may not be effective at preventing future arrhythmias. Cardiac transplantation and left ventricular assist devices play important roles in patients with both arrhythmias and intractable ischemia or severe heart failure and in patients whose arrhythmias cannot be controlled with any less drastic form of therapy.

C. Surgical or Catheter Ablation

Direct surgical or catheter approaches have been developed to eliminate or ablate the myocardial areas where the reentry circuit responsible for ventricular tachycardia arises. Both approaches involve induction of tachycardia using programmed stimulation, mapping to determine critical portions of the tachycardia circuit, and either resection or ablation at the sites identified. Map-guided surgical resection procedures are no longer commonly performed due to the high mortality associated with these operations. Although catheter ablation has been successfully used in patients with sustained ventricular tachycardia, the highest success rates have been in patients with well-tolerated tachycardias or no structural heart disease. At present, the most frequent use of catheter ablation in cardiac arrest patients is as an adjunct treatment to reduce the frequency of arrhythmias in patients who also have ICDs. New ablation approaches designed to isolate large areas of arrhythmogenic myocardium may be effective in some patients with rapid and unstable arrhythmias.

Catheter ablation of an accessory atrioventricular connection will be curative in patients with cardiac arrest in association with preexcited atrial arrhythmias. In patients with ventricular tachycardia caused by macroreentry in the His-Purkinje system, ablation of the right bundle or left bundle will eliminate further episodes but often compromises AV conduction.

D. Implantable Cardioverter-Defibrillators

The first ICD was implanted for clinical use in 1980. Primitive by today's standards, the early devices clearly demonstrated the validity of the concept that a totally implanted device could be used to terminate life-threatening arrhythmias automatically. Advances in defibrillator technology have extended the applications of these devices, and ICD therapy is now considered the main therapeutic option for cardiac arrest survivors and for primary prevention in many high-risk patients.

An ICD has two basic components: the ICD generator and a lead system for pacing and shock delivery. An ICD generator contains sensing circuits, memory storage, capacitors, voltage enhancers, a telemetry module, and a control microprocessor. Advances in miniaturization and complexity in all of these components have permitted a tremendous reduction in the size of the generator itself despite increased functionality. Current devices have extensive programming options including, antitachycardia pacing, single- and dual-chamber rate-responsive pacing for bradycardia, biphasic defibrillation waveforms, enhanced arrhythmia detection features, innovations in lead systems, and cardiac resynchronization. The most important function of an ICD is to detect and terminate life-threatening ventricular arrhythmias (Figure 15–2). To accomplish this, the device is set to monitor heart rate, and various zones are considered to be ventricular tachycardia or ventricular fibrillation. When a heart rate in these zones is detected, programmable algorithms may be used to exclude supraventricular arrhythmias. Antitachycardia pacing is often used in an attempt to terminate ventricular tachycardia, but if this fails, the device will charge and deliver a high-energy shock (see Figure 15–2). The original systems required a thoracotomy to place epicardial patches, and as a result, the implant procedure itself was associated with substantial morbidity and mortality rates. After transvenous leads were developed that allowed successful defibrillation and the generator size was reduced, subcutaneous implants in the pectoral region became standard and implant morbidity was substantially reduced. Current systems are typically implanted by electrophysiologists using local anesthesia in a cardiac laboratory.

From the point of their introduction, there was little doubt that ICDs were very effective for terminating episodes of ventricular tachycardia and ventricular fibrillation. Initially, they were implanted chiefly in patients who did not respond to antiarrhythmic drug therapy as assessed by repeat ECG monitoring or electrophysiologic testing. As the limitations of antiarrhythmic drugs became more apparent, ICDs began to be seen as the primary treatment option. Three large randomized secondary prevention trials have compared ICD therapy with antiarrhythmic therapy

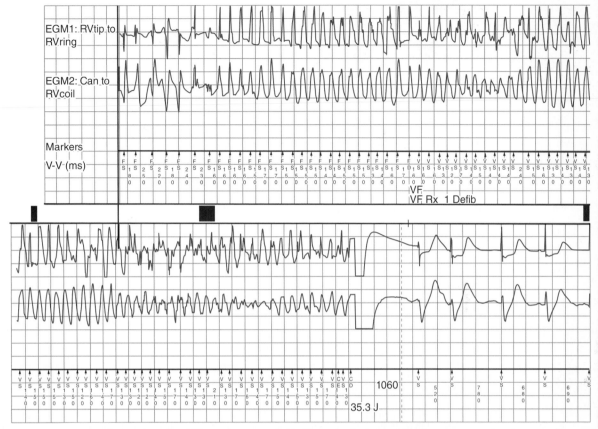

▲ **Figure 15–2.** Typical stored implantable cardioverter-defibrillator (ICD) electrogram from an episode of ventricular fibrillation (VF). A continuous two-panel printout of the stored electrogram from an aborted VF episode is shown. The top four tracings represent the bipolar electrogram from the RV lead, a far field electrogram from the RV coil to the ICD can, marker channels, and V-V intervals. The recording starts when the onset of VF is detected. Once the diagnosis is confirmed, the device charges, reconfirms that the arrhythmias is still present, and then terminates the episode with a 35.3-J shock.

in survivors of cardiac arrest or hemodynamically unstable ventricular tachycardia (Table 15–2). In the Antiarrhythmics Versus Implantable Defibrillator (AVID) study, 1016 patients were randomly assigned to either drug therapy (amiodarone or, rarely, sotalol) or an ICD. Survival analysis showed a decrease in total mortality rates of 39%, 27%, and 31% at follow-up points of 1, 2, and 3 years, respectively. The Cardiac Arrest Study Hamburg (CASH) randomly assigned 346 cardiac arrest survivors to either an ICD or drug therapy with one of three agents: amiodarone, metoprolol, or propafenone. The propafenone arm was terminated early due to an excessive mortality rate among those patients. At 2-year follow-up, the mortality rate was 37% lower in the ICD group than in the combined metoprolol and amiodarone group. In the Canadian Implantable Defibrillator

Study (CIDS), 659 patients with cardiac arrest, sustained ventricular tachycardia, or inducible ventricular tachycardia with unexplained syncope were treated with either an ICD or amiodarone. The mortality rate at 2-year follow-up was 19.7% lower in the ICD group. These three studies provide convincing evidence that an ICD should be first-line therapy in a cardiac arrest survivor.

ICD therapy has a number of limitations, however. Although efforts are made to distinguish between supraventricular and ventricular arrhythmias, this is not always successful, and inappropriate shocks for supraventricular arrhythmias are common. An ICD terminates arrhythmias by using either antitachycardia pacing or direct-current shocks. The latter produce significant discomfort, and patients who receive multiple shocks report significant

Table 15–2. Implantable Cardioverter-Defibrillator Trials

Trial	# of Patients	Age (years)	LVEF	Follow-Up (months)	Mortality Control (%)	Mortality ICD (%)	Relative RR (%)	Absolute RR (%)	NNT (36 months)
Secondary Prevention									
AVID	1016	65	0.35	18	24	16	31	8.2	9
CIDS	659	64	0.34	36	30	25	23	4.3	23
CASH	228	58	0.45	57	44	36	23	8.1	20
Primary Prevention									
MADIT	196	63	0.26	27	39	16	54	22.8	3
MADIT II	1232	64	0.23	20	20	14	31	5.4	10
DEFINITE	458	58	0.21	29	14	8	35	5.2	24
SCD-HeFT	1676	60	0.25	46	28	22	23	6.8	23
CABG-Patch	900	64	0.27	32	21	23	7 (increase)	1.7 (increase)	
DINAMIT	674	62	0.31	30	17	19	8 (increase)	1.7 (increase)	
IRIS	898	63	0.35	37	26	26	4 (increase)	0	

AVID, Antiarrhythmics Versus Implantable Defibrillator; CABG-Patch, Coronary Artery Bypass Graft-Patch Trial; CASH, Cardiac Arrest Study Hamburg; CIDS, Canadian Implantable Defibrillator Study; DEFINITE, Defibrillators in Nonischemic Cardiomyopathy Treatment Evaluation; DINAMIT, The Defibrillator in Acute Myocardial Infarction Trial; ICD, implantable cardioverter-defibrillator; IRIS, Immediate Risk Stratification Improves Survival; LVEF, left ventricular ejection fraction; MADIT I and II, Multicenter Automatic Implantable Defibrillator Trials I and II; NNT, number needed to treat; RR, risk reduction; SCD-HeFT, Sudden Cardiac Death in Heart Failure Trial.

negative effects on their quality of life. Although an ICD may be programmed to use various pacing strategies that may decrease shock frequency, these steps are not always effective, and antiarrhythmic drugs are often required as adjunctive therapy. Sotalol, amiodarone, and β-adrenergic blockers are the agents most commonly used to decrease shock frequency in patients with an ICD. Disease progression often limits the usefulness of an ICD, and the most effective use of ICDs in patients with far advanced disease is controversial. Hardware deterioration, although rarely life-threatening, continues to be a problem and may lead to the need for multiple invasive procedures. Finally, ICD therapy is very costly. Estimates of added cost over drug therapy per quality of life-year saved in the AVID and CIDS populations exceeded $100,000.

Tracy CM, et al. 2012 ACCF/AHA/HRS focused update of the 2008 guidelines for device-based therapy of cardiac rhythm abnormalities: a report of the American College of Cardiology Foundation/American Heart Association Task Force on Practice Guidelines. *Heart Rhythm.* 2012;9(10):1737–53. [PMID: 22975672]

▶ Identification of Patients at Risk

Even in communities with the most advanced systems for emergency response and out-of-hospital resuscitation, only a fraction of patients are resuscitated and survive to hospital discharge without significant residual deficits. In many areas, it is logistically impossible to rescue more than a small fraction of persons who suffer cardiac arrest. It is, therefore, important to be able to identify patients at high risk for sudden death and to determine the specific interventions that would be effective in this population.

A. Risk Assessment Studies

The most comprehensive assessments of factors that predict risk for future sudden death have been undertaken in populations of patients with recent myocardial infarction. In general, laboratory or clinical findings of residual ischemia, ventricular dysfunction, and electrical instability have been associated with an adverse prognosis. A number of findings have been identified as markers for chronic electrical instability. The presence of frequent or complex ventricular premature beats (VPBs) is a risk factor for sudden death after myocardial infarction. An increase in risk can be identified in patients with as few as 3–6 VPBs per hour on a 24-hour ambulatory recording. Poor day-to-day reproducibility in both the frequency and patterns of spontaneous ventricular arrhythmias limits the value of this finding in individual patients. Other findings during ambulatory monitoring may be useful. A decrease in the normally observed variability in R-R intervals during ambulatory ECG monitoring is a marker for heightened adrenergic tone and an increased risk of sudden death. The signal-averaged ECG is used to detect abnormal delays of ventricular activation that would be indistinguishable from noise in a routine ECG. These late potentials are frequently seen in patients with sustained monomorphic ventricular tachycardia and are predictors of mortality in patients after myocardial infarction. Microvolt alternation in T-wave amplitude during exercise is another finding thought to be a marker of increased risk. Decreased baroreceptor sensitivity and abnormal heart rate variability have also been used to identify high-risk patient subgroups. All proposed noninvasive tests have been limited by a fairly low positive predictive accuracy, and their utility for making individual patient decisions is controversial. Current guidelines for ICD implantation are evidence-based, with arrhythmia history, left ventricular ejection fraction, and New York Heart Association (NYHA) functional class, the bases for the indications.

B. Primary Prevention of Sudden Death

Primary prevention of sudden death remains an elusive goal. Although many risk factors have been identified, it has been difficult to show in clinical trials that therapy directed at any single risk factor is effective. β-Adrenergic blocking agents, cholesterol-lowering drugs, and angiotensin-converting enzyme (ACE) inhibitors have been shown to decrease both sudden and nonsudden deaths in patients with heart failure or after myocardial infarction, but these agents are not thought to treat arrhythmias in a specific fashion. Clinical trials have shown that class I antiarrhythmic drugs did not decrease sudden death mortality rates. In fact, the most definitive study—the Cardiac Arrhythmia Suppression Trial (CAST)—showed a higher mortality rate among patients who were randomized to drug therapy after it was shown that their spontaneous VPBs could be suppressed. Several studies using empirically prescribed amiodarone have reported improved survival after myocardial infarction, but the largest, placebo-controlled studies—the European and Canadian Amiodarone Myocardial Infarction Trials (EMIAT and CAMIAT) and the Sudden Cardiac Death–Heart Failure Trial (SCD-HeFT)—did not show any benefit. Dofetilide and azimilide have been tested in patients after myocardial infarction, and dofetilide in patients with chronic heart failure. Treatment with these two drugs showed no change in mortality rates. Cardiac resynchronization therapy in patients with advanced heart failure and a wide QRS has been shown to improve NYHA functional

Table 15–3. Indications and Contraindications for Implantable Cardioverter-Defibrillator Therapy

I. Indications for Secondary Prevention
 A. Documented episode of cardiac arrest due to ventricular fibrillation (VF), not due to a transient or reversible cause
 B. Documented sustained ventricular tachyarrhythmia (VT), either spontaneous or induced by an electrophysiology (EP) study (patients with syncope), not associated with an acute myocardial infarction (MI) and not due to a transient or reversible cause
II. Indications for Primary Prevention
 A. Documented familial or inherited conditions with a high risk of life-threatening VT, such as long QT syndrome or hypertrophic cardiomyopathy
 B. Coronary artery disease with a documented prior MI, a measured left ventricular ejection fraction (LVEF) < 35%, and inducible, sustained VT or VF at EP study. (The EP test must be performed more than 4 weeks after the qualifying MI.)
 C. Documented prior MI and a measured LVEF < 30%
 D. Patients with ischemic dilated cardiomyopathy, documented prior MI, New York Heart Association (NYHA) class II and III heart failure, and measured LVEF < 35%
 E. Patients with nonischemic dilated cardiomyopathy > 3 (preferably 9) months, NYHA class II and III heart failure, and measured LVEF < 35%
 F. Patients who meet all current Centers for Medicare and Medicaid Services coverage requirements for a cardiac resynchronization therapy (CRT) device and have NYHA class IV heart failure
III. Exclusions
 A. NYHA classification IV without CRT
 B. Cardiogenic shock or symptomatic hypotension while in a stable baseline rhythm
 C. Had a coronary artery bypass graft or percutaneous transluminal coronary angioplasty within past 3 months
 D. Had an enzyme positive MI within past 40 days
 E. Clinical symptoms or findings that would make them a candidate for coronary revascularization
 F. Any disease, other than cardiac disease (eg, cancer, uremia, liver failure), associated with a likelihood of survival less than 1 year
 G. Patients must not have irreversible brain damage from preexisting cerebral disease

Modified from Pub 100-03 Medicare National Coverage Determinations. Chapter 1, Part 1, Section 20.4 (Rev. 29, 03-04-05).

class, decrease hospitalizations, and reduce sudden and nonsudden cardiac deaths.

Randomized trials have indicated that ICD therapy for primary prevention of sudden death is effective in many populations. Summary data from a number of clinical trials are shown in Table 15–2, and the current indications for ICD insertion accepted by the Centers for Medicare and Medicaid Services (CMS) are shown in Table 15–3. The most recent trials have used entry criteria based primarily on left ventricular ejection fraction (below 30% or 35%) and

NYHA functional class. Most primary prevention trials have reported relative risk reductions in a range similar to those seen in the secondary prevention trials (20–30%) with three notable exceptions. The CABG-Patch Trial, the Defibrillators in Acute Myocardial Infarction Trial (DINAMIT), and the Immediate Risk Stratification Improves Survival (IRIS) study failed to show benefit in patients who received their ICD either at the time of surgical coronary revascularization or within 40 days of an acute myocardial infarction. These trials resulted in the specific exclusion of these conditions in the current CMS guidelines (Table 15–3).

Holzmeister J, et al. Implantable cardioverter defibrillators and cardiac resynchronization therapy. *Lancet.* 2011;378:722–30. [PMID: 21856486]

Roberts-Thomson KC, et al. The diagnosis and management of ventricular arrhythmias. *Nat Rev Cardiol.* 2011;8:311–21. [PMID: 21343901]

Theuns DAMJ, et al. Effectiveness of prophylactic implantation of cardioverter-defibrillators without cardiac resynchronization therapy in patients with ischaemic or non-ischaemic heart disease: a systematic review and meta-analysis. *Europace.* 2010;12:1564–70. [PMID: 20974768]

Syncope

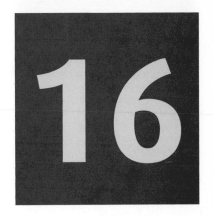

Michael H. Crawford, MD

ESSENTIALS OF DIAGNOSIS

- ▶ Sudden, unexpected, and transient loss of consciousness.
- ▶ Spontaneous and full recovery.

▶ General Considerations

Syncope can be defined as a sudden, transient loss of consciousness and postural tone that fully resolves spontaneously without specific intervention (eg, cardiopulmonary resuscitation [CPR], electrical or chemical cardioversion). The common pathophysiologic mechanism responsible for most syncopal spells is a transient reduction in cerebral blood flow and cerebral hypoperfusion. Reduced cerebral blood flow from cardiovascular and neurocardiogenic causes accounts for most cases in which a diagnosis can be made. Even when cerebral blood flow is normal, a reduced delivery of such essential cerebral nutrients as oxygen and sugar can occasionally cause altered consciousness.

Syncope is a common condition experienced by up to 50% of adults in a lifetime. It is responsible for about 3% of hospital admissions and 4% of emergency department visits. Physicians are frequently consulted to evaluate this symptom and—more commonly—presyncope, dizziness, or light-headedness, which may have a similar pathogenesis.

Syncope has many causes (Table 16–1), most of which have a benign prognosis. Because cardiac causes are associated with greater morbidity and mortality, early recognition of structural heart disease or other cardiogenic causes is important in order to prevent sudden death or injury.

▶ Pathophysiology & Etiology

A. Cardiac Causes

1. Obstruction to blood flow—Any obstructive structural lesion of the left or right side of the heart can critically reduce the cerebral blood flow. Exertional symptoms are common with obstructive lesions because cardiac output does not rise normally with exercise and cerebral perfusion is not maintained. Obstruction to left ventricular outflow occurs with aortic valve stenosis, mitral stenosis, left atrial myxoma, prosthetic aortic or mitral valve dysfunction, and hypertrophic cardiomyopathy. The ventricular arrhythmias that can occur with valvular heart disease may be responsible for both exertional and nonexertional syncope as well as sudden death.

Lesions that obstruct flow through the right side of the heart include right atrial myxoma, pulmonary stenosis, tricuspid stenosis, pulmonary hypertension, and pulmonary emboli. Limitations to right ventricular outflow diminish the cardiac output and the ability to increase the output with exertion. Exertional syncope is common with severe pulmonary hypertension and severe pulmonic stenosis.

Nonexertional syncope can be the result of pulmonary emboli (hypoxia and obstruction of right ventricular outflow) and aortic dissection with pericardial tamponade, which impedes right ventricular filling and decreases cardiac output.

2. Electrical disturbances

A. BRADYARRHYTHMIAS AND ATRIOVENTRICULAR BLOCK—Both bradyarrhythmias and tachyarrhythmias can cause transient decreased cardiac output with resultant cerebral hypoperfusion. Bradycardias result in symptoms when the rate is so slow that the compensatory increase in stroke volume is inadequate to maintain blood pressure. Periods of ventricular asystole as short as 5 seconds can cause syncope (from the ensuing cerebral hypoperfusion). Mechanisms of symptomatic ventricular bradycardia and asystole include sinus node disease (sinus exit block, sick sinus syndrome, marked sinus bradycardia, or sinus arrest) and second- or third-degree atrioventricular (AV) block. Syncope from Mobitz II second-degree AV block with paroxysms of several consecutive P waves that fail to conduct to the ventricle

Table 16–1. Major Causes of Syncope

Cardiac
　Obstruction to blood flow
　　Valvular stenosis
　　Hypertrophic cardiomyopathy
　　Prosthetic valve dysfunction
　　Atrial myxoma
　　Congenital heart disease
　　Pericardial tamponade
　　Pulmonary hypertension
　　Pulmonary emboli
　　Pump failure (myocardial infarction or ischemia)
　Arrhythmias (decreased cardiac output)
　　Bradyarrhythmias
　　　Sinus bradycardia
　　　Sick sinus syndrome
　　　Atrioventricular block (Adams-Stokes attacks)
　　　Pacemaker malfunction
　　　Drug-induced bradyarrhythmia
　　Tachyarrhythmias
　　　Ventricular tachycardia
　　　Supraventricular tachycardia
　　　Torsades de pointes
Neurocardiogenic
　Vasovagal
　Orthostatic
　Carotid sinus hypersensitivity
　Situational (tussis, micturition, defecation, deglutition)
Other Causes
　Seizures
　Drugs
　Hypoglycemia
　Hypoxia
　Hypovolemia
　Cerebral vascular insufficiency
　Extracranial vascular disease
　Neuralgia
　Psychogenesis
　Hyperventilation

diastole significantly and thus decrease ventricular filling (preload). Concomitant peripheral vasodepression with resultant hypotension may also play a role in the pathophysiology of syncope with supraventricular arrhythmias.

Ventricular tachycardia occurs most frequently in patients with organic heart disease, particularly coronary artery disease with previous myocardial infarction. Ventricular tachycardia is an important and ominous cause of syncope because ventricular tachycardia usually precedes ventricular fibrillation. Symptoms and prognosis are related to the degree of underlying myocardial dysfunction and the rate and duration of the arrhythmia.

Supraventricular arrhythmias are more likely to cause palpitations and presyncope than true syncope. Although they occur often in young patients with structurally normal hearts, they are also prevalent in structurally abnormal hearts. As with ventricular arrhythmias, the severity of the symptoms is related to the ventricular rate of the arrhythmia and the degree of underlying myocardial dysfunction. Mechanisms associated with syncope include atrial arrhythmias (fibrillation, flutter, tachycardia) with rapid ventricular response, AV nodal reentrant tachycardia, and supraventricular arrhythmias associated with accessory pathways.

Torsades de pointes is a rapid polymorphic ventricular arrhythmia classically known to cause syncope in association with class I antiarrhythmic drugs. Because this arrhythmia can also cause sudden cardiac death, it is very important to understand the reversible conditions that can precipitate it. Most cases of torsades de pointes are associated with acquired long QT syndromes that can occur with several drugs (class Ia and III antiarrhythmics, erythromycin, certain antihistamines, and tricyclic antidepressants), electrolyte abnormalities (hypomagnesemia, hypokalemia, and hypocalcemia), myocardial ischemia, and central nervous system disorders. Rarely, long QT syndrome occurs congenitally, in hereditary forms of prolongation of the QT interval (with or without associated deafness).

B. Neurocardiogenic Causes

1. Vasovagal syncope—This is the most common mechanism of syncope in young, otherwise healthy individuals, constituting approximately 60% of cases. The underlying mechanism is a paradoxical autonomic reflex resulting in profound hypotension (vasodepression) that is often associated with bradycardia (vasovagal). The underlying pathophysiology of vasovagal syncope has been elucidated with the aid of tilt-table testing (see the section on Diagnostic Studies). This technique provides a controlled means of reproducing vasovagal syncope and serves as a means to guide medical therapy. Before the development of tilt-table testing, the diagnosis of vasovagal syncope was largely a matter of exclusion.

Despite extensive study by numerous investigators, several controversies still remain regarding the underlying pathophysiology of vasovagal syncope. When one stands, a significant amount of venous pooling occurs, which can

is called an **Adams-Stokes** attack. Medications can also cause syncope, and any patient with syncope from bradycardia must be thoroughly questioned regarding medications. Calcium channel blockers, digoxin, β-blockers (including optical formulations), sympatholytics, primary antiarrhythmics, and other medications can all decrease heart rate and increase AV block—enough to cause symptoms in susceptible patients.

Pacemaker malfunction is another possible cause. If a pacemaker was previously implanted for sinus node disease or high-degree AV block and the patient has a recurrence of syncope, there may be a pacemaker system problem, such as battery failure or lead fracture.

B. TACHYARRHYTHMIAS—Transient decreased cardiac output during ventricular or supraventricular tachycardias results when the ventricular rate is fast enough to decrease shift from 300 to 800 mL of blood away from the central circulation. To counteract this gravitational effect, baroreceptors in the carotid sinus, aortic arch, and left ventricle sense decreased stretch (low pressure) and send afferent neural messages to the vasomotor center in the brainstem's medulla, which in turn sends efferent stimuli to increase peripheral sympathetic and cardiac tone (vasoconstriction and increased heart rate and contractility) and decrease vagal tone. This is the normal neural reflex arc that maintains cerebral arterial pressure and prevents hypotension or syncope with orthostatic changes.

It is believed that this reflex arc goes awry in susceptible individuals, resulting in a mixed response of vasodepression (hypotension) and cardiac inhibition (bradycardia). This symptomatic reflex arc, commonly known as a vasovagal episode, can occur as pure vasodepression or, rarely, pure cardiac inhibition; the classic mixed response is most common, with hypotension often preceding the bradycardia.

Vasovagal syncope is often, but not always, preceded by predisposing factors such as fear, pain, injury, fatigue, prolonged standing, or such medical procedures as venipuncture. During the initial phase, it is believed that blood pressure and heart rate increase in response to circulating catecholamine increase, sympathetic nerve stimulation, and vagal withdrawal. This is abruptly followed by hypotension, bradycardia, and syncope caused by inhibition of sympathetic vasoconstrictor and cardiac stimulatory activity and increases in vagal tone.

Although the exact pathophysiology is not understood, two conditions are thought to bring on the paradoxical reflex in susceptible individuals: reduced left ventricular filling (an empty ventricle) from decreased venous return and increased left ventricular pressure from increased contractility caused by cardiac stimulation from circulating catecholamines. A vigorously contracting empty ventricle is thought to paradoxically increase left ventricular pressure (mimicking hypertension), which is sensed by left ventricular stretch receptors (C fibers). This afferent neural arc to the nucleus tractus solitarius in the medulla results in an efferent arc that paradoxically decreases sympathetic and increases vagal tone, causing hypotension and bradycardia, respectively. Because both the sinus node and AV node are richly innervated with autonomic nerves, bradycardia can be caused by both vagal depression of sinus node automaticity and decreased AV nodal conduction with AV block. Assuming a supine posture provides spontaneous resolution because the gravitational effects on cerebral blood flow are immediately neutralized. Figure 16–1 shows a two-lead ambulatory recording of a classic vasovagal episode in a patient with previously undiagnosed syncope.

Vasovagal syncope is usually considered a benign form that can often be treated with patient education and avoidance of the precipitant. Some individuals, however, have frequent severe spells that result in injuries and, rarely, sudden death. Several therapies (discussed later) are available for patients who require intervention.

2. Carotid sinus hypersensitivity—The carotid sinus has baroreceptors located in the internal carotid artery just above the bifurcation of the common carotid artery. These are sensitive to stretch and pressure and give rise to afferent impulses to the vasomotor center in the medulla. In susceptible individuals, particularly the elderly, activation of this reflex results in vagal efferent stimulation, which causes marked bradycardia or AV block (the cardioinhibitory response) with vasodepression (from efferent sympathetic inhibition). In contrast to vasovagal syncope, the cardioinhibitory response is usually dominant. Syncope from carotid sinus hypersensitivity usually is suggested by historical factors: precipitation with turning the head, shaving the neck, or wearing a tight shirt collar. Spontaneous attacks can also occur. Full consciousness is usually regained in less than a minute after attaining a supine position. When syncope from carotid sinus hypersensitivity is suspected, carotid sinus massage (CSM) can be used to diagnose this condition; hypersensitivity is generally defined as cardiac asystole of 3 seconds or more or a decline in systolic blood pressure of at least 50 mm Hg.

3. Situational—The pathophysiologic mechanisms of syncope associated with micturition, defecation, coughing, and swallowing are not precisely elucidated. It is suggested that the vagal-sympathetic autonomic reflex (hypotension and bradycardia) is involved, with afferent neural stimulation coming from the involved viscera. The Valsalva maneuver (used during micturition, defecation, and coughing) is thought to contribute to hypotension by decreasing venous return, which decreases cardiac output.

In micturition syncope, which classically occurs on waking, a combination of physiologic changes that occur during sleep (eg, sudden decompression of the bladder, decreased heart rate and blood pressure) may contribute to syncope. Tussive syncope classically occurs in middle-aged men who drink alcohol, smoke, have chronic lung disease, and experience paroxysms of severe cough; it is thought to be largely due to decreased venous return caused by the Valsalva-like action of coughing. Deglutition syncope is believed to be entirely due to dysfunction of the afferent-efferent reflex arc and is associated with structural abnormalities of the esophagus (eg, diverticula, diffuse esophageal spasm, achalasia, stricture) and heart (eg, acute rheumatic carditis, myocardial infarction).

C. Orthostatic Hypotension

Volume depletion, medications, and autonomic dysfunction (primary and secondary) can all lead to cerebral hypoperfusion and syncope in the standing position. Primary chronic autonomic dysfunction is associated with Shy-Drager syndrome, Parkinson disease, and other rare dysautonomias. Secondary autonomic dysfunction with syncope has been described with diabetes mellitus, anemia, amyloidosis, multiple sclerosis, and human immunodeficiency virus (HIV) infection. Medications that commonly cause

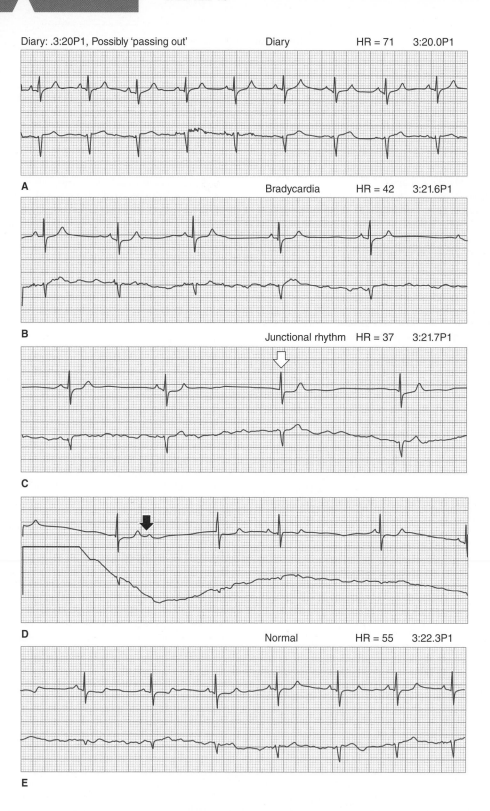

Diary: .3:20P1, Possibly 'passing out'   Diary   HR = 71   3:20.0P1

A

Bradycardia   HR = 42   3:21.6P1

B

Junctional rhythm   HR = 37   3:21.7P1

C

D

Normal   HR = 55   3:22.3P1

E

orthostatic hypotension include diuretics, antihypertensives (eg, angiotensin-converting enzyme [ACE] inhibitors, β-blockers, calcium channel blockers), and ethanol.

Essential to the diagnosis of orthostatic hypotension is evaluation of postural changes in blood pressure. Normal reflex mechanisms maintain blood pressure on standing (see discussion of neurocardiogenic syncope). The inability to maintain cerebral flow when standing or sitting upright, with resultant hypotension, dizziness, or syncope, is called orthostatic hypotension. Quantitatively, it has been defined as a 20 mm Hg or greater decline in systolic pressure or a 10 mm Hg or greater decline in diastolic pressure on assuming an upright position. Because this finding is frequent and asymptomatic in the elderly, the clinical diagnosis of syncope from orthostatic hypotension requires the presence of symptoms with blood pressure changes.

▶ Clinical Findings

A. History & Physical Examination

According to several prospective studies, the initial clinical evaluation establishes the cause of syncope or suggests the necessary diagnostic test in up to 85% of the patients in whom a diagnosis will eventually be made. A detailed history and physical examination are therefore essential parts of the initial clinical evaluation. Relevant historical information includes all details leading up to the event, precipitating factors (micturition, cough, exertion), premonitory symptoms (aura), onset (sudden or slow), associated symptoms (palpitations, chest pain, headache), activity (at rest or with exercise), position (standing, sitting, changing position), and details about the episode (injury, incontinence, rapid recovery versus postictal state) and the frequency and severity of the events. The history should include factors suggestive of cardiac or other systemic illnesses, such as a family history of cardiac illness, arrhythmias, syncope, sudden death, or pacemaker implantation. Because about 10% of syncope is caused by the use of medications and recreational drugs, information regarding their use, prescribed dosages, and the amount actually taken is very important. All witnesses to the event (family, friends, bystanders) should be thoroughly interviewed because they can often supply details that the patient cannot. These witnesses may be able to provide information about the patient's complaints just prior to the event and observations during both the event

(eg, pulse rate and rhythm, color, presence of spontaneous breathing, seizures, or seizure-like activity) and recovery. Electrocardiographic (ECG) recordings made by paramedics at the scene or recorded en route to the hospital and in the emergency department may provide important clues.

All patients need a complete cardiac, peripheral vascular, and neurologic examination, including an assessment of positional blood pressure and heart rate. Cardiac murmurs may be suggestive of structural heart disease, such as valvular stenosis. Differential blood pressure and pulse intensity may suggest aortic dissection or subclavian steal syndrome. Focal neurologic findings may point to seizure, stroke, or transient ischemic attack. The development of similar symptoms with upright posture and a corresponding decrease in blood pressure implicate orthostatic hypotension.

Several bedside maneuvers can be used to provoke syncope or presyncopal symptoms in appropriate patients. Arm flexion and extension may be used to provoke symptoms of subclavian steal syndrome; neck flexion and extension may elicit the symptoms of vertebrobasilar insufficiency. Open-mouthed hyperventilation for 1–3 minutes may elicit symptoms described in the history. CSM (when not contraindicated by presence of bruits or known carotid arteriosclerotic disease) can be performed at the bedside with ECG and blood pressure monitoring. Although the technique is not standardized, carotid massage is usually performed with the patient in the supine position, with 5 seconds of firm massage of each carotid body. Note that simultaneous bilateral massage is never done. A positive test is defined as at least 3 seconds of asystole with hypotension or reproduction of symptoms. Because of the high false-positive rate for CSM in the elderly, the diagnosis of carotid sinus hypersensitivity should only be considered if clinical events are associated with activities that press or stretch the carotid sinus.

Toxicology screens and medication levels may provide useful information and should be ordered if suggested by the patient's or the witness's history. Figure 16–2 outlines a suggested diagnostic approach.

Moya A, et al. Task force for the diagnosis and management of syncope, European Society of Cardiology, European Heart Rhythm Association, Heart Failure Association, Heart Rhythm Society, for the diagnosis and management of syncope. *Eur Heart J*. 2009;30:2631–71. [PMID: 19713422]

▲ **Figure 16–1.** Consecutive two-lead rhythm strips recorded from a patient wearing an ambulatory monitor during a vasovagal near-syncope spell, illustrating the classic response. **A:** In his diary, the patient indicates that he is possibly passing out. Because heart rate and rhythm are normal, the symptom is due to initial hypotension from vasodepression. **B:** As the episode proceeds, sinus bradycardia develops from vagal cardiac inhibition. **C:** Later still, sinus rhythm is completely suppressed, resulting in a junctional escape rhythm; *open arrow* shows first junctional beat. **D:** Vagal inhibitory effect on the atrioventricular node is also shown because a sinus beat did not conduct to the ventricle (*solid arrow*). **E:** Complete resolution to normal sinus rhythm, correlated with spontaneous full recovery.

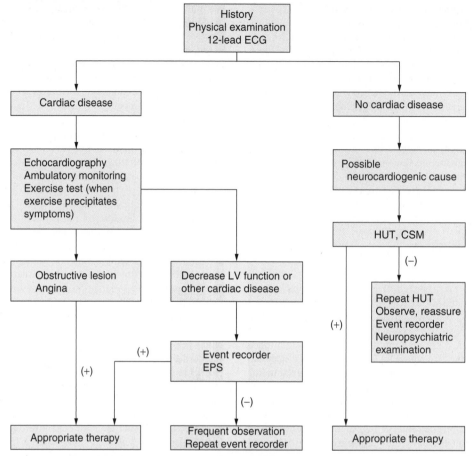

▲ **Figure 16–2.** Diagnostic approach to syncope. CSM, carotid sinus massage; ECG, electrocardiogram; EPS, electrophysiologic study; HUT, head-up tilt-table testing; LV, left ventricular.

B. Noninvasive Diagnostic Studies

1. Electrocardiography—A 12-lead ECG should be part of the routine clinical evaluation of syncope. A normal 12-lead ECG generally portends a good prognosis, with a very low incidence of either cardiogenic causes or diagnostic findings during invasive electrophysiologic testing. Unfortunately, the initial ECG rarely establishes arrhythmia as the cause unless complete heart block, ventricular tachycardia, or another abnormality is present at the time of the tracing. Given the unpredictably episodic nature of syncopal spells and the fact that most patients recover completely from them prior to the ECG, it is rare that the 12-lead ECG is diagnostic. More often, certain findings will suggest the possibility of a specific diagnosis. For example, Q waves suggestive of previous myocardial infarction correlate with abnormal electrophysiologic studies and the presence of inducible ventricular arrhythmias. Delta waves suggestive of Wolff-Parkinson-White syndrome make supraventricular

tachycardia a very likely diagnosis. A long QT interval suggests torsades de pointes, and bifascicular block correlates with abnormal electrophysiologic findings, including high-degree AV block and inducible ventricular arrhythmias.

The most common abnormalities found in patients with syncope are bifascicular block, prior myocardial infarction, left ventricular hypertrophy, sinus bradycardia, and first-degree or Wenckebach AV block. Although these findings are all nonspecific, they may suggest a cardiac cause. The ECG or rhythm strips recorded by paramedics, the emergency department, or hospital ward lead to a specific diagnosis in about 10% of patients. The most common diagnoses include ventricular tachycardia and bradyarrhythmias caused by sinus node dysfunction or high-degree AV block.

2. Echocardiography—If the history, physical examination, and ECG do not suggest the diagnosis, or if underlying heart disease is suspected, an echocardiogram is a valuable diagnostic tool. Echocardiography may diagnose the likely cause of syncope (aortic stenosis, hypertrophic heart disease); but, more commonly, it is useful in directing further evaluation. Because morbidity and mortality with syncope are directly related to the presence and severity of structural heart disease, the echocardiogram can aid the physician in assessing the patient's prognosis and the necessity for further invasive evaluation. For example, the finding of a low left ventricular ejection fraction suggests ventricular arrhythmias and would be an indication for further electrophysiologic evaluation or an implantable defibrillator. Unsuspected findings on echocardiography are reported in 5–10% of unselected patients with syncope. Although this is similar to the ECG, the cost of the study limits it to persons with no obvious cause or suspected underlying heart disease.

3. Exercise stress testing—Exercise stress testing may be useful in patients with exertional symptoms. Exertional hypotension may occur as a result of underlying structural heart disease, chronotropic incompetence, or severe conduction disease resulting in AV block with increased atrial rates. Supraventricular and ventricular arrhythmias may be provoked with exercise. Hypotension and bradycardia at the termination of exercise can be diagnostic of reflexive vasomotor instability. Also, exercise or other forms of stress testing in those who cannot exercise may detect myocardial ischemia—a potential substrate for ventricular arrhythmias.

4. Ambulatory monitoring—Prolonged ECG monitoring can be useful for documenting transient bradyarrhythmias or tachyarrhythmias. The most common method used is a Holter ambulatory ECG recording. Typically, two surface ECG leads are recorded for a period of 24–48 hours. Holter recording can be particularly helpful in diagnosing bradyarrhythmias, such as significant sinus pauses and transient high-degree AV block. When interpreting Holter recordings, clinicians must recognize that several abnormalities can occur in healthy, asymptomatic patients, and correlation with symptoms is often essential. Premature atrial and ventricular contractions, brief and paroxysmal atrial tachycardia, episodic AV Wenckebach block, sinus bradycardia, sinus pauses of up to 3 seconds especially when asleep, and nonsustained ventricular tachycardia can all be seen in

normal, asymptomatic patients. Sinus pauses of longer than 3 seconds, Mobitz II AV block, complete heart block, and frequent nonsustained ventricular tachycardia are far less prevalent.

Because the correlation of symptoms with an arrhythmia in patients with syncope provides the most valuable information, it is essential for the patient to keep an accurate diary of symptoms and activity during the recorded interval. Ambulatory monitoring is often useful in excluding arrhythmia mechanisms of syncope when patients experience syncope or presyncope without associated arrhythmias. Conversely, ambulatory monitoring may reveal significant conduction abnormalities or arrhythmias when the patient is asymptomatic. Frequent sinus pause of ≥ 3 seconds with associated atrial fibrillation indicates significant sinoatrial dysfunction. Asymptomatic Mobitz II AV block suggests distal conduction disease, with the possibility of prolonged AV block resulting in Adams-Stokes attacks. Nonsustained ventricular tachycardia in patients with significant left ventricular dysfunction (ejection fraction < 40%) correlates with a risk of sudden death from sustained ventricular arrhythmias and warrants further electrophysiologic evaluation (see section on Invasive Electrophysiology Studies).

A significant limitation of Holter ambulatory ECG recording is how infrequently patients experience either syncope or associated symptoms during the test. The results of studies suggest that Holter monitoring captures the heart rhythm during spontaneous syncope in only 4–10% of patients. For this reason, external ambulatory loop recorders have been used extensively for the evaluation of syncope. These devices record a single ECG lead continuously and can be worn by a patient for weeks. When activated by the patient or an observer, a rhythm strip is saved that includes several minutes surrounding the syncopal or presyncopal episode (Figure 16–3). The rhythm strip is sent to the laboratory using trans-telephonic equipment for added convenience for the patient and physician. Loop recorders are useful for evaluating patients with episodic syncope, presyncope, or dizziness, with or without associated palpitations.

For patients with infrequent symptoms, small loop recorders can be implanted under the skin and have a battery life of

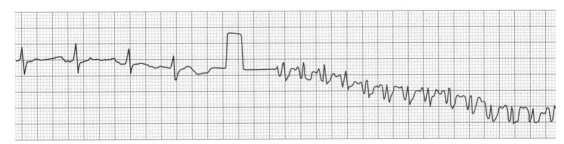

▲ **Figure 16–3.** Event recorder monitor strip received from a patient with a prior history of syncope, recurrent presyncope, and structural heart disease. The patient underwent an electrophysiology study and was found to have inducible monomorphic ventricular tachycardia that was treated with an implantable cardioverter-defibrillator.

1 year. They can be activated by the patient or a companion remotely, but newer models automatically record abnormal rhythms. This feature is especially valuable for patients who are rapidly incapacitated by their symptoms and cannot reliably activate a device. Although implantable loop recorders were once reserved as a last-resort diagnostic strategy, some physicians recommend earlier implantation because studies have shown diagnostic yields up to 87%.

5. Head-up tilt-table testing—Gravitational shifts in blood volume have long been recognized as a stimulus to neurocardiogenic syncope (also known as vasomotor, vasovagal, neurally mediated, or neurocardiogenic syncope). The use of the tilt table as a provocative maneuver in the diagnosis of unexplained syncope is decreasing because of concerns about the sensitivity, diagnostic yield, and reproducibility of the test. In patients with a normal cardiac evaluation, the pretest probability of neurocardiogenic syncope is high, so tilt-table testing is unlikely to be of value. The technique starts with monitoring the fasting patient for 10 minutes in the horizontal position, using noninvasive brachial or finger blood pressure, oxygen saturation, continuous ECG, and if somatization disorder is suspected, electroencephalogram (EEG) (true syncope can be differentiated from malingering). The patient is then tilted 60–80 degrees for up to 45 minutes; in children and adolescents, positive tests tend to occur sooner, and a period of 30 minutes is sufficient. The tilt produces a shift in blood volume distribution away from the central circulation and thorax to dependent peripheral vessels. This causes a decrease in central venous pressure, ventricular filling, stroke volume, and mean arterial blood pressure. Normally, activation of the baroreceptor-vasomotor reflex (described earlier) and renin-angiotensin system and release of catecholamines result in maintenance of blood pressure through increased heart rate and vasoconstriction. Monitoring of a normal passive tilt would show a small decrease in systolic blood pressure, with an increase in diastolic blood pressure, mean arterial pressure, and heart rate. All of these are considered normal adjustments to gravitational stress.

The test is considered positive if syncope or presyncope occurs with hypotension, with or without bradycardia. The patient is then quickly placed in the horizontal position, where normal compensatory mechanisms restore blood pressure and consciousness. The test is considered negative if symptoms and hemodynamic abnormalities fail to occur by 45 minutes of tilt. The tilt can be repeated with a provocative agent, such as the β-agonist isoproterenol, in selected patients (discussed later).

As previously discussed, various degrees of hypotension and bradycardia secondary to a paradoxical reflex that increases vagal tone and decreases sympathetic tone develop in susceptible patients. Both hypotension and bradycardia are present (a mixed response) in most patients. Hypotension usually predominates, however, and tends to occur before bradycardia (as shown in Figure 16–1). Hypotension that occurs alone, without bradycardia, is considered a purely vasodepressor response. Rarely, a patient may have a purely cardioinhibitory response (asystole).

The test has been shown to be 80–90% reproducible and specific, with a low false-positive rate (< 10%) in asymptomatic individuals. However, sensitivity ranges from 25% to 80% depending on the population studied. The 2006 American Heart Association (AHA)/American College of Cardiology Foundation (ACCF) scientific statement of the evaluation of syncope no longer recommends routine tilt-table testing for undiagnosed syncope. However, there are some patients in whom the diagnosis is unknown after a cardiac evaluation and the history is not helpful. Some of these patients would benefit from a tilt-table test, whereas in others a presumptive diagnosis of neurocardiogenic syncope is adequate.

6. Other testing—Routine laboratory tests (blood counts and chemistries) rarely reveal useful diagnostic information. Unless specifically suggested by the history and physical examination, it is not recommended in the evaluation of syncope. Likewise, EEG, computed tomography, or magnetic resonance imaging studies are of little use in patients whose history is not suggestive of a neurologic cause. These tests should be considered only in those patients whose neurologic history and physical examination are suggestive of seizure or other neurologic condition. Although routinely performed, the usefulness of transcranial Doppler ultrasonography in patients with syncope is unclear. Transient ischemic attacks rarely result in syncope without other associated symptoms. In patients with bruits on physical examination, ultrasonography is reasonable and may be useful in leading to a diagnosis.

C. Invasive Electrophysiology Studies

An invasive electrophysiology study (EPS) uses multielectrode catheters inserted percutaneously and guided under fluoroscopy or by magnetic sensors to specific cardiac locations. Electrode recording and pacing protocols are then performed to assess the patient's conduction system, including sinoatrial and AV nodal function and the distal conduction system (His-Purkinje). In addition, supraventricular and ventricular arrhythmias may be induced and their mechanisms determined in susceptible patients. In selected patients, ablation of the arrhythmic substrate with radiofrequency energy can be performed, often curing the patient of the condition.

Because patients are generally supine and sedated during EPS, one significant limitation is the inability to definitely correlate induction of arrhythmias with syncope; however, a rapid tachycardia associated with a significant decrease in systolic blood pressure generally supports the clinical importance of inducible arrhythmias. Induction of certain arrhythmias, such as atrial fibrillation, atrial flutter, polymorphic ventricular tachycardia, and ventricular fibrillation, can be a nonspecific finding. Asymptomatic patients with normal hearts can have all these induced with aggressive stimulation protocols.

The AHA/ACCF scientific statement on the evaluation of syncope does not recommend routine EPS in patients without underlying heart disease. It does recommend EPS in patients with cardiac disease and syncope that remains unexplained after appropriate evaluation, especially if the ejection fraction is reduced. In addition, EPS is reasonable in patients with recurrent unexplained syncope without structural heart disease and a negative head-up tilt test. In patients with no structural heart disease, normal ECG, normal ambulatory monitoring, and recurrent syncope not associated with injury, EPS is usually not diagnostic. EPS is not indicated in patients with a known cause of syncope for whom treatment will not be guided by electrophysiology testing.

The most significant finding at EPS is the induction of ventricular tachyarrhythmias. In addition, the induction of supraventricular tachycardias with associated hypotension is considered a positive study. Other significant findings include a prolonged corrected sinus node recovery time longer than 1000 ms, prolongation of the His-to-ventricle activation interval greater than 100 ms (normally 35–55 ms), or induction of infra-Hisian conduction block during rapid atrial pacing. These three findings are associated with significant bradyarrhythmias. Unfortunately, the diagnostic sensitivity of EPS for bradyarrhythmias is low, and further ambulatory monitoring is often necessary after a nondiagnostic EPS.

Krediet CT, et al. The history of diagnosing carotid sinus hypersensitivity: why are the current criteria too sensitive? *Europace.* 2011;13:14–22. [PMID: 21088002]

Romme JJ, et al. Diagnosing vasovagal syncope based on quantitative history taking: validation of the Calgary Syncope Score. *Eur Heart J.* 2009;30:2888–96. [PMID: 19687157]

Strickberger SA, et al; American Heart Association Councils on Clinical Cardiology, Cardiovascular Nursing, Cardiovascular Disease in the Young, and Stroke; Quality of Care and Outcomes Research Interdisciplinary Working Group; American College of Cardiology Foundation; Heart Rhythm Society; American Autonomic Society. AHA/ACCF Scientific Statement on the evaluation of syncope: from the American Heart Association Councils on Clinical Cardiology, Cardiovascular Nursing, Cardiovascular Disease in the Young, and Stroke, and the Quality of Care and Outcomes Research Interdisciplinary Working Group; and the American College of Cardiology Foundation: in collaboration with the Heart Rhythm Society: endorsed by the American Autonomic Society. *Circulation.* 2006;113(2):316–27. [PMID: 16418451]

▶ Differential Diagnosis

A. Seizure

True seizures are rarely established as the cause of a syncopal event, although they are frequently considered. A history of loss of bowel or bladder tone, witnessed convulsions, a preceding aura, and slow recovery with prolonged postictal state strongly suggest seizure. Syncope occurs frequently without a preceding aura or loss of sphincter tone and characteristically has a rapid spontaneous recovery without postictal state.

Some factors blur the distinction between these two entities: convulsions may occur with syncope (from cerebral anoxia or ischemia), the episode may be unwitnessed, the patient may not be able to recall associated symptoms, and the patient may have temporal lobe epilepsy, in which loss of consciousness is not associated with tonic-clonic movements. Temporal lobe epilepsy can also cause arrhythmias. Electroencephalography is indicated when the history cannot provide a clear distinction between syncope and seizure.

B. Metabolic Disorders and Hypoxia

Any condition that starves the cerebrum of essential nutrients (electrolytes, oxygen, glucose) or markedly changes pH can cause somnolence or coma. These conditions are not usually associated with spontaneous recovery (ie, without intervention); they tend to be longer lasting, and treatment is directed at the underlying abnormality. Hypoglycemia in outpatient diabetics, resulting from excessive insulin injection, can cause somnolence with a normal pulse and blood pressure; it is rapidly correctable with glucose.

C. Cerebral Vascular Insufficiency and Extracranial Vascular Disease

Although altered states of consciousness are known to occur with cerebral vascular events, true syncope is an uncommon presentation. Diseases of the intracranial and extracranial vessels can cause strokes and transient ischemic attacks, rarely syncope. Focal neurologic defects found during the physical examination are clues to the presence of cerebral vascular insufficiency, and differential peripheral arterial pressures or bruits suggest extracranial arterial disease. The extracranial arteries most commonly involved are the vertebrobasilar (occlusion), carotids (occlusion, emboli), aortic arch (dissection), and subclavian artery (stenosis), which may produce the subclavian steal syndrome.

D. Psychiatric Disorders with Hyperventilation and Pseudoseizure

Psychiatric illnesses are an important cause of syncope, especially in younger patients with multiple episodes and no organic heart disease. Depression, anxiety attacks, somatization disorder, panic disorder, and substance abuse (eg, alcohol, cocaine, sedatives) have all been associated with syncopal spells. In addition, pseudoseizure that may or may not be associated with true seizure disorder may be present.

Hyperventilation may cause syncope by producing hypocapnia and metabolic alkalosis, both of which stimulate cerebral arterial chemoreceptors to produce cerebral arterial vasoconstriction and decrease blood flow. Hyperventilation is frequently associated with such psychiatric illnesses as anxiety, depression, and panic attacks, but it can also occur sporadically in patients without psychiatric disease. A history of rapid breathing and perioral numbness is suggestive. A monitored hyperventilation maneuver that reproduces the patient's symptoms helps confirm the diagnosis.

▶ Treatment

Medical therapy is primarily targeted toward tachyarrhythmias, and pacemakers are generally used for bradyarrhythmias. In some situations, however, both are needed. For example, in sick sinus syndrome, a pacemaker is needed to prevent sinus bradycardia and pauses, and antiarrhythmic medications are needed to prevent the tachycardia (paroxysmal atrial fibrillation and flutter). Moreover, antiarrhythmic drugs can exacerbate bradycardia in some patients and necessitate implantation of a pacemaker to prevent medication-induced bradycardia and syncope.

A. Pharmacologic and Nonpharmacologic

Supraventricular arrhythmias can be treated with an assortment of antiarrhythmic medications (sodium channel blockers, β-blockers, potassium channel blockers, calcium channel blockers) with a wide range in therapeutic efficacy. Inherent in the medical treatment of arrhythmias, unfortunately, is a consistently high rate of side effects and the occurrence of proarrhythmia, worsening the arrhythmia or creating new arrhythmias such as torsades de pointes. Sustained ventricular arrhythmias can be suppressed with antiarrhythmic drugs; however, recent studies favor their use only in combination with an implantable cardioverter-defibrillator (ICD) in most patients.

Coronary artery, valvular, and other structural heart disease can usually be managed medically. If the disease has reached the point of causing syncope, however, it is usually severe enough to warrant surgical intervention or percutaneous revascularization.

Neurocardiogenic and situational syncope can be treated in a number of ways (Table 16–2). Education and avoidance of known precipitants are a first step. α-Agonists, such as ephedrine or midodrine, can be used to enhance vasoconstriction and counteract the vasodilation portion of the reflex arc. β-Blockers (eg, metoprolol, pindolol) have been used effectively; they are thought to work by decreasing inotropy and preventing the afferent loop of the paradoxical reflex arc. Propantheline and scopolamine have been used for their anticholinergic effects against the vagal efferent loop of the reflex. The sodium channel blocker disopyramide has been used successfully, although its mechanism of action against neurocardiogenic syncope is poorly understood. Theophylline, an adenosine antagonist, has also been used successfully (adenosine is thought to be a mediator of vasodepression in the reflex arc). Some success has been reported using the antidepressants (serotonin

Table 16–2. Medical Treatment of Neurocardiogenic Syncope

Class	Drug	Dosage Range
α-Agonists	Ephedrine	24 mg, two to four times daily
	Etilefrine	15-30 mg/day
	Midodrine	2.5 mg, two or three times daily, up to 40 mg/day
β-Blockers	Metoprolol	25-100 mg, twice daily
	Pindolol	5-30 mg, twice daily
Anticholinergics	Propantheline	7.5-15 mg, three times daily
	Scopolamine patch	1.5 mg over 3 days
Sodium channel blocker	Disopyramide CR	150–300 mg, twice daily[1]
Adenosine antagonist	Theophylline	200–450 mg, twice daily[1]
Serotonin antagonist	Sertraline	50-200 mg/day
Antidepressant	Fluoxetine	20-80 mg/day
Mineralocorticoid	Fludrocortisone	0.1 mg/day

[1]Dose can be guided by serum levels.
CR, controlled release.

reuptake inhibitors) fluoxetine and sertraline. Although the mechanism of action is not fully understood, serotonin is believed to play a central role in the development of vasovagal syncope. Volume expansion with liberalization of salt and water intake, administration of the mineralocorticoid fludrocortisone, and the use of thigh-high elastic stockings are effective because they can augment venous return. Also, isometric exercise such as handgrip and leg tensing can raise systemic blood pressure and prevent syncope if applied as soon as premonitory symptoms are appreciated.

None of these therapies has been shown to have any particular therapeutic advantage over the others. The specific therapy chosen should be based on the patient's age, lifestyle, and medication side effects. Each therapy can be given an empiric trial until an effective agent is found, or a repeat tilt-table test response can be used as a guide to long-term therapy.

When drug-induced syncope is suspected, the offending agent should be discontinued and the patient monitored closely for recurrence. In the case of documented or suspected torsades de pointes, the underlying drug; electrolyte abnormality; or thyroid, neurologic, or cardiac cause must be sought and corrected. Intravenous magnesium, lidocaine, or isoproterenol or temporary ventricular pacing can be used to stabilize a patient with torsades de pointes while the underlying problem is corrected.

B. Electrophysiologic Therapies

Implantable devices, such as the ICD and pacemakers, surgical procedures, and catheter ablation have all been used to treat syncope in appropriate patients. Besides causing syncope, ventricular tachycardia has the potential to degenerate to ventricular fibrillation. Many electrophysiologists consider syncope with ventricular tachycardia to be aborted sudden cardiac death. For this reason, patients with structural heart disease, documented ventricular tachycardia, and associated syncope are best treated with an ICD; moreover, patients with structural heart disease, syncope of unknown origin, and inducible ventricular arrhythmias during EPS are also most commonly treated with an ICD. The device continuously monitors the patient's heart rate and can apply a direct-current (DC) shock to convert ventricular fibrillation or tachycardia to sinus rhythm. ICDs have been found to reduce the likelihood of mortality in appropriate patients when compared with antiarrhythmic drugs. Although an ICD does not always prevent syncope, it effectively prevents sudden cardiac death. In addition, an ICD can terminate some ventricular tachycardias with rapid ventricular antitachycardia pacing (ATP). This therapy is painless and often unnoticed by the patient.

Ventricular tachycardia with associated ventricular aneurysm has also been successfully treated with open heart surgical ablation. With the development of nonthoracotomy ICD implantation, surgical ablation has become less common. In addition, nonsurgical catheter ablation techniques have been developed that allow for the treatment of some selected patients in the electrophysiology laboratory. In most patients, surgical or catheter ablation is used to reduce frequent appropriate ICD shocks and does not replace ICD therapy.

Single- and dual-chamber pacemakers are very effective in reducing symptomatic recurrences and preventing sudden death in patients with syncope caused by bradyarrhythmias from sinus node dysfunction, sick sinus syndrome with bradyarrhythmias and tachyarrhythmias, high-degree AV block, and carotid sinus hypersensitivity. Pacemaker therapy has been shown to have little role in treating neurocardiogenic syncope, largely because vasodepression is often the dominant component of the reflex and is not corrected by pacing. Pacemaker implantation may occasionally be appropriate for these patients if temporary pacing shows that the symptoms can be minimized (converting syncope to dizziness only) or if the episodes are purely cardioinhibitory. It may also be considered if multiple medications have been ineffective in severely diseased patients with mixed (vasodepressive and cardioinhibitory) episodes and the desired goal is to convert syncopal to presyncopal spells by abolishing the cardioinhibitory component.

In the past decade, electrophysiologic percutaneous catheter techniques using radiofrequency energy as an ablative source have been more than 95% effective in curing patients with supraventricular arrhythmias from AV nodal reentry or accessory pathways. Although successful ablation of atrial tachycardias, atrial flutter, some ventricular tachycardias, and even atrial fibrillation can be performed in selected patients, recurrence is not uncommon. In the case of atrial fibrillation with an uncontrollably rapid and symptomatic ventricular response, creation of complete heart block with catheter ablation and implantation of an activity-modulated ventricular pacemaker can effectively ameliorate symptoms.

Benditt DG, et al. Syncope: therapeutic approaches. *J Am Coll Cardiol*. 2009;53:1741–51. [PMID: 19422980]

Brignole M, et al. Prospective multicentre systematic guideline-based management of patients referred to the syncope units of general hospitals. *Europace*. 2010;12:109–18. [PMID: 19948566]

Brignole M, et al. Pacemaker therapy in patients with neurally-mediated syncope and asystole: Third International Study of Syncope of Uncertain Etiology: a randomized trial. *Circulation*. 2012;125:2566–71. [PMID: 22565936]

Romme JJ, et al. Effectiveness of midodrine in patients with recurrent vasovagal syncope not responding to non-pharmacological treatment (STAND-trial). *Europace*. 2011;13:1639–47. [PMID: 21752826]

Sheldon R, et al; POST Investigators. Prevention of Syncope Trial (POST): a randomized, placebo-controlled study of metoprolol in the prevention of vasovagal syncope. *Circulation*. 2006; 113(9):1164–70. [PMID: 16505178]

van Dijk N, et al; PC-Trial Investigators. Effectiveness of physical counterpressure maneuvers in preventing vasovagal syncope; the Physical Counterpressure Manoeuvres Trial (PC-Trial). *J Am Coll Cardiol*. 2006;48(8):1652–7. [PMID: 17045903]

▶ Prognosis

The studies to date suggest that mortality rates in patients with syncope are strongly correlated with the presence or absence of underlying structural heart disease. Dividing syncope patients into three groups is helpful for assessing their prognosis. In patients with cardiac causes of syncope, mortality is high at 1 year, ranging from 18% to 33%. In patients with noncardiac causes of syncope, 1-year mortality is much lower and ranges from 0% to 12%. Patients in whom syncope remains of unknown origin (despite an appropriate directed workup) do fairly well with a 6% 1-year mortality rate. The incidence of sudden death in the cardiac patients is also much higher than in the other two groups. Recurrence rates in all three groups are similar: up to 15% per year. Recurrences do not predict an increase in mortality, although they are associated with increased morbidity (eg, fractures, soft tissue injury).

In the emergency department, the main goal of triage is to identify high-risk patients who would benefit from hospitalization or observation with monitoring for 24–48 hours and appropriate treatment. Presumably low-risk patients could be discharged with outpatient follow-up. To facilitate this effort, several rules and scores have been developed. The easiest to use are the rules that are lists of risk factors and if one or more are present, the patient is at high risk of an untoward event. The only externally validated rule is the San Francisco Syncope Rule, which states that if any of the following five conditions is present, the patient should be admitted: congestive heart failure; hematocrit < 30%; ECG abnormalities; shortness of breath; or systolic blood pressure < 90 mm Hg (acronym CHESS). The scores assign risk points to several variables, and the derived total score is related to risk. The scores tend to focus on cardiac adverse events and were not designed for use in initial triage.

Recurrent syncope of unknown origin remains a difficult management problem. Patients with multiple atraumatic episodes and structurally normal hearts are more likely to have psychiatric illness or neurocardiogenic syncope and less likely to have electrophysiologic abnormalities at EPS. Memory-loop event recorders (to rule out bradyarrhythmias and tachyarrhythmias), tilt-table testing, and neuropsychiatric evaluation are probably the best means of evaluating these patients further. Patients with syncope of unknown origin and no structural heart disease have an excellent prognosis. They need to be reassured, but close follow-up and episodic reevaluation are also recommended. Intensive follow-up and reevaluation are needed for the patient with underlying heart disease and syncope of unknown origin. Such patients are not rare, and therapy should be directed at likely causes (such as EPS-induced sustained ventricular tachycardia). Empiric therapy (such as antiarrhythmic medication to suppress ventricular ectopy) is not without significant risk, however, and cannot be recommended as a general approach.

Costantino G, et al. Short- and long-term prognosis of syncope, risk factors, and role of hospital admission: results from the STePS (Short-Term Prognosis of Syncope) study. *J Am Coll Cardiol.* 2008;51:276–83. [PMID: 18206736]

Reed MJ, et al. The ROSE (risk stratification of syncope in the emergency department) study. *J Am Coll Cardiol.* 2010;55: 713–21. [PMID: 20170806]

Ruwald MH, et al. Prognosis among healthy individuals discharged with a primary diagnosis of syncope. *J Am Coll Cardiol.* 2013;61:325–32. [PMID: 23246392]

Sun BC, et al. External validation of the San Francisco syncope rule. *Ann Emerg Med.* 2007;49:420–7. [PMID: 17210201]

Aortic Stenosis

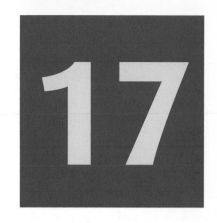

Steven J. Lester, MD

Amr E. Abbas, MD

ESSENTIALS OF DIAGNOSIS

▶ History: angina, dyspnea, syncope.

▶ Physical examination: midsystolic murmur; small and slow rising carotid pulse contour (parvus et tardus).

▶ Echocardiography: thickened immobile aortic valve leaflets; increased peak transaortic jet velocity and mean gradient; reduced valve area.

▶ General Considerations & Etiology

Over the past century, there has been a linear climb in record life expectancy and an overall aging of the human race. Therefore, we are faced with an epidemic of aging and age-associated disease, not the least of which is valvular heart disease. Aortic stenosis, the narrowing of the aortic valve orifice caused by failure of the leaflets to open normally, is now the most common indication for valve replacement in North America and Europe.

The pathogenesis of aortic stenosis is most commonly progressive calcification and degeneration of a trileaflet or congenitally bicuspid valve. Although once thought to be a degenerative process, it is now recognized that calcific aortic stenosis is in fact an active disease process that shares similarities to atherosclerosis where there is inflammation, lipid accumulation, and calcification of the leaflets. The mechanisms by which some valves degenerate and become stenotic while others remain relatively normal are unknown but are probably related to genetic polymorphisms. Those with end-stage renal disease, Paget disease, or severe familial hypercholesterolemia may present with calcific aortic stenosis at a younger age and are susceptible to more rapid progression of stenosis severity.

Rheumatic valve disease is a rare cause of aortic stenosis in industrialized nations. However, for indigenous populations within these countries as well as in developing countries, there remains a significant prevalence of rheumatic valve disease. In contrast to calcific aortic valve stenosis, the rheumatic valve shows adhesion, leaflet retraction, and commissural fusion. Along or just a few millimeters away from the free margins of the valve leaflets, small sessile nodules develop that also contribute to leaflet malcoaptation. Therefore, the rheumatic aortic valve invariably will leak. Rheumatic aortic valve disease is almost never present in isolation, and there is invariably concomitant mitral valve disease. A patient with aortic stenosis and a perfectly normal mitral valve should be considered as having another cause for their disease. Other rare causes of aortic stenosis include those associated with connective tissues diseases such as systemic lupus erythematosus and ochronosis.

▶ Clinical Findings

A. History

Those with acquired aortic stenosis generally have a long latent period before the onset of the salient clinical manifestations of the disease: effort-related dyspnea (heart failure), angina, and syncope. The most common initial clinical manifestations are a gradual decline in functional capacity and effort-related dyspnea. Regardless of the initial presenting symptom(s), it is imperative to ensure that the pathophysiologic mechanism is attributed to valve disease and not another mechanism such as concomitant coronary artery or lung disease because the onset of even mild symptoms attributed to aortic stenosis heralds a dramatic increase in the mortality rate for these patients if the valve is not replaced. Symptoms are therefore the guidepost for intervention, and understanding them is the key to understanding and managing the disease.

The primary determinants of left ventricular systolic function are contractility and afterload. The load on individual myocardial fibers can best be described as left ventricular wall stress and defined by the Laplace equation:

$$\text{Wall Stress} = \frac{\text{Pressure} \times \text{Radius}}{2 \times \text{Thickness}}$$

With acquired aortic stenosis, the obstruction will commonly progress gradually over time. Left ventricular adaptation to increases in systolic pressure is the parallel replication of sarcomeres to increase its thickness (concentric hypertrophy) in an effort to normalize wall stress and maintain systolic performance. As the severity of stenosis progresses, the increase in wall thickness may become insufficient to offset the rise in pressure ("afterload mismatch"), resulting in a rise in wall stress and a decline in ventricular function. The presence of aortic stenosis may also result in true depression of myocardial contractility, the exact mechanism of which is unclear but likely related to a loss of contractile elements secondary to reduced coronary blood flow. Thus a decline in ejection fraction results from the interplay of varying degrees between excessive afterload and true myocardial depression. Those in whom the decline in function is largely attributed to afterload mismatch are more likely to restore ventricular function following aortic valve replacement. The evaluation of left ventricular ejection phase indices should be related to the global wall tension; however, clinically it is very difficult to tease out the extent by which wall stress (afterload) and contractility are contributing to a noted decline in ejection fraction.

1. Dyspnea and exercise intolerance—The increase in left ventricular wall thickness, although imposed in an effort to maintain wall stress and systolic performance, does have maladaptive physiologic consequences. The increase in wall thickness makes it harder to fill the ventricle, and therefore, higher filling pressures are required to achieve any given volume, and end-diastolic volume will be required to increase to allow the maintenance of a normal ejection fraction (a rightward shift in the ventricular diastolic pressure volume relationship) (Figure 17–1). In alignment with the concepts of continuity disease, when the mitral valve opens, the left atrium is now exposed to the hemodynamic milieu of the left ventricle. The increased ventricular diastolic pressure is transmitted to atrium and further back into the pulmonary veins and lungs, resulting in pulmonary congestion and an increased work of breathing. Additionally, with outflow obstruction, there is a prolongation of the ejection phase; this in conjunction with an exercise-induced increase in heart rate will result in a reduction of the diastolic filling time, and the ventricle will reach its limit of "preload reserve." Once limits of preload reserve are met, stroke volume now becomes directly related to ventricular pressure (see Figure 17–1), resulting in an inability to increase cardiac output and further contributing to the presence of dyspnea and exercise intolerance.

2. Angina—Angina results from myocardial ischemia, which occurs when there is an imbalance between myocardial oxygen requirements/demand and myocardial oxygen supply. Although epicardial coronary artery disease often coexists with aortic stenosis, symptoms of angina frequently occur in those without epicardial coronary artery disease. Oxygen demand is best estimated clinically by the product of heart rate and wall stress, and as noted earlier, eventually

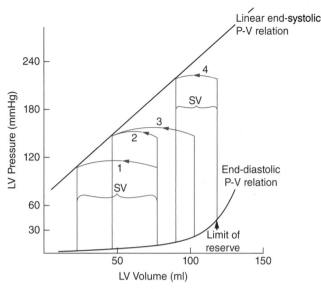

▲ **Figure 17–1.** Left ventricular (LV) pressure-volume (P-V) loops. Loop 1 is normal. As LV pressure increases, stroke volume (SV) would decrease if end-diastolic volume were fixed (loop 2). The ventricle, however, adapts by increasing end-diastolic volume to maintain a normal SV (loop 3). Eventually, the limits of preload reserve are met, whereby increases in LV pressure result in a decline in SV (SV is now directly related to LV pressure; loop 4). (Adapted with permission from Ross J. *J Am Coll Cardiol.* 1985;5[4]:811–26.)

the extent of hypertrophy cannot keep up with pressure demands of the ventricle and wall stress increases. In the absence of epicardial coronary artery disease, myocardial oxygen supply may also be decreased secondary to the rise in left ventricular end-diastolic pressure and a delayed rate of ventricular relaxation, which impairs coronary "diastolic suction," both contributing to reduced coronary perfusion and a decline in coronary flow reserve needed to offset increased oxygen demands during stress or exercise. In addition, with exercise and increased heart rates, there is reduced diastolic coronary perfusion time.

3. Syncope—Syncope is a transient loss of consciousness due to cerebral hypoperfusion. Syncope in those with aortic stenosis usually occurs during exercise. There are two primary mechanisms, not mutually exclusive, which have been theorized to cause syncope. First, the narrowed aortic valve does not permit the appropriate increase in cardiac output necessary to offset the associated reduction in total peripheral resistance associated with exercise, resulting in a drop in blood pressure. Second, the very high ventricular pressure that develops with exercise when sensed by ventricular mechanoreceptors triggers a reflexive vasodepressor response, also leading to a decline in blood pressure.

Less commonly, exercise can result in either ventricular or supraventricular arrhythmias, which can lead to a reduction in cardiac output and consequently a drop in blood pressure.

B. Physical Examination

1. Murmur—The character of a murmur can be described by its timing and shape, intensity and pitch, and location and radiation, along with changes in these characteristics imposed by transient changes in intracardiac hemodynamics.

A. TIMING AND SHAPE—The murmur of valvular aortic stenosis is a midsystolic murmur, which begins after the first heart sound and ends before the aortic (A_2) component of the second heart sound. During systole, as blood flow velocity accelerates across the valve, the intensity of the murmur increases, and as blood flow velocity decelerates, the intensity diminishes. Therefore there is a classic "crescendo-decrescendo" configuration or shape to the murmur of valvular aortic stenosis. Further insights into the configuration of the murmur may help to discern the severity of disease, where the later in systole the peak intensity occurs, generally the stenosis severity is more severe.

B INTENSITY AND PITCH—The intensity of the aortic stenosis murmur relates to the quantity and velocity of transaortic blood flow along with the ability to transmit sound through the chest. The pitch of the murmur relates to the pressure gradient and size of the "aperture" with which the blood flows through. In general, as the stenosis severity increases, the intensity and pitch of the murmur will increase. However, in those with a thick ventricle and low end-diastolic volume or in the presence of a decline in cardiac function, both of which may result in a low stroke volume, the intensity and pitch of the murmur may be lower than expected for the given severity of stenosis. Additionally, the ability to transmit the sound through the chest is impaired in those with a pericardial effusion, emphysema, or obesity. Therefore, one should be cautious in excluding significant aortic stenosis solely based on murmur intensity or pitch.

C. LOCATION/RADIATION—The murmur of aortic stenosis typically is heard loudest in the "aortic area," the right second interspace at the sternal border, and will often radiate into the carotids and along a line from the aortic area toward the left ventricular apex. At the apex, the intensity and pitch of the murmur may change to more resemble those of the murmur of mitral regurgitation; however, the shape and configuration of the murmur do not change. This is known as the Gallavardin phenomenon.

D. RESPONSE TO MANEUVERS—A transient alteration in intracardiac hemodynamics may influence the characteristics of a murmur, helping to further specify its etiology.

- Isometric handgrip: Increases systemic vascular resistance and blood pressure, decreasing the intensity of the murmur of aortic stenosis.

- Standing/Valsalva maneuver (phase II): Decreases ventricular filling, reducing the intensity of the murmur of

aortic stenosis and most all other valve murmurs except for that of hypertrophic cardiomyopathy and the duration of the murmur of mitral valve prolapse.

- Squatting: Increases ventricular filling but also increases systemic vascular resistance. Its effect on the murmur of aortic stenosis is therefore generally neutral; however, it will reduce the intensity of the murmur of hypertrophic cardiomyopathy.

- Cycle length: The intensity of the murmur of aortic stenosis may vary from beat to beat in those with atrial fibrillation or premature contractions, increasing in intensity in the beats following a longer R-R interval where diastolic filling time is increased.

2. Carotid pulse—The carotid artery pulse wave contour in those with aortic stenosis is characterized as small and slow rising (parvus et tardus). However, in older individuals with reduced arterial compliance, this finding is abrogated by increased reflected waves in the aorta. One may also appreciate a carotid shudder.

3. Heart sounds

A. SECOND HEART SOUND (S_2)—The presence of significant aortic stenosis may result in *paradoxical splitting* of the second heart sound where the A_2 component of S_2 is delayed, resulting in S_2 being more split during expiration than inspiration. Reduced movement of the aortic valve may render A_2 inaudible where only a *single* second heart sound can be appreciated.

B. FOURTH HEART SOUND (S_4)—As noted earlier, left ventricular hypertrophy imposed by the increase in wall stress reduces ventricular wall compliance. The fourth heart sound is a low-pitch sound heard coincident with late diastolic filling, due to atrial contraction, in a ventricle with reduced wall compliance and increased end-diastolic pressure.

4. Apical impulse—The apical impulse, which in aortic stenosis is generally also the point of maximal impulse, remains in its normal position but is sustained due to prolongation of the ejection time. The atrial component of ventricular filling may also be palpable. With simultaneous palpation of the apical and carotid impulses, normally one will appreciate little delay in their peaks; however, they become separated in time proportional to the severity of stenosis.

C. Diagnostic Studies

The clinical severity of aortic stenosis is largely an operational classification based on the presence or absence of symptoms, as discussed earlier. However, the indications for consideration of either a surgical or percutaneous aortic valve replacement rely on an estimate of stenosis severity.

1. Electrocardiogram—Left ventricular hypertrophy is the primary finding noted in those with aortic stenosis. Other common findings include left atrial abnormality and

ST- and T-wave abnormalities. There are, however, no electrocardiogram findings that are either sensitive or specific for aortic stenosis.

2. Chest radiography—With isolated aortic stenosis, the cardiac silhouette is generally normal in size with possible rounding of the left heart border consistent with concentric left ventricular hypertrophy. There may be signs of left atrial enlargement and pulmonary venous hypertension. The aortic shadow may become enlarged, and valve calcification may be appreciated.

3. Echocardiography—Echocardiography is the principal clinical tool used for the evaluation of aortic stenosis. Appropriate use criteria deem echocardiography appropriate when clinical evaluation provides "reasonable suspicion of valvular or structural heart disease or re-evaluation of known valvular heart disease with a change in clinical status or cardiac exam or to guide therapy." Routine surveillance in the absence of a change in clinical status or cardiac examination is deemed appropriate every 3 years in those with mild and every 1 year in those with moderate to severe valvular stenosis. The echocardiogram should include not only anatomic and hemodynamic measures of stenosis severity but also an assessment of the left ventricular response to the pressure load, insights into whether there is dilation of the ascending aorta, and assessment for the presence of coexisting valve regurgitation and other cardiac abnormalities.

A. ANATOMIC EVALUATION—Although most outcome data in those with aortic stenosis are based on measures of the hemodynamic severity and physiologic orifice area, the anatomic evaluation of the valve is gaining increased importance in the evolving era of percutaneous valve replacement in guiding patient selection and procedural planning. From primarily the transthoracic parasternal views, or transesophageal imaging if the transthoracic images are suboptimal, the number of leaflets, extent of calcification, leaflet thickening, and mobility should be evaluated. An anatomic measure of the geometric valve area can be obtained by planimetry. The fundamental limitations to accurate and reproducible measurements of the geometric orifice area are image attenuation secondary to leaflet calcification and the spatial integration of images required to ensure planimetry of the minimal opening area at the leaflet tips (Figure 17–2). It is for these reasons that the measure of geometric orifice area is reserved clinically for those circumstances where Doppler measurements are unreliable.

B. HEMODYNAMIC EVALUATION—The principal measures of the hemodynamic severity include peak transaortic jet velocity, peak instantaneous and mean pressure gradients, and valve area (effective orifice area by the continuity equation).

(1) Transaortic velocity and gradient calculations—The principle of conservation of energy states that the total amount of energy in a closed system remains constant. Energy can change its location and form but can be neither created nor destroyed. With respect to flow, as the flow stream approaches a narrowed orifice, its kinetic energy increases and potential energy decreases. Distal to the narrowed orifice, pressure is lost in part due to the dissipation of kinetic energy as heat. This creates a pressure gradient

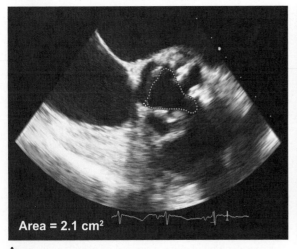

Area = 2.1 cm²

A

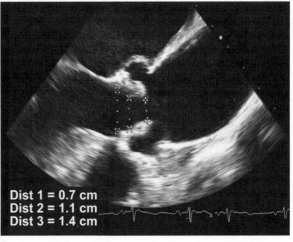

Dist 1 = 0.7 cm
Dist 2 = 1.1 cm
Dist 3 = 1.4 cm

B

▲ **Figure 17–2.** Planimetry of the aortic valve. **A:** Short axis image of the aortic valve and a calculated anatomic valve area by planimetry. Leaflet calcification and image attenuation limit accurate delineation of the leaflet borders. **B:** Long axis image of the aortic valve noting that slight alteration in the tomographic slice obtained through the aortic valve will result in marked variation in the valve area calculated by planimetry.

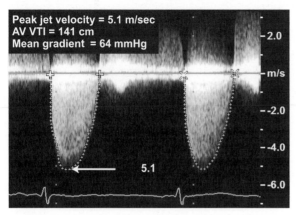

Peak jet velocity = 5.1 m/sec
AV VTI = 141 cm
Mean gradient = 64 mmHg

▲ **Figure 17-3.** Continuous wave Doppler of aortic stenosis.

across the valve orifice. Continuous wave Doppler is used to determine the maximum jet velocity through the stenotic valve. Meticulous imaging from multiple acoustic windows is required to ensure that flow velocities are acquired with a parallel intercept angle to the direction of flow limiting the error of underestimation of the peak velocity. The Bernoulli equation is then applied to the highest jet velocity obtained to calculate the peak instantaneous gradient (Figure 17–3).

Bernoulli equation:

$$\Delta P = 1/2\rho(V_2^2 - V_1^2) \quad \text{(Convective acceleration)}$$
$$+ \rho \int_1^2 (dv/dt) * ds \quad \text{(Flow acceleration)}$$
$$+ R(\mu) \quad \text{(Viscous friction)}$$

ΔP = pressure gradient; ρ = mass density of blood; V_1 and V_2 = velocity proximal and distal to obstruction, respectively; R = viscous resistance; μ = viscosity

Under most physiologic conditions, the latter two terms (flow acceleration and viscous friction) are negligible and can be ignored, and $V_2 >>> V_1$ and thus V_1 can be ignored. Therefore, under most physiologic conditions, a simplified Bernoulli equation can be applied to the peak velocity obtained to derive the peak instantaneous gradient.

Simplified Bernoulli equation: $\Delta P = 4(V_2)^2$

When either V_1 is > 1.5 m/s or V_2 is < 3.0 m/s, the proximal velocity should be included in the simplified Bernoulli equation: $\Delta P = 4(V_2^2 - V_1^2)$. The final term, $R(\mu)$, represents energy losses due to viscous friction. Failing to recall this component may result in an overestimation of gradient in those who are anemic.

The mean gradient is obtained by averaging the instantaneous gradients over the ejection period. Because it is not possible to match each point on the ejection curve between the proximal and distal velocity profiles, it is not possible to

"correct" the mean gradient when V_1 is significant, and in these circumstances, the measure of mean gradient should not be used to grade stenosis severity.

(2) Aortic valve area—Valve area calculations are based on the continuity equation, which assumes the principle of conservation of mass where flow across the left ventricular outflow tract (LVOT) is assumed equal to flow across the aortic valve (AV). Stroke volume is calculated as the product of the cross-sectional area (CSA) and velocity time integral (VTI). Therefore, aortic valve area (AVA) is calculated as:

$$AVA = (CSA_{LVOT} \times VTI_{LVOT})/VTI_{AV}$$

The calculation of flow across the LVOT assumes the outflow tract to be cylindrical in shape with its area therefore equal to π multiplied by its radius squared (πr^2); thus, an error in the calculation of LVOT diameter will be exponentially amplified. Note that the calculation of AVA is essentially the estimation of the "effective orifice area" and not the true anatomic/geometric orifice area. As blood flows toward a narrowed orifice, there is flow convergence beyond the anatomic orifice. The narrowest point of the flow stream, the vena contracta, is located just distal to the anatomic orifice, and its area is smaller than the anatomic orifice area. The ratio between the anatomic and effective orifice areas is called the contraction coefficient.

Based on the principal measures of hemodynamic severity, the American Heart Association/American College of Cardiology and European Society of Cardiology (ESC) guidelines categorize aortic stenosis, in those with normal cardiac output/transvalvular flow, as mild, moderate, or severe (Table 17–1). The aortic valve area should be indexed for body surface area in smaller individuals so as not to overestimate the severity of stenosis based on the valve area calculation. The role of indexed AVA in the obese is unclear, and it is not our practice to do so because it is difficult to integrate the relationship of weight in association to body "size" versus "adiposity."

Table 17–1. Categories of Aortic Stenosis Based on the Principal Measures of Hemodynamic Severity According to AHA/ACC and ESC Guidelines

	Transaortic Jet Velocity	Mean Gradient (mm Hg)	AVA (cm²)	Indexed AVA (cm²/m²)
Mild	2.6–2.9	< 25	> 1.5	> 0.9
Moderate	3.0–4.0	25–40	1.0–1.5	0.6–0.9
Severe	> 4.0	> 40	< 1.0	< 0.6

ACC, American College of Cardiology; AHA, American Heart Association; AVA, aortic valve area; ESC, European Society of Cardiology.

(3) Dimensionless index—As noted earlier, an error in the measure of the LVOT diameter will be exponentially amplified notwithstanding the assumption that the LVOT is cylindrical in shape. Therefore, a proposed LVOT independent measure of stenosis severity, the dimensionless index, can be helpful to either confirm or dispute stenosis severity classification based the effective orifice area calculation. The dimensionless index is defined as the ratio of the LVOT velocity to that of the transaortic jet velocity. Traditionally a value < 0.25 has been used to indicate severe aortic stenosis. The dimensionless index is however, highly variable depending on the size of the LVOT diameter and as such it has been proposed that the cut-off value for severe aortic stenosis be modified based on the LVOT diameter with values of ≤ 0.35, ≤ 0.30 and ≤ 0.25 in those with small (≤ 1.9 cm), average (2.0-2.2 cm) and large (≥ 2.3 cm) LVOT diameters, respectively.

(4) Energy loss coefficient (ELCo)—The correction coefficient increases as the extent of pressure recovery (discussed later) increases. The magnitude of pressure recovery is determined by the ratio between the effective orifice area and the cross-sectional area of the ascending aorta (measured at the sinotubular junction), most significant when the valve area is < 1.2 cm² and the aorta cross-sectional area is < 3.0 cm.

$$ELCo = (EOA \times Aa)/(Aa - EOA)$$

EOA indicates effective orifice area derived by the continuity equation, and Aa indicates cross-sectional area of the aorta measured 1 cm distal to the sinotubular junction. The ELCo then provides a value of valve area derived by Doppler echocardiography more equivalent to the valve area derived by the Gorlin equation, which is more representative of the actual energy loss caused by the stenosis and thus the burden it imposes on the ventricle.

4. Cardiac catheterization—The fundamental role of cardiac catheterization in those with aortic stenosis is to evaluate for the presence of coexisting coronary artery disease in those with symptoms of angina pectoris, helping clarify its pathophysiologic mechanism, and in whom aortic valve replacement is being considered. Cardiac catheterization should not be routinely performed for the evaluation of the hemodynamic severity of aortic stenosis but should be performed in cases where echocardiographic data is of poor quality or when there remains a discrepancy between the clinical and echocardiographic determinations of stenosis severity.

The principal measures of the hemodynamic severity of aortic stenosis as assessed by cardiac catheterization include peak-to-peak and mean pressure gradients and valve area (derived by the Gorlin equation).

A. PRESSURE GRADIENTS—The transvalvular pressure gradient is calculated by placing one catheter into the left ventricle and a second into the proximal aorta. The difference in the pressure from simultaneous recordings from each catheter represents the peak-to-peak pressure gradient. Single-catheter techniques may include a pullback gradient

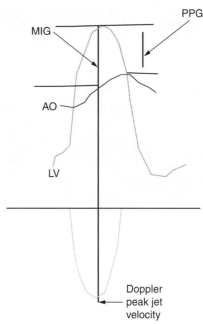

▲ **Figure 17–4.** *Top:* Simultaneous left ventricular and aortic pressure tracings; *Bottom:* Doppler echocardiography–derived transaortic velocity profile. AO, aortic pressure; LV, left ventricular pressure; MIG, maximum instantaneous gradient (the gradient that is derived by applying the Bernoulli equation to the peak jet velocity obtained by Doppler echocardiography); PPG, peak-to-peak gradient (the gradient obtained with invasive catheterization).

and the use of a Langston dual-lumen catheter. Note, Doppler echocardiography derives a maximum instantaneous gradient at a single point in time and by principal assumes that the pressure drop across the valve is irretrievably lost while the invasive measure derives a peak-to-peak gradient with the upstream pressure partially recovered. Therefore, the invasively derived measure of the peak pressure gradient is always lower than the Doppler-derived measure (Figure 17–4). Mean gradients obtained by both Doppler and cardiac catheterization correlate well but for when there is significant pressure recovery where again Doppler derived values of the mean pressure gradient will be greater than those derived by cardiac catheterization.

B. VALVE AREA—During cardiac catheterization, cardiac output is measured using primarily either the Fick or thermodilution principal, and the pressure gradient is measured as discussed earlier, with values obtained used to calculate valve area using the Gorlin equation:

$$AVA = \frac{CO/SEP \times HR}{44.3\sqrt{\Delta P_{mean}}}$$

where CO = cardiac output, SEP = systolic ejection period (in seconds), HR = heart rate, and ΔP = pressure gradient (mean). The presence of a measure of flow/cardiac output in the numerator of the Gorlin equation highlights the flow dependence on the derived values of aortic valve area. Note, that the valve area derived from the Gorlin equation is derived from recovered pressures, and as such, its value is higher than Doppler-derived valve areas by the continuity equation. The current guidelines, however, make no distinction between invasive and Doppler echocardiographic measurements in the characterization of stenosis severity by valve area and pressure gradients (see earlier discussion regarding the energy loss coefficient).

5. Cardiac computed tomography (CT)—Cardiac CT can be used to calculate the geometric valve area by planimetry and to quantify the extent and distribution of valve calcification. Although there is a weak correlation between the extent of valve calcification and hemodynamic severity of stenosis, the extent of calcification is predictive of event-free survival (survival without dyspnea, angina, syncope, heart failure, or need for valve replacement).

In contemporary clinical practice, cardiac CT, in conjunction with two- and three-dimensional echocardiography, now has an integral role in the evaluation of patients being considered for a percutaneous valve replacement primarily for:

- The evaluation of the LVOT geometry required for the appropriate selection of prosthetic valve size
- The assessment of the peripheral vasculature and suitability for arterial access
- The assessment of the geometric relationship/distance between the aortic annulus and the coronary ostia to ensure that the implanted valve, when in position, does not blanket the coronary ostia
- Characterizing the extent of valve and root calcification, which may impact both the technical success and risk of implantation
- Allowing the prediction of postimplantation aortic regurgitation

Feuchtner GM, et al. Aortic valve calcification as quantified with multislice computed tomography predicts short-term clinical outcome in patients with asymptomatic aortic stenosis. *J Heart Valve Dis.* 2006;15:494–98. [PMID: 16901041]

Leber AW, et al. Aortic valve calcium score as a predictor for outcome after tavi using the corevalve revalving system. *Int J Cardiol.* 2013;166(3):652–7. [PMID: 22197118]

Michelena HI, et al. Inconsistent echocardiographic grading of aortic stenosis: is the left ventricular outflow tract important? *Heart.* 2013;99:921-31. [PMID: 23349350]

Messika-Zeitoun D, et al. Evaluation and clinical implications of aortic valve calcification measured by electron-beam computed tomography. *Circulation.* 2004;110:356–62. [PMID: 15249504]

▶ Diagnostic Dilemmas: Area Gradient Mismatch

The principal parameters of stenosis severity, as discussed earlier, are directly related to transvalvular flow. As such, clinicians managing patients with aortic stenosis may face situations where stenosis severity is characterized as severe by area but not by gradient criteria. After excluding errors of measurement, errors of assumption, LVOT diameter related inconsistencies; low flow may account for diminished gradients despite severe aortic stenosis by AVA determination. Low-flow states (left ventricular stroke volume index < 35 mL/m^2) may be associated with either a low left ventricualr ejection fraction (EF) (*low EF area-gradient mismatch*) or a preserved EF (*normal EF area-gradient mismatch*). Less commonly, one notes the gradient in the "severe" range, while the AVA remains in the "nonsevere" range (*reverse area-gradient mismatch*). Deciphering the true severity of aortic stenosis in the presence of area-gradient mismatch is imperative to the understanding of patient prognosis and to guide therapeutic decisions.

A. Low EF Area-Gradient Mismatch

This is also known as low-flow, low-gradient (LF/LG) aortic stenosis with a depressed EF.

- Effective orifice area < 1.0 cm^2
- Left ventricular EF < 45%
- Mean pressure gradient < 30–40 mm Hg

Contemporary clinical protocol is to attempt to increase flow across the aortic valve with a dobutamine infusion and to evaluate the ventricular response and transvalvular hemodynamics. One of three scenarios will evolve:

1. True or fixed severe aortic stenosis: Those in whom dobutamine can induce a > 20% increase in stroke volume with an associated increase in transvalvular gradient and no or little change in AVA.

2. Pseudo or relative severe aortic stenosis: Those in whom dobutamine can induce a > 20% increase in stroke volume with an associated increase in AVA and no or little change in transvalvular gradient.

3. Indeterminate aortic stenosis: Those in whom dobutamine is not able to increase stroke volume (no contractile reserve) with no change in AVA or transvalvular gradient.

The changes in valve area and gradient imposed during a dobutamine infusion are largely dependent on the extent of flow augmentation achieved which can vary considerably between individuals. To overcome the inter-individual variability in flow augmentation it has been proposed to calculate an AVA at a normal flow rate. This variable is called the projected AVA (AVA_{proj}) and is derived as follows:

$$AVA_{proj} = AVA_{rest} + VC \times (250 - Q_{rest})$$

$$\text{Where: VC (valve compliance)} = \frac{AVA_{peak} - AVA_{rest}}{Q_{peak} - Q_{rest}}$$

$$\text{and Q (mean flow)} = \frac{\text{Stroke Volume (mL)}}{\text{LV Ejection time (seconds)}}$$

The AVA_{proj} may better differentiate true from pseudo aortic stenosis than traditional dobutamine stress Doppler indices. An $AVA_{proj} \leq 1.0\ cm^2$ suggests true severe aortic stenosis.

B. Normal EF Area-Gradient Mismatch

This is also known as paradoxical low-flow, low-gradient (PLF/LG) aortic stenosis.

- Effective orifice area $< 1.0\ cm^2$
- Left ventricular EF $> 50\%$ and left ventricular stroke volume index $< 35\ mL/m^2$
- Mean pressure gradient $< 30–40$ mm Hg

This scenario is the result of the interaction of a *diastolic component* whereby generally a thick ventricle with a small cavity is noted, a *myocardial component* whereby there is intrinsic myocardial dysfunction despite the persevered EF as noted with myocardial/strain imaging, and a *valvular-vascular component* imposing an increased global ventricular hemodynamic burden resulting from resistance in series by the valve stenosis and decreased systemic arterial compliance and increased vascular impedance. It has been proposed to characterize the valvular-vascular component through an index of valvuloarterial impedance (Zva). The Zva is defined as ratio of the estimated left ventricular systolic pressure (systolic blood pressure + mean pressure gradient) to the stroke volume index. The Zva can be thought of as the cost in mm Hg for each mL of blood ejected. Other hemodynamic subgroups of aortic stenosis include those with normal-flow ($> 35\ mL/m^2$) and low-gradient (NF/LG) aortic stenosis, which carries a good prognosis and considered an earlier form of the disease, and low-flow/high-gradient (LF/HG) aortic stenosis, which carries a worse prognosis intermediate between the NF/LG and the LF/LG subgroups.

Abbas AE, et al. Aortic valve stenosis: to the gradient and beyond—the mismatch between area and gradient severity. *J Interv Cardiol.* 2013;2:183-94. [PMID: 23278313]

Adda J, et al. Low-flow, low-gradient severe aortic stenosis despite normal ejection fraction is associated with severe left ventricular dysfunction as assessed by speckle-tracking echocardiography: a multicenter study. *Circ Cardiovasc Imaging.* 2012;5:27–35. [PMID: 22109983]

Briand M, et al. Reduced systemic arterial compliance impacts significantly on left ventricular afterload and function in aortic stenosis: implications for diagnosis and treatment. *J Am Coll Cardiol.* 2005;46:291–8. [PMID: 16022957]

Clavel MA, et al. Validation of conventional and simplified methods to calculate projected valve area at normal flow rate in patients with low flow, low gradient aortic stenosis; The Multicenter TOPAS (True or Pseudo Severe Aortic Stenosis) study. *J Am Soc Echocardiogr.* 2010;23:380-6.

Dumesnil JG, et al. Paradoxical low flow and/or low gradient severe aortic stenosis despite preserved left ventricular ejection fraction: implications for diagnosis and treatment. *Eur Heart J.* 2010;31:281–9. [PMID: 19737801]

Lancellotti P, et al. Clinical outcome in asymptomatic severe aortic stenosis: Insights from the new proposed aortic stenosis grading classification. *J Am Coll Cardiol.* 2012;59:235–43. [PMID: 22240128]

C. Reverse Area-Gradient Mismatch

This may be noted when inappropriate assumptions or liberties are taken when applying the simplified Bernoulli equation to Doppler-derived blood flow velocities in an effort to estimate the transvalvular gradient, such as failure to include V_1 when significant or, as noted earlier, failing to recall the viscous friction component in those with anemia. More commonly, this dilemma results secondary to the phenomenon of pressure recovery, where downstream to the obstructed orifice as the blood flow velocity/kinetic energy decreases some of the kinetic energy will be converted to potential energy with associated increases in pressure. Pressure recovery is greatest in those in whom the ascending aorta diameter measures < 3.0 cm causing discordance between Doppler and catheter-derived gradients. Pressure recovery is insignificant when the aortic diameter is > 3.0 cm. In addition eccentric jets lead to increase pressure loss across the aortic valve which leads to increased Doppler and catheter derived gradients despite a less than severe reduction in anatomic orifice area.

Clavel MA, et al. Outcome of patients with aortic stenosis, small valve area, and low-flow, low-gradient despite preserved left ventricular ejection fraction. *J Am Coll Cardiol.* 2012;60(14):1259–67. [PMID: 22657269]

▶ Treatment

Aortic stenosis is a mechanical problem requiring a mechanical solution where the only effective treatment is valve replacement. The optimal time for valve replacement is therefore at the inflection point where the procedural risk and the long-term consequences of prosthetic heart valve disease become less than medical therapy.

A. Medical Therapy

There is no effective medical therapy for aortic stenosis. Because aortic stenosis is an active disease process that shares similarities and risk factors with atherosclerosis, there has been intellectual enthusiasm for aggressive atherosclerotic risk factor modification and the use cholesterol-lowering drugs in an effort to slow stenosis progression and reduce the necessity for valve replacement. To date, studies evaluating the use of cholesterol-lowering therapies by in large have not shown salutary effects with respect to disease progression or need for valve replacement.

In those with symptomatic aortic stenosis who are not candidates for valve replacement, medical therapy is directed at the relief of symptoms because there is no therapy that prolongs life. Treatment of the patient with heart failure may include the cautious use of diuretics and angiotensin-converting enzyme (ACE) inhibitors. Initiation of such therapies should begin at low doses and slowly increased. The concern is diuretic-induced reduction in preload lowering cardiac output, resulting in a drop in systemic arterial pressure. This situation can also be imposed by ACE inhibitors. β-Blockers should be used with great caution or avoided entirely because they may unmask the left ventricle's dependence on adrenergic support for pressure generation and thereby cause heart failure. Digoxin use is reserved primarily for those with left ventricular dysfunction and/or atrial fibrillation. Hypertension should be treated with careful titration of pharmacotherapy and frequent patient monitoring to avoid hypotension.

The latest guidelines have eliminated the need for antibiotic prophylaxis to prevent infective endocarditis in those with native valvular aortic stenosis.

Chan KL, et al. Effect of lipid lowering with rosuvastatin on progression of aortic stenosis: results of the aortic stenosis progression observation: measuring effects of rosuvastatin (astronomer) trial. *Circulation.* 2010;121:306–14. [PMID: 20048204]
Cowell SJ, et al. A randomized trial of intensive lipid-lowering therapy in calcific aortic stenosis. *N Engl J Med.* 2005;352: 2389–97. [PMID: 15944423]

Rossebo AB, et al. Intensive lipid lowering with simvastatin and ezetimibe in aortic stenosis. *N Engl J Med.* 2008;359:1343–56. [PMID: 18765433]

B. Valve Replacement

1. Symptomatic patients—As noted earlier, survival in aortic stenosis abruptly declines once the classic symptoms of angina, effort syncope, or congestive heart failure appear. Fifty percent of patients with aortic stenosis in whom angina pectoris develops are dead within 5 years of its onset if aortic valve replacement is not undertaken. Half the patients with syncope will be dead within 3 years and 50% of patients with congestive heart failure will be dead within 2 years without valve replacement (Figure 17–5). The exact pathophysiologic changes that produce the onset of symptoms and begin this rapid downhill course are unknown. The development of symptoms is a class I indication for valve replacement, and following successful valve replacement, symptoms and quality of life improve, and survival in general is similar to an age-matched population. However, those who, prior to valve replacement, had severe left ventricular hypertrophy, poor functional capacity, or a large area of myocardial scar and who, after valve replacement, have untreated coexisting coronary artery disease or suboptimal prosthesis hemodynamics are at risk for a less ideal post–valve replacement

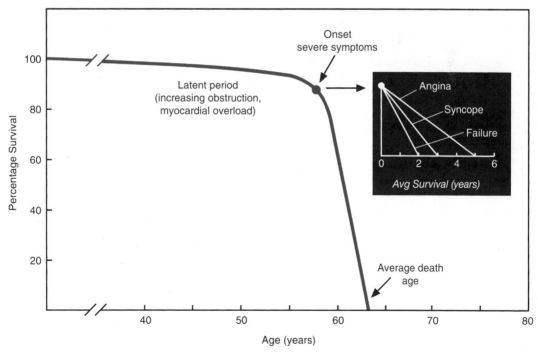

▲ **Figure 17–5.** The natural history of aortic stenosis. There is little change in survival until the symptoms of angina, syncope, or heart failure develop. (Adapted with permission from Ross J Jr, et al. *Circulation.* 1968;38[suppl V]:V-61.)

outcome. Valve replacement may be either surgical or via a transcatheter approach.

A. SURGICAL AORTIC VALVE REPLACEMENT—Surgical aortic valve replacement is done primarily through a midline sternotomy, but in those without coexisting coronary artery disease requiring bypass or a chest wall deformity, valve replacement may be approached through a "mini-sternotomy"—minimally invasive valve surgery. The advantage of the minimally invasive approach is less blood loss, a faster recovery time, and a better cosmetic outcome at the expense of less surgical "exposure." There a number of different types of valve prostheses, including mechanical, stented, and stentless heterografts, xenografts, and homografts.

Mechanical valves used in the aortic position are primarily bileaflet valves, which are durable and provide a good hemodynamic profile particularly at the larger valve sizes. The primary drawback of mechanical valves is the need for lifelong anticoagulation and the associated risk of bleeding. Heterograft valves have the primary advantage of a low thromboembolism rate without anticoagulation obviating its long-term use. For any given prosthesis size, the stentless heterograft valves have a better hemodynamic profile when compared to the more commonly used stented bioprostheses. The primary drawback of heterograft valves is their reduced durability when compared to the mechanical valves. Homografts and pulmonary autografts (Ross procedure) are rarely used in the adult population because the operation is technically more challenging and the rate of structural valve failure appears to exceed that of the heterograft valves. The decision of which type of valve prosthesis is best suited for any given patient is based on a number of patient-related factors such as the bleeding risk with anticoagulation or the need for anticoagulation in those already at high risk for thromboembolism (presence of atrial fibrillation, prior thromboembolism, or a hypercoagulable state). Those with renal failure, particularly if on dialysis, or hypercalcemia are at increased risk for structural valve failure with a bioprosthetic valve. The risk of a possible reoperation, if required, must be considered along with the complex decision facing young women considering pregnancy.

B. TRANSCATHETER AORTIC VALVE REPLACEMENT (TAVR)—Despite the dismal prognosis, many symptomatic patients either are not referred, generally because of age and the perception of surgical risk, or are declined as candidates for surgical valve replacement. TAVR now provides an option for those with severe symptomatic aortic stenosis and a life expectancy in excess of 1 year who have been deemed to have a surgical risk that would preclude aortic valve replacement. In addition, TAVR may be an alternative to surgical valve replacement in those deemed surgical candidates but who are stratified as having a very high surgical risk. As the technology evolves and experience broadens, there may be other patient populations for whom TAVR replaces the surgical approach.

Currently, TAVR is primarily performed through transfemoral arterial access. If delivery through the femoral artery is not possible, some have advocated using a subclavian approach; however, currently more common is a transapical approach through an intercostal thoracotomy. Although there are a number of transcatheter valves in development at the present time, the Edwards SAPIEN (Edwards Lifesciences Inc., Irvine, CA) and CoreValve (Medtronic Inc., Minneapolis, MN) valves are the only valves approved for clinical use. In high-risk patients not deemed surgical candidates 1 year following TAVR, there was a 20% absolute reduction in mortality, significantly fewer cardiac symptoms, and lower New York Heart Association functional class, when compared with those who received standard medical therapy. When high-risk patients were randomized to either surgical or transcatheter valve replacement, the 30-day mortality was lower with TAVR and the 1-year mortality equivalent. The incremental risk of TAVR versus either medical or surgical therapy includes vascular complications, heart block, a slight increase in neurologic events, and more perivalvular regurgitation.

Daneault B, et al. Stroke associated with surgical and transcatheter treatment of aortic stenosis: a comprehensive review. *J Am Coll Cardiol.* 2011;58:2143–50. [PMID: 22078419]

Iung B, et al. A prospective survey of patients with valvular heart disease in Europe: the euro heart survey on valvular heart disease. *Eur Heart J.* 2003;24:1231–43. [PMID: 12831818]

Leon MB, et al. Transcatheter aortic-valve implantation for aortic stenosis in patients who cannot undergo surgery. *N Engl J Med.* 2010;363:1597–607. [PMID: 20961243]

Smith CR, et al. Transcatheter versus surgical aortic-valve replacement in high-risk patients. *N Engl J Med.* 2011;364:2187–98. [PMID: 21639811]

2. Asymptomatic patients—In distinct contrast to the universal recommendation for valve replacement in those with symptomatic severe aortic stenosis, the management of the asymptomatic patient remains controversial. As noted earlier, the decision to proceed with valve replacement occurs when the risk of native aortic valve stenosis exceeds the procedural risk combined with the long-term risk of prosthetic heart valve disease. The primary concern in the strategy of watchful waiting is the risk of sudden death and the fact that symptoms are subjective and influenced by the patient's lifestyle and may be underreported.

The contemporary literature suggests that the risk of sudden death in the asymptomatic adult patient with severe aortic stenosis is approximately 1% per year. Conversely, in *low-risk* patients, there is an operative mortality of 1–3% and a 2–3% per year risk for a prosthesis-related complication such as thromboembolism, endocarditis, valve failure, bleeding (if anticoagulation is required), or death. Therefore, in general, surgical valve replacement risk exceeds any potential benefit to those with truly asymptomatic severe aortic stenosis and normal left ventricular systolic function.

Patients may either not seek medical attention immediately following the onset of symptoms or truncate their lifestyle so as to negate symptoms. Additionally, there is frequently some wait time until a valve replacement can be scheduled while the patient is symptomatic. These individuals are at increased risk, and the ideal situation is to better stratify risk in these "asymptomatic" patients and potentially offer valve replacement to those deemed at greatest risk. Features on the baseline echocardiogram including EF, left ventricular wall thickness, peak transaortic jet velocity, and the rate of hemodynamic progression are independent predictors of outcome. A noteworthy proportion of those who claim to be asymptomatic have an abnormal exercise test defined as exercise limiting symptoms and/or a fall in blood pressure below baseline, and these patients have a worse outcome. The added value of exercise-induced changes in echocardiographically derived valve hemodynamics is contentious, but reports state an incremental and independent prognostic value to an exercise-induced increase in mean gradient > 20 mm Hg even in those with a normal exercise stress test—the "truly" asymptomatic. The extent of valve calcification, very severe stenosis, and plasma brain natriuretic peptide levels may also be helpful in refining risk. Both the North American and European valve disease guidelines primarily based on expert consensus (level of evidence C) make recommendations for valve replacement in those with asymptomatic severe aortic stenosis, but there is variability in the strength of these recommendations (Table 17–2).

Lancellotti P, et al. Prognostic importance of quantitative exercise Doppler echocardiography in asymptomatic valvular aortic stenosis. *Circulation*. 2005;112:I377–82. [PMID: 16159850]

Marechaux S, et al. Impact of valvuloarterial impedance on left ventricular longitudinal deformation in patients with aortic valve stenosis and preserved ejection fraction. *Arch Cardiovasc Dis*. 2010;103:227–35. [PMID: 20656633]

Pellikka PA, et al. Outcome of 622 adults with asymptomatic, hemodynamically significant aortic stenosis during prolonged follow-up. *Circulation*. 2005;111:3290–5. [PMID: 15956131]

▶ Special Circumstances

A. Low EF Area-Gradient Mismatch (LF/LG Aortic Stenosis)

Patients with LF/LG aortic stenosis have a poor prognosis with medical management. As noted earlier, deciphering the true severity of aortic stenosis in the presence of area-gradient mismatch is imperative in the evaluation of patient prognosis and to guide the appropriate management of patients. In general, in those with true or fixed severe aortic stenosis, valve replacement should be performed and can be done with an acceptable operative risk. Those with indeterminate aortic stenosis, because of the absence of contractile reserve (the inability to increase stroke volume ≥ 20% with a dobutamine infusion), have an abysmal prognosis with medical management, but also a high operative risk reported in some series (up to 30%). However, those who survive surgery generally show an improvement in functional capacity, ventricular function, and overall survival. The management

Table 17–2. Asymptomatic Severe Aortic Stenosis: Indications for Isolated Aortic Valve Replacement

Class	ACC/AHA Guidelines	ESC Guidelines
I	Reduced LVEF < 50%	• Reduced LVEF < 50% • Abnormal exercise test showing symptoms on exercise
IIa		• Abnormal exercise test showing a fall in blood pressure below baseline • Moderate-to-severe valve calcification and a rate of peak velocity progression ≥ 0.3 m/s per year
IIb	• Abnormal exercise stress test showing either symptoms or asymptomatic hypotension • A high likelihood of rapid progression (age, calcification, and CAD) • Extremely severe stenosis (aortic valve area < 0.6 cm², mean gradient > 60 mm Hg, peak jet velocity > 5.0 m/s) with an expected operative mortality ≤ 1%	• Abnormal exercise test showing complex ventricular arrhythmias • Excessive left ventricular hypertrophy (≥ 15 mm) unless this is due to hypertension

ACC, American College of Cardiology; AHA, American Heart Association; CAD, coronary artery disease; ESC, European Society of Cardiology; LVEF, left ventricular ejection fraction.

of those with LF/LG aortic stenosis and the absence of contractile reserve is controversial. In those with significant valve calcification, a mean gradient > 20 mm Hg, and the absence of a large area of left ventricular scar, valve replacement should be considered. Note that the literature on the risks and benefits of valve replacement in these patients is based on surgical valve replacement, and over time, we may find that TAVR offers a lower procedural risk alternative for these patients.

Monin JL, et al. Low-gradient aortic stenosis: operative risk stratification and predictors for long-term outcome: a multicenter study using dobutamine stress hemodynamics. *Circulation*. 2003;108:319–24. [PMID: 12835219]

Nishimura RA, et al. Low-output, low-gradient aortic stenosis in patients with depressed left ventricular systolic function: the clinical utility of the dobutamine challenge in the catheterization laboratory. *Circulation*. 2002;106:809–13. [PMID: 12176952]

Tribouilloy C, et al. Outcome after aortic valve replacement for low-flow/low-gradient aortic stenosis without contractile reserve on dobutamine stress echocardiography. *J Am Coll Cardiol*. 2009;53:1865–73. [PMID: 19442886]

B. Normal EF Area-Gradient Mismatch (PLF/LG Aortic Stenosis)

These individuals present with a low valve area and low gradient despite a preserved left ventricular EF. There is controversy in how best to manage these patients, and the mere presence of a low gradient cannot exclude severe aortic stenosis in some of these patients who would have a poor outcome if treated medically and would benefit from valve replacement. How best to characterize and select those with PLF/LG aortic stenosis who are most likely to benefit from valve replacement remains challenging. The use of stress echocardiography (supine bicycle or dobutamine) to calculate the AVAproj may help to predict stenosis severity and guide therapeutic decision making.

Clavel MA, et al. Stress echocardiography to assess stenosis severity and predict outcome in patients with paradoxical low-flow, low-gradient aortic stenosis and preserved LVEF. J Am Coll Cardiol Img. 2013;6:175-83. [PMID: 23489531]

▶ Prognosis

As noted earlier, the prognosis of those with severe symptomatic aortic stenosis, in the absence of valve replacement, is very poor. However, the age-adjusted survival following valve replacement is excellent even in the elderly who are free of other cardiac or systemic diseases. Asymptomatic patients generally have a good prognosis, with the strongest predictor of clinical outcome (death or valve replacement) being stenosis severity. The likelihood of remaining alive without valve replacement at 2 years is approximately 20% in those with a peak jet velocity > 4.0 m/s, 66% if the jet velocity is between 3.0 an 4.0 m/s, and 84% for those with a jet velocity < 3.0 m/s. Understanding the strong impact that stenosis severity and other clinical predictors, such as functional capacity and the rate of hemodynamic progression, have on outcome is very useful when counseling patients about their prognosis and to help tailor the frequency of follow-up.

Aortic Regurgitation

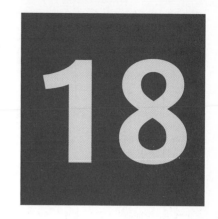

Michael H. Crawford, MD

ESSENTIALS OF DIAGNOSIS

- ▶ Following a long asymptomatic period, presentation with heart failure or angina.
- ▶ Wide pulse pressure with associated peripheral signs.
- ▶ Diastolic decrescendo murmur at the left sternal border.
- ▶ Left ventricular dilation and hypertrophy with preserved function.
- ▶ Presentation and findings dependent on the rapidity of onset of regurgitation.
- ▶ Diagnosis confirmed and severity estimated by Doppler echocardiography, aortography, magnetic resonance imaging, or computed tomography angiography.

▶ Etiology

Normally, the integrity of the aortic orifice during diastole is maintained by an intact aortic root and firm apposition of the free margins of the three aortic valve cusps. Aortic regurgitation (AR) may therefore be caused by a variety of disorders affecting the valve cusps or the aortic root (or both) (Table 18–1). With rheumatic heart disease becoming less common, nonrheumatic causes currently account for most of the underlying causes of AR, including congenitally malformed aortic valves, infective endocarditis, and connective tissue diseases. Disorders affecting the aortic root also account for a large number of patients with AR. These conditions include cystic medial necrosis, Marfan syndrome, aortic dissection, and inflammatory diseases. Even in the absence of any obvious abnormality of the aortic valve or root, severe systemic hypertension has been reported to cause significant AR.

Roberts WC, et al. Causes of pure aortic regurgitation in patients having isolated aortic valve replacement at a single US tertiary hospital (1993 to 2005). *Circulation.* 2006;114(5):422–9. [PMID: 16864725]

▶ Pathophysiology

The presentation and findings in patients with AR depend on its severity and rapidity of onset. The hemodynamic effects of acute severe AR are entirely different from the chronic type, and the two will be discussed separately.

A. Chronic Aortic Regurgitation

In response to the left ventricular volume overload associated with AR, progressive left ventricular dilation occurs. This results in a higher wall stress, which stimulates ventricular hypertrophy and which, in turn, tends to normalize wall stress. Patients with severe AR may have the largest end-diastolic volumes produced by any other heart disease and yet their end-diastolic pressures are not uniformly elevated. In keeping with the Frank-Starling mechanism, the stroke volume is also increased. Thus, despite the presence of regurgitation, a normal effective forward cardiac output can be maintained. This state persists for several years. Gradually, left ventricular diastolic properties and contractile function start to decline. The adaptive dilation and hypertrophy can no longer match the loading conditions. The left ventricular end-diastolic pressure begins to rise and the ejection fraction drops with a decline in effective forward output and development of heart failure.

B. Acute Aortic Regurgitation

In contrast to chronic AR, when sudden severe regurgitation occurs, the left ventricle has no time to adapt. The acute ventricular volume overload therefore results in a small increase in end-diastolic volume and severe elevation of end-diastolic pressure, which is transmitted to the left atrium and pulmonary veins, culminating in acute pulmonary edema. Because the ventricular end-diastolic volume is normal, the total stroke volume is not increased and the effective forward cardiac output drops. To compensate for the low output state, sympathetic stimulation occurs, which

Table 18-1. Causes of Aortic Regurgitation

Aortic cusp abnormalities
  Infectious: Bacterial endocarditis, rheumatic fever
  Congenital: Bicuspid aortic valve, Marfan syndrome
  Inflammatory: Systemic lupus erythematosus, rheumatoid arthritis,
    Behçet syndrome
  Degenerative: Myxomatous (floppy) valve, calcific aortic valve
  Trauma
  Postaortic valvuloplasty
  Diet drug valvulopathy
Aortic root abnormalities
  Aortic root dilatation: Marfan syndrome, syphilis, ankylosing spon-
    dylitis, relapsing polychondritis, idiopathic aortitis, annuloaortic
    ectasia, cystic medial necrosis, Ehlers-Danlos syndrome
  Loss of commissural support: Aortic dissection, trauma, ventricular
    septal defect
Increased pressure
  Systemic hypertension
  Supravalvular aortic stenosis

produces tachycardia and peripheral vasoconstriction, the latter further worsening AR.

▶ Clinical Findings

A. Symptoms & Signs

1. Chronic aortic regurgitation—Patients with chronic AR remain asymptomatic for a long time. Palpitations are common and may be due to either awareness of forceful left ventricular contractions or occurrence of premature atrial or ventricular beats. Angina may occur either from concomitant coronary disease or from a combination of low diastolic pressure and increased oxygen demand from ventricular hypertrophy. When left ventricular dysfunction supervenes, patients initially experience exertional dyspnea and fatigue. At a later stage, resting heart failure symptoms occur with orthopnea and paroxysmal nocturnal dyspnea.

On physical examination, visible cardiac pulsations are common. The area of the apical impulse is increased on palpation and is displaced caudally and laterally. The first heart sound is usually normal. The aortic component of the second heart sound may be decreased in conditions where cusp excursion is reduced, such as with valve calcification. An S_4 is often present due to underlying hypertrophy, and an S_3 is audible when ventricular failure occurs. On auscultation, the characteristic sound of AR is a soft, high-pitched diastolic decrescendo murmur best heard in the third intercostal space along the left sternal border at end expiration, with the patient sitting and leaning forward. In the presence of aortic root disease, the murmur may be best heard to the right of the sternum. A systolic ejection murmur may be present at the aortic area due to the high flow state. Occasionally, a diastolic rumble may be heard at the apex, referred to as the Austin Flint murmur. The mechanism underlying this murmur remains unclear. A number of different causes have been proposed, the most recent being the aortic jet encountering the mitral inflow resulting in turbulence.

The systolic arterial pressure is increased due to a large stroke volume, whereas the diastolic pressure is decreased due to runoff from the aorta into both the ventricle and peripheral arteries. This is the underlying reason for a wide pulse pressure and for a variety of associated peripheral signs in chronic significant AR (Table 18–2). However, it must be remembered that these signs are not specific for AR and may occur in any high flow state such as occurs in anemia, thyrotoxicosis, and arteriovenous malformations. With the development of heart failure, the pulse pressure narrows and the peripheral signs of AR are attenuated.

2. Acute aortic regurgitation—In contrast to chronic AR, most patients with acute severe AR are symptomatic. Initial presentation may vary depending on the underlying cause, which most commonly is aortic dissection, infective endocarditis, or trauma. In the presence of associated acute AR, clinical manifestations of severe dyspnea, orthopnea, and weakness often develop. The onset of symptoms is sudden, with rapid progression to hemodynamic collapse if left untreated.

In acute AR, the left ventricle has had no time to adapt to the volume overload state. The peripheral signs associated with chronic AR are therefore absent. Pulse pressure is usually normal, and hypotension may be present in severe cases. Bilateral rales are usually present on examination of the lungs and reflect underlying pulmonary edema. On precordial palpation, the apical impulse is not shifted. The first heart sound may be soft or absent due to the premature closure of the mitral valve. An S_3 is often present, but an S_4 is usually absent because there is little or no atrial contribution to ventricular filling due to high left ventricular end-diastolic

Table 18-2. Peripheral Signs of Aortic Regurgitation

Name of Sign	Description
Corrigan pulse	Rapid and forceful distention of arterial pulse with quick collapse
De-Musset sign	To and fro head bobbing
Müller sign	Visible pulsation of uvula
Quincke sign	Capillary pulsations seen on light compression of nail bed
Traube sign	Systolic and diastolic sounds (pistol shots) over the femoral artery
Duroziez sign	Bruits heard over femoral artery on light compression by stethoscope
Hill sign	Popliteal cuff pressure exceeding brachial pressure by 60 mm Hg or greater

pressure. The typical diastolic murmur of AR is shortened in duration, often difficult to hear, and easily missed.

Hamirani YS, et al. Acute aortic regurgitation. *Circulation.* 2012;126(9):1121–6. [PMID: 22927474]

B. Laboratory Findings

Laboratory findings depend on the underlying cause of AR. Elevated white blood cell count and erythrocyte sedimentation rate are seen in inflammatory conditions, such as infection and aortitis. Abnormal antinuclear antigen and rheumatoid factor titers may be seen in patients with rheumatologic disorders. When syphilis is suspected, serologic tests may be indicated. Plasma brain natriuretic peptide (BNP) levels are associated with prognosis in patients with AR and may contribute to the decision for surgery.

C. Diagnostic Studies

1. Electrocardiography—No specific electrocardiographic abnormalities are characteristic of AR. Signs of left atrial enlargement, left ventricular hypertrophy, and a "strain pattern" (ST depression with T-wave inversion in lateral leads) are often seen in chronic significant AR. Arrhythmias, including ventricular ectopy and ventricular tachycardia, may occur in advanced cases with left ventricular dysfunction. In acute AR, sinus tachycardia may be the only abnormality. In cases of infective endocarditis, inflammation or abscess formation may spread to the atrioventricular node, resulting in prolongation of the PR interval or development of atrioventricular block.

2. Chest radiography—Chest radiographic findings are not specific for AR and reflect an estimate of cardiac size and pulmonary vascular changes. In chronic significant AR, an increase in the size of the left heart chambers and the aorta is seen. In acute AR, the cardiac size is normal; the lung fields show increased markings due to pulmonary edema. When AR is due to aortic dissection, the chest film may show an enlarged ascending aorta. If calcification of the aortic knob is present, a helpful sign of dissection is increased separation between the outer margin of the aorta and the calcific density.

3. Echocardiography and Doppler techniques—Echocardiography is the method of choice for evaluating patients with AR. Two-dimensional echocardiography in combination with various Doppler modalities and, in selected cases, transesophageal imaging has provided a noninvasive means for not only diagnosing AR with a high sensitivity and specificity but also for assessing its etiology and severity. Furthermore, important information can be obtained on the hemodynamic impact of the regurgitant lesion, prognosis, and effectiveness of therapy.

A. DETECTION OF AORTIC REGURGITATION—Doppler techniques are extremely sensitive and specific in the detection of AR, manifested as a diastolic flow abnormality arising from the aortic valve, directed toward the left ventricle. Even trivial regurgitation can be detected, which commonly is not audible on physical examination. Although most cases of moderate-to-severe chronic AR have typical findings on physical examination, moderate lesions may occasionally be missed on examination because of the subtlety of auscultatory findings. Doppler echocardiography is also extremely valuable in patients with acute AR when the typical clinical findings of chronic AR are absent and the brief murmur can often be missed. Color Doppler echocardiography has proven to be extremely helpful in the evaluation of AR (Figure 18–1). It provides a spatial orientation of the regurgitant jet arising from the aortic root. A completely negative color Doppler examination in multiple planes virtually excludes the presence of AR. Echocardiographic imaging with M-mode and two-dimensional examinations cannot detect the presence of AR but can provide indirect clues to its presence. These include diastolic fluttering of the anterior mitral leaflet or septum depending on the impingement of the regurgitant flow on these structures. These signs, although specific, are not sensitive for the detection of AR and do not relate to the severity of regurgitation.

B. ASSESSMENT OF CAUSE—Because two-dimensional echocardiography can image cardiac structures, it provides valuable information on the cause of the AR. Structural abnormalities of the aortic valve, including calcifications or thickening, congenital deformities, vegetations, rupture, or prolapse, can be identified. Dilatation of the aortic root, calcifications, or dissection can also be evaluated. Although most of these conditions can be assessed with transthoracic echocardiography, transesophageal echocardiography has provided high-resolution images that allow for improved detection of such abnormalities, especially in technically difficult cases or in conditions such as infective endocarditis. Transesophageal echocardiography is also routinely performed when an aortic abnormality, such as aneurysm or dissection, is suspected (Figure 18–2). In patients with AR due to aortic disease, precisely defining the morphology of the valve and involvement of the aortic root is important in determining the surgical approach and deciding whether the valve can be preserved or requires replacement.

C. ASSESSMENT OF SEVERITY—In addition to the detection of AR, Doppler echocardiography combined with two-dimensional echocardiographic imaging has recently allowed an assessment of the severity of the lesion. Several methods have been proposed, including color Doppler assessment of regurgitant jet size, continuous wave Doppler using the pressure half-time method, measurements of regurgitant volume and effective regurgitant orifice area derived from two-dimensional echocardiography and pulsed Doppler techniques, and three-dimensional echocardiography to directly visualize the size of the regurgitant orifice.

With color-flow Doppler, the AR jet can be spatially oriented in the two-dimensional plane arising from the aortic

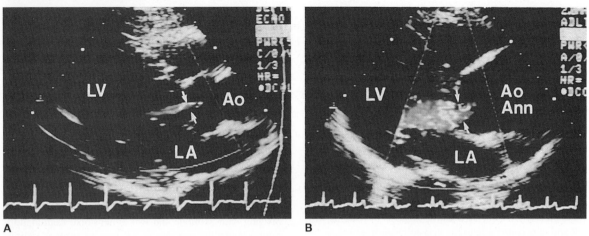

A   **B**

▲ **Figure 18–1.** Color Doppler echocardiographic frames in diastole from the parasternal long axis view in (**A**) a patient with mild aortic regurgitation and another with (**B**) severe regurgitation. The patient with severe aortic regurgitation (**B**) has a large ascending aortic aneurysm (Ao Ann). The width of the aortic regurgitation jet in the left ventricular outflow (*between arrows*) provides a good estimate of the severity of aortic regurgitation by color Doppler echocardiography. Ao, aorta; LA, left atrium; LV, left ventricle.

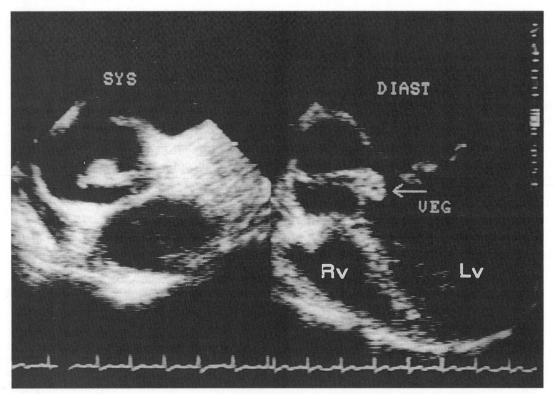

▲ **Figure 18–2.** Transesophageal echocardiographic frames in systole (SYS) and diastole (DIAST), showing a vegetation attached to the aortic valve that prolapses into the left ventricular outflow tract during diastole. In this patient, transthoracic echocardiographic imaging was difficult and failed to demonstrate the large vegetation.

Table 18–3. Grading the Severity of Aortic Regurgitation Using Doppler Techniques Combined with Echocardiography

Severity of AR	Color-Flow Doppler JH/LVOH (%)	Continuous Wave Doppler PHT (ms)	Pulsed Doppler Regurgitant Fraction (%)
Mild	< 25	> 500	< 30
Moderate	25–45	500–349	30–39
Moderately severe	46–64	349–200	40–49
Severe	> 65	< 200	> 50

AR, aortic regurgitation; JH/LVOH, ratio of aortic regurgitant jet height to left ventricular outflow height in the parasternal long axis view; PHT, pressure half-time.

valve and directed toward the left ventricle. The ratio of the AR jet diameter just below the leaflets to that of the left ventricular outflow diameter has been shown to correlate well with the severity of regurgitation when compared with the angiographic standard (Table 18–3, see Figure 18–1). Similarly, a good estimation of AR severity has been found by relating the cross-sectional area of the jet at its origin to the left ventricular outflow area. Recently, measurement of the width of the AR jet at the level of the leaflets (vena contracta) has been used to quantitatively approximate AR severity. A vena contracta of > 0.6 cm is considered a sign of severe AR. On the other hand, it is important to note that the length of the AR jet does not correlate well with AR severity. This is in part because color Doppler flow mapping is also highly dependent on the velocity of regurgitation, or the driving pressure, in addition to the regurgitant volume.

Another index of AR severity that has been useful clinically is the pressure half-time derived from continuous wave Doppler recordings of the AR jet velocity. The velocity of the regurgitant jet is related to the instantaneous pressure difference between the aorta and left ventricle in diastole by the modified Bernoulli equation: $\Delta P = 4V^2$, where ΔP is the pressure gradient in millimeters of mercury and V is the blood velocity in meters per second. The pressure half-time index is the time it takes for the initial maximal pressure gradient in diastole to fall by 50%. In patients with mild regurgitation, there is a gradual small drop in the pressure difference in diastole, whereas with severe AR, a more precipitous drop occurs (Figure 18–3). A pressure half-time greater than 500 ms is seen in mild AR, but more significant regurgitation is usually associated with a shorter pressure half-time (see Table 18–3, Figure 18–3). The severity of AR using this index may be overestimated in patients who have elevated left ventricular end-diastolic pressure.

The severity of AR can also be assessed using regurgitant volume and regurgitant fraction derived from two-dimensional

and pulsed Doppler echocardiography. This method is based on the continuity equation, which states that, in the absence of regurgitation, blood flow is equal across all valves. Stroke volume at the level of a valve annulus is calculated as the product of the cross-sectional area obtained by two-dimensional echocardiography and the time velocity integral of flow recorded by pulsed Doppler. In the presence of AR, stroke volume at the left ventricular outflow tract is higher than that across another valve without regurgitation. Therefore, AR volume can be calculated as the difference between stroke volume at the left ventricular outflow and that derived at another valve site. Dividing the regurgitant volume by stroke volume across the aortic valve gives an estimate of regurgitant fraction. A regurgitant fraction of less than 30% is usually mild, whereas regurgitant fraction greater than 50% denotes severe AR (see Table 18–3). A similar approach to estimating severity of AR can be achieved using pulsed Doppler echocardiography in the proximal descending aorta. In patients with significant AR, a large reversal of flow is observed in diastole toward the aortic arch and ascending aorta. This simple method should be used routinely to qualitatively grade the severity of regurgitation and can also be used quantitatively to derive a regurgitant fraction.

Proximal flow convergence is more difficult to identify in AR, but when it is present, the proximal isovelocity surface area method can be used to determine the effective regurgitant orifice area. This method is less accurate in eccentric jets and aortic root dilatation.

Although color-flow Doppler allows a good estimation of the severity of AR in most patients, its accuracy depends on optimization of the color Doppler examination, including gain settings, frame rate, and interrogation of multiple tomographic planes. The availability of other independent Doppler indices of AR severity further allows the corroboration of color Doppler findings. This is particularly helpful in patients with eccentric AR jets, for which severity may be difficult to assess by color-flow Doppler alone. A detailed transthoracic examination usually provides all the necessary information. When the transthoracic approach is inadequate or inconclusive, transesophageal echocardiography can be performed in this setting for the diagnosis and assessment of severity of the lesion.

Another important caveat in classifying the severity of AR is that it is in part dependent on hemodynamic status, including preload and, more importantly, afterload. Raising blood pressure may significantly increase AR severity.

D. ASSESSMENT OF HEMODYNAMIC EFFECTS—The hemodynamic effects of AR are assessed with both echocardiographic imaging and Doppler echocardiography. Two-dimensional echocardiography provides quantitation of ventricular size and function, in addition to the degree of left ventricular hypertrophy and ventricular mass. End-diastolic and end-systolic left ventricular dimensions and volumes as well as left ventricular ejection fraction provide important measures of the hemodynamic effects of AR and

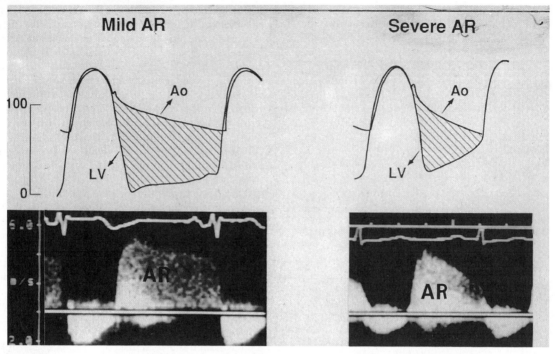

▲ **Figure 18–3.** Schematic of aortic and left ventricular pressure tracings in (*left*) a patient with mild and (*right*) another with severe aortic regurgitation and corresponding examples of continuous wave Doppler recording of aortic jet velocity in such patients. In mild aortic regurgitation, a gradual, small drop in the difference between aortic and ventricular pressures occurs in diastole, reflected by the small decrease in the velocity of the aortic regurgitation jet. In contrast, in severe aortic regurgitation, a more precipitous drop occurs in the pressure gradient and in the corresponding jet velocity. AR, aortic regurgitation; Ao, aorta; LV, left ventricle.

help identify patients at higher risk. In patients with acute AR, premature closure of the mitral valve can be demonstrated by both two-dimensional and M-mode imaging. In these situations, diastolic mitral regurgitation can also be detected by Doppler echocardiography, reflecting the rapid rise of left ventricular pressure in diastole, exceeding that of left atrial pressure. These findings indicate severe AR. In patients with chronic AR, assessment of the ventricular and atrial filling dynamics at the mitral and pulmonary venous inflow, respectively, allows for noninvasive estimation of ventricular diastolic pressure, further adding to the overall evaluation of the hemodynamic effect of AR on ventricular function. Newer modalities such as Doppler tissue imaging further enhance the accuracy of noninvasive assessment of ventricular diastolic function. Thus, in patients with chronic AR, two-dimensional echocardiography with Doppler provides serial assessment of left ventricular volumes, hypertrophy, and function and helps assess the progression of the disease and optimum timing of surgical intervention.

4. Cardiac catheterization and angiography—Prior to the introduction of Doppler echocardiography, the evaluation of the severity of AR invariably required invasive testing

by cardiac catheterization. With the improvement in the accuracy of noninvasive tests, routine cardiac catheterization is no longer necessary in most patients. At catheterization, the detection of AR is achieved with the injection of radiopaque contrast into the aortic root and the appearance of dye in the left ventricle (Figure 18–4). In addition, aortography allows evaluation of the ascending aorta for dilatation or dissection. Some of the structural abnormalities of the aortic valve may also be identified. The severity of AR is quantitatively approximated using a grading system that takes into account the intensity of contrast dye in the left ventricle and its clearance (Table 18–4). This grading system has been helpful clinically in the assessment of AR severity. However, it is important to emphasize that, similar to other diagnostic techniques, a number of technical factors may also affect interpretation. Positioning the catheter too close to the valve may itself cause regurgitation. The volume and rapidity of contrast injection, ventricular function, and type of catheter used are important factors that may affect the interpretation of AR severity.

At catheterization, the severity of AR can also be assessed by the determination of regurgitant volume and regurgitant fraction. In the absence of regurgitation or shunts, the left

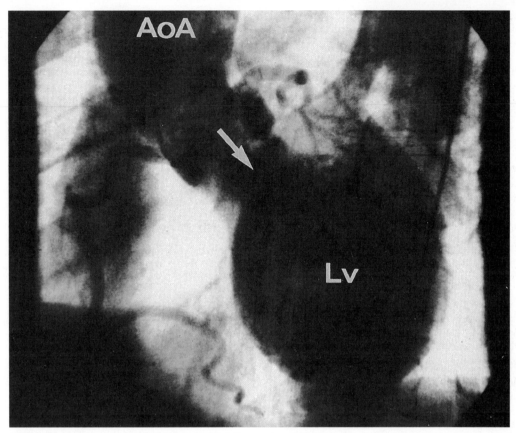

▲ **Figure 18–4.** Aortic root contrast injection in the left anterior oblique projection in a patient with severe aortic regurgitation, showing significant opacification of the left ventricle. The aortography also shows an ascending aortic aneurysm. AoA, aortic aneurysm; Lv, left ventricle.

Table 18–4. Angiographic Grading of the Severity of Aortic Regurgitation

Grade	Degree of LV Opacification	Intensity of Dye	Clearance of Dye from LV
I (mild)	Incomplete	Ao > LV	Completely cleared on each beat
II (moderate)	Complete but faint	Ao > LV	Incomplete clearance
III (moderately severe)	Complete opacification in several beats	Ao = LV	Slow
IV (severe)	Complete on first beat	Ao < LV	Slow

Ao, aorta; LV, left ventricle.

ventricular stroke volume derived from contrast ventriculography is equal to right ventricular stroke volume obtained by the Fick method or thermodilution. When isolated AR is present, subtracting left ventricular from right ventricular stroke volume gives the regurgitation volume. Regurgitant fraction is derived as the regurgitant volume divided by left ventricular stroke volume. In the presence of concomitant mitral regurgitation, a total regurgitant volume or fraction can only be assessed using this method. Because of inherent variability in the determination of stroke volume, a 10–15% error in these measurements is not infrequent and is similar to those obtained with Doppler echocardiography.

Cardiac catheterization provides an accurate assessment of the hemodynamic effect of AR. Using contrast ventriculography, preferably in biplanar projections, accurate determination of left ventricular volumes and ejection fraction can be performed. Furthermore, direct measurements of pressures in the various cardiac chambers can be recorded. In compensated chronic AR, the only abnormality that may be observed is a widened pulse pressure on the aortic pressure tracing. As decompensation occurs, left ventricular end-diastolic pressure rises. In severe, particularly acute AR, aortic and left ventricular pressures may equalize at end-diastole.

With the improvement in noninvasive testing, routine cardiac catheterization is no longer necessary in most patients for the sole assessment of the lesion. Currently, cardiac catheterization is indicated in the assessment of AR severity when noninvasive testing is equivocal or discordant with the clinical presentation and, more commonly, in the assessment of coronary artery disease prior to aortic valve surgery. Preoperative coronary angiography should be performed prior to elective surgery for AR in men older than 35 years of age, premenopausal women over 35 who have risk factors for coronary artery disease, postmenopausal women, and any patients with clinical suspicion of coronary artery disease.

5. Electrocardiographically gated multi-slice computed tomography angiography (CTA)—This test allows rapid diastolic frame rates from which the regurgitant orifice can be planimetered. Studies have shown excellent agreement with echo Doppler measures in the same patients. In addition, the size of the aorta and left ventricle can be determined as well as ejection fraction. CTA can also be used to detect significant coronary artery disease in patients with chest pain or who are being considered for surgery.

6. Magnetic resonance imaging (MRI)—Advances in MRI have recently allowed for evaluation of patients with AR. At present, three basic approaches are available: spin echo imaging, gradient echo imaging (cine-MRI), and phase velocity mapping. Spin echo imaging provides an excellent approach for depicting cardiac morphology and detecting aortic root disease. However, aortic valve visualization is poor. Using cine-MRI, AR is detected as a decrease in the signal intensity in the left ventricular outflow during diastole. In preliminary studies, the ratio of area of low-intensity signal to the area of the left ventricular outflow has provided an accurate estimate of AR severity. Regurgitant fractions have been determined by comparing right and left ventricular volumes and stroke volumes. Furthermore, using phase velocity mapping, flow in a region of interest can be assessed. Regurgitant fraction with this method can be derived by comparing flows in the ascending aorta and pulmonary artery.

The use of MRI is promising in the assessment of AR. It is particularly helpful in defining the severity and extent of AR. Imaging can be performed in any plane, without attenuation from lung or bone. However, this modality cannot be used in patients carrying metallic objects such as defibrillators or pacemakers. Its current drawbacks are lack of availability of cardiac MRI and high cost. It is an alternative to echocardiography and for centers with expertise in cardiac MRI.

7. Exercise stress testing—Exercise stress testing can be used to evaluate patients with equivocal symptoms or to guide patients who wish to participate in athletic activities. Early studies using exercise radionuclide angiography to assess ejection fraction suggested that a failure to rise or a fall in ejection fraction correlated with poor outcomes and was a criteria for considering surgery. However, when resting ejection fraction and end-diastolic left ventricular volume were considered, this exercise response in asymptomatic patients had no independent predictive value. Thus, radionuclide imaging with exercise in patients has been largely abandoned.

Alkadhi H, et al. Aortic regurgitation: assessment with 64-section CT. *Radiology.* 2007;245(1):111–21. [PMID: 17717329]

Bekeredjian R, et al. Valvular heart disease: aortic regurgitation. *Circulation.* 2005;112(1):125–34. [PMID: 15998697]

Debl K, et al. Assessment of the anatomic regurgitant orifice in aortic regurgitation: a clinical magnetic resonance imaging study. *Heart.* 2008;94(3):e8. [PMID: 17686805]

Myerson SG, et al. Aortic regurgitation quantification using cardiovascular magnetic resonance: association with clinical outcome. *Circulation.* 2012;126(12):1452–60. [PMID: 22879371]

Pizarro R, et al. Prospective validation of the prognostic usefulness of B-type natriuretic peptide in asymptomatic patients with chronic severe aortic regurgitation. *J Am Coll Cardiol.* 2011;58:1705–14. [PMID: 21982316]

Scheffel H, et al. Accuracy of 64-slice computed tomography for the preoperative detection of coronary artery disease in patients with chronic aortic regurgitation. *Am J Cardiol.* 2007;100(4):701–6. [PMID: 17697832]

▶ Treatment

The treatment of AR depends on its underlying cause, severity, cardiac function, and the presence or absence of symptoms. Mild-to-moderate AR may not require any specific treatment, whereas severe acute AR due to aortic dissection is a medical and surgical emergency.

A. Acute Aortic Regurgitation

Severe acute AR carries a high mortality rate if left untreated. It requires aggressive supportive measures, a rapid assessment of cause, and institution of definitive therapy. Because early death due to left ventricular failure and hemodynamic collapse is frequent in these patients despite intensive medical therapy, prompt surgical intervention is indicated. While the patient is being prepared for surgery, pharmacologic therapy can be initiated. Vasodilator therapy with sodium nitroprusside is the treatment of choice in acute AR because of its afterload and preload reduction. The dose is titrated to optimize forward cardiac output and pulmonary capillary wedge pressure. Positive inotropic agents such as dobutamine can be used if the patient remains hypotensive with a low systemic cardiac output.

When acute AR is associated with hemodynamic instability, the only definitive therapy is surgical correction. The timing of surgery depends on the cause and degree of hemodynamic derangement. In infective endocarditis with severe AR, it is preferable to give several days of appropriate antibiotics prior to aortic valve replacement (AVR), provided the patient is hemodynamically stable. Indications for urgent surgery are New York Heart Association (NYHA) class III–IV congestive heart failure, systemic embolization, persistent bacteremia, fungal endocarditis, or abscess formation. When AR results from aortic dissection with disruption of commissural support, urgent surgical repair is indicated.

B. Chronic Aortic Regurgitation

1. Mild-to-moderate aortic regurgitation—Patients who have mild or moderate AR and are asymptomatic and who have normal or minimally increased cardiac size require no therapy for the AR. They should be followed with clinical evaluation yearly and echocardiography at 2- to 3-year intervals. In patients with a history of rheumatic fever, prophylaxis using either penicillin or erythromycin is indicated until the age of 25 years and 5 years after the last episode. If rheumatic carditis has already occurred, lifelong prophylaxis is recommended, even following valve replacement. Any occurrence of systemic hypertension should be treated because it aggravates the degree of regurgitation. Patients with AR secondary to syphilis should receive a full course of penicillin therapy. Patients with moderate AR should avoid isometric exercise, competitive sports, and heavy physical exertion. If symptoms present in such patients, an alternative cause for the symptoms should be considered.

2. Moderate-to-severe aortic regurgitation with symptoms and normal left ventricular function—Patients with chronic significant AR and normal left ventricular ejection fraction (LVEF) (> 50%) who have NYHA class III or IV symptoms or Canadian Cardiovascular Society class II–IV angina should undergo AVR. Patients with NYHA class II symptoms should be evaluated on a case-by-case basis. If the cause or severity of symptoms is unclear, an exercise test should be done. If exercise capacity is normal, treatment should be given as for asymptomatic patients as outlined in the following section. If new, even mild symptoms appear in a patient with chronic significant AR—particularly if left ventricular size is increased or the ejection fraction is on the low side of normal—then AVR should be considered.

Medical therapy is attempted in symptomatic patients who are awaiting surgery or are not surgical candidates due to refusal, terminal medical illness, or advanced age. The aim of therapy in these patients is primarily relief of symptoms and improvement of exercise capacity. Medical therapy includes digitalis, diuretics, and vasodilator drugs. Oral vasodilators, such as hydralazine, and angiotensin-converting enzyme (ACE) inhibitors reduce afterload, allowing for greater forward cardiac output, which may improve exercise tolerance. Preload reduction with diuretics and nitrates is also helpful in reducing pulmonary congestion.

3. Moderate-to-severe aortic regurgitation with symptoms and abnormal left ventricular function—Symptomatic patients with mild-to-moderate left ventricular dysfunction (LVEF = 25–50%) should undergo AVR.

Treatment decisions for patients with more advanced left ventricular dysfunction (LVEF < 25% or left ventricular end-systolic dimension > 60 mm) is difficult. The operative risk is high, and not all patients benefit from AVR. On the other hand, outcome with medical therapy is poor as well. Patients with class II–III symptoms and recent onset of left ventricular dysfunction should be considered for surgical treatment. In patients not considered surgical candidates, aggressive medical therapy is useful in controlling symptoms. Diuretics and vasodilators are the mainstay of medical treatment. If symptoms persist, short-term inotropic support using dobutamine along with intravenous nitroprusside and diuretics may provide relief.

4. Moderate-to-severe aortic regurgitation without symptoms—The optimal timing of AVR in asymptomatic patients remains a challenging clinical decision. Clearly, patients with normal left ventricular function and good exercise capacity can live for several years without symptoms or left ventricular dysfunction, and surgery is clearly not indicated for such patients. These patients may be candidates for long-term oral vasodilator therapy. Several small studies of hydralazine, nifedipine, and ACE inhibitors have shown inconsistent results, and clinical benefits have been uncertain. However, hypertension should be treated, preferably with vasodilators. When the evidence of left ventricular dysfunction (ejection fraction < 50%) is clear, despite the absence of symptoms, AVR is recommended to prevent further left ventricular dysfunction and improve prognosis. However, once the ejection fraction is decreased, surgical risk is higher and left ventricular dysfunction may become irreversible. The ideal time to intervene is late enough in the course of the disease to justify the surgical risk and postoperative sequelae such as anticoagulation, but early enough to prevent irreversible left ventricular contractile dysfunction. To determine the optimal time for surgery in chronic asymptomatic AR, it is important to identify preoperative variables that predict postoperative left ventricular function. A number of parameters have been investigated in the hope of identifying the ideal predictor. Regurgitant volume and fraction are not predictors of postoperative outcome because they are significantly influenced by loading conditions. End-diastolic volume has modest correlation with surgical outcome. The cutoff used varies from 150 to 250 mL/m^2. An end-diastolic minor dimension of greater than 70 mm has also been associated with a poor postoperative outcome. A major limitation of end-diastolic indices is their dependence on preload, and thus, they may not reflect intrinsic myocardial contractile function. LVEF has been shown to be an important predictor of postoperative survival. An LVEF of less than 0.50 is associated with a significantly reduced 3-year survival rate (64 ± 10%) compared with an LVEF greater than 0.50 (91 ± 28%). Although LVEF has high sensitivity for identifying patients with worse postoperative outcome, it is less specific. This is understandable because LVEF reflects loading conditions in addition to the inotropic state of the myocardium. Similarly, LVEF response to exercise may be modulated by multiple factors, including peripheral resistance, preload heart rate, sympathetic tone, and type of exercise. Therefore, although a decrease in ejection fraction during exercise was previously considered to predict a poor outcome in chronic AR, recent data suggest that this is a nonspecific response. However, exercise capacity by itself is an important predictor of survival in AR.

End-systolic indices are less load-dependent and have been used to predict left ventricular function following surgery for AR. An end-systolic minor dimension greater than 55 mm or end-systolic volume greater than 60 mL/m² identifies patients with persistent left ventricular dysfunction and a poor survival rate following AVR. Recently, the ratio of left ventricular end-systolic dimension in millimeters and body surface area in square meters that exceeds 25 has been advocated as a marker of occult left ventricular dysfunction. If, in addition to an increased end-systolic ventricular size, the ejection fraction is also reduced, the survival rate drops further. Even though they are preload-independent,

end-systolic indices are still affected by afterload. The ratio of end-systolic pressure or wall stress to end-systolic volume has been advocated as an index of contractility, which is less dependent on loading conditions. In patients with chronic severe AR, abnormalities of the end-systolic pressure-volume relationship have been shown, despite a normal LVEF, reflecting depressed myocardial contractility. Such patients are more likely to have symptoms and a need for earlier valve replacement.

For asymptomatic patients with moderate-to-severe AR, a noninvasive evaluation of left ventricular size and function is recommended as well as an exercise test if functional capacity is unclear (Figure 18–5). If exercise capacity is poor or LVEF is less than 50%, surgical treatment is recommended. Those with good exercise tolerance and normal left ventricular function should be followed at 6- to 12-month intervals. Oral vasodilators may be considered in these patients. In patients who remain asymptomatic, AVR should be considered when serial testing shows decreased exercise tolerance, progressive left ventricular enlargement, or worsening left ventricular function.

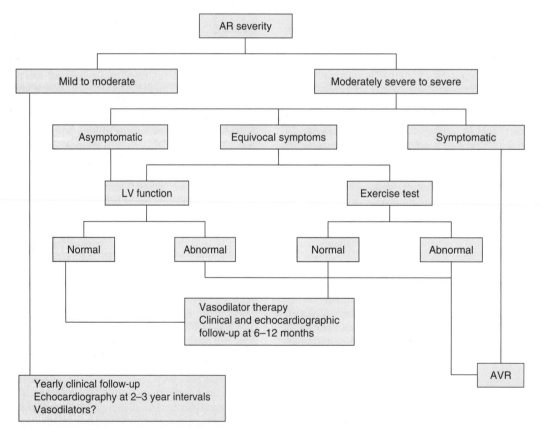

▲ **Figure 18–5.** Schematic of proposed treatment of patients with chronic significant aortic regurgitation. AR, aortic regurgitation; AVR, aortic valve replacement; LV, left ventricle.

▶ Prognosis

Asymptomatic patients with chronic AR have a stable course for many years. The mean rate of progression to surgery is approximately 4% per year. Symptoms are the major determinant of outcome in AR. The mortality rate for patients with NYHA class II–IV symptoms is over 20% per year. Even for patients with class II symptoms, the mortality rate is 6% per year compared with 3% for patients with class I symptoms. In general, good results have been observed with AVR for AR, with an average operative mortality rate of 3–4% and a 5-year survival rate of 85%. These results depend on several factors, including preoperative ventricular function, concomitant coronary artery disease, and the underlying cause of AR. Aortic valve replacement is necessary in most patients. In some cases of AR secondary to loss of commissural support, aortic valve repair can be performed. The feasibility of aortic valve repair can be determined by a transesophageal echocardiogram. In patients with excessive aortic root dilatation or aneurysm, a composite aortic graft with reimplantation of the coronary arteries is performed more frequently. Most patients show resolution of symptoms following surgery to correct AR. The end-diastolic volume is reduced immediately, with some further reduction occurring over several days after surgery. The LVEF continues to improve up to 1–2 years after surgery. There is also a gradual decline in left ventricular mass. About 20–30% of patients will have incomplete symptomatic relief and persistent left ventricular dysfunction. These findings are associated with the presence of preoperative left ventricular dysfunction, particularly if the duration of dysfunction is prolonged (> 18 months). Even though the outcome is less than optimal in patients with moderate left ventricular dysfunction, with recent surgical advances, many of them still do better with surgery than with medical management. Surgery should be considered in all symptomatic patients unless left ventricular dysfunction is very severe.

Bhudia SK, et al. Improved outcomes after aortic valve surgery for chronic aortic regurgitation with severe left ventricular dysfunction. *J Am Coll Cardiol.* 2007;49(13):1465–71. [PMID: 17397676]

Bonow RO, et al. 2008 focused update incorporated into the ACC/AHA 2006 guidelines for the management of patients with valvular heart disease. *J Am Coll Cardiol.* 2008;52:e1-e142. [PMID: 18848134]

de Waroux JB, et al. Functional anatomy of aortic regurgitation: accuracy, prediction of surgical repairability, and outcome implications of transesophageal echocardiography. *Circulation.* 2007;116(11 Suppl):I264–9. [PMID: 17846315]

Enriquez-Sarano M, et al. Clinical practice. Aortic regurgitation. *N Engl J Med.* 2004;351(15):1539–46. [PMID: 15470217]

Evangelista A, et al. Long-term vasodilator therapy in patients with severe aortic regurgitation. *N Engl J Med.* 2005;353(13):1342–9. [PMID: 16192479]

Kamath AR, et al. Survival in patients with severe aortic regurgitation and severe left ventricular dysfunction is improved by aortic valve replacement: results from a cohort of 166 patients with an ejection fraction < or =35%. *Circulation.* 2009;120 (11 Suppl);S134–8. [PMID: 19752358]

Mahajerin A, et al. Vasodilator therapy in patients with aortic insufficiency: a systematic review. *Am Heart J.* 2007;153: 454–61. [PMID: 17383279]

Tornos P, et al. Long-term outcome of surgically treated aortic regurgitation: influence of guideline adherence toward early surgery. *J Am Coll Cardiol.* 2006;47(5):1012–7. [PMID: 16516086]

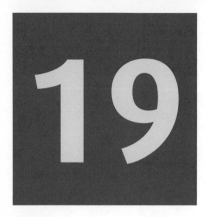

Mitral Stenosis

D. Elizabeth Le, MD

ESSENTIALS OF DIAGNOSIS

▶ Exertional dyspnea and fatigue.

▶ Opening snap, diastolic rumble murmur, loud S_1, presystolic accentuated murmur.

▶ Right ventricular heave and loud P_2 if pulmonary hypertension and right heart failure are present.

▶ A2-OS interval ≤ 80 ms in severe mitral stenosis.

▶ Sinus rhythm or atrial fibrillation, notched P wave or P mitrale in leads II and III and/or biphasic P wave in V_1, right axis deviation, high amplitude of P wave in lead II, and large R wave in V_1 on electrocardiography.

▶ Flattening of left atrial border and/or double density, elevated left main bronchus, enlarged pulmonary arteries, and Kerley B lines on chest radiography.

▶ Thickened and/or calcified mitral leaflets and subvalvular apparatus resulting in "hockey-stick" motion of the anterior leaflet and fusion of commissures resulting in fish-mouth appearance of the mitral valve on two- and three-dimensional echocardiography.

▶ Increased transmitral valve gradient and reduced mitral valve area by planimetry, pressure half-time, continuity equation, or proximal isovelocity surface area method of quantification on Doppler echocardiography.

▶ General Considerations

Mitral stenosis is a condition where the mitral valve area is reduced, causing obstruction of blood flow from the left atrium into the left ventricle during left ventricular diastole, which can lead to elevated left atrial pressure resulting in pulmonary hypertension, pulmonary edema, and right heart failure. The condition becomes clinically evident when the mitral valve area is reduced to approximately 2 cm². Mitral

stenosis occurs predominantly in adults and is one of the sequelae of rheumatic fever in about 90% of cases. Only about 50–70% patients recall having had antecedent group A β-hemolytic streptococcal tonsillopharyngitis. It has an indolent course, and the latent period can be as long as 40 years after the initial episode of rheumatic fever.

Rheumatic fever is a major public health problem in developing countries. The prevalence in developing countries is 2.2 to 2.3 per 1000 using clinical screening compared to 0.5 per 1000 in developed countries. If echocardiography is used to screen, the prevalence increases to 21.5 to 30.4 per 1000 in underdeveloped countries. Despite this fourfold difference, the prevalence in Western countries has not decreased substantially because of the increased rate of immigration from developing countries. Mitral stenosis still accounts for 10% of native valve pathology. The pattern of valvular involvement is associated with the rate of recurrent or reactivation of streptococcal infection and thus varies geographically. Individuals in developing countries are more likely to suffer from multiple episodes of rheumatic fever and thus become symptomatic at an earlier age compared to individuals in industrialized countries, who often do not present until they are ≥ 45 years old. Patients from developing countries tend to have more severe stenosis but less leaflet calcification and less atrial fibrillation. Due to the shorter latent period, younger patients tend to have more commissural thickening and pliable valves, whereas older patients with a longer latent period tend to have more calcified valves. A subgroup of patients, pregnant women, often present during the second trimester of pregnancy because increases in intravascular blood volume, cardiac output, and heart rate can make the impediment to flow more pronounced.

A. Anatomy

The mitral valve has two leaflets, anterior and posterior, which come together at the anterior and posterior commissures. The anterior leaflet occupies one-third of the saddle-shaped

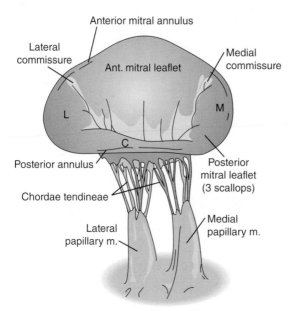

Anterior mitral annulus

Lateral commissure

Ant. mitral leaflet

Medial commissure

L

M

C

Posterior annulus

Posterior mitral leaflet (3 scallops)

Chordae tendineae

Lateral papillary m.

Medial papillary m.

▲ **Figure 19–1.** The mitral valve apparatus. The anterior mitral leaflet attaches to a smaller portion of the circumference of the annulus than the posterior mitral leaflet, but the anterior leaflet is longer. The posterior leaflet consists of three segments designated the lateral (L or P1), central (C or P2), and medial (M or P3) scallops. Both leaflets attach to both the medial and lateral papillary muscles. (From Otto CM. *Textbook of Clinical Echocardiography,* 4th ed. Philadelphia: Elsevier; 2009, with permission.)

annular circumference, and the posterior occupies two-thirds of the circumference. Primary, secondary, and tertiary chordae tendineae originate from both the anterolateral and posteromedial papillary muscles of the left ventricle and insert into margin and base of both the anterior and posterior leaflets. A competent mitral valve requires precise and concerted motion of the leaflets, chordae, and left ventricular and atrial contraction. Alteration of any components of this complex geometry can result in stenosis, insufficiency, or both (Figure 19–1).

B. Etiology

Mitral stenosis is predominantly due to organic valve pathology and less commonly due to functional valve pathology where the mitral leaflets are anatomically normal but their movement is altered. Approximately 90% of organic native valve mitral stenosis cases are associated with rheumatic fever or rheumatic heart disease, where the autoimmune response to group A streptococcal infection results in commissural thickening and fusion, valve and subvalvular apparatus thickening, calcification, and fusion, and consequently, restricted motion of the valve leaflets (Figure 19–2). Infective

endocarditis and severe mitral annular calcification account for about 3% of cases. Other conditions that have been associated with valve fibrosis are systemic lupus erythematous, rheumatoid arthritis, malignant carcinoid, and exposure to medications with direct serotonin receptors activation (ergotamine and methysergide for migraine headaches, fenfluramine and chlorphentermine for weight reduction, and pergolide and cabergoline for Parkinson disease). In < 1% of cases, mitral stenosis is due to congenital abnormalities and thus will present during infancy or childhood. These rare entities include supravalvar mitral ring, which is an abnormal connective tissue band located above the annulus or is adherent to the annulus and valve, hypoplasia of the mitral annulus, fusion of the commissures, a double orifice mitral valve, and a parachute mitral valve, where chordae from both the anterior and posterior leaflets insert into one papillary muscle. Another rare anomaly, cor triatriatum, can result in stenotic physiology without valve involvement. In this condition, a membrane or a fibromuscular band separates the left atrium into two compartments. This abnormal tissue may vary in size and shape, may have fenestrations, or can be funnel-shaped, which restricts blood flow from the left atrium into the left ventricle.

Functional native mitral valve stenosis is rare and can result from a mass, such as a left atrial myxoma or a large left atrial thrombus, advancing across the mitral annulus and occupying a portion of the mitral orifice during left ventricular diastole. Acquired mitral stenosis can also be iatrogenic where a portion of the mitral leaflet is inadvertently sutured to annular tissue during aortic or mitral valve surgery. Impingement of the anterior leaflet of the mitral valve with the CoreValve during percutaneous intervention to treat severe aortic stenosis resulting in stenosis has been reported.

Mitral stenosis can also involve prosthetic valves, where a bioprosthetic mitral valve can calcify over time with or without pannus overgrowth and cause similar pathophysiology seen in native valves. Mechanical mitral valves can also exhibit stenotic physiology when leaflet or poppet motion is impeded by thrombus, vegetation, or pannus.

C. Pathophysiology

The normal mitral valve area is 4–6 cm². Mild mitral stenosis occurs when the mitral valve area is reduced to 2 cm² and becomes severe when the area is ≤ 1 cm². In normal conditions, during early left ventricular diastole, blood flow from the left atrium into the left ventricle occurs from passive filling, is rapid, and peaks early, followed by diastasis, until active filling occurs from atrial contraction. Equalization of left atrial and left ventricular pressure occurs during mid-diastole. In the presence of mitral stenosis, the rate of passive filling is reduced and sustained throughout diastole, such that at end-diastole, left atrial pressure is higher than left ventricular pressure (Figure 19–3).

Within a cardiac cycle, the diastolic filling period (seconds per cycle) is the time between mitral valve opening and

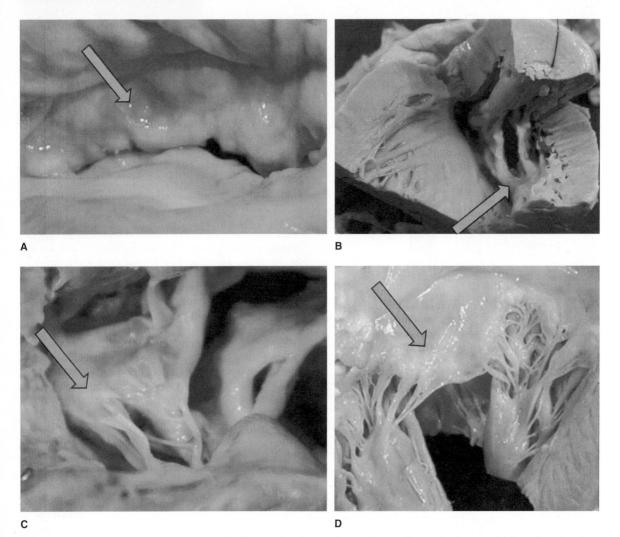

A   **B**

C   **D**

▲ **Figure 19–2.** Postmortem specimens of a rheumatic mitral valve and normal mitral valve. **A:** Thickened and nodular leaflet in rheumatic mitral valve. **B:** Calcified and fused commissure, fish-mouth shaped leaflets. **C:** Thickened, fused, and shortened subvalvular apparatus. **D:** Normal mitral leaflet and chordae tendineae. (Adapted, with permission, from Chandrashekhar Y, et al. *Lancet.* 2009;374:1271.)

closure. The diastolic filling time is determined using the following formula:

$$\text{Diastolic filling time (s/min)} = \text{Diastolic filling period (s/cycle)} \times \text{Heart rate (bpm)}$$

Mitral flow is a function of both the cardiac output and diastolic filling time and is calculated using the following equation:

$$\text{Mitral flow (mL/s)} = \frac{\text{Cardiac output (mL/min)}}{\text{Diastolic filling time (s/min)}}$$

During each minute, the diastolic filling period averages about 30–32 seconds. As heart rate increases, more time of the 1 minute is devoted to systolic ejection and isovolumetric contraction and relaxation, thus leading to a reduction in the diastolic filling period (Table 19–1). At rest, the diastolic flow across the mitral valve is about 200 mL/s. During exercise, cardiac output can triple, and along with tachycardia and the compensatory reduction in diastolic filling, transmitral flow and gradient will increase. Assuming no change in left atrial and left ventricular compliance, as the mitral valve area decreases, left atrial pressure and transmitral gradient will increase disproportionately with mitral flow

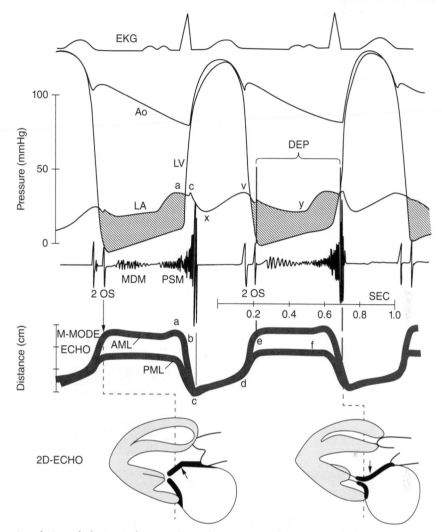

▲ **Figure 19–3.** Correlation of electrocardiogram (ECG), hemodynamic tracings, cardiac auscultation, M-mode, and two-dimensional (2D) echocardiography (ECHO) of mitral stenosis. The left atrium (LA) pressure tracing shows a prominent a wave and v wave. The atrioventricular pressure gradient (*shaded area*) is sustained throughout diastole with elevated LA pressure. The E-F slope is flat on M-mode recording of the mitral leaflets. AML, anterior mitral leaflet; AO, aorta; DFP, diastolic filling period; LV, left ventricle; MDM, mid-diastolic murmur; OS, opening snap; PML, posterior mitral leaflet; PSM, presystolic murmur. (Adapted, with permission, from Heger JW, et al. *Cardiology,* 3rd ed. Baltimore: Williams & Wilkins; 1994.)

(Figure 19–4). Chronically elevated left atrial pressure results in left atrial enlargement, which can lead to paroxysmal or permanent atrial fibrillation. Rapid atrial fibrillation reduces the diastolic filling time and cardiac output, which in turn, perpetuates the vicious circle by further increasing left atrial pressure. Chronic elevation of left atrial pressure causes a rise in pulmonary venous pressure and eventually pulmonary arterial pressure. When left atrial pressure exceeds

25 mm Hg, pulmonary edema develops. Consequently, chronic pulmonary arterial hypertension leads to right ventricular pressure overload and then volume overload when the right heart fails. Over time, the pulmonary vasculature becomes permanently damaged, leading to fixed pulmonary hypertension and elevation of pulmonary vascular resistance.

Mitral stenosis is associated with increased levels of prothrombotic metabolites. This hypercoagulable milieu poses

Table 19–1. Relation Between Heart Rate, Diastolic Filling Time, and Mitral Valve Flow with a Constant Cardiac Output of 5 L/min

Heart Rate (bpm)	Diastolic Filling Time (s/min)	Mitral Valve Flow (mL/s)
50	38	132
75	30	167
100	26	192
150	18	278
175	12	417

a high risk of left atrial and left atrial appendage thrombus formation. Other factors that independently predict thrombosis in mitral stenosis are ≥ 1 year duration of atrial fibrillation, left atrial size ≥ 4.5 cm, left atrial spontaneous echo contrast on echocardiography, and a prior thromboembolic event.

Balghith M, et al. Transcatheter aortic valve implantation (core valve) prosthesis complicated by mitral stenosis. *J Saudi Heart Assoc.* 2012;24(2):149–50.

Iung B. Mitral stenosis still a concern in heart valve diseases. *Arch Cardiovasc Dis.* 2008;101:597–9. [PMID: 19056064]

Roeder HA, et al. Maternal valvular heart disease in pregnancy. *Obstet Gynecol Surv.* 2011;66(9):561–71. [PMID: 22088233]

▶ Clinical Findings

A. Symptoms & Signs

1. Dyspnea and fatigue—The classic symptoms of mitral stenosis are dyspnea and fatigue during exercise or in the setting of any condition that results in sinus tachycardia such as hyperthyroidism, hypovolemia, anemia, fever/infection, emotional stress, pregnancy, or exposure to sympathomimetic agents. Those with more advanced disease can experience shortness of breath at rest. In addition, patients are predisposed to developing atrial fibrillation, and the loss of atrial contraction and synchronized contraction with the left ventricle during each cardiac cycle can exacerbate dyspnea on exertion or even produce shortness of breath at rest,

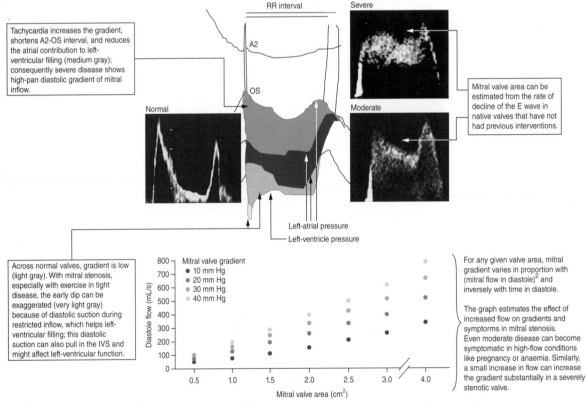

▲ **Figure 19–4.** Pathophysiology of mitral stenosis. (Adapted, with permission, from Chandrashekhar Y, et al. *Lancet.* 2009;374:1271.)

especially in patients with left ventricular dysfunction. Chest pain is rare, but patients may have intermittent or sustained palpitations from paroxysmal or permanent atrial fibrillation. One of the most devastating morbidities associated with mitral stenosis is embolic cerebral vascular accident, which occasionally can be the presenting symptom.

2. Congestive heart failure—As mitral stenosis becomes more severe, elevated left atrial pressure causes pulmonary vascular congestion. Pulmonary edema usually is manifested by dyspnea. In the early stages, pulmonary edema may occur only during exertion, and as the disease progresses, pulmonary edema occurs at rest. Occasionally, acute pulmonary edema can occur with exercise. Other signs of left heart failure include weight gain, orthopnea, and paroxysmal nocturnal dyspnea. In the late stages of mitral stenosis, there is irreversible adverse remodeling of the pulmonary vasculature, which results in elevated pulmonary artery pressure and pulmonary vascular resistance. Subsequently, right heart failure ensues when right heart hypertrophy can no longer adapt to the high pulmonary and right ventricular pressures. Symptoms of right heart failure include exercise intolerance, dyspnea, abdominal fullness, and lower extremity edema.

3. Hemoptysis—When severe mitral stenosis leads to severe pulmonary hypertension, rarely the bronchial veins can rupture and cause hemoptysis.

B. Physical Examination

1. Arterial pulses—In severe stenosis, when stroke volume is reduced, pulses are diminished.

2. Rhythm—In the early stages of mitral stenosis, patients have normal sinus rhythm. In moderate to severe mitral stenosis, elevated left atrial pressure and atrial tissue fibrosis can lead to atrial arrhythmia, predominantly in the form of atrial fibrillation, where heart sounds will be rapid and irregularly irregular.

3. Opening snap—The opening snap (OS) is due to the abrupt opening of the mitral leaflets during left ventricular diastole, where the leaflets are still relatively mobile. It may not be detected if the valve is severely calcified and restricted. The OS is heard best at the base of the heart but can also be audible at the apex. The duration between aortic valve closure and OS, the A2-OS interval, can be used to determine stenosis severity. The astute clinician can estimate the duration of this interval on auscultation. An A2-OS duration of <80 ms is indicative of severe mitral stenosis with a corresponding left atrial pressure of at least 25 mm Hg. As left atrial pressure rises, the OS occurs earlier, leading to a shorter A2-OS interval (see Figure 19–3).

4. Diastolic rumble murmur—The diastolic murmur in mitral stenosis is due to turbulent flow across the mitral valve. This murmur is low-pitch and is heard best at the apex using the bell of the stethoscope when the patient lies in the left lateral decubitus position. The diastolic murmur can also be more prominent after exercise, although tachycardia results in a shorter diastolic filling time, which may make auscultation more challenging. Maneuvers that increase venous return accentuate the diastolic murmur and shorten the A2-OS interval, whereas maneuvers that decrease venous return decrease the murmur and lengthen the A2-OS interval. The duration of the murmur, and not the amplitude, correlates with stenosis severity. In mild stenosis, the diastolic murmur is audible during late ventricular diastole when atrial systole occurs and represents "presystolic accentuation." As the valve becomes more stenotic, the diastolic murmur is present throughout diastole. In very severe stenosis, the amplitude may be diminished significantly due to extremely low flow across the valve and may be inaudible.

5. Loud S$_1$—Closure of minimally calcified and pliable mitral leaflets transmits as a loud S$_1$. However, as calcification increases, the valve is less mobile and the S$_1$ is soft.

6. Findings with pulmonary hypertension—A loud pulmonic valve closure (P$_2$) can be audible in patients who have developed passive pulmonary hypertension. There may also be a systolic murmur from tricuspid regurgitation. If right ventricular hypertrophy is also present, a right ventricular heave may be palpable. Right heart systolic dysfunction can present as hepatomegaly, peripheral edema, and ascites.

7. Other findings—If there is mixed valve disease, the holosystolic murmur of chronic mitral regurgitation is present. If there is concomitant aortic regurgitation or pulmonary insufficiency, a high-pitch blowing diastolic murmur can be appreciated. If a patient has left ventricular systolic failure, elevated jugular venous pressure, pulmonary rales, and lower extremity edema are seen.

▶ Diagnostic Studies

A. Electrocardiography

The rhythm can be sinus or atrial fibrillation. A notched P wave or "P mitrale" in leads II and III and/or a biphasic P wave in lead V$_1$ can be present, which reflect left atrial enlargement. If there is right ventricular enlargement and right ventricular failure, they manifest as right axis deviation, incomplete right bundle branch block, and tall R wave in V$_2$ or deep S wave in V$_6$. Right atrial enlargement is represented by high amplitude ($\geq$ 2.5 mm) of the P wave in lead II (Figure 19–5).

B. Chest Radiography

Left atrial appendage enlargement on radiography results in straightening of the left superior cardiac border on the posteroanterior view, which is seen more commonly than the double density, where both the left and right atrial borders are seen when the left atrium enlarges to the right. Occasionally, the left main bronchus is also elevated due to left atrial enlargement. If there is enlargement of the

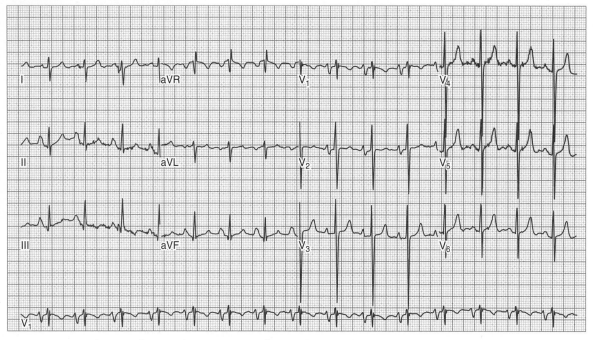

▲ **Figure 19–5.** Electrocardiogram demonstrating right axis deviation (+90° to +180°, negative amplitude in lead I, and positive amplitude in lead aVF), left atrial enlargement (notched P wave in lead II and biphasic P wave in leads V_1 and V_2), right atrial enlargement (P-wave amplitude of 4 mm in lead II), and right ventricular hypertrophy (right axis deviation > 90°, tall R in V_2, and prominent S wave in V_6) seen in mitral stenosis. (From American College of Cardiology ECG-SAPII, with permission. Copyright © 1997.)

pulmonary veins, an antler configuration is visible. In the frontal projection, when pulmonary hypertension coexists with mitral stenosis, the main pulmonary artery is enlarged and extends beyond the tangent line drawn from the aortic knob to the left ventricular apex (Figure 19–6). Chronically elevated pressure in the pulmonary veins can result in redistribution of blood flow to the upper lobes, seen as cephalization of the pulmonary vessels, and interlobular edema at the bases appearing as Kerley B lines. When pulmonary arterial hypertension ensues, pruning of the peripheral vessels is present. The left ventricular contour is usually normal, and if there is right heart failure, the right ventricle fills the retrosternal space in the lateral projection.

C. Echocardiography

1. M-mode, two-dimensional, and three-dimensional echo imaging
—Echocardiography is the imaging modality of choice to investigate the severity of mitral stenosis because it offers both anatomic and functional information. Due to commissural fusion, the anterior and posterior leaflets move anteriorly, and the E-F slope is reduced on M-mode images (Figure 19–7). Two-dimensional echo images show fusion of the commissures, thickened and calcified leaflets, and chordae tendineae. During diastole, the posterior leaflet is fixed

and the anterior leaflet opens and appears like a hockey stick in the parasternal long axis view. In the parasternal short axis view, the mitral valve has a "fish-mouth" appearance in the open position (Figure 19–8). The left atrium is enlarged and could have visible thrombus. The Wilkins echocardiography score is used to determine suitability for successful balloon valvotomy, where 1 to 4 points are assigned in each of four categories: leaflet thickening, leaflet calcification, leaflet mobility, and subvalvular apparatus thickening. A score of ≤ 8 predicts a favorable outcome.

Over the past decade, the availability of real-time, three-dimensional (3D) echocardiographic imaging allows better visualization of the stenotic valve in 3D space and provides simultaneous acquisition of orthogonal views of the mitral valve, which improves the accuracy of planimetry. 3D imaging also provides additional information on the orientation of the subvalvular apparatus, which permits detailed planning prior to interventional procedures (Figure 19–9).

2. Quantification of mitral stenosis
—The parameters used to diagnose and quantify mitral stenosis are depicted in Table 19–2. Continuous wave Doppler flow is used to measure the mean mitral gradient based on the Bernoulli equation where velocities across the mitral valve are measured and the mean pressure gradient is the $\Sigma 4v^2/n$, where

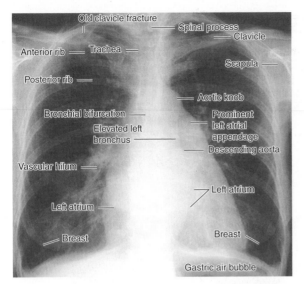

▲ **Figure 19–6.** Posteroanterior view on chest radiography of the cardiac silhouette and pulmonary structures in mitral stenosis. Left main stem bronchus is elevated. Left cardiac border is straightened with a bulging convex protrusion just beneath the aortic knob caused by left atrial appendage enlargement. Pulmonary veins are enlarged. (From C.C. Patrick, J. Lynch, and C. Carl Jaffe, Yale University, 2006, with permission.)

v is the velocity and *n* is the number of individual velocities measured. The mean gradient is determined by tracing the velocity time integral (VTI), which then is automatically calculated by ultrasound software packages. This measurement is straightforward to obtain but is dependent on heart rate, heart rhythm, and global left ventricular systolic function. The mean gradient can be low in bradycardia or in low cardiac output states (Figure 19–10).

The mitral valve area (MVA) can be measured by planimetry of the mitral orifice in the parasternal short axis view. The area can be overestimated if the imaging plane is not at the level where the orifice is the smallest or underestimated when there is significant calcification. The availability of 3D echo images has improved the accuracy and reproducibility of this technique. The advantage of this method is that it is easy to obtain if image quality is excellent (Figure 19–11A).

Using Doppler measurements, estimating the MVA by pressure half-time (PHT) is the simplest Doppler method. The PHT is the time during diastole when the transmitral gradient falls to 50% of the initial peak gradient.

$$MVA\ (cm^2) = \frac{220}{PHT\ (ms)}$$

This method is invalid immediately after balloon valvotomy and in patients with severe aortic regurgitation or in conditions with high filling pressures or decreased left ventricular compliance. In atrial fibrillation, at least five measurements should be recorded and averaged (Figure 19–11B).

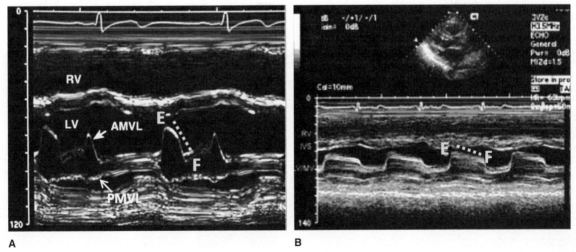

▲ **Figure 19–7.** M-mode of a normal mitral valve (**A**) and of a rheumatic mitral valve (**B**). In the normal valve, the thin leaflets separate and the E-F slope is steep; whereas in the stenotic valve, the leaflets are thickened, the posterior leaflet moves anteriorly during diastole, and the E-F slope is flat. AMVL, anterior mitral valve leaflet; LV, left ventricle; PMVL, posterior mitral valve leaflet; RV, right ventricle. (Adapted, with permission, from Otto CM. *Textbook of Clinical Echocardiography,* 4th ed. Philadelphia: Elsevier; 2009, and Armstrong WF, et al. *Feigenbaum's Echocardiography,* 7th ed. Philadelphia: Lippincott Williams & Wilkins; 2010.)

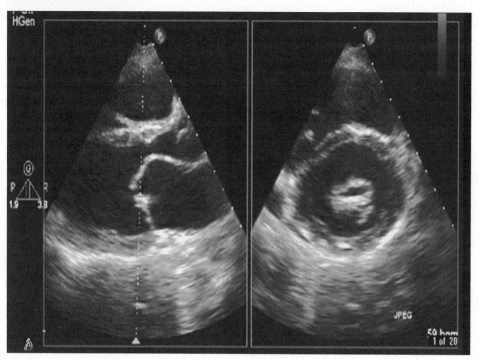

▲ **Figure 19–8.** Two-dimensional echo orthogonal views of a rheumatic mitral valve confirm that measurement of the mitral orifice is at the tip of the leaflets and is the smallest area. **Left:** In the parasternal long axis view, hockey-stick appearance of anterior leaflet and fixed posterior leaflet is seen. **Right:** In the parasternal short axis view, the opened mitral valve has a fish-mouth configuration. (Adapted, with permission, from de Augustin JA, et al. *Cardiol Clin.* 2007;25:311.)

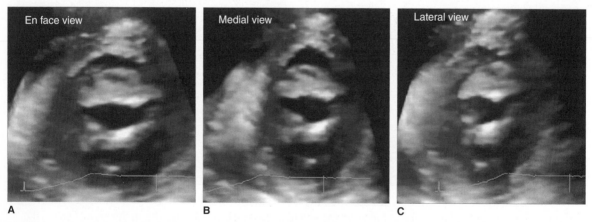

▲ **Figure 19–9.** Three-dimensional echo images of a stenotic rheumatic mitral valve in the parasternal short axis view after commissural opening. The (**A**) en face, (**B**) medial, and (**C**) lateral views showed opened commissures. (This figure was reproduced with permission and was published in Messika-Zeitoun D, et al. *Arch Cardiovasc Dis.* 2008;101:653. Copyright © 2012 Published by Elsevier Masson SAS on behalf of the Éditions françaises de radiologie. All rights reserved.)

Table 19–2. Quantification of Mitral Stenosis

Severity	MVA (cm²)	Mean Gradient (mm Hg)	PHT (ms)	PASP (mm Hg)	A2-OS Interval (ms)	NYHA HF Class
Normal	4–6	0	37–55	< 25	> 120	Normal
Mild	1.6–2.0	1–4	110–138	< 30	> 120	Normal
Moderate	1.1–1.5	5–10	147–200	30–50	80–120	II–III
Severe	≤ 1.0	≥ 10	≥ 220	> 50	< 80	II–IV

Heart rate between 60 and 80 bpm, sinus rhythm.
A2, aortic valve closure; MVA, mitral valve area; NYHA HF, New York Heart Association Heart Failure; OS, opening snap; PASP, pulmonary artery systolic pressure; PHT, pressure half-time.

The second Doppler method used to calculate MVA is based on the principle of energy conservation. The continuity equation used to calculate the cross-sectional area of the mitral valve is:

$$MVA(cm^2) = \frac{LVOT\ D^2 \times 0.785 \times VTI_{LVOT}}{VTI_{MV}}$$

where *LVOT D* is the diameter of the left ventricular outflow tract measured in the parasternal long axis view and *VTI* is the time velocity integral of the LVOT and mitral valve (MV), respectively. This method assumes that flow across the mitral valve is equivalent to flow across the aortic valve. It is inaccurate when there is significant concomitant mitral or aortic regurgitation. Mitral regurgitation can overestimate the severity of mitral stenosis, and aortic regurgitation can underestimate the severity mitral stenosis. In addition, poor visualization of the LVOT on two-dimensional imaging can significantly affect the MVA (Figure 19–11C).

The third Doppler method used in MVA calculation is the proximal isovelocity surface area (PISA) method, where

$$MVA(cm^2) = \frac{6.28 \times r^2 \times Aliasing\ velocity}{Peak\ mitral\ stenosis\ velocity} \times \frac{\alpha°}{180°}$$

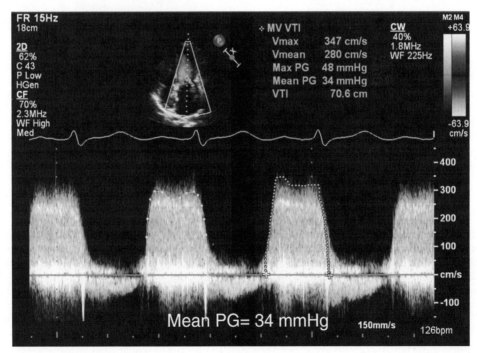

▲ **Figure 19–10.** Doppler measurement of the mean mitral gradient. (From Omran AS, et al. *J Saudi Heart Assoc.* 2011;23:51, with permission.)

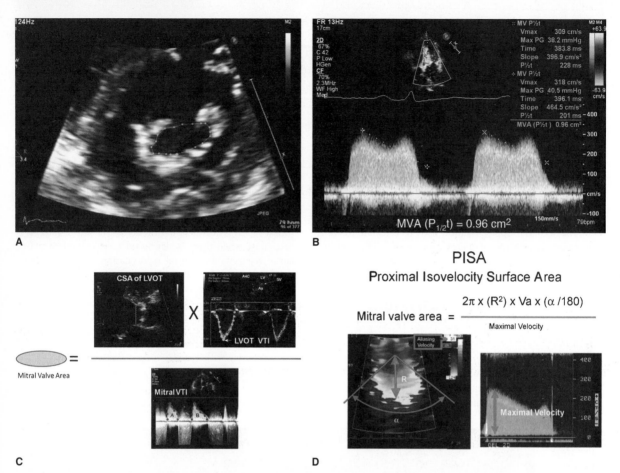

▲ **Figure 19–11.** Quantification of mitral stenosis using two-dimensional and Doppler echocardiography. **A:** Planimety of the mitral orifice. **B:** Calculation using the pressure half-time ($P_{1/2}t$) method. **C:** Calculation using the continuity equation. **D:** Calculation using the proximal isovelocity surface area (PISA) method. CSA, cross-sectional area; LVOT, left ventricular outflow tract; MVA, mitral valve area; PG, peak gradient; Vmax, maximum velocity; VTI, velocity time integral. (Panels **A** and **B** were adapted, with permission, from Omran AS, et al. *J Saudi Heart Assoc.* 2011;23:51. Panel **C** was adapted, with permission, from Baumgartner H, et al. *J Am Soc Echocardiogr.* 2009;22:1. Panel **D** was reproduced, with permission, and was published in Messika-Zeitoun D, et al. *Arch Cardiovasc Dis.* 2008;101:653. Copyright © 2012 Published by Elsevier Masson SAS on behalf of the Éditions françaises de radiologie. All rights reserved.)

This method is the most complex and technically challenging because it requires measuring the radius of PISA in the left atrium and the angle between the two mitral leaflets in the left atrium. However, since it is uses only velocity measurements, it is unaffected by factors that alter flow conditions (Figure 19–11D).

D. Exercise-Stress Echocardiography

When symptoms are discordant with two-dimensional and Doppler findings, exercise-stress echocardiography can be used to assess mitral stenosis severity since exercise increases cardiac output and gradient without changing the MVA. The mean mitral gradient and pulmonary artery systolic pressure are measured during each stage of bicycle exercise and are correlated with the perception of dyspnea. Dobutamine stress can also be employed, and a dobutamine-induced mean transmitral gradient of ≥ 18 mm Hg has a 90% accuracy rate for predicting a high-risk subpopulation. The tricuspid annulus S-wave velocity reflects right ventricular function, and its response during exercise is an independent predictor of functional capacity. A reduced S-wave velocity is a marker of poor prognosis.

E. Cardiac Computed Tomography and Magnetic Resonance Imaging

Currently, computed tomography and magnetic resonance imaging are not routinely used to assess mitral valve morphology. However, due to high image resolution of anatomic features, the role of both imaging techniques is being investigated.

F. Cardiac Catheterization

When echocardiographic data are ambiguous and/or suboptimal, often in situations when left atrial and left ventricular compliance are altered, cardiac catheterization is used to simultaneously and directly measure the left atrial and left ventricular pressures during diastole. On the left atrial pressure tracing, the "a" wave is accentuated, due to elevated pressure during atrial contraction. The left atrial pressure tracing also records an enlarged V wave, but it is not exclusively seen in mitral stenosis (Figure 19–12). If direct left atrial access is not performed, then the pulmonary capillary wedge (PCW) pressure is used as the surrogate for left atrial pressure. When PCW pressure is used, the operator must be absolutely certain that the balloon right heart catheter is in the "wedged" position by evaluating the hemodynamic waveform and, ideally, by measuring the oxygen saturation distal to the catheter, which originates from the oxygenated blood of a pulmonary vein. The diagnostic finding of mitral stenosis is the presence of a diastolic gradient when the PCW pressure or left atrial pressure is measured simultaneously with the left ventricular pressure. The magnitude of difference in gradients at end-diastole reflects the severity of obstruction. Tachycardia will increase and bradycardia will decrease the transmitral gradients. The Gorlin formula is used to calculate the MVA, where

$$MVA(cm^2) = \frac{(Cardiac\ output\ (mL/min)/Diastolic\ filling\ period\ (s)) \times Heart\ rate\ (bpm)}{Constant\ 37.9 \times \sqrt{Mean\ transmitral\ gradient\ (mm\ Hg)}}$$

This formula accurately determines MVA only in patients with isolated mitral stenosis. In those who also have mitral regurgitation, the Gorlin formula overestimates the degree of mitral stenosis because it does not account for the increased regurgitant flow across the valve. Pulmonary arterial pressure is also measured and is usually elevated proportionally with left atrial hypertension in the absence of intrinsic pulmonary disease. Similar to noninvasive measurements, in the setting of atrial fibrillation, a minimum of five measurements should be collected and averaged since the mean gradient is dependent on the R-R interval.

▶ Differential Diagnosis

Dyspnea on exertion and exercise intolerance are nonspecific symptoms that can be present in many other cardiac and noncardiac conditions. It is important to consider left and right heart cardiomyopathy; valvular pathology such as aortic stenosis, aortic insufficiency, and mitral regurgitation; pericardial disease such as chronic constrictive pericarditis; intracardiac shunting; and bradyarrhythmias and tachyarrhythmias. Obviously, numerous pulmonary processes can lead to dyspnea, including obstructive and restrictive lung disease and interstitial lung disease. Other etiologies of dyspnea and fatigue to consider are chronic anemia, hypothyroidism, thyrotoxicosis, and obesity. The likelihood of mitral stenosis should always be considered when evaluating pregnant patients with new-onset dyspnea.

Chandrashekhar Y, et al. Mitral stenosis. *Lancet.* 2009;374: 1271–83. [PMID: 19747723]
Deswarte G, et al. Longitudinal right ventricular function as a predictor of functional capacity in patients with mitral stenosis: an exercise echocardiographic study. *J Am Soc Echocardiogr.* 2010;23:667–72. [PMID: 20434881]

Messika-Zeitoun D, et al. Evaluation of mitral stenosis in 2008. *Arch Cardiovasc Dis.* 2008;101:653–63. [PMID: 19056072]
Omran AS, et al. Echocardiography in mitral stenosis. *J Saudi Heart Assoc.* 2011;23:51.

▶ Treatment

A. Lifestyle Modifications

Patients with moderate or severe mitral stenosis should be counseled to avoid strenuous activities and thereby reduce risk of tachycardia. They should also be advised to consume a low-sodium diet in order to avoid fluid retention and to prevent development of pulmonary edema.

B. Pharmacologic Therapy

1. Secondary prevention of rheumatic fever—Since recurrent rheumatic fever is associated with progression of mitral stenosis, secondary prevention with antimicrobial therapy is recommended and the duration of therapy is dependent on the individual's age, extent of initial cardiac involvement, and risk of recurrent infection. Intramuscular benzathine penicillin G (1.2 million units every 4 weeks) is recommended in most cases. In populations with a high incidence of rheumatic fever, a 3-week schedule is more effective. Patients with rheumatic fever with carditis and residual valvular disease should take antimicrobial therapy for 10 years or until age 40, whichever is longer. Those without residual cardiac disease should continue for 10 years or until age 21, whichever is longer. Individuals who had only rheumatic fever, without carditis, can take prophylactic therapy for 5 years or until age 21, whichever is longer. Alternatively, oral penicillin V 250 mg twice daily or sulfadiazine 0.5 g (< 27 kg) to 1.0 g (> 27 kg) daily can be used.

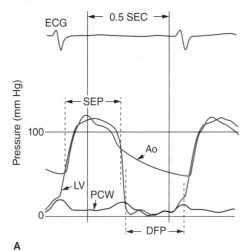

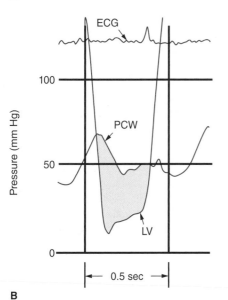

▲ **Figure 19–12.** Invasive simultaneous hemodynamic tracings of (**A**) normal left ventricular (LV), left atrial, and aortic (Ao) pressure and (**B**) pressure gradient between pulmonary capillary wedge (PCW) pressure and LV (*shaded in gray in mitral stenosis*). The LV end-diastolic pressure is atypically elevated with coincident mitral regurgitation. The PCW tracing has a large V wave. The PCW-LV pressure gradient is marked throughout diastole. DFP, diastolic filling period; SEP, systolic ejection period. (Adapted, with permission, from Carabello BA, et al. Calculation of stenotic valve orifice area. In: Baim DS, et al., eds. *Grossman's Cardiac Catheterization, Angiography, and Intervention,* 6th ed. Philadelphia: Lippincott Williams & Wilkins; 2000.)

2. Atrial fibrillation—Since tachycardia decreases the diastolic filling time, the ventricular rate should be aggressively treated with atrioventricular nodal blockers, including β-blockers, nondihydropyridine calcium channel blockers, and digoxin. When the tachycardia is refractory to atrioventricular nodal blockers, then pharmacologic cardioversion with antiarrhythmic medications or direct-current synchronized cardioversion is appropriate. In nonpregnant patients with atrial fibrillation, it is imperative that anticoagulation with warfarin be initiated with a therapeutic international normalized ratio goal of 2–3. The risk of systemic embolic events ranges from 1.5–4.7% per year without anticoagulation and decreases to about 0.7–0.8% per year on therapeutic warfarin. Successful valvotomy does not reduce the thrombotic risk, and thus patients still require indefinite anticoagulation. While tempting, there are no data to support empiric warfarin therapy in the absence of atrial fibrillation. Of note, the CHADS2 or CHA2DS2-Vasc used to estimate stroke risk associated with atrial fibrillation is not applicable in valvular or rheumatic mitral stenosis.

3. Congestive heart failure—Diuretics along with sodium restriction are used to treat pulmonary edema. In the setting of concomitant right ventricular failure, venodilators can be added.

C. Interventional Therapy

Mechanical therapy should be considered when the MVA is < 1.5 cm²/m² or when the mitral valve index is < 0.6 cm²/m². In addition, when New York Heart Association Congestive Heart Failure (NYHA) Class III/IV symptoms become refractory to optimal medical, invasive intervention should be pursued. Currently percutaneous balloon valvotomy is the preferred method for enlarging the mitral orifice in a selected patient group.

1. Percutaneous balloon valvotomy—Percutaneous balloon valvotomy is reserved for individuals with pliable valves with minimal calcification and mild or no mitral regurgitation and can be considered in those who are poor surgical candidates with the above valve morphology. It can also be performed safely in pregnant patients. All patients considered for valvotomy need to have an invasive assessment of mitral valve hemodynamic data prior to the procedure and immediately after completion of the procedure. Patient selection is absolutely essential for procedural success. The Wilkins echocardiographic score of ≤ 8 predicts a very favorable outcome. On average, the mitral gradient decreases by approximately 7–10 mm Hg, mitral orifice increases by approximately 0.7–1 cm², and cardiac output increases by about 0.6 L/min. The immediate, short-, and long-term results are excellent. For those with a score of ≤ 8, the survival rate at 12 years was 82% versus 57% in those with higher scores, and event-free survival was 38% versus 22%. At 19 years, restenosis-free survival ranges from 22 to 30%,

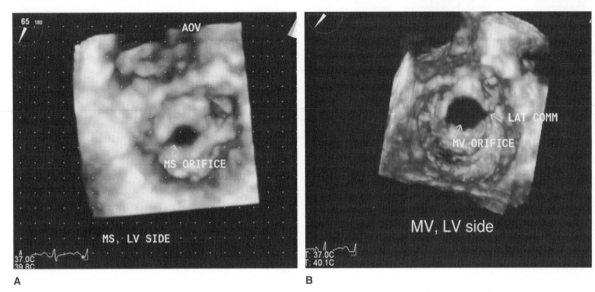

▲ Figure 19–13. Three-dimensional echocardiography images of the mitral orifice before (**A**) and after (**B**) mitral valve balloon valvotomy. AOV, aortic valve; LV, left ventricle; MS, mitral stenosis; MV, mitral valve. (From Omran AS, et al. *J Saudi Heart Assoc.* 2011;23:51, with permission.)

and event-free survival ranges from 21 to 35%. Successful valvotomy can last for decades in flexible, noncalcified valves and is comparable to surgical commissurotomy. In some patients, the stenotic mitral valve can undergo repeat balloon valvotomy. In addition, successful valvotomy can result in normalization of pulmonary artery systolic pressure, regression of tricuspid regurgitation, and improvement of left ventricular systolic function if it is reduced prior to intervention (Figure 19–13).

Even though the success rate ranges from 85 to 99% in appropriately selected patients, the procedure is associated with a 0–0.5% mortality rate, up to a 12% incidence of hemopericardium, and a 1–2% rate of systemic embolization. The most catastrophic complication of balloon valvotomy is severe mitral regurgitation, which occurs in 2–10% of cases when the heavily calcified leaflets, and not the commissures, are split. In 1.6–3% of cases, surgical treatment of mitral regurgitation is necessary. Use of transesophageal and intracardiac echocardiography during valvotomy assists in balloon placement, septal puncture guidance, and detection of complications.

2. Surgical commissurotomy—Surgical commissurotomy can be performed either by the closed or open approach. The surgical mortality rate is 2–5% in isolated mitral valve repair or replacement. After surgical commissurotomy, the post-operation mean mitral gradient and MVA can be measured noninvasively. In countries where percutaneous balloon valvotomy is not available or is cost-prohibitive, surgical commissurotomy can be performed with similar results. In populations with a high Wilkins echocardiographic score or

atrial fibrillation, compared with balloon valvotomy, surgical open mitral commissurotomy or mitral valve replacement is associated with a higher event-free survival rate of 94% versus 80% at 9 years. However, compared to the percutaneous approach, surgical commissurotomy is associated with greater morbidity, longer hospital stay, and longer recovery. Similar to the balloon valvotomy, a relatively larger mitral orifice does not reduce the risk of thrombosis.

3. Mitral valve replacement—If the valve is heavily calcified or commissurotomy does not increase the mitral orifice area sufficiently, then mitral valve replacement is indicated. A Wilkins echocardiographic score > 8 and at least moderate mitral regurgitation are independent risk factors for surgery after balloon valvotomy. The choice of a bioprosthetic valve versus a mechanical valve depends on the age of the patient, existing comorbid conditions, and ability to comply with oral anticoagulant therapy. A mechanical valve is preferable in young patients in order to avoid accelerated bioprosthetic valve calcification, especially in those who are hemodialysis dependent. In women of childbearing age who are interested in future pregnancies, a bioprosthetic valve is often selected to avoid warfarin-induced embryopathy.

Ahmari SAL, et al. Initial experience of using intracardiac echocardiography (ICE) for guiding balloon mitral valvuloplasty (BMV). *J Saudi Heart Assoc.* 2012;24:23.

Cubeddu RJ, et al. Percutaneous techniques for mitral valve disease. *Cardiol Clin.* 2010;28:139–53. [PMID: 19962055]

Fawzy ME. Mitral balloon valvuloplasty. *J Saudi Heart Assoc.* 2010;22:125.

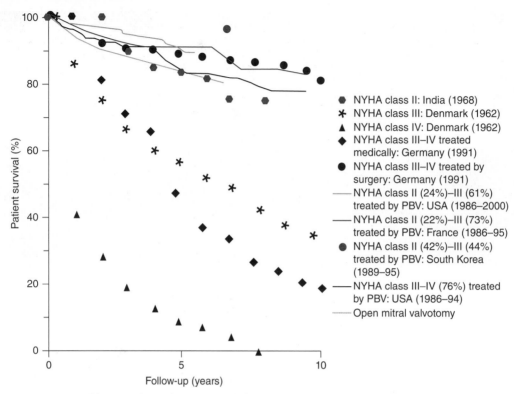

▲ **Figure 19-14.** Natural history of mitral stenosis and the effect of intervention. NYHA, New York Heart Association; PBV, percutaneous balloon valvotomy. (Adapted from Chandrashekhar Y, et al. *Lancet.* 2009;374:1271, with permission.)

Fawzy ME, et al. Long-term (up to 18 years) clinical and echo-cardiographic results of mitral balloon valvuloplasty in 531 consecutive patients and predictors of outcome. *Cardiology.* 2009;113:213–21. [PMID: 19218805]

Gerber MA, et al. Prevention of rheumatic fever and diagnosis and treatment of acute streptococcal pharyngitis: a scientific statement from the American Heart Association Rheumatic Fever, Endocarditis, and Kawasaki Disease Committee of the Council on the Young, the Interdisciplinary Council on Functional Genomics and Translational Biology, and the Interdisciplinary Council on Quality of Care and Outcomes Research: Endorsed by the American Academy of Pediatrics. *Circulation.* 2009;119:1541–51. [PMID: 19246689]

Nobuyoshi M, et al. Percutaneous balloon mitral valvuloplasty, a review. *Circulation.* 2009;119:e211–9. [PMID: 19106383]

Song JK, et al. Long-term outcomes of percutaneous mitral balloon valvuloplasty versus open cardiac surgery. *J Thorac Cardiovasc Surg.* 2010;139:103–10. [PMID: 19660411]

▶ **Prognosis**

Prognosis of uncorrected mitral stenosis is closely linked with NYHA congestive heart failure class at the time of diagnosis. The 10-year mortality rate for patients who are asymptomatic is < 20%. NYHA Class II and III patients have a mortality rate of 40%, and patients in Class IV approach a rate of 80–85%. Sixty to 70% of patients with severe mitral stenosis die from congestive heart failure, 20–30% from systemic thromboembolism, and 1–5% from infection (Figure 19–14).

Mitral Regurgitation

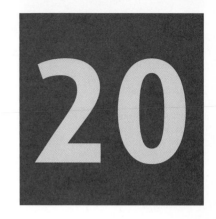

Michael H. Crawford, MD

- ▶ Dyspnea or orthopnea.
- ▶ Characteristic apical systolic murmur.
- ▶ Color-flow Doppler echocardiographic evidence of systolic regurgitation into the left atrium.

▶ General Considerations

The mitral apparatus consists of the left ventricular walls that support the papillary muscles, the chordae tendineae, mitral leaflets, annulus, and adjacent left atrial walls. Because defects in any of these components can lead to systolic regurgitation, the list of diseases that can cause mitral regurgitation includes many types of heart disease. Anything that causes left ventricular dilatation may disrupt the alignment of the papillary muscles, impairing their function and dilating the annulus, resulting in mitral regurgitation. Myocardial infarction involving the papillary muscles or the left ventricular walls that support them can impair the function of the mitral apparatus. Mitral chordae can rupture, especially in patients with hypertension or mitral valve prolapse. The most common diseases affecting the mitral leaflets are rheumatic heart disease and the myxomatous changes of mitral valve prolapse. In addition, infective endocarditis can destroy the mitral leaflets, and mitral annular calcification can impair the normal systolic contraction of the annulus, leading to mitral regurgitation. Finally, left atrial dilatation from any cause can disrupt annular function and cause mitral regurgitation. Some patients have combinations of these defects, making mitral regurgitation both more likely and more severe.

For clinical purposes, mitral regurgitation can be divided into two broad categories: organic and functional. The former refers to diseases that involve the valve leaflets and their immediate supporting apparatus, ie, chordae and annulus. The latter refers to diseases that affect the left ventricle and atrium, leaving the valve apparatus intact (Table 20–1). Most clinical studies involve patients with organic mitral regurgitation, so, unless otherwise specified, the following discussion focuses on organic mitral regurgitation.

Mitral valve prolapse is unique among the many causes of chronic organic mitral regurgitation in many ways. An increase in the middle connective tissue layer of the mitral valve causes an increase in leaflet size and elongated chordae. The resultant systolic prolapse of the valve into the left atrium may or may not be accompanied by regurgitation. In some patients, regurgitation depends on left ventricular volume. Large volumes tend to reduce prolapse and hence regurgitation; small volumes have the opposite effect.

Consequently, the presence or absence of regurgitation and its severity and timing in systole (the ventricle becomes progressively smaller during systole) are determined by a complex interplay of left ventricular volume, pressure, and contractile state. Patients with mitral valve prolapse are also unique because the condition can be hereditary connective tissue disease (eg, Marfan syndrome) or acquired (inflammation of the valve). Some patients exhibit abnormalities of connective tissue in other organs (eg, thoracic skeleton) and have demonstrable abnormalities in the autonomic nervous system. Thus, the clinical presentation of mitral valve prolapse varies from one that is similar to other forms of mitral regurgitation to a unique presentation that is dominated by extracardiac manifestations.

In **chronic mitral regurgitation,** the more common of the two general clinical presentations, the mitral regurgitation progressively worsens as the underlying heart disease worsens. In this situation, the heart has time to adapt to the mitral leak. The increased pressure in the left atrium during systole causes left atrial dilatation. If this is not adequate to decompress the left atrial pressure, the pulmonary arterial tone increases to protect the pulmonary capillaries from increased hydrostatic pressure, resulting in pulmonary

Table 20–1. Etiologic Classification of Mitral Regurgitation

Organic Mitral Regurgitation
Myxomatous changes (mitral valve prolapse)
Rheumatic heart disease
Infective endocarditis
Spontaneous chordal rupture
Collagen vascular disease
Trauma: penetrating and nonpenetrating
Functional Mitral Regurgitation
Coronary artery disease
Hypertrophic cardiomyopathy
Dilated cardiomyopathy
Left atrial dilatation

hypertension. Because the regurgitated blood returns to the left ventricle in diastole, along with the normal atrial stroke volume, the volume load on the left ventricle results in left ventricular dilatation and eccentric hypertrophy.

Initially, the loading conditions in mitral regurgitation enhance left ventricular performance because preload is increased and afterload is normal. Preload is increased by the augmentation of left ventricular diastolic volume, which increases left ventricular systolic function via the Frank-Starling mechanism. Afterload, or the left ventricular wall tension after the aortic valve opens in systole, is not increased, despite increased left ventricular volume, because much of the increased volume is regurgitated into the left atrium in early systole before the aortic valve opens and because the continued regurgitation during systole reduces forward stroke volume and blood pressure. As the severity of mitral regurgitation increases over time, the ability of the dilated left ventricle to augment systolic function reaches its limits, left ventricular systolic function falls, and heart failure ensues.

Acute mitral regurgitation presents differently because there is insufficient time for these compensatory mechanisms to develop. Sudden rupture of the chordae tendineae, for example, may result in severe acute mitral regurgitation, which markedly increases left atrial pressure. Because the left atrium has no time to dilate, the pulmonary capillary pressure rises markedly, and pulmonary edema usually ensues. The left ventricle also does not dilate adequately to handle the tremendous volume load, and forward failure occurs because of an impaired left ventricular stroke volume. Acute mitral regurgitation (caused by the abrupt failure of a component of the mitral apparatus) can precipitate or aggravate symptoms in a patient with chronic mitral regurgitation.

Nesta F, et al. New locus for autosomal dominant mitral valve prolapse on chromosome 13: clinical insights from genetic studies. *Circulation.* 2005;112(13):2022–30. [PMID: 16172273]

Magne J, et al. Ischemic mitral regurgitation: a complex multifaceted disease. *Cardiology.* 2009;112:244–59. [PMID: 18758181]

▶ Clinical Findings

A. Symptoms & Signs

1. Chronic mitral regurgitation—The medical history of patients with chronic mitral regurgitation may suggest its cause. Look for a possible history of acute rheumatic fever, coronary artery disease, or a cardiomyopathy. The most common symptom in patients with chronic mitral regurgitation is progressive dyspnea, beginning with dyspnea on exertion and progressing to paroxysmal nocturnal dyspnea and finally orthopnea. Patients may also complain of fatigue and other symptoms associated with congestive heart failure, such as edema. Chronic mitral regurgitation can lead to atrial fibrillation, and palpitations or other symptoms related to this rhythm disturbance may present in patients. Some patients with mitral valve prolapse may have atypical chest pain or inappropriate sympathetic nervous system activation (eg, inappropriate tachycardia, orthostatic hypotension).

2. Acute mitral regurgitation—The patient with acute mitral regurgitation is usually markedly symptomatic, with severe orthopnea or frank pulmonary edema. Although sudden pulmonary edema in itself may suggest the diagnosis, other features of the history may point to the cause of mitral apparatus failure, such as a history of acute myocardial infarction, uncontrolled hypertension, or symptoms of infective endocarditis.

B. Physical Examination

1. Chronic mitral regurgitation—In chronic mitral regurgitation, the heart rate may be increased because of atrial fibrillation or heart failure. The carotid pulse is usually brief and of low amplitude, and blood pressure examination shows a narrow pulse pressure. These findings reflect the reduced forward stroke volume. In the presence of heart failure, the respiratory rate may be increased and rales, pleural effusion, edema, increased jugular venous pressure, or ascites may be present. Left ventricular enlargement may result in an enlarged apical impulse. The first and second heart sounds are usually normal, but the pulmonic component of the second heart sound may be increased if pulmonary hypertension is evident. A third heart sound is common because of the left ventricular volume overload, but it does not necessarily indicate heart failure. A fourth heart sound is unusual unless associated coronary artery disease or hypertension is present. The characteristic murmur of chronic mitral regurgitation is usually holosystolic and heard best at the apex, with radiation to the axilla. Occasionally, in patients with posterior leaflet defects, the direction of the regurgitant jet may be anterior, and the murmur is heard in the aortic area. With anterior leaflet defects, the direction of the mitral jet may be posterior and transmitted to the back, where it can be heard up and down the spine. Some reports even note hearing this murmur with the stethoscope on the top of the head. In patients with mitral valve prolapse, the murmur can be crescendo and late systolic. This type of murmur, in fact, almost always represents mitral regurgitation. Often, the late systolic crescendo murmur of mitral valve prolapse is preceded by a midsystolic click from the sudden tensing of the prolapsing leaflets when the end of chordal tethering is reached. Some patients may manifest only a midsystolic click. Occasionally, mitral murmurs will be honking or musical in quality, presumably from a prolapsing leaflet that vibrates in the regurgitant stream. Some patients occasionally have other murmur configurations, whereas others with echocardiographically documented mitral regurgitation have no audible murmur, especially if the regurgitation is mild.

Because murmur configuration and radiation vary in mitral regurgitation, dynamic auscultation is of a great deal of value at the bedside for differentiating this murmur from other heart murmurs. Handgrip exercise is the favored bedside maneuver because it frequently increases the intensity of a mitral regurgitation murmur. In patients with poor grip strength, transient arterial occlusion with two blood pressure cuffs, one on each arm, is useful for producing the same effect (Table 20–2, and Chapter 5). The murmur of mitral valve prolapse behaves like that of mitral regurgitation from any cause, but it has a few unique features. Any maneuver that increases left ventricular volume will (as noted earlier) decrease the amount of mitral valve prolapse and decrease the amount of mitral regurgitation, thereby lessening the intensity of the murmur. Thus, rapid squatting will diminish the murmur of mitral valve prolapse and move the timing of the click-murmur complex later in systole (Figure 20–1).

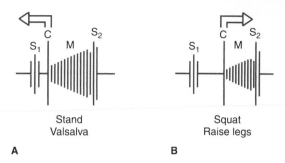

▲ **Figure 20–1.** Change in the position of the click (C)-murmur (M) complex during systole and the intensity of the murmur as a result of bedside maneuvers. **A:** Maneuvers that lengthen the murmur and increase intensity. **B:** Maneuvers that shorten the murmur and reduce its intensity. Note that the position of the midsystolic click also changes with these maneuvers.

Conversely, maneuvers that decrease left ventricular volume increase the intensity and duration of the murmur of mitral valve prolapse. Thus, standing rapidly from a squatting position will make the murmur louder and move the click-murmur complex toward early systole. Extreme left ventricular volume increases can eliminate the click-murmur and mitral regurgitation, and extreme decrease can result in a pansystolic murmur without a click. Consequently, the auscultatory findings in mitral valve prolapse vary greatly, which can make accurate clinical diagnosis difficult.

2. Acute mitral regurgitation—In acute mitral regurgitation, the physical findings are different. The marked increase in left atrial pressure, caused by regurgitation into a noncompliant left atrium, may raise left atrial pressure in late systole to the point that there is no longer any gradient for regurgitant flow. The murmur thus becomes an early systolic murmur rather than the holosystolic murmur characteristic of patients with chronic mitral regurgitation. In fact, when the acute mitral regurgitation is very severe, the murmur may not be audible. In mild-to-moderate acute mitral regurgitation, the murmur responds like the murmur of chronic mitral regurgitation with dynamic auscultation. More severe acute regurgitation is associated with high catecholamine tone and a lack of responsiveness to bedside maneuvers. Other characteristic features of acute mitral regurgitation include a fourth heart sound caused by vigorous atrial contraction following exaggerated expansion during ventricular systole (atrial diastole). In the presence of pulmonary hypertension, the pulmonary second sound increases, and murmurs of pulmonic and tricuspid regurgitation may be present. As mentioned earlier, acute mitral regurgitation invariably results in pulmonary edema. Consequently, the patient will have an increased respiratory rate, diffuse rales, evidence of plural effusion, increased heart rate, a narrow pulse pressure with low systolic blood pressure, and signs

Table 20–2. Differentiation of Systolic Murmurs Based on Changes in Their Intensity from Physiologic Maneuvers

	Origin of Murmur					
Maneuver	Flow	TR	AS	MR/VSD	MVP	HOCM
Inspiration	– or ↑	↑	–	–	–	–
Stand	↓	–	–	–	↑	↑
Squat	↑	–	–	–	↓	↓
Valsalva maneuver	↓	↓	↓	↓	↑	↑
Handgrip/TAO	↓	–	–	↑	↑	↓
Post-PVC	↑	–	↑	–	–	↑

AS, aortic stenosis; Flow, benign flow murmur; HOCM, hypertrophic obstructive cardiomyopathy; MR, mitral regurgitation; MVP, mitral valve prolapse; PVC, premature ventricular contraction; TAO, transient arterial occlusion; TR, tricuspid regurgitation; VSD, ventricular septal defect; ↑, increase in murmur intensity; ↓, decrease in murmur intensity; —, no predictable change.

of acute right-heart failure, such as increased jugular venous pressure.

3. Mixed valvular disease—Patients with rheumatic valvular disease often have mixed mitral disease, which is defined as at least 2+ (on a scale of 1–4; see following section on Echocardiography) mitral regurgitation, with a mean mitral valve diastolic gradient of more than 10 mm Hg. The clinical course of mixed mitral valve disease is similar to that of mitral regurgitation, and such patients should be treated similarly. Aortic regurgitation frequently occurs with mitral regurgitation, either because of left ventricular dilatation or because the same disease process affects the aortic valve (eg, Marfan syndrome). This places an additional volume load on the left ventricle and usually accelerates the patient's clinical deterioration.

When aortic stenosis and mitral regurgitation occur together, it is sometimes difficult to ascertain whether the same disease process (eg, rheumatic disease) involved both valves or whether the pressure load of significant aortic stenosis altered left ventricular geometry, performance, or both, resulting in functional mitral regurgitation. Diagnostic imaging studies usually resolve this issue and help direct therapy.

C. Diagnostic Studies

1. Electrocardiography—Patients with chronic mitral regurgitation may have evidence of left ventricular hypertrophy, left atrial abnormality, and sometimes, right ventricular enlargement. Patients with coronary artery disease might have evidence of myocardial infarction or ischemia. Electrocardiographic (ECG) exercise testing is usually done only to confirm the patient's physical limitations, because ECG changes in the face of a left ventricular volume load are not likely to be accurate for the diagnosis of coronary artery disease. Ambulatory ECG monitoring is occasionally done in patients with palpitations to document atrial fibrillation or other intermittent rhythm disorders.

2. Chest radiography—In cases of chronic mitral regurgitation, an enlarged left ventricle and left atrium would be expected. In severe regurgitation, right-heart enlargement and pulmonary hypertension may be evident. Patients in heart failure will show pulmonary congestion and pleural effusions. In acute mitral regurgitation, there are often signs of pulmonary congestion without enlargement of the heart.

3. Echocardiography—The color-flow Doppler identification of a systolic regurgitant jet across the mitral valve into the left atrium is diagnostic of mitral regurgitation. There are several ways of estimating the severity of mitral regurgitation by analyzing the characteristics of the regurgitant jet on color-flow Doppler. The first method is the depth of penetration of the jet into the left atrium. A penetration of 1 cm or less is considered mild; 2–3 cm, moderate; and 4 cm or more, severe. If the jet is very narrow, the actual volume of regurgitant flow may not be as great as occurs with a more

voluminous flow disturbance that penetrates to the same depth. Some investigators have therefore suggested also taking the area of the jet into consideration. One problem with this assessment system, however, is that if the jet impinges on a wall of the left atrium, it appears to penetrate less and be of a smaller area than if it is free in the atrial cavity. There is thus a tendency to underestimate the severity of mitral regurgitation when the jet hits the atrial wall. In addition, a regurgitant jet of any size occurring in a large left atrium will not appear as impressive as the same size jet in a small left atrium. The size of the leak in the mitral valve can be determined by evaluating the jet in a cross-sectional plane at the level of the mitral valve. This method gives an estimate of the size of the hole through which the jet is originating. These qualitative criteria for mitral regurgitation severity can be highly subjective.

For these reasons, there has been interest in more quantitative methods for estimating the severity of mitral regurgitation. The proximal isovelocity surface area observed where flow acceleration and convergence occur on the left ventricular side of the mitral leaflets allows the estimates of regurgitant volume and effective regurgitant orifice area. Fluid dynamics theory states that flow through an isovelocity surface is equal to the velocity times the surface area, which yields instantaneous regurgitant flow. This technique uses the color-flow Doppler color change interfaces observed with accelerating velocity through the orifice to estimate isovelocity surface area. Pulsed Doppler echocardiography can be used to quantitate regurgitant volume. The principle used is that of flow continuity. Systolic flow out the left ventricular outflow tract represents the forward stroke volume. This can be determined by multiplying the outflow tract area (measured on the two-dimensional echocardiographic image) times the outflow tract systolic velocity–time integral. Flow across the mitral valve in diastole represents the total stroke volume (forward plus regurgitant flow) and can be determined by multiplying mitral annulus area times the diastolic velocity–time integral. Regurgitant volume is the difference between total and forward stroke volume. Typically, the regurgitant volume is reported as the regurgitant fraction, which is the regurgitant stroke volume divided by the total stroke volume. Unfortunately, the calculation of regurgitant stroke volume has many possible sources of error, the largest of which is measuring the flow areas—mitral annular and outflow tract. Thus, individuals without valvular regurgitation can have regurgitant fractions of up to 20%. Also, the calculation of regurgitant flow is time-consuming and requires considerable skill. Effective regurgitant orifice area can be estimated as the ratio of regurgitant volume to the regurgitant jet velocity–time integral by pulsed Doppler.

Assessment of pulmonary venous flow velocity by pulsed Doppler echocardiography can also be of value in estimating the severity of mitral regurgitation. Normal pulmonary venous flow velocity is biphasic, with a predominant systolic forward velocity and a lesser diastolic forward velocity in older adults. Systolic forward velocity is reduced in patients with mitral regurgitation, and often the diastolic velocity predominates. In severe mitral regurgitation, the systolic flow in the pulmonary vein signal may reverse. Systolic flow reversal is highly specific for severe regurgitation, but sensitivity is low. Unfortunately, pulmonary venous flow velocity patterns vary considerably in patients with mitral regurgitation, and the predictive value for regurgitation severity is low. In many laboratories, all these factors are integrated to produce a composite estimate of the severity of regurgitation, usually on a scale of 1 to 4, with 4 being severe mitral regurgitation. Table 20–3 exhibits the criteria for grading the severity of mitral regurgitation.

Echocardiography can be used to evaluate the anatomy of the mitral apparatus to determine where the defect lies and what its cause may be. For example, patients with rheumatic mitral valve disease have thickening of the mitral leaflets, especially at the tips, with rolled edges and regurgitation along the commissural fissure lines. Patients with mitral valve prolapse have voluminous mitral leaflets that prolapse into the left atrium in the latter part of systole. Patients with coronary artery disease have wall motion abnormalities near the papillary muscle attachments. Ruptured and flail chordae tendineae are readily detected by echocardiography, as is mitral annular calcification.

The echocardiogram is also useful for assessing the compensatory changes in the cardiovascular system resulting from mitral regurgitation. The degree of left ventricular and left atrial enlargement is related to the severity of the mitral regurgitation and its chronicity. Left ventricular systolic performance is an important determinant of prognosis in mitral regurgitation (see Prognosis). Doppler estimation of pulmonary artery pressures from pulmonic or tricuspid regurgitant jets is valuable for estimating the effect of mitral regurgitation on the pulmonary circulation. An assessment of right-heart chamber sizes and function is additional useful information. Echocardiography can be deployed during bicycle exercise to assess exercise-induced changes in mitral regurgitation severity and pulmonary artery systolic pressure (PASP). Increases in either suggest a worse prognosis. Exercise echocardiography is especially useful for detecting physical limitations in asymptomatic patients with severe mitral regurgitation. Color-flow Doppler echocardiography can detect trivial or mild mitral regurgitation in up to half of otherwise healthy adults. The incidence increases with age and with the rigor with which the operator interrogates the valve. In the absence of anatomic abnormalities, small degrees of regurgitation are probably benign effects of aging. In most cases, mild mitral regurgitation found by echocardiography is not associated with a murmur on physical examination.

Table 20–3. Echocardiographic Grading of Mitral Regurgitation Severity

Grading System	Mild	Mild to Moderate	Moderate to Severe	Severe
Angiographic grade	1+	2+	3+	4+
Specific signs	Jet area < 4 cm²			Jet area > 40% of LA area
	Jet area to LA area < 20%			Visual orifice width > 0.7 cm
	Visual orifice width < 0.3 cm			Flow reversed in pulmonary veins
	No or minimal flow convergence			Major flail segment of leaflet
				Papillary muscle rupture
Supportive signs	Systolic dominant PV flow to A wave dominant mitral inflow			Dense continuous wave Doppler signal
	Low-density continuous wave Doppler MR signal			E wave dominant mitral inflow, E > 1.2 m/s
	Normal LV and LA size			Enlarged LV and LA
				Normal LV function
Quantitative measurements				
Regurgitant volume, mL/beat	< 30	30–44	45–59	≥ 60
Regurgitant fraction, %	< 30	30–39	40–49	≥ 50
Effective orifice area, cm²	< 0.2	0.2–0.29	0.3–0.39	≥ 40

LA, left atrium; LV, left ventricle; MR, mitral regurgitation; PV, pulmonary vein.

Transesophageal echocardiography (TEE) can provide the anatomic details of leaflet anatomy needed to plan surgical repair. The probe is rotated progressively to identify the scallops of the two mitral valve leaflets in midesophageal long axis views. The rotation of the color-flow jet helps confirm the incompetent scallops. In addition, annular size can be determined and the subvalvular apparatus interrogated. TEE during surgery can be of value to the surgeon. Also, three-dimensional echocardiography is useful for identifying the culprit scallops especially with TEE.

4. Cardiac catheterization—Cardiac catheterization is rarely needed to diagnose mitral regurgitation, nor is it usually needed to assess the severity of the regurgitation, left ventricular size and function, or any resultant pulmonary hypertension. Coronary angiography is useful, however, for establishing artery disease as the likely cause of mitral regurgitation as well as the risk from surgical correction of mitral regurgitation from any cause.

Hemodynamic evaluation at the time of cardiac catheterization in patients with moderate-to-severe mitral regurgitation will show an increase in pulmonary artery pressures, increases in the pulmonary capillary wedge pressure (PCWP), and possibly a reduction in forward cardiac output. The PCWP tracing often displays a large v wave, which is more than 50% greater than the height of the a wave. Although much has been made of the diagnostic value of large v waves in the PCWP tracing (especially in the intensive care unit setting), it must be remembered that any cause of left atrial pressure elevation will elevate the height of the v wave. It is only when the v wave is elevated out of proportion to the a wave that the diagnosis of mitral regurgitation is likely (> 150% of the a wave).

Left ventricular angiography is graded with a 1–4+ system, where 1+ is mild and 4+ is severe, indicating regurgitation of the angiographic dye into the pulmonary veins (see Table 20–3). This assessment method correlates well with the color-flow Doppler system. In addition, left ventricular angiography is useful for estimating left ventricular volume and ejection fraction. Cardiac catheterization can exclude the presence of other diseases, such as ventricular septal defect (VSD), hypertrophic obstructive cardiomyopathy (HOCM), and aortic stenosis, that might be confused with mitral regurgitation. Certain aspects of the patient's hemodynamics, such as the presence of pulmonary hypertension, are of prognostic value in mitral regurgitation.

La Canna G, et al. Real-time three-dimensional transesophageal echocardiography for assessment of mitral valve functional anatomy in patient with prolapse-related regurgitation. *Am J Cardiol.* 2011;107:1365–74. [PMID: 21371680]

Magne J, et al. Exercise-induced changes in degenerative mitral regurgitation. *J Am Coll Cardiol.* 2010;56(4):300–9. [PMID: 20633822]

O'Gara P, et al. The role of imaging in chronic degenerative mitral regurgitation. *JACC Cardiovasc Imaging.* 2008;1:221–37. [PMID: 19356431]

Supino PG, et al. Prognostic value of exercise tolerance testing asymptomatic chronic nonischemic mitral regurgitation. *Am J Cardiol.* 2007;100(8):1274–81. [PMID: 17920370]

▶ Differential Diagnosis

Because the symptoms seen in chronic mitral regurgitation are not specific for this condition, the physical examination is crucial for the differential diagnosis. The murmur of **tricuspid regurgitation,** for example, can occasionally be heard at the apex, especially if the right ventricle is enlarged and displaced leftward. Differentiating features include the increase in the intensity of the murmur with inspiration, the large v waves in the jugular pulse, a right ventricular lift, and a pulsatile liver. It should be noted that tricuspid regurgitation can result from pulmonary hypertension caused by mitral regurgitation, so some patients have both murmurs. In this situation, the murmur of tricuspid regurgitation is best assessed at the left or right sternal border, and that of mitral regurgitation at the apex. It may be difficult, however, to distinguish between the two murmurs in patients where both are moderately severe.

The murmur of **aortic stenosis** is often confused with mitral regurgitation, especially when the mitral regurgitant murmur is atypical or radiates to the aortic area. The murmur of aortic stenosis is usually lower in pitch than that of mitral regurgitation; it radiates to the neck and is often accompanied by an S_4 sound. In aortic stenosis, the left ventricular apical impulse amplitude often increases but is less likely to be laterally displaced, as is found in patients with mitral regurgitation. On dynamic auscultation, there is no change in the murmur of aortic stenosis with handgrip exercise, as is the case with mitral regurgitation, but the murmur of aortic stenosis does increase in the beat following a premature ventricular contraction, whereas that of mitral regurgitation does not.

A **VSD,** especially a muscular defect low in the septum, may mimic the murmur of mitral regurgitation. Because dynamic auscultation will not distinguish between these two left ventricular regurgitant murmurs, other signs must be used. The patient with VSD usually has a large right ventricle, and a vibration (thrill) over the anterior chest may be palpable. The murmur of **HOCM** can also be confused with mitral regurgitation. The major differential features are that the murmur of HOCM increases with the Valsalva maneuver, whereas the murmur of mitral regurgitation decreases; the murmur of HOCM decreases with handgrip, and the murmur of mitral regurgitation increases. In addition, the patient with HOCM usually has a prominent fourth heart sound. However, because many patients with HOCM also have mitral regurgitation, the ability to distinguish it from mitral regurgitation is difficult in some patients.

The murmur of **mitral valve prolapse** can be difficult to distinguish from the murmur of HOCM because both murmurs change in intensity and in a similar direction with the stand and squat and Valsalva maneuvers.

In this situation, other features of each disease, such as the midsystolic click with mitral valve prolapse and the left ventricular hypertrophy evident on palpation of the chest, or the fourth heart sound in the patient with HOCM, are useful for differentiating the two conditions by physical examination. The major differential diagnosis of acute mitral regurgitation is acute VSD because both may occur in the setting of acute myocardial infarction. A palpable vibration is more common with VSD, but perhaps the best differentiation is that the patient with acute VSD has much less dyspnea than does the patient with acute mitral regurgitation. The response to dynamic auscultation is the same in these two conditions.

▶ Treatment

A. Pharmacologic Therapy

1. Vasodilators—Vasodilators are useful in acute mitral regurgitation to decrease aortic pressure and impedance, favoring forward over regurgitant flow during systole. This decreases left ventricular size and left ventricular and atrial pressures, improves forward cardiac output, and decreases the amount of regurgitation. Studies of acute regurgitation with vasodilators, such as hydralazine, nifedipine, and nitroprusside, have demonstrated this effect in the hemodynamics laboratory and, thus, their usefulness for managing acute mitral regurgitation. Studies on the pharmacologic treatment of patients with chronic mitral regurgitation are scant, and the available data are not particularly encouraging. Because afterload is not increased in patients with well-compensated chronic mitral regurgitation, lowering it further may not improve forward flow and would more likely reduce it. Many patients experience vasodilator side effects, and if forward cardiac output is not improved, the patient's overall hemodynamic status is actually worsened. Thus, until further data are obtained, there is no evidence to support vasodilator therapy for asymptomatic patients with chronic mitral regurgitation. In mildly symptomatic patients who presumably have left ventricular dilation and dysfunction, but who want to avoid surgery, vasodilators could be tried. Markedly symptomatic patients, however, are better treated surgically. Patients with systemic hypertension and those with functional mitral regurgitation due to systolic dysfunction should be treated with vasodilators.

2. Digoxin—Digoxin is useful in atrial fibrillation for controlling the heart rate. Whether it is of any value for improving forward output with mitral regurgitation in patients with normal sinus rhythm is unknown. If there are other indications for using the drug, however, it is not known to be harmful to the overall hemodynamic status of patients with mitral regurgitation.

3. Oral anticoagulation—Oral anticoagulation is indicated for patients in atrial fibrillation and those with concomitant mitral stenosis. Whether patients with moderate-to-severe mitral regurgitation, with large left ventricles and large left atria, who are in normal sinus rhythm and have normal left ventricular function would benefit from anticoagulants is controversial. Eccentric regurgitant jets may produce areas of stasis in the left atrium, according to color-flow Doppler studies. Furthermore, patients with moderate-to-severe mitral regurgitation are always at risk for developing atrial fibrillation. Although an argument can be made for long-term anticoagulation in such patients, no clinical trials support this approach.

4. Antibiotic prophylaxis—Only patients with prosthetic heart valves now require antibiotics to prevent the development of bacterial endocarditis. Patients in whom rheumatic heart disease is the likely cause of mitral regurgitation should also have rheumatic fever antibiotic prophylaxis.

B. Surgical Treatment

Patients with acute, severe, or decompensated chronic severe mitral regurgitation will need urgent surgical therapy—if it is appropriate to their general medical condition. Such patients can usually be stabilized with intravenous vasodilators, such as hydralazine or nitroprusside, and other therapies for heart failure, such as diuretics. If there is no response to pharmacologic therapy, an intra-aortic balloon pump is indicated. This mechanical approach will reduce arterial and left ventricular pressure in systole, favoring forward flow rather than regurgitant and increased diastolic aortic pressure, and may improve left ventricular contractility. Most patients will stabilize on this therapy, allowing for an appropriate evaluation (eg, coronary angiography), thereby maximizing the benefits of surgery.

Patients with either acute or chronic moderately severe mitral regurgitation will eventually need surgical therapy. The issue is the appropriate timing of surgery. If the physician waits until the symptoms are marked because of left heart failure with depressed left ventricular systolic function and severe pulmonary hypertension, not much symptomatic improvement is achieved after surgery, and left ventricular function remains depressed. On the other hand, if surgery is performed earlier, the patient may become relatively asymptomatic, with normal left ventricular function. Considerable effort has been directed at determining prognostic indicators for avoiding a poor response to surgical therapy. Prospective studies have shown that the following are all markers of a poor prognosis following surgery: an ejection fraction of 60% or less, an end-systolic volume index of 50 mL/m^2 or more, an end-systolic dimension on echocardiography of 40 mm or more, significant pulmonary hypertension (PASP > 50 mm Hg or peak exercise PASP > 60 mm Hg), and atrial fibrillation. Although it seems logical that surgery should therefore be performed before these indicators are obtained in a patient, even one who is asymptomatic, this decision analysis has never been tested in clinical trials (Table 20–4).

In patients with aortic and mitral regurgitation, if the mitral valve is not obviously diseased and the mitral regurgitation is mild to moderate (1–2+), replacing the aortic valve

Table 20–4. General Indications for Considering Mitral Valve Surgery in Patients with Chronic Severe Organic Mitral Regurgitation

Symptoms such as dyspnea
Left ventricular ejection fraction ≤ 60%
Left ventricular end-systolic dimension ≥ 40 mm
Left ventricular end-systolic volume index ≥ 50 mL/m²
Atrial fibrillation
Pulmonary artery systolic pressure > 50 mm Hg at rest or > 60 mm Hg with exercise

will often diminish left ventricular size enough to reduce or eliminate the mitral regurgitation. Sometimes a mitral annular ring will be required to reduce mitral annular size. In cases where the mitral valve leaflets and chordae are diseased or the regurgitation is severe, valve repair or replacement will be necessary—at the cost of a higher likelihood of operative mortality or postoperative morbidity. Severe aortic stenosis is often accompanied by mild-to-moderate mitral regurgitation. In this situation, the reduction in left ventricular pressure produced by aortic valve replacement usually reduces the mitral regurgitation, and further mitral surgery can be avoided.

The pulmonary hypertension that often accompanies mitral regurgitation may lead to tricuspid and pulmonic regurgitation. The latter usually resolves when the pulmonary pressure is reduced by mitral valve surgery, and pulmonary valve replacement is rarely necessary. Tricuspid regurgitation, if mild-to-moderate and associated with moderately severe pulmonary hypertension, will usually resolve after successful mitral surgery. If the tricuspid regurgitation is moderately severe, but the leaflets are not diseased, a tricuspid ring may be effective; if tricuspid valve disease is present, repair or replacement will be necessary. One clinical indicator for the need for tricuspid valve repair or replacement is a mean right atrial pressure of more than 15 mm Hg; however, the decision for this is often made during surgery, after the mitral procedure has been completed.

The onset of heart failure symptoms should prompt consideration of surgical treatment. Symptoms such as dyspnea, fatigue, and edema develop in some patients before the echocardiographic signs of severe mitral regurgitation develop. The importance of other symptoms, such as a history of arrhythmias or recurrent systemic emboli, is less certain. If the hemodynamic indicators are absent, other therapies for these conditions should be attempted first, before surgery.

Other factors to be taken into account when deciding when to perform surgery are the type of operation—valve repair or replacement—and the type of prosthetic valve, should one be needed. It is now possible in many patients with mitral regurgitation to repair rather than replace the mitral valve. Patients with mitral valve prolapse, ruptured chordae tendineae, or a ruptured papillary muscle are especially likely to respond to reparative surgery, whereas patients with markedly deformed valves and fused chordae from rheumatic heart disease or patients with infective endocarditis are less likely to be helped by mitral valve repair and often require valve replacement. Repair is preferable, especially for the patient with normal sinus rhythm because there is no need for long-term anticoagulation therapy following surgery. In addition, mitral valve repair is generally associated with better preservation of left ventricular systolic function following surgery and is therefore highly advantageous for patients with a low left ventricular ejection fraction and a repairable mitral valve. Thus, if it is likely that mitral valve repair can be done, there is less reluctance about operating in asymptomatic patients that otherwise meet criteria for surgery.

If valve replacement is necessary, ventricular function can be preserved by leaving the chordae intact; chordal tethering of the papillary muscles is presumed to improve left ventricular performance. With valve replacement, the choice between a mechanical and a bioprosthetic valve may influence the timing of surgery.

In general, mechanical prosthetic valves are preferred because of their better long-term reliability. Bioprosthetic valves can be chosen when valve longevity is not an issue or when patients want to try to avoid anticoagulation therapy. The latter would apply mainly to young women with normal sinus rhythm who want to become pregnant. They will be much easier to treat without anticoagulation therapy—a feasible goal with a bioprosthetic valve. These patients must realize, however, that this valve will need to be replaced in approximately 10–15 years, as a result of deterioration. This should give these patients time for several pregnancies, if they so desire.

Generally, patients with a mechanical valve and no contraindications to anticoagulation therapy should be treated with such agents. The incidence of systemic emboli is higher with mitral than with aortic prosthetic valves. Without anticoagulation, there is a 1–3% per year chance of systemic emboli with a bioprosthetic valve in the mitral position, so aspirin therapy is recommended for patients with bioprosthetic valves. The use of warfarin for 3 months after bioprosthetic mitral valve replacement is sometimes done until the endothelium grows over the sewing ring, reducing the risk of thrombus development. Patients with other risks for thrombus formation, such as atrial fibrillation, should also receive warfarin.

Percutaneous approaches to mitral valve repair and replacement are developing rapidly. One approach is to put a clip at the tip of the mitral leaflets creating a double orifice valve similar to the surgical Alfieri technique. Initial studies suggest that it may be ideal for patients with severe functional mitral regurgitation due to dilated cardiomyopathy, where surgical risk is high. Another is to deliver an annuloplasty ring percutaneously, reducing the annulus size. Finally, stent-mounted tissue valves can be deployed in the mitral area. At this time, these devices have not been released for routine use in the United States, but they hold great promise for the future.

Carabello BA. The current therapy for mitral regurgitation. *J Am Coll Cardiol.* 2008;52(5):319–26. [PMID: 18652937]

Feldman T, et al. Percutaneous repair or surgery for mitral regurgitation. *N Engl J Med.* 2011;364(15):1395–406. [PMID: 21463154]

Glower DD, et al. Surgical approaches to mitral regurgitation. *J Am Coll Cardiol.* 2012;60(15):1315–22. [PMID: 22939558]

Webb JG, et al. Percutaneous transvenous mitral annuloplasty: initial human experience with device implantation in the coronary sinus. *Circulation.* 2006;113(6):851–5. [PMID: 16461812]

▶ Prognosis

Patients with chronic mitral regurgitation have an average survival curve similar to that of patients with chronic aortic regurgitation and chronic mitral stenosis. The cause of the chronic mitral regurgitation in individual patients influences the prognosis. In general, patients with coronary artery disease as the cause have a poor prognosis, those with the myxomatous changes of mitral valve prolapse have the best prognosis, and those with rheumatic heart disease have an intermediate prognosis. The onset of infective endocarditis can markedly alter the prognosis. In addition, any sudden deterioration of mitral valve function that leads to acute worsening of the mitral regurgitation lessens the prognosis.

The prognosis in acute mitral regurgitation, when it is associated with acute pulmonary edema and severe symptoms, is guarded; it also depends on the cause. For example, patients with acute severe mitral regurgitation from acute myocardial infarction have a much worse prognosis than do otherwise healthy individuals who rupture a chorda. In general, most patients with acute mitral regurgitation require immediate surgical attention, and their prognosis is not as good as that for patients with chronic mitral regurgitation.

Bonow RO, et al. ACC/AHA 2006 guidelines for the management of patients with valvular heart disease: executive summary. A report of the American College of Cardiology/American Heart Association Task Force on Practice Guidelines (writing committee to revise the 1998 Guidelines for the Management of Patients with Valvular Heart Disease): developed in collaboration with the Society of Cardiovascular Anesthesiologists: endorsed by the Society for Cardiovascular Angiography and Interventions and the Society of Thoracic Surgeons. *Circulation.* 2006;114(5):e84–231. [PMID: 16880336]

Enriquez-Sarano M, et al. Mitral regurgitation. *Lancet.* 2009; 373(9672):1382–94. [PMID: 19356795]

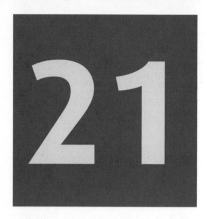

21

Tricuspid & Pulmonic Valve Disease

Brian D. Hoit, MD

Michael H. Crawford, MD

TRICUSPID VALVE DISEASE

ESSENTIALS OF DIAGNOSIS

Tricuspid regurgitation

▶ Prominent *v* wave in jugular venous pulse.

▶ Systolic murmur at left lower sternal border that increases with inspiration.

▶ Characteristic Doppler echocardiographic findings, including right ventricular (RV) volume overload (RV enlargement, paradoxical septal motion, and diastolic flattening of the interventricular septum), right atrial enlargement, and systolic turbulence in the right atrium.

Tricuspid stenosis

▶ Prominent *a* wave and reduced *y* descent in jugular venous pulse.

▶ Diastolic murmur at left lower sternal border that increases with inspiration.

▶ Characteristic Doppler echocardiographic findings, including a thickened and domed valve with restricted motion, right atrial enlargement, and increased diastolic velocity across the tricuspid valve.

▶ General Considerations

Clinical interest in tricuspid valve disorders has increased because of several distinct but interrelated events in clinical cardiology. First, high-resolution, noninvasive imaging techniques have been developed and validated, allowing clinicians to easily assess the morphology and function of the tricuspid valve. Second, the frequency of tricuspid valve endocarditis has increased significantly, owing largely to an increasing population of injection drug users, patients

with implanted cardiac devices or long-term central venous catheters, and, to a lesser extent, a growing number of immunocompromised patients. Third, several reparative percutaneous and surgical techniques with acceptable morbidity and mortality rates now exist. In addition, investigations in both animals and humans have demonstrated the influence of right-heart disease on cardiovascular performance vis-á-vis series and parallel interactions with the left ventricle.

▶ Pathophysiology & Etiology

The tricuspid valve has three leaflets that are unequal in size (anterior > septal > posterior). The papillary muscles are not as well defined as those of the left ventricle and are subject to considerable variation in both their size and leaflet support. Like the mitral valve, the leaflets, annulus, chordae, papillary muscles, and contiguous myocardium contribute individually to normal valve function and can be altered by pathophysiologic processes (Table 21–1).

A. Tricuspid Regurgitation

Tricuspid regurgitation most frequently occurs with a structurally normal tricuspid valve (functional tricuspid regurgitation), which is the result of a dilated right ventricle and tricuspid annulus and papillary muscle dysfunction.

Functional tricuspid regurgitation is usually observed in patients with disease of the left heart (eg, left ventricular [LV] dysfunction, mitral valve disease), pulmonary vascular and parenchymal disease, right ventricular (RV) infarction, arrhythmogenic RV dysplasia, and congenital heart disease.

By contrast, **organic tricuspid regurgitation** occurs when the intrinsic structure of the valve is anatomically abnormal.

Rheumatic tricuspid regurgitation almost always coexists with mitral valve involvement and is due to associated pulmonary hypertension. Although two-thirds of patients with rheumatic mitral valve disease have pathologic evidence of tricuspid valve involvement, clinically significant tricuspid disease, which generally affects young and middle-aged

Table 21–1. Causes of Tricuspid Valve Disease

Tricuspid Regurgitation	Tricuspid Stenosis
Functional (structurally normal tricuspid valve)	Rheumatic
	Carcinoid heart disease
Rheumatic	Tumors
Infective endocarditis	Congenital (eg, Ebstein anomaly)
Congenital (eg, tricuspid valve prolapse, Ebstein anomaly)	Regional cardiac tamponade
	Systemic lupus erythematosus
Carcinoid heart disease	Whipple disease
Systemic lupus erythematosus	Fabry disease
Catheter-induced	Infective endocarditis
Trauma	Endomyocardial fibrosis
Tumors	Endocardial fibroelastosis
Orthotopic heart transplantation	Methysergide therapy
Endomyocardial fibrosis	Antiphospholipid syndrome
Antiphospholipid syndrome	

women, is much less common. Rheumatic tricuspid involvement is usually mild and generally is shown clinically as pure regurgitation or mixed regurgitation and stenosis, caused by the fibrosis of the valve leaflets and chordae tendineae; contracture of the leaflets and commissural fusion produce regurgitation and stenosis, respectively.

Tricuspid valve endocarditis occurs primarily in injection drug users and patients with chronic intravascular hardware, left-to-right shunts, burns, and immunocompromised states. Infective endocarditis is more common in injecting drug users who are human immunodeficiency virus (HIV) positive than in those who are HIV negative. Infective endocarditis is typically caused by virulent pathogens that infect structurally normal valves. *Staphylococcus aureus* is the most common organism; the next most common pathogens are streptococci and enterococci. *Pseudomonas* and *Candida* species also predominate, and polymicrobial infections are not uncommon. Geographic location should also be considered when attempting to identify the responsible pathogens. Fungal endocarditis should be considered when vegetations are large; they occasionally cause obstruction. Abscesses may involve the annulus and septum, and chordal rupture or valve perforations may cause tricuspid regurgitation.

Carcinoid tumors are a rare cause of both tricuspid and pulmonic valve disease. The vasoactive substances (principally serotonin) produced by these tumors are believed to be causal, and patients with carcinoid valvular disease have higher serum levels of serotonin and increased urinary excretion of its metabolite, 5-hydroxyindoleacetic acid (5-HIAA), than those without cardiac disease. Left-sided valve involvement is unusual due to inactivation of these vasoactive molecules by monoamine oxidase in the lungs, but can be seen in patients with right-to-left shunts or bronchial tumors. The valve exhibits pathognomonic plaque-like deposits of fibrous tissue (which may also deposit on the endocardium); leaflet distortion leads to regurgitation, stenosis, or both. Tricuspid regurgitation is the most common lesion and is detected by echocardiography in virtually all patients with carcinoid tricuspid valve disease. Cardiac involvement is progressive and causes significant morbidity and mortality in such patients, but early detection and surgical management may prolong survival. Long-term survival has been reported after tricuspid valve replacement, but carcinoid plaques may deposit on the bioprosthetic leaflets.

Tricuspid valve prolapse, owing to myxomatous degeneration, is seen almost exclusively in patients with mitral valve prolapse and occurs in as many as 50% of cases. Isolated involvement has been confirmed, however, by both echocardiography and necropsy. Anterior leaflet prolapse is most common, followed by septal and posterior leaflet prolapse. The associated tricuspid regurgitation is usually mild. Although tricuspid valve prolapse may be a marker of generalized connective tissue disease and a poor prognostic indicator in patients with mitral valve prolapse, its clinical significance remains undefined. Like mitral valve prolapse, the precise incidence of tricuspid valve prolapse is difficult to determine because of inconsistent clinical, echocardiographic, and angiographic definitions.

Tricuspid regurgitation is a frequent component of **Ebstein anomaly** of the tricuspid valve because of the apical displacement of septal and posterior tricuspid leaflets. This results in "atrialization" of a variable portion of the right ventricle and a range of abnormalities involving the anterior leaflet and atrial septum. The downward displacement of the tricuspid valve frequently causes a tricuspid regurgitant murmur (heard best in the apical area). This uncommon congenital abnormality is associated with right-to-left intra-atrial shunting, RV dysfunction, supraventricular arrhythmias, and sudden death.

Tricuspid regurgitation of at least moderate severity may complicate as many as 25% of cases of **systemic lupus erythematosus**; significant tricuspid regurgitation is usually due to the pulmonary hypertension produced by lupus pulmonary disease. Libman-Sacks endocarditis that involves the tricuspid valve is far less common. However, Libman-Sacks endocarditis has been associated with antiphospholipid antibodies, which has been shown to cause valvular thickening, isolated tricuspid involvement, and the development of nonbacterial vegetations. The cause of the valve disease is poorly understood, but intravalvular capillary thrombosis is believed to be a factor. Most patients present with combined tricuspid regurgitation and stenosis, and the regurgitation is typically moderate or severe. Pulmonary hypertension is usually present and contributes to the valvular dysfunction.

Although **catheter-induced** tricuspid regurgitation occurs in approximately 50% of cases with catheters across the valve, the regurgitation is quantitatively small, clinically unimportant, and usually disappears when the catheter is removed. Tricuspid regurgitation can occur as a late complication of successful mitral valve replacement (MVR). In one series, Doppler-detected moderate-to-severe regurgitation occurred in two-thirds of patients at a mean of over 11 years following MVR; over one-third of these patients had clinically evident tricuspid regurgitation. Other causes include blunt and penetrating trauma (rupture of papillary muscles, chordal disruption or detachment, leaflet rupture, complete valve destruction), primary or secondary cardiac tumors, orthotopic heart transplantation, and endomyocardial fibrosis.

B. Tricuspid Stenosis

Tricuspid stenosis is an uncommon lesion that is usually rheumatic in origin and almost exclusively accompanies mitral stenosis. Isolated rheumatic tricuspid stenosis is rare, and subvalvular disease is usually less severe in tricuspid than in mitral stenosis. Isolated carcinoid tricuspid stenosis is also rare; tricuspid regurgitation is more frequent and often occurs with pulmonic stenosis. Right atrial (RA) myxomas and obstructing metastatic tumors may produce hemodynamic changes that are indistinguishable from tricuspid stenosis. Tricuspid stenosis may be congenital and is infrequently predominant in Ebstein anomaly. Extrinsic compression of the tricuspid valve by a loculated pericardial effusion is an uncommon cause of tricuspid stenosis. Other unusual causes include systemic lupus erythematosus, Whipple disease, Fabry disease, antiphospholipid syndrome, infective endocarditis, endocardial fibroelastosis, and as a sequela to methysergide therapy. It should be noted that prosthetic tricuspid valves, like all prosthetic valves, are inherently stenotic.

Arora R, et al. Prevalence of tricuspid valve disease in rheumatic heart disease. *J Am Coll Cardiol.* 2012;59:E1263.

Mutlak D, et al. Echocardiography-based spectrum of severe tricuspid regurgitation: the frequency of apparently idiopathic tricuspid regurgitation. *J Am Soc Echocardiogr.* 2007;20:405–8. [PMID: 17400120]

Perez-Villa F, et al. Severe valvular regurgitation and antiphospholipid antibodies in systemic lupus erythematosus: a prospective, long-term, follow-up study. *Arthritis Rheum.* 2005;53(3):460–7. [PMID: 15934103]

▶ Clinical Findings

A. Symptoms & Signs

Tricuspid valve disease can be difficult to recognize clinically. The symptoms may be overshadowed by associated illness, such as systemic lupus erythematosus, infective endocarditis, trauma, or neoplasia. The dominant presenting features may be symptoms that are usually not considered cardiac in origin: abdominal discomfort, ascites, jaundice, wasting, and inanition. In addition, patients with associated cardiovascular disease may have nonspecific symptoms (exertional dyspnea and fatigue in mitral stenosis) that obfuscate the diagnosis and deflect the suspicion of tricuspid valve disease. In patients with mitral stenosis, for example, tricuspid valve disease protects the pulmonary circulation and exertional dyspnea, pulmonary edema, and hemoptysis are less commonly reported, although a history of excessive fatigue may be elicited. Most often, however, the history is insufficient to diagnose tricuspid valve disease, and only a careful physical examination provides the necessary clues.

B. Physical Examination

1. Jugular venous pulse—Because the internal jugular veins lack effective valves, they should be inspected for an estimate of RA pressure (Figure 21–1 shows a normal jugular venous pulse). There are three waves (*a, c,* and *v*) and two descents, *x* and *y* (which correspond to the *a* and *v* waves, respectively). The *a* wave and the initial descent are produced by atrial contraction and relaxation, respectively. The *x* descent is interrupted by a *c* wave that is caused by isovolumetric contraction of the right ventricle and resultant bowing of the tricuspid valve toward the right atrium. The continuation of the *x* descent (sometimes called *x'*) is caused by the descent of the arteriovenous (AV) ring toward the apex during RV ejection. The right atrium fills and, because the tricuspid valve is closed, RA pressure rises, causing the *v* wave. The rapid fall in volume and pressure when the valve opens produces the *y* descent. Except for a small but variable delay, the jugular venous pulse and RA pressure contours are similar.

When inspecting the jugular venous pulse, the examiner should pay careful attention to the magnitude of the central venous (mean RA) pressure, the dominant wave (*a* or *v*), and changes in pulse contour with respiration. Tricuspid valve disease is typically associated with increased central venous pressure.

A. TRICUSPID REGURGITATION—The *x* descent of the jugular venous pulse is interrupted by an early *v* wave (*c-v* wave) with a rapid *y* descent (Figure 21–2). These findings are characteristically augmented during inspiration. The neck veins are distended, and the earlobes may pulsate. Because venous distention may obscure the jugular pulse contour, it is important to elevate the patient's head. RV volume overload leads to prominent pulsations over the left lower sternal border.

B. TRICUSPID STENOSIS—In tricuspid stenosis (Figure 21–3), inspection of the jugular veins reveals a dominant *a* wave (assuming sinus rhythm), which increases with inspiration, and a slow and shallow *y* descent due to resistance to early RV diastolic filling.

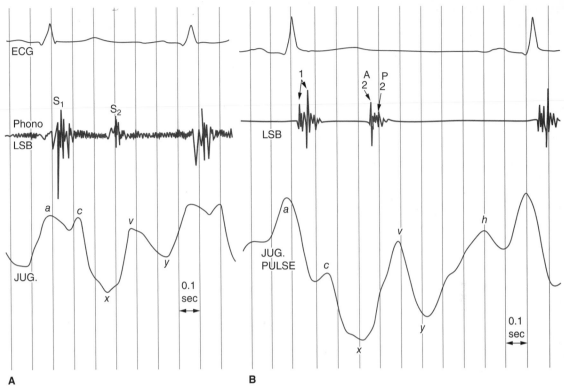

▲ **Figure 21–1.** Normal jugular venous pulse tracings at fast (**A**) and slow (**B**) heart rates. The *a* wave is the dominant reflection. At slow heart rates, an *h* wave signifying the end of right ventricular filling can be seen. LSB, left sternal border. (Reproduced, with permission, from Tavel ME. *Clinical Phonocardiograpy and External Pulse Recoding.* Yearbook Medical Publishers, 1978.)

2. Cardiac auscultation

A. TRICUSPID REGURGITATION—Tricuspid regurgitation is classically associated with a holosystolic murmur that is best heard at the right or left midsternal border, but when the right ventricle is markedly dilated, the location of the murmur may move toward the left and suggest mitral regurgitation. The auscultatory hallmark of tricuspid regurgitation is an inspiratory augmentation from increased systemic venous return and tricuspid valve flow (Figure 21–4). Under such circumstances as severe tricuspid regurgitation, markedly increased RA pressures, and RV systolic failure, the murmur may not increase with inspiration. Although usually described as holosystolic, the timing of the murmur may be early, mid, or late systolic. The murmur may be decrescendo when tricuspid regurgitation is severe and acute, and its character reflects the presence of a giant *c-v* wave; there may be a middiastolic flow rumble that resembles tricuspid stenosis. The murmur of tricuspid regurgitation is usually not accompanied by a thrill, and there is little radiation of the murmur. When the tricuspid valve is wide open in systole, there may be no murmur. An S_3, which can vary in intensity and with inspiration, is often

associated with an extremely dilated right ventricle. An S_4 may also be heard if there is significant RV hypertrophy.

B. TRICUSPID STENOSIS—The tricuspid opening snap is difficult to distinguish from the mitral opening snap, and auscultatory findings may be difficult to distinguish from existing mitral stenosis. Unlike mitral stenosis, however, the diastolic rumble of tricuspid stenosis has a higher pitch, increases with inspiration, is usually loudest at the lower left sternal border, and follows the opening snap of mitral stenosis. The tricuspid stenosis murmur is often scratchy, ends before the first heart sound, and has no presystolic crescendo in patients with normal sinus rhythm. A diastolic murmur from relative tricuspid stenosis may be heard with large atrial septal defects and severe tricuspid regurgitation. In patients with normal sinus rhythm, a presystolic hepatic pulsation may be felt; this is due to reflux from atrial contraction against the stenotic valve. Both tricuspid stenosis and regurgitation can, if chronic, lead to ascites, peripheral edema, jaundice, wasting, and muscle loss. Tricuspid valve disease, which is often diagnosed or suspected at the bedside, can almost always be confirmed with echocardiography.

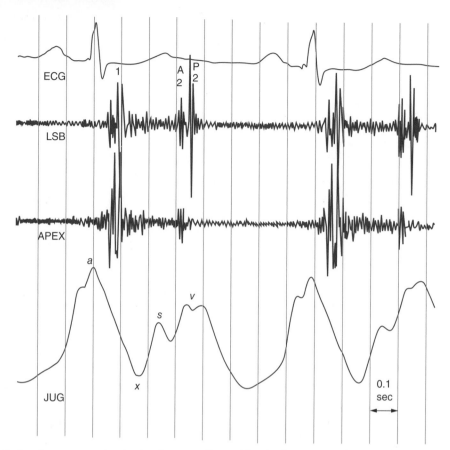

▲ **Figure 21–2.** Jugular venous pulse tracing from a patient with mitral stenosis and tricuspid regurgitation secondary to pulmonary hypertension. Note the shallow *x* descent, the midsystolic *s* wave, and the respiratory increase in the *v* wave. (Reproduced, with permission, from Tavel ME. *Clinical Phonocardiography and External Pulse Recording.* Yearbook Medical Publishers, 1978.)

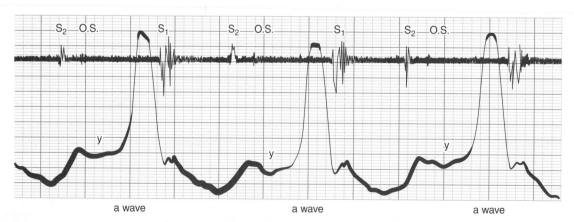

▲ **Figure 21–3.** Jugular venous pulse tracing and phonocardiogram from a patient with rheumatic tricuspid stenosis. Note the striking *a* waves and the shallow *y* descents. A loud S_1 and opening snap (O.S.) are evident on the accompanying phonocardiogram.

INSPIRATION   INSPIRATION

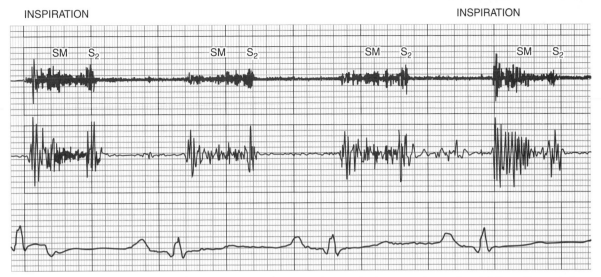

▲ **Figure 21–4.** Phonocardiogram from a patient with tricuspid regurgitation secondary to heart failure. The systolic murmur increases with inspiration, seen most clearly on the lower phonocardiographic tracing. Note that the murmur does not extend to the second heart sound.

C. Diagnostic Studies

The diagnostic evaluation of suspected tricuspid valve disease includes electrocardiography (ECG), plain chest film, echocardiography, and cardiac catheterization. Limited experience with cine magnetic resonance imaging (MRI) and computed tomography (CT) suggests that, except in certain instances (such as the evaluation of carcinoid heart disease), these techniques offer no clear advantage over echocardiography.

1. Electrocardiography—P waves characteristic of RA enlargement with no evidence of RV hypertrophy suggest isolated tricuspid stenosis. Most often, however, the rhythm is atrial fibrillation. When pulmonary hypertension is the cause of tricuspid regurgitation, the ECG may show evidence of RV hypertrophy with right axis deviation and tall R waves in V_1 to V_2 and RA enlargement (Figure 21–5A). Atrial fibrillation is also common, and incomplete right bundle branch block and Q waves in V_1 are occasionally seen. Preexcitation frequently accompanies Ebstein anomaly (Figure 21–5B).

2. Chest radiography—In tricuspid stenosis, the chest film is characterized by cardiomegaly, with a prominent right-heart border caused by RA enlargement, and a dilated superior vena cava and azygos vein. Pulmonary vascular markings may be notably absent. The chest film in tricuspid regurgitation shows cardiomegaly from RA and RV enlargement; pleural effusions and elevated diaphragms from ascites may be seen. In general, a dilated heart in the absence of pulmonary congestion or pulmonary hypertension should suggest either tricuspid valve disease or pericardial effusion. Massive RA enlargement suggests Ebstein anomaly.

3. Echocardiography—Echocardiography is the most useful noninvasive diagnostic test for evaluating tricuspid valve disease. Two-dimensional and Doppler echocardiographic examinations can identify associated disease of the left ventricle and other cardiac valves (eg, mitral stenosis), show the anatomic sequelae of chronic tricuspid valve disease (eg, dilated right heart chambers), and detect structural abnormalities of the tricuspid valve (eg, a thickened tricuspid valve with decreased mobility, compression of the tricuspid annulus, or involvement by tumor or prolapsing or displaced leaflets and vegetations; Figure 21–6). Three-dimensional echocardiography can be helpful in defining the anatomy of the tricuspid valve.

A. TRICUSPID REGURGITATION—In tricuspid regurgitation, the echocardiographic findings usually show RV volume overload with a dilated right ventricle, paradoxical septal motion, and diastolic flattening of the interventricular septum. Color-flow Doppler echocardiography can visualize the tricuspid regurgitant jet. The tricuspid valve diastolic gradient can be quantified using continuous wave Doppler, and pulmonary arterial pressure can be estimated from the pulmonary artery acceleration time or the peak velocity of the tricuspid regurgitant jet. Two-dimensional echocardiography distinguishes between primary disease of the left heart and RV disease, both of which cause functional tricuspid regurgitation, and organic disease of the tricuspid valve. Contrast found in the inferior vena cava and hepatic veins following injection of agitated saline into an arm vein implies significant tricuspid regurgitation. On the other hand, a tricuspid valve annulus less than 3.4 cm in diameter during diastole virtually excludes significant tricuspid regurgitation.

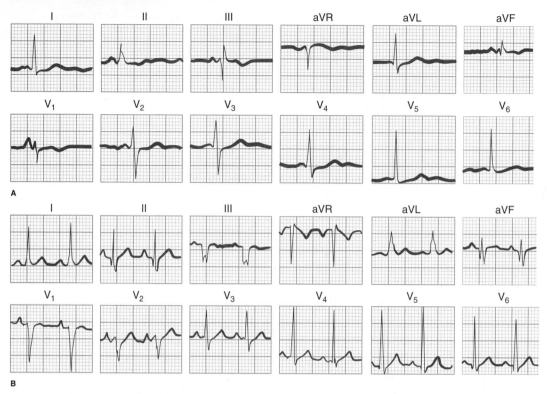

▲ **Figure 21–5.** Electrocardiograms from patients with tricuspid valve disease. **A:** Mitral stenosis and isolated tricuspid stenosis. The tall initial P-wave forces in lead V₁ indicate right atrial enlargement. There is no electrocardiographic evidence of right ventricular hypertrophy. (Reproduced, with permission, from Chou TE. *Electrocardiography in Clinical Practice,* 3rd ed. Philadelphia: WB Saunders; 1991.) **B:** Patient with Ebstein anomaly and preexcitation. Delta waves create a pseudoinfarct pattern. P-wave amplitude in leads II and V₂ is consistent with right atrial enlargement. (Used with permission from Chou TE.)

The temporal and spatial distribution of systolic turbulence in the right atrium, using color-flow mapping, can be a means of estimating the severity of the regurgitation. Systolic reversal of the Doppler signal in the hepatic veins indicates significant tricuspid regurgitation. Doppler techniques that quantitatively estimate effective regurgitant orifice, regurgitant volume, and regurgitant fraction have been developed and validated. It should be recognized that Doppler-detected tricuspid regurgitation occurs commonly in normal individuals. In such cases, the Doppler signal tends not to be holosystolic, and systolic turbulence occupies only a small area of the right atrium.

B. Tricuspid stenosis—As shown in Figure 21–7, the stenotic tricuspid valve is thickened and domed and has restricted motion. The echocardiographic appearance alone may be misleading because many patients with two-dimensional echocardiographic findings that suggest tricuspid stenosis have normal tricuspid valve diastolic pressure gradients. Although the right atrium is usually dilated, the right ventricle is not enlarged in isolated tricuspid stenosis.

The severity of the stenosis is determined with continuous wave Doppler. Accurate peak instantaneous and mean gradients across the stenotic tricuspid valve are readily calculated using the modified **Bernoulli equation,** which relates a pressure drop (dP) to the velocity (V) across a stenosis ($dP = 4V^2$). The pressure half-time method for calculating valve orifice area, used successfully for the mitral valve, has not been validated for the tricuspid valve. A tricuspid valve area less than 1.0 cm² indicates severe tricuspid stenosis.

4. Cardiac catheterization

A. Tricuspid regurgitation—Opacification of the right atrium following injection of radiographic contrast into the right ventricle detects and estimates the severity of the regurgitation. Although right ventriculography requires a catheter across the tricuspid valve, there is no significant contrast leak into the right atrium under normal circumstances. Right atrial and ventricular pressures are elevated, and the RA pressure may become "ventricularized" as a result of a large

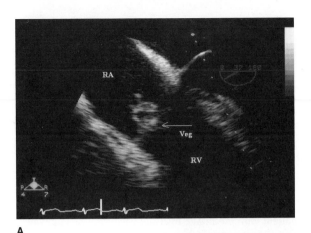

A

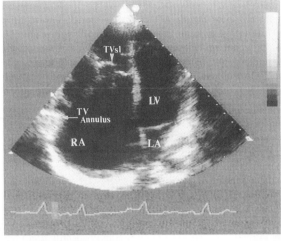

B

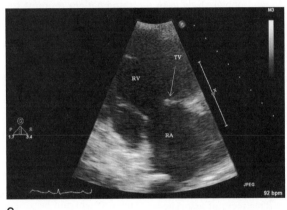

C

▲ **Figure 21–6.** Two-dimensional echocardiograms illustrating abnormalities of the tricuspid valve leaflets. **A:** Infective endocarditis. RA, right atrium; RV, right ventricle; Veg, tricuspid valve vegetation. **B:** Ebstein anomaly. Note the displacement of the septal leaflet (TVsl) relative to the tricuspid valve annulus. LV, left ventricle; RA, right atrium. **C:** Carcinoid syndrome. Note the thickened and rigid tricuspid leaflets (*arrow*).

c-v wave and an absent *x* descent (Figure 21–8A). **Kussmaul sign** (increased RA pressure with inspiration or the absence of a normal fall in RA pressure) may be seen when the regurgitation is severe.

B. TRICUSPID STENOSIS—In tricuspid stenosis, the mean RA pressure is increased; characteristically, the *a* wave is prominent and the *y* descent is slow. The hallmark of tricuspid stenosis is a diastolic gradient between the right atrium and right ventricle that increases with inspiration (Figure 21–8B). The gradients are frequently small; however, their detection is enhanced by recording RA and RV pressures simultaneously with two optimally damped catheters and equally sensitive transducers. Because of the low gradient, calculation of the valve area is unreliable. Injection or rapid volume infusion of atropine to increase

the heart rate can increase the diastolic gradient and facilitate the diagnosis.

American College of Cardiology; American Heart Association Task Force on Practice Guidelines (Writing Committee to revise the 1998 guidelines for the management of patients with valvular heart disease); Society of Cardiovascular Anesthesiologists; Bonow RO, et al. ACC/AHA 2006 guidelines for the management of patients with valvular heart disease: a report of the American College of Cardiology/American Heart Association Task Force on Practice Guidelines (writing Committee to Revise the 1998 guidelines for the management of patients with valvular heart disease) developed in collaboration with the Society of Cardiovascular Anesthesiologists endorsed by the Society for Cardiovascular Angiography and Interventions and the Society of Thoracic Surgeons. *J Am Coll Cardiol.* 2006;48(3):e1–148. [PMID: 16875962]

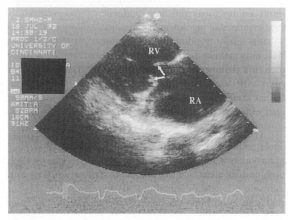

A

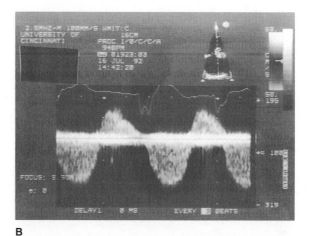

B

▲ **Figure 21–7. A:** Two-dimensional echocardiogram from a patient with rheumatic tricuspid valve disease, showing a thickened and domed tricuspid valve (*arrows*). The right atrium (RA) is considerably dilated, and the right ventricle (RV) is enlarged. **B:** Continuous wave Doppler study from the same patient confirms tricuspid stenosis and regurgitation. The high-velocity signal above the baseline during diastole represents right ventricular inflow; the signal below the baseline during systole represents tricuspid regurgitation.

▶ Treatment

A. Medical

Tricuspid regurgitation is usually well tolerated in the absence of pulmonary hypertension. When pulmonary arterial pressures increase, cardiac output falls, leading to symptoms of right-heart failure (edema, fatigue, dyspnea). Restriction of sodium and the use of potent loop diuretics decrease RA pressure. Medical therapy is also aimed at the cause of pulmonary hypertension. Treatment of associated systemic diseases is a critically important aspect of the therapeutic paradigm; it is, however, beyond the scope of this discussion. Symptomatic tricuspid stenosis is treated surgically.

B. Surgical

Surgery on the tricuspid valve may involve repair, reconstruction, excision, or replacement with a prosthetic valve. The decision to operate on the stenotic tricuspid valve is a straightforward one; the decision to operate on a regurgitant valve is more challenging. The surgeon must determine whether the regurgitation is functional or organic (ie, associated with a structurally normal or abnormal tricuspid valve), and if it is functional, the response of the pulmonary arterial pressure to the primary procedure should be anticipated. For example, repair may be unnecessary for functional tricuspid regurgitation if there is a high likelihood of a postoperative fall in pulmonary arterial pressure. In addition, repair of the functionally regurgitant tricuspid valve in patients with severe right ventricular dysfunction is unlikely to improve their status. However, the response of tricuspid regurgitation to reduced pulmonary artery pressure can be difficult to

predict, and, as mentioned previously, significant tricuspid regurgitation often complicates successful MVR despite reduced pulmonary artery pressures. Given the high morbidity and mortality associated with reoperation to correct tricuspid regurgitation following MVR, the presence of any degree of preoperative tricuspid regurgitation, especially organic regurgitation, warrants consideration of concurrent tricuspid valve repair. Moreover, because "functional" tricuspid regurgitation may be due to unrecognized annular involvement and because annular dilation may be progressive, "prophylactic" tricuspid annuloplasty has been recommended when the annular diameter exceeds 21 mm/m^2. Interestingly, in patients with chronic pulmonary thromboembolic disease, pulmonary thromboendarterectomy dramatically reduces functional tricuspid regurgitation without a change in tricuspid annular diameter.

The decision whether to repair or replace the tricuspid valve with a prosthesis depends on the suitability of valve repair, the associated surgical procedures, and the underlying disease. Thrombosis is a more frequent problem with tricuspid than with mitral prostheses. Thus, primary valve repair, when possible, is the preferred procedure. Repair of the stenotic tricuspid valve involves identifying and separating the fan chordae (the chords that support the leaflets in the area of the commissure), leaflet decalcification, and chordal or papillary muscle division.

Annuloplasty procedures correct dilatation of the tricuspid valve annulus. The dilatation, which is not symmetric, typically involves the annulus around the anterior and posterior leaflets (posterior more than anterior). The procedure involves sizing and selectively plicating the anterior and posterior annuli. Although the routine use of an annuloplasty

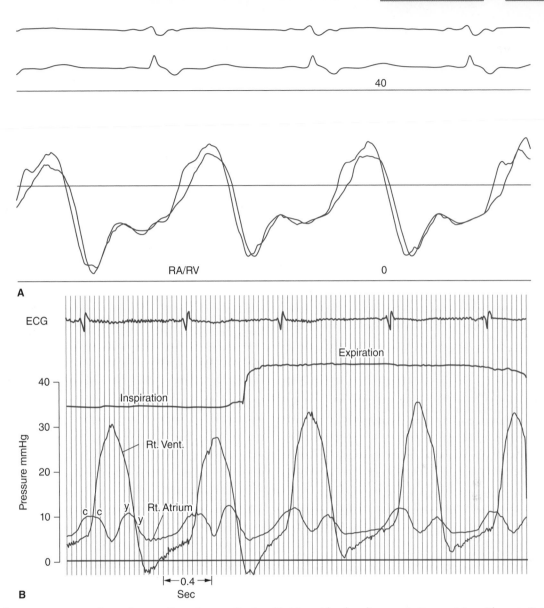

▲ **Figure 21–8.** Hemodynamic recordings from patients with tricuspid valve disease. **A:** Severe tricuspid regurgitation. There is "ventricularization" of the right atrial (RA) pressures, which are indistinguishable from right ventricular (RV) pressures. **B:** Simultaneous and equally sensitive recordings of RA and RV pressures from a patient with rheumatic tricuspid stenosis. Note the RA-RV gradient throughout diastole, which increases with inspiration. (Reproduced, with permission, from Fowler N, et al. *Diagnosis of Heart Disease.* New York: Springer-Verlag; 1991.)

ring is considered superior to nonring methods and is recommended by some groups, this position is not universally accepted.

When the tricuspid valve cannot be repaired and replacement is necessary, a bioprosthesis is often used because of the lower risk of thrombosis, although recent changes in valve design have significantly lowered the risk of thrombosis with

mechanical prostheses. Bioprosthetic valves are also more prone to late failure than mechanical prostheses. If anticoagulation is necessary for other reasons, a St. Jude prosthesis is preferred by some surgeons—especially for younger patients. Also, there is a risk of complete heart block requiring permanent pacing with tricuspid valve replacement. Recent studies indicate that long-term outcomes (mortality, thrombosis, structural deterioration) for bioprosthetic and mechanical valves are similar.

The primary indications for surgery in patients with tricuspid valve endocarditis are uncontrollable infection, septic emboli, or refractory congestive heart failure. Because virulent organisms are the rule, they are not, per se, an indication for surgery. Total excision of the tricuspid valve is an attractive option in injection drug users, considering both recidivism and the threat of prosthetic valve endocarditis. As noted earlier, tricuspid regurgitation without pulmonary hypertension is well tolerated; however, 20% of these patients ultimately may require valve replacement for right-heart failure. Debridement and valve repair have been suggested as alternative procedures to valve excision.

Successful percutaneous balloon valvuloplasty has been reported for native valve tricuspid stenosis and stenotic bioprosthetic tricuspid valves, but experience is limited. There are no published studies to compare percutaneous balloon valvotomy with surgical valvuloplasty, and only limited long-term results have been published.

Antunes MJ, et al. Management of tricuspid valve regurgitation. *Heart.* 2007;93(2):271–6. [PMID: 17228081]

Bonow RO, et al. American College of Cardiology/American Heart Association Task Force on Practice Guidelines. 2008 focused update incorporated into the ACC/AHA 2006 guidelines for the management of patients with valvular heart disease: a report of the American College of Cardiology/American Heart Association Task Force on Practice Guidelines. *J Am Coll Cardiol.* 2008;52(13):e1–142. [PMID: 18848134]

Marquis-Gravel G, et al. Retrospective cohort analysis of 926 tricuspid valve surgeries: clinical and hemodynamic outcomes with propensity score analysis. *Am Heart J.* 2012;163:851–8.e1. [PMID: 22607864]

Pfannmüller B, et al. Isolated tricuspid valve surgery in patients with previous cardiac surgery. *J Thorac Cardiovasc Surg.* August 28, 2012 [Epub ahead of print] [PMID: 22939859]

Raikhelkar J, et al. Isolated tricuspid valve surgery: predictors of adverse outcome and survival. *Heart Lung Circ.* 2013;22: 211–20. [PMID: 23103071]

Taramasso M, et al. The growing clinical importance of secondary tricuspid regurgitation. *J Am Coll Cardiol.* 2012;59:703–10. [PMID: 22340261]

Vahanian A, et al. Guidelines on the management of valvular heart disease: The Task Force on the Management of Valvular Heart Disease of the European Society of Cardiology. *Eur Heart J.* 2007;28(2):230–68. [PMID: 17259184]

Vassileva CM, et al. Tricuspid valve surgery: the past 10 years from the Nationwide Inpatient Sample (NIS) database. *J Thorac Cardiovasc Surg.* 2012;143:1043–9. [PMID: 21872283]

▶ Prognosis

The natural history of tricuspid valve disease is a function of the associated valvular lesions and the underlying disease. Isolated lesions are rare, and their natural history is unknown.

Regardless of etiology, tricuspid regurgitation is associated with decreased survival, and mortality increases as severity of regurgitation increases. In general, the results of tricuspid valve surgery depend on the types of valve lesions, the corrective procedures, the degree and reversibility of LV and RV function, and the pulmonary vascular resistance. Residual tricuspid regurgitation usually occurs when the pulmonary vascular resistance remains elevated. Many patients have small-to-moderate tricuspid valve gradients after tricuspid valve replacement; like residual tricuspid valve leaks, these are usually not clinically important. Although most surgeons favor repair over replacement, the superiority of this approach is difficult to prove.

Yang W, et al. Vena contracta width as a predictor of adverse outcomes in patients with severe isolated tricuspid regurgitation. *J Am Soc Echocardiogr.* 2011;24:1013–9. [PMID: 21820277]

PULMONIC VALVE DISEASE

ESSENTIALS OF DIAGNOSIS

Pulmonic regurgitation

▶ Diastolic murmur at the left upper sternal border that increases with inspiration.

▶ Split S_2 with a loud P_2.

▶ Characteristic Doppler echocardiographic findings, including valvular abnormalities (depending on etiology), right ventricular enlargement, and diastolic turbulence in the right ventricular outflow tract.

Pulmonic stenosis

▶ Systolic murmur at the left second intercostal space preceded by a systolic click.

▶ Split S_2 with a soft P_2.

▶ Characteristic Doppler echocardiographic findings, including thickened and domed leaflets, and increased systolic velocities across the pulmonic valve.

▶ General Considerations

The technologic advances made in the fields of noninvasive cardiac imaging, interventional cardiology, and cardiac surgery over the past few decades have had a noticeable effect on the diagnosis and management of pulmonic valve disease.

▶ Pathophysiology & Etiology

The normal pulmonic valve is a semilunar valve with anterior, left, and right leaflets. The function and texture of the valve leaflets, as well as the size of the valve annulus, can be adversely affected in a variety of diseases.

A. Pulmonic Regurgitation

Trivial to mild pulmonic regurgitation occurs in almost everyone at any age, but more severe pulmonic regurgitation commonly occurs in the setting of pulmonary hypertension. The regurgitation is caused by dilatation of the pulmonic valve ring, and any cause of pulmonary hypertension can precipitate pulmonic regurgitation. **Idiopathic dilation** of the pulmonary trunk and **Marfan syndrome** also cause pulmonic regurgitation via a similar distortion of the valve ring. **Infective endocarditis** is unusual, but when present, often causes pulmonic regurgitation, with vegetations causing dysfunction of the leaflets themselves. Although the pulmonic valve is the least likely to be seeded in endocarditis, the rising number of injecting drug users, immunocompromised persons, and patients with subclinical pulmonic stenosis represent a growing population at risk. Pulmonic regurgitation can also occur as a consequence of surgical treatment for **tetralogy of Fallot** or balloon valvuloplasty of **congenital pulmonic stenosis**. The pulmonic regurgitation is generally mild and hemodynamically insignificant, but in rare cases, it can progress to RV dilation, necessitating pulmonic valve replacement. **Rheumatic heart disease** is an infrequent cause of pulmonic regurgitation, and it invariably occurs in the setting of multiple valve disease. Other rare causes of pulmonic regurgitation include chest trauma, carcinoid tumors, syphilis, and catheter-related valve dysfunction.

B. Pulmonic Stenosis

Pulmonic stenosis is a congenital disorder in over 95% of cases. Congenital pulmonic stenosis is usually caused by a valvular lesion, although subvalvular (infundibular hypertrophy) and supravalvular (rare intracardiac tumors, congenital rubella syndrome) lesions do occur. Valvular pulmonic stenosis is most often due to fibrosis of the valve with thickening of the leaflets. The leaflets dome into the pulmonary trunk during systole, producing a narrow central aperture. Less commonly, the valve leaflets are dysplastic and rubbery with a small valve annulus. Bicuspid pulmonic valves also occur. The pathologic distinctions made earlier do have some clinical relevance, as dysplastic valves are less responsive to balloon dilatation than dome-shaped valves. **Isolated congenital pulmonic stenosis** is the most commonly encountered congenital pulmonic valve disease in adulthood, and it typically causes valvular pulmonic stenosis. **Tetralogy of Fallot** also causes pulmonic stenosis with a bicuspid valve, and **Noonan syndrome** can be associated with dysplastic pulmonic stenosis. Other congenital syndromes associated with pulmonic stenosis include double-outlet right ventricle, atrioventricular canal defect, and univentricular atrioventricular connection.

The most common acquired form of pulmonic stenosis occurs with **carcinoid heart disease.** The proposed mechanism for carcinoid valve disease has been discussed earlier in this chapter. The whitish carcinoid plaques adhere to the valve leaflets and can cause both pulmonic stenosis and pulmonic regurgitation. Rheumatic heart disease is a rare cause of pulmonic stenosis and, when present, is generally seen with multiple valve disease. Large vegetations on an infected pulmonic valve can rarely cause pulmonic stenosis.

▶ Clinical Findings
A. Symptoms & Signs

As with tricuspid disease, the symptoms of pulmonic valve disease can be subtle and overshadowed by coexisting illnesses. Patients with pulmonic regurgitation are often asymptomatic unless symptoms of pulmonary hypertension and RV failure eventuate. Patients with pulmonic stenosis are also frequently asymptomatic. Symptoms can appear gradually as the pulmonic valve pressure gradient increases and include exertional dyspnea, chest pain, and fatigue.

B. Physical Examination

1. Jugular venous waveform—The presence of pulmonic stenosis is suggested by a prominent jugular venous *a* wave in the setting of a relatively normal central venous pressure.

2. Cardiac auscultation

A. PULMONIC REGURGITATION—The pulmonic component of S_2 is usually loud because most patients have pulmonary hypertension, and the second heart sound is often split due to prolonged RV emptying. RV S_3 and S_4 gallops are sometimes heard in the left parasternal area. In the absence of pulmonary hypertension, the murmur of pulmonic regurgitation is a low-pitched, crescendo–decrescendo diastolic murmur that is best heard near the left second or third intercostal space. The murmur is augmented during inspiration. However, in patients with significant pulmonary hypertension, the murmur assumes a different quality. The dilatation of the pulmonic valve annulus allows for a more forceful regurgitant jet, resulting in a high-pitched, decrescendo murmur that is best heard at the left parasternal border near the second or third intercostal space, otherwise known as the **Graham Steell murmur.**

B. PULMONIC STENOSIS—The second heart sound is also split with pulmonic stenosis, and this splitting is proportional to the degree of stenosis. Unlike in pulmonic regurgitation, the pulmonic component of S_2 is soft in pulmonic stenosis, and an S_4 can frequently be appreciated over the lower left sternal border. A high-frequency systolic click can be heard near the left upper sternal border that precedes the late-peaking crescendo–decrescendo systolic murmur that typifies pulmonic stenosis. Unlike the murmur, the click becomes softer during inspiration due to enhanced late diastolic pulmonic valve opening with the increased RV filling. The murmur can be associated with a thrill, and an RV impulse is frequently palpable.

C. Diagnostic Studies

The diagnostic evaluation of pulmonic valve disease should include an ECG, chest film, and a transthoracic echocardiogram. Cardiac catheterization is generally unnecessary given the high degree of agreement between echocardiographic and catheterization data in pulmonic valve disease.

1. Electrocardiography—Pulmonic regurgitation and pulmonic stenosis can both cause ECG evidence of RV enlargement. Typical findings include right bundle branch block, right axis deviation, and RV hypertrophy. Mild or moderate pulmonic stenosis frequently presents with a normal ECG.

2. Chest radiography—Nonspecific enlargement of the right ventricle and pulmonary arteries can be seen with pulmonic regurgitation. Characteristically, pulmonic stenosis is associated with dilatation of the main pulmonary artery.

3. Echocardiography—In pulmonic regurgitation, the pulsed Doppler technique is used to accurately detect the presence and severity of pulmonic regurgitation. In addition, the presence of pulmonary hypertension, RV hypertrophy and dilation, and coexistent valve disease can be detected. Transesophageal echocardiography has a role in the evaluation of suspected pulmonic valve endocarditis.

Echocardiography determines the nature, location, and severity of the stenosis. Pulmonary stenosis is diagnosed almost exclusively by Doppler echocardiography, and, as with pulmonic regurgitation, data regarding the status of the ventricles and other valves can also be obtained. Transesophageal studies may be useful when the location of the stenosis is unclear from the surface study.

4. Cardiac catheterization—Cardiac catheterization is recommended in adolescents and young adults with congenital pulmonic stenosis for evaluation of the valvular gradient if the Doppler peak jet velocity is greater than 3 m/s and balloon valvotomy is feasible.

5. Magnetic resonance imaging (MRI)—MRI provides excellent images of the pulmonary outflow tract and valve and is especially useful for planning percutaneous bioprosthetic valve placement. It can also visualize the main pulmonary artery anatomy to assess for branch stenosis. In addition, it provides for accurate assessment of RV size and function. Finally, it can assess both stenosis and regurgitation quantitatively.

Karamitsos TD, et al. The role of cardiovascular magnetic resonance in the evaluation of valve disease. *Prog Cardiovasc Dis.* 2011;54:276–86. [PMID: 22014494]

▶ Treatment

Pulmonic regurgitation rarely requires specific treatment. Treatment of predisposing cardiac conditions, such as pulmonary hypertension, endocarditis, or left-sided valve disease, often improves the pulmonic regurgitation. As mentioned previously, certain patients may progress to right-heart failure from pulmonic regurgitation following repair of tetralogy of Fallot. These patients may require valve replacement, often with a bioprosthetic valve or pulmonary allograft.

Pulmonic stenosis has been managed with great success by balloon valvuloplasty. Treatment is based on severity of disease: balloon valvotomy is recommended if the RV–to–pulmonary artery peak-to-peak gradient is greater than 30 mm Hg at catheterization in the symptomatic patient, and greater than 40 mm Hg in the asymptomatic patient. Patients with dysplastic valves may not respond to balloon valvuloplasty and may require valve replacement with a bioprosthetic valve. Percutaneous stented pulmonary valve implantation is an alternative to surgical replacement of pulmonic stenosis and regurgitation in selected patients.

Holmes DR, et al. Transcatheter valve therapy. *J Am Coll Cardiol.* 2011;58:445–55. [PMID: 21715122]

▶ Prognosis

The prognosis of pulmonic valve disease is generally excellent. With pulmonic regurgitation, clinicians must consider the comorbidities involved (particularly pulmonary hypertension) that may influence prognosis. Patients with congenital pulmonic stenosis can expect a life expectancy comparable to that of the general population.

Harrild DM, et al. Long-term pulmonary regurgitation following balloon valvuloplasty for pulmonary stenosis. *J Am Coll Cardiol.* 2010;55:1041–7. [PMID: 20202522]

Parent JJ, et al. Outcomes of pulmonary balloon valvuloplasty for isolated pulmonary valve stenosis in children. *J Am Coll Cardiol.* 2012;59(Suppl):E813.

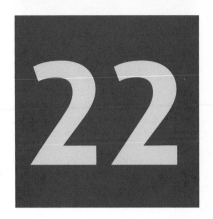

Infective Endocarditis

Michael H. Crawford, MD

▶ Fever.

▶ Blood cultures positive for bacteria or fungi.

▶ Characteristic cardiac lesions on echocardiography.

▶ General Considerations

Infective endocarditis is one of several infections in which endothelium is the initial site of infection. Healthy endothelium possesses an effective system of defense against both hemostasis and infection. Infection of the endothelium of blood vessels occurs only at sites markedly altered by disease or surgery, such as the severely atherosclerotic aorta or the suture lines of vascular grafts. By contrast, infection of the cardiac valve leaflet endothelium (endocardium) is not rare and occurs even in the absence of identifiable preexisting valve disease.

▶ Pathophysiology & Etiology

A. Cardiac Infection—Vegetations

1. Precursor lesion and bacteremia—Valve infection probably begins when minor trauma, with or without accompanying valve disease, impairs the antihemostatic function of valve endocardium. Infection usually first appears along the coapting surface of the leaflets, suggesting a role for valve opening and closing. This hypothesis is supported by the observation that the ranking of valves in order of frequency of infection corresponds to the ranking of valves according to the force acting to close the valve (mitral > aortic > tricuspid > pulmonic).

This minor trauma may cause the formation of a microscopic thrombus on the leaflet surface. A small noninfected thrombus on the leaflet is called **nonbacterial thrombotic**

endocarditis **(NBTE).** The next step is infection of the fibrin matrix of the thrombus by blood-borne organisms, which appear briefly in blood under many circumstances, such as brushing one's teeth. When transient bacteremia coincides with the presence of an NBTE lesion, organisms may adhere to the valve leaflet and begin to proliferate.

This theory for the pathogenesis of endocarditis is supported by observations regarding the circumstances under which endocarditis occurs and the particular organisms involved. Patients with endocarditis often tell of a preceding event that likely resulted in transient bacteremia. The common infecting organisms are those that gain entry to the blood because they colonize body surfaces and are adapted for attachment and proliferation in the NBTE lesion (see Clinical Syndromes).

2. Growth of vegetations—Vegetations begin near the coaptation line of the leaflet on the side that contacts the opposite leaflet during valve closure. Mitral valve vegetations are typically attached within 1–2 cm of the leaflet tip on the left atrial side and prolapse into the left atrium during systole. Aortic valve vegetations usually occur on the left ventricular (LV) side of the mid or distal portions of the aortic cusps and prolapse into the LV outflow tract during diastole. A similar distribution of lesions occurs on the tricuspid and pulmonic valves.

Although the course of cardiac lesions in endocarditis varies, in a typical sequence of events (without treatment), the infection progresses by enlargement of the vegetation and extension of its region of attachment toward the base of the leaflet. Valve regurgitation almost always develops, as a result of either destruction of the leaflet tip or scarring and retraction of the leaflet. Erosion of the leaflet may lead to perforation (usually associated with clinically significant regurgitation). Weakening of the leaflet's spongiosum layer may result in a deformity called a leaflet aneurysm. Mitral or tricuspid chordal involvement may cause rupture and acute severe regurgitation. In rare cases (primarily in mitral bioprosthetic endocarditis; see Management of High-Risk

Endocarditis), a large vegetation may cause hemodynamically significant valve obstruction.

3. Metastatic vegetations—These vegetations may form when the regurgitant jet of blood from an infected valve strikes an endocardial surface in the receiving chamber (wall or chordae), producing a small area of denuded endothelium. The thrombus that forms at this site also becomes infected, constituting a secondary vegetation. Such metastatic vegetations most often appear on the ventricular side of the anterior mitral leaflet where it is struck by a regurgitant jet from aortic valve endocarditis. Another common location is on the mitral chordae, also from aortic regurgitation. Metastatic lesions on the mural endocardium of the cardiac chambers can occur as well.

4. Abscess and fistula formation—Organisms eventually invade the valve annulus and adjacent myocardium. Abscess formation can take multiple forms and may occur with or without fistula formation. Aortic annular abscess is an infective mass that burrows into or around the outside of the annulus. The abscess may extend upward to the sinus of Valsalva or ascending aorta (a type of mycotic aneurysm). This extension may lead to a fistulous communication between the aorta and the left atrium or (rarely) the right atrium. In other patients, the abscess extends down through the fibrous trigone and forms a fistula to the LV outflow tract.

A band of fibrous tissue at the base of the anterior mitral leaflet (the intervalvular fibrosa) separates the aortic annulus from the left atrial wall. Infection extending down from the posterior aortic annulus may produce an aneurysm in this area, which may in turn fistulize to the left atrium, aortic root, or into the pericardial space. Infection extending down from the anterior aortic annulus may invade the septal myocardium, causing a block in the conduction system.

When mitral valve infection extends to the base of the anterior leaflet, abscess formation involving the fibrous trigone may track upward and become fistulous. Infection from the posterior leaflet may extend to form a myocardial abscess in the LV posterior wall or a fistula around or through the mitral annulus between the left atrium and left ventricle. Infection may even penetrate through to the pericardial space, producing purulent pericarditis.

B. Extracardiac Disease

At any time during cardiac infection, extracardiac complications may supervene and dominate the clinical picture. Although these manifestations are emphasized in the medical literature, it should be kept in mind that many patients with endocarditis do not have them, especially at the time of presentation. The extracardiac disease in endocarditis results from immunologic phenomena and the shedding of bacteria and fragments of infected thrombus from the valve vegetations.

1. Immune disease—The bacteremia accompanying endocarditis persists over long periods of time and represents a prolonged antigenic challenge to the immune system. Various antibodies and immune complexes appear in the blood—more so with longer duration of illness. Rheumatoid factors (anti-IgG or IgM antibody) are rarely of interest for their diagnostic value. Other antibodies, such as those that form circulating immune complexes and activate complement, are of major importance because they cause microvascular damage, most frequently glomerulonephritis and vasculitic skin lesions.

2. Systemic and pulmonary emboli—The embolization of fragments of vegetation is a frequent and potentially catastrophic complication of endocarditis. The clinical consequences are highly variable and depend on many factors, including the size of the embolus, the site at which it lodges in the vasculature, the type and quantity of organisms carried, the point during treatment at which embolism occurs, and the host response. Small emboli are likely to present as metastatic infection; the most dreaded of these is brain abscess. Septic embolization may also lead to abscesses in the kidney, liver, bone, and (from the right heart) lung.

Large emboli present with signs and symptoms of major vascular obstruction. For endocarditis of the left heart, the most frequent and serious extracardiac complication is embolism to the brain; these strokes tend to be large, complicating subsequent management and often causing death. Emboli may also cause infarction of the spleen, liver, kidney, and the myocardium. Embolism to large arteries of the extremities is unusual and occurs primarily in fungal endocarditis.

3. Mycotic aneurysms—When infection of the arterial wall results in localized dilatation and progresses to abscess formation, mycotic aneurysms can occur. The cause is thought to be embolization of vegetation that does not obstruct blood flow enough to present clinically as embolism. These lesions frequently occur at vessel branch points. The mycotic aneurysm may produce signs and symptoms many weeks after the diagnosis of endocarditis, and recognition may be difficult. Their effects are especially devastating in the central nervous system. Aneurysms may act as a protected site of infection and cause persistent fever or bacteremia despite appropriate antibiotic therapy. Alternatively, if antibiotic therapy has sterilized the aneurysm, it may present months or years later as unexplained hemorrhage.

C. Clinical Syndromes

Endocarditis can assume any of a wide variety of forms because of the many possible combinations of infecting organisms, portals of entry, and other factors such as the patient's immune status and the presence of concomitant diseases. Although the list of organisms capable of causing endocarditis is very long (and the list of possible combinations of organisms and other factors is even longer), there are several common and distinctive clinical syndromes.

Table 22–1. Characteristics of Acute and Subacute Endocarditis[1]

Acute	Subacute
Symptom onset to diagnosis: 1 week	Symptom onset to diagnosis: 4 weeks
Acute malaise	Weight loss
Shaking chills	Fatigue
Fever (may be high)	Night sweats
Leukocytosis	Low or no fever
Normal gamma globulins	Normal white cell count or leukopenia
Rheumatoid factor +	Elevated gamma globulins
	Rheumatoid factor +

[1]Elevated erythrocyte sedimentation rate and anemia common to both syndromes.

A distinction between the acute and subacute forms of endocarditis has been found to be of some clinical value. The differing characteristics of patients with these two forms are shown in Table 22–1. Many patients with endocarditis cannot be easily placed into one or the other of these two categories.

1. Viridans streptococcal endocarditis—The bacterial species classified as viridans streptococci account for approximately 25% of cases of endocarditis. These organisms can be divided into three groups: normal human oral flora (*Streptococcus mitis, Streptococcus sanguinis, Streptococcus anginosus, Streptococcus mutans, Streptococcus salivarius,* and other nutritionally variant species), inhabitants of the lower gastrointestinal and genitourinary tracts (nonenterococcal group D organisms, of which *Streptococcus bovis* is important), and *Streptococcus pneumoniae,* or pneumococcus, which infrequently causes endocarditis and causes a syndrome very different from the other viridans streptococci. The first two groups of streptococci cause almost no other disease in humans, except for endocarditis. This predilection appears to stem from bacterial cell wall proteins that bind to fibronectin, platelets, laminin, and other components of blood clots.

Viridans streptococci usually grow slowly, and the patient typically has a febrile illness of at least 10 days' duration and modest intensity; many cases fit the clinical syndrome of subacute bacterial endocarditis. Although valve destruction may be extensive, it is gradual, and abscess formation in the heart or elsewhere is uncommon. Infection of a normal valve by viridans streptococci is probably unusual. The renal disease accompanying endocarditis caused by these organisms is usually mild and rarely causes significant renal insufficiency. Viridans streptococcal endocarditis is therefore often treatable medically and has a relatively good prognosis if antibiotic treatment is begun before complications occur.

Endocarditis from *S bovis* is strongly associated with underlying colorectal disease, especially malignancy. Colonization of the gastrointestinal tract by this organism increases with age and with malignancy for reasons that are not well understood. After initial endocarditis treatment, a patient with this disease should undergo colonoscopy.

Extra vigilance for complications is needed when treating patients with endocarditis from certain other streptococci. *Streptococcus anginosus* and *Streptococcus milleri* tend to cause abscesses in the brain and other major organs, and nutritionally variant streptococci are associated with higher morbidity and mortality rates than are the other viridans organisms—again for reasons that are not understood.

Complications from viridans streptococcal endocarditis are almost never due to failure to sterilize vegetations. Nevertheless, the sensitivity of these organisms to penicillin is not uniform, and testing for resistance is essential for establishing an appropriate antibiotic regimen.

2. Staphylococcus aureus endocarditis—*S aureus* is a relatively common cause of endocarditis, accounting for approximately 33% of all cases. In hospitals serving a large population of injecting drug users, this may be the most common cause of endocarditis. Although *S aureus* frequently enters the circulation from the skin or nares, a culprit lesion may not be apparent on examination of these areas. Less than 25% of episodes of *S aureus* bacteremia in hospitalized patients are caused by endocarditis.

Unlike patients with streptococcal endocarditis, those with endocarditis caused by *S aureus* are likely to seek medical attention soon after the onset of bacteremia, which generally produces a febrile illness with marked constitutional symptoms and often rigors. This picture is especially common in injecting drug users. *S aureus* tends to cause valve destruction more rapidly than do other organisms; approximately 30% of cases result in extensive left-heart valve involvement complicated by abscess or fistula formation or pericarditis. *S aureus* endocarditis of the aortic valve is the most common cause of aortic annular abscess, often signaled by the appearance of PR interval prolongation. Mitral annular and myocardial abscesses are also associated with this organism.

Central nervous system involvement is present in 20% or more of cases and manifests as cerebral embolization, intracranial hemorrhage from mycotic aneurysm rupture, and microscopic or macroscopic brain abscesses. Other significant complications include septic arthritis, osteomyelitis, and major organ abscesses. Renal involvement, as indicated by an active urine sediment, is present in almost all cases, and frank renal impairment occurs in approximately 20%. The renal dysfunction caused by *S aureus* rarely progresses to dialysis or permanent renal failure.

S aureus is the most lethal of the organisms commonly causing endocarditis, with mortality rates of approximately 30% in non–injecting drug users and greater than 50% in patients with prosthetic valves. Injecting drug users have a much lower mortality rate (approximately 5%).

3. Enterococcal endocarditis—This form accounts for approximately 5% of cases of endocarditis—almost all from *Enterococcus faecalis*. Enterococcal endocarditis tends to occur in elderly men undergoing diagnostic manipulation or surgery involving areas colonized by this organism, such as the gastrointestinal and genitourinary tracts; in injecting drug users; or in women following obstetric procedures. An acute or insidious syndrome may be present in patients with enterococcal endocarditis, although the findings typical of subacute bacterial endocarditis are unusual.

Enterococcal endocarditis is especially difficult to treat because of antibiotic resistance (discussed later). It is markedly different from and far more serious than streptococcal endocarditis. Overall mortality is only slightly less than that for staphylococcal endocarditis, and the incidence of major complications and need for valve replacement is approximately 30–40%.

4. Endocarditis from gram-negative bacteria—Gram-negative bacteria rarely cause endocarditis, with the exception of three groups of organisms: *Pseudomonas aeruginosa*, the HACEK organisms (*Haemophilus* spp., *Actinobacillus, Cardiobacterium, Eikenella, Kingella*), and the enteric organisms (*Escherichia coli, Proteus, Klebsiella*, and *Serratia marcescens*). *Pseudomonas* and *Serratia* are occasional causes of endocarditis in injecting drug users.

The HACEK organisms are relatively slow growing and usually cause a subacute clinical syndrome. Organisms such as *Haemophilus* and *Cardiobacterium* are thought to account for cases of culture-negative endocarditis. Despite the often mild symptoms and signs of endocarditis caused by these organisms, valve destruction may be extensive by the time of diagnosis. The HACEK organisms are associated with endocarditis that causes major vessel embolism from large vegetations. Enteric organisms tend to produce an acute clinical syndrome similar to that caused by *Pseudomonas*.

5. Fungal endocarditis—Fungal endocarditis is associated with settings of immune compromise and procedures that give the organism access to the bloodstream, such as surgery, intravenous catheter placement, and injecting drug use. *Candida* species (especially *C albicans*), *Histoplasma capsulatum*, and *Aspergillus* account for approximately 80% of cases of fungal endocarditis. Other less common causative organisms include *Mucor* and *Cryptococcus*. Clinicians must recognize when patients are at risk for fungal endocarditis because the signs and symptoms of the disease often escape notice or lead to misdiagnosis. Risk factors are listed in Table 22–2. In most patients with fungal endocarditis of a native valve, the infection is related to a fundamental immune system impairment. Fungal superinfection should be considered when a patient with bacterial endocarditis relapses either late in the antibiotic course or after completing treatment. This observation is especially true for bacterial infection of a prosthetic valve. *Candida* species infection

Table 22–2. Risk Factors for Fungal Endocarditis

History of an implanted cardiac device (eg, prosthetic valve, pacemaker, AICD)
Indwelling vascular catheter and prolonged hospitalization
Prolonged treatment with broad-spectrum antibiotics
Immunosuppression (eg, steroid or cytotoxic drugs, radiation, malnutrition, untreated malignancy)
Injecting drug use

AICD, automatic implantable cardioverter-defibrillator.

is usually hospital-acquired, whereas histoplasmosis may be a community-acquired infection. Fungal endocarditis in injecting drug users is almost always due to non-*albicans* species of *Candida*.

The clinical syndrome of fungal endocarditis is more difficult to recognize than that of bacterial endocarditis. This may be due partly to the postsurgical state or multisystem disease common in these patients. It has also been suggested that fever and murmurs develop later in the course of fungal disease than in bacterial endocarditis and that leukocytosis and such peripheral manifestations as petechiae are less frequent. The development of symptoms is often insidious, extending over weeks or months. Cardiac involvement is generally limited to the development of vegetations; invasion of the myocardium occurs with a lower frequency than in bacterial endocarditis. The vegetations usually lead to leaflet destruction and valve regurgitation; they may be large and may occasionally cause valve orifice obstruction. The most likely complication of fungal infective endocarditis is embolism, including occlusion of large peripheral arteries from embolization. Table 22–3 lists the approximate frequency of causative organisms in native valve endocarditis.

6. Prosthetic valve endocarditis—The risk of developing endocarditis is higher with prosthetic heart valves than

Table 22–3. Native Valve Endocarditis: Causative Organisms

Organism	% of Cases
Viridans streptococci	28
Other streptococci	23
Enterococci	4
Staphylococcus aureus	28
Coagulase-negative staphylococcus	7
Gram-negative bacteria	4
Other	5
No growth	5

Table 22–4. Prosthetic Valve Endocarditis: Causative Organisms

Early (< 60 days postsurgery)	%	Late (> 60 days postsurgery)	%
Staphylococcus epidermidis	33	Streptococci	30
Gram-negative bacteria	19	Staphylococcus epidermidis	26
Staphylococcus aureus	17	Staphylococcus aureus	12
Diphtheroids	10	Gram-negative bacteria	12
Candida albicans	8	Enterococci	6
Streptococci	7	Diphtheroids	4
Enterococci	2	Candida albicans	3
Aspergillus	1		

with severely diseased native valves, approximately 0.5% per patient-year. Despite some overlap, there is a clear difference between the causes of disease that develops within 2 months of implantation and the causes of disease that occurs later (Table 22–4). The difference is probably due to infection occurring during surgery in early prosthetic endocarditis, with organisms from the skin of the patient and operating room personnel (Staphylococcus epidermidis and S aureus) accounting for more than half the cases. The incidence of early prosthetic endocarditis has been greatly reduced by the routine use of prophylactic antibiotics for several days after operation. Prosthetic infection after 2 months usually involves the same mechanism as does native valve endocarditis, except that the causative organisms are those adapted to nonbiologic material.

Infection of a bioprosthesis involves primarily the sewing ring. Vegetations similar to those of native valve endocarditis can occur when the prosthesis is biologic, but infection more often begins in the area of attachment of the sewing ring to the annulus. Vegetations may form in this area, but—most important—early in the disease, abscesses often form along the suture line, resulting in fistulization, paravalvular regurgitation, and partial or complete detachment (dehiscence) of the prosthesis.

Infection of a mechanical prosthesis centers on the sewing ring. The inward growth of an infective mass from the ring frequently causes the occluder to become stuck in a partially open or closed position. The lesions caused by sewing ring infection of mechanical prostheses are otherwise similar to those of bioprostheses.

Two important differences distinguish prosthetic valve endocarditis from native valve infection. Prosthetic valve infection may be extensive without the clinical signs, such as a murmur of regurgitation, heart failure, or embolism, usually seen in advanced native valve infection. When prosthetic valve dysfunction does occur (especially in a mechanical prosthesis), it tends to be abrupt and severe, as when the occluder becomes fixed in a half-open position. (Other differences are discussed later in this chapter.)

7. Endocarditis in the injection drug user—The patient usually has an intense febrile illness of several days' duration, starting within 24–48 hours of the last injection. The mode of infection is a needle contaminated by skin flora, and an intravenous injection site may show an abscess or thrombophlebitis. The most likely causative organism is S aureus, which, overall, causes 70% of endocarditis in injecting drug users and which, in this setting, has a benign prognosis with only a 2–5% mortality rate. Many other organisms can cause endocarditis in injection drug users, including gram-negative bacilli, especially P aeruginosa, C albicans, enterococci, and S marcescens, as well as viridans streptococci. The prevalence of specific causative organisms varies widely in different urban areas. Endocarditis from these organisms tends to be less acute than that caused by S aureus, but only rarely is it truly subacute.

Infection of the tricuspid valve is almost unique to injecting drug users and occurs in approximately 60% of cases of endocarditis in this population. Significant tricuspid regurgitation may not be clinically apparent. In as many as 40% of cases, the left heart valves alone are infected. Despite its proximity to the portal of entry in injecting drug users, the pulmonic valve is rarely involved, probably because of the low pressure gradient and low wear and tear of this valve. Chest pain and dyspnea should prompt consideration of septic pulmonary emboli, which occur in 30% of tricuspid valve endocarditis. This complication usually presents as chest pain accompanied by scattered fluffy pulmonary infiltrates. On serial chest films, these lesions may appear migratory because of simultaneous resolution of older infiltrates and appearance of new ones. Infiltrates may also progress to cavitation.

8. Endocarditis and human immunodeficiency virus (HIV)—HIV infection and acquired immunodeficiency syndrome (AIDS) do not increase the risk of infective endocarditis. The increased frequency of endocarditis in patients with HIV is due to the prevalence of injecting drug use in this population. HIV/AIDS patients appear to have an increased susceptibility to Salmonella endocarditis, a relatively antibiotic-responsive infection. Otherwise, the types of causative organisms seen are not altered by HIV status. The clinical syndrome and natural history of the disease in HIV-positive patients is also unchanged, except that patients with advanced AIDS (CD4 count < 200 cells/mcL) tend to have a more fulminant course and increased mortality rates.

9. Hospital-acquired endocarditis—Hospital-acquired endocarditis is uncommon; overall approximately 5% of positive blood cultures in hospitalized patients are due to infective endocarditis (exceptions include streptococcal viridans and nutritionally variant streptococci). Prosthetic valves are at far greater risk than native valves: endocarditis develops in 15–20% of patients with prosthetic valves who become bacteremic. Hospital-acquired endocarditis is marked by an increased likelihood of the presence of unusual or antibiotic-resistant organisms and an infected indwelling catheter as the likely portal of entry. Endocarditis occurs only rarely in postsurgical patients, usually after prolonged sepsis.

The usual causative organisms are coagulase-negative *Staphylococcus*; *S aureus; Enterococcus;* and enteric gram-negative organisms, such as *Pseudomonas* and *Serratia.* Fungi, especially *Candida,* and fastidious organisms should also be suspected when endocarditis occurs in debilitated, leukopenic patients and those previously treated with long courses of antibiotics. Hospital-acquired endocarditis should be suspected when fever develops in a hospitalized patient who has positive blood cultures without an apparent source. Potential culprit catheters should be removed and cultured, followed by transesophageal echocardiography (TEE) if an additional risk factor for endocarditis exists. Examples of risk factors in this setting include a prosthetic valve, native valve disease predisposing to infection, or *S aureus* bacteremia. If the findings of TEE are normal, and other sources of infection have been ruled out, a short (2-week) course of antibiotics is usually appropriate. Surveillance blood cultures during and after treatment and a repeat TEE should be considered if uncertainty regarding the response to treatment persists. In the case of exposure of a prosthetic valve to bacteremia, blood culture surveillance should be extended for at least 2 months.

10. Pacemaker or implanted defibrillator endocarditis— Pacemaker endocarditis is infection of the lead or of parts of the heart in contact with the lead (tricuspid valve, right ventricular endocardium). Mortality is high, up to 25%, and the diagnosis is often missed due to the indolent nature of the infection. Most cases are due to contamination at the time of implant; hematogenous infection of a lead is rare. Most cases have evidence of present or prior infection at the implant site. The delay from the most recent pacemaker procedure to the diagnosis of endocarditis may be as long as 2 years or as little as 6 weeks. In addition to fever and positive blood cultures, infection causes septic pulmonary emboli in about one-third of cases. Transesophageal echocardiography is the diagnostic test of choice, with a sensitivity of over 90%. The findings on transthoracic echocardiography (TTE) are often falsely normal.

Staphylococci are the usual infecting organisms, with *S epidermidis* accounting for 70% of cases and *S aureus* for most of the rest. As with prosthetic valve endocarditis, *S aureus* is the most likely culprit when endocarditis develops soon after implant, whereas *S epidermidis* is more likely when endocarditis develops later. *Staphylococcus* species produce a slime-like "sleeve" along the lead that protects

bacteria from the patient's immunologic defense as well as from antibiotic therapy. Treatment requires removal of the lead, and usually the entire system. Lead removal can be accomplished percutaneously with reasonable safety if the masses attached to the lead are small (< 1 cm). Surgery is indicated if the lead is fixed, if a large mass (> 1 cm) is present (with dislodgement likely to result in severe pulmonary embolism), or if tricuspid valve involvement is extensive. Lead removal is followed by 6 weeks of antibiotic therapy. The pacemaker-dependent patient is given an epicardial lead; reimplant of a transvenous system can be considered after 2 months with negative surveillance blood cultures.

▶ Clinical Findings

A. Diagnostic Criteria

In the current era, with the availability of sensitive blood culture techniques and TEE, the clinician will rarely need to rely on a formal schema for the diagnosis of endocarditis. The most useful schema is the Duke criteria, which involve two "major" criteria (definite echocardiographic evidence of endocarditis, positive blood cultures) and six "minor" criteria (predisposing cardiac condition, fever, vascular phenomena, immunologic phenomena, suggestive echocardiogram, ambiguous blood cultures) to reach a probable diagnosis. This approach was useful because of the low sensitivity and specificity of clinical features by themselves. Now TEE and blood cultures independently have a diagnostic sensitivity of greater than 90%, and TEE has a specificity of greater than 90%. Diagnostic uncertainty may arise when the result of TEE is ambiguous or when adequate blood cultures are not obtained before starting antibiotics. In many such situations, a diagnosis can be reached by gathering more data. For example, if the TEE fails to show endocarditis-specific valve disease and the patient is doing well, discontinuing antibiotics in order to repeat cultures should be considered. Many of the common features of endocarditis—fever, a cardiac murmur, and a set of positive blood cultures—occur frequently in other diseases and are occasionally absent in patients with endocarditis. Other diseases frequently mimicked by endocarditis include malignancy, autoimmune disease, and septicemia. In addition, patients with endocarditis may come to the physician because of a complication of endocarditis so dramatic as to distract attention from the underlying infection. Typical settings in which this error occurs include heart failure, stroke, and myocardial infarction.

The recognition of possible **prosthetic valve endocarditis** may be difficult because the signs of infection may be very subtle. In early prosthetic endocarditis, the symptoms and signs may be incorrectly ascribed to other diseases. Fever and bacteremia during the first few weeks after prosthetic implantation should be considered to indicate prosthetic valve endocarditis until proven otherwise. This is especially important because early prosthetic valve endocarditis appears to follow a more fulminant course than either late prosthetic or native valve endocarditis. These patients often have other potential causes of bacteremia, however, and an effort to prove infection from another site should be pursued vigorously. Transesophageal echocardiography probably has a sensitivity of approximately 80% for prosthetic valve endocarditis and should be performed whenever an alternative explanation for fever or bacteremia is not readily apparent. If the TEE findings are normal but bacteremia persists (especially if the organism is a frequent cause of prosthetic endocarditis), prosthetic infection should be presumptively treated. Fluoroscopy to rule out dehiscence has been replaced by TEE.

Fungal endocarditis is also often difficult to diagnose. Blood cultures are negative in approximately half of cases caused by *C albicans,* the majority of histoplasmosis cases, and almost all cases caused by *Aspergillus.* Histologic examination and culture should be performed whenever possible on specimens of embolic material, oropharyngeal lesions (especially for histoplasmosis), skin lesions (for *Candida* species and *Aspergillus*), liver, bone marrow, and urine (for histoplasmosis). In addition, a careful eye examination should be performed in patients with suspected fungal endocarditis because of the high frequency of anterior uveitis and chorioretinitis.

Tricuspid valve endocarditis (as seen in injecting drug users) produces a distinctive picture because of the frequent occurrence of septic pulmonary emboli. Scattered fluffy infiltrates seen on chest film are accompanied by pleuritic chest pain. Less often, the presentation may mimic pneumonia or include pleural effusion. The murmur of tricuspid regurgitation may be inaudible or soft because right-heart pressures are normally low, even when tricuspid infection is extensive.

B. Symptoms & Signs

Constellations of certain symptoms should arouse suspicion of endocarditis. One combination of symptoms often seen is constitutional symptoms (eg, fatigue, malaise, headache, arthralgias or myalgias, nausea, anorexia, weight loss) and fever, which can range from mild feverish feelings and night sweats to shaking chills. When these symptoms are chronic or mild, other diagnoses are often considered, such as malignancy and autoimmune disease.

A high suspicion of endocarditis is warranted when this picture is associated with any symptom pointing to the circulatory system, such as complaints associated with left- or right-heart failure (dyspnea, orthopnea, cough, peripheral edema), vascular occlusion (stroke, systemic embolism), and chest pain (Table 22–5).

C. Physical Examination

The physical examination is not essential for the diagnosis of endocarditis. Most of the physical findings caused by endocarditis are not specific for this diagnosis and should be interpreted in the context of the overall examination and the patient's history. There are also no physical findings that,

Table 22–5. Frequency of Symptoms and Signs in Endocarditis

Frequency	Symptom	Sign
High (> 40% of patients)	Fever	Fever
	Chills	Murmur
	Weakness	Skin lesions or emboli
	Dyspnea	Petechiae
Moderate (10–40% of patients)	Sweats	Osler or Janeway lesions
	Anorexia/weight loss	Splinter hemorrhages
	Cough	Splenomegaly
	Stroke	Major complication: stroke, heart failure, pneumonia, meningitis
	Rash	
	Nausea/vomiting	
	Headache	
	Chest pain	
	Myalgias/arthralgias	
Low (< 10% of patients)	Abdominal pain	New or changing murmur
	Delirium/coma	Retinal lesions
	Hemoptysis	Renal failure
	Back pain	

when absent, are useful for ruling out the diagnosis. A prominent murmur or skin lesion may arouse a clinical suspicion of endocarditis, but a murmur of valve regurgitation may be absent in patients with endocarditis. Vegetations may be present but may cause only slight regurgitation.

The examination is absolutely essential, however, to the treatment of endocarditis. The initial examination assists the clinician in assessing the severity of the illness. During treatment (or observation for more definite evidence of endocarditis), serial physical examinations are vital for identifying important changes in the patient's status because physical findings may signal the need for surgery.

1. Fever—Fever is usually present when the patient seeks medical attention, although it may be intermittent or already resolved through inappropriate antibiotic treatment. It may be infrequently masked by severe comorbid conditions, such as alcoholic cirrhosis, leukopenia, or malnutrition. The diversity of endocarditis does not permit generalizations about the temporal pattern or degree of fever. Fever may be low grade (37.5–38.5°C) and accompanied by only malaise and anorexia, or it may be hectic with rigors, sweats, and temperature higher than 40°C. Recurrence of fever during treatment of endocarditis is a very important problem (see section on Failure of antibiotic therapy).

2. Cardiac examination—The cardiac examination in the patient with suspected or known endocarditis focuses on identifying which heart valves are infected, the hemodynamic severity of the resultant regurgitation (or stenosis), and the adequacy of the patient's circulatory state.

At the time of initial evaluation of a patient with suspected endocarditis, the value of a detected murmur may be low because there may be no reliable information about the patient's prior cardiac condition. Systolic murmurs, for example, are common in the general population and very frequent in older or hospitalized patients; they are usually due to LV outflow or degenerative sclerosis of the aortic valve. Because endocarditis rarely causes valve stenosis, a systolic murmur related to endocarditis is almost always regurgitant.

Specific auscultatory features occasionally may be useful for determining how a valve has been damaged by infection. In mitral valve endocarditis, the examination may help identify which mitral leaflet has become partially flail. If the mitral regurgitant murmur radiates to the patient's back, the jet is likely to be directed posteriorly as a result of anterior leaflet prolapse into the left atrium. If the murmur radiates to the upper parasternal area (mimicking aortic stenosis), the posterior leaflet is likely to have lost its support.

It is essential that the examiner carefully note and document the cardiac findings as soon as the diagnosis of endocarditis is suspected. In addition to murmurs, the clinician should pay close attention to those aspects of the examination related to hemodynamic consequences of valvular dysfunction. Signs of pulmonary edema, dysfunction of either ventricle, and a low output state should be sought.

3. Skin and extremities—Assessment of the severity of extracardiac disease in endocarditis begins with a careful examination of the skin and peripheral circulation for evidence of vasculitis and emboli. Although these findings are not specific for the diagnosis of endocarditis, in the context of probable endocarditis, they strongly support that diagnosis. Their appearance during antibiotic therapy may signal the need for a change in the treatment plan.

A. PETECHIAE—Examine the soft palate, buccal mucosa, conjunctiva, and the skin of the extremities for petechiae, which are often transient, appearing in crops and fading in 2–3 days.

B. SPLINTER HEMORRHAGES—These brown streaks are 1–2 mm in length and found under the fingernails and toenails. Lesions in the proximal nail bed are moderately specific for endocarditis, whereas similar lesions under the distal nails are commonly found in healthy persons who work with their hands.

C. ROTH SPOTS—Vasculitis affecting small arteries of the retina may, on rare occasions, produce retinal infarction. The resulting funduscopic lesion, usually seen near the optic disc, is a pale retinal patch surrounded by a darker ring of hemorrhage.

D. OSLER NODES—These painful indurated nodules are 2–15 mm in diameter and appear on the palms and soles and often involve the distal phalanges. They are usually multiple and, like petechiae, tend to occur in crops and fade over 2–3 days. Osler nodes are thought to be caused by either vasculitis or septic embolization.

E. JANEWAY LESIONS—These painless, flat red macules are similar in size and location to Osler nodes that usually persist longer than a few days. Their pathogenesis is uncertain but is suspected to be vasculitis.

F. BLUE-TOES SYNDROME—Embolization of small vegetation fragments may cause ischemia in the distal arterial distribution of an upper or lower extremity. The affected finger or toe is tender, mottled, and cyanotic; over a period of days to weeks, the area becomes black and develops dry gangrene. Management is usually conservative (see Embolism section, later in this chapter). Acute arterial occlusive ischemia of a larger portion of an extremity raises the possibility of fungal endocarditis and is usually managed by embolectomy.

4. Neurologic examination—Cerebral embolization in endocarditis signals a poor prognosis and has a major impact on the overall management approach. The neurologic examination is an integral part of the evaluation of any patient with known or suspected endocarditis. During antibiotic treatment, symptoms that may be of neurologic origin justify careful repeat examination, often with computed tomography (CT).

5. Abdominal examination—Splenomegaly occurs in patients with endocarditis as part of generalized hyperplasia of the reticuloendothelial system. Its presence usually indicates endocarditis of at least 10 days' duration. Marked splenomegaly may be accompanied by abdominal pain from splenic infarction.

D. Diagnostic Studies

1. Detection of blood-borne infection—Bacteremia or fungemia invariably occurs at some point during endocarditis. The presence of the organism in the blood is generally of low grade and continuous because of the vegetations in the circulating bloodstream. Bacteremia may be intermittent or of variable intensity, however, especially if abscess formation has occurred or if the patient is under treatment.

The method of obtaining blood cultures depends on the severity of the patient's illness, as judged from the clinical syndrome and results of TEE. The preferred method in cases of suspected endocarditis is to obtain two or three sets of aerobic and anaerobic cultures, each from a separate venipuncture site, over 12 or more hours. This approach should be used if the suspicion of endocarditis is low, the patient appears well enough to tolerate a 12-hour delay of antibiotic therapy, or the TEE is normal or inconclusive.

Initiation of antibiotic therapy, however, should not be delayed if the suspicion of endocarditis is high and the patient is acutely ill, with a temperature more than 40°C, tachycardia, discomfort, or hypotension; the TEE is abnormal; or complications of endocarditis, such as embolism or congestive heart failure, have already occurred. Under these conditions, the cultures should be obtained over 30 minutes, followed immediately by antibiotic therapy.

Blood cultures have been found positive for an infecting organism in 70–95% of cases of endocarditis reported in studies since 1970. Proper technique and timing of blood cultures can improve the positive yield. Potential causes of negative blood cultures in patients with endocarditis are shown in Table 22–6. When blood cultures remain negative at 24–48 hours in a patient with probable endocarditis, the most important concern is infection from unusual organisms, such as the fungi, HACEK organisms, *Coxiella burnetii* (Q fever), *Chlamydophila psittaci,* or *Bartonella* and *Abiotrophia* species (nutritionally variant streptococci). The laboratory should be notified of the suspected diagnosis, and infectious disease consultation obtained.

If antibiotics have already been started for another diagnosis, modification of the blood culture technique can increase the positive yield. The importance of recovering the causative organism may warrant stopping all antibiotics. Blood cultures then should be drawn according to the routine outlined earlier, usually with an additional two blood cultures drawn at 24 hours.

If the suspicion of endocarditis remains moderate or high after the initial blood culture sets are drawn, empiric antibiotic therapy should also begin. The antibiotics should be changed according to the blood culture results as soon as these become available. If the initial blood cultures are negative after 24 hours but endocarditis is still suspected, three more sets should be obtained and processed under the guidance of an infectious disease specialist.

2. Serologic testing—Serologic testing can be helpful for identifying certain causes of endocarditis when blood cultures

Table 22–6. Causes of Negative Blood Cultures in Endocarditis

Failure to obtain more than one set of blood cultures
Failure to hold blood cultures for longer than 1 week
Prior antibiotic prescription (normally within 2-3 days of culture)
Organism grows slowly in standard culture (eg, HACEK organisms, nutritionally variant streptococci)
Organism fails to grow in standard culture (eg, fungi, rickettsiae, Q fever, psittacosis, nutritionally variant streptococci)
Intermittent bacteremia or fungemia (rare)

are negative. Histoplasmosis antigen is highly specific for systemic infection by this organism. Positive antibody titers for Q fever (*C burnetii*) or *Brucella* in a patient with culture-negative endocarditis identify these organisms as the cause. Although not essential to the diagnosis of endocarditis, nonspecific serologic testing is supportive and can be useful in certain situations. A positive rheumatoid factor is commonly found in patients with endocarditis of longer than 2 weeks' duration. This laboratory abnormality is not specific for endocarditis. When blood cultures are positive but other evidence of endocarditis is lacking or equivocal, a positive rheumatoid factor should prompt careful follow-up and retesting (eg, repeat TEE) for further evidence of endocarditis. Under some circumstances, these positive serologic tests may even warrant extension of antibiotic therapy to treat presumed endocarditis.

3. Echocardiography

A. Transesophageal echocardiography—Patients with suspected endocarditis should undergo TEE as soon as possible. With its detailed images of the heart valves and related structures, TEE is highly sensitive and specific for the diagnosis of endocarditis and is essential to defining the extent of disease. A TEE that shows a mass with the characteristics of a vegetation has a specificity of more than 90% for endocarditis (in the absence of a history of endocarditis, since it is difficult to distinguish between old and new vegetations). A normal TEE does not rule out endocarditis, but it has a negative predictive accuracy of at least 90%. Because false-normal TEE studies can occur, however, a patient with a normal study but a high clinical suspicion of endocarditis should be either observed carefully or treated, depending on the clinical severity of the illness. The TEE should be repeated if needed.

(1) Classification—Transesophageal echocardiographic studies in patients with suspected endocarditis may be classified according to the probability of the disease. A useful scheme is based on four categories: normal, possible, probable, and almost certain. In the **normal** category, no substrate for endocarditis or other abnormalities is present.

The TEE findings are classified as **possible endocarditis** in the presence of valve disease, such as a prosthetic heart valve, rheumatic or degenerative valvular sclerosis, or valve regurgitation likely to be pathologic, that predispose the patient to endocarditis—but without evidence of lesions. The classification of **probable endocarditis** is used when less specific lesions are found. Examples of such abnormalities include localized leaflet thickening or a nonmobile leaflet-related mass (especially if the lesion has the reflectance of soft rather than sclerotic tissue), mitral or aortic valve prolapse, chordal rupture, intracardiac thrombi, and paravalvular regurgitation in patients with prosthetic valves.

Patients with no history of endocarditis who have a lesion very strongly associated with infective endocarditis fall into the **almost certain** category. In such cases, TEE shows an intracardiac mass with typical vegetation characteristics—a pedunculated mass attached near the leaflet tip and prolapsing during valve closure into the lower pressure chamber. Vegetations have soft-tissue reflectance (like myocardium) and vibratory or rotatory motion independent of the motion of the leaflet. Vegetations apparent on TEE vary in length from 1 or 2 mm to several centimeters.

Other lesions considered almost certain for endocarditis would be an abscess or fistula, a metastatic vegetation, and an aneurysm of the intervalvular fibrosa. An abscess appears on TEE as an echolucent space adjacent to a valve annulus or prosthetic sewing ring. The abscess often appears to be separated from adjacent structures by thin septa, and jets of blood flowing into the abscess during systole or diastole (depending on abscess location) may be shown by color Doppler interrogation. The abscess is considered a fistula when there is communication with two or more adjacent cardiac chambers or blood vessels. Metastatic vegetations appear on echocardiography as vibratory or rotatory masses attached to an endocardial surface at a site with a regurgitant jet.

It should be noted that this TEE classification scheme is appropriate only in patients with other reasons to suspect endocarditis (eg, unexplained fever, positive blood cultures) and no prior history of endocarditis.

(2) Diagnostic accuracy—Possible causes of false TEE results are shown in Table 22–7. Of particular importance is the possibility that TEE findings may be normal because endothelial infection may be in the vasculature rather than in the heart. Because vascular infection is rare in the absence of prior vascular surgery, the diagnosis is usually suspected based on the patient's history. Nevertheless, the TEE examination in patients with suspected endocarditis routinely includes the thoracic aorta. Transesophageal echocardiography may identify severe atherosclerosis with mobile atheroma or thrombi. Although these abnormalities

are not nearly as specific for infection as are intracardiac vegetations, the clinical picture may justify antibiotic treatment.

In general, less than 10% of TEE results are falsely abnormal. By causing thickened, prolapsing leaflets and ruptured chordae, a myxomatous mitral valve can closely mimic endocarditis. A benign leaflet tumor, called a **papillary fibroelastoma,** may give the appearance of a vegetation. Several other abnormalities seen by TEE have lower specificity for the diagnosis of endocarditis than do typical vegetations; examples include para-aortic cavities (potentially representing either an abscess or an aneurysm of the sinus of Valsalva) and paraprosthetic regurgitation. Clinical context is often crucial to the interpretation of these findings. The paraneoplastic syndrome of myxomas may mimic endocarditis, although usually location and morphologic features of myxomas distinguish them from thrombi or vegetations. Intracardiac thrombi may be innocent bystanders in a patient with a clinical syndrome suggesting endocarditis, or they may be secondarily infected.

Lambl excrescences are thin, strand-like structures extending 1–10 mm from the valve leaflet margins. Because they prolapse and exhibit hypermobility, Lambl excrescences can be mistaken for small vegetations. Nodules of Arantius are similar extensions, not more than a few millimeters in length, from the center of the aortic cusp margin. When the aortic valve is closed, a TEE may show these nodules prolapsing from the center of the valve.

In addition to detecting vegetations, TEE usually provides a detailed picture of the extent of cardiac infection; it is very accurate at assessing the exact size and location of vegetations. Several complicated forms of cardiac involvement are usually identifiable by TEE. Because many of these complex lesions require surgery, TEE should be performed as soon as possible in a patient with a moderate or high suspicion of endocarditis.

Blood cultures should be drawn either before or 15 minutes after TEE to avoid the transient bacteremia that infrequently occurs during the procedure. Prophylaxis for endocarditis is not indicated prior to TEE.

B. Transthoracic echocardiography—The initial diagnostic value of TTE is limited in patients with possible endocarditis because of its low sensitivity: a large number of false-abnormal results occur, particularly in patients with prosthetic valves. On the other hand, a TTE showing typical vegetations is at least 90% specific for the diagnosis of endocarditis. TTE, however, cannot provide the detailed information regarding the anatomic extent of infection available from TEE.

Despite these limitations, TTE has a valuable ancillary role in patients with known endocarditis. It is well suited to assessing cardiac chamber dilatation, left and right ventricular dysfunction, and the patient's hemodynamic status. Presystolic closure of the mitral valve on TTE is a sign of elevated LV end-diastolic pressure and is an indication that the patient with aortic insufficiency should be considered

Table 22–7. Causes of False Results of Transesophageal Echocardiography

False-Abnormal
Myxomatous mitral valve disease
Papillary fibroelastomas
Partially flail leaflet
Healed vegetations
Mitral valve strands
Nodules of Arantius (aortic valve)
Lambl excrescences

False-Normal
Aortic valve prosthesis
Mitral valve mechanical prosthesis (includes shadowing of aortic valve by a mitral prosthesis)
Calcified aortic root shadowing tricuspid or pulmonic valves
Mitral annular calcification
Aortic atheroma or aneurysm infection
Study done too early in disease course

for surgery. Similarly, right atrial and pulmonary artery pressures can be estimated by transthoracic Doppler examination. Additional Doppler data are essential to assessing the severity and hemodynamic sequelae of mitral regurgitation, including elevated left atrial pressure. Changes in the patient's clinical status during treatment often can be readily diagnosed by comparison of serial TTE studies. For these reasons, it is advisable to perform transthoracic study at the same time as the initial TEE. One useful strategy is to discuss the results of TTE with the referring physician while the patient is still in the laboratory, and then proceed to TEE if appropriate.

4. Electrocardiography and chest radiography—The electrocardiogram (ECG) is occasionally useful in alerting the clinician to the severity of endocarditis. In patients with known or suspected aortic valve endocarditis, the PR interval should be monitored closely for prolongation, an indication of aortic annular abscess formation. Less frequently, the ECG may show increased QRS voltage and a precordial strain pattern in patients with either severe aortic or mitral regurgitation and marked LV enlargement. The chest radiograph is primarily useful in evaluating the patient with suspected endocarditis to assess the presence and severity of pulmonary edema and to detect septic pulmonary emboli in patients with possible right-heart endocarditis.

Cecchi E, et al. Are the Duke criteria really useful for the early bedside diagnosis of infective endocarditis? Results of a prospective multicenter trial. *Ital Heart J.* 2005;6(1):41–8. [PMID: 15773272]

Crawford MH, et al. Clinical presentation of infective endocarditis. *Cardiol Clin.* 2003;21(2):159–66. [PMID: 12874890]

Li JS, et al. Proposed modifications to the Duke criteria for the diagnosis of infective endocarditis. *Clin Infect Dis.* 2000;30(4):633–8. [PMID: 10770721]

Sachdev M, et al. Imaging techniques for diagnosis of infective endocarditis. *Cardiol Clin.* 2003;21(2):185–95. [PMID: 12874892]

Thuny F, et al. Risk of embolism and death in infective endocarditis: prognostic value of echocardiography: a prospective multicenter study. *Circulation.* 2005;112(1):69–75. [PMID: 15983252]

▶ Management

A. Initial Decisions

Management of newly diagnosed endocarditis requires the physician to make two decisions promptly. The first is whether to initiate empiric antibiotic therapy based on available clinical information or to await the exact identity and antibiotic sensitivities of the infecting organism and then to select the optimal regimen. The second decision is whether valve surgery is indicated immediately or can be deferred to allow assessment of the patient's response to antibiotic therapy.

Both decisions depend on the extent of cardiac infection (usually characterized by TEE), the severity of the patient's symptoms and signs of infection, the patient's circulatory status, the seriousness of extracardiac complications, and the available data about the organism.

Once initial treatment is under way, the physician must maintain a high level of vigilance for evidence of an inadequate response to treatment or the development of complications that will require additional medical or surgical intervention.

B. Antibiotic Therapy

The goal of antibiotic therapy is to sterilize vegetations. For most causative organisms, this is an achievable goal and will cure the patient if cardiac abscess and metastatic infection to other organs have not occurred. Vegetations, however, provide proliferating organisms with an environment that is protected against both the patient's immune system and antibiotics. Organisms grow under the surface of the vegetation where phagocytes cannot penetrate, and bacterial metabolism is slowed within the nutrient-poor vegetation, contributing to antibiotic resistance. For these reasons, antibiotic treatment is directed toward achieving bactericidal concentrations of drug within the vegetation over an extended period. It must be noted that certain important aspects of antibiotic dosing, especially in seriously ill patients, are beyond the scope of this text, and infectious disease consultation is advised.

1. Principles of antibiotic therapy

A. IN VITRO SENSITIVITY TESTING—For organisms with variable antibiotic sensitivity (eg, streptococci), the choice of drug and the dosage depend on in vitro sensitivity testing of the strain infecting the patient. An organism's sensitivity to an antibiotic is quantified by the minimum inhibitory concentration (MIC) and minimum bactericidal concentration (MBC). The MIC is defined as the minimum concentration of antibiotic that prevents proliferation of the organism in a standardized culture system. The MBC is the minimum concentration that kills 99.9% of the bacteria at 24 hours in a similarly standardized system. These tests are widely used to guide treatment of endocarditis.

B. DRUG COMBINATIONS—Combinations of drugs with additive, or synergistic, killing power are used frequently for treating endocarditis. A common combination is a β-lactam antibiotic (the penicillins and cephalosporins) with an aminoglycoside. This combination is synergistic because the β-lactam drug damages the bacterial cell wall, which allows more rapid penetration of the aminoglycoside into the cell.

C. PARENTERAL TREATMENT—Antibiotic treatment must be given parenterally to ensure high and consistent serum drug levels and compliance. Outpatient intravenous drug therapy can be undertaken only under specific conditions (see section on Outpatient Treatment), and oral therapy is almost never sufficient.

D. PROLONGED TREATMENT—The duration of antibiotic administration is almost always for a month or more. Prolonged exposure of the patient to antibiotics can lead to frequent side effects and serious toxicity (monitoring antibiotic therapy is discussed in the following section).

2. Empiric antibiotic therapy—Empiric antibiotic therapy is the initiation of antibiotics for the purpose of treating endocarditis without identifying the causative organism. Ideally, empiric therapy is needed only briefly until culture and sensitivity data are available. It requires treating the patient for the worst-case organism and can subject the patient to the additional risk of receiving multiple antibiotics over a prolonged period. This approach should be avoided whenever the patient's clinical status allows waiting for blood culture results, and the physician should make every effort to draw blood cultures consistent with a tolerable delay in the initiation of appropriate therapy.

Empiric therapy may be necessary if the patient has the syndrome of acute endocarditis, appears with symptoms of significant toxicity, or shows signs of septic shock; if the patient shows signs and symptoms of left-heart failure and is likely to need surgery in the near future; or if the patient's echocardiogram (preferably TEE) shows evidence of extensive cardiac involvement. Although data on the prognostic implications of specific TEE findings are still incomplete, extensive involvement probably includes a vegetation longer than 2–3 cm, valve dysfunction likely to be hemodynamically significant, more than one infected valve, leaflet perforation, annular abscess, and pericarditis. The choice of antibiotic for empiric therapy may be guided by considering the most likely infecting organisms based on the clinical presentation.

3. Outpatient treatment—Outpatient parenteral antibiotic therapy, now widely used, can provide an excellent outcome. Careful patient selection and management are mandatory. The first 2 weeks of treatment should almost always be as an inpatient because complications are most likely during this time. If the patient has a low-virulence organism, if valve involvement is limited to vegetations attached to leaflets and vegetations are not large (< 15 cm), and the first 2 weeks have been uncomplicated, then outpatient treatment should be considered. Endocarditis due to viridans streptococci and the HACEK group can be treated as an outpatient. At present, it is less certain that infection with *S aureus,* especially of the aortic valve, can be safely treated this way, due to the frequency of abscess and subvalve extension.

In addition to a specialized team of nurses managing the infusion and assessing the patient daily, a physician experienced in the treatment of endocarditis should be available for a same-day visit in the event of evidence of complications (discussed further later under the Management of Complications section). The patient should live close to

a hospital and have drug levels, blood cultures, and other blood work monitored as with an inpatient.

4. Monitoring antibiotic therapy

A. DRUG LEVELS—Monitoring the levels and effects of antibiotics is important in managing endocarditis because the patient's prolonged exposure to high doses of antibiotics increases the frequency of adverse drug effects. The use of aminoglycosides requires monitoring of serum levels at peak (1–2 hours after infusion is started) and trough (immediately before the next dose). A peak level for gentamicin or vancomycin of less than 5 mcg/mL is associated with treatment failure for many organisms and may warrant adjustment of the dose or the dosing interval. At a trough level of more than 2 mcg/mL, gentamicin carries an increased risk of nephrotoxicity, and the dose should be reduced. Monitoring these levels assumes even greater importance in the setting of renal insufficiency, especially if renal function is changing. Although vancomycin and flucytosine levels should always be monitored for the same reasons, levels for β-lactam antibiotics are available but rarely needed.

B. ADVERSE EFFECTS—The most common adverse effects are a pruritic maculopapular rash and low-grade fever seen with β-lactam antibiotics. The rash may signify delayed hypersensitivity and may be accompanied by hepatic or renal dysfunction. Liver biochemical tests (aspartate aminotransferase and alkaline phosphatase) and creatinine should be checked in this situation. If these tests are abnormal, substitution of another drug is required. If not, it is preferable to continue the antibiotic and treat the symptoms. Patients taking β-lactam antibiotics should have a routine complete blood count every 3 or 4 days during therapy to detect anemia, thrombocytopenia, and leukopenia. The sodium content of β-lactam antibiotics may require diuretic therapy in patients with heart failure.

Patients taking aminoglycosides should have the serum creatinine checked routinely at 3- to 4-day intervals. Equally useful for detection of renal dysfunction is the periodic examination of urine for white cell or granular casts. Ototoxicity is an idiosyncratic reaction unrelated to aminoglycoside levels that occurs in 10–20% of cases.

Diarrhea may occur during antibiotic therapy; this is usually due to overgrowth of gut organisms competing with those sensitive to the antibiotic (eg, *Clostridium difficile* colitis).

C. Management of Complications

1. Failure of antibiotic therapy—Changes in the cardiac examination during antibiotic treatment are particularly important in detecting failure of medical therapy. Changes in a regurgitant murmur almost always indicate valve dysfunction, and the appearance of a new murmur may signal metastatic infection of another valve. Such new findings almost always warrant repeat echocardiography (usually TEE) and blood cultures. There may also be an increase in the resting sinus rate and the appearance of heart failure. In aortic valve endocarditis, an abrupt increase in the pulse pressure should raise suspicion of worsening or new aortic regurgitation.

Failure of antibiotic therapy is usually heralded by persistent or recurrent fever. Persistent fever is defined as continuing for more than a week during antibiotic treatment. Recurrent fever develops after an afebrile period of several days and occurs at least a week after initiation of antibiotics. Persistent infection is only one cause of fever in this setting; others include hypersensitivity to antibiotics and other drugs, phlebitis, silent emboli (especially pulmonary and splenic), intercurrent urinary or upper respiratory tract infection, or simply a delayed response to antibiotic therapy. Blood cultures should be obtained and efforts made to rule out these possibilities. If blood cultures are negative, and the patient shows no other evidence of deterioration, watchful waiting is appropriate.

Positive blood cultures after more than 1 week of antibiotic therapy strongly suggest persistent infection. The cause may be either antibiotic resistance or a protected site of infection. The site may be an intracardiac annular or myocardial abscess or an extracardiac site of metastatic infection, septic embolization, or mycotic aneurysm. Repeat TEE is strongly indicated. Careful comparison to the studies obtained at the time of initial diagnosis may detect intracardiac suppurative complications; there is a sensitivity range of 80–90%. If TEE findings are abnormal, urgent surgery is indicated. If they are normal, a careful history and physical examination coupled with CT or a technetium, gallium, or indium scan will often reveal an infective focus.

2. Worsening valve dysfunction and heart failure—At any time during the course of endocarditis, heart failure signs and symptoms may appear as a result of worsening regurgitation and failure of ventricular compensatory mechanisms. In fact, heart failure may appear despite effective antibiotic therapy—and even after bacteriologic cure. The onset of heart failure may be insidious and difficult to recognize, or it may be abrupt and catastrophic. Frequent appraisal of the patient's status by history and physical examination is the best way to ensure early detection of heart failure. Any change in the patient's regurgitant murmur during antibiotic therapy usually signifies progression of valvular dysfunction and the likely need for surgery. A persistent tachycardia or slowly increasing heart rate is a useful sign of impending heart failure prior to the appearance of the typical signs such as rales, S_3, and pulmonary vascular redistribution on chest radiograph. In patients with aortic valve endocarditis, the appearance of a widened pulse pressure usually indicates increased valve regurgitation.

Serial TTE or TEE is useful in confirming a suspected change in the patient's hemodynamic status; it may even identify the cause. Worsening of the mitral regurgitant lesion is suggested by an increase in size of the color-flow Doppler jet or an increase in the radius of the flow convergence region on the LV side of the regurgitant orifice. A rise in transmitral early filling velocity (E wave) and a fall in forward systolic pulmonary venous flow (S wave) may indicate a rise in mean left atrial pressure.

In the case of aortic regurgitation, jet enlargement over time is also a useful indicator of worsening regurgitation. Additional indications of severe aortic regurgitation include closure of the mitral valve on M-mode echocardiography prior to the onset of the QRS and shortening of the pressure half-time of the aortic insufficiency velocity, both from a rapid rise of LV pressure to a high level in late diastole. For either mitral or aortic regurgitation, the presence or development of a hyperdynamic left ventricle (increased ejection fraction, stroke volume, or both) and progressive LV dilatation on two-dimensional echocardiography are useful indirect indications of an excessive regurgitant burden. The appearance of pulmonary or right atrial hypertension, as estimated from tricuspid jet velocity and inferior vena caval dynamics, is another sign of hemodynamic decompensation. Transesophageal echocardiography has the additional major advantage of being able to detect the intracardiac complications accounting for the change in the patient's hemodynamic status.

If heart failure is mild, surgery should be deferred while diuretics, digoxin, and afterload-reducing drugs are given to optimize the patient's hemodynamic status. If the patient responds readily to therapy, surgery might be optional. In most cases, however, surgery should be undertaken as soon as feasible because it is almost certain that valve repair or replacement will be required eventually (for the hemodynamic lesion, if not for infection), and the patient's surgical risk is lowest at this early stage. One clear exception to surgery for mild heart failure is sodium overload (related to antibiotic therapy) and suspected valve dysfunction not confirmed by echocardiography.

If heart failure is moderate or severe, valve surgery should be undertaken immediately while drug therapy is used to stabilize the patient. Because of the difficulty in predicting the rate of progression of valve dysfunction, delaying surgery for hemodynamic optimization is ill-advised. Rapid development of heart failure may signal the occurrence of a major intracardiac complication, such as leaflet perforation, chordal rupture, or fistula formation. Preoperative or intra-operative TEE is usually helpful in guiding surgical planning in this setting.

3. Embolism—Embolism most often occurs early in the course of antibiotic therapy but can occur at any time, even after biologic cure. Suspected cerebral embolism should be evaluated immediately by CT; if necessary, cerebral angiography should be performed in order to rule out an intracranial mycotic aneurysm. Nonhemorrhagic infarcts may warrant measures to reduce cerebral edema.

If the patient is already receiving anticoagulant therapy prior to development of endocarditis, anticoagulation is usually continued. After cerebral embolism in a patient with endocarditis, however, anticoagulation therapy is usually discontinued (if possible) for 14–30 days to reduce the likelihood of massive intracerebral bleeding. If stroke occurs in mechanical prosthetic valve endocarditis, the balance of risks and benefits of continuing anticoagulation is unknown. In patients with stroke from endocarditis, serial neurologic examinations and (if a change is suspected) repeated CT scans are indicated to permit early detection of brain abscess.

Because no clinically useful means (including echocardiography) has been found to identify patients at high risk for embolism, valve surgery in endocarditis is not indicated to prevent embolism. Even the probability of embolism recurring after one episode is not necessarily high enough to warrant surgery for prevention. On the other hand, surgery may be advised if the patient has had more than one episode and has a persistent vegetation.

Peripheral embolization is managed conservatively and without anticoagulation whenever possible. Vascular surgery to restore the circulation may be indicated if major organ embolization becomes life-threatening. Embolectomy is generally indicated in culture-negative endocarditis in order to make a causative diagnosis; likely organisms include *Aspergillus, Candida*, and the HACEK group. Embolectomy is necessary, strictly for treatment, in fungal endocarditis in order to remove as much infection as possible from the circulation.

4. Mycotic aneurysm—A complaint of severe headache or visual disturbance (especially homonymous hemianopsia) in a patient with endocarditis should prompt an urgent CT scan for the possibility of an expanding intracranial mycotic aneurysm. This catastrophic complication may also present as a subarachnoid or intracerebral hemorrhage, usually massive. If the scan is negative, cerebral angiography is often necessary to confirm or rule out the diagnosis. Treatment is surgical removal as soon as the patient's condition will allow.

5. Myocardial infarction—Chest pain in the course of infective endocarditis is most likely due to myocardial infarction, pericarditis, or septic pulmonary embolization. Myocardial infarction during infective endocarditis is almost always caused by coronary embolization, although it may occasionally complicate purulent pericarditis or myocardial abscess. In the latter setting, inflammatory thrombosis of the artery probably occurs. Treatment is noninterventional. Anticoagulation is probably not indicated because its benefits for reducing myocardial ischemia in this setting are unknown and the risks of potential cerebral embolization are significant.

6. Pericarditis—The possibility of purulent pericarditis complicating infective endocarditis should be evaluated by TTE. If pericardial fluid is seen, prompt pericardiocentesis is needed. A transudate may be present; in this infrequent case, management can be conservative. Usually a purulent exudate will be found, necessitating surgical drainage or pericardiectomy. Most important, purulent pericarditis may signal the presence of an intracardiac abscess. Transesophageal echocardiography

is indicated, and if an abscess is found, surgical drainage and valve surgery should be performed. Fortunately, the treatment of these related problems can be performed in a single operation. If an underlying myocardial abscess is not found, a pericardial window may be sufficient therapy. Continued observation is indicated because of the risk of subsequent additional cardiac or pericardial suppurative complications.

D. Management of High-Risk Endocarditis

1. Prosthetic valve endocarditis—Far higher morbidity and mortality rates are associated with prosthetic valve endocarditis than with native valve endocarditis. Infection of a prosthesis by fungi carries a mortality rate of more than 90%, whereas prosthetic infection from streptococci has a mortality rate of approximately 30%. In addition, the mortality rate from prosthetic valve endocarditis early after implantation is around twice that of late infection (after 2 months). Survival is improved by early operation in most cases, when the patient's surgical risk is acceptable. Surgical replacement is necessary in 85% of cases of biologic valve endocarditis and in almost all cases of mechanical prosthetic infection. Indications for surgery in prosthetic valve endocarditis are summarized in Table 22–8.

Medical treatment can be attempted in mechanical valve endocarditis when the surgical risk is high and the only evidence of valve involvement (using TEE) is a vegetation in the area of the sewing ring. In such cases, frequent serial TEE may be useful to monitor valve function and the response of the infected mass to treatment. Initial medical treatment of bioprosthetic endocarditis may be attempted when infection is due to a low-risk organism (such as *Streptococcus*) and involvement is limited to a vegetation on either the prosthetic leaflets or sewing ring. Repeated TEE is very useful if the patient does not respond to antibiotics. Blood cultures should be obtained every 4–7 days during treatment and weekly for a month following apparently successful treatment.

2. Fungal endocarditis—Overall mortality rates for fungal endocarditis are more than 80%; they are especially high in cases caused by *Aspergillus* and *Candida* species. Treatment requires the close collaboration of the primary physician, cardiologist, surgeon, and infectious disease specialist.

Table 22–8. Indications for Surgery in Prosthetic Valve Endocarditis

Mechanical prosthesis (almost all cases)
Bioprosthesis if:
　New paravalvular regurgitation or fistula
　Sewing-ring abscess or dehiscence
　Infection from *Staphylococcus epidermidis* or *aureus*, *Enterococcus*, gram-negative bacteria, fungi
Blood cultures still positive after 1 week of antibiotics
Embolism or other major complication

Treatment is almost always a combination of valve replacement and a full course of an antifungal agent. Late relapses are common and require prolonged surveillance for years following successful completion of antifungal therapy. In addition to serologic tests and blood cultures, TEE is useful in monitoring the patient during and after treatment. Some clinicians have advocated long-term suppressive therapy with an oral azole agent for patients who survive the surgical and medical therapies for the acute infection.

3. Endocarditis from gram-negative bacteria—

Pseudomonas endocarditis carries a mortality rate of almost 80% because of the frequent inability to sterilize vegetations by medical treatment. Among the causes for this inability is the frequent emergence of antibiotic-resistant bacterial strains during therapy. Surgery is usually performed as soon as possible after the diagnosis of *Pseudomonas* endocarditis of the left-sided valves. Surgery is also frequently indicated for endocarditis caused by the HACEK organisms, but here the reason is extensive valvular destruction by the time of diagnosis. In contrast to *Pseudomonas,* infection from HACEK organisms is readily cured by antibiotics. The treatment of endocarditis from enteric gram-negative bacteria is similar to that for *Pseudomonas* in that antibiotic therapy may fail, leading to a need for valve replacement. In vitro antibiotic sensitivity testing is crucial to antibiotic therapy of gram-negative bacteria.

E. Surgery

The indications for valve replacement or repair during infective endocarditis (discussed in the preceding section) are summarized in Table 22–9. The indications and timing of valve surgery are guided by several important principles. Surgical morbidity and mortality rates are much higher if the patient is in even mild heart failure, is hypotensive, or has a low cardiac output when sent to the operating room. Similarly, uncontrolled infection, with its attendant systemic stress and peripheral dilatation, confers a higher surgical risk. In the absence of these factors, surgical risk is generally low despite active infective endocarditis. Surgery should not be delayed with the intention of prolonging preoperative antibiotic therapy. It has

Table 22–9. Indications for Valve Surgery in Native Valve Endocarditis

Absolute Indications
Intracardiac abscess or fistula
Left heart failure from severe regurgitation or (rarely) obstruction
Endocarditis caused by fungi and resistant gram-negative organisms
Relative Indications
Mild heart failure in otherwise uncomplicated case
Recurrent embolization with persistent vegetation
Purulent pericarditis
Bacteremia despite optimal antibiotic therapy
Recurrent life-threatening septic pulmonary emboli
Severe tricuspid regurgitation with a low output state

never been shown that either the risk of reinfection of the new prosthetic valve or surgical complications are reduced by longer preoperative antibiotic treatment.

The anatomic location and extent of valve involvement and other factors may allow valve debridement and repair rather than replacement. The advantages of valve repair are that future anticoagulation is not needed, and subsequent valve replacement carries a lower risk. The disadvantages of valve repair are the greater possibility of residual infected tissue and significant valve regurgitation. Valve repair is not considered in the presence of abscess or fistula near the valve or when significant leaflet erosion has occurred. As part of a repair, however, leaflet perforation can be patched and chordal support reconstructed. In general, valve repair is feasible when excision of the infected leaflet with a 2-mm margin of normal tissue will still leave enough normal leaflet to preserve valvular competence. Preoperative or intraoperative TEE is usually indicated for surgical planning and guidance.

F. Follow-Up after Endocarditis

Long-term survival of the patient following an episode of endocarditis is much lower than that of the general population. Overall survival following native valve endocarditis is approximately 80% at 5 years and 50% at 10 years. Survival is considerably lower after prosthetic valve endocarditis. The patient remains at risk for three consequences of the disease: relapse of the original infection, noninfective sequelae of the infection, and recurrent endocarditis.

Failure to eradicate infection completely is usually apparent within 15 days after antibiotics are discontinued, although relapse has been reported up to 6 months after apparently successful treatment. Relapse rates tend to be low with viridans streptococci (< 5%), intermediate with enterococci (8–20%), and high with *Pseudomonas* and fungi (> 20%). Relapse of *S aureus* endocarditis is not common (5%) but should prompt a search for an extracardiac source. Treatment of a relapse includes a reassessment of the extent of cardiac infection, and surgery warrants careful consideration. If a trial of antibiotic therapy is given, the patient should be carefully monitored during therapy to determine the need for surgery.

After successful treatment of infection, the patient remains at risk for the development of heart failure, stroke, and rupture of a mycotic aneurysm. A new baseline TTE should be obtained after treatment completion. If the patient had moderate or severe valve regurgitation or an episode of heart failure prior to hospital discharge, the probability of late heart failure is greatly increased. The risk of embolic stroke is very low after the first 4 weeks of antibiotic treatment but may persist for an unknown length of time. Rupture of a mycotic aneurysm after treatment is also rare but should be considered when a patient with stroke has a history of prior endocarditis.

Although estimates vary, recurrent endocarditis, defined as a repeat episode after more than 6 months, occurs in approximately 5–8% of cases. Controversy exists regarding the tendency for the infecting organism and the involved valve to be similar to those of the original episode. The recurrent episode probably carries a higher mortality rate than the original one. Risk factors for recurrent endocarditis include injecting drug use, congenital heart disease, rheumatic and myxomatous disease, and periodontitis. Any new febrile illness requires three sets of blood cultures before starting antibiotic therapy.

Andrews MM, et al. Patient selection criteria and management guidelines for outpatient parenteral antibiotic therapy for native valve infective endocarditis. *Clin Infect Dis.* 2001;33(2):203–9. [PMID: 11418880]

Baddour LM, et al; Committee on Rheumatic Fever, Endocarditis, and Kawasaki Disease; Council on Cardiovascular Disease in the Young; Councils on Clinical Cardiology, Stroke and Cardiovascular Surgery and Anesthesia; American Heart Association; Infectious Diseases Society of America. Infective endocarditis: diagnosis, antimicrobial therapy, and management of complications: a statement for healthcare professionals from the Committee on Rheumatic Fever, Endocarditis, and Kawasaki Disease, Council on Cardiovascular Disease in the Young, and the Councils on Clinical Cardiology, Stroke and Cardiovascular Surgery and Anesthesia, American Heart Association: endorsed by the Infectious Diseases Society of America. *Circulation.* 2005;111(23):e394–434. [PMID: 15956145]

Cabell CH, et al; International Collaboration on Endocarditis Merged Database (ICE-MD) Study Group Investigators. Use of surgery in patients with native valve infective endocarditis: results from the International Collaboration on Endocarditis Merged Database. *Am Heart J.* 2005;150(5):1092–8. [PMID: 16291004]

Delahaye F, et al. Indications and optimal timing for surgery in infective endocarditis. *Heart.* 2004;90(6):618–20. [PMID: 15145858]

Moreillon P, et al. Infective endocarditis. *Lancet.* 2004; 363(9403): 139–49. [PMID: 14726169]

Olaison L, et al. Current best practices and guidelines. Indications for surgical intervention in infective endocarditis. *Cardiol Clin.* 2003;21(2):235–51. [PMID: 12874896]

Hypertrophic Cardiomyopathy

23

Karthik Ananthasubramaniam, MD

ESSENTIALS OF DIAGNOSIS

Note: Not all criteria are needed for diagnosis of hypertrophic cardiomyopathy.

▶ Asymmetric hypertrophied nondilated ventricle with septal to posterior wall end-diastolic thickness ≥ 1.3 cm not explained by other etiologies.

▶ Ejection murmur that increases with Valsalva with or without concomitant mitral regurgitation murmur and preserved aortic second sound.

▶ Increased gradients causing obstruction across left ventricular outflow tract and/or mid ventricle with characteristic late peaking "dagger"-shaped Doppler velocity profile.

▶ Mitral systolic anterior motion with varying degree of mitral regurgitation.

▶ Midsystolic aortic valve closure.

▶ Impaired diastolic function with decrease in tissue Doppler (early diastolic velocity [E']) and longitudinal strain.

▶ General Considerations

A. Definition & Prevalence

Hypertrophic cardiomyopathy (HCM) is a disorder of the myocardium caused by mutations of the sarcomere or sarcomere-associated proteins. It mainly manifests as symmetric or asymmetric left ventricular hypertrophy (LVH) > 1.5 cm (Figure 23–1) in a nondilated ventricle unexplained by other cardiac or systemic causes of hypertrophy (see Table 23–1 for differential diagnosis of LVH). HCM has numerous alternate names such as idiopathic hypertrophic subaortic stenosis (IHSS) or asymmetrical septal hypertrophy (ASH). However, HCM is the widely preferred term for this condition as

segmental hypertrophy can occur in any segment of the ventricle, not just the septum. Coexistent right ventricular (RV) hypertrophy and RV outflow obstruction occur less commonly in biventricular involvement.

HCM is relatively common (1 in 500) in the general population with about 750,000 people affected in the United States. Although it is the most common cause of sudden death in the young (< 35 years old) in North America, most people afflicted with HCM live a normal life. Contrary to the long mistaken notion that HCM was a uniformly fatal disease associated with a shortened life span, HCM patients may live well into their sixth to eighth decades, with patients older than age 90 with HCM being reported. Moreover, the first clinical recognition of HCM may occur when patients are in their sixth to eighth decade of life; usually these patients have milder forms of the disease with the most serious complications being uncommon after age 60. The natural history of HCM can take many paths: sudden cardiac death, symptomatic HCM heart failure, end-stage cardiomyopathy, atrial fibrillation, and stroke. However, if intervened upon in a timely manner, HCM can potentially have no effect on normal longevity.

B. Genetics & Histopathology

The genetics of HCM involve an autosomal dominant pattern of inheritance, with 60–70% of patients having an affected family member. HCM is more common in males than females. Common genes affected include β-myosin heavy chain, myosin binding protein C, troponin I, and troponin T, but numerous others have been described. Mutations of the sarcomeric proteins lead to histopathologic evidence of myocardial disarray, which then leads to pathologic hypertrophy and patchy fibrosis of the myocardium. Intramural vessels are also frequently abnormal in HCM with thrombotic obliteration causing ischemia, which may propagate fibrosis regardless of presence of epicardial coronary disease. The genetic basis of ventricular hypertrophy does not always correlate with prognosis. Patients with

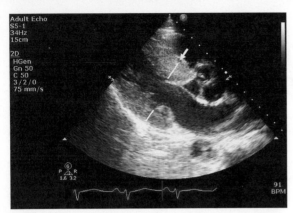

▲ **Figure 23–1.** Parasternal long axis view in diastole showing asymmetric septal hypertrophy (*white arrow*) compared to the inferolateral wall.

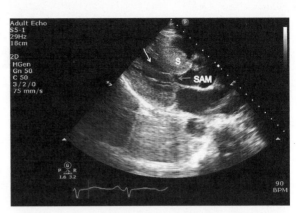

▲ **Figure 23–2.** Parasternal long axis view still frame in a patient with obstructive hypertrophic cardiomyopathy. Asymmetric septal hypertrophy (S) is noted along with systolic anterior motion (SAM; *blue arrow*) and hypertrophied and anteriorly displaced papillary muscle (*white arrow*) causing further narrowing of left ventricular midcavity and outflow tract.

tropomyosin mutations have only a mild degree of ventricular hypertrophy, with little or no left ventricular (LV) outflow tract obstruction, but they still carry a disproportionately high risk for sudden death.

C. Phenotype of Hypertrophic Cardiomyopathy

The extent and location of hypertrophy in HCM are highly variable. Asymmetric hypertrophy is most common (septal 90%, midventricular 1%, posteroseptal and lateral wall 1%, apical 3%, symmetric 5%). ASH is defined as septal-to-posterior wall ratio > 1.3 and, in hypertensive patients, > 1.5. Massive hypertrophy > 30 mm is a risk factor for sudden death. Abnormal mitral valve and its apparatus are commonly seen in HCM. Elongated mitral leaflets and abnormal/anteriorly displaced papillary muscles and direct insertion of chordae tendineae or papillary muscles to anterior mitral leaflet can be seen (Figure 23–2). All these factors may contribute to outflow obstruction.

Table 23–1. Differential Diagnosis of Left Ventricular Hypertrophy

Athlete's heart
Systemic hypertension
Subaortic membrane/ridge
Aortic stenosis
Supravalvular stenosis
Right ventricular hypertrophy
Fabry disease
Glycogen storage disease (PRKAG2 cardiomyopathy, Danon disease, Pompe disease)
Mucopolysaccharide storage disease
Amyloidosis
Sarcoidosis

▶ Pathophysiology

The following processes contribute to the pathophysiology of HCM.

1. Abnormal diastolic function
2. Outflow tract obstruction
3. Mitral regurgitation
4. Myocardial ischemia
5. Arrhythmias
6. Abnormal autonomic function

A. Diastolic Dysfunction

Diastolic filling abnormalities, invariably present in almost all patients with HCM, may precede hypertrophy, and as it worsens, an increased dependence on atrial contribution to ventricular filling occurs. Thus arrhythmias, like atrial fibrillation, are poorly tolerated by patients with HCM and should be promptly treated with sinus rhythm preferentially restored if feasible. Mitral inflow parameters demonstrate varying degrees of dysfunction, most commonly impaired relaxation, whereas restrictive filling patterns are less common but manifest in advanced disease states. Myocardial abnormalities documented by tissue Doppler, speckle tracking echocardiography-based strain, and LV twist and torsion abnormalities have been demonstrated in HCM. Figure 23–3 demonstrates impaired relaxation in mitral inflow, delayed propagation slope on color M-mode, and abnormal tissue Doppler, all indicative of diastolic dysfunction in a patient with HCM.

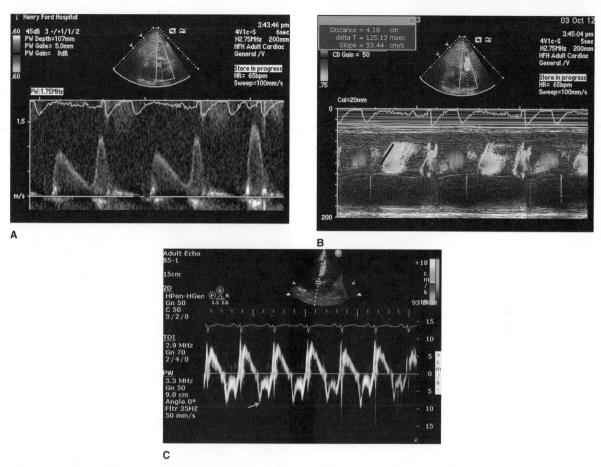

▲ **Figure 23–3. A:** Diastolic mitral inflow profile in a 32-year-old patient with hypertrophic cardiomyopathy (HCM) indicating impaired relaxation pattern. **B:** Color M-mode flow propagation abnormalities in HCM from same patient. *Black slanted line* indicates propagation slope of <50 cm/s, indicating impaired relaxation. **C:** Pulsed tissue Doppler of the septal annulus in a 40-year-old patient with HCM and preserved left ventricular ejection fraction showing low e′ velocities suggesting underlying myocardial dysfunction.

B. Outflow Obstruction

HCM can be broadly categorized into obstructive and non-obstructive types based on presence or absence of gradient (Figure 23–4). About two-thirds of patients with HCM have outflow tract obstruction manifesting as resting or provocable gradient of ≥ 30 mm Hg. However, only 25–30% of patients demonstrate obstruction at rest. Simple maneuvers such as the Valsalva maneuver, standing, or administration of amyl nitrite can provoke or exacerbate outflow tract obstruction and gradients and should be a routine part of clinical and echocardiographic evaluation when HCM is suspected (Table 23–2, Figure 23–5). Outflow obstruction can contribute to exercise intolerance, angina, syncope, and decreased survival. Patients with obstructive HCM are at higher risk of adverse events (heart failure and death) than those without obstruction. The combination of hypertrophied septum bulging into LV outflow tract and abnormal mitral valve motion in systole (systolic anterior motion [SAM]) contribute to outflow obstruction.

Although the exact cause of SAM is debated, two perspectives exist. One is a causal mechanism of SAM precipitated by chordal slackening/anterior displaced mitral valve apparatus leading to "drag forces," and the other implicates SAM as a consequence of Venturi effect of accelerated flow across the left ventricular outflow tract (LVOT) (Figure 23–6). The severity of obstruction and timing of SAM onset are linearly related. An important caveat is that SAM can be seen in non-HCM states, such as a hyperdynamic small-ventricle, volume-depleted state, post mitral valve repair, and as a nonspecific finding confined to the chordal apparatus (chordal SAM).

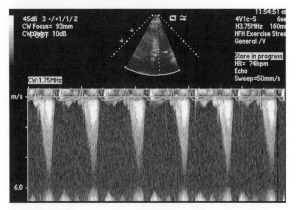

▲ **Figure 23–4.** Continuous wave Doppler across left ventricular outflow tract at rest demonstrates "dagger-shaped" late peaking velocity consistent with outflow tract obstruction.

Thus, although patients in many different pathophysiologic states may exhibit HCM physiology (gradients, SAM), this does not equate to a diagnosis of HCM.

C. Mitral Regurgitation

The main etiology of mitral regurgitation (MR) in HCM is malcoaptation of the mitral leaflets secondary to SAM. SAM-related MR is posteriorly directed starting in mid-late systole (Figure 23–7). If a nonposterior jet of MR is seen, then intrinsic mitral valve disease should be suspected. Concomitant primary mitral valve disease is reported in about 20% of patients with HCM (mitral valve prolapse, ruptured chordae, mitral annular calcification, and anomalous or anteriorly displaced papillary muscle) (see Figure 23–2). If SAM is relieved by either myectomy or septal ablation, posterior MR tends to resolve or diminish. Nonposterior MR may require surgical repair or replacement of the valve,

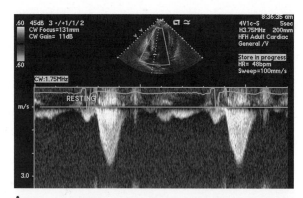

A

B

C

▲ **Figure 23–5.** Hypertrophic cardiomyopathy outflow tract gradient (**A**) at rest, (**B**) standing, and (**C**) with Valsalva.

which may be one reason why surgical myectomy is favored over ablation as a treatment strategy for HCM.

A comprehensive echocardiography assessment of MR is important in HCM. The assessment of peak outflow gradients can be challenging in some patients with HCM in the setting of MR due to contamination of both jets (Figure 23–8). Careful observation of jet profile, coexistent inflow profile,

Table 23–2. Factors Influencing Obstruction in Hypertrophic Cardiomyopathy

Obstruction worsens (gradient increases and murmur increases)
1. Tachycardia
2. Hypovolemia
3. Standing
4. Valsalva
5. Inotropes, diuretics, vasodilators

Obstruction lessens (gradient decreases and murmur decreases)
1. Negative inotropes
2. Bradycardia
3. Vasoconstrictors
4. Squatting
5. Isometric handgrip

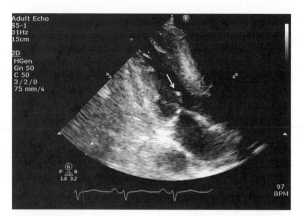

▲ **Figure 23–6.** Apical three-chamber still frame showing systolic anterior motion of mitral valve encroaching on the left ventricular outflow tract creating outflow obstruction physiology (*white arrow*).

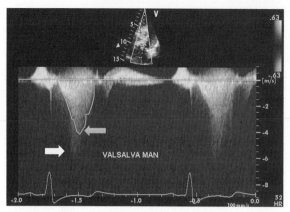

▲ **Figure 23–8.** Continuous wave Doppler evaluation of a patient with hypertrophic cardiomyopathy during Valsalva provocation. Two distinct flow patterns are seen: one of the outflow obstruction, which has a late peak (*blue arrow*), and a superimposed Doppler profile signal of mitral regurgitation (*white arrow*), making assessment of peak outflow obstruction velocity challenging.

and evaluation of peak gradients from different windows will help to differentiate outflow gradients from MR.

D. Myocardial Ischemia

The combination of significant LVH with or without outflow obstruction sets the stage for substantial increase in myocardial oxygen demand and can precipitate angina secondary to myocardial ischemia in HCM. Angina has been reported in approximately 30% of HCM patients, although ischemic perfusion defects on myocardial perfusion imaging can be present in a large majority of patients with HCM. Although epicardial coronary disease may cause angina/perfusion

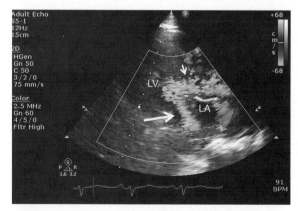

▲ **Figure 23–7.** Parasternal long axis view still frame with color illustrating consequence of systolic anterior motion and left ventricular outflow tract (LVOT) obstruction, which leads to turbulent flow across LVOT (*small arrow*) during left ventricular (LV) systole and posterior directed jet of mitral regurgitation (*large thick arrow*) into left atrium (LA).

defects, a supply-demand mismatch in conjunction with abnormal microvasculature is likely the major contributor.

E. Abnormal Autonomic Tone

About 25% of HCM patients demonstrate abnormalities of autonomic function, which if present, portend a poorer prognosis. Abnormalities with exercise, such as systolic drop in blood pressure of ≥ 20 mm Hg, or failure to augment blood pressure can occur from factors such as outflow obstruction and inappropriate vasodilatation despite an appropriate increase in cardiac output.

▶ Clinical Findings

A. Physical Examination

A general exam is not helpful in diagnosing HCM except when associations with other diseases such as Friedrich ataxia or Noonan syndrome are present. The cardiovascular clinical exam findings of HCM are usually striking unless there is no obstruction at rest. Radial pulse is of brisk character. There is a characteristic brisk carotid upstroke with an abrupt deceleration due to obstruction. The apical impulse is described as bifid and sustained due to the initial powerful contraction followed by obstruction and then by continued contraction of the left ventricle. A systolic thrill may be felt. The first and second heart sounds are normal. An S_4 may be heard due to atrial contraction against a noncompliant left ventricle.

The systolic murmur in HCM is a harsh crescendo-decrescendo heard all over the precordium but usually is not transmitted to the carotids. The murmur increases in intensity with Valsalva, standing, and inhalation of amyl nitrite, due to a drop in preload and decrease in LV cavity size and vasodilation (amyl nitrite), which can worsen outflow obstruction. The murmur intensity decreases with squatting and passive leg raising. A second murmur of mid-late MR can be heard, induced by SAM of mitral valve. The combination of powerful ejection followed by obstruction and subsequent mitral insufficiency can be aptly described as the "eject-obstruct-leak" triad of hypertrophic obstructive cardiomyopathy (HOCM). The key differentiation of HCM murmur is from aortic stenosis (AS). However, the pulse of AS is low amplitude and slow (parvus et tardus) compared to brisk in HCM. Ejection click (with bicuspid etiology) and aortic regurgitation murmur are more common in AS and not typically seen in HCM. Aortic second sound is abnormal in AS and normal in HCM. Finally, AS murmur decreases with Valsalva in contrast to HCM murmur, which increases.

B. Diagnostic Tests

1. Electrocardiogram—More than 90% of patients with HCM exhibit 12-lead electrocardiography (ECG) abnormalities. Such abnormalities can precede echocardiographic

findings and become more prevalent as age increases. Common abnormalities include LVH with strain, prominent Q waves, left atrial enlargement, and left axis deviation. ST elevation or depression or T-wave inversions can also be seen. Specific patterns such as deep symmetric T-wave inversions in lateral precordial leads (suggestive of apical variant HCM) are also well recognized (Figure 23–9). In general, ECG abnormalities are present in > 80% of obstructed HCM compared to approximately 50% in nonobstructive types of HCM. Preexcitation patterns are also seen in some patients with HCM, and atrial fibrillation has been documented in up to 25–30% of elderly HCM patients.

2. Echocardiogram—Echocardiography (echo) plays an integral role in diagnosis, follow-up, and management of patients with HCM. Abnormalities can be demonstrated on M-mode echo; two-dimensional (2D) echo; color, pulsed and continuous wave, and tissue Doppler; and strain imaging. Key findings of HCM by echo include the following.

A. M-MODE—Midsystolic notching of aortic valve is seen in HCM (Figure 23–10). SAM of mitral valve can also be assessed, and extent of SAM and SAM-septal contact distance as a marker of severity can be assessed (Figure 23–11).

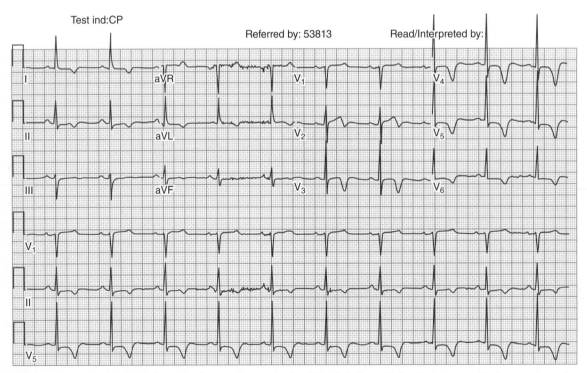

▲ **Figure 23–9.** Twelve-lead electrocardiogram in a patient with palpitations. Note deep symmetric T-wave inversions in the precordial leads. There are also T-wave abnormalities in the limb leads. In the absence of hypertension, these should raise suspicion of hypertrophic cardiomyopathy. Subsequent echocardiography and cardiac magnetic resonance imaging confirmed diagnosis of apical hypertrophic cardiomyopathy.

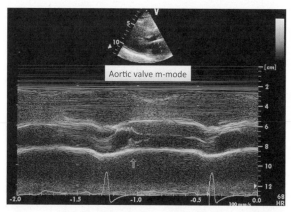

▲ **Figure 23–10.** Midsystolic notching of the aortic valve (*arrow*) is indicative of dynamic left ventricular outflow obstruction.

RV and LV septal and posterior wall thickness and chamber sizes can be determined.

B. 2D ECHO—Asymmetric septal hypertrophy is the most common pattern, although other patterns can be seen (see Figure 23–1). RV hypertrophy may also be present. Because echo can underestimate or miss hypertrophy confined to the lateral wall and apex, comprehensive multiple nonforeshortened views of LV are needed. Echo contrast imaging can be useful to assess apical variant HCM. Mitral valve abnormalities can be seen as described previously. SAM can be assessed, and all chamber sizes can be evaluated. Recently enlarged left atrium (indexed volume > 34 mL/m²) has been shown to be an independent adverse prognosticator in HCM. A nonspecific increased backscatter of hypertrophied myocardium causing a "ground-glass" appearance can be

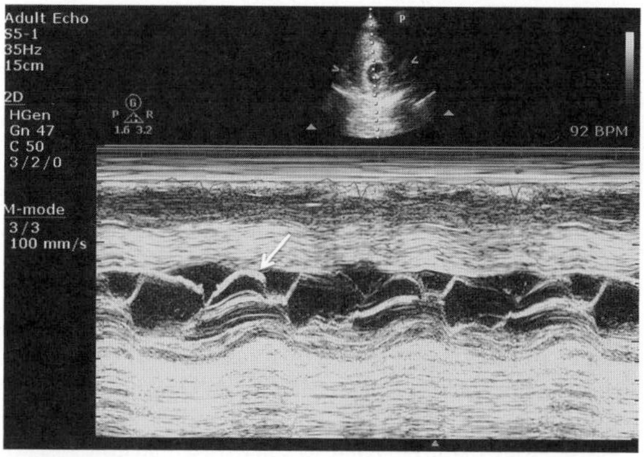

seen. However, this is not specific for HCM and can be seen in other infiltrative diseases.

C. DOPPLER—Pulsed wave and continuous wave Doppler assessment is integral in establishing the level of outflow obstruction and peak gradients, respectively. The modified Bernoulli equation $(4V^2)$ is used to determine peak gradient. The classic late peaking "dagger-shaped" velocity profile can be seen when outflow obstruction is present (see Figure 23–4). A peak gradient of > 30 mm Hg is considered as evidence for resting outflow obstruction. Gradients should be assessed at rest and with provocation by Valsalva or standing (see Figure 23–5B). If echo features suggest HCM but no obstruction is demonstrable at rest or Valsalva, exercise echo with peak/immediate postexercise gradient assessment could unmask HOCM (latent obstruction). Color Doppler and continuous wave Doppler can be used to comprehensively assess severity and mechanism of MR. It is important to reliably distinguish the MR signal from the LVOT obstruction signal to avoid overestimation of severity of outflow obstruction. Diastolic function and tissue Doppler abnormalities of myocardial function should be assessed. In particular, recent studies have shown that average E′ velocities by tissue Doppler of < 13.5 cm/s predicted genotype-positive HCM with a sensitivity of 75% and specificity of 86%. Reduced longitudinal peak systolic deformation (strain) averaged across all walls < 10.6% (in absolute value) predicted HCM with a sensitivity of 85% and specificity of 100% and helped differentiate it from hypertensive LVH. A combination of septal/posterior wall ratio > 1.3 and systolic strain assessment yields a predictive accuracy for HCM of 96%. The estimation of filling pressures using E/E′ at best correlates moderately with invasive wedge pressure measurements, although low E′ in itself has independent adverse prognostic value in HCM. Delayed untwisting of LV has been demonstrated by torsion analysis using speckle tracking techniques, again reflecting diastolic dysfunction-related abnormalities seen in HCM.

3. Cardiac magnetic resonance imaging—Cardiac magnetic resonance imaging (CMRI) is rapidly becoming a key component in enhancing diagnostic accuracy, morphology, and more importantly, prognostication due to tissue characterization of fibrosis in HCM. With its superior spatial resolution and indefinite choice of imaging planes, it has demonstrated enhanced accuracy in assessing HCM features and identifying patterns of hypertrophy not well seen on echocardiography. Approximately 6% of patients missed by echo (mainly anterolateral hypertrophy) are diagnosed with HCM by CMRI, and 57% of apical aneurysms missed by echo are identified on CMRI in the apical variant. Assessment of LV mass and end-diastolic wall thickness is more accurate with CMRI than echo. Figures 23–12 and 23–13 show CMRI delineation of septal hypertrophy in HCM.

CMRI also provides superb assessment of mitral valve apparatus morphologic abnormalities and gives unparalleled assessment of the right ventricle. However, echo is

▲ **Figure 23–11.** Systolic anterior motion of mitral valve on M-mode echocardiography. The duration and extent of mitral–septal contact correlate with extent of outflow obstruction.

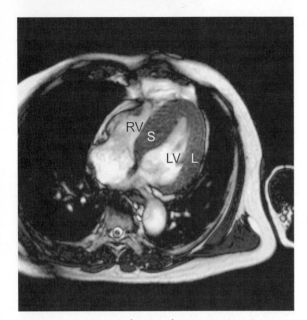

▲ **Figure 23–12.** Steady-state free precession cine sequence still frame view of left ventricle (LV) and right ventricle (RV) showing significant asymmetric septal hypertrophy (S) compared to lateral wall (L). Note outstanding delineation of the LV blood to endocardial interface enabling accurate measurements of thickness of myocardial walls.

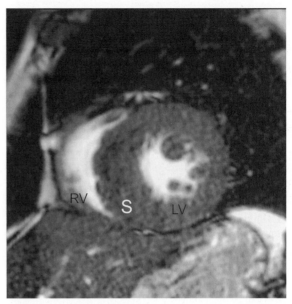

▲ **Figure 23–13.** A still frame from a steady-state free precession short axis cardiac magnetic resonance study in a patient with suspected hypertrophic cardiomyopathy. There is severe asymmetric left ventricular (LV) hypertrophy involving the septum (S). Multiple papillary muscle heads are also noted in LV cavity. RV, right ventricle.

superior to CMRI in the functional assessment of severity of obstruction and diastolic function assessment. The presence of patchy myocardial fibrosis in HCM detected by late gadolinium enhancement techniques in CMRI is increasingly recognized as an adverse prognosticator for arrhythmias and mortality. Characteristic patterns include delayed enhancement detected at RV insertion points into the left ventricle, although multiple areas of fibrosis can be seen in the left and/or right ventricle with predominance in the hypertrophied zones of the ventricle (Figure 23–14). CMRI is also excellent to evaluate success of interventions, such as surgical myectomy or percutaneous alcohol septal ablation. It can be used to assess extent of procedural success and scar formation following septal ablation. Most recently, CMRI has been used to characterize presence of "myocardial crypts" or recesses in different areas of the myocardium in phenotype-negative but genotype-positive family members of probands with HCM. Whether these represent early manifestations of an HCM phenotype yet to develop remains to be established, as does any long-term significance.

Bruder O, et al. Myocardial scar visualized by cardiovascular magnetic resonance imaging predicts major adverse events in patients with hypertrophic cardiomyopathy. *J Am Coll Cardiol.* 2010;56:875–87. [PMID: 20667520]

Maron MS, et al. Clinical profile and significance of delayed enhancement in hypertrophic cardiomyopathy. *Circ Heart Fail.* 2008;1:184–91. [PMID: 19808288]
O'Hanlon R, et al. Prognostic significance of myocardial fibrosis in hypertrophic cardiomyopathy. *J Am Coll Cardiol.* 2010;56: 867–74. [PMID: 20688032]

4. Cardiac computed tomography angiography, cardiac nuclear perfusion imaging, and positron emission tomography—Cardiac computed tomography angiography (CCTA), cardiac nuclear perfusion imaging, and positron emission tomography (PET) are not routinely used in assessment of HCM but may be useful in select cases. Retrospective gated CCTA can provide LV function assessment apart from LV morphology and coronary anatomy. It can also accurately delineate septal perforator course noninvasively as a road map for septal ablation. Single-photon emission computed tomography (SPECT) and PET can demonstrate characteristic intense uptake of radioisotope in hypertrophied zones of myocardium and also demonstrate perfusion abnormalities mainly related to microvascular flow reserve abnormalities in HCM Quantitative PET-determined coronary flow reserve abnormalities along with ischemic perfusion defects have been shown to predict adverse outcomes in HCM in limited studies. However, there is no evidence

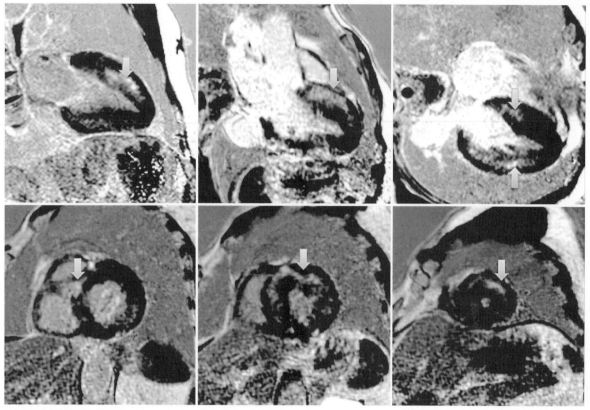

▲ **Figure 23–14.** Gadolinium-based delayed enhancement CMRI showing abnormal enhancement in multiple areas of the myocardium denoting fibrosis. Note the noncoronary predominant mid-myocardial distribution of hyperenhancement seen in nonischemic etiologies.

that routine CCTA or PET adds incremental information in diagnostic accuracy or risk stratification to warrant routine use in all patients with HCM.

5. Cardiac catheterization—Echo with Doppler forms the crux of diagnosis of HCM, and invasive hemodynamics is usually not necessary. However, if clinical and echo findings are discrepant or the exact severity of obstruction cannot be accurately determined by echo, then catheterization may be needed. A carefully conducted study with continuous documentation of pullback gradients will outline the level and severity of obstruction. A classic "spike and dome" arterial pulse waveform can be recorded representing the rapid ejection followed by sudden obstruction. Pulmonary capillary wedge pressure may be elevated, reflecting high filling pressures from diastolic dysfunction, stiff ventricle, and noncompliant atrium. Depending on the severity of MR, a prominent "v" wave can be recorded. Also the Brockenbrough-Braunwald-Morrow sign can be demonstrated by inducing premature ventricular beats. Following a ventricular extrasystole, an increase occurs in LV systolic pressure, decrease in ascending aortic pressure, and increase

in gradient. Importantly, a drop in pulse pressure is seen in HCM compared to AS where pulse pressure does not change (Figure 23–15).

6. Exercise echocardiography—Exercise echocardiography is recommended to provoke obstruction, which is either absent or minimal at rest (< 30 mm Hg), particularly in patients with features of nonobstructive HCM. Furthermore, exercise can unmask abnormal hemodynamic responses such as failure to augment systolic blood pressure or a drop in systolic blood pressure with exercise. Other abnormal signs with exercise include poor exercise capacity, ventricular arrhythmias, ST depression, and/or ischemic wall motion abnormalities (regardless of presence of epicardial disease). Exercise echocardiography has a class 2A indication in the 2011 American College of Cardiology/American Heart Association (ACC/AHA)'s HCM guidelines for evaluation of provocable gradients and exercise hemodynamics. Symptomatic patients with HCM with gradients at rest or with provocation ≥ 50 mm Hg usually require therapy (medical and/or invasive), and hence, exercise testing is not indicated in such patients. However, once medical therapy is

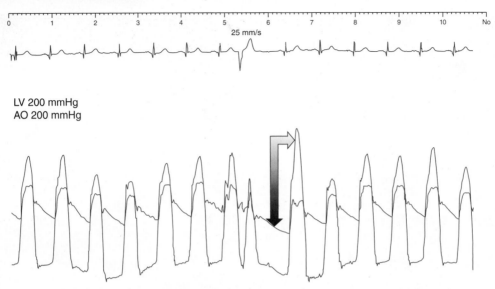

▲ **Figure 23–15.** Brockenbrough-Braunwald-Morrow sign. Following a premature ventricular beat, there is an increase in the gradient but a decrease in aortic and pulse pressure in hypertrophic cardiomyopathy during cardiac catheterization (*double arrow*).

maximized in patients with HOCM, repeat exercise echocardiography may be helpful to reevaluate symptoms, exercise hemodynamics, and effects of medical therapy on reduction of outflow obstruction/gradients. Although dobutamine can induce outflow obstruction and gradients, it is not recommended for testing in HCM as it can provoke a similar response even in normal individuals.

7. Genetic testing—The most practical current application for genetic testing in HCM is screening of asymptomatic family members of patients with HCM. If a known mutation exists in HCM patients, focused genetic testing can be done for that mutation in the family. If genetic testing is unyielding, surveillance imaging may be needed. Adolescents and athlete family members should undergo echo annually, and nonathlete family members should undergo echo every 5 years.

C. Diagnostic Considerations in Hypertrophic Cardiomyopathy Variants

1. Apical HCM—This form of HCM is more frequently reported in the Asian populations and is associated with deep symmetric T-wave inversions in the anterior precordial leads (see Figure 23–9). Echo reveals a predominant pattern of hypertrophy distributed toward the apex with relative sparing of the base, although concomitant basal hypertrophy may also be present. In conjunction with the normal contractility, the marked narrowing of the hypertrophied apex in systole produces the "ace of spades" appearance on echo. Apical variant HCM can be missed in echo due to foreshortened views or poor visualization of hypertrophy with low-frequency transducers. Use of higher

frequency transducers, color Doppler to delineate full extent of blood flow, and contrast echo can overcome these limitations. CMRI is an excellent alternative to echo and is a superior technique to diagnose apical HCM due to lack of any limitations that occur with echo (Figure 23–16). In general, isolated apical HCM is devoid of outflow obstruction, and these patients have a more benign prognosis than the classical HCM patients.

2. Midventricular HCM—This variant involves predominant hypertrophy of the mid ventricle, resulting in midcavitary obstruction and separation of the ventricle into two compartments in systole. Flow acceleration and obstructive gradients can be demonstrated in the mid ventricle where most obstruction exists, although concomitant outflow obstruction may be present. Abnormal early diastolic color flow can be seen during isovolumic relaxation due to differential intraventricular pressure gradients across the obstruction. Coexistent hypertension may exacerbate midventricular hypertrophy. In the pure midventricular HCM, SAM may be absent and no outflow obstruction may be detected. Continuous wave Doppler can delineate maximal obstructive midventricular gradients (Figure 23–17A). Long-standing obstruction in mid ventricle can cause apical necrosis with aneurysm formation due to chronic subendocardial ischemia (Figure 23–17B). This subset of patients is more prone to ventricular arrhythmias and thrombus formation. CMRI is an excellent technique to demonstrate these apical aneurysms, which can often be missed by echo.

3. Hypertensive HCM in the elderly—First described in the 1980s, this entity is increasingly recognized more

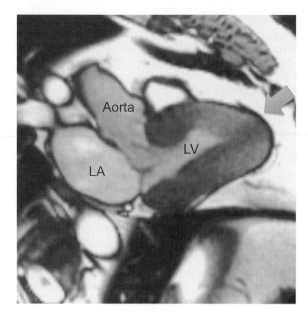

▲ **Figure 23–16.** Steady-state free precession left ventricular (LV) outflow tract view still frame showing marked LV myocardial hypertrophy with obliteration of apex in systole (*arrow*). Note characteristic "ace of spades" appearance of LV myocardium in systole. LA, left atrium.

frequently given the growing population of elderly patients with hypertension. Whether this represents a variant of HCM or mimics the physiology of HCM is still debated. Most patients have a long history of hypertension, small hypertrophied ventricles, narrow LVOT with mitral annular calcification, and some anterior displacement of the mitral annulus. This constellation can set the stage for acceleration of flow, SAM, and outflow obstruction, although midventricular obstruction may also be present. Treatment is similar to HCM with regard to relief of outflow obstruction with negative inotropic drugs and adequate control of hypertension. Avoidance of excessive diuresis and preload reduction is also a key component.

4. End-stage HCM—Seen in < 5% of patients, end-stage HCM features ventricular dilation, advanced diastolic dysfunction, and a course predominated with symptoms of systolic and diastolic heart failure. Medical treatment consists of angiotensin-converting enzyme (ACE) inhibitors or angiotensin receptor blockers, β-blockers, diuretics, and spironolactone, as well as nonpharmacologic strategies such as implantable cardioverter-defibrillator (ICD) and biventricular pacing if indicated. In refractory cases, heart transplantation should be considered. Survival after heart transplantation in HCM is comparable to the general population.

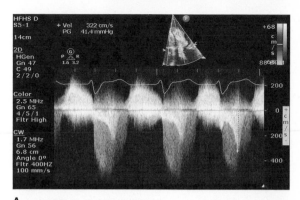

A

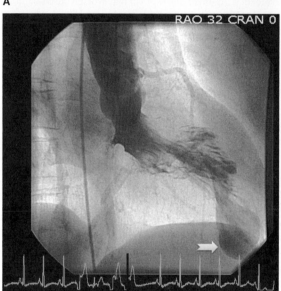

B

▲ **Figure 23–17. A:** An example of a continuous wave Doppler signal across the left ventricle LV showing the mitral regurgitation signal and concomitant late peaking signal of midcavitary obstruction with a peak gradient of 41 mm Hg. **B:** A still frame left ventriculogram in a patient with severe mid ventricular HCM with apical aneurysm and outpouching.

▶ **Management**

The therapeutic strategies in HCM can be divided into pharmacologic and nonpharmacologic strategies.

A. Pharmacologic Strategies

Pharmacologic therapy for HCM is focused on decreasing inotropy, augmenting diastolic filling time, and reducing dynamic outflow obstruction. Resting gradients are not useful to gauge effectiveness of therapy. Negative inotropic agents such as β-blockers and rate-slowing calcium channel blockers can help diminish gradients and outflow obstruction in HOCM and also decrease myocardial oxygen demand. High doses, such as 200 mg of propranolol or metoprolol or 240–360 mg of verapamil or diltiazem, may be effective. Caution should be used when high resting outflow gradients are present when initiating verapamil because peripheral vasodilatation may occur, leading to syncope. Disopyramide, a class Ia antiarrhythmic agent with potent negative inotropic effect, can be used as an adjunct to standard therapies. Amiodarone, which has β-blocking properties, has been shown to have a favorable effect on prognosis in selected patients with HCM. Pure vasodilators (eg, dihydropyridines, nitrates, hydralazine) should be avoided. β-Agonists and digoxin may worsen obstruction by augmenting contractility and should be avoided. Excessive diuresis should also be avoided because it may exacerbate obstruction, although diuretics will be needed to relieve pulmonary congestion in the setting of pulmonary edema. Exercise echocardiography can be used to assess efficacy of treatment and decrease provocable gradients on therapy. In nonobstructive variants of HCM, treatments can be targeted for diastolic dysfunction with judicious use of diuretics as needed for elevated filling pressures. In advanced HCM with dilated and dysfunctional ventricles ("burnt out" or end-stage HCM), standard heart failure therapies are indicated as discussed earlier. Atrial fibrillation occurs in 25–30% of elderly patients with HCM, is poorly tolerated, and requires electrical cardioversion and/or aggressive rate control. HCM patients with atrial fibrillation are at high risk for stroke and should receive anticoagulation therapy. Radiofrequency ablation can be offered to some patients with drug-refractory atrial fibrillation. Finally, if the HCM patient continues to remain symptomatic despite medical treatment, more aggressive nonpharmacologic therapies should be explored regardless of degree of residual outflow obstruction.

B. Nonpharmacologic Therapies

Nonpharmacologic strategies include surgical septal myectomy, alcohol septal ablation, and dual-chamber pacing.

1. Surgical septal myectomy—Septal myectomy is widely regarded as the best treatment for HCM with regard to relief of outflow obstruction. In brief, the procedure involves removal of the basal portion of the ventricular septum to enable a wider outflow tract for exit of blood, thus relieving outflow obstruction. Modifications of this procedure include wider zones of resection of the ventricular septum up to the level of papillary muscles, resection and/or reimplantation of abnormal papillary muscle heads, and mitral valve repair or replacement if needed for associated primary mitral valve disease. Mortality rate for isolated myectomy is < 0.5% in experienced centers, with > 90% of patients experiencing symptomatic relief. Complications occur in < 1% and include heart block, ventricular septal defect, aortic regurgitation, and conduction delays, most commonly left bundle branch block.

2. Alcohol septal ablation—The basic principle underlying alcohol septal ablation is to identify a septal perforator branch (usually from the left anterior descending coronary artery) that supplies the hypertrophied portion of the basal septum and inject absolute ethanol (1–3 mL) via a percutaneous approach and induce a local transmural infarction in that zone (usually an overage of 10% of the overall LV wall). This has been shown to reduce outflow gradient and concomitant MR similar to myectomy. An immediate fall in outflow gradient is observed with successful septal ablation in > 90% of patients. Continued improvement may be seen over ensuing months as the scar forms and retracts and the outflow tract widens. Preprocedural determination of limited zone of supply of the perforator branch to the obstructing portion of septum is crucial and is achieved usually with injection of echo contrast agents selectively during angiography into the septal branch. If the contrast agents light up adjacent areas of the heart or right ventricle portion of the septum, alcohol should not be infused. Ideal candidates for this procedure usually include older patients whose comorbidities preclude surgical myectomy. The likelihood of permanent pacemaker implantation is four to five times higher with septal ablation than with myectomy. Massive septal hypertrophy is unlikely to benefit from septal ablation. The hemodynamic and functional improvement over 3–5 years has been shown to be similar overall for septal ablation and myectomy. Similarly, there appears to be no difference in the medium-term incidence of sudden cardiac death (SCD) or all-cause mortality between myectomy and septal ablation. However, the incidence of sustained ventricular arrhythmias and SCD after septal ablation is reported at 3–10% (regardless of underlying HCM risk) in contrast to myectomy, which has much a lower incidence of sustained ventricular arrhythmias (0.2–0.9%/year). Thus, long-term follow-up studies comparing the two techniques are required to conclusively decide whether the scar created with septal ablation carries long-term risk of SCD.

3. Dual-chamber pacing—The physiologic principle underlying dual-chamber pacing (DDD) is the induction of asynchronous contraction of the septum induced by RV pacing. This causes the septum not to bulge into the outflow tract in early-mid systole and thus decreases the outflow obstruction and gradients. However, DDD pacing is now considered to be of not much benefit because most symptomatic improvement reported by patients in initial studies has been deemed to be a placebo effect in subsequent randomized trials. Nevertheless, it could be considered as a treatment option in selected elderly patients above 65 years old or in those who already have an ICD in place where a trial of pacing can assess whether there is gradient reduction and symptom improvement. However, there is no benefit from DDD pacing in reducing risk of SCD, and it has no role in nonobstructive HCM. Figure 23–18 summarizes all treatment options as well as genetic counseling recommendations for HCM.

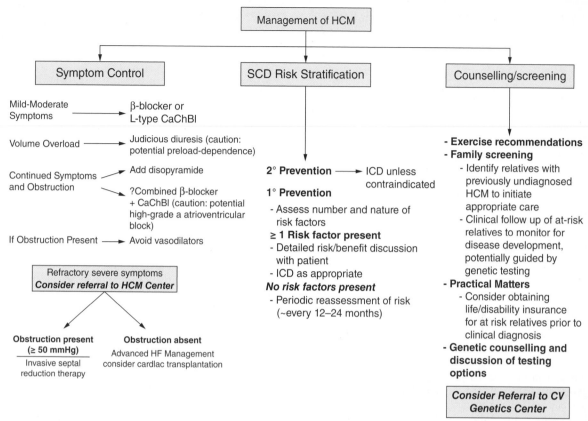

▲ Figure 23–18. Flow diagram outlining proposed approach to management of hypertrophic cardiomyopathy (HCM). CaChBl, calcium channel blocker; CV, cardiovascular; HF, heart failure; ICD, implantable cardioverter-defibrillator; SCD, sudden cardiac death.

C. Prevention of Sudden Cardiac Death in Hypertrophic Cardiomyopathy

A subset of patients with HCM is at increased risk of SCD (1%/year). The only effective prevention strategy against SCD for these patients is an ICD. Although ICD recommendations for secondary prevention are usually straightforward, the decision as to when to recommend ICD in a primary prevention setting is challenging. Existing evidence suggests a 4%/year ICD intervention rate when used for primary prevention in appropriate high-risk patients. Some of the risk factors for SCD in patients are provided below to help guide decisions in identifying the high-risk patient who may need close follow-up and/or ICD therapy as part of primary prevention.

In the list below, the first nine risk factors for SCD are considered established risk factors. The 2011 ACC/AHA's HCM Guidelines consider ICD implantation reasonable (Class 2A Level of Evidence C) for risk factors indicated with an asterisk.

1. Young (age < 30 years)
2. Massive septal hypertrophy (> 30 mm)*
3. Family history of sudden death*
4. Nonsustained ventricular tachycardia on Holter or exercise-induced nonsustained ventricular tachycardia and other SCD risk markers*
5. Sustained ventricular tachycardia or supraventricular tachycardia
6. Certain gene mutations (Arg403Gln)
7. Recurrent unexplained syncope with HCM*
8. Bradyarrhythmias (occult conduction system disease)
9. Inappropriate blood pressure response (failure to increase by at least 20 mm Hg systolic or a drop of 20 mm Hg systolic with exercise) and other SCD risk markers*
10. Severity of LVOT obstruction (conflicting evidence)
11. Late gadolinium enhancement with CMRI (emerging evidence, not established risk factor)
12. LV apical aneurysm (limited evidence)

Bockstall KE, et al. A primer on arrhythmias in patients with hypertrophic cardiomyopathy. *Curr Cardiol Rep.* 2012;14(5):552–62. [PMID: 22825919]

Maron BJ, et al. Implantable cardioverter-defibrillators and prevention of sudden cardiac death in hypertrophic cardiomyopathy. *JAMA*. 2007;298:405–12. [PMID: 17652294]

D. Hypertrophic Cardiomyopathy and Athlete's Heart

Physiologic LV remodeling with LVH mimicking HCM can sometimes be seen in athletes, which makes decision making regarding pathologic versus physiologic LVH challenging. Borderline increase in LV thickness (13–15 mm) is usually seen in elite/endurance athletes (long-distance cycling, cross-country skiing, rowing), but LV thickness > 15 mm should raise concern for HCM. Women athletes seldom develop LV thickness > 12 mm, beyond which pathologic hypertrophy should be suspected. Echo plays a key role in helping differentiate physiologic from pathologic hypertrophy. Normal-to small-sized ventricle, diastolic function impairment, tissue Doppler and strain abnormalities, and abnormal mitral valve apparatus all favor HCM. Cardiopulmonary exercise testing may also help because athletes will have high levels of VO_{2max} with excellent exercise capacity compared to HCM, where these parameters will be impaired. CMRI may also help as a complementary imaging modality to make more accurate estimations of LV wall thickness, cavity size, and presence of delayed enhancement. Despite all of these potential parameters used for differentiation between these two entities, sometimes conclusive diagnosis may be elusive and a period of deconditioning for 3 months may be needed with repeat assessment of LV wall thickness/mass. There will be regression of LV thickness and mass in physiologic but not pathologic hypertrophy. Athletes with HCM should not participate in high-intensity or contact sports regardless of whether they have obstruction. However, they can participate in light to moderate intensity sport activity (eg, golf).

Myerson M, et al. Pre-participation athletic screening for genetic heart disease. *Prog Cardiovasc Dis*. 2012;54:543–52. [PMID: 22687598]

E. Special Considerations in Hypertrophic Cardiomyopathy

1. Endocarditis prophylaxis—Current ACC/AHA guidelines do not recommend routine antibiotic prophylaxis for HOCM patients unless prior history of endocarditis exists. Overall risk of endocarditis is considered low in HCM unless significant outflow obstruction and abnormal mitral valve structure coexist.

2. Pregnancy and HCM—Asymptomatic HCM is not a contraindication for pregnancy but requires counseling prior to planning and careful observation during pregnancy. Pregnant HCM patients stable on β-blockers can have these continued with monitoring of fetus for bradycardia. Severely symptomatic HCM patients who are pregnant require high-risk obstetrics/cardiology care. Pregnancy is discouraged for HCM patients with heart failure due to high maternal and fetal morbidity and mortality.

Gersh BJ, et al. 2011 ACCF/AHA guideline for the diagnosis and treatment of hypertrophic cardiomyopathy: executive summary: a report of the American College of Cardiology Foundation/American Heart Association Task Force on Practice Guidelines. *Circulation*. 2011;124:2761–96. [PMID: 22068435]

Restrictive Cardiomyopathy

24

James A. Goldstein, MD

ESSENTIALS OF DIAGNOSIS

▶ Predominant biventricular diastolic dysfunction with lesser impairment of systolic performance.

▶ Symptomatic presentation:

• Chronic biventricular "backward failure" manifest as dyspnea and peripheral edema (often hepatomegaly and ascites).

• Reduced preload limits cardiac output (fatigue).

▶ Echocardiography: small stiff ventricles, preserved systolic function (until late stages), dilated atria and diastolic dysfunction by Doppler.

▶ Many disorders manifest restrictive "physiology" and must be excluded (eg, hypertrophic cardiomyopathy and constrictive pericarditis).

▶ Cardiac magnetic resonance imaging powerful: delineates myocardial infiltration, inflammation, and fibrosis and assesses pericardium, thereby helping establish underlying disorder.

▶ Tissue biopsy may be necessary for definitive diagnosis in some disorders (eg, amyloidosis).

▶ Overview

Restrictive cardiomyopathies (RCM) are indolent disabling diseases resulting from pathophysiologic processes that induce predominant diastolic chamber dysfunction with lesser impairment of systolic performance. RCM is characterized by small stiff ventricles with progressive impairment of diastolic filling, leading to the hemodynamic conundrum of low preload but high filling pressures (Figure 24–1). This pattern of diastolic dysfunction leads to dilated atria and elevated mean atrial pressures, resulting clinically in biventricular "backward failure" manifest as pulmonary venous

congestion (dyspnea) as well as systemic venous pressure elevation (peripheral edema). Systolic function is preserved in most cases, depending on the underlying cause (at least in the presenting stages of most of the underlying diseases). However, despite intact systolic function, the restrictive constraints on true ventricular preload limit stroke volume, thereby resulting in low cardiac output (fatigue) and ultimately hypoperfusion.

The abnormal diastolic properties of the ventricle are typically attributable to abnormalities of the myocardium (infiltration, inflammation, or fibrosis) or the endomyocardial surface (inflammation and scarring). The RCM classification (Figure 24–2) may be most easily considered based on underlying pathophysiologic process as *infiltrative* (eg, amyloidosis), *storage* (eg, hemochromatosis), *inflammatory* (eg, hypereosinophilic syndrome), *noninfiltrative* (eg, diabetic), or *idiopathic*. Identification of specific infiltrative processes may have prognostic and therapeutic implications. Of note, secondary restrictive physiology can develop at a late stage in hypertrophic, dilated, valvular, hypertensive, and ischemic heart disease.

The vast majority of the underlying disease processes are slowly progressive, but by the time patients develop cardiac symptoms, the disease is advanced pathologically and heart failure progresses rapidly over a short period of time, and the majority die within a few years following diagnosis.

▶ Pertinent Aspects of Normal Hemodynamics

An appreciation of the physiology of the venous circulations and the dynamic effects of intrathoracic pressure (ITP) and respiratory motion on cardiovascular physiology is critical to understanding the hemodynamic pathophysiology of RCM and differentiating it from other conditions, particularly constrictive pericarditis (CP). Under physiologic conditions, venous return to both atria is biphasic, with a systolic peak determined by atrial relaxation ("X" descent of the atrial and jugular venous pressure [JVP] waveforms) and a diastolic peak determined by tricuspid valve (TV) resistance and right

RCM: Stiff Ventricles

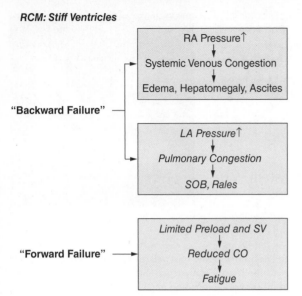

"Backward Failure"

RA Pressure↑
↓
Systemic Venous Congestion
↓
Edema, Hepatomegaly, Ascites

LA Pressure↑
↓
Pulmonary Congestion
↓
SOB, Rales

"Forward Failure" →

Limited Preload and SV
↓
Reduced CO
↓
Fatigue

▲ **Figure 24–1.** Pathophysiology of restrictive cardiomyopathy (RCM). CO, cardiac output; LA, left atrium; RA, right atrium; SOB, shortness of breath; SV, stroke volume.

ventricular (RV) compliance ("Y" descent). Respiratory oscillations exert complex effects on cardiac filling and dynamics, with disparate effects on the right and left heart attributable to differences in their anatomic relationships to the respective venous return systems relative to the intra-pleural space. Normally, inspiration induces decrements in ITP (−25 to −30 mm Hg), which are transmitted through the pericardium to the cardiac chambers. On the right heart, these decrements in ITP enhance the filling gradient from the extrathoracic systemic veins, thereby augmenting venous return and increasing right heart filling and output. In con-trast, the left heart and its tributary pulmonary veins are entirely intrathoracic. Therefore, inspiratory decrements in ITP are evenly distributed, and thus, mitral valve (MV) flow and left ventricular (LV) filling are essentially unchanged throughout the respiratory cycle.

▶ Pathophysiology

The pathognomonic feature of RCM is stiffness of the ventricular walls, which impairs diastolic filling, result-ing in limited ventricular preload (and therefore stroke volume) despite increased diastolic filling pressures. Echocardiography (echo) documents small ventricles, often with thick walls. By invasive hemodynamic assessment, RCM is characterized by elevated ventricular diastolic pressures

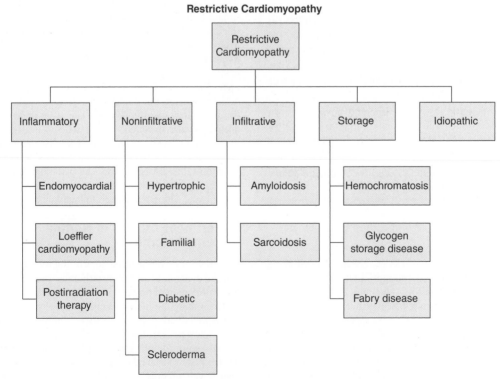

Restrictive Cardiomyopathy

Restrictive Cardiomyopathy

| Inflammatory | Noninfiltrative | Infiltrative | Storage | Idiopathic |

- Endomyocardial
- Loeffler cardiomyopathy
- Postirradiation therapy

- Hypertrophic
- Familial
- Diabetic
- Scleroderma

- Amyloidosis
- Sarcoidosis

- Hemochromatosis
- Glycogen storage disease
- Fabry disease

▲ **Figure 24–2.** Classification of restrictive cardiomyopathies.

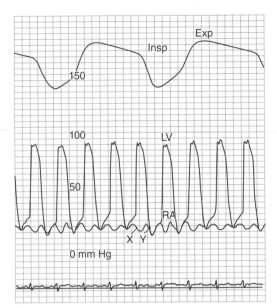

▲ **Figure 24–3.** Simultaneous recordings of left ventricular (LV) and right atrial (RA) pressures. Note the marked "W" or "M" pattern in the RA pressure tracing with prominent X and Y descents and with no fall with inspiration (Kussmaul sign). The nasal respirometer tracing is also shown. Exp, expiration; Insp, inspiration. (From Higano ST, et al. *Cath Cardiovasc Inter.* 1999;46: 473–86.)

(Figures 24–3 and 24–4), often with a mild diastolic "dip and plateau" or "square root" pattern, a nonspecific indicator of stiff noncompliant chambers, a phenomenon also seen in other conditions such as CP (discussed later). Echo-Doppler demonstrates classic features of impaired diastolic function (impaired myocardial relaxation with increased early LV filling velocity, decreased atrial filling velocity, and decreased isovolumic relaxation time). Ventricular systolic function is typically preserved until the later stages of the underlying disease. Biatrial enlargement reflects ventricular noncompliance and may also result from primary atrial myocardial involvement by the disease process (eg, amyloidosis). Atrial filling pressures are elevated, and the X and Y descents tend to be relatively blunted; in cases in which the atria are primarily involved by the restrictive process, the A wave may be depressed (see Figure 24–3). In RCM, a pattern of "elevated and equalized" chamber diastolic filling pressures indicating pancardiac "stiffness" is common, but this nonspecific pattern is also seen in other diseases, particularly pericardial constraint conditions (eg, CP). However, in RCM, left-sided pressures are typically somewhat higher than right due to the greater intrinsic stiffness of the LV. This difference may be amplified by maneuvers that augment ventricular filling such as volume infusion, leg-raising, or post–premature ventricular contraction increased filling time. Disproportionate

left heart stiffness may also result in moderate pulmonary hypertension (a subtle distinguishing feature from CP).

In RCM, inspiratory changes in ITP are fully transmitted through the pericardium to the cardiac chambers. However, chamber noncompliance contributes to a relative lack of respiratory variation in cardiac filling, and therefore, mitral and tricuspid flow velocity during respiration are typically decreased. Because of the lack of pericardial constraint and a relatively noncompliant interventricular septum, there is minimal ventricular interdependence, and thus inspiratory effects on ventricular systolic pressures are concordant (ie, there is little change in peak ventricular systolic pressures with respiration and they move in the same direction) (see Figure 24–4); as will be discussed, the pressure pattern in CP is "discordant." As RCM progresses and right-sided chambers become less distensible, the respiratory swings in pressure diminish further. At its most severe, noncompliance to inflow results in the "Kussmaul sign," an inspiratory increase in venous return that cannot be accommodated by the stiff right heart, resulting in inspiratory elevation of JVP (see Figure 24–3). Doppler flow patterns show blunting of the expected physiologic respiratory increases in flow across the TV and minimal change across the MV.

Higano ST, et al. Hemodynamic rounds series II: hemodynamics of constrictive physiology: influence of respiratory dynamics on ventricular pressures. *Catheter Cardiovasc Interv.* 1999;46: 473–86. [PMID: 10216021]

Kushwaha S, et al. Restrictive cardiomyopathy. *N Engl J Med.* 1997;336:267–76. [PMID: 8995091]

Mogensen J, et al. Restrictive cardiomyopathy. *Curr Opin Cardiol.* 2009;24:214–20. [PMID: 19593902]

Oh JK, et al. Diagnostic role of Doppler echocardiography in constrictive pericarditis. *J Am Coll Cardiol.* 1994;23:154–62. [PMID: 8277074]

▶ Clinical Findings

Patients with RCM suffer symptoms attributable to biventricular diastolic dysfunction. Systemic venous congestion related to right heart noncompliance typically predominates, characterized by pedal edema, abdominal swelling, and gastrointestinal symptoms related to hepatic/bowel congestion (loss of appetite). Physical exam reveals elevated jugular venous pressure often with Kussmaul sign, peripheral edema, and ascites; with advancing disease, hepatomegaly, ascites, and anasarca develop. Patients typically are limited by dyspnea on exertion attributable to left heart diastolic dysfunction. At the bedside, patients will exhibit signs of right heart failure (eg, elevated JVP with edema, ascites), but the precordial exam will be quiet with no evidence of an RV heave, thus pointing away from other causes of right heart failure such as pulmonary hypertension, dilated cardiomyopathy, or TV regurgitation (all of which will manifest an RV heave/lift in the left parasternal area).

Respiratory Patterns in CP vs RCM

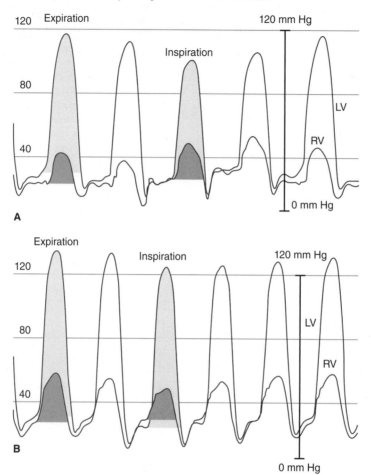

▲ **Figure 24–4.** Left ventricle (LV) and right ventricle (RV) high-fidelity manometer pressure traces from two patients during expiration and inspiration. Note that both patients have early rapid filling and elevation and end-equalization of the LV and RV pressures at end expiration. **A:** A patient with surgically documented constrictive pericarditis. During inspiration, there is an increase in the area of the RV pressure curve (*orange-shaded area*) compared with expiration. The area of the LV pressure curve (*yellow-shaded area*) decreases during inspiration as compared with expiration. **B:** A patient with restrictive myocardial disease documented by endomyocardial biopsy. During inspiration, there is a decrease in the area of the RV pressure curve (*orange-shaded area*) as compared with expiration. The area of the LV pressure curve (*yellow-shaded area*) is unchanged during inspiration as compared with expiration. (From Talreja DR, et al. *J Am Coll Cardiol.* 2008;51:315.)

In the early stages of RCM, systolic function is typically preserved, although deterioration in contractility may be observed as the disease progresses; the severity and patterns of dysfunction depend on the specific etiology and severity of the underlying disease entity. Despite preserved systolic ventricular function, impaired diastolic filling limits ventricular preload, thereby rendering the stiff heart limited in its ability to increase cardiac output with exercise, resulting in fatigability. Low output combined with autonomic insufficiency characteristic of some RCMs (eg, amyloidosis) renders patients susceptible to symptoms of orthostatic

hypotension. Atrial dilation often leads to atrial fibrillation, which further exacerbates diastolic dysfunction due to high heart rate and loss of atrial contraction.

▶ Etiologies

A. Myocardial Disorders

1. Idiopathic or primary RCM—Idiopathic or primary RCM, often due to hereditary contractile protein mutations, represents approximately 50% of cases and occurs more commonly in older women than men. Wall thickness is commonly increased by echocardiography, and biopsy typically reveals myocyte hypertrophy often with patchy endocardial fibrosis involving both ventricles. Idiopathic diagnosis can only be established in the absence of other identifiable causes (ie, storage, infiltrative, and inflammatory diseases), many of which induce thick ventricular walls and infiltrative/storage damage on biopsy.

2. Infiltrative disorders

A. Cardiac amyloid—Amyloidosis is the prototypical RCM, arising from a group of disorders resulting in multisystem infiltrative disease with organ involvement, including heart, dependent on the underlying amyloid precursor protein entity. Cardiac amyloid is typically silent until tissue infiltration is extensive, leading to RCM with symptomatically progressive biventricular diastolic dysfunction. Imaging modalities, biochemical tests, and tissue samples establish definitive diagnosis. Echo documentation of thick walls, small cavities, and granular speckled "hyperrefractile" myocardial pattern is nearly diagnostic. Cardiac magnetic resonance imaging (MRI) shows diffuse late gadolinium enhancement throughout both ventricles, particularly the subendocardium. To exclude amyloid of the AL type, monoclonal gammopathy may be evident on urine and serum protein electrophoresis, although immunofixation and assays for serum free light chains are more sensitive. Amyloid deposits can be documented by biopsy of myocardium (by histology, Congo Red staining delineates amyloid deposits between cardiac myocytes); tissue specimens can also be obtained from fat pad or rectum. The general treatment approach is as with any RCM. The mainstay is diuretics to decongest within the limits tolerated by hypotension. These patients are at high risk of thromboembolism, especially with atrial fibrillation, but even in its absence, anticoagulation should be strongly considered. Untreated patients with AL amyloid have a median survival < 6 months after onset of heart failure. Aggressive chemotherapy and stem cell transplantation, followed by cardiac transplantation, have shown promising potential in a small number of cases, but transplantation mortality rate is high and randomized data are lacking.

B. Hemochromatosis—Cardiac iron overload, due to heritable disorder or chronic and excessive iron administration, is always associated with involvement of multiple organs, giving rise to the classic clinical presentation of heart failure, cirrhosis, impotence, and diabetes. At pathology, hearts are dilated and ventricular walls thickened. Echo shows a nonspecific mixed pattern of systolic and diastolic dysfunction. The condition is commonly complicated by and may be announced by arrhythmias. Laboratory evaluation is usually diagnostic (marked elevations of plasma iron, serum ferritin, and transferrin saturation, but lower normal total iron binding capacity). Cardiac MRI is a sensitive marker of iron deposition and predictive of future events. Endomyocardial biopsy is definitive, but usually not necessary when biochemical testing is diagnostic. Chelation

therapy is appropriate and may limit further damage but is unlikely to reverse existing organ dysfunction.

C. Sarcoidosis—This systemic inflammatory condition results in multiorgan noncaseating granulomatous infiltration, typically in the lungs, reticuloendothelial system, and skin. The heart is involved in 20–30% of cases at autopsy, with patchy granulomatous infiltration in discrete areas of the ventricular walls with a predilection for the posterior LV free wall, basal septum, and conduction system. Cardiac infiltrate may result in fibrotic scars and "microaneurysm" formation. Cardiac sarcoid most commonly presents clinically with conduction block or malignant arrhythmias and less commonly with heart failure due to RCM. The electrocardiogram (ECG) may reveal atypical infarction patterns and various degrees of AV block. Echo varies according to disease activity, with wall thickening due to granulomatous expansion but later wall thinning due to fibrosis. Segmental hypokinesia most commonly localizes to mid and basal segments of the LV free wall and upper septum. Owing to patchy involvement, endomyocardial biopsy provides diagnostic evidence in only 25–50% of autopsy-confirmed cases. Cardiac MRI and positron emission tomography (PET) are more sensitive and correlate with disease severity. If treated early, when inflammation predominates and fibrosis is less advanced, anti-inflammatory therapy (steroids and cyclophosphamide [Cytoxan]) may improve cardiac function. In those with arrhythmias, pacemaker and defibrillator therapy should be considered.

D. Storage disorders due to heritable diseases—RCMs may result from heritable metabolic disorders resulting in myocardial accumulation or infiltration of abnormal metabolic products, producing classic RCM. The recent availability of enzyme replacement in some disorders makes early diagnosis increasingly essential. The most common are glycogen storage disorders (Gaucher and Fabry disease) resulting from lysosomal accumulation in the heart and other organs. Gaucher disease commonly presents with RCM in childhood and is responsive to enzyme replacement therapy or, in extreme cases, hepatic transplantation. In Fabry disease, cardiac involvement is typically manifest in the third or fourth decade of life; the thick ventricular walls mimic hypertrophic cardiomyopathy; differentiation by MRI may be helpful. Other less common heritable storage disorders that may result in RCM include the mucopolysaccharidoses, myocardial oxalosis (related to underling primary hyperoxaluria), and Friedreich ataxia (an autosomal recessive neurodegenerative disorder associated with RCM and/or dilated cardiomyopathy in 90–100% of cases).

B. Endomyocardial Disease

There are two variants of endomyocardial disease, with different pathogenesis but shared and overlapping features. Endomyocardial fibrosis (EMF) refers to a specific syndrome with characteristic geographic epidemiologic features. Other cardiomyopathy syndromes with similar pathologies include

Loeffler endocarditis (also called hypereosinophilic endomyocarditis) and other diseases that induce fibrotic changes of the endocardium (eg, carcinoid heart disease).

1. Endomyocardial fibrosis—EMF occurs primarily in tropical regions and in subtropical zones, presents at a young age, and is the most common form of RCM worldwide. EMF is characterized by fibrosis of the apical endocardium of the ventricles. The clinical manifestations are classic RCM.

2. Loeffler "hypereosinophilic" endomyocarditis—This group of disorders results from sustained overproduction of eosinophils, leading to eosinophilic infiltration and mediator release, which damages multiple organs. Diagnosis is established by eosinophil counts > 1500 for at least 6 months. The disease may be primary, but it is essential to search for secondary and potentially treatable causes including leukemia, reactive disorders such as parasite infection, allergies, granulomatous syndromes, hypersensitivity, and neoplastic disorders. Eosinophil-mediated heart damage, detected by echo or MRI, evolves through three stages: (1) an acute necrotic stage; (2) an intermediate phase characterized by thrombus formation along the damaged endocardium; and (3) a fibrotic stage. Treatment is aimed at the underlying disease.

3. Carcinoid heart disease—Carcinoid tumors metastatic to the liver elaborating circulating serotonin (and 5-hydroxyindolacetic acid, its primary metabolite) induce fibrous endocardial plaques in 50% of patients. By echo, plaques are typically seen on the endocardium downstream of the TV, commonly resulting in stenotic and regurgitant valvular lesions (especially TV). The observation that the right heart is preferentially affected reflects inactivation of these toxic substances in the lung. Management of the underlying carcinoid is the focus of treatment. Identical pathology results from exposure to the anorectic drug fenfluramine and its related medications.

Ammash NM, et al. Clinical profile and outcome of idiopathic restrictive cardiomyopathy. *Circulation.* 2000;101:2490–6. [PMID: 10831523]

Falk RH. Cardiac amyloidosis: a treatable disease, often overlooked. *Circulation.* 2011;124:1079–85. [PMID: 21875922]

Seward JB, et al. Infiltrative cardiovascular diseases. Cardiomyopathies that look alike. *J Am Coll Cardiol.* 2010;55:1769–79. [PMID: 20413025]

Yilmaz A, et al. Comparative evaluation of left and right ventricular endomyocardial biopsy: differences in complication rate and diagnostic performance. *Circulation.* 2010;122:900–9. [PMID: 20713901]

▶ Differentiating Restrictive Cardiomyopathy from Other Disorders

Cardiac chambers with thick walls, small ventricular cavities with intact systolic function, and dilated atria are also typical of conditions with myocyte hypertrophy such as congenital hypertrophic cardiomyopathy (HCM) or acquired hypertensive and valvular heart disease. Coronary artery disease, especially in diabetics, can also mimic clinical RCM. Careful history, physical examination, noninvasive testing, and arteriography can exclude these acquired conditions, whereas differentiating HCM may pose challenges.

Differentiating RCM versus CP poses one of the most challenging clinical hemodynamic conundrums and deserves special consideration. These two conditions are remarkably similar in their hemodynamic pathophysiology, share nearly identical clinical presentation characterized by systemic and pulmonary congestion due to biventricular diastolic dysfunction with limited cardiac output, and appear quite similar by echocardiography, with small ventricles, dilated atria, and intact systolic function. However, they are distinctly different entities in terms of clinical course, management, and prognosis. CP is "curable" through surgical pericardiectomy, whereas RCM is treated by palliative measures and rarely if ever cured. Because of this important distinction, accurate differentiation is crucial.

First, it is essential to appreciate the subtle similarities and differences in hemodynamic pathophysiology of CP compared to RCM. CP is the result of inflammatory fibrocalcification leading to a thick, inelastic pericardium that encases the heart, inducing biventricular diastolic dysfunction. As in RCM, this process is typically indolent and slowly progressive, with clinical manifestations appearing often years after the initial insult. There is substantial overlap in hemodynamic features, which reflect similarities in pathophysiology rather than differences in disease mechanism. In CP, early ventricular filling is resistance free; however, as the ventricles fill, they abruptly meet the inelastic resistance of the stiff pericardium, at which time filling pressure rises rapidly to an elevated plateau, inscribing an RV "dip and plateau" or "square root" waveform pattern, similar to RCM (see Figure 24–4). In CP, atrial filling pressures are elevated, reflecting both ventricular noncompliance and atrial constraint. The right atrium Y descent is sharper in CP, reflecting the initial rapid, resistance-free early RV filling. In CP, diastolic filling pressures are elevated and equalized, reflecting the common constraining effects of the pericardium. In RCM, the intrinsic cardiac disease more often results in "nearly equalized patterns" with disproportionate elevation of left heart filling pressures. Hemodynamic challenges including rapid volume loading, leg elevation, or exercise to effect a disproportionate rise in LV diastolic pressure suggest RCM but are not diagnostic. The presence of mild-moderate pulmonary hypertension favors the diagnosis of RCM, but may occur in constriction due to preexistent left heart or intrinsic pulmonary disease.

The effects of respiration on cardiac dynamics differ between RCM and CP in subtle but complex ways, findings that may help differentiate these conditions. In CP, increased pericardial resistance more tightly couples the two ventricles and increases their interdependence. Pericardial constraint limits total cardiac volume; consequently, an increase in filling on one side of the heart impedes

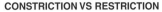

contralateral filling through intensified septal-mediated interactions. In CP, the inelastic fibrocalcific pericardial shell isolates the heart from the lungs, and therefore, respiratory changes in ITP are not fully transmitted to the cardiac chambers, resulting in dissociation of respiratory effects on ITP and intracardiac flows in the right heart versus the left heart. This represents an important difference compared to RCM. In CP, the inspiratory gradient created between the extrathoracic systemic veins and intrathoracic but extrapericardial cavae augments venous return to the right heart, but the constrictive pericardial shell neither fully facilitates inspiratory augmentation of right heart filling, nor accommodates whatever meager increments in filling occur. The result is an inspiratory increase in jugular venous and right heart filling pressures known as the Kussmaul sign (also seen in RCM). Anatomic–pathophysiologic relationships in the left heart are different: The pulmonary veins are entirely intrathoracic, the LA is not fully encased within the pericardium due to the pericardial reflection around the pulmonary veins, but the LV is fully constrained within the pericardium. Therefore, the inspiratory decrement in ITP is exerted upon the pulmonary veins, but not transmitted to the LV, resulting in reduced transmitral pressure gradient and flow. Because the rigid pericardium fixes total cardiac volume and induces tight ventricular coupling, there is a reciprocal relation between left and right heart filling. This results in inspiratory decrease in LV filling, which allows a small relative increase in tricuspid inflow and RV filling, leading to opposite directional increase in RV but decrease in LV changes in inspiratory ventricular systolic pressures, called "ventricular discordance" (see Figure 24–4), which is indicative of enhanced ventricular interaction and a strong indicator of CP. Analogous findings are evident in Doppler flow velocities including >25% expiratory increase in mitral E velocity and expiratory decrease in hepatic vein diastolic flow velocity and >25% increase in diastolic flow reversals compared with inspiratory velocity. In contrast, in RCM, inspiratory changes in ITP are fully transmitted through the pericardium to the cardiac chambers, but chamber noncompliance limits respiratory augmentation of cardiac filling, which, together with lack of pericardial constraint and a noncompliant interventricular septum, minimizes ventricular interdependence. The result is blunted respiratory flow velocities by Doppler and "concordant" ventricular systolic pressures. These disparate patterns with respiration have been proposed to differentiate CP versus RCM (see Figure 24–4). However, the overall specificity and sensitivity of these hemodynamic criteria, both alone and in combination, have not been sufficient to provide a basis for definitive diagnosis in individual patients.

▶ Clinical Algorithms to Differentiate Constriction from Restriction

Since the clinical presentation of these two entities is often similar, separating them on the basis of anatomic and

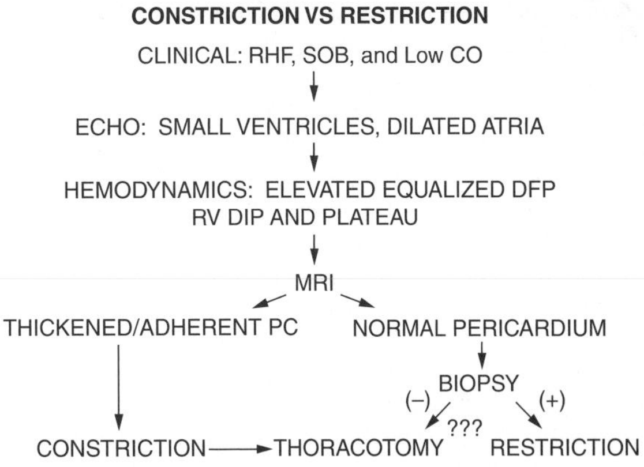

CONSTRICTION VS RESTRICTION

CLINICAL: RHF, SOB, and Low CO

↓

ECHO: SMALL VENTRICLES, DILATED ATRIA

↓

HEMODYNAMICS: ELEVATED EQUALIZED DFP
RV DIP AND PLATEAU

↓

MRI

THICKENED/ADHERENT PC   NORMAL PERICARDIUM

(−) BIOPSY (+)

CONSTRICTION → THORACOTOMY ??? RESTRICTION

▲ **Figure 24–5.** Clinical algorithm to differentiate constrictive pericarditis versus restrictive cardiomyopathy. CO, cardiac output; DFP, diastolic filling pressure; ECHO, echocardiography; MRI, magnetic resonance imaging; PC, pericardium; RHF, right heart failure; RV, right ventricle; SOB, shortness of breath.

physiologic derangements is essential and requires the use of techniques that visualize the cardiac chambers and the pericardium, in conjunction with modalities that delineate the physiologic manifestations of the anatomic abnormalities. Most important, the single distinctive feature differentiating CP from RCM is anatomic, not physiologic: In patients with CP, the pericardium is almost always thickened and motion of the heart within the pericardium constrained, whereas in RCM patients, this is not the case. Therefore, anatomic documentation of pericardial thickness in patients with constrictive-restrictive physiology is crucial in differentiating these conditions (Figure 24–5). However, it must be emphasized that the finding of pericardial thickening should not be construed as the equivalent of a physiologic disorder because a thickened pericardium does not necessarily constrict. For example, pericardial thickening can be present in patients without physiologic constriction, particularly with tuberculosis or after open-heart surgery. Conversely, there can be physiologic pericardial constriction with normal-appearing pericardium by advanced cardiac imaging modalities.

Traditional and advanced cardiac imaging provides valuable information. The chest x-ray in CP may reveal pericardial calcification. In both conditions, the ECG is nonspecific but often reveals diffuse low voltage with nonspecific ST-T changes. By echocardiography, most RCMs exhibit thick walls, whereas CP does not. RCMs, particularly amyloid, result in the paradox of thick walls by echo but small volts by ECG, a pattern not seen in CP. Cardiac MRI is a powerful tool to evaluate patients with RCM in general and to distinguish it from CP. MRI provides data regarding not only chamber size, wall thickness, and ventricular function, but also the presence or absence of myocardial infiltration, inflammation, or fibrosis, patterns which inform the diagnosis of specific forms of RCM. After establishing that the myocardium appears normal, the delineation of pericardial thickness provides a basis for a therapeutic algorithm to definitively delineate CP versus RCM (see Figure 24–5). MRI provides insight not only regarding pericardial thickness, but also the dynamic nature of myocardial-pericardial interactions, specifically whether the pericardial layers are adherent to the heart and whether the heart slides normally in a smooth independent pattern within the pericardium during cardiac motion. Documentation of a thickened pericardium adherent to the epicardium and lack of independent motion are sufficient to diagnose CP, although RCM and CP may coexist (eg, radiation induced).

In patients with a clinical presentation and echo-Doppler findings consistent with either diagnosis, invasive hemodynamics should be performed with documentation of pericardial thickness "in hand." Employing this strategy, if pericardial imaging is confirmatory and hemodynamic findings consistent, biopsy is unnecessary and surgical exploration and pericardiectomy are warranted. In patients without these findings, assiduous clinical search for disease entities that result in RCM (eg, amyloidosis, hemochromatosis, scleroderma) will often result in delineation of the underlying etiology. Although clinical features and biochemical testing (eg, serum/urine protein electrophoresis, iron studies) may be sufficient, endomyocardial biopsy may be necessary to confirm its presence in the heart. However, if imaging fails to demonstrate constrictive features, then endomyocardial biopsy can be performed at the time of cardiac catheterization. Finally, it is important to emphasize that some patients with severe pericardial constriction proven at surgical exploration may have normal pericardial thickness by imaging techniques. Accordingly, in patients with severe clinical manifestations, lack of increased pericardial thickness, and normal endomyocardial biopsy, thoracoscopy or minimally invasive exploratory thoracotomy with provisional planned pericardiectomy should be considered.

Goldstein JA. Cardiac tamponade, constrictive pericarditis and restrictive cardiomyopathy. *Curr Prob Cardiol.* 2004;29:503–67. [PMID: 15365561]

Talreja DR, et al. Constrictive pericarditis in the modern era. *J Am Coll Cardiol.* 2008;51:315–. [PMID: 18206742]

Yilmaz A, et al. Comparative evaluation of left and right ventricular endomyocardial biopsy: differences in complication rate and diagnostic performance. *Circulation.* 2010;122:900–9. [PMID: 20713901]

▶ Treatment

Since few cases of RCM have treatable primary disease etiologies, management is based on diuretics to ameliorate pulmonary and systemic venous congestion. Frustratingly, optimal diuretic doses in RCM may reduce ventricular preload, leading to decreased cardiac output and symptoms of fatigability and light-headedness and even signs of hypotension and hypoperfusion. The development of atrial fibrillation and concomitant loss of atrial contractile contribution to filling of these stiff ventricles may worsen existing diastolic dysfunction and low output; in addition, rapid ventricular response may further compromise cardiovascular function. Thus, it is important to maintain sinus rhythm if feasible. However, digoxin should be used with caution, since it is potentially arrhythmogenic, particularly in patients with amyloidosis; other medications such as amiodarone should be considered. Atrial fibrillation renders patients prone to thromboemboli, and amyloid patients are at particular risk; therefore, anticoagulation should be strongly considered. When systolic dysfunction ensues, vasodilators may be tried, but caution should be employed due to predilection to orthostatic hypotension. Depending on the cause, cardiac transplantation may be considered but is often contraindicated because of the underlying primary disease.

▶ Prognosis

Typically, by the time a patient develops symptoms attributable to RCM, the disease is pathologically advanced and largely irreversible (with few exceptions; eg, acute inflammatory stages of sarcoid responsive to immunosuppression). Clinical progression is typically rapid over a short interval, and although RCM carries a variable prognosis dependent on etiology, the majority of patients die within a few years. The prognosis in amyloid is particularly grim (although the familial transthyretin-related form is more protracted compared with the immunoglobulin-associated disease).

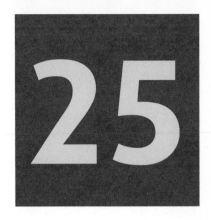

Myocarditis

Michael H. Crawford, MD

ESSENTIALS OF DIAGNOSIS

▶ New congestive heart failure with a history of an antecedent viral syndrome.

▶ Elevated cardiac biomarkers.

▶ Electrocardiogram shows sinus tachycardia, nonspecific ST-T changes, atrial or ventricular arrhythmias, or conduction abnormalities.

▶ Echocardiogram demonstrates chamber enlargement, wall motion abnormalities, systolic or diastolic dysfunction, or mural thrombi.

▶ Endomyocardial biopsy reveals an inflammatory infiltrate with adjacent myocyte injury.

▶ General Considerations

Myocarditis is defined simply as an inflammatory process with necrosis that involves the myocardium. In the past, the myocardial injury was believed to be a direct result of the cytotoxic effects of the relevant organisms. Even as early as 1806, however, it was thought that a persistent inflammatory process following such an infection (eg, diphtheria) of the myocardium led to progressive cardiac damage and dysfunction. When the term "myocarditis" was first introduced in 1837 as inflammation or degeneration of the heart, the diagnosis could be made only postmortem. Fortunately, endomyocardial biopsy now allows the sampling of human myocardial tissue during life and thus the accurate antemortem diagnosis of myocarditis.

▶ Pathophysiology

The histologic hallmark of myocarditis is a focal patchy or diffuse inflammatory infiltrate with adjacent myocyte injury. The inflammation may not be restricted to the myocardium but may also involve the adjacent endocardium, pericardium, and valvular structures.

Myocarditis is most commonly initiated by viral infection (Table 25–1). Initiation of the pathophysiologic abnormalities, however, may result from a variety of insults, including drugs, toxins, hypersensitivity reactions, collagen vascular diseases, and autoimmune reactions. The most common viruses associated with myocarditis in the United States and Western Europe in immunocompetent persons are adenoviruses, coxsackievirus B (enterovirus), parvovirus B19, herpes simplex, influenza A, and cytomegalovirus (CMV). Other viruses, bacteria, rickettsiae, spirochetes, fungi, protozoans, or metazoans can also produce myocarditis; such causes are uncommon, however (see Table 25–1). Successful identification of the most common offending pathogens depends on knowledge of the geographic region's relevant endemic and epidemic infectious diseases, the person's immunization status and immunocompetence, and the sophistication and availability of public health services.

Several mechanisms of myocardial damage have been proposed. (1) Direct injury of myocytes by the infectious agent. (2) Myocyte injury caused by a toxin such as that from *Corynebacterium diphtheriae*. (3) Myocyte injury as a result of infection-induced immune reaction or autoimmunity.

The autoimmunity hypothesis is the most widely accepted theory. It is believed that the viral infection triggers a cell-mediated immunologic response that ultimately causes myocardial injury; the myocardial injury persists despite viral clearance.

In the murine model, coxsackievirus B3 causes an infectious phase, which lasts 7–10 days, and is characterized by active viral replication. During this phase, initial myocyte injury takes place, causing the release of antigenic intracellular components (such as myosin) into the bloodstream. Subsequently, after viral clearance, a second phase of myocyte damage will start. This phase is immune-mediated by CD8 lymphocytes and autoantibodies against various myocyte components. Antimyosin antibodies were isolated

Table 25-1. Important Causes of Myocarditis

Infectious	
Viral	**Bacterial**
Coxsackie A and B	β-Hemolytic streptococci
Influenza A and B	Corynebacterium diphtheriae
Echovirus	Neisseria meningitides
Arbovirus	Staphylococcus aureus
Cytomegalovirus	Mycoplasma pneumoniae
HIV	Salmonella typhi
Hepatitis	Mycobacterium tuberculosis
Epstein-Barr virus	Borrelia burgdorferi
Mumps	Rickettsia rickettsii
Poliomyelitis	Campylobacter jejuni
Herpes simplex	Chlamydia trachomatis
Herpes zoster	Listeria monocytogenes
Human herpes virus 6	Legionella pneumophila
Parvovirus B19	Coxiella burnetii
Rabies	
Rubella	
Rubeola	
Vaccinia	
Protozoal	**Metazoal**
Trypanosoma cruzi	Echinococcus
Toxoplasma gondii	Trichinella spiralis
Fungal	
Noninfectious	
Toxic	**Hypersensitivity**
Anthracyclines	Drugs
Catecholamines	Vaccines
Interleukins	
Alpha-2 interferon	
Trastuzumab	
Autoimmune	
Giant cell myocarditis	
Hypereosinophilic syndrome	
Kawasaki disease	
Sarcoidosis	
Rheumatologic diseases	
Other	
Thyrotoxicosis	
Arsenic, copper, iron	
Radiotherapy	

from mice that developed myocarditis following coxsackievirus B infection, as well as from patients with myocarditis. Antigenic mimicry, the cross reactivity of antibodies to both virus and myocardial proteins, occurs when an infectious agent shares an identical antigen with the normal myocyte. This mechanism is documented in animal models, and it may play a role in humans. Myocyte injury may be a direct result of CD8 lymphocyte infiltration. The local release of cytokines, such as interleukin-1, interleukin-2, interleukin-6, tumor necrosis factor (TNF), and nitric oxide may play a role in determining the T-cell reaction and the subsequent degree of autoimmune perpetuation. These cytokines may also cause reversible depression of myocardial contractility without causing cell death.

The popularity of the autoimmune hypothesis deemphasizes the role of the virus. Animal studies show, however, that viral proliferation itself might cause myocarditis. Some studies demonstrate the persistence of viral genomic fragments in myocardial cells of patients with active myocarditis and in some patients with dilated cardiomyopathy. Although these fragments may not be infectious, viral RNA may still serve as a persistent antigen to drive the immunologic response.

Exposure to cardiotropic viruses, presumably followed by a viral infection of the myocardium, is common. Based on the detection of serum antibodies to cardiotropic viruses, approximately 70% of the adult population has had prior exposure. Nonetheless, resultant abnormalities in cardiac function or symptomatic heart failure are unusual. The host factors predisposing to these deleterious immune responses are as yet undefined. Immunocompromised patients, such as pregnant women and patients with acquired immunodeficiency syndrome (AIDS), are predisposed to myocarditis. The susceptibility to viral myocarditis may also be age-related or, based on familial occurrence, genetically predetermined.

Kindermann I, et al. Update on myocarditis. *J Am Coll Cardiol.* 2012;59:779–92. [PMID: 22362396]

Mahrholdt H, et al. Presentation, patterns of myocardial damage, and clinical course of viral myocarditis. *Circulation.* 2006;114(5):1581–90. [PMID: 17015795]

▶ Clinical Findings

A. Symptoms & Signs

Myocarditis is most commonly asymptomatic, with no evidence of left ventricular dysfunction. The clinical manifestations of myocarditis are protean, when they are present. Myocardial involvement may be overshadowed or completely masked by the constitutional symptoms of the illness or other organ dysfunction. Cardiac symptoms may result from systolic or diastolic left ventricular dysfunction or from tachyarrhythmias or bradyarrhythmias. Patients frequently seek medical attention days to weeks after an acute febrile illness, particularly a flu-like syndrome. Common constitutional symptoms include fever, malaise, fatigue, arthralgias, myalgias, and skin rash.

Chest discomfort is a common symptom and is typically pericardial in nature; ischemic or atypical pain may also occur. Occasionally, patients have the syndrome of acute myocardial infarction with ischemic chest pain, electrocardiographic (ECG) abnormalities, elevated cardiac isoenzymes, or evidence of left ventricular wall motion abnormalities. Viral coronary arteritis and vasospasm have been implicated as the cause of this syndrome, but the epicardial coronary arteries are usually widely patent.

The acute onset of symptoms of congestive heart failure in a young person or in a patient without known coronary artery disease often suggests the diagnosis of myocarditis. Classic symptoms of congestive heart failure, including dyspnea, fatigue, decreased exercise tolerance, palpitations, and right heart failure, may be present. This constellation of signs and symptoms may be indistinguishable from dilated cardiomyopathy. It should be noted that because the metabolic demands on the heart associated with fever or a viral illness may initiate the first episode of congestive heart failure in patients with asymptomatic left ventricular dysfunction or reduced cardiac reserve, heart failure following a viral syndrome does not necessarily imply myocarditis.

Patients may also present with other symptoms that have been described in myocarditis: dizziness, syncope, or palpitations caused by atrial and ventricular arrhythmias and conduction disturbances. Myocarditis may present as sudden death, as a result of malignant ventricular arrhythmias or complete heart block; systemic and pulmonary thromboemboli have also been noted.

B. Physical Examination

The findings on physical examination vary widely. The patient may appear ill because the other manifestations of a viral illness dominate the clinical picture, and myocardial involvement may become evident only later in the course of the illness. Preexisting heart disease can also obscure the findings of myocarditis on examination.

Tachycardia, hypotension, and fever are associated with myocarditis. The tachycardia may be disproportionate to the degree of fever, and the heart rate is frequently elevated both at rest and with effort. Bradycardia is seen rarely, and a narrow pulse pressure is occasionally detected. Murmurs of mitral or tricuspid regurgitation are common, but diastolic murmurs are rare. The intensity of S_1 may be decreased and the intensity of pulmonic closure increased, and S_3 and S_4 gallops may also be heard.

In more severe cases, congestive heart failure with distended neck veins, pulmonary rales, wheezes, gallops, and peripheral edema may be detected. Pleural and pericardial rubs are common in acute viral myocarditis, and a rhythm disturbance or conduction delay may be evident. Circulatory collapse and shock may occur, but these are rare.

C. Diagnostic Studies

1. Electrocardiography—ECG abnormalities are common in patients with myocarditis. These ECG changes are often nonspecific and transient, usually appearing only in the first 2 weeks of the illness. The most common abnormality is sinus tachycardia. While the presence of ST segment and T-wave changes suggests the diagnosis of myocarditis during a viral syndrome, subtle ECG changes may be caused solely by fever, hypoxia, hyperkalemia, and other metabolic abnormalities associated with the syndrome. Atrioventricular (AV) and intraventricular conduction delays are also common. Left bundle branch block occurs in approximately 20% of patients with active myocarditis. Complete AV block is not an uncommon finding and is often diagnosed after the patient presents with syncope. Heart block is usually transient but may occasionally require a temporary pacemaker. Supraventricular tachycardia is common, particularly with associated congestive heart failure or pericarditis. Ventricular ectopy may be the only clinical finding that suggests myocarditis. Other reported abnormalities include axis shifts and repolarization abnormalities.

2. Chest radiography—The chest radiograph may be normal, or it may demonstrate mild to moderate cardiomegaly from dilatation of the left or right ventricular cavity (or both). The cardiac silhouette may also be globular when a pericardial effusion is present, however. Evidence of venous congestion and pulmonary edema may be seen in more severe cases, and pulmonary infiltrates from concomitant pneumonia may be present.

3. Echocardiography—Echocardiography is a convenient and noninvasive method of evaluating chamber sizes, valvular function, and myocardial contractility. Left ventricular systolic dysfunction is commonly seen in patients with congestive heart failure. Regional wall motion abnormalities mimicking a myocardial infarction are surprisingly common; however, global hypokinesis may also occur. The left ventricular cavity may be normal in size or minimally enlarged; it may be markedly enlarged in those with fulminant disease. Mitral or tricuspid regurgitation may be present. Interestingly, an increase in wall thickness mimicking hypertrophic cardiomyopathy may be seen early in the course of the disease, presumably secondary to edematous inflammation. Mural thrombi occur in approximately 15% of cases. Echocardiography is also helpful in demonstrating abnormalities of diastolic filling that mimic restrictive cardiomyopathy and in distinguishing ventricular dilatation from pericardial effusion. Echocardiograms are commonly obtained serially to monitor the course of the illness and to evaluate therapy. Echocardiographic changes may persist, improve, or even worsen after clinical resolution of acute myocarditis.

4. Magnetic resonance imaging—Acute myocarditis can be detected by gadolinium-enhanced cardiovascular magnetic resonance imaging (MRI) using three primary imaging techniques. T2-weighted images readily detect myocardial edema, which is characteristic of inflammation. Early gadolinium enhancement in T1-weighted images identifies an increase in tissue blood volume due to vasodilatation from inflammation. Late gadolinium enhancement reflects myocardial fibrosis or necrosis, which is typical of the later stages of myocarditis. The best diagnostic accuracy compared to myocardial biopsy is when multiple criteria are used. If two of these three MRI abnormalities are found, the sensitivity in pooled studies is about 90%, specificity about 70%, and accuracy about 80%. Finding decreased left ventricular function, increased left ventricular cavity size, and increased myocardial volume are also supportive findings. MRI may help localize the areas where biopsy specimens should be taken. MRI is most often positive when biopsy specimens show definite myocarditis. Borderline biopsy criteria cases are less likely to be detected by MRI, and no MRI parameter predicts the presence of viral genomics by polymerase chain reaction (PCR).

5. Cardiac catheterization—Cardiac catheterization is not routinely performed in all cases of myocarditis; however, it may help in the diagnosis when the presentation mimics myocardial infarction. Characteristic hemodynamic findings of myocarditis include an elevated left ventricular end-diastolic pressure, a depressed cardiac output, and increased ventricular volumes. Ventriculography may also confirm abnormalities seen on echocardiography or MRI. Coronary angiogram typically demonstrates normal coronary arteries.

6. Endomyocardial biopsy—Myocardial biopsy is considered the gold standard for the diagnosis of myocarditis. It is an invasive procedure, although it only involves minimal morbidity and discomfort. The Stanford-Caves reusable bioptome is typically introduced to the right ventricular cavity. Newer, single-use bioptomes and sheaths can be introduced through right and left jugular, subclavian, or femoral veins and femoral arteries. Four to six tissue fragments are obtained, usually from the right side of the intraventricular septum, but cardiovascular MRI can be used to direct the bioptome to areas of focal disease. The major risk of myocardial biopsy is cardiac puncture. It occurs in less than 1% of cases but is often fatal. Computed tomography or three-dimensional echocardiography guidance can reduce the risk of right ventricular free wall puncture.

The histologic criteria for the diagnosis of myocarditis are defined as an inflammatory infiltrate of the myocardium with injury to the adjacent myocytes not typical for the ischemic damage associated with coronary artery disease. The diagnosis of borderline myocarditis is made when the infiltrate is not accompanied by myocyte injury. In large trials, only about 10% of patients with unexplained congestive heart failure met the criteria for active myocarditis. Many patients with negative biopsies have the classic clinical presentation of myocarditis. One explanation for the low yield of endomyocardial biopsy is that the inflammation may be focal or patchy. Another reason might be that some patients

have purely humoral or cytokine-mediated forms of myocarditis with little or no cellular infiltrate. Furthermore, the histologic changes may be transient with rapid resolution. It should be noted that endomyocardial biopsy may rule in, but never rule out active myocarditis.

In recent years, the role of endomyocardial biopsy has changed. It is no longer mandatory and essential in the evaluation of unexplained heart failure because the information it provides will rarely determine specific therapy. This became particularly evident after publication of the results of the Myocarditis Treatment Trial, which failed to show any benefit of the immunosuppressive therapy. It remains important to consider biopsy in some special cases of myocarditis, particularly in patients who do not respond to conventional therapy. Some patients in this group may have giant cell myocarditis, which requires a more aggressive approach with immunosuppressive therapy and consideration for early transplantation. Current guidelines suggest that biopsy may be appropriate in cases of unexplained new-onset (< 2 weeks) heart failure. After 2 weeks, no response to treatment or suspicion of special diagnoses, such as eosinophilic myocarditis, are considered valid indications for biopsy.

7. Other tests—An elevated erythrocyte sedimentation rate (ESR) is detected in approximately 60% of patients with active myocarditis. If the ESR is elevated, it may help monitor the course of the illness and effectiveness of therapy. The accuracy of this test may be affected by coexisting hepatic congestion or hepatitis; these conditions decrease the synthesis of fibrinogen and lower the ESR.

Mild to moderate leukocytosis occurs in approximately 25% of patients, along with neutrophilia or lymphocytosis and occasionally eosinophilia, particularly in parasitic illnesses. The percentage of eosinophils may also increase in the recovery phase of myocarditis.

The creatine phosphokinase-myocardial band (CK-MB) fraction is elevated in approximately 6% of patients, with the degree of elevation being proportional to the degree of myocyte injury. Cardiac troponin-I (Tn I) is a sensitive and specific marker for myocyte injury and is increased in about one-third of patients with myocarditis.

Measurement of serum antibody titers to various cardiotropic viruses is useful for establishing exposure to these agents. The titers may be neutralizing antibodies, complement-fixing antibodies, or hemagglutination-inhibiting antibodies. Because a fourfold rise in titer over a 4–6 week period is required to document an acute infection, serial blood samples must be obtained. It must be kept in mind that an elevated antibody titer or rise in dilution only implies infection with the offending organism. Proof of active myocarditis also requires a positive biopsy result. Cultures of throat washings, urine, and feces may help identify a viral pathogen. Unfortunately, viral cultures are usually negative, and serologic studies are often nondiagnostic. In addition, viral recovery is usually possible only during the acute phase of the illness when active replication is occurring. Because this phase is not associated with viral injury, the diagnostic yield of culture of myocardial samples obtained by endomyocardial biopsy is minimal. Other laboratory analyses that may be useful include a monospot test, Epstein-Barr virus titers, hepatitis serology, and urine and serum for CMV.

The detection of viral genomic material in endomyocardial biopsies using recombinant DNA techniques is a promising diagnostic tool. Two methods are used: PCR and in situ hybridization. Plus-strand RNA indicates persistent viral state, and minus-strand RNA indicates active viral replication. Unfortunately, studies have been inconsistent, with viral detection ranging between 10% and 60% of patients with dilated cardiomyopathy and myocarditis, compared with almost no viral detection in the control groups. Some studies have noted a relationship between viral persistence and progressive myocardial dysfunction. At the present time, routine viral study of endomyocardial biopsy is not recommended and remains investigational with the possibility of clinical application in the future.

Cooper LT, et al; American Heart Association, American College of Cardiology; European Society of Cardiology; Heart Failure Society of America; Heart Failure Association of the European Society of Cardiology. The role of endomyocardial biopsy in the management of cardiovascular disease: a scientific statement from the American Heart Association, the American College of Cardiology, and the European Society of Cardiology. Endorsed by the Heart Failure Society of America and the Heart Failure Association of the European Society of Cardiology. *J Am Coll Cardiol*. 2007;50(19):1914–31. [PMID: 17980265]

De Cobelli F, et al. Delayed gadolinium-enhanced cardiac magnetic resonance in patients with chronic myocarditis presenting with heart failure or recurrent arrhythmias. *J Am Coll Cardiol*. 2006;47(18):1649–54. [PMID: 16631005]

Friedrich MG, et al. Cardiovascular magnetic resonance in myocarditis: a JACC White Paper. *J Am Coll Cardiol*. 2009;53: 1475–87. [PMID: 19389557]

Gutberlet M, et al. Suspected chronic myocarditis at cardiac MR: diagnostic accuracy and association with immunohistologically detected inflammation and viral persistence. *Radiology*. 2008;246(2):401–9. [PMID: 18180335]

Kühl U, et al. High prevalence of viral genomes and multiple viral infections in the myocardium of adults with "idiopathic" left ventricular dysfunction. *Circulation*. 2005;111(7):887–93. [PMID: 15699250]

Kühl U, et al. Viral persistence in the myocardium is associated with progressive cardiac dysfunction. *Circulation*. 2005;112(13):1965–70. [PMID: 16172268]

Mahfoud F, et al. Virus serology in patients with suspected myocarditis: utility or futility? *Eur Heart J*. 2011;32(7):897–903. [PMID: 21217143]

Mahrholdt H, et al. Cardiovascular magnetic resonance assessment of human myocarditis: a comparison to histology and molecular pathology. *Circulation*. 2004;109(10):1250–8. [PMID: 14993139]

▶ Treatment

Patients with suspected acute myocarditis should be hospitalized and monitored closely for evidence of worsening congestive heart failure, arrhythmias, conduction disturbances, or emboli. Bed rest is essential, and activities that increase cardiac workload should be strongly discouraged. In the animal model, exercise has been shown to both intensify the inflammatory process in the myocardium and increase morbidity and mortality. Activities should be restricted until clinical improvement occurs or a follow-up biopsy documents the resolution of inflammation.

Antipyretics, other than nonsteroidal anti-inflammatory drugs (NSAIDs), should be given to febrile patients, and analgesics are helpful in dealing with pleuropericardial chest pain. Hypoxia, decrease in cardiac output, and tachycardia warrant the administration of supplemental oxygen. If anemia is present, correcting it may improve cardiopulmonary function. The use of tobacco and alcohol should be strongly discouraged.

Patients with congestive heart failure should be treated by restricting sodium and fluids and by administering diuretics, angiotensin-converting enzyme (ACE) inhibitors or angiotensin receptor blockers, β-blockers, and spironolactone. Patients with fulminant disease manifesting as cardiogenic shock will require more aggressive therapy with intravenous vasodilators and inotropic agents such as dobutamine or milrinone. Occasionally, cases may be refractory to conservative measures and require mechanical circulatory support. Favorable reports have used extracorporeal membrane oxygenation, intra-aortic balloon, and ventricular assist devices. Recent reports have demonstrated that early aggressive approach with mechanical circulatory support might help as a "bridge to recovery." As a last resort, cardiac transplantation may be considered in patients with acute myocarditis if all other measures have failed and the patient's condition is rapidly deteriorating. Unfortunately, an increased morbidity and mortality in transplant rejection results from the activated immunologic system that the donor heart encounters.

Antiarrhythmic agents are warranted in patients with tachyarrhythmias or ventricular arrhythmias. It is best to avoid agents with strong negative inotropic effects. Patients with symptomatic bradyarrhythmias or high-grade conduction blocks will benefit from the implantation of a pacemaker.

Anticoagulation therapy is indicated in patients with systemic or pulmonary emboli or mural thrombi detected by echocardiography or ventriculography. Patients with active myocarditis and even mild left ventricular dysfunction should probably receive anticoagulation (animal models have demonstrated a propensity toward mural thrombi). Anticoagulation may be contraindicated in patients with coexisting pericarditis.

Immunosuppressive therapy has been reported in few studies with disappointing results. Controlled trials of prednisone plus cyclosporine or azathioprine did not show significant differences in left ventricular ejection fraction or left ventricular diastolic diameter at 1 year. Also, no significant difference in survival occurred during the follow-up period.

Intravenous immune globulin was suggested to be useful by some reports. In those with persistent viral genome, interferon-β has been reported to eliminate viruses and improve left ventricular function, although immunosuppressive therapy is generally not indicated except in special cases.

The prognosis in giant cell myocarditis is very poor, and immunosuppressive therapy may be helpful. Another situation where immunosuppressive therapy may be indicated is myocarditis associated with underlying immune diseases, such as systemic lupus erythematosus. In a small percentage of myocarditis patients, the disease may recur after initial resolution; in these patients, immunosuppressive therapy may help in decreasing the recurrences.

Chandra D, et al. Usefulness of percutaneous left ventricular assist device as a bridge to recovery from myocarditis. *Am J Cardiol.* 2007;99(12):1755–6. [PMID: 17560889]

Cooper LT. Myocarditis. *N Engl J Med.* 2009;360(15):1526–38. [PMID: 19357408]

Sagar S, et al. Myocarditis. *Lancet.* 2012;379:738–47. [PMID: 22185868]

▶ Prognosis

Most patients with myocarditis have self-limited, asymptomatic disease without residual cardiac dysfunction. Symptomatic patients have a poorer prognosis. Patients may spontaneously recover at any point during the illness, the degree of ventricular dysfunction may stabilize, or it may progress to dilated cardiomyopathy and heart failure, especially in the face of such causes as AIDS or giant cell myocarditis. Unfortunately, a small percentage of patients will die suddenly and unexpectedly, regardless of therapy. The overall prognosis is poor, with an estimated cumulative mortality rate at 5 years of about 50%. Progressive heart failure is the predominant cause of death. Interestingly, patients with fulminant myocarditis have a better long-term prognosis than patients with mild acute or chronic presentations. These patients should therefore be supported aggressively with vasopressor therapy and mechanical circulatory support, if necessary, to give them the best chance of surviving the initial critical phase, since the likelihood of long-term recovery is high.

Magnani JW, et al. Survival in biopsy-proven myocarditis: a long-term retrospective analysis of the histopathologic, clinical, and hemodynamic predictors. *Am Heart J.* 2006;151(2):463–70. [PMID: 16442915]

▶ Specific Forms of Myocarditis

A. Chagas Disease, or American Trypanosomiasis

Chagas disease is endemic in the rural areas of Central and South America. A few cases have been reported in the Southwestern United States among immigrants from endemic areas. It is estimated that 18–20 million people worldwide are infected with the protozoan *Trypanosoma cruzi,* the organism that causes Chagas disease; of those infected, 50,000 die each year. *T cruzi* is transmitted by reduviid insects (Triatominae family). The insect becomes infected when it bites an animal or human carrier. Humans acquire the trypanosomes when the insects bite them during sleep. Alternatively, the insect might deposit its feces on the skin; trypanosomes then gain access to the bloodstream by the person rubbing the abraded skin or the conjunctivae.

Acute Chagas disease will develop in approximately 1% of the people bitten by reduviid bugs. Myocarditis may develop in this phase; however, patients usually recover within several weeks to several months. The patient may have an erythematous, pruritic skin lesion (chagoma) at the inoculation site. Unilateral, painless, palpebral edema with local lymphadenopathy (Romaña sign) is particularly common in children. After resolution of the acute phase, many patients enter a latent period during which a subclinical cardiomyopathy may develop. Approximately 30% of these patients progress to chronic Chagas disease, manifested as visceral organ enlargement (megaesophagus and megacolon) and cardiac disease, which is characterized by unrelenting congestive heart failure, malignant arrhythmias, heart block, thromboembolic phenomena, and sudden death. Cellular and humoral immune responses to *T cruzi*–altered host's cells appear to be responsible for myocardial injury. Characteristic ECG changes include right bundle branch block, with or without a left anterior fascicular block, and variable degrees of AV block. Echocardiography may demonstrate dilated ventricles, wall motion abnormalities, and specifically apical aneurysms. Active myocarditis can be demonstrated by endomyocardial biopsy using the Dallas criteria. Complement fixation test (Machado-Guerreiro test) and indirect immunofluorescent antibody assay are helpful in the diagnosis of chronic Chagas disease.

Treatment of Chagas disease is difficult and primarily symptomatic. Heart failure is treated in the usual manner, and the use of anticoagulants and antiarrhythmic agents (amiodarone) may be warranted. Heart block may necessitate pacemaker placement. For life-threatening ventricular arrhythmia, implantable cardioverter-defibrillator (ICD) implantation is indicated. Antiparasitic agents such as nifurtimox, benzimidazole, or itraconazole may be beneficial in both acute and untreated chronic Chagas disease. Cardiac transplantation may be an option in some cases; however, parasitemia is a common result of immunosuppression, and nifurtimox prophylaxis should be considered.

B. Human Immunodeficiency Virus

Infection with human immunodeficiency virus (HIV) is one of the leading causes of acquired heart diseases. The cardiac complications tend to occur late in the disease and with lower CD4 counts. The HIV-related cardiac manifestations are likely to become more prevalent as therapy and longevity improve. Evidence of cardiac involvement is found at autopsy in more than 50% of patients dying with

AIDS. There is a wide spectrum of cardiac manifestations in HIV patients, including pericardial, myocardial, and valvular involvement. Myocarditis in HIV patients is common. Causes may be a direct effect of HIV on the myocardium, or an autoimmune process induced by HIV alone or in conjunction with other viruses. About 20% of HIV-related myocarditis is caused by multiple infectious organisms, such as coxsackievirus group B, Epstein-Barr virus, CMV, adenovirus, *Toxoplasma gondii*, and *Histoplasma capsulatum*. HIV itself is responsible for the remaining 80% of cases. HIV cardiomyopathy is probably more related to HIV than to opportunistic infections.

Clinical presentation may be asymptomatic left ventricular systolic dysfunction or congestive heart failure. Echocardiography shows increased left ventricular dimensions and decreased function. Myocardial biopsy reveals patchy lymphocytic infiltrate; the lymphocytes consist of T cells—mostly CD8, CD2, CD3, and rarely CD4.

Prognosis in HIV cardiomyopathy is grim, and the mortality rate is high independent of CD4 count. Rapid-onset congestive heart failure carries a worse prognosis, with 50% mortality in 6–12 months. Treatment is similar to that for other forms of cardiomyopathy. Intravenous immunoglobulins have been used with some success in acute congestive heart failure and in myocarditis in HIV-infected patients.

C. Toxoplasmosis

Active myocarditis may result from acute infection by the intracellular protozoan *T gondii*. This form is primarily diagnosed in immunocompromised persons, such as HIV patients, but may also occur following cardiac transplantation. The infection can be transmitted by the donor heart. Endomyocardial biopsy reveals edema, organisms within the myocytes in areas of focal myocyte necrosis, and a mixed inflammatory infiltrate containing eosinophils. Toxoplasmic cysts may also be seen, and a rise in antibody titer may be detected. The infection is usually asymptomatic, although heart failure, arrhythmias, and conduction abnormalities may occur. If detected early, pyrimethamine and sulfadiazine may be curative.

D. Cytomegalovirus

Symptomatic myocarditis caused by CMV infection usually occurs only in immunosuppressed patients, such as those with neoplasms, HIV disease, or transplanted organs. Asymptomatic myocarditis is known to occur in the general population but is usually self-limited. Endomyocardial biopsy may demonstrate viral inclusions within myocytes, and viral DNA can be found within the myocardium. A focal lymphocytic infiltration with fibrosis is characteristic. Treatment is with intravenous ganciclovir.

E. Lyme Myocarditis

Infection with the tick-borne spirochete *Borrelia burgdorferi* causes Lyme disease, which manifests primarily with myalgias, arthralgias, headache, fever, adenopathy, and erythema chronicum migrans. Symptomatic, but usually transient, cardiac involvement develops in approximately 10% of infected patients. Conduction abnormalities or fluctuating degrees of AV block may be present. Syncope secondary to complete heart block is common and may require temporary transvenous pacing. Left ventricular dysfunction is rare. Endomyocardial biopsy may reveal active myocarditis. Spirochetes have been isolated from the myocardium in some patients. It is unclear whether the myocarditis of Lyme disease is a direct result of spirochetal infection or the immunologic response to it. The course of the disease is usually benign, and complete recovery is the rule.

Treatment with penicillin or doxycycline is recommended, but it is unknown if this treatment alters the course of the cardiac disease.

F. Giant Cell Myocarditis

Giant cell myocarditis is a rare form of myocarditis characterized by multinucleated giant cells within the myocardium, particularly at the margins of necrosis. The precise cause is as yet unknown, although it has been associated with several autoimmune diseases, such as ulcerative colitis, Crohn disease, and myasthenia gravis. This form of myocarditis is rapid in onset and usually associated with fever and widespread ECG changes. Conduction abnormalities, including high-grade AV block and ventricular tachyarrhythmias, are more commonly seen in giant cell myocarditis than in viral myocarditis. The disease course is characterized by a progressive downhill trend regardless of medical therapy. Early recognition of this form of myocarditis is important, as the prognosis is far worse than viral myocarditis. It should be suspected in young patients with rapidly progressive heart failure that is refractory to conventional therapy. Myocardial biopsy is usually diagnostic.

Immunosuppressive therapy with a combination of cyclosporine, azathioprine, and corticosteroids appears to be beneficial, possibly prolonging the time to transplant or death. Cardiac transplantation should be considered early despite the possibility of disease recurrence in the transplanted heart.

G. Sarcoidosis

This systemic granulomatous disease is of unknown origin. The pathologic hallmark of this disease is noncaseating granuloma. The granuloma consists of activated helper-inducer T lymphocytes, macrophages, and multinucleated giant cells. The granulomas trigger a fibrotic response, resulting in organ damage.

The disease may be widespread or limited to a single organ. The lymphoid, pulmonary, cardiovascular, hepatobiliary, and hematologic systems are most commonly involved, with the lungs being affected in over 90% of patients. Cardiac sarcoidosis is more common than previously recognized and is less likely to be diagnosed antemortem than pulmonary sarcoidosis. Frequently, the initial presentation is sudden death. In myocardial sarcoidosis, portions of the myocardial wall are replaced by sarcoid granulomas. Based on the degree of myocardial involvement, the presenting signs and symptoms vary from first-degree AV block to fulminant heart failure. About 25% of deaths due to cardiac sarcoidosis are from heart failure, whereas sudden death accounts for about a third of the deaths. The diagnosis of cardiac sarcoidosis can be challenging, so evidence of other organ involvement should be sought. Chest radiography, ECG, and echocardiography are helpful diagnostic tools. Myocardial perfusion scintigraphy may demonstrate small diffusely scattered perfusion defects consistent with the granulomas (Swiss cheese heart). Due to the scattered nature of the granulomas, endomyocardial biopsy lacks sensitivity and seldom aids the diagnosis despite high specificity. Treatment of sarcoidosis has not been studied by controlled trials; however, corticosteroids can improve cardiac symptoms and reverse ECG changes in over half of the treated patients. Antiarrhythmic drugs and automatic internal defibrillator placement may be indicated to decrease the risk of sudden death.

Heart Failure with Reduced Ejection Fraction

26

Liviu Klein, MD, MS

ESSENTIALS OF DIAGNOSIS

▶ Dyspnea on exertion and at rest, orthopnea, paroxysmal nocturnal dyspnea, and fatigue.

▶ Elevated jugular venous pressure, basilar rales or coarse rales throughout both lung fields with wheezing, cardiomegaly, S_3 gallop, hepatomegaly, and bilateral peripheral pitting edema.

▶ Dilated left ventricle with a reduced ejection fraction on transthoracic echocardiography.

▶ Elevated left ventricular filling pressures on cardiac catheterization.

▶ General Considerations

Heart failure (HF) is a complex clinical syndrome resulting from any structural or functional myocardial dysfunction that leads to an impaired ability to circulate blood at a rate sufficient to maintain the metabolic needs of internal organs and peripheral tissues. The myocardial dysfunction is often the consequence of long-standing ischemia due to coronary artery disease or loss of myocardial mass due to prior infarction, long-standing myocardial stress due to suboptimally treated hypertension or valvular disease, or direct long-term toxin exposure (alcohol abuse, illicit substance use, or chemotherapeutic agents); rarely, fulminant infections (especially viral) can lead to autoimmune myocardial damage, and in some cases, there is no apparent cause (idiopathic cardiomyopathy, usually related to inherited or spontaneous gene mutations).

The cardinal manifestations of HF are dyspnea and fatigue (which may limit exercise tolerance) and fluid retention (which may lead to pulmonary/hepatic/splanchnic congestion and peripheral edema). Both abnormalities impair the functional capacity and quality of life of affected patients, but they may not necessarily dominate the clinical picture at the same time.

The prevalence of HF in the United States is around 5.8 million patients, of which approximately 45% have reduced ejection fraction/systolic dysfunction. There are over half a million cases of HF being newly diagnosed every year, and this incidence is expected to rise to over 700,000 new cases per year by 2040, mainly due to the aging of the population, as HF incidence doubles with each successive decade above age 45 for both men and women.

At age 40, the lifetime risk for HF is as high in women as in men, and is approximately one in five. Although over 75% of HF patients have antecedent hypertension or coronary artery disease, the population attributable risk (PAR) is different in men and women; the PAR for HF associated with coronary artery disease is 39% in men and 18% in women, whereas the PAR associated with hypertension is 39% in men and 59% in women, emphasizing the crucial need for population-based strategies to prevent the development of HF.

Multiethnic epidemiologic studies showed that the highest risk for developing HF is in African Americans (highest in young women and middle-aged men), followed by Hispanics/Latinos, Caucasians, and Chinese. This higher risk likely reflects differences in the prevalence of hypertension and diabetes mellitus and in socioeconomic status between different ethnicities.

Although the survival after HF diagnosis has improved, the 5-year mortality is still close to 50%, and over a quarter million deaths every year have antecedent HF. HF is one of the leading causes of hospitalization in the United States, with over one million hospitalizations a year (a figure that has not changed over the past decade). Indeed, 85% of patients diagnosed with HF will be hospitalized within 5 years of diagnosis, and over 40% will be hospitalized at least four times. HF accounts for over 12 million office visits and 6.5 million hospital days each year in the United States, with an estimated total cost of $39 billion, making it a major contributor to total health-care expenditure and the number one health expenditure for Medicare.

Bahrami H, et al. Differences in the incidence of congestive heart failure by ethnicity: the Multi-Ethnic Study of Atherosclerosis. *Arch Intern Med.* 2008;168:2138–45. [PMID: 18955644]

Chen J, et al. National trends in heart failure hospital stay rates, 2001 to 2009. *J Am Coll Cardiol.* 2013;61:1078–88. [PMID: 23473413]

Curtis LH, et al. Incidence and prevalence of heart failure in elderly persons, 1994-2003. *Arch Intern Med.* 2008;168:418–24. [PMID: 18299498]

Go AS, et al; American Heart Association Statistics Committee and Stroke Statistics Subcommittee. Heart disease and stroke statistics–2013 update: a report from the American Heart Association. *Circulation.* 2013;127:e6–e245. [PMID: 23239837]

▶ Pathophysiology

When an excessive workload is imposed on the heart by increased systolic blood pressure (pressure overload, such as in chronic hypertension or aortic stenosis), increased diastolic volume (volume overload, such as in progressive dilated idiopathic cardiomyopathy or chronic aortic or mitral regurgitation), or loss of myocardium (acutely in the setting of myocardial infarction, or chronically in the setting of flow-limiting coronary artery disease), normal myocardial cells hypertrophy in order to increase the contractile force of the unaffected areas. The biochemical, electrophysiologic, and contractile changes that ensue lead to alterations in the mechanical properties of the myocardium. Eventually, the compensatory force of the normal myocardial contraction decreases as cell loss and hypertrophy continue, leading to increased ventricular volume ("cardiac remodeling") and significant geometric ventricular alterations (ellipsoid to spherical shape). After the initial compensatory phase, the increase in ventricular volume is associated with further reductions in the ejection fraction (progressive systolic dysfunction) and with abnormalities in the peripheral circulation from activation of various neurohormonal compensatory mechanisms.

In the United States, coronary artery disease is the underlying etiology for systolic HF in more than half of the cases and a major contributor in another 15–20%. Transient ischemic events may cause prolonged systolic dysfunction that persists even after the ischemic event has resolved (myocardial stunning). The sustained reduction in the coronary blood flow leads to tissue hypoperfusion that is sufficient to maintain viability, but insufficient to maintain a normal contractility (myocardial hibernation). However, hibernation cannot be maintained indefinitely, and myocardial necrosis will ensue if coronary blood flow is not restored. Ischemia and hibernation may lead to myocyte apoptosis, which may result in progression of left ventricular systolic dysfunction characterized by a reduction in cardiac output and/or an increase in wall stress.

These functional and structural myocardial changes result in compensatory activation of neurohormonal systems, such as the renin–angiotensin–aldosterone system (RAAS), the adrenergic system, and the hypothalamic–neurohypophyseal system. The mechanisms for RAAS activation in HF include renal hypoperfusion with decreased filtered sodium reaching the macula densa and decreased stretch of the juxtaglomerular apparatus leading to increased renin release. Renin cleaves four amino acids from circulating angiotensinogen to form the biologically inactive angiotensin I. Angiotensin-converting enzyme (ACE) cleaves two amino acids from angiotensin I to form the biologically active angiotensin II, which binds to vascular angiotensin receptors causing vasoconstriction of the efferent postglomerular arterioles (promoting reabsorption of sodium, urea, and water) and to cardiac angiotensin receptors causing myocyte hypertrophy, apoptosis, and interstitial fibrosis. Increased circulating levels of angiotensin II also promote the release of aldosterone from the adrenal zona glomerulosa, resulting in sodium reabsorption and potassium excretion in the distal nephron, along with myocardial fibroblast proliferation and collagen deposition. The abnormal hypertrophy and fibrosis increase the passive stiffness of the ventricles and arterial bed, interfering with ventricular filling and reducing arterial compliance and, along with myocyte slippage and interstitial growth, result in ventricular remodeling. Finally, angiotensin II may increase the release of arginine vasopressin via a mechanism that does not rely on changes in osmolality, leading to renal free water reabsorption and dilutional hyponatremia seen with severe HF.

In patients with HF, the inhibitory input from high-pressure carotid sinus and aortic arch baroreceptors and low-pressure cardiopulmonary mechanoreceptors decreases, while nonbaroreflex peripheral chemoreceptors and muscle metaboreceptors excitatory input increases, with a net increase in sympathetic nerve traffic and blunted parasympathetic nerve traffic, and a resultant loss of heart rate variability and increased peripheral vascular resistance. As a result of the increase in sympathetic tone, there is an increase in circulating levels of norepinephrine from a combination of increased release from adrenergic nerve endings and its consequent "spillover" into the plasma, with reduced uptake of norepinephrine by adrenergic nerve endings. In patients in early stages of HF, norepinephrine increases heart rate and contractility and may support cardiac function. However, in later stages of HF, cardiac response to norepinephrine is blunted, partly because of the decreased β-receptor density seen in patients with chronic severe HF, where a shift occurs from the normal density (β1/β2 ratio of 70–80%/20–30%) to a more even distribution of 60%/40%. In addition, α-adrenergic receptors increase in the failing heart so that the end result is a more balanced distribution of myocardial α, β1, and β2 receptors. Chronic adrenergic stimulation has been shown to induce expression of proinflammatory cytokines, such as tumor necrosis factor-α, interleukin-1, and interleukin-6. Increased cytokine levels may result in the skeletal muscle myopathy characteristic of HF and cause myocardial inflammation, cell proliferation, and apoptosis, thereby worsening the HF syndrome. Tumor necrosis factor-α also activates transcription factors and enzymes involved in signal transduction, and it induces a number of genes, including the fetal gene program. Peripheral arteriolar tone is also increased in patients with HF (via α-adrenergic receptor stimulation), producing an increase in blood pressure and ventricular afterload and vasoconstriction of the renal efferent arterioles that causes significant sodium and water retention and increases production of renin, angiotensin II, and aldosterone, emphasizing the tight interplay between the adrenergic system and the RAAS. Indeed, ACE inhibition in patients with HF has been found to reduce peripheral sympathetic nerve impulse traffic and cardiac adrenergic drive, and the beneficial effects of ACE inhibitors appear to be especially prominent in patients with increased adrenergic activation. Conversely, β-blockade reduces the secretion of renin, therefore reducing the levels of angiotensin and aldosterone.

Arginine vasopressin is synthesized in the hypothalamus, and its release from the hypophysis is enhanced by osmolar stimuli as well as elevated concentrations of norepinephrine and angiotensin II. Increased release of arginine vasopressin in HF causes vasoconstriction and myocardial fibrosis (through binding to vasopressin 1 receptors) and water retention with dilutional hyponatremia (through binding to vasopressin 2 receptors).

The vasodilator peptides, such as atrial natriuretic peptide (ANP) and β-natriuretic peptide (BNP), are overexpressed in HF (as result of increased wall stress) and lead to a lowering of the right atrial, pulmonary artery, and pulmonary artery wedge pressures. In addition, systemic vascular resistance declines and cardiac output improves, circulating aldosterone and norepinephrine levels decrease, and natriuresis and glomerular filtration increase. However, in many patients with HF, the natriuretic peptides become ineffective despite high circulating levels. The profound activation of the RAAS and adrenergic system may overcome the ability of natriuretic peptides to increase sodium excretion or reduce afterload. In addition, most of the circulating natriuretic peptides in advanced HF patients are secreted as biologically inactive ("defective") molecules. Finally, changes in renal hemodynamics and a combination of receptor downregulation and increased cyclic guanosine monophosphate phosphodiesterase activity lead to a decreased natriuretic peptide response with consequent increase in salt retention and further deterioration of renal function and increased vasoconstriction.

The development of myocardial hypertrophy, as consequence of neurohormonal activation, initially represents an important adaptive mechanism to hemodynamic stress and is characterized by structural changes at the myocyte level that are translated into alterations in chamber size and geometry. In addition to myocyte alterations, the cardiac fibroblasts and the increased production of extracellular matrix participate in the remodeling process. Increased hemodynamic stress results in changes in myocardial gene expression leading to an impairment of contractile function. In patients with HF, a marked increase in the ventricular end-diastolic pressure may be responsible for changes in the shape of the left ventricle from an ellipsoid to a more spherical configuration. These changes in ventricular geometry result in papillary muscle rearrangement and secondary mitral insufficiency. In addition, the elevated ventricular end-diastolic pressures cause subendocardial ischemia that is perpetuated by compensatory tachycardia, which shortens the diastole and decreases the coronary filling time. This is reflected at a biochemical level by increased production of lactate, adenosine triphosphate, and creatine phosphate and at a histologic level through fibrosis, lowering the threshold for malignant ventricular arrhythmias.

The myocardial fibrosis and chamber dilatation lead to electrical dyssynchrony by fibrosis of the conduction system that, in turn, results in mechanical dyssynchrony (observed in about 40% of the systolic HF patients). When mechanical dyssynchrony is present, contraction and relaxation of the lateral wall occurs earlier than that of the interventricular septum, leading to decreased stroke volume and cardiac output and eventually to secondary mitral regurgitation.

In systolic HF patients, the decreased cardiac output leads to renal hypoperfusion, and the fluid retention leads to increased venous congestion, resulting in further reduction in the renal blood flow and relative renal vasoconstriction, which further exacerbate the sodium and water retention. In addition, the elevated cytokine levels and relative resistance of the bone marrow to erythropoietin lead to anemia in many HF patients. In these patients, peripheral perfusion decreases as a result of a decreased vascular resistance, leading to neurohormonal activation with subsequent reduction in renal blood flow and kidney function, ultimately resulting in expansion of plasma volumes. The increased plasma volume results in increased cardiac work, which leads to left ventricular hypertrophy and ultimately worsens the cardiac function, which in turn worsens renal function, completing the vicious circle (cardio-renal-anemia syndrome).

The chronic elevation in the left ventricular filling pressures that occurs in the setting of left ventricular remodeling and dilatation will lead to an increase in pulmonary venous pressures and a passive increase in pulmonary artery pressures. Due to the chronic elevation in pulmonary arterial pressures (secondary pulmonary hypertension), the pulmonary vascular resistance increases, increasing the right ventricular afterload and leading to deterioration in the right ventricular function over time (right HR). This eventually leads to a decrease in both right and left ventricular stroke volume, which is associated with signs and symptoms of both congestion (dyspnea, peripheral edema, hepatomegaly, elevated jugular venous pressures) and low cardiac output (mental status changes, renal dysfunction, fatigue).

Eventually, the progressive compensatory mechanisms described earlier are overwhelmed and the patients become symptomatic and present to medical attention, often in a hospital setting. In most patients, the condition is progressive, and further deterioration occurs at a myocardial/renal/hepatic/skeletal muscle level, and patients end up having recurrent hospitalizations. There is clear evidence that each hospitalization for HF leads to further myocardial necrosis (evidence by troponin release) and renal injury, which in turn will worsen the overall prognosis and lead to progressive HF and death.

In rare circumstances, a hyperkinetic circulatory state associated with vasodilatation occurs (usually due to an increased demand on the heart from another condition, such as anemia, or thyrotoxicosis) and can trigger HF when superimposed on an underlying heart disease. Fortunately, this is often reversible by prompting treating the associated triggering condition.

Braunwald E. Heart failure. *J Am Coll Cardiol HF*. 2013;1:1–20.

Damman K, et al. The cardiorenal syndrome in heart failure. *Prog Cardiovasc Dis*. 2011;54:144–53. [PMID: 21875513]

Haddad F, et al. Pulmonary hypertension associated with left heart disease: characteristics, emerging concepts, and treatment strategies. *Prog Cardiovasc Dis*. 2011;54:154–67. [PMID: 21875514]

Shah AM, et al. In search of new therapeutic targets and strategies for heart failure: recent advances in basic science. *Lancet*. 2011;378:704–12. [PMID: 21856484]

Triposkiadis F, et al. The sympathetic nervous system in heart failure physiology, pathophysiology, and clinical implications. *J Am Coll Cardiol*. 2009;54:1747–62. [PMID: 19874988]

▶ Clinical Findings

One of the first principles in the clinical evaluation is to determine whether the patient is indeed presenting with HF, since the presenting signs and symptoms are often nonspecific. Despite a careful history and physical examination, additional diagnostic information may be necessary to support the diagnosis and to determine the mechanism of the symptoms, the severity of the condition, and the prognosis for the individual patient.

A. Symptoms & Signs

The cardinal symptoms of HF are dyspnea and fatigue that occur with exertion and/or at rest, although some patients may present with acute pulmonary edema. **Dyspnea** is a subjective feeling of air hunger and is the most frequent symptom in HF patients. Initially, dyspnea on exertion will be noted by a change in the extent of physical activity that causes the shortness of breath. As the HF worsens, the intensity of exertion required to produce dyspnea will decrease, and eventually the dyspnea will be present at rest. Interestingly, the severity of dyspnea decreases after right ventricular failure develops.

Paroxysmal nocturnal dyspnea occurs after the patient has been in the supine position for some time. The patient wakes up suddenly with a sensation of choking and air hunger and assumes an upright posture to relieve the symptoms. Paroxysmal nocturnal dyspnea usually precedes orthopnea, may be associated with bronchospasm and wheezing (cardiac asthma), and is caused by a mobilization of interstitial fluid from infradiaphragmatic locations during recumbency with a resultant increase in the circulating blood volume and increased pulmonary venous pressure.

Orthopnea (dyspnea occurring within a few minutes after the patient assumes a supine position) has the same cause as paroxysmal nocturnal dyspnea, but represents a more severe cardiac dysfunction. While elevating the head of the bed, sitting up, or standing can improve the symptoms, the most severely affected patients usually sleep sitting upright.

Another manifestation of pulmonary congestion is a dry or nonproductive **cough** (especially at night) that is usually relieved by treating the elevated left-sided filling pressures.

As with dyspnea, the mechanism of **fatigue** in patients with systolic HF is unclear. Although the fatigue was attributed for many years to a low cardiac output, there is mounting evidence of contribution of abnormal skeletal muscle metabolism with shifts in fiber distribution (increase in the percentage of the fast-twitch, glycolytic, easily fatigable fibers) and muscle atrophy, even in the presence of a normal cardiac output. Chronic fatigue begets further inactivity, which leads to further deconditioning and a greater extent of disability.

Other disabling symptoms in HF patients include extreme **thirst** (associated with activation of the arginine–vasopressin system), **nocturia** (due to enhanced urine formation in the recumbent position when renal vasoconstriction decreases and venous return to the heart increases), **oliguria** (usually associated with either increased venous congestion or markedly reduced cardiac output), **cerebral symptoms**—memory impairment, confusion, insomnia—(usually markers of reduced cardiac output), and **ascites and abdominal fullness**, accompanied by **right upper quadrant pain, early satiety, and nausea** (usually related to passive hepatic and splanchnic congestion).

B. Physical Examination

Although most patients with HF appear well nourished, those with more advanced disease (especially in the setting of chronic splanchnic congestion) frequently appear malnourished. This appearance arises from poor caloric intake (due to early satiety and nausea) and impaired absorption of fat and, occasionally, a protein-losing enteropathy, in combination with an increased metabolism due to elevated levels of norepinephrine and tumor necrosis factor-α. The combination of reduced intake and increased energy expenditure leads to a reduction of tissue mass and, in some cases, to **cardiac cachexia**.

Patients with systolic HF frequently show evidence of increased sympathetic activity such as **diaphoresis, pallor** and coldness of the limbs, **peripheral cyanosis** of the digits, abnormal distention of the superficial veins, and compensatory **sinus tachycardia** (when the cardiac output is decreased).

Cheyne-Stokes respiration (alternating phases of hyperpnea and apnea in a crescendo-decrescendo manner) can be seen in patients with systolic HF and represents an altered neurogenic control of respiration, facilitated by a combination of pulmonary congestion, prolonged circulation time from lung to the brain, and decreased sensitivity of the respiratory center to hypercapnia and hypoxia.

Pulmonary rales can be heard at the lung bases, and they are a result of the transudation of fluid into the alveoli that subsequently moves into the airways. In pulmonary edema, coarse rales and wheezes are heard all over the lung fields and may be accompanied by frothy sputum. With progressive fluid accumulation, pleural effusions (hydrothorax) occur and will increase the severity of dyspnea by further reducing pulmonary vital capacity. **Dullness on percussion** is the characteristic sign, and shifting dullness can be found when the patient moves from the sitting to the lateral decubitus position. Breath sounds over the area of effusion are diminished or absent. Hydrothorax usually is reabsorbed slowly as diuresis ensues, but in many cases, the pleural effusion lags behind for many days after the symptoms disappear.

Symmetric pitting edema is common in systolic HF patients and involves the dependent portions of the body with higher venous pressure: feet and ankles of ambulatory patients and the sacral area of bedridden ones. With progressive, untreated disease, the edema becomes massive and generalized (anasarca), involving the genital area, the upper extremities, and the thoracic and abdominal walls. Occasionally, in massive overload, skin breakdown and extravasation of fluid can occur. Chronic edema results in increased pigmentation, reddening, and induration of the skin of the lower extremities (**stasis dermatitis**).

An important part of the volume status assessment is detecting the abnormal **distention of the internal jugular veins**. Patients should be examined while they are lying down, with the torso and head tilted at 45 degrees. A persistent elevation of the jugular venous pressure is one of the earliest and most reliable signs of HF and is a powerful prognostic indicator of increased risk of HF hospitalizations and all-cause mortality. The inability of the right ventricle to accept transient increases in venous return (**positive hepatojugular reflux**) is observed during transient compression (30–60 seconds) of the upper abdomen. Passive hepatic congestion is identified by epigastric fullness, **hepatomegaly** and tenderness on palpation, and dullness to percussion of the right upper quadrant. As with the hydrothorax, these findings may persist after other signs of HF have disappeared because it takes longer for hepatic congestion to disappear. Occasionally, systolic pulsations of the liver may be felt in patients with severe tricuspid regurgitation.

Although rarely used, the hemodynamic response to the **Valsalva maneuver** is simple to perform and carries one of the best combinations of specificity (91%) and sensitivity (69%) for the detection of elevated left ventricular filling pressures. The maneuver is performed with the blood pressure cuff inflated 15 mm Hg over the systolic blood pressure. While the physician auscultates over the brachial artery, the patient is asked to perform a forced expiratory effort against a closed airway (the Valsalva maneuver). In a normal response, the Korotkoff sounds disappear during sustained maneuver and reappear after release of the maneuver. An abnormal response, in which blood pressure sounds either do not reappear after the maneuver (absent overshoot) or are maintained throughout the maneuver (square wave), is found in patients with systolic HF and elevated left ventricular filling pressures.

Cardiomegaly, with a laterally displaced and sustained point of maximal impulse, can be found on physical examination, but this is a nonspecific finding. The decrease in ventricular compliance becomes apparent by the presence of a late diastolic atrial sound (S_4 gallop). A protodiastolic sound (S_3 gallop), better heard in more tachycardic patients, is caused by acute deceleration of ventricular inflow after the early filling phase and is a marker of increased left ventricular filling pressures. Together with elevated jugular venous pressure, the presence of a third heart sound is a powerful predictor of outcome and is associated with an increased risk of death and hospitalization for HF. **Systolic murmurs** are common in HF patients and are secondary to functional mitral or tricuspid regurgitation that results from ventricular dilatation.

Pulsus alternans (a regular rhythm of alternating strong and weak pulsations) is common in patients with systolic HF and is due to an alternation in the stroke volume of the left ventricle. If persistent, it usually implies advanced HF and a chronic low output state.

It is important to emphasize that HF remains a clinical diagnosis. While the symptoms, signs, and clinical findings can, in isolation, be ascribed to other conditions, a systematic integrated approach establishes the diagnosis of HF. Several scoring systems have been used in epidemiologic and clinical studies to diagnose HF, and the Framingham Heart Study criteria have been shown to have the best sensitivity and specificity (Table 26–1). Once the HF is diagnosed, it is important to determine the clinical profile (Figure 26–1) and the severity of symptoms (New York Heart Association functional class), which will dictate the subsequent therapy.

C. Laboratory Testing

Patients with new-onset HF should undergo routine laboratory tests when the condition is first diagnosed. This is also recommended for patients with chronic HF and acute decompensation, when there is a change in therapeutic intervention, or in periodic monitoring for clinical stability. A basic metabolic profile can show hyponatremia (marker of advanced HF or excessive diuretic use) and signs of renal dysfunction (elevated urea and creatinine). Congestion

Table 26–1. Clinical Framingham Heart Study Criteria for Heart Failure

Major Criteria	Minor Criteria
Paroxysmal nocturnal dyspnea or orthopnea	Dyspnea on exertion
Elevated jugular venous pressure	Night cough
Hepatojugular reflux	Tachycardia > 120 bpm
Pulmonary rales	Hepatomegaly
S_3 gallop	Bilateral lower extremity edema
Enlarging heart silhouette on consecutive chest x-rays	Pulmonary vascular engorgement on chest x-ray
Pulmonary edema on chest x-ray	Pleural effusion on chest x-ray
Weight loss on diuretics (> 10 lb in 5 days)	
Increased venous pressure > 16 cm H_2O (assessed via a central line)	

Presence of two major or one major and two minor criteria is required for heart failure diagnosis.

of the liver is often associated with abnormalities of liver function tests, while hyperglycemia and abnormalities in thyroid-stimulating hormone levels can identify concomitant precipitating conditions (such as diabetes or hyper- or hypothyroidism). The recognition of anemia and iron deficiency in patients with systolic HF is important, as early treatment may reverse these abnormalities.

Determining the level of BNP or of its amino-terminal fragment (NT-proBNP) provides important diagnostic utility for diagnosing HF in the acute clinical setting. BNP levels over 100 pg/mL and NT-proBNP levels higher than 450 pg/mL in younger patients or higher than 900 pg/mL in patients older than 50 years are highly sensitive and specific for HF when the clinical diagnosis is in doubt. Although several studies have shown the incremental prognostic value of serial natriuretic peptide level determination, the efficacy of natriuretic peptide–guided therapy in systolic HF patients remains controversial.

Serum cardiac troponins (at levels that do not meet myocardial infarction criteria) are detected in over half of systolic HF patients (including in those without significant coronary artery disease) and are usually a sign of volume overload and elevated left ventricular filling pressures. Detectable serum troponin levels carry powerful prognostic information and may help in tailoring of therapy (eg, initiation and rapid

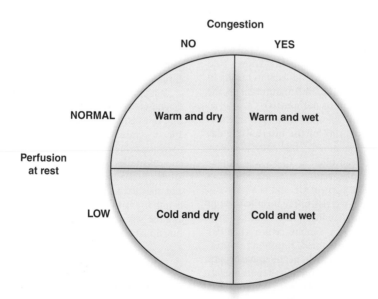

▲ **Figure 26–1.** Presentation of heart failure based on assessment of congestion and perfusion. ACE, angiotensin-converting enzyme.

Signs and symptoms of congestion: orthopnea, paroxysmal nocturnal dyspnea, jugular venous distension, positive hepatojugular reflux, pulmonary rales, hepatomegaly, symmetric pedal edema, and Valsalva maneuver square wave.

Evidence of impaired perfusion: sleepiness, cool extremities, narrow pulse pressure, low serum sodium, increased serum creatinine, and hypotension with ACE inhibitors.

titration of vasodilators and avoidance of positive intravenous inotropes in hospitalized patients).

D. Diagnostic Studies

1. Electrocardiography—An electrocardiogram should be routinely obtained and examined for evidence of underlying structural alterations (eg, left ventricular hypertrophy, prior myocardial infarctions), for rhythm abnormalities as a cause or consequence of HF decompensation (eg, atrial fibrillation/flutter, frequent ventricular ectopic beats, or sustained arrhythmias), and for the presence of conduction abnormalities (eg, left bundle branch block) that may lead to electrical dyssynchrony. The QT interval should be noted because many therapies can prolong it and provoke lethal arrhythmias. In patients who have undergone cardiac resynchronization therapy (CRT), changes in the QRS complex duration or morphology may provide information about underlying pacing or programming changes.

2. Chest radiography—Careful examination of the cardiac silhouette, as well as the pulmonary vasculature, remains part of routine evaluation in all patients with systolic HF. Cardiomegaly (cardiothoracic ratio > 50%) can be found in almost all patients with chronic HF, but may be absent in those with acute HF due to acute myocarditis or myocardial infarction. In systolic HF, there is progressive vasoconstriction of pulmonary vessels in the lower lobes and redistribution of the pulmonary flow to the upper lobes. Interstitial and perivascular edema develop when the left-sided filling pressures increase above 25 mm Hg and the bronchovascular markings at the bases become prominent. Kerley lines, spindle-shaped linear opacities at the periphery of the lung bases, occur in the later stages of HF. Pleural effusions can also be seen. After lowering of the pulmonary capillary pressure, there may be a delay of 48 hours before improvement and clearing of pulmonary findings can be seen on chest radiograph.

3. Echocardiography—Echocardiographic evaluation is an essential diagnostic tool for assessing cardiac structure and function. It should be used early in the initial phase of the HF diagnosis in order to define the syndrome (systolic versus diastolic HF), and at any time there is a clinical change that would lead to a change in management. A careful observer will examine the right and left ventricular size/volume, wall motion abnormalities (including aneurysms), hypertrophy, left ventricular diastolic function, left-/right-sided filling pressures, stroke volume, ejection fraction, presence of intracardiac thrombus or shunt, and valvular pathology (morphology, regurgitation, stenosis). A comprehensive examination can elucidate the cardiac component of the HF symptoms and may lead to targeted treatments (eg, diuresis versus vasodilatation versus need for inotropic support).

4. Cardiac magnetic resonance imaging (cMRI)—This newer imaging tool provides in-depth anatomic information and can provide information on the myocardial structure (scarring, fatty infiltration, or iron overload), helping in the noninvasive diagnosis of infiltrative cardiomyopathies (eg, sarcoidosis, amyloidosis), iron overload cardiomyopathies (eg, hemochromatosis), acute myocarditis, or genetic cardiomyopathies (eg, arrhythmogenic right ventricular cardiomyopathy, left ventricular noncompaction cardiomyopathy). In addition, in patients with coronary artery disease, it can relay information on myocardial viability that can be used to decide on percutaneous or surgical revascularization. The major limitations are the use of a magnetic field (which can interfere with cardiac implantable electrical devices that many systolic HF patients have), its relative high cost (limiting its use to major medical centers), and the claustrophobic feeling that many patients experience.

5. Cardiopulmonary exercise stress testing (CPET)—CPET has been shown to add substantial precision in the initial evaluation of patients with HF and in their prognosis over time, especially when advanced therapies are considered. Measurements of the peak oxygen consumption (peak V_{O_2}) and the slope of the ratio of ventilation (V_E) to carbon dioxide production (V_{CO_2}) (V_E/V_{CO_2}) are powerful predictors of prognosis. A peak V_{O_2} less than 14 mL/kg/min in patients intolerant of β-blockers (12 mL/kg/min on patients on β-blockers) or less than 50% predicted are considered indications for heart transplantation or left ventricular assist devices as destination therapy. Additionally, valuable information regarding chronotropic competence can be gathered from the CPET.

6. Cardiac catheterization—Because coronary artery disease is the main cause of systolic HF in the United States, coronary angiography is necessary whenever the suspicion for coronary artery disease as etiologic or aggravating factor of HF is suspected. Research has clearly shown that misdiagnosis of ischemic heart disease among patients with HF is common if angiographic evaluation is not undertaken as part of the initial workup. In addition, surgical revascularization in ischemic systolic HF has been shown to improve cardiovascular outcomes.

Right heart catheterization may be important in patients who are doing poorly with severe congestion, ascites, or signs and symptoms of low cardiac output or when constrictive physiology or restrictive cardiomyopathy is suspected. Most right-sided heart catheterizations performed in patients with HF today are used to help guide therapy rather than to make a specific diagnosis.

7. Endomyocardial biopsy—The role of diagnostic endomyocardial biopsy in patients with systolic HF has diminished. Although cMRI has replaced many of its uses, endomyocardial biopsy is still used in patients with suspected fulminant myocarditis, giant cell myocarditis, sarcoidosis, amyloid heart disease, or hemochromatosis. In addition, routine surveillance for rejection after cardiac transplantation still uses endomyocardial biopsies (at least for the first 6–12 months).

8. Genetic testing—Clinical genetic testing in HF has become available in many commercial testing laboratories. At the present time, the best use of genetic testing remains identification of at-risk individuals for inherited cardiomyopathies that will require careful evaluation and close monitoring (eg, hypertrophic cardiomyopathy, arrhythmogenic right ventricular dysplasia). In addition, for specific diseases (eg, transthyretin amyloidosis, some of the idiopathic dilated cardiomyopathies), genetic tests are available for confirmatory purposes. In the future, it is possible that pharmacogenomics-guided therapy will be used to better select HF therapies most likely to benefit a specific patient.

Arena R, et al. Cardiopulmonary exercise testing in the clinical evaluation of patients with heart and lung disease. *Circulation.* 2011;123:668–80. [PMID: 21321183]

Braunwald E. Biomarkers in heart failure. *N Engl J Med.* 2008;358:2148–59. [PMID: 18480207]

Karamitsos TD, et al. The role of cardiovascular magnetic resonance imaging in heart failure. *J Am Coll Cardiol.* 2009;54: 1407–24. [PMID: 19796734]

▶ Treatment

A. Prevention

The burden of HF can be affected only by drastically decreasing its incidence, and as such, it is crucial to identify the primary drivers for this problem and develop/implement population-level preventive strategies. To aid in this goal, the American College of Cardiology/American Heart Association adopted a new stage-based system for the classification of HF in 2001 (Table 26–2). In this approach, stage A included patients without structural cardiac disorders or HF symptoms, but with risk factors that clearly predispose carriers toward the development of HF (eg, hypertension, coronary artery disease, diabetes). Stage B included patients without HF symptoms, but with structural cardiac abnormalities (eg, left ventricular hypertrophy, prior myocardial infarction, valvular heart disease) that if untreated could progress to symptomatic HF. Stages C and D included the symptomatic HF patients. This new classification added a useful dimension to the understanding of HF by recognizing that there are established risk factors and structural prerequisites for the development of the clinical syndrome and that therapeutic interventions performed even before the appearance of left ventricular dysfunction or symptoms can prevent the development of HF.

Because nearly 33% of adults in the United States have hypertension and due to the high PAR of hypertension in HF in both men and women, aggressive control of blood pressure is the most effective approach to reduce the incidence of HF. Primary prevention trials have shown up to a 50% reduction in the incidence of HF in patients with hypertension who are treated with thiazide diuretics, ACE inhibitors, angiotensin II receptor blockers (ARBs), and most β-blockers and calcium channel blockers.

The roles of coronary artery disease and myocardial infarction as major antecedents of systolic HF have been well established. Therapy with ACE inhibitors has been shown to reduce the risk of developing HF in patients with stable coronary artery disease, while therapy with ACE inhibitors, ARBs, β-blockers, and mineralocorticoid receptor blockers (MRBs) have been shown in several randomized trials to reduce the risk of progression to symptomatic HF in patients with myocardial infarction and asymptomatic left ventricular systolic dysfunction.

Diabetes mellitus has been consistently associated with a two- to fivefold increase in the risk of HF, especially in women. Although several studies have shown an 8–16% increase in the risk of hospitalizations for HF for every 1% increase in hemoglobin A1c, the optimal treatment strategy (eg, insulin versus metformin versus sulfonylureas versus thiazolidinediones) is currently unknown.

B. Nonpharmacologic Treatment

1. Dietary measures—It is widely believed that HF management should include dietary sodium and fluid restriction, recommendations endorsed by all national and international guidelines. Most current recommendations are for 2000–3000 mg/day sodium for all HF patients and for less than 2000 mg/day with some degree of fluid restriction (1500–2000 mL/day) for HF patients with volume overload. Given the possibility that increased sodium intake leads to increased fluid retention in HF, it has been assumed that a low-sodium diet would improve outcomes in HF patients. However, the data on which these recommendations are drawn are limited, and the few clinical trials conducted to date have produced inconsistent findings. The new American Heart Association recommendations for 1500 mg/day sodium appear to be appropriate for patients with stage A and B, because of the data linking sodium intake with incidence of hypertension and HF. However, there are insufficient data to support a certain level of sodium or fluid intake in symptomatic HF patients (stages C and D).

2. Physical activity and exercise training—For decades, exercise testing and exercise training were considered dangerous in patients with systolic HF because of concerns about exacerbating HF symptoms, potential deleterious effects on ventricular function, and the possibility of severe ventricular arrhythmias and cardiac arrest. Recent work has shown that exercise training in these patients is associated with improved response to pharmacologic vasodilators, improved endothelial function, improved skeletal muscle metabolism and performance, and attenuation of the activation of the overactive muscle ergoreflex. The large randomized trial, Heart Failure: A Controlled Trial Investigating Outcomes of Exercise Training (HF-ACTION), showed that in patients with symptomatic systolic HF exercise training was safe (no increase in arrhythmias over usual care) and was associated with a significant decrease in hospitalizations for

Table 26–2. Staging System in the Classification of Heart Failure

ACC/AHA Staging	Clinical Heart Failure	Symptoms (NYHA Functional Class)	Population Estimate from NHANES (millions)[1]	Population Estimate: Adults > Age 45 from Olmsted County (%)[2]
D **Refractory, end-stage** (Marked symptoms despite maximal therapy)	Yes	IIIB-IV	0.2	0.2
C **Symptomatic HF** (Shortness of breath, fatigue, reduced exercise tolerance)	Yes	I-IIIA	5.1	11.8
B **Asymptomatic HF** (Prior myocardial infarction, left ventricular hypertrophy, valvular disease, etc.)	No	None	10	34
A **High Risk for Developing HF** (Hypertension, coronary disease, diabetes, obesity, etc.)	No	None	60	22
None	No	None	237	32

ACC, American College of Cardiology; AHA, American Heart Association; HF, heart failure; NHANES, National Health and Nutrition Examination Survey; NYHA, New York Heart Association.
[1]From Go AS, et al; on behalf of the American Heart Association Statistics Committee and Stroke Statistics Subcommittee. Heart disease and stroke statistics–2013 update: a report from the American Heart Association. *Circulation.* 2013;127:e6-245
[2]From Olmsted country, adapted from Ammar KA, et al. Prevalence and prognostic significance of heart failure stages: application of the American College of Cardiology/American Heart Association heart failure staging criteria in the community. *Circulation.* 2007;115: 1563–70.

HF and an improvement in the patients' well-being and in exercise capacity. Thus, all patients with systolic HF should be prescribed an exercise training program in addition to evidence-based pharmacologic therapy.

3. Treatment of sleep-disordered breathing—Sleep-disordered breathing is common in systolic HF patients and is associated with adverse prognosis. Continuous positive airway pressure is the major treatment, especially if obstructive rather than central sleep apnea predominates, and its use has been associated with improvement in symptoms and ejection fraction. Adequate suppression of central sleep apnea by positive airway pressure may also be associated with improved survival. Bilevel positive airway pressure may be preferable over continuous pressure in patients who experience expiratory pressure discomfort. Adaptive (or auto) servo ventilation, which adjusts the positive airway pressure depending on the patient's airflow or tidal volume, may be useful in HF patients if continuous pressure is found ineffective.

4. Ultrafiltration—The mechanical removal of fluid from the vasculature is accomplished by applying hydrostatic

pressure across a semipermeable membrane, resulting in isotonic plasma water separation from blood; thus, large amounts of fluid can be removed without affecting serum concentration of electrolytes and other solutes. Several small studies in HF patients have shown that ultrafiltration was associated with relief of congestive symptoms, improved exercise capacity, lower intracardiac filling pressures, and improved pulmonary function and neurohormonal levels. In recent years, ultrafiltration gained immense popularity in the treatment of hospitalized patients with HF and volume overload, and it has been increasingly used even in outpatient settings in HF patients at risk for readmission. However, in the recently published Cardiorenal Rescue Study in Acute Decompensated Heart Failure (CARESS-HF) trial, the use of a stepped diuretic algorithm was superior to a strategy of ultrafiltration for the preservation of renal function, with a similar amount of weight loss. Due to the possible side effects related to the ultrafiltration therapy, it should be reserved only for inpatients with HF and volume overload with preserved renal function who are not responding adequately to high-dose diuretic therapy.

Bart BA, et al; Heart Failure Clinical Research Network. Ultrafiltration in decompensated heart failure with cardio-renal syndrome. *N Engl J Med.* 2012;367:2296–304. [PMID: 23131078]

Gupta D, et al. Dietary sodium intake in heart failure. *Circulation.* 2012;126:479–85. [PMID: 22825409]

O'Connor CM, et al; HF-ACTION Investigators. Efficacy and safety of exercise training in patients with chronic heart failure: HF-ACTION randomized controlled trial. *JAMA.* 2009;301:1439–50. [PMID: 19351941]

Sharma BK, et al. Adaptive servoventilation for treatment of sleep-disordered breathing in heart failure: a systematic review and meta-analysis. *Chest.* 2012;142:1211–121. [PMID: 22722232]

C. Pharmacologic Treatment: Life-Saving Therapies

The pharmacologic treatment of symptomatic systolic HF has evolved substantially in the past 40 years, with neurohormonal antagonists becoming the mainstay of treatment due to marked improvements in morbidity and mortality.

1. ACE inhibitors—Inhibition of ACE in HF results in an increase in the cardiac output, with concomitant decrease in ventricular filling pressures and pulmonary and systemic vascular resistances, without an increase in the heart rate. Over time, ACE inhibition leads to a decrease in left ventricular end-systolic and end-diastolic dimensions, a reduction in the incidence of ventricular arrhythmias, and continuous and sustained improvements in symptoms (occurring as early as 2 weeks), exercise duration, and quality of life. The most significant benefit of therapy with ACE inhibitors is the 20% increase in survival seen in all patients with systolic HF and in all patients with left ventricular systolic dysfunction after myocardial infarction, even in those without symptoms or signs of HF.

ACE inhibitors should be used in conjunction with β-blockers and MRBs as part of the "triple therapy" in order to achieve the maximal symptomatic improvement and survival benefit, and with a diuretic to maintain the sodium balance and prevent the development of fluid overload. The highest tolerated ACE inhibitor dose should be achieved, as clinical trials have shown improved HF outcomes at higher doses. Once the drug has been titrated (Table 26–3), patients can usually be maintained on long-term therapy with little difficulty. The need to decrease the ACE inhibitor dose due to hypotension and/or renal dysfunction may signal the development of end-stage HF and the need for advanced therapies (ie, ventricular assist devices, heart transplantation). Renal function and serum potassium should be assessed within 2 weeks of initiating therapy and every 3 months thereafter.

The main adverse effects of the therapy are related to the angiotensin suppression (hypotension, increase in serum creatinine and potassium) and bradykinin potentiation (cough and angioedema). The initial hypotension responds to a decrease in the dose of diuretic, liberalization of salt intake, or initiation of a lower dose of ACE inhibitor. Hypotension can be delayed and prolonged with longer acting ACE inhibitors (enalapril and lisinopril), leading to decreased systemic perfusion and compromise of renal and cerebral functions, but is shorter in duration with captopril, which rarely compromises organ perfusion. Some patients may be very sensitive to the hypotensive effects of ACE inhibitors, particularly end-stage HF patients who are dependent on the RAAS for blood pressure maintenance. In general, treatment should be reassessed if serum creatinine increases above 3 mg/dL or if serum potassium increases above 5.5 mEq/L. Patients should not be given ACE inhibitors if they are pregnant, have a history of angioedema or anuric renal failure during a previous exposure to this class, or are severely hypotensive and at risk of immediate cardiogenic shock.

2. ARBs—These agents block the angiotensin II receptor and inhibit the effects of angiotensin II produced not only through the classical ACE pathway, but also by the chymase pathway. Available ARBs block the angiotensin II type 1 receptors (associated with myocardial hypertrophy and remodeling) and enhance the activation of angiotensin II type 2 receptors, causing vasodilation. In addition, these effects are achieved without accumulation of bradykinin, which is considered to be responsible for some of the adverse reactions associated with the use of ACE inhibitors, such as cough or angioedema. Although the hemodynamic effects of ARBs are similar to those of ACE inhibitors, the randomized clinical trials have shown a consistent mortality benefit only in patients with systolic HF who are intolerant of ACE inhibitors. Candesartan was the only ARB that showed in clinical trials a 15% reduction in mortality when added to an ACE inhibitor. Use of ARBs in higher doses (see Table 26–3) in addition to ACE inhibitors and β-blockers is associated with symptomatic improvement and an overall modest 15% reduction in HF hospitalizations.

3. MRBs—Despite treatment with ACE inhibitors or ARBs, patients with HF demonstrate elevated aldosterone levels, due to alternative stimuli for aldosterone synthesis (eg, adrenocorticotropic hormone or endothelin), potassium-dependent aldosterone secretion, and reduced aldosterone clearance. Spironolactone is a renal competitive aldosterone antagonist, inhibiting its effect by competing for the aldosterone-dependent sodium–potassium exchange site in the distal tubule cells. Eplerenone is a selective MRB that prevents the binding of aldosterone and is devoid of the painful gynecomastia seen in about 10% of men taking spironolactone. Multiple clinical trials have shown that use of MRBs in addition to ACE inhibitors and β-blockers in patients with systolic HF and a variety of symptoms (New York Heart Association functional class II–IV) leads to a 15–30% decrease in mortality (including a 20% decrease in sudden cardiac death immediately after a myocardial infarction), improvement in HF symptoms, and a 30–40%

Table 26–3. Target Doses of Renin–Angiotensin–Aldosterone System Inhibitors in Heart Failure

Agent	Starting Dose (mg)	Target Dose (mg)	Frequency	Trial(s)
ACE inhibitors				
Captopril	6.25	50	Three times daily	SAVE
Enalapril	5	10	Twice daily	SOLVD P/T
Fosinopril	10	40	Daily	FEST
Lisinopril	2.5	40	Daily	ATLAS
Ramipril	2.5	5	Twice daily	AIRE
Trandolapril	1	4	Daily	TRACE
ARBs				
Candesartan	4	32	Daily	CHARM
Losartan	25	150	Daily	HEAAL
Valsartan	40	160	Twice daily	VALHEFT
MRBs				
Eplerenone	12.5	50	Daily	EMPHASIS-HF, EPHESUS
Spironolactone	25	25	Daily	RALES

ACE, angiotensin-converting enzyme; AIRE, Acute Infarction Ramipril Efficacy; ARB, angiotensin II receptor blocker; ATLAS, Assessment of Treatment with Lisinopril and Survival; CHARM, Candesartan in Heart failure: Assessment of Reduction in Mortality and Morbidity; EMPHASIS-HF, Eplerenone in Mild Patients Hospitalization and Survival Study in Heart Failure; EPHESUS, Eplerenone Postacute Myocardial Infarction Heart Failure Efficacy and Survival; FEST, Fosinopril Efficacy/Safety Trial; HEAAL, Heart Failure Endpoint Evaluation of Angiotensin II Antagonists Losartan; MRB, mineralocorticoid receptor blocker; RALES, Randomized Aldactone Evaluation Study; SAVE, Survival and Ventricular Enlargement Trial; SOLVD P/T, Studies of Left Ventricular Dysfunction Prevention/Treatment; TRACE, Trandolapril Cardiac Evaluation; VALHEFT, Valsartan Heart Failure Trial.

decrease in hospitalizations for HF. Due to these significant benefits in a variety of systolic HF patients, MRBs and not ARBs should be the drugs of choice in the initial triple therapy with ACE inhibitors and β-blockers. The use of MRBs should be restricted to those patients with an estimated glomerular filtration rate above 30 mL/min/1.73 m² and with serum potassium below 5 mEq/L; potassium levels should be monitored within a week of initiation and at least every 4 weeks for the first 3 months and every 3 months thereafter. Although low, the risk of hyperkalemia is real with these agents and can lead to a significant increase in morbidity and mortality.

4. β-Adrenergic receptor blockers—β-Blockers act by inhibiting the adverse effects of the sympathetic nervous system activation in patients with systolic HF. Long-term benefits of β-blockade include an increase in ejection fraction, a decrease in left ventricular volumes and in mitral regurgitation, and a reversion of the left ventricle to a more elliptical shape. Administration of β-blockers is associated with an early deterioration in cardiac function (consistent with the negative inotropic effects), followed

by return to baseline values after 1 month and an increase in the ejection fraction after 3 months of treatment with further improvement for up to a year. Although the exercise capacity may not be improved by objective assessments (CPET), β-blockers, when added to ACE inhibitors, lead to marked symptomatic improvement, translated in robust 18% decreases in hospitalizations for HF and 35% improvement in survival. Only three β-blockers (bisoprolol, carvedilol, and metoprolol succinate) have been consistently shown to improve symptoms and survival in clinical trials, and therefore, only these should be used in patients with systolic HF. As in the case of ACE inhibitors, use of the highest tolerated β-blocker doses is recommended due to improvement in outcomes. In direct comparison studies, carvedilol was associated with better survival than metoprolol tartrate; in addition, the incidences of myocardial infarction, stroke, atrial fibrillation, and diabetes were lower with the use of carvedilol. In patients with reactive airway disease, bisoprolol has been shown to improve the peak expiratory flow and be better tolerated compared to the other approved β-blockers.

Table 26–4. Target Doses of β-Blockers in Heart Failure.

Agent	Starting Dose (mg)	Target Dose (mg)	Frequency	Trial(s)
Bisoprolol	2.5	10	Daily	CIBIS I, II, III
Carvedilol	3.125	25	Twice daily	CAPRICORN, COPERNICUS, U.S. carvedilol trials
Metoprolol succinate	25	200	Daily	MERIT-HF
Nebivolol[1]	1.25	10	Daily	SENIORS

[1]Approved for use for systolic heart failure patients in Europe only. CAPRICORN, Carvedilol Post-Infarct Survival Control in Left Ventricular Dysfunction; CIBIS, Cardiac Insufficiency Bisoprolol Study; COPERNICUS, Carvedilol Prospective Randomized Cumulative Survival; MERIT-HF, Metoprolol CR/XL Randomised Intervention Trial in Congestive Heart Failure; SENIORS, Study of the Effects of Nebivolol Intervention on Outcomes and Rehospitalisation in Seniors with Heart Failure.

β-Blockers should be prescribed to all patients with asymptomatic left ventricular systolic dysfunction and stable systolic HF unless they have a contraindication. Patients should be clinically stable, receive ACE inhibitors and MRBs, and receive diuretics as needed to control the fluid retention associated with adrenergic blockade. β-Blockers should be initiated at very low doses (in euvolemic, noninotrope-dependent patients) and increased gradually, typically at 2-week intervals, to achieve the target doses from published clinical trials (Table 26–4).

Treatment with β-blockers can be associated with fatigue and weakness, which usually resolve in a few weeks. Symptomatic bradycardia is a serious adverse effect that requires a decrease in the dose or sometimes cardiac pacing. Hypotension is a side effect seen especially with nonselective blockers such as carvedilol. Usually, it occurs within the first 48 hours of initiation of therapy and subsides with repeated dosing without any change in the dose. Administration of ACE inhibitors and diuretics at a different time of day than the β-blockers can minimize the hypotension and dizziness. Administration of β-blockers is contraindicated in patients with severe bronchospasm, systolic blood pressure below 85 mm Hg, symptomatic bradycardia, or advanced heart block in the absence of a pacemaker.

5. Hydralazine-nitrates combination—Nitrates have a greater effect on venous capacitance (venodilation) than on the arterial system, while hydralazine is a direct-acting smooth muscle relaxant that seems to dilate arterioles predominantly. Long-term administration of isosorbide dinitrate has been associated with significant improvements in

hemodynamic parameters, exercise capacity, and relief of symptoms in moderate-to-severe systolic HF. When used in combination with nitrates, hydralazine has shown a short-term increase in cardiac output and decrease in ventricular filling pressure. Patients who have dilated left ventricles appear to have a better hemodynamic and clinical response than do patients with lesser degrees of enlargement. The combination therapy was tested in African Americans with systolic HF in the African-American Heart Failure Trial (A-HeFT) and was associated with a significant 43% improvement in survival and a 33% decrease in HF hospitalizations, when used in addition to ACE inhibitors, β-blockers, and spironolactone. These results led to the first approval of a combination drug pill based on self-identified ethnicity. When the endothelial nitric oxide synthase (through which the combination of drugs is thought to work) was genotyped, the benefits of the therapy were evident only in those patients who were homozygous for glutamic acid in position 298 (GLU298GLU). Although 80% of African Americans have this genomic variant (as shown in A-HeFT), studies have shown that up to 40% of Caucasians have the same genotype, leading to intriguing possibilities for future pharmacogenomically targeted therapies. Unfortunately, the therapy is not easily tolerated due to side effects. Nitrates can produce headaches, while hydralazine can be associated with flushing, palpitations, nausea, vomiting, myocardial ischemia, and lupus-like syndrome.

Yancy CW, et al. 2013 American College of Cardiology Foundation/American Heart Association guidelines for the management of heart failure: a report of the American College of Cardiology Foundation/American Heart Association Task Force on Practice Guidelines. *J Am Coll Cardiol*. 2013; S0735-1097(13)02114-1. [PMID: 23747642]

Konstam MA, et al; HEAAL Investigators. Effects of high-dose versus low-dose losartan on clinical outcomes in patients with heart failure (HEAAL study): a randomised, double-blind trial. *Lancet*. 2009;374:1840–8. [PMID: 19922995]

Krum H, et al. Medical therapy for chronic heart failure. *Lancet*. 2011;378:713–21. [PMID: 21856485]

McNamara DM, et al. Endothelial nitric oxide synthase (NOS3) polymorphisms in African Americans with heart failure: results from the A-HeFT trial. *J Card Fail*. 2009;15:191–8. [PMID: 19327620]

Zannad F, et al; EMPHASIS-HF Study Group. Eplerenone in patients with systolic heart failure and mild symptoms. *N Engl J Med*. 2011;364:11–21. [PMID: 21678313]

D. Pharmacologic Treatment: Symptomatic Therapies

1. Diuretics—**Diuretics** provide rapid symptomatic relief of congestive symptoms by promoting excretion of sodium and water and lowering plasma volume, thus reducing congestion in the pulmonary and systemic vascular beds and improving symptoms and functional capacity. Diuretics are tightly bound to plasma proteins and are actively secreted into the proximal tubular lumen. Loop diuretics inhibit the sodium/potassium/chloride symporter in the ascending loop of Henle; thiazide-type diuretics affect the sodium/chloride transporter in the distal convoluted tubules; whereas potassium-sparing diuretics work at sites in the collecting duct to inhibit the sodium/potassium transporter. The loop diuretics increase sodium excretion by 20–25% and enhance free water clearance. Orally dosed furosemide has variable bioavailability (10–100% in patients with HF), whereas bumetanide and torsemide are absorbed more completely, with 80% bioavailability after oral dosing. Although thiazide diuretics have bioavailability of 60–70%, their action is limited if the glomerular filtration falls below 40 mL/min/1.73m^2 (with the exception of chlorothiazide and metolazone). Furosemide and thiazides are renally excreted, whereas the liver metabolizes torsemide and bumetanide. Thiazides and distal tubule diuretics have longer half-lives that allow them to be given once daily or even every other day. Because the plasma half-life of loop diuretics ranges from 1 to 4 hours, once a dose of a loop diuretic has been administered, its effect dissipates before the next dose is given. During this time, the nephron avidly reabsorbs sodium, resulting in rebound sodium retention that nullifies the prior natriuresis. In order to counteract this, the loop diuretics have to be given twice daily. Despite rapid symptomatic improvement, several retrospective analyses of systolic HF trials have linked non–potassium-sparing diuretics with an increase in mortality. Therefore, the lowest dose that achieves the desired effect should be used.

Diuretics should be used in all patients with evidence of volume overload; in an acutely decompensated state, a higher dose or combination of oral diuretics or intravenous diuretics is needed to achieve euvolemia. Using too low a diuretic dose causes fluid retention, which can diminish the response to ACE inhibitors and increase the risk of treatment with β-blockers. Use of inappropriately high doses of diuretics leads to volume contraction and increased risk of hypotension and renal insufficiency with ACE inhibitors. Diuretic resistance can be overcome by the intravenous administration of diuretics (intermittent bolus or continuous infusions have the same efficacy), the use of diuretic combinations (eg, loop and thiazide), or use of intravenous diuretics with low dose dopamine. Volume depletion (resulting in hypotension and/or renal failure), hypokalemia, hypomagnesemia, and thiamine deficiency are the most common side effects of diuretics. Diuretics may also cause metabolic alkalosis, carbohydrate intolerance, hyperuricemia, hypersensitivity reactions, and acute pancreatitis.

2. Digoxin—Digoxin exerts its effects by inhibition of sodium-potassium adenosine triphosphatase in the myocardium (resulting in an increase in myocardial contraction), in the vagal afferent fibers (sensitizing the cardiac baroreceptors and reducing the sympathetic outflow), and in the kidney (reducing the renal tubular reabsorption of sodium). These observations have led to the hypothesis that

the beneficial effects of digoxin in HF are due to the attenuation of the activation of neurohormonal systems. Clinically, the beneficial effects in patients with systolic HF and sinus rhythm include improved HF symptoms, increased exercise time, modestly increased ejection fraction, enhanced cardiac output, and decreased HF hospitalizations. The benefits of digoxin are higher in patients with more symptomatic HF (New York Heart Association functional class IV), cardiomegaly (greater cardiothoracic ratio on chest x-ray), or an ejection fraction below 25%. However, due to its narrow therapeutic index, digoxin has a bidirectional effect with improvement in HF mortality and increase in the non-HF (presumed arrhythmic) mortality. Retrospective analyses of the Digitalis Investigation Group (DIG) trial have suggested an increased mortality with serum concentration above 1 ng/mL, especially in women. Due to these considerations, digoxin has been reserved in systolic HF patients in sinus rhythm who are still symptomatic despite triple therapy with ACE inhibitors, β-blockers, and MRBs. In patients with systolic HF and atrial fibrillation, digoxin can be used to decrease the ventricular response, usually associated with improved symptoms. Although more rare than in prior decades, digitalis intoxication may occur in patients hospitalized for HF. Common findings are nausea, vomiting, anorexia, malaise, drowsiness, headache, insomnia, altered color vision, or arrhythmia. Cardiac arrhythmias (most commonly premature ventricular beats, junctional tachycardia, paroxysmal atrial tachycardia with block, bidirectional ventricular tachycardia) can be caused by digitalis and are facilitated by hypokalemia. Digoxin toxicity is usually confirmed by the reversal of symptoms or cessation of arrhythmias after withdrawal of digoxin therapy. Severe toxicity can be reversed quickly with digoxin immune Fab.

Felker GM, et al. Diuretics and ultrafiltration in acute decompensated heart failure. *J Am Coll Cardiol.* 2012;59:2145–53. [PMID: 22676934]

E. Pharmacologic Treatment: Other Therapies

1. Oral phosphodiesterase-5 inhibitors—Due to the chronic elevation in left ventricular filling pressures, a large number of systolic HF patients will develop secondary pulmonary hypertension. While the presence of fixed pulmonary hypertension has been shown to be a poor prognostic factor in patients undergoing heart transplantation, recent studies have suggested that improvement in pulmonary artery pressures with **oral phosphodiesterase-5 inhibitors** (ie, sildenafil, tadalafil) may lead to improvements in symptoms in HF patients. Although this hypothesis has been recently rejected in the Evaluating the Effectiveness of Sildenafil at Improving Health Outcomes and Exercise Ability in People with Diastolic Heart Failure (RELAX) study, a large randomized trial will address the question in patients with systolic HF and pulmonary hypertension. Until the results of the PDE5 Inhibition with Tadalafil Changes

Outcomes in Heart Failure (PITCH-HF) trial become available, it is prudent to use these drugs in patients with systolic HF and pulmonary hypertension, only if they are compensated and have a pulmonary capillary wedge pressure close to normal.

2. Antiarrhythmic agents—More than 80% of systolic HF patients have frequent and complex ventricular arrhythmias as documented by Holter monitoring, and 50% have frequent nonsustained ventricular tachycardia. In addition, 35–40% of patients have paroxysmal or persistent atrial fibrillation that can lead to HF exacerbation. Systolic HF patients frequently require some antiarrhythmic drugs in order to stabilize these arrhythmias. Due to the structural heart disease seen in HF, only some of the class III antiarrhythmics (dofetilide and amiodarone) are safe to use. Although clinical trials have shown that amiodarone per se does not improve prognosis in systolic HF patients, they have also shown that it is a rather safe option. It can be administered acutely to control ventricular response in HF patients with atrial fibrillation, and its long-term use may restore and maintain sinus rhythm. Amiodarone may also be used to suppress symptomatic ventricular tachycardia in combination with β-blockers, especially in patients who are receiving frequent defibrillator shocks. Close monitoring for side effects is required. Dofetilide was shown to be effective in restoring sinus rhythm in patients with systolic HF and atrial fibrillation without adverse effects on overall survival. Treatment with dofetilide also decreased the overall and HF hospitalizations in the Danish Investigations of Arrhythmia and Mortality on Dofetilide (DIAMOND) study. However, dofetilide dosing has to be closely titrated, based on creatinine clearance and QT interval, requiring 72-hour inpatient monitoring. Dronedarone is a benzofuran-derivative class III antiarrhythmic drug with pharmacologic properties similar to amiodarone and should not be used in patients with systolic HF due to the increased mortality risk associated with the drug.

3. Antithrombotic therapy—In patients with systolic HF and sinus rhythm, antithrombotic therapy has traditionally been considered for those with very low ejection fraction. However, a multitude of clinical trials have failed to show a clear benefit of this strategy in preventing strokes in these patients. As such, the decision to use an antiplatelet or anticoagulant must be individualized, taking into account the comorbidities of the patient (eg, presence of concomitant coronary artery disease or peripheral vascular disease). All patients with systolic HF and atrial fibrillation (even paroxysmal) should be anticoagulated with warfarin or newer antithrombotic agents (apixaban, dabigatran, or rivaroxaban) in order to prevent strokes.

4. Statins (3-hydroxy-3-methyl-glutaryl-coenzyme A reductase inhibitors)—Statins are the cornerstone of primary and secondary prevention for patients with coronary artery disease or vascular disease. Paradoxically, even though 70% of systolic HF patients have coronary artery disease, the role of statins in systolic HF is only marginal. Two large randomized clinical trials testing the role of rosuvastatin in this setting failed to show a benefit on mortality. Patients with underlying coronary artery disease experienced a reduction in cardiovascular hospitalizations, presumably by averting small myocardial infarctions due to plaque destabilization. As such, statins should only be used in patients with systolic HF and clinical coronary artery disease.

5. Omega-3 polyunsaturated fatty acids—The use of omega-3 polyunsaturated acids in systolic HF patients leads to small improvements in left ventricular ejection fraction, reduction in left ventricular end systolic volumes and functional capacity, and a small 10% decrease in cardiovascular mortality and 7% decrease in risk for cardiovascular hospitalizations. The dose used in clinical trials of 1 g (850–882 mg eicosapentaenoic acid and docosahexaenoic acid as ethyl esters in the average ratio of 1:1.2) is much smaller than the dose used to treat hypertriglyceridemia and, therefore, more likely to be tolerated by patients.

6. Intravenous iron therapy—Iron deficiency is quite frequent in patients with systolic HF, and several small studies and one large randomized trial showed improvements in symptoms, exercise capacity, and quality of life with intravenous ferric carboxymaltose. **Intravenous iron therapy** (there are several preparations available) is relatively safe and should be used for all patients with systolic HF who are iron deficient even in the absence of anemia (ferritin level < 100 mcg/L or 100–299 mcg/L if the transferrin saturation is < 20%).

Although anemia is common and portends poor prognosis in systolic HF, treatment with **darbepoetin** was not associated with improved survival or decrease in hospitalization in these patients. Moreover, patients treated with darbepoetin experience more thromboembolic events, and thus, the erythropoiesis-simulating agents should not be used or should be used very cautiously in systolic HF patients. In patients with decompensated HF and hemoglobin level < 10 g/dL, careful transfusion with packed red blood cells, while giving diuretics, has been shown to improve outcomes.

GISSI-HF Investigators, et al. Effect of n-3 polyunsaturated fatty acids in patients with chronic heart failure (the GISSI-HF trial): a randomised, double-blind, placebo-controlled trial. *Lancet.* 2008;372:1223–30. [PMID: 18757090]

Homma S, et al; WARCEF Investigators. Warfarin and aspirin in patients with heart failure and sinus rhythm. *N Engl J Med.* 2012;366:1859–69. [PMID: 22551105]

Kjekshus J, et al; CORONA Group. Rosuvastatin in older patients with systolic heart failure. *N Engl J Med.* 2007;357:2248–61. [PMID: 17984166]

Køber L, et al.; Dronedarone Study Group. Increased mortality after dronedarone therapy for severe heart failure. *N Engl J Med.* 2008;358:2678–87. [PMID: 18565860]

Redfield MM, et al; for the RELAX Trial. Effect of phosphodiesterase-5 inhibition on exercise capacity and clinical status in heart failure with preserved ejection fraction: a randomized clinical trial. *JAMA*. 2013;309:1268–77. [PMID: 23478662]

Swedberg K, et al; for the RED-HF Committees and Investigators. Treatment of anemia with darbepoetin-alfa in systolic heart failure. *N Engl J Med*. 2013 Mar 28;368(13):1210-9. [PMID: 23473338]

F. Pharmacologic Treatment: Specific Therapies in Hospitalized Patients

The majority of hospitalized patients with systolic HF are volume overloaded and may require **vasodilators** in order to decrease the filling pressures and improve dyspnea. For faster action, intravenous options such as sodium nitroprusside, nitroglycerin, or nesiritide are available. Due to the frequent titration needed, sodium nitroprusside and nitroglycerin can only be used in the intensive care setting. Nesiritide (recombinant BNP) is an agent with vasodilator, natriuretic, and diuretic effects that does not require titration and that can be used in telemetry units. Although proven to be safe, it has been shown to only marginally improve symptoms in patients with decompensated systolic HF, and as such, its use has been very limited.

A minority of hospitalized systolic HF patients presents with very low cardiac output ("cold" profile) and require **intravenous inotropes** in order to maintain perfusion and diuresis. The two most frequently used agents are dobutamine and milrinone. Dobutamine augments cardiac contractility primarily via stimulation of β-adrenergic receptors and is a modest vasodilator, whereas milrinone exerts potent inotropic and direct vasodilator effects via phosphodiesterase inhibition in the myocardium and vasculature. While these agents are fairly effective, their use is associated with further myocardial injury (evidence of troponin release even in nonischemic cardiomyopathy), and they can precipitate fatal ventricular arrhythmias. Their use is best reserved for patients in need of a bridge to mechanical circulatory support or transplant or in those patients where palliative home hospice is entertained.

Mebazaa A, et al. Levosimendan vs. dobutamine for patients with acute decompensated heart failure: the SURVIVE randomized trial. *JAMA*. 2007;297:1883–91. [PMID: 17473298]

O'Connor CM, et al. Effect of nesiritide in patients with acute decompensated heart failure. *N Engl J Med*. 2011;365:32–43. [PMID: 21732835]

G. Electrical Treatment

The majority of patients with systolic HF experience ventricular arrhythmias, and as many as 50% of all deaths in this population are sudden in nature. Findings from large clinical trials have clearly shown that **implantable cardioverter-defibrillators** (ICDs) are the most effective therapy available to prevent sudden cardiac death in these patients at risk, and ICD treatment has become standard therapy for primary and secondary prevention of sudden cardiac death in addition to optimal medical therapy in patients with left ventricular ejection fraction below 35%. Only about 10% of patients implanted with ICDs have appropriate discharges (highlighting the poor predictive value of current selection algorithms based solely on ejection fraction), with another 20% of patients experiencing inappropriate shocks (leading to an increase in mortality), and with the vast majority not using them at all. Fortunately, better discrimination algorithms for supraventricular tachycardia and the optimal use of ventricular antitachycardia pacing have markedly decreased the frequency of inappropriate shocks in these patients.

In addition, a third of systolic HF patients experience intraventricular conduction abnormalities (eg, left bundle branch block) that lead to mechanical dyssynchrony and adversely affect the cardiac performance. Several clinical trials have shown that **CRT** as standalone treatment or combined with ICD in patients with systolic HF and ejection fraction below 35% significantly improves the ejection fraction, decreases ventricular volumes, improves HF symptoms, improves exercise tolerance, and decreases the hospitalization rate for HF, as well as cardiovascular and all-cause mortality. These benefits are seen across the spectrum of HF patients (New York Heart Association functional class I–IV) and are more evident in patients in sinus rhythm, with a left bundle branch block pattern, QRS duration greater than 150 ms, and an ejection fraction below 35%. Proper patient selection to meet these strict criteria, together with selection of a viable (noninfarcted) lateral wall and optimal placement of the coronary sinus pacing lead can markedly decrease the frequency of CRT "nonresponders" (estimated at about 40% of the population implanted). The value of periodic CRT optimization by adjusting the atrioventricular and intraventricular timing for pacing (either via device-specific algorithms or echocardiography) is still a matter of debate, although in several studies, it has been shown to improve symptoms and ventricular remodeling parameters.

Holzmeister J, et al. Implantable cardioverter defibrillators and cardiac resynchronisation therapy. *Lancet*. 2011;378:722–30. [PMID: 21856486]

Moss AJ, et al. Cardiac-resynchronization therapy for the prevention of heart-failure events. *N Engl J Med*. 2009;361:1329–38. [PMID: 20178156]

H. Surgical Treatment

Cardiac surgical approaches for patients with systolic HF have changed and matured over the last decade due to improved surgical techniques and as a result of several randomized clinical trials. Until recently, uncertainty still existed about the role and benefits of revascularization in patients with ischemic systolic HF. However, the Surgical Treatment of Ischemic Heart Failure (STICH) trial showed a 19% decrease in cardiovascular mortality and a 15% decrease in cardiovascular hospitalizations in patients undergoing **coronary artery bypass surgery** in addition to optimal medical therapy when compared to optimal medical therapy alone. Thus, patients with ischemic systolic HF should be evaluated for surgical (or possibly percutaneous) revascularization.

Many HF patients with decreased systolic function and coronary artery disease have apical aneurysms as result of prior myocardial infarctions. Based on case series, surgical aneurysm reduction was thought to be beneficial by making the left ventricular contraction more efficient; however, data from the STICH trial showed that the improvement in ventricular volume with **surgical ventricular restoration** did not translate into a measurable clinical benefit for the patients.

A large number of systolic HF patients develop functional mitral regurgitation as results of left ventricular enlargement. While data are more convincing for concomitant **mitral valve repair** at the time of coronary bypass surgery, several large case series showed that even in nonischemic patients, mitral valve repair with an undersized complete rigid annuloplasty ring and without alteration of the subvalvular apparatus can be performed safely with low operative mortality. At the present time, it is unknown if this operation will translate into reverse remodeling or improved clinical outcomes. Recently, percutaneous plication or repair of the mitral valve has become possible and may replace surgical approaches in the future.

Patients with advanced systolic HF who are not amenable to conventional pharmacologic, electrical, or surgical therapies should be considered for advanced surgical options. Although with the current advances in immunosuppression therapy, the 1-year survival after **cardiac transplantation** approaches 90% and 50% of patients survive more than 12 years, only about 2200 adult patients will get transplanted every year due to the lack of available organs. The strict evaluation of candidates for heart transplantation will address comorbid diseases such as pulmonary hypertension, kidney disease, diabetes, chronic obstructive lung disease, and cancers in an attempt to identify the candidates most likely to benefit long term from this therapy.

Left ventricular assist device implantation has been used as a bridge to recovery (in patients with acute myocarditis or postpartum cardiomyopathy), a bridge to transplant (for patients likely to wait extended period of time for an available organ) or destination therapy. The devices in current commercial use, ThoratecHeartMate II and HeartWare HVAD, are second- and third-generation devices that have good reliability and have transformed the field of mechanical circulatory support. While the surgical operation itself has become fairly standardized, the long-term postoperative care is complex, and the use of assisted circulation is associated with risk of complications such as gastrointestinal bleeding, right-sided HF, renal insufficiency, infection, and thromboembolic events.

Aaronson KD, et al; HeartWare Ventricular Assist Device (HVAD) Bridge to Transplant ADVANCE Trial Investigators. Use of an intrapericardial, continuous-flow, centrifugal pump in patients awaiting heart transplantation. *Circulation*. 2012;125: 3191–200. [PMID: 22619284]

Di Salvo TG, et al. Mitral valve surgery in advanced heart failure. *J Am Coll Cardiol*. 2010;55:271–82. [PMID: 20117430]

Hunt SA, et al. The changing face of heart transplantation. *J Am Coll Cardiol*. 2008;52:587–98. [PMID: 18702960]

Jones RH, et al; STICH Hypothesis 2 Investigators. Coronary bypass surgery with or without surgical ventricular reconstruction. *N Engl J Med*. 2009;360:1705–17. [PMID: 19329820]

Slaughter MS, et al; HeartMate II Investigators. Advanced heart failure treated with continuous-flow left ventricular assist device. *N Engl J Med*. 2009;361:2241–51. [PMID: 19920051]

Velazquez EJ, et al; STICH Investigators. Coronary-artery bypass surgery in patients with left ventricular dysfunction. *N Engl J Med*. 2011;364:1607–16. [PMID: 21463150]

▶ Disease Management

Disease management programs are an important part of the care for systolic HF patients and include a broad range of health services, such as home health care, visiting nurses, and rehabilitation. The goal of these programs is to offer a combination of treatment, complication prevention, and education (about medications, diet, symptoms, etc.) in a variety of settings. Research has shown that patients enrolled in these programs receive more customized treatment and that these program may reduce the overall cost of HF care by preventing hospitalizations.

Sochalski J, et al. What works in chronic care management: the case of heart failure. *Health Aff*. 2009;28:179–89. [PMID: 19124869]

▶ Prognosis

Prognostication is critical in patient management, and patients deserve careful, thoughtful, and compassionate analysis of the data and information that will guide them through the important challenges of self-care. Although many demographic and clinical variables have been shown to predict survival in epidemiologic studies and clinical trials, the clinician is faced with the almost impossible task of juggling all of these variables at the hospital bedside or in the office when seeing a patient. During day-to-day management of individuals with systolic HF, the physician should focus attention on readily available clinical information that includes symptom severity (usually New York Heart Association functional classification, distance walked in 6 minutes, or oxygen consumption on CPET), left ventricular ejection fraction, routine biochemical markers (serum sodium, creatinine, blood urea nitrogen, and uric acid levels), and select neurohormones such as BNP. Several algorithms have been developed and tested to assist in determining which patients might benefit from advanced HR options such as assist devices or cardiac transplantation. The models that are most commonly used are the Heart Failure Survival Score (using presence of ischemia, resting heart rate, left ventricular ejection fraction, presence of a QRS duration > 200 ms, mean resting blood pressure, peak oxygen uptake, and serum sodium level) and the Seattle Heart Failure Model (using 25 different demographic and clinical variables). Both models have been extensively validated and can give a fairly accurate survival estimate. When such evaluation indicates a poor prognosis, the clinician needs to have an in-depth discussion with the patient and their family, where all the options (including palliative care) should be discussed.

Allen LA, et al. Discordance between patient-predicted and model-predicted life expectancy among ambulatory patients with heart failure. *JAMA.* 2008;299:2533–42. [PMID: 18523222]

Kalogeropoulos AP, et al. Utility of the Seattle Heart Failure Model in patients with advanced heart failure. *J Am Coll Cardiol.* 2009;53:334–42. [PMID: 19161882]

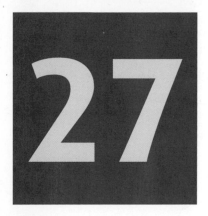

Heart Failure with Preserved Ejection Fraction

Sanjiv J. Shah, MD

▶ Symptoms and signs of heart failure with preserved left ventricular ejection fraction (LVEF > 50%).

▶ Presence of an underlying cause of heart failure with preserved ejection fraction (eg, comorbidities such as hypertension, coronary artery disease, diabetes, chronic kidney disease; or underlying valvular heart disease, restrictive cardiomyopathy, or specific myocardial diseases such as amyloidosis).

▶ Objective evidence of elevated left ventricular filling pressure (at rest or with exercise) on echocardiography or cardiac catheterization.

▶ General Considerations

Heart failure with preserved ejection fraction (HFpEF) is an increasingly common, debilitating syndrome of the elderly, and one that carries a high rate of morbidity and mortality. HFpEF accounts for > 50% of all hospitalizations for heart failure, and while a recent patient-level meta-analysis found that patients with heart failure and reduced ejection fraction (HFrEF) have a worse prognosis compared to HFpEF, two earlier large epidemiologic studies found that patients with HFpEF have a mortality rate that is nearly identical to HFrEF. Regardless of underlying ejection fraction, survival for all heart failure (HF) patients is poor, especially after HF hospitalization.

HFpEF is the preferred term for patients with a normal ejection fraction who have the syndrome of HF, because HFpEF highlights the fact that HF is a syndrome and not a distinct clinical or pathophysiologic entity. Many investigators and experts have used the term "diastolic heart failure" for HFpEF in the past. However, this term is not ideal for two main reasons. First, there is ample evidence that patients with HFpEF have abnormalities in systolic function (as

defined by tissue Doppler imaging) despite a normal ejection fraction, and many patients with HFrEF have abnormal diastolic function. Second, in the clinical setting, patients with HF are currently classified into two categories: low ejection fraction (< 50%) and preserved ejection fraction (> 50%). By calling HFpEF "diastolic HF," clinicians may not consider the entire differential diagnosis of HFpEF (of which pure diastolic dysfunction is only one cause). HFpEF has also previously been called "HF with preserved systolic function" or "HF with normal systolic function." As stated earlier, it is now clear that many patients with HFpEF have abnormalities in systolic function; therefore, HFpEF is a better term.

Finally, HFpEF has the advantage of being an easy mnemonic for patients to remember. HFpEF sounds like "HUFF-PUFF," which helps patients understand this syndrome, in which dyspnea and fatigue are two of the most common symptoms.

Borlaug BA, et al. Heart failure with preserved ejection fraction: pathophysiology, diagnosis, and treatment. *Eur Heart J*. 2011;32(6):670–9. [PMID: 21138935]

Maeder MT, et al. Heart failure with normal left ventricular ejection fraction. *J Am Coll Cardiol*. 2009;53(11):905–18. [PMID: 19281919]

Meta-analysis Global Group in Chronic Heart Failure (MAGGIC). The survival of patients with heart failure with preserved or reduced left ventricular ejection fraction: an individual patient data meta-analysis. *Eur Heart J*. 2012;33(14):1750–7. [PMID: 21821849]

▶ Pathophysiology

Since HFpEF is heterogeneous, there is no single mechanism that can explain the pathophysiology of the HFpEF syndrome. In some patients with HFpEF, such as those who have the signs and symptoms of HF due to severe valvular disease or pericardial disease (ie, constrictive pericarditis), pathophysiology is relatively straightforward and well-defined. However, in most patients with HFpEF, pathophysiologic abnormalities cannot be ascribed to a single well-defined mechanism. Instead, these patients typically have one or more of the following underlying pathophysiologic processes: (1) diastolic dysfunction due to impaired left ventricular (LV) relaxation, increased LV diastolic stiffness, or both; (2) LV enlargement with increased intravascular volume, which may be due to extracardiac factors such as renal insufficiency; (3) abnormal ventricular-arterial coupling with increased ventricular systolic stiffness and increased arterial stiffness; (4) right HF due to pulmonary venous hypertension with or without superimposed pulmonary arterial hypertension; and (5) chronotropic incompetence. In addition, LV hypertrophy and coronary artery disease are especially important in the pathophysiology of patients with HFpEF.

A. Diastolic Dysfunction

Diastolic dysfunction occurs when the ventricle loses its normal ability to suction blood from the left atrium. When the ventricle relaxes abnormally, filling is delayed and left atrial emptying is incomplete. An abnormally stiff ventricle worsens the problem by also impeding left atrial emptying. The end result is abnormally high left atrial and LV diastolic pressures. The LV loses its suction and instead of "pulling" blood from the left atrium and pulmonary veins, it now relies heavily on left atrial contraction so that the LV can fill and distend appropriately and recoil in systole. This is one reason why atrial fibrillation is tolerated so poorly in patients with advanced LV diastolic dysfunction with resultant elevation of left atrial pressure, pulmonary vascular congestion, and poor cardiac output.

In patients with HFpEF who have substantial diastolic dysfunction as a cause of their symptoms, the end-diastolic pressure-volume relationship is shifted up and to the left (Figure 27–1). In these patients, even small increases in central blood volume or vascular (arterial or venous) tone can result in significant increases in left atrial volume and pulmonary venous pressures. Patients with an upward and leftward shift in the LV end-diastolic pressure–volume relationship tend to have a high relative wall thickness (high LV mass/volume ratio); increased fibrosis and scar of the LV myocardium due to ischemia, infarction, infiltrative disease, or radiation; and impaired active relaxation of the myocardium (due to abnormal myocyte calcium homeostasis).

B. Left Ventricular Enlargement and Increased Intravascular Volume

LV enlargement is a key predictor of HF, regardless of ejection fraction. However, patients with isolated diastolic HF are often thought to have small LV volumes. This apparent discrepancy can be explained by the underlying cause of HFpEF and diastolic HF. It is likely that patients with significant coronary disease or myocardial ischemia (even in the absence of epicardial coronary disease) suffer from increased

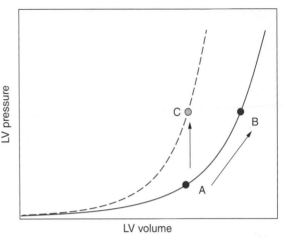

▲ **Figure 27–1.** In patients who have a noncompliant left ventricle (LV), the end-diastolic pressure-volume relationship (EDPVR) is displaced upward and to the left; therefore, there is diminished capacity to fill at low LV filling pressures. A = normal LV compliance; B = stiff, noncompliant LV with upward and leftward-shifted EDPVR; C = normal LV compliance with volume overload (note that the EDPVR curve does not shift but LV filling pressure is increased). It is difficult to distinguish scenario A from scenario C on echocardiography alone (ie, both scenarios could result in grade II diastolic dysfunction on echocardiography). Thus, "diastolic dysfunction" determined by echocardiography can help diagnose elevated LV filling pressures (and impaired LV relaxation), but it is harder to diagnose reduced LV compliance by echocardiography alone.

LV enlargement. In addition, many patients with LV enlargement have increased intravascular volume due to comorbidities such as chronic kidney disease, anemia, and obesity. Thus, LV enlargement and increased intravascular volume cause symptoms of HFpEF by a pathophysiologic mechanism that is distinct from pure LV diastolic dysfunction.

C. Abnormal Ventricular-Arterial Coupling

Ventricular-arterial coupling describes the interaction between ventricular stiffness and central arterial stiffness. In healthy patients, young and old, arterial and ventricular elastance (stiffness) are matched in order to maintain optimal cardiac efficiency. However, with increasing age, ventricular stiffness is elevated and results in decreased contractile reserve, thereby rendering elderly patients susceptible to HF, blood pressure lability, and decreased exercise tolerance. Some patients with HFpEF appear to be particularly susceptible to abnormal ventricular-arterial coupling. These patients have the age-related increases in ventricular stiffness described earlier, but instead of matched ventricular and arterial stiffness, ventricular stiffness rises out of proportion of arterial stiffness, which results in poor cardiac efficiency. These patients tend to have high pulse pressure, and they tend to be most sensitive to diuretics whereby small changes in blood volume result in large changes in blood pressure (either significantly hypertensive or hypotensive).

D. Right Heart Failure

Elevated pulmonary artery systolic pressure (PASP) on echocardiography is present in > 75% of patients with HFpEF and is a marker of worse outcomes in HFpEF. In addition, elevated PASP is the echocardiographic finding that has the best test characteristics for differentiating patients with HFpEF from those with systemic hypertension without HF. It is not surprising that elevated PASP and pulmonary hypertension are common in HFpEF since elevated left atrial pressure (at rest and/or with exercise) is present almost universally in these patients. Elevated left atrial pressure results in increased pulmonary venous pressures, thereby causing pulmonary hypertension. Significant systemic hypertension, which also occurs commonly in HFpEF, also contributes to the high PASP. Thus, pulmonary venous hypertension, defined invasively as mean pulmonary artery pressure (mPAP) > 25 mm Hg with a pulmonary capillary wedge pressure (PCWP) > 15 mm Hg, is common in HFpEF and contributes to right ventricular hypertrophy, dysfunction, and eventual right HF. Some patients (most likely < 5–10% of HFpEF) develop superimposed pulmonary arterial hypertension (on top of pulmonary venous hypertension) either as an extension of their severe pulmonary venous hypertension or due to other risk factors such as chronic thromboembolic disease, chronic hypoxemic lung disease, or obstructive sleep apnea. The best invasive marker for differentiating pulmonary venous hypertension from superimposed pulmonary arterial hypertension is not the transpulmonary gradient (mPAP-PCWP) or pulmonary vascular resistance; rather, it is the pulmonary vascular gradient (pulmonary artery diastolic pressure [PADP]-PCWP). If the PADP-PCWP gradient is > 5–10 mm Hg, pulmonary arterial hypertension is present; if the PADP and PCWP are equalized (ie, PADP-PCWP < 5 mm Hg), only pulmonary venous hypertension is present, and there is no significant superimposed pulmonary arterial hypertension.

E. Chronotropic incompetence

Up to 20–30% of patients with HFpEF have evidence of chronotropic incompetence. The inability to increase heart rate with exercise causes exercise intolerance. Patients with advanced HFpEF in particular, such as those with restrictive cardiomyopathy, severe LV hypertrophy, or severe coronary artery disease, have a very stiff LV and are unable to augment stroke volume with exercise. Thus, these patients rely upon increasing heart rate to augment cardiac output with exercise. If chronotropic incompetence is present, exercise capacity will be very limited in these types of patients.

F. Left Ventricular Hypertrophy

LV hypertrophy contributes substantially to the pathophysiology of HFpEF and is an important risk factor. LV hypertrophy limits coronary flow reserve, increases LV diastolic stiffness, and impairs LV relaxation. Patients with LV hypertrophy suffer from an inability to adequately utilize the Frank-Starling mechanism. Therefore, inadequate preload and chronotropic incompetence can lead to decreased cardiac output, with resultant lightheadedness, dizziness, and exercise intolerance. Finally, because of increased LV wall thickness, the subendocardium is especially vulnerable to ischemia in patients with and without epicardial coronary disease due to decreased coronary blood flow during exercise. Subendocardial ischemia can cause both systolic and diastolic dysfunction in these patients and further exacerbate HFpEF.

G. Coronary Artery Disease

Approximately 50% of patients with HFpEF have concomitant coronary artery disease. In these patients, coronary disease is often severe, involving multiple epicardial coronary arteries. Patients with prior myocardial infarction, ongoing ischemia, or stable chronic coronary disease can all present with HFpEF. Myocardial ischemia causes calcium sequestration in diastole, which results in impaired LV relaxation and increased LV filling pressures. In areas of prior infarction or ongoing ischemia, regional systolic dysfunction and dyssynchrony can further exacerbate abnormal loading conditions and create a mixture of systolic and diastolic dysfunction. Furthermore, patients with chronic coronary artery disease often have LV remodeling with resultant ventricular enlargement, a known risk factor for increased mortality and HF, regardless of ejection fraction. Preservation of ejection fraction can occur in some patients with prior infarction due to hypertrophy and hyperdynamic function of noninfarcted areas.

Patients with coronary disease suffer from a vicious cycle of abnormalities that contribute to HFpEF. As noted earlier, ischemia can cause impaired LV relaxation and increased LV filling pressures. Impaired LV relaxation in turn can also adversely affect coronary blood flow and coronary flow reserve, which exacerbates ischemia. Increased LV filling pressures results in extravascular compression of the small intramyocardial coronary vessels, which can cause subendocardial ischemia. Increased LV end-diastolic pressure can also result in poor epicardial coronary blood flow. Thus, ischemia begets worsening LV diastolic function, which begets more ischemia.

Borlaug BA, et al. Impaired chronotropic and vasodilator reserves limit exercise capacity in patients with heart failure and a preserved ejection fraction. *Circulation*. 2006;114(20):2138–47. [PMID: 17088459]

Guazzi M, et al. Pulmonary hypertension due to left heart disease. *Circulation*. 2012;126(8):975–90. [PMID: 22908015]

Kliger C, et al. A clinical algorithm to differentiate heart failure with a normal ejection fraction by pathophysiologic mechanism. *Am J Geriatr Cardiol*. 2006;15(1):50–7. [PMID: 16415647]

Lam CS, et al. Pulmonary hypertension in heart failure with preserved ejection fraction: a community-based study. *J Am Coll Cardiol.* 2009;53(13):1119–26. [PMID: 19324256]

Maurer MS, et al. Left heart failure with a normal ejection fraction: identification of different pathophysiologic mechanisms. *J Card Fail.* 2005;11(3):177–87. [PMID: 15812744]

Shah SJ. Evolving approaches to the management of heart failure with preserved ejection fraction in patients with coronary artery disease. *Curr Treat Options Cardiovasc Med.* 2010;12(1):58–75. [PMID: 20842482]

Zile MR, et al. Diastolic heart failure—abnormalities in active relaxation and passive stiffness of the left ventricle. *N Engl J Med.* 2004;350(19):1953–9. [PMID: 15128895]

▶ Clinical Findings

The first step in caring for a patient with HFpEF is to ensure the correct diagnosis (see later section on Differential Diagnosis). Several criteria for the diagnosis of HFpEF exist. All require signs and symptoms of HF and objective evidence of preserved LV ejection fraction ($\geq 50\%$).

A. Risk Factors

1. Age—Patients with HFpEF are almost universally elderly, and aging has several effects on cardiovascular structure and function that are pertinent to HFpEF patients. Aging reduces the diastolic filling rate as a result of prolonged relaxation, which results in left atrial overload and pulmonary venous hypertension. Arterial stiffness increases with age, resulting in increased afterload and load-dependent diastolic dysfunction. In addition, stiffening of the central arteries (which is especially common in women) leaves them less capable to handle changes in blood volume, thereby increasing susceptibility to hypotension, lightheadedness, and dizziness. Finally, aging reduces exercise capacity by increasing ventricular end-systolic chamber elastance (stiffness), which results in decreased ability to augment contractility with exercise.

2. Hypertension—Hypertension is the most important risk factor for HFpEF and is present in most patients with HFpEF. Hypertensive emergency with flash pulmonary edema is a common presentation of HFpEF. Hypertension leads to LV hypertrophy, which causes impaired relaxation, poor coronary flow reserve, and increased diastolic stiffness, all of which exacerbate HFpEF. Hypertension is also a potent risk factor for epicardial coronary disease, which often complicates HFpEF. Ischemia causes both increased LV stiffness and impaired LV relaxation. Many patients with HFpEF have symptoms of chronic angina. Alternatively, recurrent HF may be an anginal equivalent in many patients with concomitant HFpEF and coronary disease.

3. Obstructive sleep apnea—Obstructive sleep apnea is a common comorbidity in patients with HFpEF, and it can result in worsening LV hypertrophy and pulmonary hypertension. In addition, patients with HFpEF may also have sleep-disordered breathing (such as Cheyne-Stokes respirations) due to their HF. Finally, increased upper airway edema due to generalized HF may actually cause obstructive sleep apnea, a finding that has been shown to improve with diuretic therapy. All of the above contribute to nocturnal microarousals and hypoxia, which result in poor sleep quality, which in turn worsens daytime fatigue and exercise intolerance. Therefore, there should be a low threshold to perform overnight polysomnography on the patient with HFpEF.

4. Other clinically important risk factors—Other clinically important risk factors for HFpEF include coronary artery disease, diabetes, chronic kidney disease, obesity, atrial fibrillation, anemia, and chronic obstructive pulmonary disease. All of these comorbidities have their own signs and symptoms that can complicate presentations of HFpEF and add to diagnostic, prognostic, and therapeutic complexities.

B. Symptoms & Signs

Symptoms and signs of HFpEF are identical to those in patients with HFrEF (systolic HF) and include dyspnea, fatigue, peripheral pitting edema, and jugular vein distention (see Chapter 26). Exercise intolerance and acute decompensated HF are two common presentations of HFpEF.

1. Exercise intolerance—Exercise intolerance is one of the main symptoms of HFpEF and one of the most debilitating. In patients with HFpEF, there are many reasons for exercise intolerance, including the following:

- Almost all patients with HFpEF have increased LV diastolic or left atrial pressures, or both. These pressure increases are transmitted to the pulmonary veins, which can cause decreased lung compliance, which is exacerbated by exercise.

- Increased LV diastolic pressure during exercise can limit subendocardial blood flow at a time when there are increased myocardial demands, thereby worsening diastolic function. Poor myocardial perfusion is even worse in patients with LV hypertrophy, which is very common in patients with HFpEF.

- Patients with HFpEF have an abnormal stroke volume response to tachycardia with blunted increase in cardiac output with exercise. Inadequate cardiac output can increase lactate production and worsen muscle fatigue.

2. Acutely decompensated HFpEF—The most common factor in acute decompensation is uncontrolled, severe hypertension. Other common clinical findings associated with acute decompensated HFpEF include arrhythmias; noncompliance with medications or salt restriction, or both; acute coronary syndrome; renal insufficiency; valvular regurgitation or stenosis; and infection (eg, pneumonia, urinary tract infection). It is important to recognize the clinical factors associated with acute decompensation because preventing hospitalization is one of the most important goals in patients with HFpEF.

C. Diagnostic Studies

The diagnosis of HFpEF involves two steps: (1) making sure the patient has the HF syndrome (ie, evidence of elevated left-sided filling pressures) and a preserved ejection fraction (ie, LV ejection fraction ≥ 50%); and (2) determining the underlying cause of HFpEF once it is diagnosed. Echocardiography is a key diagnostic test because it allows the determination of LV ejection fraction, cardiac structural and functional abnormalities, and the comprehensive assessment of LV diastolic function, which can help rule in the presence of HF. Table 27–1 lists a standardized battery of diagnostic and prognostic tests for patients being evaluated for HFpEF.

1. Echocardiography—Echocardiography is the most important tool in diagnosing diastolic dysfunction and evaluating for other etiologies of HFpEF, such as valvular, pericardial, and coronary disease. All patients with possible or confirmed HFpEF should undergo comprehensive Doppler echocardiography with tissue Doppler imaging. Besides assessment of diastolic function (see below), all patients should be evaluated for increased LV mass and increased relative wall thickness (= [septal thickness + posterior wall

Table 27–1. Diagnostic Evaluation of Heart Failure with Preserved Ejection Fraction

Cardiac imaging
 Two-dimensional/M-mode echocardiography
 Doppler echocardiography
 Tissue Doppler imaging
 Contrast-enhanced cardiac MRI
Laboratory testing
 Complete blood count with evaluation of anemia (if present)
 Comprehensive chemistry panel (including liver function tests,
  albumin, total protein)
 Fasting glucose, hemoglobin A_{1c}
 Fasting lipid panel
 B-type natriuretic peptide (or NT-proBNP)
 Urine microalbumin
 Serum immunofixation and urine protein electrophoresis
Exercise testing
 Cardiopulmonary exercise testing
 Noninvasive evaluation of coronary artery disease (eg, stress
  echocardiography)
 Diastolic stress echocardiography
Cardiac catheterization
 Coronary angiography (if pretest probability is high or if stress test
  is abnormal)
 Invasive hemodynamic testing to confirm elevated LV diastolic
  pressure, evaluate for constriction versus restriction, evaluate for
  pulmonary hypertension, and dynamic testing (systemic or
  pulmonary vasodilator challenge, fluid challenge, exercise
  testing)
 Endomyocardial biopsy (in selected cases)
Other
 Pulmonary function testing
 Overnight polysomnography

thickness]/LV end-diastolic dimension > 0.45). Assessment of PASP; right atrial pressure (from size and collapsibility of the inferior vena cava); and right ventricular size, function, and wall thickness is important in evaluation of pulmonary hypertension.

It is critically important to understand that no one abnormality on echocardiography can diagnose diastolic dysfunction, and age must be factored into the diagnosis, since almost all parameters of diastolic function are age-dependent. Only the proper combination of echocardiographic abnormalities can make the diagnosis of diastolic dysfunction. Figure 27–2 displays an algorithm for the diagnosis of diastolic dysfunction, which requires comprehensive assessment of diastolic function, including mitral inflow, tissue Doppler imaging of the mitral annulus, left atrial volume, and pulmonary venous flow. The first step in evaluating diastolic function by echocardiography is to examine mitral inflow. In most patients, the ratio of early (E) to late (A) mitral inflow velocities (E/A ratio) < 0.8 signifies impaired relaxation (grade I diastolic dysfunction), especially if the patient is younger than 70 years and tissue Doppler e' velocity is < 10 cm/s at the lateral annulus. In these patients, exercise stress echocardiography (see below) can help evaluate the functional significance of impaired LV relaxation. If the E/A ratio is > 1.5 and early mitral deceleration time is < 150 ms in an elderly patient, the diagnosis is grade III diastolic dysfunction. These patients universally should have an e' velocity < 10 cm/s at the lateral mitral annulus.

If the E/A ratio is 0.8–1.5 or if the E/A ratio is > 1.5 and early mitral deceleration time is > 150 ms, the question of normal versus pseudonormal mitral inflow arises. In these cases, an E/e' ratio > 15 or e' velocity < 10 cm/s usually signifies pseudonormal mitral inflow (grade II diastolic dysfunction). In these patients, left atrial volume index should be increased (> 28 mL/m²). Absence of left atrial enlargement should cause reconsideration of the diagnosis of diastolic dysfunction. In patients who do not meet these criteria, further evaluation with Valsalva maneuver, pulmonary venous flow, or flow propagation velocity can all be used to help differentiate normal versus pseudonormal mitral inflow. Increased left atrial volume index and LV mass index can both provide clues to the presence of diastolic dysfunction in these patients. Even with all of these criteria for LV diastolic dysfunction, there is a subset of patients in whom diastolic function is indeterminate. In addition, there are patients in whom diastolic function is difficult or impossible to assess noninvasively. These patients include those with moderate or greater mitral regurgitation, any degree of mitral stenosis, severe mitral annular calcification, a mitral annuloplasty ring, or mitral valve prosthesis. In patients with atrial fibrillation, although diastolic function grade is difficult to determine, an E/e' ratio > 11, using e' velocity from the septal mitral annulus, signifies elevated LV filling pressures.

It is important to note that although Doppler echocardiography is a powerful noninvasive tool for the assessment

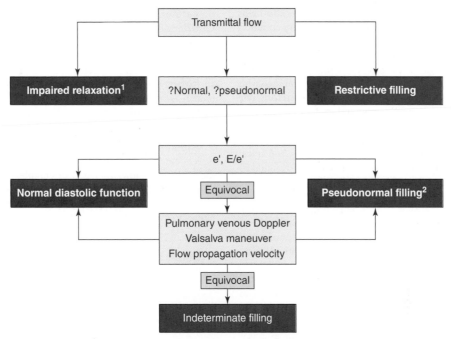

▲ **Figure 27–2.** Echo-Doppler categorization of diastolic function in patients with normal left ventricular ejection fraction. (Reproduced, with permission, from Mottram PM, et al. Assessment of diastolic function: what the general cardiologist needs to know. *Heart.* 2005;91:681–95. © BMJ Publishing Group Ltd & British Cardiovascular Society 2005. All Rights reserved.)

of diastolic function, diastolic dysfunction is not synonymous with diastolic HF. Many asymptomatic patients have abnormal diastolic function, but since they do not have signs and symptoms of HF, they should not be diagnosed incorrectly with diastolic HF. In addition, all Doppler echocardiographic variables for the assessment of diastolic function, except perhaps tissue Doppler e′ velocity, are extremely load sensitive, and therefore convey more information about preload and afterload than true intrinsic diastolic stiffness. Therefore, it is always important to consider all clinical data, including clinical history and physical examination, when making the diagnosis of diastolic HF or HFpEF.

2. B-type natriuretic peptide (BNP)—BNP may also have a role in the diagnosis of HFpEF. The Breathing Not Properly Study showed that a BNP > 100 pg/mL had a high sensitivity and negative predictive value for the diagnosis of HFpEF. Therefore, the diagnosis of HFpEF is unlikely in patients presenting to the emergency department with dyspnea and a BNP < 100 pg/mL. However, there is considerable overlap of BNP values in patients with and without HFpEF, especially in elderly women, since BNP increases with age, worsening renal function, and in women. To complicate matters, morbid obesity has been associated with low

BNP values, which may be due to BNP clearance receptors on adipocytes and decreased BNP production. Furthermore, in a study of HFpEF outpatients, all of whom had elevated PCWP, BNP was normal (ie, < 100 pg/mL) in 29%. Therefore, BNP, like Doppler echocardiography findings, must be considered within the context of the patient, and cannot be used as a stand-alone diagnostic test for HFpEF.

3. Exercise testing—Since exercise intolerance is a key symptom in HFpEF, exercise testing is extremely valuable in these patients. Although many patients who are being evaluated for HFpEF may not be able to withstand a Bruce protocol exercise test given their advanced age and multiple comorbidities, low-intensity and bicycle stress protocols are very feasible. There are two exercise tests that are helpful in evaluating patients with HFpEF: cardiopulmonary exercise testing (CPET) and diastolic stress echocardiography. Studies have shown that on CPET, patients with HFpEF have reduced exercise tolerance, low peak workload, and low peak oxygen consumption (Vo_2). Exertional dyspnea is prominent in HFpEF, and a Vo_2 provides objective evidence of reduced exercise tolerance. In addition, CPET is useful in differentiating cardiac from pulmonary components of dyspnea and decreased exercise tolerance. Often, CPET is coupled with pulmonary function testing, which also helps evaluate for pulmonary dysfunction, which is very common in elderly patients with HFpEF.

Stress echocardiography for the evolution of diastolic function aims to look for increases in LV filling pressures with exercise. The diastolic evaluation stress can be combined with traditional exercise stress echocardiography. Therefore, one test can diagnose coronary disease and exercise-induced LV diastolic dysfunction. Patients are either tested with a treadmill or bicycle stress protocol. Baseline images are obtained in the parasternal long axis, parasternal short axis, and apical two-chamber, four-chamber, and three-chamber (long-axis) views for assessment of wall motion. Baseline images should also include Doppler assessment of early mitral inflow (E) and tissue Doppler imaging of the septal mitral annulus (e′). At peak stress, wall motion analysis should come first, after which the patient should undergo repeat assessment of mitral inflow and mitral annular velocities. In patients with exercise-induced diastolic dysfunction, LV filling pressures remain elevated for several minutes, which is advantageous since the heart rate must come down to below 100 bpm in order to prevent E and A (and e′ and a′) merging on mitral inflow and tissue Doppler imaging, respectively. At peak exercise, an E/e′ ratio > 13 (using e′ at the septal annulus) suggests exercise-induced increase in LV filling pressures and is diagnostic of exercise-induced diastolic dysfunction.

4. Stress testing for the evaluation of coronary artery disease—All patients with HFpEF should undergo evaluation for coronary artery disease. Exercise stress echocardiography is ideal since patients can be evaluated for the presence of coronary artery disease and exercise-induced diastolic dysfunction with one test. However, adenosine or dipyridamole pharmacologic stress imaging is the test of choice in patients who cannot exercise and in institutions where nuclear myocardial perfusion imaging is superior. Dobutamine stress echocardiography can be performed, but in patients with significant LV hypertrophy, this test may have reduced sensitivity for the detection of wall motion abnormalities.

5. Cardiac catheterization—In patients with a high pretest probability for coronary artery disease and in patients with abnormal results of stress testing, coronary angiography should be performed. LV diastolic pressures should be measured in all patients to confirm the diagnosis of elevated LV pressures. Simultaneous right- and left-heart catheterization can be extremely valuable in the assessment of patients with HFpEF and is often underutilized. Invasive assessment in the cardiac catheterization laboratory is currently the gold standard for hemodynamic assessment, allows accurate assessment of cardiac output, and can be very helpful in evaluating for restrictive cardiomyopathy, constrictive pericarditis, or pulmonary hypertension. In addition, dynamic maneuvers such as exercise, fluid challenge, nitroprusside challenge, and pulmonary vasodilator testing (with inhaled nitric oxide or intravenous adenosine) can be valuable in specific circumstances.

6. Cardiac magnetic resonance imaging (MRI)—Cardiac MRI can be extremely helpful in the evaluation of patients with HFpEF. Cardiac MRI is the gold standard for assessment of LV volumes, left atrial volume, and LV mass. In addition, cardiac MRI can evaluate for focal areas of fibrosis (hyperenhancement), aortic enlargement and dissection (which is important since most patients with HFpEF have significant hypertension), infiltrative cardiomyopathies, and pericardial thickness/enhancement.

7. Endomyocardial biopsy—In cases where cardiac MRI or echocardiography shows significant LV hypertrophy but the patient has low-voltage QRS complexes on electrocardiogram or the patient does not have a long-standing history of hypertension, it is important to perform endomyocardial biopsy to evaluate for infiltrative cardiomyopathies.

Anjan VY, et al. Prevalence, clinical phenotype, and outcomes associated with normal B-type natriuretic peptide levels in heart failure with preserved ejection fraction. *Am J Cardiol.* 2012;110(6):870–6. [PMID: 22681864]

Burgess MI, et al. Diastolic stress echocardiography: hemodynamic validation and clinical significance of estimation of ventricular filling pressure with exercise. *J Am Coll Cardiol.* 2006;47(9):1891–900. [PMID: 16682317]

Guazzi M, et al. Cardiopulmonary exercise testing in the clinical and prognostic assessment of diastolic heart failure. *J Am Coll Cardiol.* 2005;46(10):1883–90. [PMID: 16286176]

Kasner M, et al. Utility of Doppler echocardiography and tissue Doppler imaging in the estimation of diastolic function in heart failure with normal ejection fraction: a comparative Doppler-conductance catheterization study. *Circulation.* 2007;116(6):637–47. [PMID: 17646587]

Leong DP, et al. Heart failure with normal ejection fraction: the complementary roles of echocardiography and CMR imaging. *JACC Cardiovasc Imaging.* 2010;3(4):409–20. [PMID: 20394903]

Nagueh SF, et al. Recommendations for the evaluation of left ventricular diastolic function by echocardiography. *J Am Soc Echocardiogr.* 2009;22(2):107–33. [PMID: 19187853]

▶ Differential Diagnosis

When considering the differential diagnosis in a patient with HFpEF, it is important to first make sure that the diagnosis of HF is correct. Mimickers of HF include pulmonary disease, obesity, and anemia, all of which can cause shortness of breath and exercise intolerance. Edema, whether confined to the lower extremity or more generalized, has a large differential diagnosis beyond HF, and includes venous insufficiency or obstruction (eg, venous thrombosis), liver disease, renal disease (eg, nephrotic syndrome), thyroid disease, and protein-losing enteropathies.

Once the diagnosis of HF is confirmed, it is important to make sure that the LVEF has been accurately measured and that ejection fraction is truly preserved. A multiplanar imaging modality (most commonly two-dimensional echocardiography) with quantitative measurement of ejection fraction (ie, biplane method of discs) is essential for ensuring accurate quantitation of global LV systolic function. An increasingly common group of patients with HF are those with a prior history of severe systolic dysfunction (often with LVEF < 25%) who have recovered ejection fraction with medical or device therapies, but who continue to have mild-to-moderate symptoms of HF. These patients, who may have episodic or reversible LV systolic dysfunction, such as patients with tachycardia-induced, alcoholic, viral, or tako-tsubo cardiomyopathy, appear to be distinct from traditional forms of HFpEF.

Once patients are categorized as true HFpEF, the differential diagnosis is broad. Table 27–2 lists the various causes of HFpEF. It is also important to recognize common comorbidities in patients with HFpEF, which may act in concert to cause signs and symptoms of HF. The most important comorbidities include hypertension, diabetes, coronary artery disease, chronic kidney disease, obesity, anemia, and atrial fibrillation, and it is common for multiple comorbidities to coexist in a single patient with HFpEF. Furthermore, many patients have more than one of the aforementioned etiologies of HFpEF. For example, it is not uncommon for an elderly patient to have HFpEF with hypertension, diabetes, chronic kidney disease, severe coronary artery disease, and moderate mitral regurgitation.

When evaluating the underlying cause of HFpEF in the individual patient, it is important to consider the full differential diagnosis before simply concluding that the patient has "garden-variety" HFpEF (ie, HFpEF due to aging and an amalgamation of hypertension, diabetes, obesity, and/or other comorbidities). All patients should be evaluated by echocardiography for the diagnoses of infiltrative cardiomyopathy and constrictive pericarditis. Clues on echocardiography for infiltrative cardiomyopathy include: (1) severe (grade III) diastolic dysfunction (especially if present in a young patient without end-stage renal disease or severe coronary artery disease); (2) low-voltage QRS on electrocardiography with increased LV wall thickness on echocardiography; and (3) severely reduced longitudinal tissue velocities. Clues for the diagnosis of constrictive pericarditis include: (1) history of radiation to the chest wall, cardiac surgery, connective tissue disease, acute pericarditis, or rheumatic heart disease; (2) markers of diastolic dysfunction on mitral inflow and pulmonary vein flow with preserved or increased tissue Doppler e' velocities; (3) increased respiratory variation in the mitral inflow Doppler tracing; and (4) diastolic interventricular septal "bounce."

Table 27–2. Etiologies of Heart Failure with Preserved Ejection Fraction

HFpEF with abnormal diastolic function
Hypertensive heart disease
Coronary artery disease
Prior myocardial infarction
Inducible myocardial ischemia
Severe, chronic, stable multivessel coronary disease
Restrictive cardiomyopathy
Radiation-induced cardiac injury
Infiltrative diseases (amyloidosis, sarcoidosis, hemochromatosis)
Metabolic storage diseases (eg, Fabry disease)
Endocardial fibrosis
Primary diabetic cardiomyopathy (in the absence of hypertension and coronary disease)
Idiopathic
Hypertrophic cardiomyopathy
Obstructive
Nonobstructive
Other causes of HFpEF
Primary valvular heart disease
Aortic stenosis
Aortic regurgitation
Mitral stenosis
Mitral regurgitation
Mimickers of obstructive valvular disease (eg, left atrial myxoma, cor triatriatum)
Pericardial disease
Constrictive pericarditis
Cardiac tamponade
Primary right ventricular dysfunction
Pulmonary arterial hypertension
Right ventricular myocardial infarction
Arrhythmogenic right ventricular dysplasia
Congenital heart disease
High-output cardiac failure
Severe anemia
Thyrotoxicosis
Cirrhosis
Arteriovenous fistulae

▶ Prevention

HFpEF often represents the culmination of several underlying comorbidities such as hypertension, diabetes, coronary artery disease, chronic kidney disease, and obesity. Therefore, it is imperative to aggressively treat these risk factors in patients who may be at risk for HFpEF. Aggressive control of hypertension is probably the most important factor in preventing HFpEF and is a class I American College of Cardiology/American Heart Association recommendation for treatment and prevention of HFpEF.

The Valsartan in Diastolic Dysfunction (VALIDD) trial showed that improvement in diastolic function is related to decreases in blood pressure irrespective of type of antihypertensive therapy, and these findings underscore the importance of aggressive blood pressure control in patients with hypertension in order to improve diastolic function. Many studies have shown that lowering blood pressure reduces HF events, and VALIDD adds to these studies by showing improvement in diastolic function with aggressive control of hypertension. Furthermore, the ALLHAT-HFpEF substudy showed that chlorthalidone outperformed other antihypertensives in reducing incident HFpEF.

Poor control of diabetes has been associated with increased incidence of HF (regardless of type of HF). Although there is a tight association between poor glycemic control and incidence of HF, it is unclear whether tight control of diabetes will reduce HFpEF. In the absence of randomized controlled data, patients with diabetes should be treated aggressively with tight glycemic control, although vigilance is needed to prevent hypoglycemic episodes. Tight glycemic control results in prevention of microvascular complications, particularly diabetic nephropathy, which can result in fluid overload and HF.

Treatment of ischemia is an attractive target for prevention of HFpEF. However, there is little data on whether or not there is a benefit of revascularization. In the Coronary Artery Surgery Study (CASS) database, patients with HFpEF had a higher mortality compared with those with preserved ejection fraction but no HF. Despite these findings, there were no differences in survival between patients with HFpEF in CASS who underwent surgical revascularization and those who underwent medical therapy for multivessel coronary disease. Therefore, patients with symptomatic angina and significant coronary disease should be treated with medications or revascularization, or both, but whether doing so will prevent HFpEF remains to be seen.

Davis BR, et al. Heart failure with preserved and reduced left ventricular ejection fraction in the antihypertensive and lipid-lowering treatment to prevent heart attack trial. *Circulation*. 2008;118(22):2259–67. [PMID: 19001024]

Solomon SD, et al. Effect of angiotensin receptor blockade and antihypertensive drugs on diastolic function in patients with hypertension and diastolic dysfunction: a randomised trial. *Lancet*. 2007;369(9579):2079–87. [PMID: 17586303]

▶ Treatment

A. Nonpharmacologic Therapy

All patients should keep a diary of daily weight and blood pressure. These two parameters are of extreme importance in evaluating for underdiuresis and overdiuresis. When patients are educated about looking for increased weight gain and increasing blood pressure, they can alert their health care provider in a timely fashion in order to allow for intervention prior to progression of HF, which invariably leads to hospitalization.

Several studies have now shown that patients with HFpEF benefit from exercise training. Thus, in symptomatic HFpEF patients who can exercise, prescribed exercise training should be considered.

An innovative wireless hemodynamic monitor (CardioMEMS), implanted percutaneously in the pulmonary artery, was shown in the CHAMPION trial (N = 550) to reduce HF hospitalizations compared to placebo in HFpEF (16% vs. 33%, $P < 0.0001$). The CHAMPION trial has been the only clinical trial to show a clear benefit in HFpEF, and although not yet U.S. Food and Drug Administration

approved, devices like CardioMEMS may play a big role in HFpEF management in the future.

Finally, catheter-based renal denervation therapy has resulted in significant lowering in blood pressure and regression of LV hypertrophy in patients with resistant hypertension. Although clinical trials of renal denervation in HFpEF are lacking, this therapy may be very important in the future for prevention and treatment of HFpEF.

Abraham WT, et al. CHAMPION Trial Study Group. Wireless pulmonary artery haemodynamic monitoring in chronic heart failure: a randomised controlled trial. *Lancet*. 2011; 377(9766):658–66. [PMID: 21315441]

Kitzman DW, et al. Exercise training in older patients with heart failure and preserved ejection fraction: a randomized, controlled, single-blind trial. *Circ Heart Fail*. 2010;3(6):659–67. [PMID: 20852060]

Sobotka PA, et al. The role of renal denervation in the treatment of heart failure. *Curr Cardiol Rep*. 2012;14(3):285–92. [PMID: 22392370]

Taylor RS, et al. Effects of exercise training for heart failure with preserved ejection fraction: a systematic review and meta-analysis of comparative studies. *Int J Cardiol*. 2012 Jun 2. [Epub ahead of print] [PMID: 22664368]

B. Pharmacologic Therapy

Treatment of HFpEF remains empiric. Compared to HFrEF, there is a relative paucity of randomized controlled trial data to guide treatment. To date, only few large randomized trials have specifically studied patients with HFpEF. The major trials include DIG-PEF, CHARM-Preserved, I-PRESERVE, PEP-CHF, and SENIORS.

In the DIG trial, digoxin did not decrease mortality, and although there was a trend toward decreased hospitalization, there was also a trend toward increased unstable angina. Digoxin increases systolic energy demand and adds to calcium overload in diastole and may be deleterious to patients with HFpEF; therefore, it is generally not recommended. If digoxin is necessary for rate control in patients with HFpEF who have atrial fibrillation, digoxin concentration should be kept at 0.5–0.9 ng/mL since higher concentrations were associated with increased mortality in the DIG trial.

In the CHARM-Preserved trial of mostly male patients with ejection fraction > 40%, candesartan, an angiotensin receptor blocker, was associated with a slight decrease in hospitalization but no difference in mortality when compared with placebo. The large I-PRESERVE trial (N = 4128) enrolled HFpEF patients who more closely matched with those encountered in clinical practice (60% female with a mean age of 72 years). However, I-PRESERVE, which studied irbesartan versus placebo, also found no improvement in outcomes with angiotensin receptor blocker therapy in HFpEF.

The PEP-CHF trial, which studied perindopril (an angiotensin-converting enzyme inhibitor [ACEI]), and SENIORS, which studied nebivolol (a vasodilating β-blocker), both included patients with HF and preserved or relatively preserved ejection fraction, and both did not show major benefits in terms of improved hard outcomes.

Despite these disappointing results, a few recent clinical trials in patients with HFpEF demonstrate that there may be beneficial therapies on the horizon. In a small randomized controlled trial (N = 44) of sildenafil in patients with HFpEF, pulmonary venous hypertension, and superimposed pulmonary arterial hypertension (ie, PADP-PCWP gradient > 5 mm Hg), sildenafil resulted in improved cardiac structure/function and improved exercise capacity. In PARAMOUNT, a phase 2 randomized controlled trial (N = 301) of a novel class of drug (angiotensin receptor neprilysin inhibitor LCZ696), patients with HFpEF randomized to the LCZ696 had greater reduction, compared to placebo, in N-terminal proBNP and left atrial volume at 3 months. LCZ696 was well tolerated, and there were also less serious adverse outcomes in the LCZ696 arm, although this finding did not reach statistical significance (15% vs. 30%, P = 0.32).

Since extensive randomized controlled trial data for HFpEF are not available, treatment of HFpEF relies on extrapolation of therapies for HFrEF, nonspecific relief of congestion, and ameliorating the underlying disease processes and comorbidities. Table 27–3 lists the most important treatment priorities for patients with HFpEF, as outlined below.

For symptomatic relief, the most important first step is to reduce the congestive state. Salt restriction and vasodilator therapy (ACEI, angiotensin receptor blockers, or hydralazine/nitrates) make up the cornerstone of treatment. Diuretics and other forms of fluid removal (eg, dialysis, ultrafiltration) are often needed, but as the acute congestive episode resolves, it is important to minimize diuretic therapy, since overdiuresis activates a heightened neurohormonal response and aggravates the cardiorenal syndrome.

From an electrophysiologic standpoint, it is important, whenever possible, to maintain atrial contraction and atrioventricular synchrony. Therefore, patients with atrial fibrillation or atrial flutter should undergo cardioversion or ablation. When necessary, patients should undergo pacemaker therapy to ensure atrioventricular synchrony or to treat chronotropic incompetence.

In some patients with HFpEF, it is ideal to promote bradycardia and avoid tachycardia. Tachycardia increases myocardial oxygen demand and decreases coronary perfusion time, which promotes diastolic dysfunction due to ischemia even in the absence of epicardial coronary disease. In addition, the time allotted for LV relaxation is decreased and diastolic filling time is decreased when tachycardia is present. By inducing relative bradycardia (eg, heart rate 50–60 bpm), coronary perfusion is optimized, and LV relaxation and diastolic filling time are both increased. Patients who benefit most from this type of treatment are most likely those who have impaired LV relaxation and prolonged early mitral inflow deceleration times. In patients with more severe, end-stage HFpEF, such as severe restrictive cardiomyopathy, increased heart rate may be the most important

Table 27–3. Treatment of Heart Failure with Preserved Ejection Fraction: General Principles

Treat underlying causes and precipitating factors
Treat congestion and edema
  Diuretics
  Ultrafiltration or dialysis (when diuretics are insufficient)
  Sodium restriction
  Vasodilator therapy
Aggressively treat hypertension
  Use vasodilating β-blockers (eg, carvedilol), ACEIs or angiotensin receptor blockers, and thiazide diuretics whenever possible
  Avoid clonidine
Control heart rate and rhythm
  Goal heart rate ~60 bpm (use caution in patients with advanced diastolic dysfunction or restrictive cardiomyopathy who require increased heart rates to maintain cardiac output because of fixed stroke volume, and also consider the diagnosis of chronotropic incompetence in patients who do not tolerate heart rate–lowering agents)
  Maintain sinus rhythm (cardioversion, ablation)
  Pacemaker therapy (when necessary) to maintain atrioventricular synchrony or for patients who have chronotropic incompetence
Treat comorbidities
  Myocardial ischemia (medications, revascularization)
  Dyslipidemia (preferably with statins for pleiotropic benefit)
  Anemia
  Chronic kidney disease
Nonpharmacologic therapy
  Instruct patients to keep diary of daily weight and blood pressure
  Prescribe exercise training (cardiac rehabilitation) in mild-to-moderate heart failure to improve functional status and decrease symptoms
  Treat obstructive sleep apnea, sleep-disordered breathing, and nocturnal hypoxia

factor maintaining cardiac output, since stroke volume is often decreased and fixed. These patients invariably have a very high early mitral inflow velocity and short deceleration time. Although tachycardia should be avoided, heart rates of 80–90 bpm are often required in order to maintain adequate cardiac output. In these patients, overzealous β-blockade or nondihydropyridine calcium channel blocker therapy can result in a precipitous decline in cardiac output.

Most patients with HFpEF will benefit from rate control therapy with medications such as β-blockers and nondihydropyridine calcium channel blockers (verapamil, diltiazem). A good rule of thumb to follow when choosing β-blockers is that metoprolol succinate is a good agent in patients who have problems with rate control (eg, atrial fibrillation) and those with low or normal blood pressure. In patients who have severe hypertension, carvedilol is the agent of choice since it has potent antihypertensive effects due to its α-adrenergic blockade properties. Most patients with HFpEF have significant hypertension; thus carvedilol is typically a first-line drug for most HFpEF patients. In the COHERE registry, which was an observational study, treatment with carvedilol resulted in improved outcomes compared to other β-blockers, regardless of the underlying LV ejection fraction.

As stated earlier, all patients should be evaluated for myocardial ischemia, and when present, ischemia should be treated aggressively with revascularization, β-blockers, nitrates, and dihydropyridine calcium channel blockers. Hypertension should be treated aggressively with goal blood pressure < 130/80 mm Hg. Control of hypertension is the only proven therapy for prevention of HFpEF, and therefore is essential in all patients. HFpEF patients commonly have severe hypertension, and when they are referred, they may be taking four or five or more antihypertensive medications. The number of medications should be kept to a minimum in order to avoid the dangers of polypharmacy and adverse drug–drug interactions. In addition, minimizing medications will often promote increased patient compliance. Patients with HFpEF and severe hypertension are often taking medications such as clonidine and minoxidil, while other medications with proven cardiovascular benefits, such as β-blockers and ACEIs, are not titrated to maximum doses. Therefore, patients with significant hypertension should ideally be treated with a vasodilating β-blocker and maximum dose of an ACEI or angiotensin receptor blocker, unless contraindicated. Most patients will also benefit from a thiazide diuretic such as chlorthalidone. Routine use of more potent thiazides, such as metolazone, should be avoided since these medications often exacerbate the cardiorenal syndrome. Aldosterone antagonists can be very useful in HFpEF patients both for controlling blood pressure and for improving diuresis. However, these patients should be monitored closely for hyperkalemia. The utility of spironolactone in HFpEF is currently being evaluated in the TOPCAT randomized controlled trial.

In patients with severe, resistant hypertension who cannot be treated adequately with a combination of β-blockers, ACEIs, and thiazide diuretics, the following steps should be taken: (1) ensure medication compliance, (2) ensure euvolemia since fluid overload will exacerbate hypertension, and (3) look for causes of secondary hypertension. Using these steps, most patients will have adequately controlled blood pressure with two or three medications. In patients who need an additional agent, the combination of hydralazine and nitrates is a good option given their beneficial effects in HF. If tolerated and not associated with increased lower extremity edema, dihydropyridine calcium channel blockers may also be used to treat severe hypertension. These agents are often useful in patients who have significant chronic kidney disease since they may not be able to take ACEIs, angiotensin receptor blockers, or aldosterone antagonists.

Besides beneficial antihypertensive effects, β-blockers, ACE inhibitors, and angiotensin receptor blockers attenuate neurohormonal activation, which may be beneficial in HFpEF. In addition, ACEIs, angiotensin receptor blockers,

and spironolactone may prevent fibrosis and may promote regression of LV hypertrophy. Statins may have pleiotropic benefit in HF, and all HFpEF patients with dyslipidemia or coronary risk factors should be treated with a statin. Interestingly, in a large study of Medicare beneficiaries discharged with a primary diagnosis of HF and documentation of preserved ejection fraction, statins were associated with increased survival irrespective of total cholesterol, coronary disease, diabetes, hypertension, or age.

1. Categorization of HFpEF subtype—As stated earlier, HFpEF is a heterogeneous syndrome. Once the HFpEF syndrome is diagnosed, patients can be further categorized clinically into etiologic and pathophysiologic subtypes in order to help guide therapy above and beyond the recommendations listed above. Table 27–4 summarizes these HFpEF subtypes and provides guidance to HFpEF subtype-specific treatment options.

2. Caveats—Some patients with HFpEF live a delicate balance between symptomatic congestion (due to inadequate diuresis) and poor cardiac output (due to overdiuresis). The latter causes lightheadedness, dizziness, fatigue, and worsening renal dysfunction due to decreased renal perfusion. Patients with HFpEF who have a classic physiologic picture of isolated "diastolic HF" rely on increased LV filling pressures to maintain cardiac output, and they tend to be very sensitive to overdiuresis, with small decreases in LV diastolic pressure resulting in large decreases in stroke volume. Therefore, it is important to start low and go slow with diuretic therapy. Many patients typically require frequent visits in order to find a diuretic regimen that results in optimal symptom control without exacerbating the cardiorenal syndrome.

In patients with hypertrophic cardiomyopathy, nondihydropyridine calcium channel blockers (verapamil, diltiazem) can be beneficial and therefore may be used as first-line therapy before β-blockade. Thiazide diuretics can exacerbate hyperglycemia and hyperuricemia, which are often present in elderly patients with HFpEF. Positive inotropes should be avoided in general because they promote calcium influx into cardiac myocytes, which worsens diastolic function. In addition, many of these patients have hypercontractile ventricles with small LV volumes. Therefore, positive inotropes frequently cause cavity obliteration with resultant obstruction of forward flow and decreased cardiac output. In patients with HFpEF who have non-ST elevation acute coronary syndromes, mortality is increased and patients are often undertreated. Therefore, all efforts should be made to treat this high-risk group (including an early invasive approach) using evidence-based guidelines.

Aside from treatment of hypertension, coronary disease, and atrial fibrillation (as listed earlier), it is important to treat other underlying comorbidities such as diabetes, metabolic syndrome, obesity, chronic kidney disease, and anemia. In addition, many patients with HFpEF have concomitant chronic obstructive pulmonary disease, which should also

Table 27–4. Treatment of Heart Failure with Preserved Ejection Fraction: Treatment Approaches by Subtype

"Garden variety" HFpEF: See Table 27-3 for general recommendations; several medications are often required for control of blood pressure. Treatment of comorbidities is essential.

Coronary artery disease HFpEF: These patients typically have multivessel coronary artery disease and/or a history of prior coronary artery bypass graft. Treatment of these patients involves revascularization (if indicated to improve symptoms), β-blocker, ACEI or angiotensin receptor blocker, statin, nitrate, and antiplatelet therapy.

Atrial arrhythmia-predominant HFpEF: In these patients, blood pressure is typically easy to control, but atrial arrhythmias can be difficult to control and result in HF exacerbations. Here, treatment with long-acting metoprolol succinate, a nondihydropyridine calcium channel blocker, and/or amiodarone (or other antiarrhythmic, if not contraindicated) can be helpful. Some patients may require further intervention with either catheter-based or surgical treatment of atrial arrhythmias.

Right heart failure HFpEF: These patients typically have right ventricular dysfunction and pulmonary hypertension that predominates their clinical course. Right heart catheterization should be performed to exclude pulmonary arterial hypertension or superimposed pulmonary arterial hypertension (on top of pulmonary venous hypertension). In patients with advanced right ventricular failure, cardiac output is reduced and systemic blood pressure can be low. Treatment is challenging and often requires a combination of diuretics (or ultrafiltration for refractory cases), digoxin (for right ventricular inotropy), and phosphodiesterase-5 inhibition (eg, sildenafil). Midodrine, an α-agonist, can be useful to support the systemic blood pressure if hypotension occurs during diuresis.

Hypertrophic cardiomyopathy (HCM)-like HFpEF: These patients are typically elderly with long-standing hypertension. They have echocardiographic characteristics that mimic HCM (moderate or severe LV hypertrophy [with or without asymmetric septal hypertrophy] and LV outflow tract or intracavitary obstruction). These patients should be treated like younger patients with genetic HCM. Treatment includes metoprolol succinate and/or nondihydropyridine calcium channel blockers, control of atrial arrhythmias, and avoidance of vasodilators. Diuretics should be used sparingly and with caution to avoid hypotension or syncope.

High-output HFpEF: Treatment of the underlying cause of the high-output state is essential. Diuretics will be the mainstay of treatment for fluid overload.

Rare causes of HFpEF: Treat the underlying cause of HFpEF, and understand the caveats of treatment (eg, for cardiac amyloidosis, the most common cause of infiltrative cardiomyopathy, besides working up and treating the underlying type of amyloidosis, certain drugs [eg, digoxin, nondihydropyridine calcium channel blockers, ACEIs/angiotensin receptor blockers] should be avoided, and all patients should be evaluated for anticoagulation given the high risk of atrial thrombi).

be treated aggressively in order to improve symptoms of breathlessness.

3. Drugs to avoid—In all patients with HFpEF, it is important to avoid polypharmacy at all costs since adverse events increase and compliance decreases with increased numbers of medications. In addition, medications should always be carefully scrutinized as causes of signs and symptoms of HF. For example, calcium channel blockers and thiazolidinediones (eg, pioglitazone) can cause significant edema, nonsteroidal anti-inflammatory drugs (NSAIDs) can cause renal failure, and hydroxychloroquine (which is frequently used in rheumatologic diseases such as systemic lupus erythematosus and rheumatoid arthritis) can cause a restrictive cardiomyopathy. In the elderly cohort of patients with HFpEF, medications for Parkinson disease are common, and these agents have been shown to cause valvular disease. Certain foods and herbal supplements can also be deleterious in patients with HFpEF. Licorice can cause mineralocorticoid excess, ginseng interferes with warfarin, and ginseng also falsely elevates digoxin levels. Treatment of gout is difficult since NSAIDs are contraindicated in patients with HFpEF and colchicine is dangerous because many of these patients are elderly and have abnormal kidney function. In these patients, corticosteroid injection directly into the involved joint, a short pulse of oral corticosteroids, and colchicine 0.6 mg three times a week or allopurinol for maintenance therapy may be the best treatment options.

Ahmed A, et al. Effects of digoxin on morbidity and mortality in diastolic heart failure: the ancillary digitalis investigation group trial. *Circulation*. 2006;114(5):397–403. [PMID: 16864724]

Bennett KM, et al. Heart failure with preserved left ventricular systolic function among patients with non-ST-segment elevation acute coronary syndromes. *Am J Cardiol*. 2007;99(10):1351–6. [PMID: 17493458]

Yusuf S, et al. Effects of candesartan in patients with chronic heart failure and preserved left-ventricular ejection fraction: the CHARM-Preserved Trial. *Lancet*. 2003;362(9386):777–81. [PMID: 13678871]

▶ Prognosis

Once hospitalized for HF, patients with HFpEF have a high mortality. Five-year mortality is high and is similar to HFrEF. Two large epidemiology studies of patients hospitalized with HFpEF have shown that survival is only 30–40% after 5 years. A patient-level meta-analysis, which included both epidemiologic studies and clinical trials and inpatient and outpatient settings, found that survival of patients with HFrEF was worse than HFpEF, although both types of HF were associated with high mortality rates.

Despite the abundance of studies now showing a high rate of mortality in HFpEF, the cause of death remains unclear. Predictors of death in patients hospitalized with HFpEF include increased age, male gender, increased serum creatinine, decreased hemoglobin, decreased blood pressure, increased respiratory rate, and hyponatremia. In addition, diabetes, peripheral arterial disease, cancer, dementia, and end-stage renal disease requiring hemodialysis are all independent predictors of death in HFpEF. In the CHARM trial echocardiographic substudy, evidence of moderate or greater diastolic dysfunction was strongly associated with adverse outcomes. In the DIG trial, worsening HF and arrhythmias were the leading causes of death in all HF patients, regardless of ejection fraction. However, noncardiovascular causes of death were more frequent in patients with HFpEF, due to their advanced age. Several studies, including analyses of the CHARM-Preserved and I-PRESERVE trials, as well as a retrospective analysis of the Duke Databank for Cardiovascular Disease, have found that sudden cardiac death occurs in HFpEF with a frequency ranging from 8–28%.

Cause of death in HFpEF is most likely multifactorial. Although some patients may die of HF and pulmonary edema, most patients do not die of LV pump failure, and as stated earlier, many may die due to arrhythmias or sudden cardiac death. Even more may die due to important age-related comorbidities such as cancer and dementia. Until we learn more about cause of death in patients with HFpEF, it is important for health care providers to understand the importance of comorbidities in the prognosis of these patients. Therefore, although evaluation of treatment of HFpEF is extremely important, attention to comorbidities and a multidisciplinary approach to patients with HFpEF will likely lead to the best possible outcome in these patients.

Bhatia RS, et al. Outcome of heart failure with preserved ejection fraction in a population-based study. *N Engl J Med.* 2006;355(3):260–9. [PMID: 16855266]

Bursi F, et al. Systolic and diastolic heart failure in the community. *JAMA.* 2006;296(18):2209–16. [PMID: 17090767]

Fonarow GC, et al; OPTIMIZE-HF Investigators and Hospitals. Characteristics, treatments, and outcomes of patients with preserved systolic function hospitalized for heart failure: a report from the OPTIMIZE-HF Registry. *J Am Coll Cardiol.* 2007;50(8):768–77. [PMID: 17707182]

Owan TE, et al. Trends in prevalence and outcome of heart failure with preserved ejection fraction. *N Engl J Med.* 2006;355(3):251–9. [PMID: 16855265]

Persson H, et al. Diastolic dysfunction in heart failure with preserved systolic function: need for objective evidence: results from the CHARM Echocardiographic Substudy-CHARMES. *J Am Coll Cardiol.* 2007;49(6):687–94. [PMID: 17291934]

Shah SJ, et al. Heart failure with preserved ejection fraction: treat now by treating comorbidities. *JAMA.* 2008;300:431–3. [PMID: 18647986]

Zile M, et al. Mode of death in patients with heart failure and a preserved ejection fraction: results from the irbesartan in heart failure with preserved ejection fraction (I-PRESERVE) trial. *Circulation.* 2010;121:1393–405. [PMID: 20231531]

Pericardial Diseases

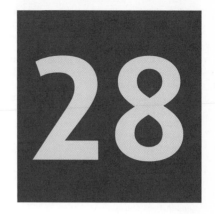

Massimo Imazio, MD

▶ General Considerations

A. Normal Pericardial Anatomy & Physiology

The pericardium consists of two layers: a serous visceral layer, which is intimately adherent to the heart and epicardial fat, and a fibrous parietal layer. The pericardium encloses the greater part of the surface of the heart, the juxtacardial portions of the pulmonary and systemic veins, and the proximal segments of the great vessels. A significant portion of the left atrium, however, is not enclosed within the pericardium. The pericardium is not essential for sustaining life or health, as evidenced by preservation of cardiac function even if the pericardium is congenitally absent or surgically removed. The pericardium plays a role in normal cardiovascular function, however, and can be involved in a number of important disease states. The normal functions of the pericardium include maintaining an optimal cardiac shape, promoting cardiac chamber interaction, preventing the overfilling of the heart, reducing friction between the beating heart and adjacent structures, providing a physical barrier to infection, and limiting displacement during the cardiac cycle.

B. Pericardial Pressure & Normal Function

The bulk of current evidence indicates that with normal cardiac volumes, the effective pericardial pressure ranges from 0–1 mm Hg to (at most) 3–4 mm Hg. The pericardial space between the parietal and visceral layers normally contains 15–50 mL of fluid, and the reserve volume of the pericardium is relatively small. The pericardium has a limited distensibility essentially determined by the histologic composition of the parietal pericardium with a limited amount of elastic fibers and more collagen fibers. However, if pericardial fluid accumulates slowly, a remodeling of pericardial connective tissue may allow pericardial distension with accumulation of 1000–1500 mL of fluid, and occasionally up to 2000 mL. Normally, acute tamponade occurs with accumulation of < 250 mL. The pressure–volume relation

of normal pericardium is a J-shaped curve. After an initial short shallow portion, which allows the pericardium to prevent cardiac chamber dilatation in response to physiologic events such as posture changes, there is a minimal increase in pericardial pressure. Thereafter, the pressure increase is extremely steep for sudden, acute changes of volume. Thus, an acute increase of 100–200 mL may greatly elevate pericardial pressure to 20–30 mm Hg and be responsible for cardiac tamponade. On the contrary, a slowly increasing pericardial volume is accompanied by only modest increase of pericardial pressure until 1000–2000 mL before the development of cardiac tamponade.

▶ Etiology & Pathogenesis

Pericardial diseases are relatively common in clinical practice and may have different presentations either as isolated disease or manifestation of a systemic disorder. Although the etiology is varied and complex (Table 28–1), the pericardium has a relatively nonspecific response to these different causes. On this basis, there are few main clinical presentations including pericarditis, pericardial effusion, cardiac tamponade, and constrictive pericarditis. Causes are essentially divided as infectious or noninfectious.

A. Infectious Pathogens

1. Viruses—Viruses are considered the most common causes of pericardial diseases in developed countries. An unidentified virus almost certainly underlies most cases of acute idiopathic pericarditis. The possibility of a viral cause is suggested when pericarditis occurs in the absence of other factors. Frequently, a prodromal syndrome consistent with a viral infection is present (ie, upper respiratory tract syndrome, pneumonia, or gastroenteritis). The viral agents most commonly associated with pericarditis include coxsackie viruses, Epstein-Barr virus, parvovirus, and human immunodeficiency virus (HIV). Although a wide range of viral agents have been implicated, no specific antiviral

Table 28–1. Etiology of Pericardial Diseases

Infectious causes:
Viral (coxsackievirus, influenza, **Epstein-Barr virus,** cytomegalovirus, adenovirus, varicella, rubella, mumps, hepatitis B virus, **hepatitis C virus, HIV, parvovirus B19,** and human herpes virus 6)
Bacterial (tuberculosis, *Coxiella burnetii,* other bacterial rare may include pneumo-, meningo-, gonococcosis, *Haemophilus,* streptococci, staphylococci, *Chlamydia, Mycoplasma, Legionella, Leptospira, Listeria*)
Fungal (rare: *Histoplasma* more likely in immunocompetent patients; aspergillosis, blastomycosis, *Candida* more likely in immunosuppressed host)
Parasitic (very rare: *Echinococcus, Toxoplasma*)

Noninfectious causes:
Autoimmune:
Pericardial injury syndromes (postmyocardial infarction syndrome, *postpericardiotomy syndrome,* posttraumatic including forms after iatrogenic trauma; *postinterventions*: eg, coronary percutaneous intervention, pacemaker lead insertion, and radiofrequency ablation).
Systemic autoimmune and autoinflammatory diseases (systemic lupus erythematosus, Sjögren syndrome, rheumatoid arthritis, systemic sclerosis, systemic vasculitides, Behçet syndrome, sarcoidosis, familial Mediterranean fever)
Neoplastic:
Primary tumors (rare, above all pericardial mesothelioma)
Secondary metastatic tumours (common, above all *lung and breast cancer, lymphoma*)
Metabolic (uremia, myxedema, other rare)
Traumatic and Iatrogenic
Direct injury (penetrating thoracic injury, esophageal perforation, iatrogenic)
Indirect injury (nonpenetrating thoracic injury, radiation injury)
Drug-related (procainamide, hydralazine, isoniazid, and phenytoin as lupus-like syndrome, penicillins as hypersensitivity pericarditis with eosinophilia, doxorubicin and daunorubicin [often associated with a cardiomyopathy, may cause a pericardiopathy])

therapy has been shown to be effective in immunocompetent patients.

2. Bacterial pericarditis—Bacterial infection of the pericardium can occur following thoracic surgery; as a result of a contiguous pleural, mediastinal, or pulmonary infection; as a complication of bacterial endocarditis; or as a result of systemic bacteremia. Direct extension from pneumonia or empyema with staphylococci, pneumococci, and streptococci accounts for most cases. However, the most important bacterial agent is *Mycobacterium tuberculosis,* especially in developing countries. In developed countries, bacterial pericarditis is rare (< 5%). Preexisting pericardial effusions and immunosuppressed states are important predisposing factors. HIV infection is often associated with tuberculous pericarditis and effusions in underdeveloped countries (eg, countries in Africa).

3. Tuberculous pericarditis—Although several decades of effective antituberculous therapy and public health measures have brought about a declining rate of tuberculous pericarditis, this condition remains a major problem in immunocompromised persons and in developing countries, especially in association with HIV infection. Thus, HIV-associated tuberculosis is a common cause of symptomatic pericardial effusion.

4. HIV and acquired immunodeficiency syndrome (AIDS)—The most common pericardial abnormality encountered in AIDS is an asymptomatic pericardial effusion. Before highly active antiretroviral therapies, symptomatic pericardial effusion with or without chest pain, friction rub, and electrocardiogram (ECG) changes was caused by a variety of opportunistic infections and neoplasms in patients with HIV infection and AIDS. The most common infectious pathogens identified in symptomatic pericardial effusion are *M tuberculosis* and *Mycobacterium avium-intracellulare.* The HIV virus itself can cause an effusion. Lymphomas and Kaposi sarcoma are the most common neoplasms associated with effusion. Pericarditis or symptomatic pericardial effusion in a patient with AIDS should therefore prompt an immediate search for infection or neoplasm. Pericardial effusion in HIV disease usually occurs in the context of full-blown AIDS and is strongly associated with a shortened survival time independent of the CD4 count. The mortality rate at 6 months for patients with effusion was nine times greater than for patients without effusion. After the introduction of highly active antiretroviral therapy, the etiologic spectrum of the HIV-infected patient has become similar to that of noninfected patients.

B. Iatrogenic Causes

Iatrogenic causes of pericardial diseases are emerging in developed countries due to the aging of the population and widespread use of percutaneous interventions. Such forms are usually reported as **postcardiac injury syndromes,** reflecting the fact that the offending agent may involve not only the pericardium but also the myocardium and whole heart.

1. Surgery-related syndromes—Several distinct pericardial syndromes may occur after heart surgery.

Cardiac tamponade may occur during in-hospital recuperation, most commonly in the first 24 hours due to hemopericardium. It is identified by the hemodynamic perturbations typical of tamponade. The sudden cessation of previously brisk bleeding from drains should alert the physician to the possibility of clogging. Therapy consists of prompt surgical exploration and evacuation.

Cardiac tamponade is less common after the first 24 hours, with fewer typical clinical manifestations, and symptoms may consist largely of nonspecific generalized complaints. Two-dimensional echocardiography establishes the presence of a significant effusion and may delineate its anatomic distribution. Pericardial effusions in this setting are often loculated and may compress only one cardiac chamber. The approach to drainage is largely dictated by the location of the effusion.

Early pericarditis, consisting of fever, chest pain, pericardial friction rubs, and typical ECG features, is common. In most cases, the syndrome resolves spontaneously, and nonsteroidal anti-inflammatory drugs (NSAIDs) with or without colchicine are effective treatment. Corticosteroids are also very efficacious in this setting.

Postpericardiotomy syndrome is reported in 10–40% of patients, depending on the type of surgery and the adopted diagnostic criteria. This syndrome, which usually occurs during the first several postoperative weeks, consists of fever, pleuritis, and pericarditis. Diagnosis proceeds by exclusion, and treatment consists of administering NSAIDs and colchicine; sometimes corticosteroids are used, especially to avoid interference of aspirin or a NSAID with oral anticoagulant therapy.

Constrictive pericarditis occurs rarely as a complication of cardiac surgery. Its incidence is estimated to only be 0.2–0.3% of cardiac operations. However, cardiac surgery is emerging as an important cause of constrictive pericarditis because so many cardiac surgeries are performed in the United States annually. The risk of constriction has been estimated at 2–5% in patients with acute pericarditis due to a postcardiac injury syndrome. Constrictive pericarditis has been reported to occur at times ranging from 2 weeks to 21 years after the surgery. Because of the relative rarity of this complication, it has been difficult to identify specific predisposing procedural factors; however, bleeding in the pericardium is presumed to be a major trigger. Occasionally, constrictive pericarditis appears within days or weeks after surgery. These cases appear to respond well to a course of corticosteroids. With this exception, the mainstay of therapy for postsurgical constrictive pericarditis is pericardiectomy.

2. Trauma—Traumatic hemorrhagic pericardial effusions, which can result from blunt or penetrating injuries of the chest, can also be caused by a variety of iatrogenic causes such as cardiac catheterization and coronary interventional procedures, pacemaker insertion, arrhythmia ablation procedures, endoscopy, and closed chest cardiac massage. The rapidity with which pericardial fluid can accumulate can quickly cause hemodynamic compromise. Hypotension in this setting should prompt both an immediate echocardiographic search for pericardial fluid and swift evacuation of any significant effusions. Delayed manifestations may include recurrent pericardial effusions and, in rare cases, constrictive pericarditis.

3. Radiation therapy—The incidence of pericardial injury from therapeutic radiation is related to dose, duration, and technical features. Pericardial damage from radiation may appear during the course of therapy or following it. The syndrome that appears during radiation therapy is acute pericarditis. The onset of clinical manifestations in the delayed

form is usually within 12 months but may take many years. The clinical features of the late form range from asymptomatic pericardial effusions to acute pericarditis or constrictive pericarditis. Radiation therapy is now one of the leading causes of constrictive pericarditis.

C. Connective Tissue Disorders

Connective tissue vascular diseases are a common cause of pericardial diseases. A number of rheumatic diseases can involve the pericardium. This is most likely to occur in patients with known systemic lupus erythematosus, Sjögren syndrome, or rheumatoid arthritis, but can also occur in progressive systemic sclerosis, mixed connective tissue disease, polyarteritis, giant cell arteritis, polymyalgia rheumatica, other systemic vasculitides, acute rheumatic fever, and familial Mediterranean fever. Rarely, occasional patients with gout may suffer attacks of pericarditis during an episode of arthritis.

Symptomatic pericarditis can occur with all of these disorders, during the active phase of the systemic disease. In other cases, pericardial involvement may be subclinical with a clinically silent pericardial effusion. In unselected series of patients, acute pericarditis occurred in 2–7% of cases. However, in many cases, the diagnosis of a connective tissue disease was already known at the time of the diagnosis of pericarditis.

D. Other Causes

1. Myocardial infarction—Clinical evidence of pericarditis can be found in 7–20% of patients within the first week after myocardial infarction, although autopsy series suggest a significantly higher incidence of clinically silent, localized fibrinous pericarditis. The incidence is greatest with large, ST segment elevation myocardial infarctions. Anticoagulant therapy and antiplatelet therapy administered in conjunction with percutaneous revascularization procedures do not appear to increase the incidence of pericardial effusions after myocardial infarction. While it is theoretically possible that these drugs may increase the chance of hemorrhage into the pericardial space if an effusion does occur, they are not generally considered to be contraindicated in the setting of early postmyocardial infarction pericarditis. Thrombolytic therapy has been associated with a decreased incidence of pericarditis in placebo-controlled studies. In contemporary series of patients with ST segment elevation acute myocardial infarctions (AMIs) treated with primary percutaneous coronary intervention, pericarditis has become less common. Early post-AMI pericarditis has been reported in 4–5% with an increasing prevalence according to presentation delay: < 2% for < 3 hours, 5–6% for 3–6 hours, and 10–15% for > 6 hours. Identified risk factors for early post-AMI pericarditis include presentation times > 6 hours and primary percutaneous coronary intervention failure. Although pericarditis is associated with a larger infarct size, in-hospital and 1-year mortality and major adverse cardiac events are similar in patients with and without pericarditis.

Dressler syndrome (postmyocardial infarction syndrome) occurs from 1 to 6 weeks after myocardial infarction and consists of fever, pleuropericardial pain, malaise, and evidence of pleural and pericardial effusions. The syndrome has been considered a **contraindication to anticoagulant therapy** since a real increase of the likelihood of pericardial hemorrhage and tamponade has not been demonstrated. However, there is little data to support this precaution. The incidence of this syndrome has been decreasing in recent years. Dressler syndrome has become rare in the primary percutaneous coronary intervention era and is reported in < 0.5% of cases. It is believed to have an autoimmune cause due to sensitization to myocardial cells at the time of necrosis. Antimyocardial antibodies have been demonstrated in patients with Dressler syndrome.

2. Malignancy—A variety of hematologic and solid malignancies (especially lung and breast cancer, lymphomas) can cause pericardial metastases that are more frequently revealed during autopsy rather than during life. Malignant tumors can spread to the pericardium through the lymphatics (mainly lung and breast carcinomas, and other carcinomas with lung metastases), through the coronary arteries (leukemia, lymphomas, and melanomas), or by direct local invasion (lung or mediastinal neoplasms). Neoplastic involvement of the pericardium can cause pericarditis, pericardial effusion with or without cardiac tamponade, and constrictive pericarditis. Primary tumors of the pericardium are rare; most are mesotheliomas and may be relatively frequent in some areas where asbestos is extracted or used in industry. Neoplastic pericarditis is responsible for 4–7% (approximately 5%) of unselected cases of pericarditis.

Typically, the diagnosis of malignancy has already been established in the patient with a malignant pericardial effusion, and other sites of metastatic spread are evident. On rare occasions, tamponade from the malignant effusion is the first manifestation of tumor. It is important to distinguish malignant effusions from other causes of effusion, such as radiation, infection, and uremia, because the management and prognosis of malignant and nonmalignant effusions in cancer patients differ substantially.

3. Renal failure—Pericardial involvement in patients with renal failure can take several forms. Pericardial effusions can be found on an echocardiogram in many patients with chronic kidney disease who are asymptomatic. These effusions, which are typically small, are related more closely to the patient's volume status than other variables and usually warrant no intervention beyond clinical vigilance.

The incidence of uremic pericarditis has been decreasing for years, a trend attributable to earlier and more intensive dialysis. Uremic pericarditis typically occurs before the initiation of long-term dialysis; its development is related, in part, to the elevation of absolute levels of blood urea nitrogen (BUN) and serum creatinine, and it almost always responds to dialysis. Although uremic pericarditis can lead to tamponade, it is more commonly associated with the slow accumulation of large, low-pressure pericardial effusions.

4. Drug-related causes—A number of pharmacologic agents have been implicated in pericardial disease. Pericarditis can occur as a feature of drug-induced systemic lupus erythematosus syndrome caused by procainamide, hydralazine, diphenylhydantoin, reserpine, methyldopa, and isoniazid. In addition to their propensity for causing myocardial inflammation, anthracycline antineoplastic agents can cause acute pericarditis. Methysergide can cause pericardial constriction as part of the syndrome of mediastinal fibrosis, and pericarditis can be part of a hypersensitivity reaction to penicillin. Minoxidil has been reported to cause pericarditis and tamponade; the mechanism is unknown.

5. Hypothyroidism—Pericardial effusion can be found in one-third of patients with myxedema. The frequency of pericardial involvement is related to both the severity and duration of hypothyroidism. The accumulation of pericardial fluid in this condition appears to be a result of a combination of increased capillary permeability and retarded lymphatic drainage. Because the pericardial fluid accumulates slowly, tamponade is rare. If pericardiocentesis is required before the diagnosis of hypothyroidism is made, the diagnosis can be suspected if the fluid is yellow and contains a high level of cholesterol. Pericardial disease in hypothyroidism reliably responds to thyroid hormone replacement therapy.

Imazio M. The post-pericardiotomy syndrome. *Curr Opin Pulm Med.* 2012;18(4):366–74. [PMID: 22487945]

Imazio M. Pericardial involvement in systemic inflammatory diseases. *Heart.* 2011;97(22):1882–92. [PMID: 22016400]

Imazio M, et al. Aetiological diagnosis in acute and recurrent pericarditis: when and how. *J Cardiovasc Med (Hagerstown).* 2009;10(3):217–30. [PMID: 19262208]

Imazio M, et al. Medical therapy of pericardial diseases: part II: noninfectious pericarditis, pericardial effusion and constrictive pericarditis. *J Cardiovasc Med (Hagerstown).* 2010;11(11): 785–94. [PMID:20925146]

Imazio M, et al. Post-cardiac injury syndromes. An emerging cause of pericardial diseases. *Int J Cardiol.* 2012;S0167-5273(12):01158–8. [PMID: 23040075]

Imazio M, et al. Risk of constrictive pericarditis after acute pericarditis. *Circulation.* 2011;124(11):1270–5. [PMID: 21844077]

ACUTE PERICARDITIS

 ESSENTIALS OF DIAGNOSIS

▶ Central chest pain aggravated by coughing, inspiration, or recumbency.

▶ Pericardial friction rub on auscultation.

▶ Characteristic ECG changes (widespread ST segment elevation or PR depression).

▶ Pericardial effusion (new or worsening).

► General Considerations

Acute pericarditis is an inflammatory condition of the pericardium that can be caused by virtually any of the conditions just discussed. As discussed earlier, a viral infection is the most common cause in developed countries (North America and Western Europe), while tuberculosis is the most common cause of pericarditis and pericardial diseases in developing countries and all over the world. This epidemiologic background should be kept in mind when managing a single patient, since immigration may lead to an increase of less common infectious causes, especially tuberculous pericarditis.

► Clinical Findings

A. Symptoms & Signs

The primary symptom of acute pericarditis is chest pain whose location, intensity, and nature are variable. The pain may be described as sharp or dull. Most often it is precordial or retrosternal in location and may be referred to the trapezius ridge, which is almost pathognomonic for pericarditis. It is characteristically aggravated by inspiration, coughing, or recumbency and lessened by sitting upright and leaning forward. Although it typically takes an hour or two to develop fully, the pain can sometimes appear remarkably abruptly. Many patients relate prodromal symptoms suggestive of a viral infection (respiratory infections or gastroenteritis). Bacterial pericarditis may present with fever, chills, night sweats, and dyspnea.

B. Physical Examination

Patients with pericarditis may be febrile (but high fever > 38°C is usually associated with a bacterial or immune-mediated form) and show tachycardia. The pericardial friction rub—the characteristic auscultatory finding—is typically scratchy and may have three components corresponding to atrial contraction, ventricular systole, and early diastole. It is not unusual for only one or two components to be audible; the systolic component is most consistently present. It has been reported in about one-third of patients. Exercise may facilitate the identification of all three components. Because the friction rub may be evanescent, varying widely in intensity even in the course of a single day, repeated auscultation is important. Furthermore, because posture can affect the pericardial rub, auscultation with the patient in several positions (eg, supine, sitting) is often helpful. When the intensity of the rub is modulated significantly by respiration, it is termed a "pleuropericardial friction rub."

C. Diagnostic Studies

Evaluation of a patient with suspected pericarditis should routinely include an ECG, complete blood count, markers of inflammation (ie, erythrocyte sedimentation rate and C-reactive protein), markers of myocardial lesion (ie, troponins), echocardiography, and a chest radiograph. Additional diagnostic laboratory tests should be tailored to the clinical presentation. High-risk features at presentation include high fever (> 38°C), subacute course, large pericardial effusion, cardiac tamponade, and lack or incomplete response to empiric anti-inflammatory therapy after 7–10 days (Figure 28–1). Echocardiography is a sensitive test for detecting pericardial effusion; however, pericardial effusion can occur in the absence of pericardial inflammation, and pericarditis may occur without a pericardial effusion. About 60% of patients with acute pericarditis show pericardial effusion at presentation, generally mild (< 1 cm). The clinical diagnosis of acute pericarditis is made with the presence of at least two of four clinical diagnostic criteria: (1) pericarditic chest pain, (2) pericardial rubs, (3) typical ECG findings (widespread ST segment elevation or PR depression) (Figure 28–2), and (4) pericardial effusion.

1. Electrocardiography—Serial ECGs are valuable in diagnosing pericarditis. Four stages of ECG changes have been described (Table 28–2). In stage I, the changes accompany the onset of chest pain and consist of widespread ST segment elevation (Figure 28–2). The ST segment is concave upward (in distinction to the elevation in myocardial infarction). ST segment elevation is typically present in all leads except aVR and V_1, where ST segment depression is often present. The T waves are upright in the leads with ST elevation. The stage I pattern of pericarditis may be difficult to distinguish from the normal variant of early repolarization. A differentiating point that may be useful is the ST:T ratio in V_6. A T-wave apex four times (or greater) higher than the height of the ST segment is more likely to indicate early repolarization; if this ratio is less than 4, pericarditis is more likely. In addition, pericarditis causes changes in the ECG that distinguish it from early repolarization. In stage II, typically occurring several days later, the ST segments return to baseline, and the initially upright T waves flatten. In stage III, the T waves invert, and the ST segments may become depressed—changes that may persist indefinitely. Finally, in stage IV, which may occur weeks or months later, the T waves revert to normal. All four stages can be serially identified in about 50% of patients.

2. Other tests—Laboratory evidence of inflammation, such as mild leukocytosis and an elevated erythrocyte sedimentation rate and C-reactive protein, is common in acute pericarditis. These findings are less consistent in pericarditis associated with uremia or connective tissue disorders. Cardiac enzymes may be slightly elevated when the inflammatory process involves subepicardial myocardium. Alternatively, some cases occur in conjunction with a true viral myocarditis with more substantial elevations in creatine kinase and troponin I. Although the chest radiograph most often reveals no abnormalities in uncomplicated pericarditis, it may occasionally show evidence of pericardial effusion (discussed in the following section). Cases with acute pericarditis (according to clinical criteria) and troponin elevation, but normal ventricular function and wall motion, are usually referred to as **myopericarditis**. They

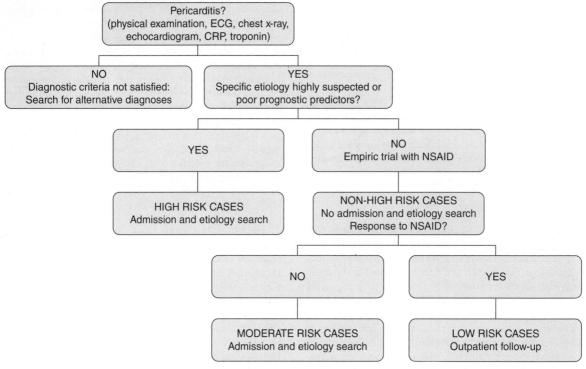

▲ **Figure 28-1.** Triage of acute pericarditis. Red flags include high fever (> 38°C), subacute course, large pericardial effusion, cardiac tamponade, and lack or incomplete response to empiric anti-inflammatory therapy after 7–10 days. If at least one is present, patient should be admitted to hospital and complete etiology search performed. Otherwise, low-risk pericarditis may be managed as outpatient. CRP, C-reactive protein; ECG, electrocardiogram; NSAID, nonsteroidal anti-inflammatory drug. (Reprinted from Imazio M, et al. *Circulation.* 2010;121(7):916–28.)

have a generally good prognosis, and management mimics that reported for acute pericarditis. When myocardial inflammatory involvement is prevalent (as generally manifested by troponin elevation, wall motion abnormalities, and/or mildly reduced ventricular function), the term generally used in the literature is **perimyocarditis** (Figure 28–3). The only way to make the diagnosis of bacterial pericarditis is to analyze pericardial fluid, which should include Gram staining, acid-fast staining, fungal staining, and culture to identify the responsible organism. In suspected tuberculous pericarditis, polymerase chain reaction can be used to detect *M tuberculosis* DNA in the pericardial fluid.

▶ **Treatment**

The management of pericarditis associated with an identifiable etiology is directed primarily to the underlying cause. In the usual case of idiopathic acute pericarditis, treatment with any of the NSAIDs usually suppresses the clinical manifestations within 24–48 hours—and frequently more rapidly. Because of its excellent side-effect profile, ibuprofen, 600 mg orally three times a day for 10–14 days, has been recommended.

Aspirin, 750–1000 mg three times a day, is equally efficacious and may be favored in patients who already are take or need this drug for other indications (ie, ischemic heart disease). An alternative regimen, especially useful in systemic inflammatory diseases, is indomethacin, 50 mg three times a day (Table 28–3). The initial dose is given every 8 hours to achieve good symptom control throughout the whole day. Tapering may be considered when the patient is asymptomatic and markers of inflammation are normalized. C-reactive protein may be helpful to confirm the clinical suspicion of pericarditis and to individualize the length of the initial dose as recently demonstrated in acute pericarditis. Colchicine, which has an excellent track record in the prophylaxis of recurrent pericarditis (see below), should be added to aspirin or NSAID if tolerated and there are no contraindications. The loading dose may be avoided to improve patient tolerance. Weight-adjusted doses of 0.6 mg once daily for patients ≤70 kg or 0.6 mg twice daily for patients > 70 kg for 3 months have been recommended. At these low doses, the drug is safe and well tolerated. Gastrointestinal intolerance, especially diarrhea, is the main side effect, and has been reported in 8% of cases.

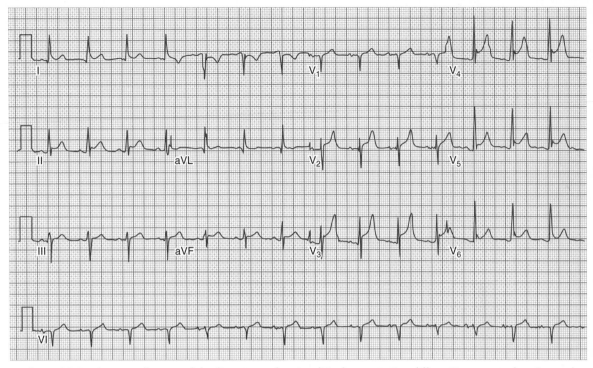

▲ **Figure 28-2.** Electrocardiogram of the first stage of pericarditis demonstrating diffuse ST segment elevation and upright T waves.

A short course of corticosteroids is very effective in ameliorating the pain of acute pericarditis. However, their use is rarely required, and recent evidence suggests they may increase the chance of recurrence. Accordingly, corticosteroids should be avoided unless absolutely necessary to control severe symptoms that do not respond to other measures. If used, low to moderate doses (ie, prednisone 0.2–0.5 mg/kg/day; that is, a prednisone dose of 25 mg for the average man of 70 kg) should be used instead of high doses (ie, prednisone 1 mg/kg/day). Specific indications for the use of corticosteroids include pregnancy, systemic inflammatory diseases when steroids are needed, and postpericardiotomy syndromes to avoid interference of aspirin or NSAID with concomitant oral anticoagulant therapies.

In about 85–90% of patients, a single course of NSAID therapy will effectively control the illness, and pericarditis will resolve without sequelae. In about 30% of patients, a recurrence may develop over a period of weeks or months after the initial episode, generally within 18 months from the index attack. Recurrences can be managed with repeated courses of an NSAID, usually adding colchicine for 6 months at the doses recommended for acute pericarditis. In difficult cases of recurrent pericarditis, prolonged colchicine therapy has

Table 28-2. Serial Electrocardiographic Changes in Pericarditis

Stage	ST Segment	T Waves
I	Elevated	Upright
II	Isoelectric	Upright → flat
III	Isoelectric	Inverted
IV	Isoelectric	Upright

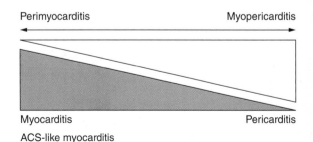

▲ **Figure 28-3.** Spectrum of myopericardial inflammatory syndromes ranging from pure pericarditis to pure myocarditis through intermediate stages: prevalent pericarditis (myopericarditis) or prevalent myocarditis (perimyocarditis). ACS, acute coronary syndrome.

Table 28–3. Empiric Anti-inflammatory Therapy of Pericarditis

Drug	Attack Dose and Tapering
Aspirin	975 mg every 8 hours for 1–2 weeks then tapered (ie, 650 mg every 8 hours for 1–2 weeks, then 325 mg every 8 hours for 1–2 weeks)
Ibuprofen	600 mg every 8 hours for 1–2 weeks, then tapered every week (ie, 600 mg + 400 mg + 600 mg for 1 week, then 600 mg + 400 mg + 400 mg for 1 week, then 400 mg every 8 hours for 1 week)
Indomethacin	50 mg every 8 hours for 1–2 weeks, then tapered every week (ie, 50 mg + 25 mg + 50 mg for 1 week, then 50 mg + 25 mg + 25 mg for 1 week, then 25 mg every 8 hours for 1 week)
Prednisone	0.2–0.5 mg/kg/day for 2–4 weeks, then slow tapering
Colchicine	1.2 mg every 12 hours for 1–2 days, then 0.6 mg every 12 hours for 6–12 months (halved doses if < 70 kg: 0.6 mg twice a day for 1–2 days, then 0.6 mg once a day for 6–12 months)

demonstrated efficacy in prophylaxis and should be strongly considered. While corticosteroids in general should also be avoided in chronic, recurrent pericarditis, occasional patients can best be managed with corticosteroids. Full doses are kept for 2–4 weeks and then slowly tapered (ie, reducing the dose of 2.5 mg every 2–4 weeks) (Table 28–4). Rarely, immunosuppressive drugs, especially azathioprine, may be helpful in these patients, but with a weaker reported evidence base.

Intravenous antimicrobial therapy should be started as soon as the diagnosis of purulent pericarditis is suspected. Although high intrapericardial antibiotic levels are achievable, prompt percutaneous or surgical drainage is essential. Cardiac tamponade may occur rapidly and resemble septic shock. In countries where tuberculosis is not endemic, only patients with proven or very likely tuberculous pericarditis should be treated.

In rare cases, frequent and severe recurrences despite aggressive medical therapy have prompted pericardiectomy. Pericardiectomy is generally disappointing, and further recurrences have been reported with incomplete removal of the pericardium, as generally occurs. However, the efficacy of pericardiectomy in this circumstance is unknown, and in one small series was reported to only rarely be effective.

The most feared complication of pericarditis is the development of constrictive pericarditis. The risk is related to the etiology and not the number of recurrences. Idiopathic and viral pericarditis has a low risk (< 1%); immune-mediated (systemic inflammatory diseases and postcardiac injury syndromes) and neoplastic pericardial diseases have an intermediate risk (2–5%), whereas the highest risk has been reported for bacterial etiologies, especially tuberculosis and purulent forms (20–30%). The risk of constrictive evolution is negligible in idiopathic recurrent pericarditis.

Imazio M, et al. Colchicine for pericarditis: hype or hope? *Eur Heart J.* 2009;30(5):532–9. [PMID: 19190012]

Imazio M, et al. Controversial issues in the management of pericardial diseases. *Circulation.* 2010;121(7):916–28. [PMID: 20177006]

Imazio M, et al. Corticosteroids for recurrent pericarditis: high versus low doses: a nonrandomized observation. *Circulation.* 2008;118(6):667–71. [PMID: 18645054]

Imazio M, et al. Management of pericardial diseases during pregnancy. *J Cardiovasc Med (Hagerstown).* 2010;11(8):557–62. [PMID: 20389257]

Imazio M, et al. Myopericarditis: etiology, management, and prognosis. *Int J Cardiol.* 2008;127(1):17–26. [PMID: 18221804]

Imazio M, et al. Prevalence of C-reactive protein elevation and time course of normalization in acute pericarditis: implications for the diagnosis, therapy, and prognosis of pericarditis. *Circulation.* 2011;123(10):1092–7. [PMID: 21357824]

Lotrionte M, et al. International collaborative systematic review of controlled clinical trials on pharmacologic treatments for acute pericarditis and its recurrences. *Am Heart J.* 2010;160(4):662–70. [PMID: 20934560]

Table 28–4. Prednisone Tapering for Patients with Recurrent Pericarditis

Prednisone Daily Dose (mg)	Tapering: Daily Dose to Be Reduced at Weekly Intervals as Indicated Below[1]
> 50	10 mg/day every 1–2 weeks
25–50	5–10 mg/day every 1–2 weeks
15–25	2.5 mg/day every 2–4 weeks
< 15	1.25–2.5 mg/day every 2–6 weeks

[1]Every decrease should be done only if the patient is asymptomatic and markers of inflammation are within the normal reference values.

PERICARDIAL EFFUSION

 ESSENTIALS OF DIAGNOSIS

▶ Echocardiographic demonstration of pericardial fluid.

▶ General Considerations

Pericardial effusion can develop as a result of pericarditis or an injury of any kind to the pericardium. It can be encountered in the absence of pericarditis in many clinical settings, such as uremia, cardiac trauma or chamber rupture, malignancy, AIDS, and hypothyroidism.

▶ Clinical Findings

A. Symptoms & Signs

Clinical manifestations of pericardial effusion are directly related to the absolute volume of the effusion and the rapidity of accumulation. Small, incidental effusions rarely, if ever, cause symptoms or complications, and patients with slowly developing pericardial effusions can accumulate large volumes of fluid without symptoms. With a very slowly accumulating effusion, the pericardium can accommodate 1–2 L or more of fluid without a clinically significant elevation of intrapericardial pressure. Many of these large effusions are discovered incidentally when a chest radiograph is performed. Some may become clinically manifest by compression of adjacent structures or by causing dysphagia, cough, dyspnea, hiccups, hoarseness, nausea, or a sense of abdominal fullness. It is exceedingly rare for a specific cause of large, incidentally discovered effusions to be identified. In contrast, more rapid accumulation of even modest fluid volumes can be associated with increased intrapericardial pressures and life-threatening hemodynamic compromise.

B. Physical Examination

On examination, signs of pericardial effusion are absent in patients who have small effusions without increased pressure. Large effusions may muffle the heart sounds or cause left lower lobe lung dullness to percussion of the chest (Ewart sign) as a result of compression of lung parenchyma or dullness to percussion of the sternum.

C. Diagnostic Studies

1. Electrocardiography—The ECG may be entirely normal. Large effusions can cause both reduced voltage (Figure 28–4) and electrical alternans—alternating QRS voltage as a result of a swinging motion of the heart that characteristically occurs at a frequency of half the heart rate. If pericarditis coexists with effusion, the usual findings may be present.

2. Chest radiography—An increase in the cardiac silhouette combined with clear or oligemic lung fields suggests the presence of a significant pericardial effusion (> 250–300 ml) (Figure 28–5), although the chest radiograph can appear entirely normal in the presence of a small to moderate effusion. Very rapidly accumulating fluid may result in only the subtlest of changes in the cardiac silhouette. With slowly accumulating fluid, the cardiac silhouette may assume a globular shape that has been likened to a water bottle with clear lungs. Radiographic differentiation of pericardial effusion and cardiac enlargement may not be possible. Occasionally, the presence of an effusion may cause increased separation of the pericardial fat-pad layers.

3. Echocardiography—Transthoracic echocardiography is the fastest and most accurate means of diagnosing and estimating the size of a pericardial effusion, but it is not accurate in assessing pericardial thickness. The effusion appears as an echo-free space between the moving epicardium and the stationary parietal pericardium. Although M-mode echocardiography can identify as little as 15 mL of pericardial fluid, two-dimensional echocardiography has the advantage of demonstrating the full distribution of the effusion and

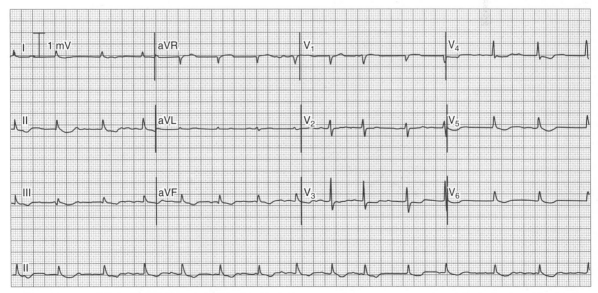

▲ **Figure 28–4.** Reduced QRS voltages (the amplitudes of QRS complexes are < 5 mm in the limbs leads, and < 10 mm in all but one of the precordial leads) and atrial fibrillation in a patient with a chronic, large pericardial effusion.

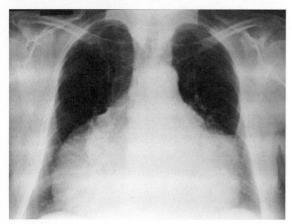

▲ **Figure 28–5.** Large pericardial effusion on chest x-ray with water bottle heart shape.

identifying a loculated effusion. Quantification of the volume of effusion by echocardiography is not always precise. Semiquantitative assessment is practical. Large pericardial effusions (> 20 mm) have been associated with a higher risk of nonidiopathic etiologies and complications during follow-up (Figure 28–6). Small effusions (< 10 mm) tend to be imaged only posteriorly, whereas an anterior echo-free space, however, may reflect subepicardial fat rather than pericardial effusion. Larger effusions are usually distributed both anteriorly and posteriorly. A moderate effusion is considered with the widest diastolic echo-free space between 10 and 20 mm. On occasion, large effusions (> 20 mm) are associated

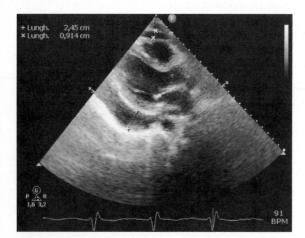

▲ **Figure 28–6.** Semiquantitative assessment of pericardial effusion. The largest diastolic width of echo-free space is measured by M-mode or two-dimensional echocardiography using different echocardiographic views, also off-axis if needed. The largest size is used to estimate the effusion as mild (< 10 mm), moderate (10–20 mm), or large (> 20 mm).

with an excessive swinging motion of the heart within the fluid-filled pericardium. Transesophageal echocardiography is particularly useful in quantifying the anatomic distribution of effusions, especially when loculated, and is superior to transthoracic echocardiography in imaging the thickness of the pericardium.

4. Cardiac magnetic resonance imaging and computed tomography—Both of these modalities provide highly accurate imaging of pericardial effusions but, in most cases, are not necessary if echocardiographic images are technically satisfactory. However, they are the most accurate methods for delineating the size of effusions, their anatomic distribution, and the thickness of the pericardium. Thus, they are often valuable adjuncts to echocardiography and may help to characterize the nature of the effusion.

In clinical practice, most cases with pericardial effusion (> 60%) have a known underlying medical condition or systemic disease that may explain the presence of the effusion. Pericarditis with elevation of markers of inflammation should be ruled out, and if present, the management of the effusion should follow the recommendations for pericarditis. In the absence of inflammation and systemic conditions, large effusions with cardiac tamponade are associated with a high risk of neoplastic etiologies, especially lung cancer, that should be ruled out (Figure 28–7).

▶ **Treatment**

The management of a pericardial effusion is largely dictated by its size, the presence or absence of hemodynamic compromise from increased intrapericardial pressure (see next section), and the nature of the underlying disorder (discussed earlier). In most cases, a small or incidentally discovered effusion warrants no specific intervention. At the same time, it should be recalled that once an effusion reaches a certain magnitude, even small additional amounts of fluid can cause a marked increase in intrapericardial pressure and rapid clinical deterioration; these patients must be monitored closely. Very large, chronic effusions (> 3 months) discovered accidentally usually do not progress. However, some of these (up to one-third) will eventually result in cardiac tamponade. Therefore, elective, closed pericardiocentesis may be recommended in these cases. Interestingly, these effusions typically do not recur following removal of the fluid.

Dudzinski DM, et al. Pericardial diseases. *Curr Probl Cardiol.* 2012;37(3):75–118. [PMID: 22289657]

Imazio M. Contemporary management of pericardial diseases. *Curr Opin Cardiol.* 2012;27(3):308–17. [PMID: 22450720]

Imazio M, et al. Medical therapy of pericardial diseases: part I: idiopathic and infectious pericarditis. *J Cardiovasc Med (Hagerstown).* 2010;11(10):712–22. [PMID: 20736783]

Imazio M, et al. Medical therapy of pericardial diseases: part II: noninfectious pericarditis, pericardial effusion and constrictive pericarditis. *J Cardiovasc Med (Hagerstown).* 2010;11(11): 785–94. [PMID: 20925146]

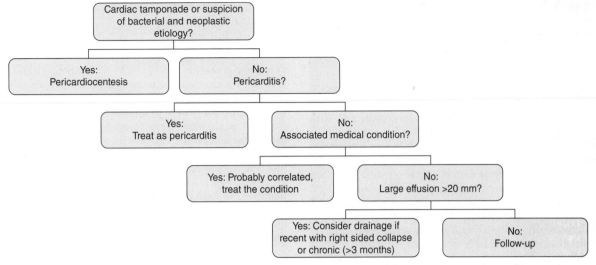

▲ **Figure 28–7.** Triage for pericardial effusions of unknown origin. (Reprinted from Imazio M, et al. *Circulation.* 2010;121(7):916–28.)

Imazio M, Adler Y. Management of pericardial effusion. *Eur Heart J.* 2013;34:1186-97. [PMID: 23125278]

Imazio M, et al. Triage and management of pericardial effusion. *J Cardiovasc Med (Hagerstown).* 2010;11(12):928-35. [PMID: 20814314]

Refaat MM, et al. Neoplastic pericardial effusion. *Clin Cardiol.* 2011;34(10):593-8. [PMID: 21928406]

CARDIAC TAMPONADE

 ESSENTIALS OF DIAGNOSIS

▶ Increased jugular venous pressure with an obliterated y descent.

▶ Pulsus paradoxus.

▶ Echocardiographic evidence of right atrial and ventricular collapse.

▶ Equal diastolic pressures in all four cardiac chambers.

▶ General Considerations

Cardiac tamponade exists when increased intrapericardial pressure from accumulation of fluid compromises the filling of the heart, thereby impairing cardiac output. Whether the intrapericardial pressure rises to a level that impedes filling depends on both the rapidity of accumulation and the volume of the effusion. Severe tamponade may thus ensue in the setting of a traumatic effusion where a modest volume of blood fills the pericardial space in a brief time. Conversely, in settings such as myxedema or chronic idiopathic effusions, a slowly accumulating effusion may reach a remarkably large volume without raising the intrapericardial pressure.

▶ Clinical Findings

A. Symptoms & Signs

Patients with cardiac tamponade may complain of dyspnea and chest discomfort, but dyspnea has been reported as the symptom with the highest sensitivity (85–90%). In more severe cases, consciousness may be impaired, and there may be signs of reduced cardiac output and shock. The systemic arterial pressure is typically low, although it may be surprisingly well-preserved on occasion; pulse pressure is usually diminished. The patient with tamponade is typically tachycardic and tachypneic, although bradycardia may ensue in terminal stages. Patients with tamponade are almost always more comfortable sitting upright. If pericarditis coexists, typical pain and a friction rub may be present.

1. Pulsus paradoxus—Pulsus paradoxus, defined as an abnormally large decline (> 10 mm Hg) in systolic arterial pressure during inspiration, is present in most cases. This is the most accurate physical sign with a high sensitivity (70–90%) and specificity (70–80%). The term is actually something of a misnomer because the paradoxical pulse represents an exaggeration of the normal small decline in systolic arterial pressure that occurs during inspiration. In the presence of cardiac tamponade, the volume that can be occupied by cardiac chambers becomes fixed. During inspiration, the increase of venous return and thus right ventricle volume can occur only at the expenses of a reduced left ventricular volume. This phenomenon is also referred as ventricular interdependence. On echocardiography, mitral peak E waves show a marked respiratory variation > 25% of their values.

Pulsus paradoxus is evaluated through careful auscultation of the Korotkoff sounds as the cuff pressure is slowly released. It is measured as the difference in cuff pressure from the point at which sounds are initially heard intermittently during expiration and the point at which the sounds are audible throughout the respiratory cycle and with each ventricular systole. A pulsus paradoxus greater than 10 mm Hg is considered abnormal. In severe tamponade, the peripheral pulse reveals an obvious decrease in the stroke volume and may even disappear on inspiration. The presence of an abnormal pulsus paradoxus is not essential to the diagnosis of cardiac tamponade, and it may be absent in clinical situations where tamponade coexists with cardiac volume overload lesions, such as atrial septal defect or aortic insufficiency. The absence of a pulsus paradoxus in these settings should not dissuade the physician from the correct diagnosis. In addition, pulsus paradoxus can be present when the inspiratory decrease in intrapleural pressure is exaggerated, as in obstructive airway disease. Reversed pulsus paradoxus—a fall in pressure with expiration—can be seen in patients on positive pressure respirators.

2. Jugular venous pressure—The venous pressure is usually markedly elevated, and examination of the jugular venous pulse wave reveals obliteration of the normal y descent. In patients with low-pressure tamponade (see section on cardiac catheterization), the venous pressure may actually be normal or only mildly elevated.

3. Other findings—Diminished heart sounds can be heard in one-third of cases; a pericardial friction rub may be heard but is absent in most patients. The concept of an inverse relation between the intensity of a pericardial rub (when present) and the size of the effusion cannot be used in assessing individual patients; the relationship is too variable to be reliable.

B. Diagnostic Studies

1. Electrocardiography—ECG may offer no specific diagnostic clues, although the ECG abnormalities described in pericarditis and pericardial effusion may be seen. The development of electrical alternans almost always indicates a hemodynamically significant effusion. However, low QRS voltages and electrical alternans have a low reported sensitivity (< 50%).

2. Chest radiography—Chest radiography offers no specific diagnostic signs of tamponade. As mentioned earlier, the cardiac silhouette may be remarkably normal in size in cases where a modestly sized effusion accumulates rapidly. A pericardial fat pad sign is diagnostic of pericardial effusion but does not necessarily indicate tamponade. The lung fields are frequently oligemic. Occasionally, the chest radiograph

offers clues to important coexisting conditions, such as aortic dissection or malignancy.

3. Echocardiography—Echocardiography is an invaluable adjunctive tool. It confirms the presence of pericardial fluid and can provide evidence of increased intrapericardial pressure. The most useful echocardiographic sign is diastolic collapse of the right atrium and right ventricle. Although these changes are neither completely sensitive nor specific, they first occur when the pericardial pressure transiently exceeds the intracardiac chamber pressure. They can therefore be useful in identifying patients whose pericardial pressure level should be of concern. Echocardiography is also extremely useful as a guide in pericardiocentesis. The cardiac chambers are small in tamponade, and as discussed earlier, in extreme cases, the heart swings anteroposteriorly within the effusion. Distention of the caval vessels that does not diminish with inspiration is another useful sign.

Doppler velocity recordings demonstrate exaggerated respiratory variation in right- and left-sided venous and valvular flow, with marked inspiratory increases on the right and decreases on the left (> 25%). Loss of the y descent in the jugular venous pressure is caused by reduced systemic venous inflow during early diastole. Correspondingly, Doppler evaluation reveals that most caval and pulmonary venous inflow occurs during ventricular systole. These flow patterns were found to have a sensitivity of 75% and a specificity of 91% for diagnosing tamponade. The absence of chamber collapse is especially useful in excluding tamponade in patients with effusions, but its presence is less well-correlated with tamponade than abnormal venous flow patterns. Newer techniques such as tissue Doppler do not yet have a well-defined, additive role in cardiac tamponade. Inferior vena cava plethora with reduced or absent respiratory changes of size have been typically reported in cardiac tamponade.

4. Cardiac catheterization—In the patient with tamponade, cardiac catheterization reveals a depressed cardiac output as well as elevated and equal or near-equal filling pressures in all four chambers (difference < 5 mm Hg). Examination of the atrial pressure waveforms reveals the loss of the normal y descent. The initial presentation and hemodynamic profile of tamponade may, however, be altered by a concomitant state of intravascular volume depletion, a scenario that has been called **low-pressure cardiac tamponade.** This term underscores an important feature of the pathophysiology of pericardial effusions; the hemodynamic effect is a function of both the intrapericardial pressure and the intravascular volume. Although this syndrome typically occurs in patients undergoing dialysis for chronic renal failure, it can be encountered in any setting of increased intrapericardial fluid and intravascular volume depletion. In these patients, the effusions are ordinarily insufficient to cause major hemodynamic embarrassment; they become significant when intravascular volume is depleted. The diagnosis should be considered in patients

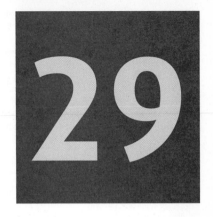

Pulmonary Embolic Disease

Sandeep A. Saha, MBBS

Rajni K. Rao, MD

ESSENTIALS OF DIAGNOSIS

▶ Otherwise unexplained dyspnea, tachypnea, or chest pain.

▶ Clinical, electrocardiogram, or echocardiographic evidence of acute cor pulmonale.

▶ Positive chest computed tomography angiography scan with contrast.

▶ High-probability ventilation-perfusion lung scan or high-probability perfusion lung scan with a normal chest radiograph.

▶ Positive venous ultrasound of the legs with a convincing clinical history and suggestive lung scan.

▶ Diagnostic contrast pulmonary angiogram.

▶ General Considerations

The term "venous thromboembolism" (VTE) encompasses both pulmonary embolism (PE) and deep venous thrombosis (DVT) and accounts for more than 250,000 hospitalizations per year in the United States. VTE constitutes one of the most common causes of cardiovascular and cardiopulmonary illnesses in Western civilization. PE causes or contributes to at least 50,000 deaths per year in the United States, a rate that has probably remained constant for the past three decades. However, a significant proportion of cases of PE remain undiagnosed, partly due to the variable nature of its clinical presentation and partly due to the lack of access of appropriate diagnostic testing modalities at the point of initial care. With the increasing use of computed tomographic pulmonary angiography (CT-PA) in mainstream clinical practice, a larger proportion of PE cases are now being diagnosed. In fact, the estimated incidence of PE has approximately doubled after the introduction of CT-PA in routine clinical practice, from 62.1 to 112.3 cases

per 100,000 individuals. For those who survive PE, further disability includes the potential development of chronic pulmonary hypertension or chronic venous insufficiency. After a VTE event, patients and their physicians are concerned about the presence of an occult carcinoma, the risk of a recurrent PE after anticoagulation therapy has been discontinued, and whether the patients' family members are at risk for VTE.

▶ Etiology

"Primary" PE occurs in the absence of surgery or trauma. Patients with this condition often have an underlying hypercoagulable state, although a specific thrombophilic condition may not be identified. A common scenario is a clinically silent tendency toward thrombosis, which is precipitated by a stressor such as prolonged immobilization, oral contraceptives, pregnancy, or hormone replacement therapy. Recently, there has been an increased appreciation of the risks of VTE among patients with medical illnesses, including cancer (which itself may be associated with a hypercoagulable state), congestive heart failure, and chronic obstructive pulmonary disease.

The prevalence of "secondary" PE is high among patients undergoing certain types of surgery, especially orthopedic surgery of the hip and knee, gynecologic cancer surgery, major trauma, and craniotomy for brain tumor. PE in these patients may occur as late as a month after discharge from the hospital.

A. Thrombophilia

A thorough history should be obtained, including history of prior VTE, family history of VTE, history of frequent miscarriages, past history of cancer, recent history of heparin use (suggestive of heparin-induced thrombocytopenia), and history of prothrombotic conditions (myeloproliferative disease, nephrotic syndrome, collagen-vascular disease, and congestive heart failure). An acquired or inheritable

Table 29–1. Thrombophilic Risk Factors for Venous Thromboembolism

Common
  Factor V Leiden
  Prothrombin gene mutation
  Anticardiolipin antibodies (including lupus anticoagulant) as a
    feature of the antiphospholipid antibody syndrome
  Hyperhomocysteinemia (usually due to folate deficiency)
Uncommon
  Antithrombin III deficiency
  Protein C deficiency
  Protein S deficiency
  Mutations of cystathionine β-synthase or methylene tetrahydrofo-
    late reductase (MTHFR)
  High concentrations of factors VIII or XI (or both)

risk factor is found in 50% of patients who present with an initial VTE. Principal thrombophilic risk factors for VTE are listed in Table 29–1. The two most common genetic mutations that predispose to VTE are the factor V Leiden and the prothrombin gene. Both are autosomal dominant. Whether factor V Leiden predisposes to recurrent VTE after anticoagulation is discontinued remains controversial. The prothrombin gene mutation is associated with an increased risk of recurrent VTE after discontinuation of anticoagulation, especially in patients who have coinherited the factor V Leiden mutation.

Laboratory screening for inherited thrombophilia does not always impact the treatment plan and therefore is not always indicated. Regardless of whether a risk factor is identified, just the history of having had a VTE event is the most significant risk factor for predicting future recurrence. Screening for deficiencies of antithrombin III, protein C, and protein S is a low-yield strategy that produces positive findings in less than 5% of patients. Heparin decreases the antithrombin III level, whereas warfarin, pregnancy, and oral contraceptives decrease the protein C and S levels, thereby resulting in potentially spurious diagnoses of these hypercoagulable states. There are no data that support screening for or treating hyperhomocysteinemia in the setting of VTE. A positive finding of inherited thrombophilia does not necessarily imply that the patient is at higher risk for recurrent VTE or would benefit from extended duration of anticoagulation. Therefore, the 2012 American College of Chest Physicians (ACCP) guidelines do not find that testing for inherited thrombophilic disorders should be a major determinant of VTE treatment. However, in patients with a strong family history of VTE, or based on strong patient preferences, screening can be considered for the patient and first-degree relatives, particularly if it may impact decisions about oral contraceptive use.

In contrast to screening for inheritable disorders, because malignancy is a hypercoagulable state and because VTE may be the first presenting symptom of malignancy, age-appropriate cancer screening after VTE is prudent.

B. Women's Health

PE poses a special threat for women because VTE is associated with the use of oral contraceptives, pregnancy, and hormone replacement therapy.

One-third of pregnancy-related VTE occurs postpartum. The risk of DVT is present throughout pregnancy and is highest during the third trimester. After delivery, two of the most important risk factors for VTE are increased maternal age and cesarean section. Emergency cesarean section increases the VTE risk by about 50% compared with elective cesarean section.

Among women with a history of VTE during pregnancy or puerperium in one study, the prevalence of factor V Leiden was 44% and the prevalence of the prothrombin gene mutation was 17%. Compared with controls, the Leiden mutation increased the risk of VTE ninefold, and the prothrombin gene mutation increased the risk by a factor of 15. The combination of the Leiden and prothrombin gene mutations increased the VTE risk to more than 100 times that seen in the controls. Irrespective of factor V Leiden, pregnancy itself causes hypercoagulability because it induces a relative state of activated protein C resistance.

Hormone replacement therapy also predisposes to VTE. In 1996, three separate large data sets implicated hormone replacement therapy as doubling, tripling, or even quadrupling the risk of VTE. As with oral contraceptives, the risk of VTE peaks during the first year of hormone replacement therapy.

Wiener RS, et al. Time trends in pulmonary embolism in the United States: evidence of overdiagnosis. *Arch Intern Med.* 2011;171(9):831–37. [PMID: 21555660]

▶ Clinical Findings

PE is often difficult to diagnose due to the variable nature of its clinical presentation. Acute PE can manifest clinically as massive, submassive, or nonmassive based on the severity of the clinical presentation, although this distinction is somewhat vague and does not necessarily correlate with clinical outcomes. Acute massive PE is a life-threatening condition characterized by sudden onset of chest pain, hypotension, hypoxemia, and distended neck veins, and it needs to be differentiated quickly from other potentially lethal conditions including acute myocardial infarction, tension pneumothorax, or pericardial tamponade. Despite the availability of radionuclide lung scanning, chest computed tomography (CT) scanning, and pulmonary angiography, many pulmonary emboli are not discovered until postmortem examination. Appreciation of the clinical settings that make patients susceptible to PE and maintenance of a high degree of clinical suspicion are, therefore, of paramount importance.

A. Symptoms & Signs

The most common symptoms or signs of PE are nonspecific: dyspnea, tachypnea, chest pain, or tachycardia. Patients with life-threatening or massive PE are apt to have dyspnea, syncope, or cyanosis rather than chest pain. Less than one-third of patients with PE have symptoms of a DVT. Massive PE should be suspected in hypotensive patients who have evidence of, or predisposing factors for, venous thrombosis and clinical findings of acute cor pulmonale (acute right ventricular failure), such as distended neck veins, an S_3 gallop, a right ventricular heave, tachycardia, or tachypnea. The definition of massive PE proposed by the American Heart Association is: an acute PE with sustained hypotension (systolic blood pressure < 90 mm Hg for at least 15 minutes or requiring inotropic support, not due to a cause other than PE, such as arrhythmia, hypovolemia, sepsis, or left ventricular dysfunction), pulselessness, or persistent profound bradycardia (heart rate < 40 bpm with signs or symptoms of shock). Submassive PE has been defined as an acute PE without systemic hypotension (systolic blood pressure > 90 mm Hg) but with either evidence of right ventricular dysfunction or myocardial necrosis. Low-risk or nonmassive PE is defined as an acute PE without the presence of hemodynamic instability, right ventricular dysfunction, or myocardial necrosis.

Patients with severe chest pain or hemoptysis usually have anatomically small PE near the periphery of the lung. This is where innervation is greatest and where pulmonary infarction is most likely to occur from a dearth of collateral bronchial circulation.

Decision algorithms have been developed to help determine the probability of PE based on clinical symptoms and signs and to guide the selection of diagnostic tests in order to make a rapid and accurate diagnosis and thus initiate treatment without delay. To this end, an integrated diagnostic approach for cases of suspected PE, as shown in Figure 29–1, has been shown to be useful. The diagnostic workup should begin by quantifying the clinical suspicion with a precise clinical scoring algorithm.

Traditionally, the clinical likelihood of PE has been estimated subjectively by "gestalt" as low, moderate, or high. However, to better define the clinical probability of PE in a given patient, quantitative clinical scoring systems have been devised in order to provide the clinician with a standardized and objective approach.

One of the most widely used clinical scoring systems is the Ottawa Scoring System (also known as the modified Wells index), which has a maximum of 12.5 points (Table 29–2). The greatest emphasis is placed on the presence of signs or symptoms of DVT (3 points) and whether an alternative diagnosis is unlikely (3 points). If the score exceeds 4 points, the overall likelihood of PE being confirmed with imaging tests is 41%. However, if the score is 4 points or less, the likelihood of PE is only 8%. Although this scoring system has the advantage of simplicity and rapidity, it offers a somewhat subjective approach with regard to the important, heavily weighted category of "alternative diagnosis unlikely."

In clinical settings such as outpatient clinics or emergency departments where the overall prevalence of PE is low but many patients have symptoms such as chest pain or shortness of breath, the Pulmonary Embolism Rule-out Criteria (PERC) may be used to exclude a PE without additional diagnostic testing. The eight factors that constitute the PERC are age < 50 years, heart rate < 100 bpm, oxygen saturation ≥ 95%, no hemoptysis, no estrogen use, no prior history of PE or DVT, no unilateral leg swelling, and no surgery or trauma needing hospitalization within the past 4 weeks. If a patient does not have any of the PERC criteria *and* has a low clinical suspicion of PE using clinical gestalt

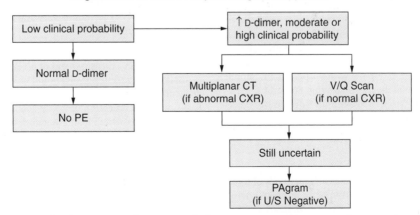

Brigham and Women's Hospital Integrated Approach

▲ **Figure 29–1.** Strategy for diagnosing pulmonary embolism. CT, computed tomography; CXR, chest x-ray film; PAgram, pulmonary angiogram; PE, pulmonary embolism; U/S, ultrasound.

Table 29-2. Ottawa (Modified Wells) Scoring System

Signs or Symptoms	Points
Hemoptysis	1.0
Malignancy (on treatment, treated in the last 6 months or palliative)	1.0
Heart rate > 100 bpm	1.5
Immobilization or surgery in the previous 4 weeks	1.5
Previous DVT or PE	1.5
Clinical signs and symptoms of DVT (minimum of leg swelling and pain with palpation of the deep veins)	3.0
An alternative diagnosis is less likely than PE	3.0
Risk level	**Score**
Low	0-1
Intermediate	2-6
High	≥7

DVT, deep vein thrombosis; PE, pulmonary embolism.

or the modified Wells index, then the diagnosis of PE can likely be excluded without additional diagnostic testing. This approach has been validated in a multicenter cohort study of > 8000 emergency department patients, but it should only be used in a setting where the prevalence of acute PE is low.

B. Diagnostic Studies

1. Nonimaging studies

A. ELECTROCARDIOGRAPHY—Electrocardiograms (ECG) may show evidence of acute cor pulmonale, manifested by a new $S_1 Q_3 T_3$ pattern, new incomplete right bundle branch block, right axis deviation, or right ventricular ischemia or strain with ST segment depressions in the right precordial leads. However, these changes are usually only seen in patients with acute massive PE, and therefore, absence of these ECG changes in a patient with suspected PE should not preclude additional diagnostic testing. Some ECG findings that have been associated with an adverse prognosis in patients with acute PE include atrial arrhythmias, right bundle branch block, Q waves in the inferior leads III and aVF, and ST segment changes and T-wave inversions in the precordial leads.

B. ARTERIAL BLOOD GASES—Neither measurement of room air arterial blood gases nor calculation of the alveolar-arterial oxygen gradient is useful in excluding the diagnosis of PE. Among patients in whom PE is suspected, neither test helped differentiate patients with a confirmed PE at angiography from those with a normal pulmonary angiogram. Therefore, arterial blood gases should not be obtained as a screening test for suspected PE.

C. PLASMA D-DIMER ENZYME-LINKED IMMUNOSORBENT ASSAY—Endogenous fibrinolysis, although ineffective in preventing PE, almost always causes the release of D-dimers from fibrin clot in the presence of established PE. However, an elevated D-dimer test is not specific and may occur in a variety of other conditions including acute comorbid illnesses, such as acute myocardial infarction, metastatic cancer, sepsis, or recent surgery. A normal (< 500 ng/mL) result virtually excludes the diagnosis of PE: among patients with a normal D-dimer level, the likelihood of PE is < 5%. Despite its sensitivity, in patients with a very high clinical suspicion of PE, the D-dimer should not be used in isolation to exclude PE. The combination of low clinical suspicion, ideally quantified with a validated scoring system, and a normal D-dimer enzyme-linked immunosorbent assay makes PE exceedingly unlikely.

D. TROPONIN LEVELS—Screening for troponins is now the standard blood test for cardiac injury, and it is obtained routinely when acute myocardial infarction or unstable angina is suspected. Circulating troponin indicates irreversible myocardial cell damage and is much more sensitive than creatine kinase or its myocardial muscle isoenzyme. Cardiac markers of injury should not be used, however, as a primary diagnostic test for acute PE. Nevertheless, elevation of cardiac troponin is an adverse prognostic factor in patients with acute PE and is associated with a markedly increased mortality rate and requirement for inotropic support and mechanical ventilation. Troponin elevation also correlates with ECG evidence of right ventricular strain. This suggests that release of troponin from the myocardium during PE may result from acute right ventricular microinfarction due to pressure overload, impaired coronary artery blood flow, or hypoxemia caused by the PE. A meta-analysis of 20 observational studies showed that patients with acute PE with elevated troponin T or troponin I levels had a fivefold higher risk of short-term mortality and a ninefold increased risk of death due to PE.

E. BRAIN NATRIURETIC PEPTIDE (BNP) LEVELS—As with cardiac troponins, measurement of BNP levels or N-terminal proBNP (NT-proBNP) levels should not be used to diagnose an acute PE. However, elevation of BNP or NT-proBNP levels may be a reflection of right ventricular dysfunction in the setting of an acute PE and therefore may have prognostic value. In a meta-analysis of 16 studies of patients with acute PE, in-hospital or short-term mortality was increased sixfold in those with a BNP level > 100 pg/mL and 16-fold among those with an NT-proBNP level > 600 ng/L.

2. Imaging studies

A. CHEST RADIOGRAPHY—Chest radiography can help exclude diseases such as lobar pneumonia, pneumothorax,

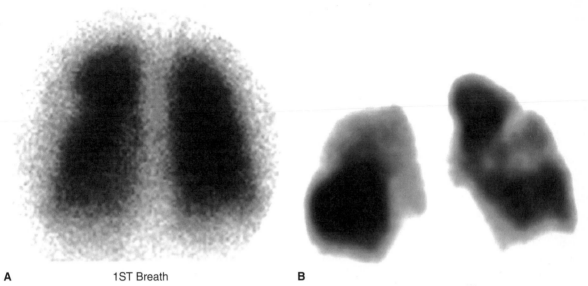

A   1ST Breath   **B**

▲ **Figure 29–2.** Lung scan for a 63-year-old woman who presented with idiopathic pulmonary embolism. The lung scan showed (**A**) normal ventilation and (**B**) multiple segmental perfusion defects, indicating a ventilator perfusion mismatch and high probability of pulmonary embolism.

or cardiogenic pulmonary edema, which can have clinical presentations that mimic acute PE. However, patients with these disorders can also have concomitant PE.

B. Radionuclide lung scanning—This study has served as the principal diagnostic imaging test for PE but is now with increasing frequency being superseded by chest CT scanning. Lung scanning is most useful when unequivocally normal or when highly suggestive of PE (Figure 29–2). Neither intermediate nor low-probability scans (in the presence of high clinical suspicion) exclude PE. For example, with the combination of a low-probability scan and high clinical suspicion for PE, the likelihood of PE is 40%. When lung scanning is performed, the ventilation scan is being used less frequently than previously because its contribution to the diagnostic decision is only marginally better than the combination of a perfusion scan and chest radiograph.

C. Chest CT scanning—The chest CT is diagnostic of PE when an intraluminal pulmonary arterial filling defect is surrounded by contrast material. CT scanning has two major advantages over lung scanning: (1) directly visualizing thrombus and (2) establishing alternative diagnoses on CT images of the lung parenchyma that are not evident on a chest film.

Conventional chest CT scanning relies on imaging a series of consecutive sections of the chest. With the introduction of spiral chest CT scanning, patients can be scanned continually. As patients are advanced through the spiral CT scanner, the x-ray source and single-row detector array rotate around them. These scans are performed during a

single breath-hold, thereby eliminating respiratory motion artifact that previously limited thoracic imaging. Overlap data from adjacent slices are acquired, thus reducing the possibility of missed pathology. Scans are performed in less than 30 seconds, and excellent vascular opacification with the contrast agent can usually be achieved (Figure 29–3).

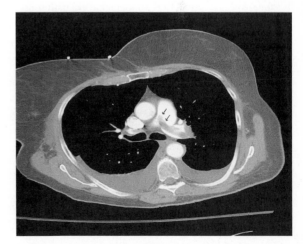

▲ **Figure 29–3.** Spiral computed tomography scan of massive bilateral pulmonary arterial filling defects (*arrows*) in the main pulmonary arteries of a 72-year-old woman who suffered acute pulmonary embolism after general surgery.

However, the major limitation has been failure to detect PEs beyond the third-order pulmonary arterial branches.

Further innovations occurred with the introduction of multidetector CT scanners, which acquire four slices simultaneously during each rotation of the x-ray source. Multidetector CT improves resolution from 5 mm to 1.25 mm and allows for better visualization of subsegmental vessels. Compared with conventional spiral CT, the sensitivity of multirow detector scanners for the diagnosis of acute PE increased from about 70% to 80–90%. In the PIOPED II study, which used multidetector CT angiography, the sensitivity and specificity were 83% and 96%, respectively. The positive predictive value was 96% with a concordant clinical assessment. The addition of CT venography to image DVTs improves the sensitivity from 83% to 90% with no change in specificity. In order to answer concerns that CT angiography could miss clinically important PEs in the branch pulmonary arteries, another randomized trial directly compared CT angiography with V̇/Q̇ scanning. In this study, CT was found to be noninferior. PE was diagnosed in more patients in the CT group than in the V̇/Q̇ scanning group. The risk of VTE during 3-month follow-up after having a negative imaging study was 0.4% for CT and 1% for V̇/Q̇ scan.

Occasionally, determining whether a pulmonary embolus represents the residua of prior PE or a new event may be challenging. A systematic review of the literature has shown that over half of patients with PE will still have a defect on either CT scan or radionuclide imaging 6 months after diagnosis.

D. Venous ultrasonography—In combination with color Doppler imaging, venous ultrasonography is known as duplex sonography and is the principal diagnostic imaging test for suspected acute DVT. Sonographic evaluation uses compression ultrasound along the full length of the femoral, popliteal, and calf veins. The transducer is held transverse to the vein and, normally, the vein collapses with gentle manual compression. The compressed vein appears as if it is winking. The main criterion for diagnosing DVT is lack of compression of a deep vein. This diagnosis can be confirmed by direct visualization of thrombus on ultrasound or by abnormal venous flow on Doppler examination (eg, loss of physiologic respiratory variation or loss of the expected augmentation of blood flow during calf compression).

Among symptomatic patients, duplex sonography is very accurate, with high sensitivity and specificity. Its sensitivity decreases when assessing asymptomatic patients. Major limitations include an inability to image pelvic vein thrombosis directly, lower sensitivity for diagnosing isolated calf DVT, and difficulty diagnosing an acute DVT superimposed upon a chronic one. Magnetic resonance imaging may be useful under these circumstances.

Importantly, many patients with PE do not have evidence of leg DVT, probably because the thrombus has already embolized to the pulmonary arteries. Therefore, PE is not necessarily ruled out if the clinical suspicion is high and imaging evidence of DVT is lacking.

E. Echocardiography—Echocardiography should not be used routinely to diagnose suspected PE because most patients with PE have normal echocardiograms. However, the echocardiogram, like the troponin level, is an excellent tool for risk stratification and prognostication. Echocardiography is useful diagnostically when the differential diagnosis includes pericardial tamponade, right ventricular infarction, and dissection of the aorta as well as PE.

Imaging a normal left ventricle in the presence of a dilated, hypokinetic right ventricle strongly suggests the diagnosis of PE (Figure 29–4). The presence of right ventricular

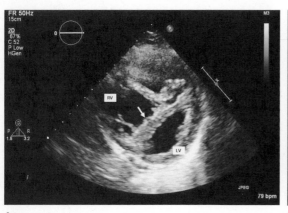 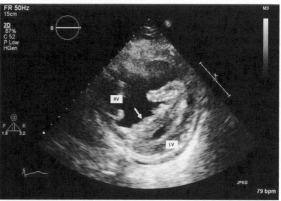

A   **B**

▲ **Figure 29–4.** Parasternal short-axis views of the right ventricle (RV) and left ventricle (LV) in (**A**) diastole and (**B**) systole. Diastolic and systolic bowing of the interventricular septum (*arrows*) into the LV is evident, which is compatible with RV volume and pressure overloads, respectively. The RV is appreciably dilatated and markedly hypokinetic, with little change in apparent RV area from diastole to systole. PE, small pericardial effusion.

Table 29–3. Abnormal Echocardiographic Findings in Pulmonary Embolism

Abnormal Finding	Description
Right ventricular dilatation and hypokinesis	Associated with leftward septal shift; the ratio of the RVEDA to LVEDA exceeds the upper limit of normal (0.6). Associated with right atrial enlargement and tricuspid regurgitation.
Septal flattening and paradoxical septal motion	Right ventricular contraction continues even after the left ventricle starts relaxing at end-systole; therefore, the interventricular septum bulges toward the left ventricle.
Diastolic left ventricular impairment with a small difference between left ventricular area during diastole and systole, indicative of low cardiac output	Due to septal displacement and reduced left ventricular distensibility during diastole; consequently, Doppler mitral flow exhibits a prominent A wave, much higher than the E wave, with an increased contribution of atrial contraction to left ventricular filling.
Direct visualization of PE	Only if PE is large and centrally located; much more easily visualized on transesophageal than on transthoracic echocardiography.
Pulmonary arterial hypertension detected by Doppler flow velocity in the right ventricular outflow tract	Shortened acceleration time, with peak velocity occurring close to the onset of ejection. Biphasic ejection curve, with midsystolic reduction in velocity.
Right ventricular hypertrophy	With mildly increased right ventricular thickness (often about 6 mm, with 4 mm as upper limit of normal); clear visualization of right ventricular muscle trabeculations.
Patent foramen ovale	When right atrial pressure exceeds left atrial pressure, the foramen ovale may open and cause worsening hypoxemia or stroke.

LVEDA, left ventricular end-diastolic area; PE, pulmonary embolism; RVEDA, right ventricular end–diastolic area.

mid-free wall akinesis with sparing of the apex (the McConnell sign) has been found to be highly specific for acute PE. Echocardiographic findings in PE patients are summarized in Table 29–3.

The pulmonary arterial systolic pressure can be estimated by measuring the peak velocity of the tricuspid regurgitant jet obtained with Doppler echocardiography. The gradient across the tricuspid valve can be estimated by using the modified Bernoulli equation, $P = 4V^2$, where V is the peak velocity of the regurgitant jet, and P represents the peak pressure difference between the right atrium and right ventricle. The estimated right atrial pressure is added to the gradient to obtain an estimate of pulmonary arterial systolic pressure. The pulmonary artery systolic pressure may be low, normal, or mildly elevated in the setting of acute PE. Significant pulmonary hypertension suggests a subacute or chronic process. The incidence of chronic thromboembolic pulmonary hypertension following a first episode of PE is low overall (~1%), but in patients with unexplained persistent dyspnea after PE, the incidence may be as high as 4% after 2 years. Echocardiography to measure pulmonary artery pressure and exclude chronic thromboembolic pulmonary hypertension should be obtained for patients with persistent unexplained dyspnea following treatment of PE.

Transesophageal echocardiography for suspected PE is best reserved for critically ill patients. Transesophageal echocardiography diagnoses PE by direct visualization of

thrombus, assesses its extent, and provides guidance regarding its surgical accessibility. Transesophageal echocardiography may also have a valuable role in detecting unexplained sudden cardiac arrest and pulseless electrical activity due to acute PE. In a series of 1246 patients who suffered cardiac arrest, 5% of cases were caused by PE; of those with PE, 63% of cardiac arrest cases were caused by pulseless electrical activity. Therefore, when pulseless electrical activity is present, the possibility of an acute PE should be considered.

F. PULMONARY ANGIOGRAPHY—Pulmonary angiography is considered to be the "gold standard" diagnostic modality for the diagnosis of acute PE. This imaging method is rapidly becoming a lost art and is being undertaken primarily for therapeutic interventions (such as suction catheter embolectomy) rather than to solve diagnostic dilemmas. Most diagnostic questions can be resolved with the new-generation chest CT scanners, which provide resolution to subsegmental branches. A constant intraluminal filling defect seen in more than one projection is the most reliable angiographic diagnostic feature for PE.

Pulmonary angiography can almost always be accomplished safely, although the risk may be increased in patients with severe pulmonary hypertension. Selective angiography should be performed, with the equivocal portion of the perfusion lung scan or chest CT scan serving as a road map. To avoid damaging the intima of the pulmonary artery, soft, flexible catheters with side holes should be used, rather than stiff catheters with end holes. Low-osmolar contrast agents minimize the transient hypotension, heat, and coughing that often occur with conventional radioactive contrast agents.

Anderson DR, et al. Computed tomographic pulmonary angiography vs ventilation-perfusion lung scanning in patients with suspected pulmonary embolism: a randomized controlled trial. *JAMA.* 2007;298(23):2743–53. [PMID: 18165667]

Becattini C, et al. Prognostic value of troponins in acute pulmonary embolism: a meta-analysis. *Circulation.* 2007;116(4):427–33. [PMID: 17606843]

Cavallazzi R, et al. Natriuretic peptides in acute pulmonary embolism: a systematic review. *Intensive Care Med.* 2008;34(12):2147–56. [PMID: 18626627]

Jaff MR, et al. Management of massive and submassive pulmonary embolism, iliofemoral deep vein thrombosis, and chronic thromboembolic pulmonary hypertension: a scientific statement from the American Heart Association. *Circulation.* 2011;123:1788–830. [PMID: 21422387]

Kearon C, et al. Antithrombotic therapy for VTE disease. Antithrombotic therapy and prevention of thrombosis, 9th ed: American College of Chest Physicians Evidence-Based Clinical Practice Guidelines. *Chest.* 2012;141:e419S. [PMID: 22315268]

Kline JA, et al. Prospective multicenter evaluation of the pulmonary embolism rule-out criteria. *J Thromb Haemost.* 2008;6(5):772–80. [PMID: 18318689]

Nijkeuter M, et al. Resolution of thromboemboli in patients with acute pulmonary embolism: a systematic review. *Chest.* 2006;129(1):192–7. [PMID: 16424432]

Stein PD, et al; PIOPED II Investigators. Multidetector computed tomography for acute pulmonary embolism. *N Engl J Med.* 2006;354(22):2317–27. [PMID: 16738268]

van Belle A, et al; Christopher Study Investigators. Effectiveness of managing suspected pulmonary embolism using an algorithm combining clinical probability, D-dimer testing, and computed tomography. *JAMA.* 2006;295(2):172–9. [PMID: 16403929]

▶ Prevention

PE is easier and less expensive to prevent than to diagnose or treat; therefore, virtually all hospitalized patients should receive prophylaxis against VTE. Unfortunately, such prophylaxis is underutilized, even for high-risk patients. Furthermore, prophylaxis, even when instituted, may not be effective. Nonetheless, prevention programs should be established at all hospitals to ensure that adequate measures are implemented. Nurses and physicians must collaborate to achieve this goal by instituting protocols that are both streamlined and standardized. In addition, quality assurance personnel should adopt a proactive stance to encourage the development of such programs.

The preventive measures should be based on an assessment of the patient's level of risk for PE and whether the optimal strategy will be nonpharmacologic, pharmacologic, or combined modalities. Because the risk of PE continues after discharge from the hospital, prophylaxis should be continued at home among those patients at moderate or high risk for VTE.

A. Nonpharmacologic Prevention

The most commonly used nonpharmacologic measures are graduated compression stockings (GCS) and intermittent pneumatic compression devices (IPC or "SCD boots"). Vascular compression with either GCS or IPC is effective among surgical patients, because it counters the otherwise-unopposed perioperative venodilation that appears causally related to postoperative venous thrombosis. Even among low-risk general surgery patients, graduated compression stockings can substantially reduce the frequency of venous thrombosis and should therefore be considered first-line prophylaxis against PE in all hospitalized patients, except those with peripheral arterial occlusive disease whose condition may be worsened by vascular compression.

IPC boots, which provide intermittent inflation of air-filled cuffs, prevent venous stasis in the legs; they also appear to stimulate the endogenous fibrinolytic system. Because it appears that GCS and IPC boots work through somewhat different—although complementary—mechanisms, these modalities can be used in combination in patients at moderate or high risk for venous thrombosis.

B. Pharmacologic Prevention

Anticoagulant drugs can be used instead of—or in addition to—nonpharmacologic prophylaxis. A number of agents are used for prophylaxis against VTE in patients at high risk for thrombosis. These include unfractionated heparin (usually administered at a dose of 5000 units subcutaneously twice or thrice daily), low-molecular-weight heparins (LMWHs) such as enoxaparin or dalteparin, and antithrombin-binding pentasaccharides such as fondaparinux. Other agents have recently been recommended for use for VTE prophylaxis in selected patient populations, such as vitamin K antagonists such as warfarin, and newer antithrombotic agents such as dabigatran, rivaroxaban, and apixaban.

The ACCP recently published clinical guidelines for the use of thromboprophylaxis in hospitalized patients. All critically ill patients should receive thromboprophylaxis with either LMWH (such as enoxaparin or dalteparin) or low-dose unfractionated heparin, unless they are actively bleeding or are at high risk of major bleeding, in which case they should receive nonpharmacologic prophylaxis with GCS or IPC devices until the bleeding risk is reduced. For acutely ill, nonsurgical hospitalized patients who are at high risk for thrombosis, pharmacologic prophylaxis is recommended with LMWH, low-dose unfractionated heparin (at a dose of 5000 units two to three times per day), or fondaparinux. For nonsurgical hospitalized patients with high risk for thrombosis who are bleeding or are at risk for major bleeding, nonpharmacologic prophylaxis should be used. Hospitalized patients at low risk for thrombosis should not receive any thromboprophylaxis, and early and frequent ambulation is desirable in these patients.

The recent ACCP clinical guidelines also provide detailed recommendations for the use of thromboprophylaxis for

Table 29–4. Food and Drug Administration–Approved Low-Molecular-Weight Regimens for Orthopedic and General Surgery Prophylaxis

Indication	Drug and Dose	Duration	Timing of Initial Dose
Hip replacement ("USA-style") with enoxaparin	Enoxaparin 30 mg q12h or 40 mg q24h	≤ 14 days	12-24 h postoperatively, providing that hemostasis has been achieved
Hip replacement ("European-style") with enoxaparin	Enoxaparin 40 mg q24h	≤ 14 days	12 h ± 3 h preoperatively
Hip replacement with dalteparin (option #1)	Dalteparin 2500 units preoperatively and first dose postoperatively, followed by 5000 units q24h	≤ 14 days	First dose within 2 h preoperatively; second dose at least 6 h after the first dose, usually on the evening of the day of surgery; omit second dose on the day of surgery if surgery is done in the evening
Hip replacement with dalteparin (option #2)	Dalteparin 5000 units q24h	≤ 14 days	First dose on the preoperative evening; second dose on the evening of the day of surgery (unless surgery is done in the evening)
Extended hip prophylaxis	Enoxaparin 40 mg q24h	An additional 3 weeks after initial hip replacement prophylaxis	After the initial hip replacement prophylaxis regimen has been completed
General surgery with enoxaparin	Enoxaparin 40 mg q24h	≤ 12 days	2 h preoperatively
General surgery with dalteparin (moderate risk for venous thromboembolism)	Dalteparin 2500 units q24h	5-10 days	1-2 h preoperatively
General surgery with dalteparin (high risk for venous thromboembolism: option #1)	Dalteparin 5000 units q24h	5-10 days	Preoperative evening
General surgery with dalteparin (high risk for venous thromboembolism: option #2)	Dalteparin 2500 units preoperatively and first dose postoperatively, followed by 5000 units q24h	5-10 days	First dose 1-2 h preoperatively; second dose 12 h later

patients undergoing orthopedic and nonorthopedic surgery. Table 29–4 lists the various pharmacologic agents that are recommended for use in patients undergoing orthopedic and general surgery. In patients undergoing total hip or total knee arthroplasty, the ACCP recommends the use of one of the following agents for thromboprophylaxis for a minimum of 10–14 days: LMWH (enoxaparin or dalteparin), fondaparinux, apixaban, dabigatran, rivaroxaban, low-dose unfractionated heparin, adjusted-dose vitamin K antagonist (warfarin), aspirin, or an IPC device. In patients undergoing major orthopedic surgery who have an increased risk of bleeding, they recommend the use of an IPC or no prophylaxis rather than pharmacologic treatment. Patients undergoing general and abdominal-pelvic surgery at very low or low risk for VTE should receive nonpharmacologic prophylaxis using IPC devices and early ambulation, whereas those at moderate to high risk for VTE but not at high risk for

major bleeding should receive pharmacologic prophylaxis with LMWH or low-dose unfractionated heparin, along with use of nonpharmacologic agents such as IPC devices in high-risk patients.

C. Future Directions

Many hospitals routinely use protocol-driven prophylaxis for all hospitalized patients, especially for medical patients hospitalized in intensive care units. The current guidelines from the ACCP, as well as guidelines published by the American College of Physicians (ACP), form the basis of most of these protocols. The emphasis on preventive strategies includes the time of hospital discharge or transfer to a skilled nursing facility or rehabilitation hospital. Orders to prescribe these prophylactic measures often are prompted by a computerized order entry system that reminds physicians about the need for prophylaxis. As studies with the use of newer antithrombotic agents are completed and reported, the safety and efficacy of these agents will be better defined, and clinical guidelines for their use in thromboprophylaxis will need to be updated accordingly.

Falck-Ytter Y, et al. Prevention of VTE in orthopedic surgery patients: antithrombotic therapy and prevention of thrombosis, 9th ed: American College of Chest Physicians Evidence-Based Clinical Practice Guidelines. *Chest.* 2012;141(2 Suppl): e278S–325S. [PMID: 22315265]

Gould MK, et al. Prevention of VTE in nonorthopedic surgical patients: antithrombotic therapy and prevention of thrombosis, 9th ed: American College of Chest Physicians Evidence-Based Clinical Practice Guidelines. *Chest.* 2012;141(2 Suppl): e227S–77S. [PMID: 22315263]

Kahn SR, et al. Prevention of VTE in nonsurgical patients: antithrombotic therapy and prevention of thrombosis, 9th ed: American College of Chest Physicians Evidence-Based Clinical Practice Guidelines. *Chest.* 2012;141(2 Suppl):e195S–226S. [PMID: 22315261]

Lederle FA, et al. Venous thromboembolism prophylaxis in hospitalized medical patients and those with stroke: a background review for an American College of Physicians Clinical Practice Guideline. *Ann Intern Med.* 2011;155(9):602–15. [PMID: 22041949]

Qaseem A, et al. Venous thromboembolism prophylaxis in hospitalized patients: a clinical practice guideline from the American College of Physicians. *Ann Intern Med.* 2011;155(9):625–32. [PMID: 22041951]

▶ Risk Stratification

Not all PEs are created equal. The most important concept in PE management is that acute PE spans a wide range of risk, from small asymptomatic emboli to massive thromboembolism with catastrophic cardiovascular collapse and death due to right ventricular failure. Therapy must be geared to patient risk. Low-risk patients will do well with anticoagulation alone, whereas high-risk patients may require thrombolysis or embolectomy in addition to anticoagulation.

The Pulmonary Embolism Severity Index (PESI) is a clinical scoring system that uses a total of 11 parameters, including demographic characteristics (age and male sex), comorbid illnesses (cancer, heart failure, and chronic lung disease), and clinical findings (heart rate, systolic blood pressure, respiratory rate, body temperature, alteration of mental status, and arterial oxygen saturation), and has been shown to independently predict mortality at 30 days in patients with acute PE. A simplified version of the PESI has also been developed and is similar in prognostic utility but easier to use in the clinical setting. The original and simplified PESI scoring systems are summarized in Table 29–5.

The most important imaging test for risk stratification is echocardiographic assessment of right ventricular function. Even if the initial systemic blood pressure is normal, patients with echocardiographic evidence of right ventricular dysfunction may develop cardiogenic shock within 24 hours;

Table 29–5. The Pulmonary Embolism Severity Index (PESI)

Clinical Variable	Point Value in Original PESI	Point Value in Simplified PESI
Age > 80 years	Age in years	1
History of heart failure	10	}1*
History of chronic lung disease	10	
Male sex	10	
Pulse ≥ 110 bpm	20	1
Respiratory rate ≥ 30 breaths/min	20	
Temperature < 36°C	20	
Arterial oxygen saturation < 90%	20	1
History of cancer	30	1
Systolic blood pressure < 100 mm Hg	30	1
Altered mental status	60	

*1 point for a history of either heart failure or chronic lung disease.

Risk Categories	Point Value in Original PESI	Point Value in Simplified PESI	30-Day Mortality (original PESI cohort)	30-Day Mortality (simplified PESI cohort)
Low risk		0		1.1%
Class I	≤ 65	–	1.1%	–
Class II	66–85	–	3.1%	–
Intermediate risk		N/A		
Class III	86–105	–	6.5%	–
High risk		≥ 1		8.9%
Class IV	106–125	–	10.4%	–
Very high risk				
Class V	≥ 126	–	24.5%	–

Adapted from: Jimenez D, et al. *Arch Intern Med.* 2010;170:1383–9.

these patients may have a high mortality rate. In contrast, the mortality rate is low in normotensive patients with normal right ventricular function on echocardiography. Pulmonary hypertension, as estimated by Doppler echocardiography, that persists for more than 5 weeks after the diagnosis of PE is associated with an adverse long-term prognosis.

Biomarkers that reflect right ventricular strain or ischemia may also be useful tools to assess risk. The combination of either an elevated BNP or an elevated troponin level in conjunction with echocardiographic evidence of right ventricular dysfunction increases the odds of an in-hospital complication by 10-fold. Elevated levels of these biomarkers should prompt an echocardiogram to look for right ventricular dysfunction.

Aujesky D, et al. Derivation and validation of a prognostic model for pulmonary embolism. *Am J Respir Crit Care Med.* 2005;172(8):1041–6. [PMID: 16020800]

Jiménez D, et al. Prognostic models for selecting patients with acute pulmonary embolism for initial outpatient therapy. *Chest.* 2007;132(1):24–30. [PMID: 17625081]

Jiménez D, et al. Simplification of the pulmonary embolism severity index for prognostication in patients with acute symptomatic pulmonary embolism. *Arch Intern Med.* 2010;170(15):1383–9. [PMID: 20696966]

▶ Treatment

The treatment of PE must be initiated as soon as possible, and the timing of initiation of therapy depends on the clinical suspicion of PE and the expected delay between ordering a diagnostic test and making a definitive diagnosis of acute PE. The clinical suspicion of acute PE should be informed by the use of a validated clinical scoring system such as the Ottawa scoring system described earlier. If there is strong clinical suspicion of acute PE, empiric treatment with a parenteral anticoagulation agent should be started while waiting for the test results to arrive. In patients with intermediate clinical suspicion for acute PE in whom the test results are expected to be delayed for 4 hours or more, empiric anticoagulation should be initiated. In patients with a low clinical suspicion for acute PE, empiric anticoagulation should not be given until the test results are obtained, provided the results are available within 24 hours. However, in patients in whom the risk of major bleeding is moderate or high, the decision to initiate anticoagulation should be made on a case-by-case basis considering the overall clinical picture, as well as the patient's preferences and values. If anticoagulation is contraindicated and an acute PE is confirmed, the patient should be considered for placement of an inferior vena cava (IVC) filter, as detailed later.

Unfractionated heparin has traditionally been the first choice for anticoagulation for acute PE. However, in recent times, the use of LMWH is recommended as preferred anticoagulation agents for most patients with acute PE, as studies have shown that these agents are either equivalent or superior in efficacy, have lower rates of adverse reactions including thrombocytopenia, have more predictable pharmacokinetics, and do not require frequent monitoring of the activated partial thromboplastin time (aPTT). Newer anticoagulant agents have also been developed over the past few years and are used as acceptable alternatives to LMWH in certain clinical situations.

A. Heparin

Although unfractionated heparin has served as the standard foundation of PE treatment for more than 40 years, this anticoagulant has important limitations. Its variable protein binding leads to an often unpredictable dose response and makes it a drug that is difficult to administer properly in everyday clinical practice. Subtherapeutic levels of heparin increase the risk of recurrent PE, while excessive levels of heparin increase the risk of major bleeding.

Unfractionated heparin for PE treatment is usually ordered as an intravenous bolus followed by a continuous intravenous infusion. The required dose is unpredictable and must be adjusted according to the aPTT. Heparin is usually administered as a bolus of 5000–10,000 units (80 units/kg) followed by a weight-based hourly infusion (18 units/kg/h), which is titrated based on the aPTT, which is measured every 4–6 hours (Table 29–6). In general, the target partial thromboplastin time is 60–80 seconds.

With the increasing use of LMWHs, the use of unfractionated heparin is now restricted to the following clinical situations: patients with acute PE and persistent hypotension (since the LMWHs have not been well studied in this subgroup); patients with increased risk of bleeding (due to its shorter half-life); patients with morbid obesity or severe anasarca (due to concern about adequate subcutaneous absorption); patients with severe renal insufficiency (since most LMWHs are renally excreted); and patients in whom thrombolytic therapy is being considered.

Patients being treated with heparin who have a subsequent drop in platelet count should be evaluated for heparin-induced thrombocytopenia. The platelet count may decline within hours or, more commonly, 5–10 days after exposure to

Table 29–6. Unfractionated Heparin Weight-Based Nomogram for Acute Venous Thromboembolism

PTT	Repeat Bolus	Stop Infusion (min)	Rate Change	Repeat PTT (h)
< 35	70 units/kg[1]	0	Increase 3 units/kg/h	6
35–59	35 units/kg[2]	0	Increase 2 units/kg/h	6
60–80 target	0	0	No change	6
81–100	0	0	Decrease 2 units/kg/h	6
> 100	0	60	Decrease 3 units/kg/h	6

[1]Maximum bolus 10,000 units.
[2]Maximum bolus 5000 units.
PTT, activated partial thromboplastin time; measured in seconds.

heparin. Patients with known or suspected heparin-induced thrombocytopenia should be treated with either direct thrombin inhibitors (such as lepirudin, argatroban, or bivalirudin) or heparinoids (such as danaparoid). Heparin, LMWH, and warfarin monotherapy should be avoided in the setting of known or suspected heparin-induced thrombocytopenia.

B. Low-Molecular-Weight Heparin

LMWHs have revolutionized the initial management of VTE (Table 29–7) and are now considered first-line agents for the initial treatment of acute PE in the majority of patients. In addition, LMWHs are the preferred agents for long-term anticoagulation for PE patients who are pregnant or have underlying cancer. The use of LMWHs to treat DVT has dramatically converted the therapy of this illness from a 5- to 6-day hospitalization to primarily outpatient or overnight in-hospital management. In the United States, two LMWHs are commonly used for the treatment of patients with symptomatic DVT, with or without PE: enoxaparin and dalteparin (Table 29–8). The U.S. Food and Drug Administration–approved outpatient therapy for DVT with the LMWH enoxaparin is 1 mg/kg actual body weight given subcutaneously twice daily, or a once-daily subcutaneous dose of 1.5 mg/kg actual body weight. Dalteparin is administered subcutaneously at a dose

Table 29–7. Comparison of Unfractionated Heparin (UFH) Versus Low-Molecular-Weight Heparin (LMWH)

Characteristic	UFH	LMWH
Molecular weight (average in daltons)	15,000	5000
Ratio of anti-Xa to anti-IIa (thrombin) activity	1	> 1
Metabolism	Hepatic	Renal
Bioavailability	Fair	Excellent
Frequency of subcutaneous administration	2–3×/day	1–2×/day
Frequency of heparin-induced thrombocytopenia	1–2%	0.1–0.2%
Osteoporosis after prolonged exposure	Rare	Very rare
Laboratory assay of anticoagulant effect	Activated partial thromboplastin time	Anti-Xa level
Reversal of anticoagulant effect	Protamine	Protamine
Spinal or epidural anesthesia	Okay	Heed the FDA warning

FDA, Food and Drug Administration.

Table 29–8. FDA-Approved Low-Molecular-Weight Heparins for the Initial Treatment of DVT (with or without Asymptomatic PE)

Enoxaparin 1 mg/kg twice daily
Enoxaparin 1.5 mg/kg once daily
Tinzaparin 175 units/kg once daily

DVT, deep venous thrombosis; FDA, Food and Drug Administration; PE, pulmonary embolism.

of 100 IU/kg actual body weight twice daily or 200 IU/kg actual body weight once daily, up to a maximum daily dose of 18,000 IU per day. Tinzaparin is administered once daily at a dose of 175 IU/kg actual body weight, but is contraindicated in patients > 70 years of age with renal insufficiency. Patients with cancer, extensive clot burden, or obesity (actual body weight > 100 kg or a body mass index of 30–40) preferably should be treated with enoxaparin at the 1 mg/kg twice-daily dose.

LMWHs appear to be safer than unfractionated heparin because osteopenia and heparin-induced thrombocytopenia occur far less often. They have a much more predictable dose response than unfractionated heparin and can usually be administered on the basis of weight alone, without any blood testing to modify the dose. They have a minimal effect on the partial thromboplastin time. Renal insufficiency (particularly a creatinine clearance [CrCl] < 30 mL/min), low body weight, massive obesity, elderly age, and pregnancy increase the risk of incorrect dosing, resulting in either over- or under-anticoagulation. Avoidance of LMWH, dose-adjustment, or monitoring of anti-factor Xa activity may be necessary in these patients (Table 29–9). Even though dose adjustment is not recommended for patients with mild to moderate renal insufficiency (CrCl ≥ 30 mL/min), spontaneous bleeding from standard weight-based dosing of LMWHs may develop in such patients.

In a meta-analysis of randomized DVT treatment trials comparing LMWHs with unfractionated heparin, LMWHs were found to be more effective and safer. Their use resulted in fewer recurrent thromboemboli, less bleeding, less thrombocytopenia, and an improved quality of life and patient satisfaction. The strategy of using LMWHs was also more cost-effective. The 2007 ACP guidelines thus recommend the initial use of LMWH in lieu of unfractionated heparin for the inpatient or outpatient treatment of DVT. The more recently published clinical guidelines by the ACCP also recommend the preferential use of subcutaneous LMWH or fondaparinux over intravenous or subcutaneous unfractionated heparin for patients diagnosed with acute PE.

C. Fondaparinux

Fondaparinux is a subcutaneously administered synthetic pentasaccharide that contains the antithrombin binding

Table 29-9. Low-Molecular-Weight Heparin Weight-Based Nomogram for Enoxaparin in the Presence of Renal Insufficiency or Marked Obesity

Renal Insufficiency Creatinine Clearance (mL/min)	Enoxaparin Dose	Anti-Xa Monitoring (Heparin Level)[1]
> 70	1 mg/kg q12h	None
35-69	0.75 mg/kg q12h	3-6 h after the third injection
< 35	1 mg/kg q24h	3-6 h after the third injection
Obese Weight	Enoxaparin Dose	Anti-Xa Monitoring (Heparin Level)[1]
< 100 kg	1 mg/kg q12h	None
100-130 kg	1 mg/kg q12h	3-6 h after the first injection
> 130 kg	130 mg q12h	3-6 h after the first injection

[1]Therapeutic level is 0.5-1.0 units/mL.

domain found in heparin and LMWH, which binds to antithrombin and inactivates factor Xa, leading to a formation of a covalent antithrombin–Xa complex. Subcutaneous fondaparinux has been shown to be noninferior to intravenous unfractionated heparin for treatment of acute PE and has the advantages of not requiring dose adjustment and a lower risk of thrombocytopenia.

Fondaparinux has almost complete bioavailability after subcutaneous administration, a predictable anticoagulant response, and a long half-life, making it amenable to once-daily, fixed-dose administration. Fondaparinux is given at a dose of 7.5 mg subcutaneously once daily for patients with a body weight of 50–100 kg, 5 mg once daily for those with body weight < 50 kg, and 10 mg once daily for those with body weight > 100 kg.

However, fondaparinux is cleared almost exclusively by the kidneys and is thus contraindicated in patients with renal insufficiency (CrCl < 30 mL/min). The dose should be reduced by 50% in patients with mild to moderate renal insufficiency (CrCl 30–50 mL/min). Most patients do not need monitoring of factor Xa levels while on fondaparinux, but in those who do, fondaparinux-specific factor Xa assays are needed. If uncontrollable bleeding occurs with the use of fondaparinux, recombinant factor VIIIa may be used since protamine sulfate is ineffective.

D. Thrombolysis

PE thrombolysis remains a controversial treatment option because large clinical trials using survival as an end point have not been conducted. Nevertheless, successful

Table 29-10. Pulmonary Embolism Patients at High Risk (in the Absence of Systemic Arterial Hypotension and Cardiogenic Shock)

Physical findings of right ventricular dysfunction (eg, distended neck veins, accentuated P_2, tricuspid regurgitation murmur)
Electrocardiographic manifestations of right ventricular strain (eg, new right bundle branch block, new T-wave inversion in leads V_1-V_4)
Right ventricular dilatation and hypokinesis or akinesis on echocardiogram
Patent foramen ovale
Free-floating right-heart thrombi
Doppler echocardiographic pulmonary arterial systolic pressure > 50 mm Hg
Elevated troponin level
Age > 70 years
Cancer
Congestive heart failure
Chronic obstructive pulmonary disease

thrombolysis usually reverses right heart failure rapidly and safely, thereby preventing a downhill spiral of cardiogenic shock. Thrombolysis may also prevent chronic pulmonary hypertension over the long term and thus improve exercise tolerance and quality of life. It is certain that thrombolysis should be considered only for those patients at high risk for an adverse clinical outcome with anticoagulation alone. Although no precise indications currently exist in the absence of massive PE with cardiogenic shock, the clinician should be wary of conservative management in the presence of risk factors for a poor prognosis (Table 29-10). The ACCP guidelines, as well as American Heart Association (AHA) guidelines (AHA Class IIa indication), recommend consideration of thrombolysis in the setting of massive acute PE with acceptable bleeding risk.

However, thrombolysis for submassive PE remains controversial. Thrombolysis for submassive PE with adverse prognostic features (hemodynamic instability, respiratory insufficiency, severe right ventricular dysfunction, or major myocardial necrosis) is an AHA Class IIb indication. The ACCP guidelines also state that in selected patients with acute PE who do not have hypotension but have a high risk of developing hypotension and carry a low bleeding risk, thrombolytic therapy should be considered. However, clinical evaluation of a patient who is at risk of developing hypotension can be very challenging. Echocardiography helps identify a subgroup of PE patients with impending right ventricular failure who appear to be at high risk for adverse clinical outcomes if treated with heparin alone. Right ventricular dysfunction can also be inferred when right ventricular dilatation is seen on CT scan. In addition, ECG evidence of right ventricular dilation and dysfunction (pseudoinfarct pattern or T-wave inversion in the anterior precordial leads); ultrasonographic evidence of residual DVT burden in the lower limbs; persistent hypoxia; elevated levels of serum biomarkers such as BNP, NT-proBNP, and cardiac troponins T and I; and the presence of comorbid illnesses that lead to a lower cardiopulmonary reserve suggest an adverse clinical outcome in patients with acute PE, and thrombolytic therapy can be considered in these patients if bleeding risk is low. The combination of elevated cardiac biomarkers (which likely indicate right ventricular infarction or strain) along with echocardiographic evidence of right ventricular dysfunction predicts a poor outcome in acute submassive PE.

A careful assessment of the risks of bleeding must be made before the decision to use thrombolytic therapy is made. Contraindications to the use of systemic thrombolytic therapy in patients with acute PE include the presence of an intracranial neoplasm, recent intracranial surgery or head trauma within the past 2 months, history of internal bleeding within the past 6 months, history of a hemorrhagic stroke, history of nonhemorrhagic stroke within the past 2 months, any surgery within the past 10 days, history of a bleeding diathesis, thrombocytopenia ($< 100,000/mm^3$), or uncontrolled hypertension (systolic blood pressure > 200 mm Hg or diastolic blood pressure > 110 mm Hg).

If a decision to use thrombolytic therapy is made, the ACCP recommends the use of shorter infusion time (2 hours) and use of a peripheral vein rather than a central venous catheter for administration of the thrombolytic agent. The preferred agent is alteplase (t-PA), but streptokinase or urokinase may also be used.

There are a number of invasive catheter-based approaches for delivery of thrombolytic agents directly into the pulmonary embolus rather than systemically, including intraembolic thrombolytic delivery, catheter suction, rheolytic and rotational devices, and ultrasound-enhanced thrombolysis. These are sophisticated techniques that may necessitate transport of the patient to a facility with an experienced interventional radiology department. Studies of these approaches are very limited, and the success rates are heavily dependent upon the expertise and familiarity with a certain approach of the treating interventional radiologist. Patients undergoing these procedures usually need to be monitored in an intensive care unit setting for several days and are vulnerable to complications related to vascular access, injury to the great vessels, arrhythmias, exposure to iodinated contrast, and of course, major bleeding. The ACCP guidelines suggest the use of catheter-directed thrombus removal in patients with acute PE associated with hypotension in whom systemic thrombolysis is contraindicated or has failed or in patients who are in shock that is likely to cause death before systemic thrombolysis can take effect and that it should only be performed in centers with adequate resources and expertise in these techniques.

E. Embolectomy

Patients at high risk for an adverse outcome with anticoagulation alone should be considered for embolectomy if they have contraindications to thrombolytic therapy. Embolectomy can be performed as a catheter-based procedure in the interventional laboratory or in the operating room. Clinical success has been reported, but randomized trials are lacking. Catheter embolectomy has a very limited application because it cannot successfully remove large amounts of thrombus, due to limitations in available catheter devices.

Surgical embolectomy for acute PE should be considered for patients who would otherwise receive thrombolytic therapy but who have contraindications to this treatment modality. The operation is best performed by median sternotomy with continuous transesophageal echocardiogram monitoring. The embolus should be removed under direct visualization, never "blindly." With experience, all lobar and most segmental pulmonary artery branches can be visualized. It is crucial to refer high-risk PE patients as soon as their prognosis with anticoagulation has been established. Taking a "watch and wait" approach and delaying referring until the onset of cardiogenic shock requiring pressors yields poor results.

To manage severe *chronic* thromboembolic pulmonary hypertension (CTEPH) due to a prior PE, a separate and more technically challenging operation can be performed—a pulmonary thromboendarterectomy. This operation is recommended by the ACCP guidelines by an experienced thromboendarterectomy team for selected patients with CTEPH who have central disease. If successful, this operation can reduce and possibly cure pulmonary hypertension. This surgery requires careful dissection of the old thrombus, which has turned whitish and hardened, from the walls of the pulmonary arteries. Complications include pulmonary arterial perforation and hemorrhage; pulmonary steal syndrome, in which blood rushes from previously well-perfused lung tissue to newly perfused tissue; and reperfusion pulmonary edema. For patients who are not candidates for pulmonary thromboendarterectomy, balloon pulmonary angioplasty can be considered.

F. Inferior Vena Cava Filters

There are two unequivocal indications for placing an IVC filter for patients with acute PE associated with acute proximal DVT: (1) concomitant major bleeding requiring transfusion, intracranial hemorrhage, or any absolute contraindication to the use of anticoagulant therapy; and (2) recurrent PE despite prolonged intensive anticoagulation. Other situations in which an IVC filter may be considered are patients with massive PE or CTEPH in whom another embolic event would be devastating; a proximal DVT in a patient with poor cardiopulmonary reserve; or DVT in a patient with a high bleeding risk. Although IVC filters reduce the frequency of PE, they do not halt the thrombotic process and are associated with a doubling of the rate of DVT. If the contraindication to anticoagulation is expected to be short-term, a retrievable IVC filter can be placed, and removal can be assessed periodically after 3–12 months. If the patient becomes a candidate for anticoagulation after an IVC filter has been placed, the patient should be preferentially anticoagulated and filter removal should be considered.

G. Warfarin

Warfarin is the standard oral anticoagulant used in the United States. For most patients with acute PE, treatment is initiated with a heparin (either LMWH or unfractionated heparin) or fondaparinux, and then transitioned to warfarin for long-term treatment. Warfarin dosing is adjusted according to a standardized prothrombin time by using the international normalized ratio (INR). For PE and DVT, the target INR is ordinarily between 2.0 and 3.0. The current ACCP guidelines recommend the use of vitamin K antagonists such as warfarin as the preferred choice for long-term therapy for patients with acute PE who do not have cancer. Warfarin can be started on the same day or after the initiation of heparin or fondaparinux, and patients should have an overlap of at least 5 days or until the INR has been within the therapeutic range for at least 24 hours. Warfarin should not be initiated before the administration of heparin or fondaparinux, because it can cause a transient hypercoagulable state and has been associated with a threefold increased risk of recurrent PE or DVT when used alone without "bridging."

Unfortunately, warfarin treatment is limited by a narrow therapeutic window. Too little anticoagulant effect leads to thromboembolism, and excessive anticoagulation leads to bleeding. The drug is plagued by a long list of interactions with other drugs that either decrease or increase warfarin's anticoagulant effect. The consumption of vitamin K–containing foods such as green leafy vegetables decreases the anticoagulant effect, whereas the ingestion of alcohol increases the likelihood of hemorrhage.

Optimal warfarin dosing can be facilitated by understanding the following factors. First, use of acetaminophen in high doses may lead to an unintended increase in the INR. Second, warfarin should be initiated in a dose of about 5 mg once daily for an average-sized adult, rather than initiating much higher loading doses. Third, since 2–3% of patients have a genetic mutation that results in slow metabolism of warfarin, the INR should be tested after several doses of warfarin, rather than waiting for 5 days after initiation of therapy. Pharmacogenetic testing to help guide initial warfarin dosing is being studied and may become common practice in the future. Finally, for patients who require long-term anticoagulation, point-of-care fingerstick INR testing machines can be prescribed for home use for patients who are able to be trained to self-adjust their warfarin doses based on the results of the INR.

Although warfarin is the most commonly used drug for long-term outpatient anticoagulation, for select patient populations, such as those with cancer, difficult to control INR values, or recurrent embolism despite therapeutic INR, long-term LMWH may be preferable to warfarin.

When the INR exceeds 5.0 in the absence of clinical bleeding, warfarin should be withheld and oral vitamin K administered, usually in a dose of 2.5 mg. Although oral vitamin K is preferable, it may be given subcutaneously when gastrointestinal absorption is uncertain. Occasionally, patients will require immediate reversal of excessive anticoagulation. This can be accomplished by the emergency administration of fresh frozen plasma, usually 2 units. However, to ensure continued reversal, vitamin K should be administered concomitantly.

H. Newer anticoagulants

Rivaroxaban is an oral factor Xa inhibitor and has been shown to be noninferior to a standard treatment approach (enoxaparin followed by warfarin or acenocoumarol titrated to an INR of 2.0–3.0) in one clinical trial of patients with acute PE. Although the risk of major bleeding was lower with rivaroxaban in this trial, the absolute benefit was small, and the open-label design of the trial led to the potential for bias. Dabigatran etexilate is a direct thrombin inhibitor that has been approved for use for stroke prophylaxis in patients with nonvalvular atrial fibrillation but has not yet been adequately studied as a treatment for acute PE. Current guidelines do not yet recommend the use of these drugs as first-line agents for the treatment of acute PE.

I. Adjunctive Measures

Occasionally, PE patients will require ventilatory assistance for respiratory failure or will rarely require pulmonary artery catheterization to determine optimal fluid management. Most patients with acute PE, however, can be cared for in an intermediate-care or step-down unit. Most will benefit from supplemental oxygen. Opioids usually do not relieve the chest discomfort. Nonsteroidal anti-inflammatory agents are often effective, and combining them with anticoagulation usually does not pose an undue risk of bleeding complications.

Patients with PE and concomitant DVT of the leg should wear below-knee GCS (ideally 30–40 mm Hg or, if not tolerated, 20–30 mm Hg), to provide leg support while ambulating, for a minimum of 1 year after DVT diagnosis. The stockings help prevent distention of the vein wall and may mitigate the syndrome of chronic venous insufficiency—most often characterized by leg swelling and discomfort—that most DVT patients experience.

J. Duration of Treatment of Acute Pulmonary Embolism

The optimal duration of anticoagulation for patients with acute PE remains extremely controversial. The ACP guidelines recommend that anticoagulation be continued for 3–6 months for VTE due to transient risk factors (such as postoperative state) and for > 12 months or indefinitely for recurrent VTE. For first-time idiopathic VTE (ie, PE that occurs without relation to cancer, surgery, or trauma), the optimal duration of anticoagulation is not known, but a minimum of 3 months is suggested for most patients. Although several trials have shown that extended duration (beyond 3–12 months) of anticoagulant therapy for idiopathic VTE does reduce the rate of VTE recurrence, the follow-up has only been for 4 years, and therefore, the risk-benefit ratio needs to be determined on a case-by-case basis.

The recent ACCP guidelines have provided detailed recommendations with regard to the treatment approach as well as the optimal duration of anticoagulant therapy in patients with acute PE. Once the decision to initiate treatment for acute PE has been made, the ACCP recommends the use of parenteral anticoagulation with LMWH, subcutaneous fondaparinux, or unfractionated heparin administered either intravenously or subcutaneously. Subcutaneous LMWH or fondaparinux is the preferred first-line agent for initial treatment, and if LMWH is being used, once-daily dosing is preferred (enoxaparin 1.5 mg/kg actual body weight or dalteparin 200 IU/kg ideal body weight, up to a maximum of 18,000 IU/day).

For patients with acute PE provoked by surgery, the recommended duration of anticoagulation is 3 months. In patients with acute PE provoked by a nonsurgical transient risk factor such as prolonged immobilization, the duration of therapy should be 3 months. In patients with an unprovoked acute PE, anticoagulation should be given for at least 3 months, and extended therapy beyond 3 months should be considered for those with low to moderate bleeding risk. In patients with a second unprovoked VTE (PE or DVT), extended anticoagulation therapy for > 3 months should be given for those with low to moderate bleeding risk, and those with high bleeding risk should be treated for 3 months. Patients with active cancer who develop PE and have a low to moderate bleeding risk should receive extended anticoagulation therapy for > 3 months. The risks and benefits of extended anticoagulation should be assessed at periodic intervals, and the patient's preferences and values should be incorporated in the decision-making process. Further research is required to identify those patients prospectively who are at highest risk for recurrence after discontinuation of anticoagulation.

A special group of patients are those with the antiphospholipid antibody syndrome as they may benefit from extended duration or more intense anticoagulation.

K. Venous Thromboembolism in Pregnancy

The risk of VTE is increased fivefold during pregnancy. There is insufficient evidence to definitively guide the management of VTE during pregnancy, as most of the evidence comes from retrospective studies. Warfarin should be avoided in early pregnancy because it may lead to embryopathy between 6 and 12 weeks of gestation. On the other hand, unfractionated heparin and LMWH are not associated with embryopathy because they do not cross the placenta. However, prolonged unfractionated heparin use may lead to osteoporosis, may lead to heparin-induced thrombocytopenia, and is inconvenient to use due to the need for frequent aPTT testing to titrate the dose. LMWHs are more convenient to use, are associated with a lower risk of thrombocytopenia, and may also carry a lower risk of osteoporosis when compared to unfractionated heparin. However, the correct dosing of LMWH may also be difficult to determine by weight during pregnancy; thus, anti-factor Xa levels may need to be monitored periodically to ensure adequacy of dosing. Single-dose, prefilled vials of LMWH that are preservative-free should be preferably used in pregnant patients, as some preservatives used in multidose vials may have adverse fetal effects.

The ACCP guidelines recommend the use of LMWH over unfractionated heparin for both prevention and treatment of VTE during pregnancy. LMWH should be stopped at least 24 hours before induction of labor or induction of epidural anesthesia or cesarean section. Heparin can be started 6 hours after vaginal delivery or 12 hours after a cesarean section if there is no significant bleeding risk. Patients may then be transitioned to warfarin with discontinuation of heparin once the INR is within the therapeutic range.

▶ Counseling

Although PE can be as devastating emotionally and physically as myocardial infarction, the burden on individual patients may be even greater because the general public does not have as good an understanding of PE, particularly in terms of the potential incomplete recovery from it and long-term disability it engenders. Young patients with PE repeatedly voice a common theme. Although they appear healthy, they have actually suffered a life-threatening illness. Because of their youth and healthy appearance, others may not empathize with their fears and feelings about the illness. Virtually all patients with PE will wonder why they were stricken with the illness and whether they harbor an underlying coagulopathy (or "bad" gene) that predisposed them. When anticoagulation is discontinued after an adequate course of therapy, patients are often fearful of recurrent PE. It is therefore essential to have an open discussion about the various treatment options available, the adverse effect profile of the drugs used, and the recommended duration of treatment using evidence-based clinical guidelines, and also to understand the patient's values and expectations for treatment, in order to make balanced, collaborative treatment choices that both the patient and the treating clinician can agree on. A close collaboration with an experienced clinical pharmacist is also of benefit to assist with long-term management of patients on anticoagulant therapy. Regular assessments and ongoing discussions with the patient about the risks and benefits of ongoing treatment are essential, especially in those on long-term anticoagulation.

Campbell IA, et al. Anticoagulation for three versus six months in patients with deep vein thrombosis or pulmonary embolism or both: randomised trial. *BMJ*. 2007;334(7595):674. [PMID: 17289685]

Hron G, et al. Identification of patients at low risk for recurrent venous thromboembolism by measuring thrombin generation. *JAMA*. 2006;296(4):397–402. [PMID: 16868297]

Jaff MR, et al. Management of massive and submassive pulmonary embolism, iliofemoral deep vein thrombosis, and chronic thromboembolic pulmonary hypertension: a scientific statement from the American Heart Association. *Circulation* 2011;123:1788–830. [PMID: 21422387]

Logeart D, et al. Biomarker-based strategy for screening right ventricular dysfunction in patients with non-massive pulmonary embolism. *Intensive Care Med*. 2007;33(2):286–92. [PMID: 17165016]

Palareti G, et al; PROLONG Investigators. D-dimer testing to determine the duration of anticoagulation therapy. *N Engl J Med*. 2006;355(17):1780–9. [PMID: 17065639]

Schwarz UI, et al. Genetic determinants of response to warfarin during initial anticoagulation. *N Engl J Med*. 2008;358(10):999–1008. [PMID: 18322281]

Segal JB, et al. Management of venous thromboembolism: a systematic review for a practice guideline. *Ann Intern Med*. 2007;146(3):211–22. [PMID: 17261856]

Snow V, et al; American College of Physicians; American Academy of Family Physicians Panel on Deep Venous Thrombosis/Pulmonary Embolism. Management of venous thromboembolism: a clinical practice guideline from the American College of Physicians and the American Academy of Family Physicians. *Ann Intern Med*. 2007;146(3):204–10. [PMID: 17261857]

Pulmonary Hypertension

Christopher F. Barnett, MD, MPH
Teresa De Marco, MD

ESSENTIALS OF DIAGNOSIS

Pulmonary hypertension

▶ A loud pulmonic valve closure sound (P_2), a right-sided S_4, or a right ventricular heave.

▶ Electrocardiographic evidence of right ventricular hypertrophy.

▶ Presence of sustained elevation in mean pulmonary artery pressure ≥ 25 mm Hg.

Pulmonary arterial hypertension

▶ A subset of pulmonary hypertension.

▶ Elevated mean pulmonary artery pressure ≥ 25 mm Hg.

▶ Pulmonary arterial wedge pressure ≤ 15 mm Hg.

Pulmonary hypertension (PH) is a description of the finding of a mean pulmonary artery pressure (mPAP) greater than 25 mm Hg and may occur in many settings. PH most commonly results from a variety of cardiac and pulmonary diseases that increase pulmonary artery pressure (PAP) either passively or through vasoconstriction. The term pulmonary arterial hypertension (PAH) describes a specific group of diseases characterized by a mPAP greater than 25 mm Hg and normal left heart filling pressures (pulmonary artery wedge pressure [PAWP] < 15 mm Hg) resulting from vasoconstriction and arteriopathy of the precapillary pulmonary arterioles. PAH may be idiopathic or associated with one or more underlying diseases such as connective tissue disease, human immunodeficiency virus (HIV) infection, or portal hypertension. In patients clinically suspected of having PH, echocardiography is often the first test performed to estimate PAP and evaluate right ventricular function. Further comprehensive testing is required to make a diagnosis and establish the etiology of PH.

PH commonly occurs in patients with left heart disease and hypoxemic lung disease. The development of PH in

patients with heart or lung disease is an ominous sign and is generally associated with decreased survival. Treatment in this case is directed at the underlying condition (ie, bronchodilators, supplemental oxygen, valve repair, or heart failure treatment). Use of PAH-specific therapy in this setting is generally not beneficial and may worsen symptoms and mortality. In patients with PAH, increased pulmonary vascular resistance from vasoconstriction and arteriopathy results in increased PAP, leading rapidly to right heart failure and death. In this setting, PAH-specific therapy improves symptoms, exercise tolerance, and survival. Selection of therapies for patients with PAH is complex and requires understanding of any associated diseases, the severity of the patient's symptoms, as well as toxicities and drug interactions of PAH therapy. Early referral to a specialty center for patients with PAH is often crucial for confirmation of diagnosis, early initiation of appropriate therapy, and monitoring of response to treatment. Significant advances have been made over the past decade in improving clinicians' understanding of the clinical profile, pathobiology, and treatment of PAH.

▶ General Considerations

PH is defined as a sustained elevation in the mPAP of 25 mm Hg or greater at rest. This is in contrast to a normal mPAP of 12–16 mm Hg. In healthy humans, the small arteriovenous pressure gradient generated by blood flow across the pulmonary circulation results from the large total vascular surface area and high pulmonary vascular compliance. The pulmonary vascular resistance (PVR) is quantified using **Ohm's law** [PVR = (mPAP − PAWP)/cardiac output (CO)] and describes the relationship between the pressure gradient and blood flow.

▶ Classification & Pathogenesis

The World Health Organization has proposed a system to categorize PH into five groups on the basis of underlying etiology (Table 30–1). PH can also be categorized on a hemodynamic

30

Table 30–1. Classification System for Pulmonary Hypertension

Group 1: Pulmonary arterial hypertension
- Idiopathic
- Familial
- Associated with:
  Connective tissue disease
  Congenital systemic-to-pulmonary shunts (including repaired shunts)
  Portal hypertension
  HIV infection
  Drugs and toxins
  Schistosomiasis
  Other (thyroid disorders, glycogen storage disease, Gaucher disease, hereditary hemorrhagic telangiectasia, hemoglobinopathies, myeloproliferative disorders, splenectomy)
- Associated with significant venous or capillary involvement
  Pulmonary veno-occlusive disease
  Pulmonary capillary hemangiomatosis
- Persistent pulmonary hypertension of the newborn

Group 2: Pulmonary hypertension with left-sided heart disease
- Left-sided atrial or ventricular heart disease
- Left-sided valvular heart disease

Group 3: Pulmonary hypertension associated with lung disease and/or hypoxemia
- Chronic obstructive pulmonary disease
- Interstitial lung disease
- Sleep-disordered breathing
- Alveolar hypoventilation disorders
- Long-term exposure to high altitude

Group 4: Pulmonary hypertension due to chronic thrombotic and/or embolic disease
- Chronic thromboembolic pulmonary hypertension
- Nonthrombotic pulmonary embolism (tumor, parasites, foreign material)

Group 5: Miscellaneous
- Sarcoidosis, histiocytosis X, lymphangiomatosis, compression of pulmonary vessels (adenopathy, tumor, fibrosing mediastinitis)

basis at right heart catheterization (Figure 30–1). PH is characterized based on the mPAP: mild (25–40 mm Hg), moderate (41–55 mm Hg), or severe (> 55 mm Hg).

A. Pulmonary Arterial Hypertension

Pathologic abnormalities in PAH are localized to the precapillary pulmonary arterioles, resulting in a characteristic hemodynamic profile that can be identified during right heart catheterization (RHC) (see Figure 30–1). PAH is defined by a sustained elevation of the mPAP $\geq$ 25 mm Hg and a PAWP or left ventricular end-diastolic pressure $\leq$ 15 mm Hg (normal PAWP, 8–12 mm Hg).

PAH is caused by a disparate group of diseases that have in common vasoconstriction and arteriopathy with remodeling of the precapillary pulmonary arterioles (see Table 30–1). PAH results in progressive cardiopulmonary deterioration, right heart failure, and death. While the prognosis for patients with PAH varies with the underlying cause, overall

survival is poor. Figure 30–2 shows survival characteristics in patients with different subtypes of PAH.

The prevalence of PAH in the United States is estimated to be between 50,000 and 100,000 cases. Of these, only 15,000 to 25,000 are appropriately diagnosed and treated. Multicenter registry data suggest that most patients with PAH are women (with a 2:1 female-to-male ratio), with a mean age of 50 years. Seventy-five percent of patients with PAH have symptoms at rest or with minimal exertion. The mean duration of symptoms prior to diagnosis is 27 months.

Three processes contribute to pulmonary artery (PA) luminal narrowing in PAH: vasoconstriction, arterial remodeling, and thrombosis in situ (Figure 30–3). In susceptible individuals, pulmonary vascular injury leads to disruption of the homeostatic balance present in the healthy pulmonary arteries. Upregulation of vasoconstrictive and proproliferative mediators (ie, endothelin-1, serotonin, and thromboxane) and downregulation of vasodilatory and antiproliferative mediators (ie, nitric oxide, prostacyclin, and smooth muscle cell potassium channels) lead to increased vasoconstriction and disordered cell proliferation. In situ thrombus formation occurs as a result of increased platelet activation, increased blood stasis, upregulation of plasminogen activator inhibitor-1, and reduced fibrinolytic activity. The cellular processes that have been implicated in the pathogenesis of PAH are summarized in Figure 30–4.

PAH is termed idiopathic if no disease associated with PAH is present and heritable if there is an underlying genetic predisposition or familial occurrence of PAH. Idiopathic and heritable PAH are rare disorders with a prevalence of 15 cases per million per year and an incidence of 1–2 cases per million per year. Idiopathic and heritable PAH afflict predominantly young women, with a mean age at diagnosis of 35 years. These are progressive disorders with a high mortality (median life expectancy 2.8 years from diagnosis).

Mutations in the bone morphogenetic protein receptor (*BMPR*)-2 gene have been identified in approximately 50% of patients with heritable PAH. Those who inherit the mutation have a 10% risk of developing PAH. The genetic pattern of inheritance is autosomal dominant with incomplete penetrance and anticipation (subsequent generations manifest the disease at an earlier age). A mutation in the activin receptor-like kinase type-1 (ALK-1 or endoglin) often with coexistent hereditary hemorrhagic telangiectasia may have also been identified in patients with PAH. Both BMPR-2 and ALK-1 are members of the transforming growth factor β signaling pathway.

Diseases associated with PAH include collagen vascular diseases (especially systemic sclerosis), congenital systemic-to-pulmonary shunts, portal hypertension, HIV infection, drug (notably anorexigens) and toxin exposures, and other disorders as delineated in Table 30–1.

For those patients in whom PAH develops secondary to collagen-vascular disease, the prognosis is extremely poor. In patients with PAH associated with systemic sclerosis, for instance, the 1-year survival is approximately 50%.

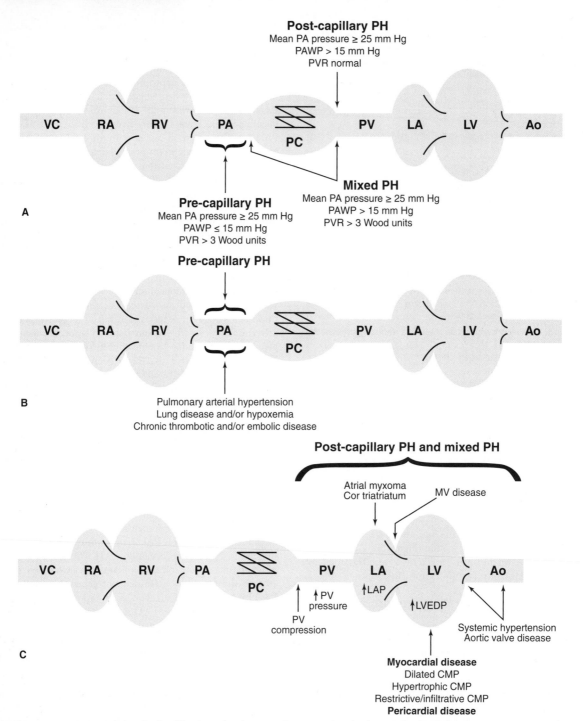

▲ **Figure 30–1.** Hemodynamic classification of pulmonary hypertension (PH). **A:** Pulmonary hypertension may result from pathology in precapillary or postcapillary pulmonary circulation. **B:** Common causes of precapillary PH. **C:** Common causes of postcapillary and mixed PH. Ao, aorta; CMP, cardiomyopathy; LA, left atrium; LV, left ventricle; LVEDP, left ventricular end-diastolic pressure; PA, pulmonary artery; PAWP, pulmonary arterial wedge pressure; PC, pulmonary capillaries; PV, pulmonary veins; PVR, pulmonary vascular resistance; RA, right atrium; RV, right ventricle; VC, vena cava.

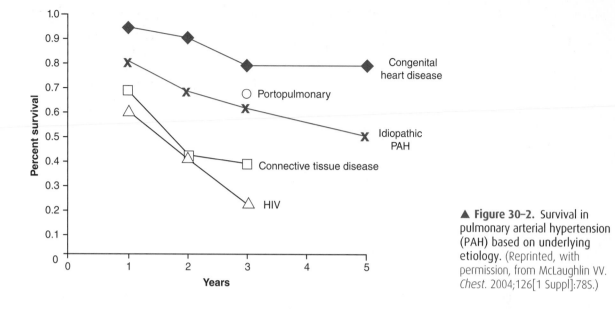

▲ **Figure 30–2.** Survival in pulmonary arterial hypertension (PAH) based on underlying etiology. (Reprinted, with permission, from McLaughlin VV. *Chest.* 2004;126[1 Suppl]:78S.)

Congenital systemic-to-pulmonary shunts result from ventricular or atrial septal defects, anomalous pulmonary venous drainage, patent ductus arteriosus, or an aorto-pulmonary window. Systemic-to-pulmonary shunts expose the pulmonary vasculature to a persistent high-flow state. This can lead to PA endothelial dysfunction, mediator activation, and reactive vasoconstriction. Vascular remodeling ensues and can progress to the point that shunt reversal occurs (Eisenmenger syndrome). Shunt reversal worsens hypoxemia and further exacerbates PAH. PAH may also develop many

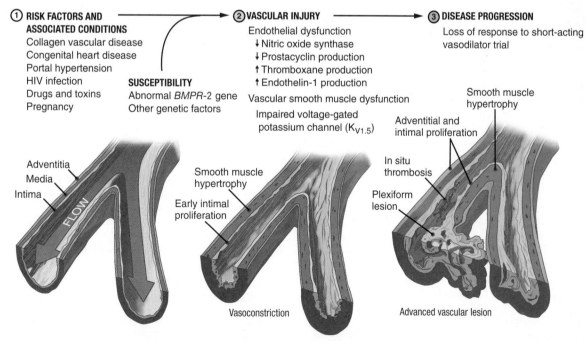

▲ **Figure 30–3.** Pathogenesis of pulmonary arterial hypertension. (Reproduced, with permission, from Gaine S. *JAMA.* 2000;284:3160.)

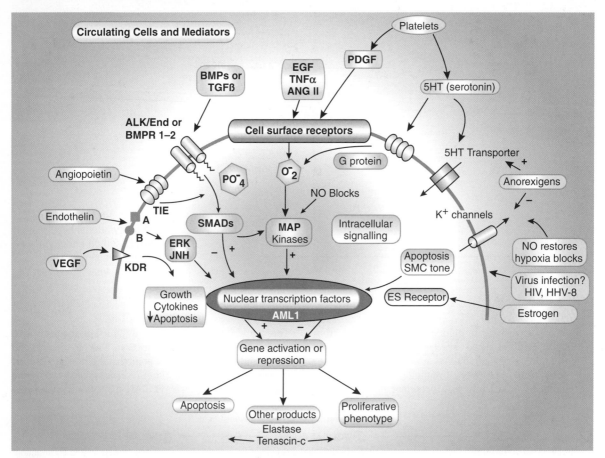

▲ **Figure 30-4.** Some cellular processes implicated in the pathogenesis of pulmonary arterial hypertension. VEGF indicates vascular endothelial growth factor; its receptor is KDR. Endothelin is vasoactive and acts through calcium channels and ERK/Jun kinases. TIE is the angiopoietin receptor, a system found to be upregulated in pulmonary vascular disease. Alk1 and BMPR1-2 are TGF receptors. Alk1 mutations cause hereditary hemorrhagic telangiectasia and some cases of pulmonary hypertension. Epidermal growth factor, tumor necrosis factor, angiotensin II, and platelet-derived growth factor are all proliferative stimuli that act through tyrosine kinase receptors. SMADs are regulatory proteins that activate nuclear transcription factors and interact with MAP kinases. AML1 is a nuclear transcription factor. (Reprinted, with permission, from Newman JH. *Circulation.* 2004;109:2947.)

years after repair of a congenital shunt as a long-term consequence of vascular injury sustained prior to shunt repair.

PAH develops in approximately 5–10% of patients with portal hypertension. Porto-pulmonary hypertension can interfere with eligibility for liver transplantation because it is associated with high perioperative mortality.

It is estimated that PAH develops in 1 of every 200 patients with HIV infection. Those patients with HIV in whom PAH develops have a particularly poor prognosis (see Figure 30-2). Methamphetamine use is also associated with the development of PAH. The diet drug fenfluramine, which has been removed from the U.S. market, has also been associated with increased likelihood of PAH.

The disorders discussed thus far, while distinct, result in pulmonary endothelial and vascular smooth muscle cell dysfunction, maladaptive arterial remodeling, and increased vascular resistance. While prognosis of PAH varies based on the underlying disease, presence of PAH significantly increases the morbidity and mortality of all associated conditions.

B. Pulmonary Hypertension with Left-Sided Heart Disease

Elevation of left-sided cardiac filling pressures can lead to PH through passive congestion and retrograde transmission of elevated pressure to the PA tree. This is termed "postcapillary pulmonary hypertension" (see Figure 30–1A, C). Postcapillary PH is characterized hemodynamically by an mPAP ≥ 25 mm Hg, PAWP > 15 mm Hg, and a normal PVR. Elevation of left-sided cardiac filling pressures may result from aortic or mitral valve dysfunction, myocardial disease, pericardial disease, atrial myxoma with obstruction, or pulmonary vein compression. With chronic elevation of pulmonary venous pressures, upregulation of inflammatory cytokines, as well as vasoconstrictive and proproliferative mediators, results in reactive vasoconstriction. Elevation of PA pressure can therefore exist out of proportion to left-sided filling pressures. This entity is referred to as mixed PH or "reactive PH" and is characterized hemodynamically by an mPAP ≥ 25 mm Hg, PAWP > 15 mm Hg, and a PVR > 3 Wood units (240 dynes $\times$ s $\times$ cm^{-5}).

Since the PVR is normal in pure postcapillary PH, optimal management of left-sided heart disease with appropriate therapies that reduce the left-sided cardiac filling pressure (ie, surgery for valvular dysfunction, diuretics, angiotensin-converting enzyme inhibitors, hydralazine) will result in normalization of the PAP. This may not be the case if mixed PH has developed, as is seen in patients with severe end-stage heart failure undergoing transplant evaluation. Targeted vasodilator therapy can often improve reactive PA vasoconstriction in this setting. However, "fixed" mixed PH that is refractory to vasodilator therapy from vascular arterial remodeling can pose a significant problem in patients undergoing heart transplantation. Acute right heart failure may occur when an unconditioned donor right ventricle is exposed to irreversibly high PVR after transplantation.

C. Pulmonary Hypertension Associated with Lung Diseases and Hypoxemia

PH is also associated with diseases that affect the lung parenchyma such as chronic obstructive pulmonary disease (COPD) and interstitial lung disease (ILD). PH secondary to lung disease is hemodynamically precapillary in origin (see Figure 30–1A, B). Several factors contribute to the development of PH in this setting. Disruption of capillary networks results in a decrease in the overall surface area of the pulmonary vascular bed and thereby increases PVR. Hypoxemia directly triggers pulmonary vasoconstriction and indirectly contributes to pulmonary vascular remodeling by resulting in upregulation of proproliferative mediators. Hyperviscosity secondary to hypoxia-induced erythrocytosis can worsen PH. Sleep-disordered breathing, alveolar hypoventilation disorders, and prolonged exposure to high altitude are other causes of PH associated with hypoxemia.

Treatment of these disorders is based on correction of the underlying disorder, provision of supplemental oxygen, and management of cor pulmonale. Although some benefits from PAH-specific therapy have been observed in ILD patients, these treatments also worsen hypoxemia because they inhibit physiologic pulmonary vasoconstriction and worsen ventilation-perfusion mismatch. Use of PAH-specific therapy in this setting is generally discouraged.

D. Pulmonary Hypertension due to Chronic Thrombotic or Embolic Diseases

A massive, sudden pulmonary embolus (PE) may significantly increase PAP and cause hemodynamic collapse secondary to acute right ventricular failure. This scenario leads to death in approximately 20–40% of patients with acute PE. The presence of severe PH in this setting portends a poor prognosis and predicts an increased likelihood of chronic thromboembolic PH (CTEPH). In fact, most patients with pulmonary embolism experience complete resolution of thromboemboli within 30 days.

CTEPH occurs in up to 4% of patients following acute PE or 10% following recurrent PE. However 50% of patients diagnosed with CTEPH have no history of a thromboembolic event. Why some patients develop CTEPH is not well understood, but surgical specimens show evidence of persistence and organization of thromboembolic material as well as vascular remodeling characterized by intimal thickening with deposition of collagen and hemosiderin, atherosclerosis, and calcification. Vasculopathy and pathologic remodeling of unobstructed downstream pulmonary arterioles similar to that which occurs in idiopathic PAH also develops possibly secondary to abnormal blood flow.

Mortality in patients with CTEPH is high but, in selected patients, can be improved markedly with surgical pulmonary thromboendarterectomy (PTE). Excluding CTEPH as a cause of PH requires evaluation with a ventilation-perfusion scan followed by confirmatory conventional pulmonary angiography. Computed tomography (CT) pulmonary angiography is not adequately sensitive to definitively exclude the diagnosis. Early referral to a center that can perform PTE is needed.

E. Miscellaneous

This category of PH encompasses a diverse group of disorders that are hemodynamically precapillary in origin and includes sarcoidosis, histiocytosis X, lymphangiomatosis, and pulmonary vein compression.

F. Pathophysiologic Consequences of Pulmonary Hypertension

Elevations in PAP eventually result in right ventricular systolic failure from chronic pressure overload (Figure 30–5). In response, the right ventricle undergoes hypertrophic remodeling to maintain CO and compensate for increased afterload. Early on, the right ventricle can have supernormal function and normal-to-reduced chamber dimensions. Chronic right ventricular pressure overload results in persistent upregulation of proproliferative neurohormones, endothelin-1, and cytokines. These mediators contribute to

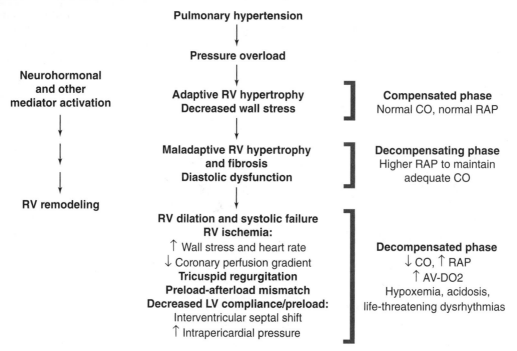

▲ **Figure 30–5.** Pathophysiology of right ventricular dysfunction in pulmonary hypertension. AV-DO$_2$, arteriovenous oxygen differential; CO, cardiac output; LV, left ventricular; RAP, right atrial pressure; RV, right ventricular.

the development of maladaptive hypertrophy with fibrosis and diastolic dysfunction.

If exposure to elevated PA pressure continues, the right ventricle dilates. This is an ominous sign because it signifies the presence of increased right ventricular wall stress. Increased wall stress, when coupled with increased heart rate, results in increased myocardial oxygen demand. This develops in concert with a reduction in the epicardial-to-endocardial coronary perfusion gradient secondary to increased right ventricular end-diastolic pressure. In sum, these changes result in a myocardial oxygen supply-demand mismatch and right ventricular ischemia. Right ventricular ischemia worsens systolic function, increases end-diastolic pressure, and promotes further ventricular enlargement. Tricuspid regurgitation secondary to annular dilatation often occurs and serves to further reduce effective right ventricular forward output.

Right ventricular dilation, in the setting of an intact pericardium, results in a shift of the interventricular septum toward the left ventricle. This, especially when coupled with increased intrapericardial pressure, impedes left ventricular filling (preload). In turn, when left ventricular filling is impaired, systemic CO is reduced.

Multiple mechanisms contribute to the development of hypoxemia in PH, even when intrinsic pulmonary disease (COPD, CTEPH) is absent. Pulmonary vascular remodeling

and in situ thromboses disrupt normal capillary-alveolar gas exchange and raise the alveolar-to-arterial oxygen gradient. Increased pulmonary pressures can increase right atrial pressure and cause shunting through a patent foramen ovale. Because a patent foramen ovale is present in up to 30% of adults, right-to-left shunting should be considered in patients with PH and hypoxemia.

De Marco T, et al. Managing right ventricular failure in pulmonary arterial hypertension. *Adv Pulm Hypertension.* 2005;4(4):16–26.

Humbert M, et al. Pulmonary arterial hypertension in France: results from a national registry. *Am J Respir Crit Care Med.* 2006; 173(9):1023–30. [PMID: 16456139]

McLaughlin VV, et al. Pulmonary arterial hypertension. *Circulation.* 2006;114(13):1417–31. [PMID: 17000921]

Moraes DL, et al. Secondary pulmonary hypertension in chronic heart failure: the role of the endothelium in pathophysiology and management. *Circulation.* 2000;102(14):1718–23. [PMID: 11015353]

Newman JH, et al; National Heart, Lung and Blood Institute/ Office of Rare Diseases. Pulmonary arterial hypertension: future directions: report of a National Heart, Lung and Blood Institute/Office of Rare Diseases workshop. *Circulation.* 2004; 109(24):2947–52. [PMID: 15210611]

Pengo V, et al; Thromboembolic Pulmonary Hypertension Study Group. Incidence of chronic thromboembolic pulmonary hypertension after pulmonary embolism. *N Engl J Med.* 2004; 350(22):2257–64. [PMID: 15163775]

Schermuly RT, et al. Mechanisms of disease: pulmonary arterial hypertension. *Nat Rev Cardiol.* 2011;8(8):443–55. [PMID: 21691314]

Simonneau G, et al. Updated clinical classification of pulmonary hypertension. *J Am Coll Cardiol.* 2009;54(1 Suppl):S43–54. [PMID: 19555858]

▶ Clinical Findings

A. Symptoms & Signs

One of the major difficulties in PH management is the failure to make an early diagnosis. It takes an average of 2.5 years from symptom onset to PH diagnosis. This results, in part, from the fact that PH often presents with a subtle, nonspecific symptom complex. PH most commonly manifests as dyspnea on exertion or fatigue, but it can also manifest as chest pain or syncope (often with exercise). Once right ventricular failure occurs, lower extremity edema and ascites become manifest. The New York Heart Association (NYHA) and World Health Organization have proposed systems for categorizing the severity of symptoms secondary to PH (Table 30–2).

B. Physical Examination

Careful examination of the patient with PH can reveal clues not only about the presence or severity of PH but also about the underlying cause. A loud pulmonic valve closure (P_2) or an early systolic ejection click may be heard as a consequence of marked elevation in PA pressures. With right ventricular hypertrophy and enlargement, a left parasternal lift can be palpated. Another manifestation of right ventricular hypertrophy with diastolic dysfunction is the right ventricular S_4 gallop. A right-sided S_3 is also appreciable in patients with

significant elevation in the right ventricular end-diastolic pressure.

Often the holosystolic murmur of tricuspid regurgitation (although frequently without the classically described respiratory variation) and the less common diastolic murmur of pulmonic insufficiency are noted in patients with PH. Jugular venous distention, peripheral edema, and ascites become manifest in advanced PH with right heart failure. Cool extremities and diminished peripheral pulses are indicative of low CO and peripheral vasoconstriction in severe right ventricular failure.

A murmur of mitral or aortic stenosis, a left-sided S_3, or severe bronchial wheezing and diminished breath sounds may be clues to the presence of left-sided heart disease or pulmonary parenchymal disease, respectively. Jaundice and spider angiomata may point to the presence of cirrhosis and portal hypertension. Connective tissue diseases may present not only with signs of PH but also with Raynaud phenomenon, arthritis, rashes, or other skin changes (ie, sclerodactyly).

C. Diagnostic Studies

1. Electrocardiography—The electrocardiogram (ECG) in patients with significant PH typically suggests right ventricular hypertrophy. There is often a distinct correlation between the amplitude of the R wave in V_1, the R/S ratio in V_1, and the severity of the PH. Classic ECG findings include right axis deviation and right atrial enlargement. Incomplete or complete right bundle branch block is also common. The ECG criteria for right ventricular hypertrophy and a typical ECG in a patient with PH are shown in Table 30–3 and Figure 30–6, respectively. The ECG is not sensitive enough to serve as a screening tool for PH.

2. Chest radiography—Radiographic examination of the chest in a patient with PAH may show enlargement of the main pulmonary artery and its major branches, with distal pruning of peripheral arteries. The retrosternal space is often filled by the hypertrophic right ventricle on lateral projection. Pulmonary venous congestion and left atrial or left ventricular enlargement suggest the presence of a left-sided cause of PH. Hyperinflated lung fields or bullous changes point to a chronic pulmonary disorder with secondary PH. A classic chest radiograph of a patient with PAH is shown in Figure 30–7.

Table 30–2. New York Heart Association (NYHA) and World Health Organization (WHO) Functional Classes in Pulmonary Hypertension

Class	Symptoms/Function
NYHA I/WHO I	No limitation in physical activity. Ordinary physical activity does not cause undue dyspnea, fatigue, chest pain, or near-syncope.
NYHA II/WHO II	Slight limitation in physical activity. Ordinary physical activity causes undue dyspnea, fatigue, chest pain, or near-syncope.
NYHA III/WHO III	Marked limitation in physical activity. Less than ordinary physical activity causes undue dyspnea, fatigue, chest pain, or near-syncope.
NYHA IV/WHO IV	Inability to carry out any physical activity without symptoms. Patients manifest signs of right heart failure. Dyspnea and/or fatigue may be present at rest.

Table 30–3. Electrocardiographic Criteria for Right Ventricular Hypertrophy

Right axis deviation (axis > +90 degrees)
R-S amplitude in lead V_1 > 1.0 mm
R-wave amplitude in V_1 ≥ 7 mm
S-wave amplitude in V_1 < 2 mm
qR pattern in precordial lead V_1
R-wave amplitude in lead V_1 + S-wave amplitude in V_5 or V_6 > 10.5 mm
R-S amplitude in V_5 or V_6 ≤ 1.0 mm

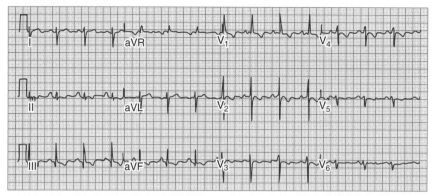

▲ **Figure 30–6.** Electrocardiogram in a patient with pulmonary arterial hypertension and right ventricular hypertrophy.

3. Echocardiography—Two-dimensional and Doppler echocardiography are essential to the noninvasive assessment of patients with suspected PH. Echocardiography can demonstrate cardiac structural changes such as right atrial or right ventricular enlargement, right ventricular hypertrophy, and PA enlargement. Flattening or leftward shift of the interventricular septum can also be identified. If the shift occurs during systole, it suggests ventricular pressure overload. If it occurs during diastole, it suggests volume overload. Leftward shift of the septum throughout the cardiac cycle suggests both right ventricular pressure and volume overload (Figure 30–8A, B). The left ventricle is often small and underfilled in PH, with normal systolic function (Figure 30–8B).

Echocardiography is also useful to assess the severity of tricuspid regurgitation (TR) and estimate pulmonary artery systolic pressure (PASP). PASP is estimated by entering the peak velocity of the TR jet right into the modified Bernoulli equation and adding the right atrial pressure estimated by evaluating respiratory change in the inferior vena cava diameter (PASP = $4v^2$ + right atrial [RA] pressure) (Figure 30–8C). Noninvasive PA pressure assessment is not only important in establishing a diagnosis of PH but also in monitoring response to therapy. Echocardiography-estimated PASP may by inaccurate when the peak velocity cannot be accurately assessed due to minimal TR, an eccentric TR jet, or severe TR. In patients with risk factors for PH and who have

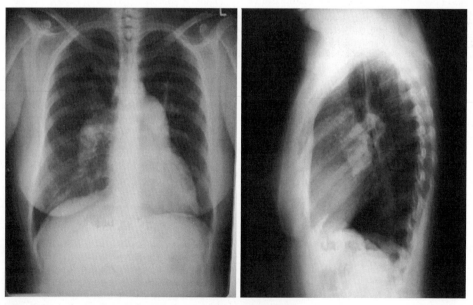

▲ **Figure 30–7.** Chest radiograph in pulmonary arterial hypertension demonstrating enlargement of the central pulmonary arteries with peripheral pruning of the pulmonary vasculature. Also notable is the reduction in the retrosternal air space on the lateral view and the distinct lack of pulmonary pathology.

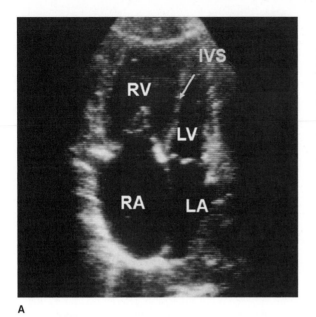

A

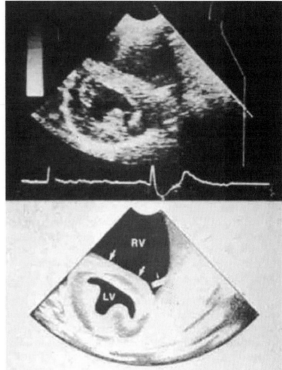

B

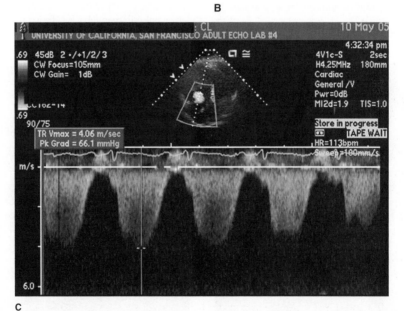

C

▲ **Figure 30–8.** Transthoracic echocardiogram of a patient with pulmonary arterial hypertension. **A:** This apical four-chamber view demonstrates RA and RV enlargement. There is leftward shifting (flattening) of the interventricular septum. **B:** This parasternal short-axis view demonstrates RV enlargement, a small LV cavity, and leftward shifting (flattening) of the interventricular septum. **C:** This continuous wave Doppler recording shows how the tricuspid regurgitation velocity is obtained by echocardiography and used to estimate the pulmonary artery systolic pressure (PASP = $4V^2$ + RAP). RV, right ventricle; IVS, interventricular septum; LV, left ventricle; RA, right atrium; LA, left atrium; RAP, right atrial pressure.

signs and symptoms concerning for PH, low estimated PASP may not exclude PH.

Echocardiography can also be helpful in detecting left-sided heart disease. A dilated, hypocontractile left ventricle, valvular disease, or left atrial myxoma can be identified or excluded on a routine echocardiogram. Color-flow and agitated saline injection can also be used to assess for the existence of congenital intracardiac or intrapulmonary shunts.

4. Lung scintigraphy—Ventilation-perfusion (V/Q) lung scintigraphy is necessary during the evaluation of patients with PH to exclude CTEPH as the etiology of PH. In PAH, the V/Q scan may reveal a normal perfusion pattern, or it may show diffuse, patchy ("mottled") perfusion defects. Parenchymal lung disease can also result in perfusion scan abnormalities, but typically, these are matched by ventilatory defects. In CTEPH, however, the lung perfusion scan demonstrates one or more segmental defects mismatched by the ventilation scan (Figure 30–9). An abnormal V/Q scan should prompt conventional pulmonary angiography to confirm the diagnosis of CTEPH.

5. Pulmonary function testing—Pulmonary function testing is helpful in PH because it can establish the diagnosis of underlying obstructive or restrictive pulmonary disease. Interpretation of pulmonary function test results should be tempered by an awareness that PAH can reduce diffusing capacity of carbon monoxide. If the total lung capacity is less than 70% of predicted, a high-resolution CT scan should be considered to evaluate for ILD.

6. Computed tomography and magnetic resonance imaging—CT scans and magnetic resonance imaging (MRI) of the chest can provide useful information in parenchymal lung disorders and several other conditions that can cause PH. Chest CT or MRI scans can demonstrate characteristic findings in patients with fibrosing mediastinitis and cystic fibrosis, as well as infiltrative or granulomatous lung diseases. Findings on CT pulmonary angiography may suggest a diagnosis of CTEPH; however, the test is not sensitive enough to exclude the diagnosis of CTEPH.

7. Cardiac catheterization and pulmonary angiography—RHC represents the gold-standard test to establish the diagnosis of PH, ascertain its etiology, establish severity and prognosis, evaluate vasoreactivity, and assist in guiding therapy. RHC should be performed by a clinician with experience in the evaluation and management of patients with PH.

During RHC, a full cardiopulmonary hemodynamic profile is established by recording the right atrial, right ventricular, PA, and PAWP, as well as measuring the CO. The PVR ([mPAP – PAWP]/CO) is also determined during RHC. Arterial and venous oxygen saturations obtained during RHC are used to detect and determine the severity of shunts. Abnormalities of the left heart, such as aortic or mitral valve disease or left heart failure, will be suggested during RHC by the presence of an elevated PAWP. In patients with characteristics associated with diastolic heart failure (elderly with diabetes, hypertension, left ventricular hypertrophy, or left atrial enlargement), administration of a fluid bolus or

Low probability

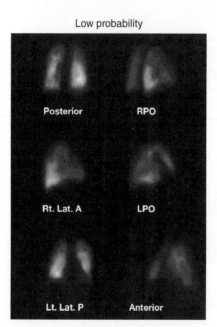

Chronic thromboembolic disease

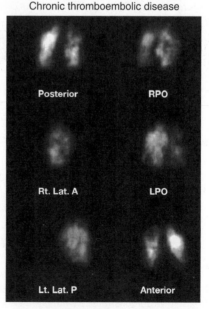

▲ **Figure 30–9.** Perfusion lung scans from a normal patient and a patient with chronic thromboembolic disease. The scan on the left shows uniform perfusion. The scan on the right shows multiple perfusion defects consistent with the diagnosis of chronic thromboembolic disease. LPO, left posterior oblique; RPO, right posterior oblique.

exercise during RHC should be considered to exclude the presence of occult diastolic dysfunction.

Vasoreactivity testing is an important component of RHC in PAH. Acute vasoreactivity is tested using inhaled nitric oxide or intravenous prostacyclin or adenosine. A reduction in mean PA pressure > 10 mm Hg with a final mPAP ≤ 40 mm Hg suggests that reversible vasoconstriction, rather than fixed vascular remodeling, is the major mechanism for PAH. Less than 15% of patients with idiopathic PAH will respond to acute vasodilator testing, but a positive vasoreactivity trial identifies a subset of patients with superior overall prognosis and high likelihood of benefit from high-dose calcium channel blocker therapy.

Pulmonary angiography is not routinely performed in patients with PH. When ventilation-perfusion scintigraphy or CT pulmonary angiography suggests chronic thromboembolic disease, pulmonary angiography and angioscopy are needed to confirm the diagnosis and determine the extent and location of thromboembolic disease. Findings on pulmonary angiography determine if patients with CTEPH are operative candidates.

8. Lung biopsy—A lung biopsy is infrequently required to determine the cause of PH. Lung biopsy can identify injected particulate matter in injection drug users, can establish the diagnosis of pulmonary veno-occlusive disease, and may identify causative pathogens in ILD. Due to its substantial morbidity, however, lung biopsy is seldom used. If lung biopsy is obtained in an individual with reversible PH, medial smooth muscle hypertrophy may be noted. In more advanced cases, necrotizing arteritis and plexiform lesions can be seen (Figure 30–10).

9. Functional capacity and exercise testing—The use of the World Health Organization's functional classification and symptom-limited exercise testing can be very helpful in the evaluation of patients with PH. Exercise testing, particularly the 6-minute walk test, has been shown to predict mortality and allows for objective assessment of symptom burden. Baseline functional capacity and exercise testing utilizing the 6-minute walk test should be measured prior to initiation of therapy and serially to monitor response to treatment.

10. Other studies—If sleep apnea is suspected, a full sleep study can be diagnostic. Liver biochemical testing and hepatic ultrasound are used to exclude liver cirrhosis and portal hypertension. Screening for connective tissue diseases (eg, scleroderma, rheumatoid arthritis, systemic lupus erythematosus, mixed connective tissue disease, polymyositis) should be performed with appropriate serologic and immunogenetic studies. Thyroid function and HIV testing should also be performed. Parasitic disease (schistosomiasis or filariasis) should be suspected and tested for in patients from endemic areas with PH. Tissue biopsy, complement fixation, blood smear, and skin testing are diagnostic tests of choice in such patients.

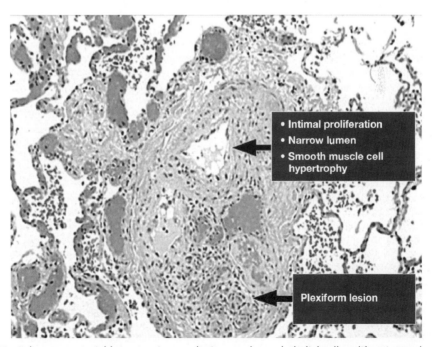

- Intimal proliferation
- Narrow lumen
- Smooth muscle cell hypertrophy

Plexiform lesion

▲ **Figure 30–10.** Pulmonary arterial hypertension results in vascular endothelial cell proliferation and smooth muscle cell hypertrophy. Plexiform lesions can develop and predispose to in situ thrombosis. (Reprinted, with permission, from the American Medical Association; Gaine S. *JAMA*. 2000;284:3160–8.)

Cockrill BA, et al. Comparison of the effects of nitric oxide, nitroprusside, and nifedipine on hemodynamics and right ventricular contractility in patients with chronic pulmonary hypertension. *Chest.* 2001;119(1):128–36. [PMID: 11157594]

Fleischmann D, et al. Three-dimensional visualization of pulmonary thromboemboli in chronic thromboembolic pulmonary hypertension with multiple detector-row spiral computed tomography. *Circulation.* 2001;103(24):2993. [PMID: 11413092]

McGoon M, et al; American College of Chest Physicians. Screening, early detection, and diagnosis of pulmonary arterial hypertension. ACCP evidence-based clinical practice guidelines. *Chest.* 2004;126(1 Suppl):14S–34S. [PMID: 15249493]

Miyamoto S, et al. Clinical correlates and prognostic significance of six-minute walk test in patients with primary pulmonary hypertension. Comparison with cardiopulmonary exercise testing. *Am J Respir Crit Care Med.* 2000;161(2 Pt 1):487–92. [PMID: 10673190]

▶ Differential Diagnosis

The differential diagnosis for PAH includes a number of well-defined causes of PH (see Table 30–1). Diagnostic efforts should be pursued vigorously, since PAH can progress rapidly and is associated with substantial morbidity and mortality. An algorithmic approach to diagnosis has been proposed by the American College of Chest Physicians and is shown in Figure 30–11.

Suspicion for PAH should be raised on the basis of clinical history and physical examination, as previously outlined. Initial diagnostic testing should include a baseline ECG and chest radiograph. Two-dimensional and Doppler echocardiography are recommended to noninvasively assess PASP and evaluate biventricular structure and function. Color-flow and agitated saline injection should be utilized to assess for the existence of congenital intracardiac or intrapulmonary shunts.

If echocardiography suggests that PH is present and no clear left-sided or congenital lesions have been identified, an evaluation for thromboembolic disease should be conducted. If evidence of CTEPH is present on V/Q scintigraphy, pulmonary angiography is performed to confirm the diagnosis and to evaluate for PTE candidacy.

Pulmonary disease can be assessed with chest radiograph, arterial oxygen saturation measurement, pulmonary function testing, and chest CT scan. If sleep apnea or sleep-disordered breathing is suspected, a thorough sleep study should be conducted. A serologic workup for common connective tissue diseases, thyroid disease, liver disease, and HIV is also required.

Assessment of functional capacity and symptom burden should be conducted using the World Health Organization's functional classification and 6-minute walk test. Exercise capacity correlates well with overall prognosis, and baseline 6-minute walk test values can help later evaluation of treatment response. RHC is also recommended at this stage in order to document right atrial pressure, pulmonary arterial pressure, and PAWP. CO, PVR, and vasoreactivity testing should also be assessed during RHC. If a patient has an elevated mPAP on RHC and no cause of PH has been identified, the diagnosis of idiopathic PAH has been made. Genetic testing should be discussed with the patient and family members.

▶ Treatment

A. Pulmonary Arterial Hypertension

Improvement in cardiopulmonary hemodynamics, exercise capacity, functional class, survival, and prevention of clinical worsening are the goals of PAH treatment. General measures in the management of PAH include symptom-limited, regular exercise to maintain skeletal muscle conditioning and overall cardiovascular fitness. Intense exercise should be avoided, especially if the patient with PAH has a history of exercise-induced syncope or presyncope. Patients should avoid high altitudes, and supplemental oxygen should be provided for air travel. Since patients with PAH have reduced cardiopulmonary reserve, immunization against influenza and pneumococcus is recommended.

Pregnancy in PAH deserves special attention. Patients with PAH should be counseled to avoid pregnancy because it is associated with significant (30%) mortality. Birth control should be discussed and contraceptive methods prescribed in women of childbearing age. Hemoglobin levels should be monitored regularly. In patients with Eisenmenger syndrome, erythrocytosis should be treated with phlebotomy only if symptoms of hyperviscosity develop. Patients with PAH should refrain from smoking and adhere to a sodium-restricted diet in the setting of right heart failure.

Patients with PAH require supplemental oxygen if they exhibit arterial oxygen desaturation at rest or with minimal exertion. Patients with PAH, particularly idiopathic PAH, should receive oral anticoagulant therapy with a goal international normalized ratio (INR) of 1.5 to 2.5. This recommendation is based on several nonrandomized clinical trials showing improved survival in patients with idiopathic PAH treated with warfarin.

Diuretic therapy is the mainstay of treatment for symptomatic PAH with volume overload. Digoxin may also help improve right-sided hemodynamics and is the preferred rate-controlling agent in the setting of atrial tachyarrhythmia. Digoxin has also been shown to reduce circulating catecholamine levels in patients with chronic PAH. However, no other data exist regarding the efficacy of cardiac glycosides (ie, digoxin) in PAH with right ventricular failure. Digoxin toxicity, especially in patients with severe hypoxia, renal insufficiency, or hypokalemia, is well recognized and warrants vigilance.

In patients with PAH and decompensated right heart failure, strategies to improve clinical status and restore end-organ perfusion include (1) afterload reduction with pulmonary vasodilators, such as oxygen, inhaled nitric oxide, prostanoids, endothelin receptor antagonists, and phosphodiesterase inhibitors; (2) preload reduction with diuretics or ultrafiltration; and (3) augmentation of right ventricular

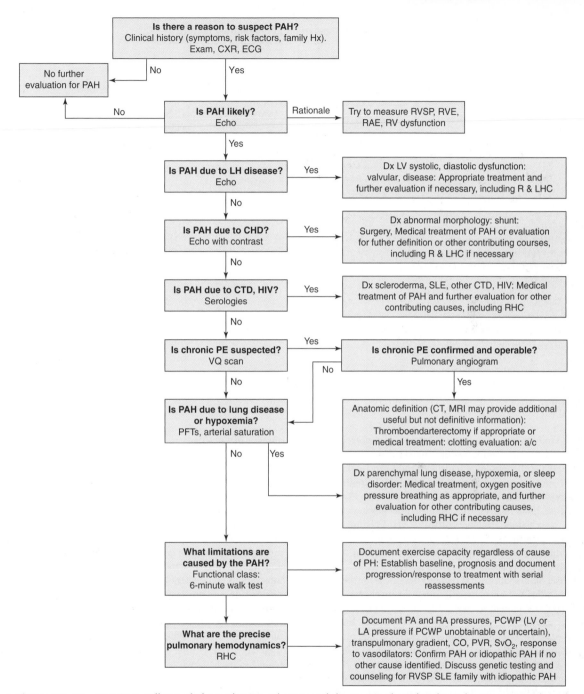

▲ **Figure 30–11.** American College of Chest Physicians' proposed diagnostic algorithm for pulmonary arterial hypertension. CHD, congenital heart disease; CTD, connective tissue disease; a/c, anticoagulation; CO, cardiac output; Dx, diagnosis; Echo, echocardiography; Hx, history; LH, left heart; LA, left atrial; LV, left ventricular; PCWP, pulmonary capillary wedge pressure; PE, pulmonary embolism; PFT, pulmonary function test; PVR, pulmonary vascular resistance; RAE, right atrial enlargement; RHC, right catheterization; R&LHC, right and left heart catheterization; RV, right ventricular; RVE, right ventricular enlargement; mixed venous oxygen saturation; TRV, peak velocity of tricuspid regurgitation jet. (Reproduced, with permission, from McGoon M, et al. *Chest.* 2004;126:14S.)

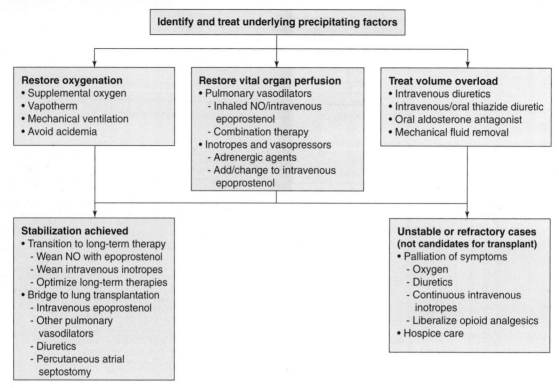

```
┌──────────────────────────────────────────────────────────┐
│    Identify and treat underlying precipitating factors     │
└──────────────────────────────────────────────────────────┘
```

Restore oxygenation
• Supplemental oxygen
• Vapotherm
• Mechanical ventilation
• Avoid acidemia

Restore vital organ perfusion
• Pulmonary vasodilators
  - Inhaled NO/intravenous
    epoprostenol
  - Combination therapy
• Inotropes and vasopressors
  - Adrenergic agents
  - Add/change to intravenous
    epoprostenol

Treat volume overload
• Intravenous diuretics
• Intravenous/oral thiazide diuretic
• Oral aldosterone antagonist
• Mechanical fluid removal

Stabilization achieved
• Transition to long-term therapy
  - Wean NO with epoprostenol
  - Wean intravenous inotropes
  - Optimize long-term therapies
• Bridge to lung transplantation
  - Intravenous epoprostenol
  - Other pulmonary
    vasodilators
  - Diuretics
  - Percutaneous atrial
    septostomy

**Unstable or refractory cases
(not candidates for transplant)**
• Palliation of symptoms
  - Oxygen
  - Diuretics
  - Continuous intravenous
    inotropes
  - Liberalize opioid analgesics
• Hospice care

▲ **Figure 30–12.**

function with inotropic therapy. Intravenous inotropes such as low-dose dobutamine or dopamine (1–2 mcg/kg/min) are of particular benefit in patients with right ventricular failure and hypotension in whom diuretic therapy is ineffective or in whom renal failure has developed (Figure 30–12).

Until 1996, high-dose calcium channel blockers were the only vasodilators available to treat PAH. Calcium channel blocker therapy may reduce PA pressure and right ventricular afterload, thereby improving right ventricular hemodynamics and increasing CO. Vasoreactivity testing identifies a subset of idiopathic PAH patients (less clear for the general PAH cohort) who may benefit from calcium channel blocker therapy. If a patient with PAH has a favorable response to acute vasodilator testing, a hemodynamically monitored trial of an oral calcium channel blocker, such as nifedipine, amlodipine, or diltiazem, may be undertaken. If a reduction in PA pressures occurs with preservation of CO, then the patient can be considered for long-term therapy. Verapamil is contraindicated due to its significant negative inotropic properties. Response to calcium channel blocker therapy should be assessed during a repeat RHC.

There are several limitations to calcium channel blocker therapy. Use of a calcium channel blocker is not advisable in patients with severe right ventricular failure or hypotension. Calcium channel blocker therapy is contraindicated in the absence of a positive vasoreactivity trial or a favorable hemodynamic response. Lastly, only a small percentage (< 7%) of patients with PAH who have acute vasoreactivity will have a sustained response to long-term calcium channel blocker therapy; therefore, close monitoring during calcium channel blocker therapy is needed.

Fortunately, the following drugs have been approved as alternatives for the treatment of PAH: oral bosentan and ambrisentan, oral sildenafil and tadalafil, inhalational iloprost and treprostinil, subcutaneous/intravenous treprostinil, and intravenous epoprostenol. These agents target the endothelin, nitric oxide, and prostacyclin pathways (Figure 30–13). These pathways are thought to mediate vascular tone and arterial remodeling. When used appropriately, these pulmonary vasodilators can improve symptoms and exercise capacity. Most of these agents delay time to clinical worsening. Only epoprostenol has been shown to improve survival in a randomized trial (Table 30–4).

Endothelin-1 is secreted by vascular endothelial cells and is a potent vasoconstrictor and mediator of smooth muscle cell proliferation. In addition, endothelin-1 enhances vascular fibrosis, increases platelet aggregation, promotes cardiac myocyte hypertrophy, and increases aldosterone production. Endothelin-1 is secreted in response to a variety of stimuli, including hypoxemia, endothelial sheer and pulsatile stress,

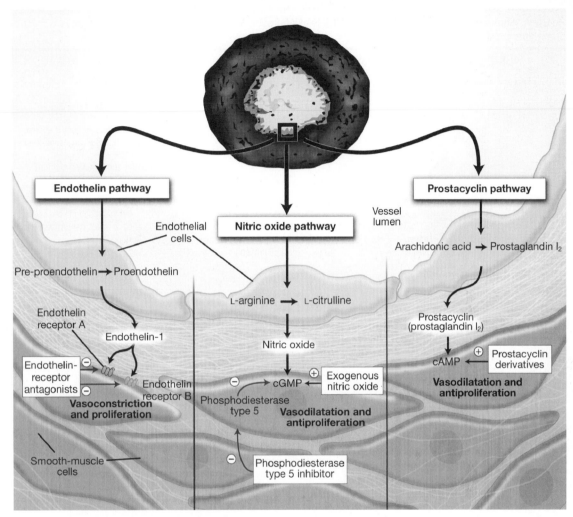

▲ **Figure 30–13.** Therapeutic targets for pulmonary arterial hypertension treatment. cAMP, cyclic adenyl monophosphate; cGMP, cyclic guanyl monophosphate. (Reprinted, with permission, from Humbert M, et al. *N Engl J Med.* 2004;351:1425.)

and neurohormonal activation, as well as PH-related growth factors and cytokines.

Bosentan is an endothelin-A and -B receptor antagonist approved for the treatment of functional class III and IV PAH. Bosentan has been shown to increase 6-minute walk distance, decrease symptom burden, and delay clinical worsening in patients with idiopathic PAH and patients with associated PAH secondary to scleroderma (see Table 30–4). Bosentan also appears to have benefit in symptomatic patients with PAH secondary to congenital heart disease and Eisenmenger syndrome.

Transaminitis develops in approximately 11% of patients treated with bosentan, and monthly liver function testing

in patients treated with bosentan is required. Transaminitis is usually reversible with cessation of treatment. A drop in hemoglobin is common and is usually not clinically significant; however, periodic monitoring of hemoglobin is recommended. Bosentan is highly teratogenic, and treated patients of childbearing potential must reliably utilize approved contraception and undergo monthly pregnancy testing. Side effects associated with bosentan include nasal congestion, flushing, anemia, and lower extremity edema.

Ambrisentan is a selective endothelin-A receptor antagonist that has recently been approved in the United States for PAH for functional class II and III patients. Ambrisentan significantly improves exercise capacity, delays time to clinical

Table 30–4. Summary of Randomized Controlled Trials of Approved Drugs for the Treatment of Pulmonary Arterial Hypertension

Drug	Study Characteristics	Positive Results	Disadvantages
Endothelin Receptor Antagonists			
Oral bosentan (nonselective)	*Name:* BREATHE-1 *Design:* Double-blind *Number:* 213	Improved 6-minute walk distance Improved dyspnea Delayed clinical worsening	Hepatic toxicity Teratogenic Fluid retention, peripheral edema, anemia, nasal congestion, sinusitis, flushing Monthly transaminase monitoring required
Oral ambrisentan (selective)	*Name:* ARIES-1 *Name:* ARIES-2 *Design:* Double-blind *Number:* 202 and 192, respectively	Improved 6-minute walk distance (30–51 m) Delayed clinical worsening Improved cardiopulmonary hemodynamics Transaminase monitoring not required	Teratogenic Fluid retention, peripheral edema, anemia, nasal congestion, sinusitis, flushing
Phosphodiesterase-5 Inhibitors			
Oral sildenafil	*Name:* SUPER-1 *Design:* Double-blind *Number:* 278	Improved 6-minute walk distance Improved dyspnea Improved cardiopulmonary hemodynamics	No delay in clinical worsening end point Headache, flushing, dyspepsia, epistaxis, visual disturbance Important drug–drug interactions
Oral tadalafil	*Name:* PHIRST *Design:* Double-blind *Number:* 405	Improved 6-minute walk distance Improved time to clinical worsening Improved cardiopulmonary hemodynamics Improved quality of life	Headache, myalgias, flushing, dyspepsia, epistaxis, visual disturbance Important drug–drug interactions
Prostanoids			
Epoprostenol (prostacyclin)	*Design:* Open-label *Number:* 81	Improved 6-minute walk distance Improved dyspnea Improved cardiopulmonary hemodynamics Improved survival	Indwelling central line Pump malfunction Flushing, jaw pain, thrombocytopenia headache, dizziness, nausea/vomiting/diarrhea, abdominal pain, hypotension, rash
Treprostinil (prostacyclin analogue, intravenous or subcutaneous)	*Design:* Double-blind *Number:* 470	Improved 6-minute walk distance Improved dyspnea Improved cardiopulmonary hemodynamics	Indwelling central line or subcutaneous catheter Pain, erythema at infusion site (subcutaneous) Flushing, jaw pain, thrombocytopenia headache, dizziness, nausea/vomiting/diarrhea, abdominal pain, hypotension, rash
Inhaled treprostinil (prostacyclin analogue)	*Name:* Triumph *Design:* Double-blind *Number:* 470	Improved 6-minute walk distance Improved quality of life Administration 4 times daily	No delay in clinical worsening or dyspnea No change in functional class Cough, headache, nausea, dizziness, flushing, throat irritation or pain
Inhaled iloprost (prostacyclin analogue)	*Design:* Double-blind *Number:* 203	Improved composite end point of 6-minute walk distance and dyspnea	Administration 6–9 times daily Cough, headache, nausea, dizziness, flushing, throat irritation or pain

worsening, and improves cardiopulmonary hemodynamics. The incidence of transaminitis is approximately 3% at 1 year. Monthly liver function testing is no longer mandatory, but most experts still monitor liver function every 3–6 months. Importantly, ambrisentan has no significant interactions with warfarin or sildenafil. The drug is teratogenic, and so, as with bosentan, pregnancy must be avoided. Ambrisentan can cause peripheral edema, nasal congestion, and flushing.

In patients with PAH, nitric oxide bioavailability is significantly reduced. Nitric oxide is secreted by the endothelial cell and diffuses to the smooth muscle cell where it mediates vasodilation and exerts an antiproliferative effect via activation of the cyclic guanyl monophosphate (cGMP) pathway.

The nitric oxide pathway can be enhanced by administering exogenous inhaled nitric oxide. It can also be enhanced by inhibiting phosphodiesterase isoform-5, the enzyme responsible for the degradation of cGMP. Sildenafil and tadalafil are oral phosphodiesterase-5 (PDE-5) inhibitors known to dilate the PA bed without increasing left-sided filling pressures. They are approved for treatment of PAH patients with functional class II–IV symptoms. When administered long term, both agents improve exercise capacity, reduce symptom burden, and improve cardiopulmonary hemodynamics (see Table 30–4). Tadalafil but not sildenafil has been shown to delay clinical worsening. Tadalafil is dosed once daily compared to three times daily dosing for sildenafil. PDE-5 inhibitors can cause headache, flushing, dyspepsia, epistaxis, and visual changes.

Prostacyclin (PGI$_2$) is a direct pulmonary and systemic vasodilator as well as an inhibitor of vascular remodeling and platelet aggregation. Prostacyclin is secreted by the endothelial cell and exerts its vascular effect by stimulating smooth muscle cell cyclic adenyl monophosphate (cAMP). The PGI$_2$ pathway is downregulated in PAH. To enhance this pathway, exogenously synthesized epoprostenol (prostacyclin) and other prostanoids can be administered. Currently, Food and Drug Administration–approved prostanoids for PAH are administered through intravenous, subcutaneous, or inhalational routes. A summary of the pivotal trials that have led to approval of these agents for PAH is provided in Table 30–4.

Epoprostenol has a short half-life and is unstable if exposed to room temperature or light. It is degraded by gastric pH and must therefore be administered via continuous intravenous infusion. When added to conventional therapy, epoprostenol has been shown to improve exercise capacity, reduce symptom burden, improve cardiopulmonary hemodynamics, and reduce mortality in patients with PAH who have NYHA class III–IV symptoms. Major adverse effects of this agent relate to its complex delivery system and include infection, thrombosis, and pump malfunction. Due to its short half-life, brief interruption of epoprostenol infusion can result in rebound PH and cardiopulmonary collapse. Prostanoids, as a class, are known to cause headache, flushing, nausea, vomiting, diarrhea, arthralgias, myalgias, and jaw pain. Newer temperature-stable formulations of epoprostenol may simplify administration.

Treprostinil is a prostanoid that is premixed, stable at room temperature, and has a longer half-life than epoprostenol. Treprostinil can be administered subcutaneously as well as intravenously. In patients with NYHA class II–IV PAH, treprostinil improves exercise capacity, reduces symptoms, and improves cardiopulmonary hemodynamics (see Table 30–4). Inhalational iloprost has also been shown to improve clinical outcomes in patients with symptomatic PAH. Iloprost must be administered six to nine times daily to maintain efficacy. Treprostinil can also be administered by inhalation and is dosed four times daily. While iloprost and treprostinil have advantages over epoprostenol, epoprostenol is the only prostanoid shown to reduce mortality in advanced PAH.

Choosing the correct treatment regimen for the patient with PAH relies on an understanding of the underlying disease and of patient-specific factors. Disease severity, as assessed by integration of hemodynamic, clinical, and laboratory parameters, is crucial in selecting the appropriate treatment (Table 30–5; see Figure 30–11). Individual patient factors, such as comorbidities (ie, liver disease), concomitant drug therapy, or a history of medication nonadherence, may all influence treatment choice (Figure 30–14).

Invasive treatment options for PAH include atrial septostomy, lung transplantation, and combined heart-lung transplantation. Atrial septostomy has been performed as a palliative measure for patients with PAH and right heart failure or recurrent syncope. It is postulated that a right-left shunt in this setting improves left ventricular filling and CO. Atrial septostomy can, however, worsen hypoxia and increases the likelihood of paradoxical embolization. As such, it is recommended that atrial septostomy be performed only at experienced centers. Outcomes with lung and combined

Table 30–5. Prognostic Factors for Risk of Pulmonary Arterial Hypertension Disease Progression

Determinant	Higher Risk	Lower Risk
Evidence of RV failure	Yes	No
Progression	Rapid	Gradual
WHO Class	IV	II, II
6-minute walk distance	< 325 m	> 380 m
Brain natriuretic peptide	> 180 pg/mL	< 180 pg/mL
Echocardiographic findings	Pericardial effusion; significant RV dysfunction	Minimal RV dysfunction
Hemodynamics	High RAP, Low CI	Normal/near-normal RAP and CI

CI, cardiac index; RAP, right atrial pressure; RV, right ventricular; WHO, World Health Organization.

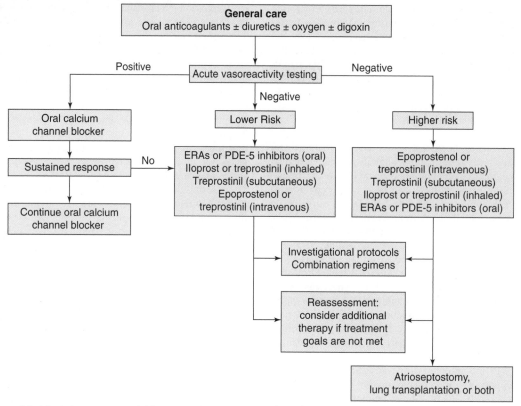

▲ **Figure 30–14.** Pulmonary arterial hypertension treatment algorithm. ERA, endothelin receptor antagonist; PDE-5, phosphodiesterase-5. (Adapted, with permission, from McLaughlin VV, et al. *Circulation*. 2006;114:1417.)

heart-lung transplantation are improving. One-year survival posttransplantation is 70%, and 5-year survival is 50%. Transplantation is reserved for PAH patients with heart failure and poor quality of life who continue to deteriorate despite maximal medical therapy.

B. Pulmonary Hypertension with Left-Sided Heart Disease

PH occurs in 25–30% of patients with left-sided heart disease and is associated with worse outcomes in this population. Treatment is dictated by the underlying disease process. Surgical or percutaneous treatment of aortic or mitral valve disease and treatment of coronary artery disease should be aggressively pursued as these interventions can improve left-sided filling pressures, reduce PA pressure, and improve symptoms. Standard therapy for systolic and diastolic heart failure is recommended. Supplemental oxygen is required for those who exhibit systemic oxygen desaturation.

Although limited data are available, oral or intravenous vasodilators (eg, nitrates or sildenafil, nitroprusside, nesiritide, milrinone) are sometimes used for the management of refractory cases of PH with left-sided heart disease. Calcium

channel blocker therapy, with the possible exception of amlodipine, is contraindicated in systolic heart failure with PH. Endothelin-receptor antagonists are also contraindicated in left-sided heart failure because they have been shown to worsen heart failure and increase mortality. Intravenous epoprostenol is also contraindicated in the treatment of advanced systolic heart failure because it has been shown to increase mortality. Mechanical circulatory-assist devices and heart-lung transplantation are other therapies available for PH due to left-sided heart disease.

C. Pulmonary Hypertension Associated with Lung Disease or Hypoxemia

PH in persons with lung disease or hypoxemia, or both, is best relieved by treating the underlying disease. In this cohort, correction of hypoxemia is especially important. Bronchodilator therapy should be optimized for patients with obstructive pulmonary disease. Continuous positive airway pressure and weight loss often aid in the treatment of PAH patients with sleep-disordered breathing. Inflammatory conditions that lead to ILD should be sought and aggressively treated with anti-inflammatory agents. Specific pulmonary vasodilator therapy is controversial for PH associated with lung disease on the basis of insufficient evidence.

Cor pulmonale, or right heart failure secondary to lung disease, often develops in patients with PH. As previously outlined for PAH, sodium restriction and diuretics are the mainstays of right heart failure therapy. Digoxin and vasodilator therapy may be considered, although outcome data are lacking. For select, severely symptomatic patients with PH and lung disease, lung transplantation can improve quality of life and survival.

D. Pulmonary Hypertension due to Chronic Thrombotic or Embolic Disease

Mortality in patients with CTEPH is high, and CTEPH should be excluded in all patients undergoing evaluation for PH. Patients with CTEPH in whom conventional pulmonary angiography demonstrates proximal surgically accessible disease may be candidates for PTE. At experienced centers, perioperative mortality following PTE is as low as 4.4%. Following PTE, most patients experience marked improvement in PAP, right heart function, NYHA class, and exercise capacity.

Residual PH occurs in approximately 10% of patients after PTE and appears to be linked to the degree of small vessel arteriopathy. Pathophysiologic similarities between PAH and CTEPH have prompted investigation into the usefulness of pulmonary vasodilator therapy for PH that persists after PTE and as bridging therapy. Encouraging data are emerging from small nonrandomized trials showing hemodynamic improvement in chronic thromboembolic PH patients with vasodilator therapy. The role for medical treatment in chronic thromboembolic PH is as yet incompletely defined and is an area of ongoing research.

Badesch DB, et al. Medical therapy for pulmonary arterial hypertension: updated ACCP evidence-based clinical practice guidelines. *Chest.* 2007;131(6):1917–28. [PMID: 17565025]

Galie N, et al; Sildenafil Use in Pulmonary Arterial Hypertension (SUPER) Study Group. Sildenafil citrate therapy for pulmonary arterial hypertension. *N Engl J Med.* 2005;353(20):2148–57. [PMID: 16291984]

Humbert M, et al. Treatment of pulmonary arterial hypertension. *N Engl J Med.* 2004;351(14):1425–36. [PMID: 15459304]

Mclaughlin VV, et al. Survival in primary pulmonary hypertension: the impact of epoprostenol therapy. *Circulation.* 2002;106(12):1477–82. [PMID: 12234951]

Rubin LJ, et al. Bosentan therapy for pulmonary arterial hypertension. *N Engl J Med.* 2002;346(12):896–903. [PMID: 11907289]

Sitbon O, et al. Long-term response to calcium channel blockers in idiopathic pulmonary arterial hypertension. *Circulation.* 2005;111(23):3105–11. [PMID: 15939821]

Thistlethwaite PA, et al. Pulmonary thromboendarterectomy surgery. *Cardiol Clin.* 2004;22(3):467–78. [PMID: 15302365]

▶ Prognosis

PH is a progressive disorder associated with a high mortality rate. The underlying cause of the PH is a key factor in determining the prognosis and natural history of the disease (see Figure 30–2). Patients with PAH associated with connective tissue disease and those with PAH and HIV have the worst prognoses. Patients with congenital heart disease, by contrast, have the best prognosis (6-month survival is 89%). Even for patients with PH due to lung disease or hypoxemia, survival rates vary widely. Patients with PH and emphysema have a 6-month survival of 81%, whereas patients with PH and interstitial lung disease have a 6-month survival of 38%.

Clinical features and hemodynamic parameters also strongly influence survival. Markers of poor prognosis in PH include advanced functional class (NYHA III–IV) (see Table 30–2), poor exercise capacity (reduced 6-minute walk distance), resting hemodynamics consistent with right ventricular failure (high right atrial pressure, low cardiac output), elevated B-type natriuretic peptide, and presence of a pericardial effusion or significant right ventricular dysfunction on echocardiogram (see Table 30–5).

Badesch DB, et al. Diagnosis and assessment of pulmonary arterial hypertension. *J Am Coll Cardiol.* 2009;54(1 Suppl):S55–66. [PMID: 19555859]

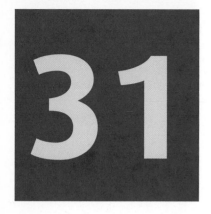

Congenital Heart Disease in Adults

Ian S. Harris, MD

Elyse Foster, MD

▶ General Considerations

Congenital cardiac anomalies are the most common birth defects in humans, affecting approximately 0.8 in 100 live births. While the incidence of congenital heart disease is expected to decline as a consequence of improved prenatal diagnosis, the number of patients surviving with congenital heart disease, both in the United States and worldwide, has increased significantly over the past three decades. Over 85% of infants born with cardiovascular anomalies now can expect to reach adulthood. Reduced mortality rates can be attributed to improved diagnostic abilities, enhanced surgical and nonsurgical therapies, and improvements in intensive care. For the first time, the number of adults with congenital heart disease exceeds the number of children with the disorders.

The increase in the number of adults with congenital heart disease requires that the physicians managing the care of these patients have improved knowledge of simple and complex anatomy and physiology. Although actual numbers are difficult to ascertain, it has been estimated that approximately 1 million adults in the United States alone currently have congenital heart disease and that the number of patients reaching adulthood with treated congenital heart disease will increase by approximately 9000 per year.

These patients fall into several broad categories: those surviving into adulthood without intervention and perhaps without clinical recognition, those surviving with curative surgical or nonsurgical intervention, and those surviving with palliative surgical or nonsurgical intervention. Nonsurgical interventions may include catheter-based valvuloplasty, stenting, coiling, or device occlusion. The patients who are today making the transition into the adult congenital heart disease population have hemodynamic and cardiac problems differing from those in previous eras. Surgical techniques have evolved, intervention occurs earlier and is often definitive rather than palliative, and a greater number of patients with complex single-ventricle physiology and various modifications of cavopulmonary anastomoses (Glenn shunt, Fontan procedure) will reach adulthood. Because of

the unique clinical conditions and needs of these patients, the American College of Cardiology and the American Heart Association have recommended that all patients with moderate or complex congenital heart disease be evaluated at least once by a physician with specialized training and expertise in adult congenital heart disease. Furthermore, it is recommended that diagnostic and interventional cardiac catheterization and electrophysiologic and surgical procedures in these patients be performed in regional adult congenital heart disease centers.

Hoffman JI, et al. Prevalence of congenital heart disease. *Am Heart J.* 2004;147(3):425–39. [PMID: 14999190]

Webb GD, et al. Thirty-Second Bethesda Conference: care of the adult with congenital heart disease. *J Am Coll Cardiol.* 2001;37(5):1166. [PMID: 11300416]

Wilson W, et al; American Heart Association Rheumatic Fever, Endocarditis, and Kawasaki Disease Committee; American Heart Association Council on Cardiovascular Disease in the Young; American Heart Association Council on Clinical Cardiology; American Heart Association Council on Cardiovascular Surgery and Anesthesia; Quality of Care and Outcomes Research Interdisciplinary Working Group. Prevention of infective endocarditis: guidelines from the American Heart Association: a guideline from the American Heart Association Rheumatic Fever, Endocarditis, and Kawasaki Disease Committee, Council on Cardiovascular Disease in the Young, and the Council on Clinical Cardiology, Council on Cardiovascular Surgery and Anesthesia, and the Quality of Care and Outcomes Research Interdisciplinary Working Group. *Circulation.* 2007;116(15):1736–54. [PMID: 17446442]

Wren C, et al. Survival with congenital heart disease and need for follow up in adult life. *Heart.* 2001;85(4):438–43. [PMID: 11250973]

▼ ACYANOTIC CONGENITAL HEART DISEASE

The most common acyanotic congenital heart defects include abnormalities of the heart valves and great vessels, ventricular or atrial communications with left-to-right shunting, and such lesions as partial anomalous pulmonary veins and anomalous coronary arteries.

CONGENITAL AORTIC VALVULAR DISEASE

 ESSENTIALS OF DIAGNOSIS

- ▶ History of murmur since infancy, coarctation repair, or endocarditis.
- ▶ Early systolic ejection click, harsh crescendo-decrescendo systolic, or early decrescendo diastolic murmur.
- ▶ Left ventricular hypertrophy.
- ▶ Abnormal bicuspid or dysplastic aortic valve with stenosis or regurgitation on Doppler echocardiography.

▶ General Considerations

Congenital aortic stenosis is the most common anomaly encountered in the adult population and constitutes approximately 7% of all forms of congenital heart disease. The male:female ratio is approximately 2–3:1. The term "bicuspid aortic valve" is actually a misnomer; a raphe caused by commissural fusion of two leaflets usually exists. The valve is often dysplastic, with thickened, rolled, and calcified leaflets. The predominant pathophysiology results from mildly obstructed nonlaminar (disturbed) flow across the abnormal valve. A left ventricle-to-aorta pressure gradient of variable severity occurs, setting the stage for the inevitable deterioration of the valve with long-term calcium deposition and progressive stenosis or regurgitation. The valve is also at risk for endocarditis, which can lead to early destruction and regurgitation. Congenital aortic valve disease frequently occurs as a developmental "triad" with coincident aortopathy and coarctation, and these conditions should be sought clinically and echocardiographically in patients with congenital aortic valve disease. Familial congenital aortic valve disease occurs occasionally. While the genetics of this are incompletely understood, mutations in the gene encoding Notch 1 have been implicated in a subset of these patients.

▶ Clinical Findings

A. Symptoms & Signs

The individual with congenital aortic stenosis is usually asymptomatic unless hemodynamically significant stenosis or regurgitation is present. Routine physical examination reveals a normal carotid pulse contour and left ventricular (LV) impulse, a normal S_2, an early systolic click or sound, and an early-peaking systolic murmur. Identifying these patients in the asymptomatic stage is important. Current guidelines do not recommend endocarditis prophylaxis for the native valve. Refraining from high-level isometric exercise is generally believed to preserve valve function and limit valve regurgitation. The presence of a diastolic murmur of aortic regurgitation in a patient with a febrile illness should alert the clinician to the possibility of endocarditis and prompt the performance of appropriate diagnostic tests (eg, blood cultures, echocardiogram).

Congenital aortic stenosis is progressive; once hemodynamically significant valvular disease develops in a patient, generally in the fifth or sixth decade of life, the symptoms and signs are identical to those of a patient with acquired aortic valvular disease. Dyspnea, chest pain, and exertional syncope are the classic presenting symptoms. When stenosis predominates, the carotid upstroke is delayed and diminished in volume, the systolic click is no longer present, S_2 is single, and the systolic murmur is crescendo-decrescendo, peaking in late systole. The murmur of aortic regurgitation is often present. The finding of upper extremity hypertension should alert the examiner to the possibility of concomitant aortic coarctation.

B. Diagnostic Studies

1. Electrocardiography and chest radiography—The major electrocardiographic (ECG) findings occur in the presence of hemodynamically significant disease and include left ventricular hypertrophy (LVH) with high QRS voltage, left-axis deviation, and repolarization changes; left atrial enlargement may also be present. The chest radiographic findings are nonspecific. With predominant valvular aortic stenosis, the cardiothoracic ratio may be normal, but LV enlargement and calcification may be evident in the region of the aortic valve on the lateral film. A dilated ascending aorta or a prominent aortic knob may be seen. The cardiac silhouette is enlarged in patients with predominant aortic regurgitation. Pulmonary vasculature may be prominent in the presence of congestive heart failure (CHF).

2. Echocardiography—In the child and younger adult, the abnormally thickened leaflets of the congenitally abnormal valve are readily seen, and the bicuspid valve with its ovoid appearance in systole is apparent (Figure 31–1). On M-mode echocardiography, the point of closure may be eccentric. Heavy calcification often obscures the original valve morphology in the older individual with stenosis. The peak systolic gradient in severe aortic stenosis is usually greater than 64 mm Hg (peak velocity > 4 m/s by continuous wave Doppler). Aortic valve area can be accurately calculated by the continuity equation. Severe aortic stenosis is defined as a valve area of less than 1.0 cm^2 or 0.5 cm^2/m^2. The LV shows concentric hypertrophy with thick walls and normal cavity dimensions, and the LV ejection fraction is usually normal. In cases with reduced ejection fraction, however, the peak gradient across the aortic valve is generally lower.

In hemodynamically significant aortic regurgitation, the high-velocity diastolic color-flow jet is broad at its site of origin below the aortic valve. Spectral Doppler imaging

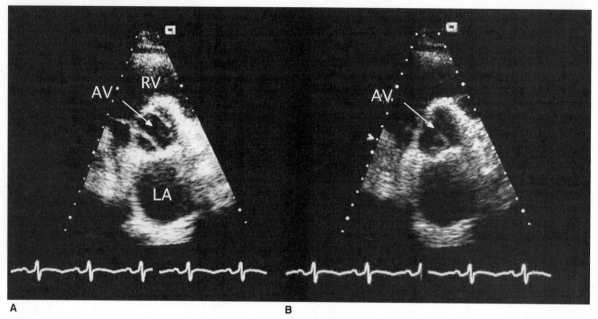

▲ **Figure 31–1.** Transesophageal echocardiographic views of a patient with bicuspid aortic valve. **A:** Systolic frame showing two leaflets of the aortic valve (AV) with an ovoid opening (*arrow*). **B:** Diastolic frame showing the single line of coaptation (*arrow*). LA, left atrium; RV, right ventricle.

demonstrates a dense diastolic velocity signal with a short pressure half-time (< 400 ms), and diastolic flow reversal can be recorded in the descending aorta. The LV shows eccentric hypertrophy with normal LV wall thickness and a dilated cavity.

In occasional patients with poor precordial windows, transesophageal echocardiography (TEE) may be required to define valve anatomy by demonstrating commissural fusion and asymmetric sinuses of Valsalva. Systolic doming of the leaflets can be easily seen in the long axis view of the LV outflow tract, which also allows measurements to be taken of the aortic valve annulus, sinuses of Valsalva, sinotubular ridge, and ascending aorta.

Cardiac magnetic resonance angiography (MRA) is a possible alternative imaging technique.

3. Cardiac catheterization—Indications for cardiac catheterization in congenital aortic valve disease have changed significantly because most of the diagnostic data are now available noninvasively. According to current guidelines, however, cardiac catheterization is indicated when noninvasive tests are inconclusive or when there is a discrepancy between noninvasive tests and clinical findings regarding severity of aortic stenosis. It is also indicated preoperatively in patients at risk for atherosclerotic coronary artery disease (men age 35 years or older, premenopausal women age 35 years or older who have coronary risk factors, and postmenopausal women) and in patients for whom a pulmonary autograft (Ross procedure)

is contemplated and if the origin of the coronary arteries was not identified by noninvasive techniques

4. Magnetic resonance imaging—Serial imaging with magnetic resonance imaging (MRI) permits accurate and reproducible follow-up of aortic dilatation and is accepted as the standard of care for follow-up of repaired coarctation, a frequent association with a bicuspid aortic valve.

▶ **Differential Diagnosis**

Valvular aortic stenosis should be distinguished from subaortic stenosis, which may be due to an obstructing fibrous membrane in discrete subaortic stenosis, which is more frequently encountered in adults, or by a tubular fibromuscular channel that usually presents in childhood. Aortic regurgitation, commonly associated with discrete membranous subaortic stenosis (in approximately 60% of cases), increases in frequency with age. Regurgitation may occur due to leaflet thickening induced by direct trauma to the aortic leaflets from the high-velocity jet or by interference with leaflet closure from the membrane. The aortic valve appearance and the severity and mechanism of aortic regurgitation must be carefully assessed.

Recurrent stenosis caused by regrowth following surgical resection of the fibromuscular ridge is sometimes encountered in the adolescent or adult. Discrete subaortic stenosis and congenital valvular aortic stenosis must also be

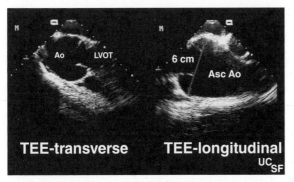

▲ **Figure 31-2.** Transesophageal echocardiographic (TEE) views of the ascending aorta (Asc Ao) measuring 8 cm in a patient with Marfan syndrome. LVOT, left ventricular outflow tract.

distinguished from dynamic LV outflow-tract obstruction caused by hypertrophic cardiomyopathy (see Chapter 23). Supravalvular aortic stenosis is frequently seen in patients with Williams syndrome.

When aortic regurgitation is the predominant lesion and ascending aorta dilatation is present, the condition must be distinguished from Marfan syndrome and other genetic aortopathies. This latter condition is characterized by dilatation of the aortic root at the level of the sinuses of Valsalva (Figure 31-2). The aortic valve leaflets are not thickened, and regurgitation is caused by failure of leaflet coaptation caused by the root dilatation. With valvular stenosis, the aorta narrows toward normal at the sinotubular junction, and the descending thoracic aorta is spared. In some patients with a bicuspid aortic valve, an underlying abnormality of the medial layer of the aorta above the valve predisposes to the dilatation of the aortic root, which may progress to aneurysm formation or rupture and places the patient at risk for aortic dissection. All components of the vessel wall, smooth muscle, elastic fibers, collagen, and ground substance can be affected and should be recognized as a potential risk in the surgical patient.

▶ Prognosis & Treatment

The natural history of aortic stenosis presenting in childhood depends largely on the severity of the stenosis at the time of diagnosis. During a 25-year follow-up period, approximately one-third of the children with a peak systolic gradient of less than 50 mm Hg who were treated medically, required surgery, in contrast to 80% of those with an intermediate gradient (50–79 mm Hg). Of those treated surgically for a gradient of more than 79 mm Hg, approximately one-fourth required reoperation; reoperation was more common in those treated with initial valvotomy (30%) than aortic valve replacement (5%). The overall 25-year survival rate is approximately 85%; sudden death accounts for approximately half of the cardiac-related deaths.

Once symptoms of aortic stenosis develop, the prognosis without valve replacement is poor; the 5-year mortality rate is approximately 90%. Although percutaneous valvuloplasty has been successful in children and adolescents, the results in adults (even those with congenitally abnormal valves) have been disappointing. Therefore, surgery with aortic valve replacement, rather than percutaneous valvuloplasty, is generally mandated. Surgery is indicated in the symptomatic patient with a valve area of less than 1.0 cm^2 (or < 0.5 cm^2/m^2). It should be considered in the asymptomatic patient with critical stenosis when the patient requires cardiac surgery (eg, coronary artery bypass surgery) for another lesion. A particularly difficult management decision ensues in the asymptomatic woman with severe aortic stenosis who is contemplating pregnancy. Valve replacement prior to pregnancy should be considered when there is evidence of LV dysfunction or reduced exercise tolerance on objective stress testing.

Patients with a bicuspid aortic valve and concomitant annuloaortic ectasia may show a more rapid progression of aortic regurgitation and require surgical intervention earlier than those patients with pure aortic stenosis.

An ideal substitute for replacing the aortic valve does not exist. Homografts and bioprosthetic valves can develop rapid calcific degeneration, causing valve dysfunction, particularly in the younger cohort of patients. Mechanical valves, although extremely durable, require anticoagulation to reduce the complication of thromboembolism. The risks associated with long-term anticoagulation have made surgical options to avoid the use of mechanical valves desirable alternatives. This is particularly germane to the choice of prosthetic valve in young women of childbearing age, in whom management of anticoagulation can be problematic. The Ross procedure (in which the autologous pulmonary valve replaces the aortic valve, and an aortic or pulmonary homograft replaces the pulmonary valve) has been increasingly performed for a variety of LV outflow tract diseases, including aortic insufficiency and valvar aortic stenosis with or without other forms of obstruction (eg, subaortic stenosis, supravalvar stenosis, and arch hypoplasia). Although the Ross procedure is more complex than simple aortic valve replacement, it can be performed with a low mortality rate in selected patients. Advantages of the pulmonary valve autograft include freedom from anticoagulation and the absence of compromise from host reactions and autograft growth, making it an attractive option for aortic valve replacement in infants and children. It is recognized, however, that the pulmonary homograft will require replacement for degenerative disease and size restriction in children. In adults who are confronting surgery for a stenotic aortic valve in the fifth or sixth decade of life, the Ross procedure has shown to be an acceptable alternative to the usual mechanical or bioprosthetic valve. However, recently recognized problems associated with the Ross procedure include progressive dilatation of the neo-aortic root, pulmonary conduit stenosis, and neo-aortic valve regurgitation. Contraindications to the Ross procedure include advanced three-vessel coronary artery disease, poor LV function, a severely calcified or dilated aortic root, or pulmonary valve pathology.

American College of Cardiology/American Heart Association Task Force on Practice Guidelines; Society of Cardiovascular Anesthesiologists; Society for Cardiovascular Angiography and Interventions; Society of Thoracic Surgeons; Bonow RO, et al. ACC/AHA 2006 guidelines for the management of patients with valvular heart disease: a report of the American College of Cardiology/American Heart Association Task Force on Practice Guidelines (writing committee to revise the 1998 guidelines for the management of patients with valvular heart disease): developed in collaboration with the Society of Cardiovascular Anesthesiologists; endorsed by the Society for Cardiovascular Angiography and Interventions and the Society of Thoracic Surgeons. *Circulation*. 2006;114(5):e84–231. [PMID: 16880336]

Knott-Craig CJ, et al. Aortic valve replacement: comparison of late survival between autografts and homografts. *Ann Thorac Surg*. 2000;69(5):1327–32. [PMID: 10881799]

Lambert V, et al. Long-term results after valvotomy for congenital aortic valvar stenosis in children. *Cardiol Young*. 2000;10(6):590–6. [PMID: 11117391]

Masani N. Transesophageal echocardiography in adult congenital heart disease. *Heart*. 2001;86(Suppl 2):II30–II40. [PMID: 11709532]

Niwa K, et al. Structural abnormalities of great arterial walls in congenital heart disease: light and electron microscopic analyses. *Circulation*. 2001;103(3):393–400. [PMID: 11157691]

Raja SG, et al. Current outcomes of Ross operation for pediatric and adolescent patients. *J Heart Valve Dis*. 2007;16(1):27–36. [PMID: 17315380]

Siu SC, et al. Bisucpid aortic valve disease. *J Am Coll Cardiol*. 2010;55(25):2789–800. [PMID: 20579534]

PULMONARY VALVE STENOSIS

ESSENTIALS OF DIAGNOSIS

▶ History of systolic murmur since infancy.

▶ Systolic ejection click and an early systolic murmur in the second left intercostal space with transmission to the back. S_2 may split widely.

▶ ECG evidence of right ventricular hypertrophy.

▶ Dilatation of main and left pulmonary arteries on chest radiograph.

▶ Right ventricular hypertrophy, systolic doming of the pulmonary valve, and a transpulmonic gradient by Doppler echocardiography.

▶ General Considerations

Pulmonary valve, or pulmonic stenosis (PS), is the second most common form of congenital heart disease in the adult. Although many cases are so mild that they require

no treatment, it often coexists with other congenital cardiac abnormalities (atrial septal defect [ASD], ventricular septal defect [VSD], patent ductus arteriosus, or tetralogy of Fallot [TOF]). Pulmonary valve stenosis is characterized by a conical or dome-shaped pliant valve with a narrow outlet at its apex. Right ventricular (RV) outflow is obstructed depending on the size of the orifice, and RV stroke volume may not rise appropriately during exercise. In response to the pressure overload, the RV hypertrophies, with an increase in wall thickness. This compensatory hypertrophy can involve the infundibulum and potentially lead to reversible dynamic subpulmonic stenosis once the valvular stenosis is relieved. If severe stenosis remains untreated, RV failure may ensue. It is important to differentiate pulmonary valve stenosis from stenoses of the peripheral pulmonary arteries and primary infundibular stenosis, often associated with VSD (see Tetralogy of Fallot). Pulmonary stenosis from a thickened, dysplastic valve is seen in patients with Noonan syndrome (a heterogeneous malformation syndrome with autosomal dominant inheritance).

▶ Clinical Findings

A. Symptoms & Signs

The patient with PS usually has exercise intolerance in the form of exertional fatigue, dyspnea, chest pain, or syncope. RV failure with systemic venous congestion occurs late in the course of the disease. If the foramen ovale is patent or a concomitant ASD exists, shunting of blood from the right atrium to the left may occur, causing cyanosis and clubbing. The volume overload of pregnancy may precipitate right heart failure in patients with severe PS, although mild and even moderate stenosis are usually well tolerated.

In significant PS, the physical examination demonstrates a parasternal RV heave, a delayed and diminished or absent P_2, and a late-peaking crescendo-decrescendo murmur that increases in volume with inspiration. If the valve is pliable, an ejection click precedes the murmur. This pulmonic ejection sound, best heard in the second left intercostal space, is the only right-sided event that decreases in intensity during inspiration and increases during expiration. As the stenosis becomes more severe, the systolic murmur will peak later in systole and the ejection click moves closer to the first heart sound, eventually becoming superimposed on it. The jugular venous pulse shows a prominent *a* wave, as a result of the diminished RV compliance, but jugular venous pressure is increased only in the late stages when RV failure occurs. Similarly, there may be an RV S_4 gallop early in the course of the disease and a right-sided S_3 in the later stages.

B. Diagnostic Studies

1. Electrocardiography and chest radiography—The ECG demonstrates evidence of right ventricular hypertrophy (RVH) with right-axis deviation, prominent R waves in the

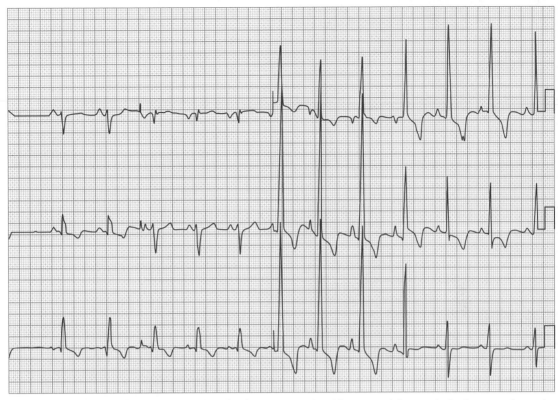

▲ **Figure 31–3.** Electrocardiograph in congenital pulmonic stenosis with severe right ventricular hypertrophy and marked right-axis deviation.

right precordial leads, and deep S waves in the left precordial leads (Figure 31–3). There may also be evidence of right atrial enlargement with peaked inferior (II, III, aVF) P waves.

The cardiac silhouette on the chest radiograph is normal in mild-to-moderate PS but may become enlarged in severe stenosis when right heart failure occurs. The main and left pulmonary arteries are often dilated. In addition to this "poststenotic dilatation," dilatation may be seen even in cases of mild PS and may be related to intrinsic abnormalities of the pulmonary artery (idiopathic pulmonary artery dilatation).

2. Echocardiography—The poor near-field resolution of transthoracic echocardiography (TTE) often limits definition of pulmonary valve morphology in the adult patient. When examined from the parasternal short-axis view, the valve may appear thickened (rarely calcified) and usually manifests systolic doming. In the absence of right heart failure, the RV dimension is normal or only mildly increased, but the RV wall thickness is increased (> 5 mm). In severe cases, the septum may be deviated toward the LV from the pressure overload of the RV. The right atrium and ventricle dilate late in the course of the disease. Saline contrast echocardiography should be performed in all patients with

pulmonary valve stenosis to exclude an ASD or a patent foramen ovale.

Color-flow Doppler imaging demonstrates high-velocity flow within the pulmonary artery and is helpful in excluding a VSD or a patent ductus arteriosus. Continuous wave Doppler demonstrates a high-velocity jet across the RV outflow tract (Figure 31–4B). This signal is best obtained from the parasternal short-axis or subcostal short-axis views where flow is axial to the Doppler beam. PS is classified as mild when the RV systolic pressure is < 50 mm Hg, moderate when the gradient is 50–79 mm Hg, and severe when the gradient is > 80 mm Hg. Unfortunately, because of the lack of range resolution, continuous wave Doppler cannot localize the level of the obstruction. The morphology of the valve by echocardiography and pulsed wave Doppler mapping may provide localizing information, but additional diagnostic procedures are often necessary.

TEE provides excellent definition of the RV outflow tract and pulmonary valve in the basal longitudinal views and excellent images of the atrial septum. As a result, noninvasive methods may now be adequate for establishing the diagnosis, even in adults.

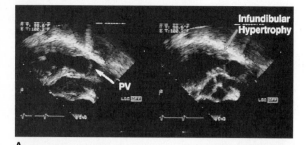

A

B

▲ **Figure 31–4. A:** Transesophageal echocardiographic views of a pregnant woman with severe pulmonary valve (PV) stenosis. The left image demonstrates the doming pulmonary valve in systole. The right frame illustrates the severe infundibular hypertrophy. **B:** Continuous wave Doppler recording from the same patient demonstrated a peak velocity of 6 m/s corresponding to a peak transvalvular gradient of 144 mm Hg.

3. Cardiac catheterization—In most patients, cardiac catheterization is therapeutic as well as diagnostic because percutaneous balloon valvuloplasty has virtually replaced surgery for treatment of pulmonary valve stenosis (see below). During right-heart catheterization, the level of the stenosis can be confirmed by pressure monitoring during pullback from the pulmonary artery and supplemented by RV angiography. In valvular stenosis, there is a rise in peak systolic pressure as the catheter tip passes from the pulmonary artery into the infundibulum. In contrast, when the stenosis is in the infundibulum, the systolic pressure increases when the catheter is pulled into the body of the RV. As mentioned earlier, in PS, secondary hypertrophy may result in some degree of infundibular stenosis, and a pressure differential may be demonstrated at both levels on pullback (Figure 31–5). If the level of obstruction is still uncertain, cine-angiography may show the hypertrophied infundibulum or, alternatively, the domed and thickened pulmonary valve. Of course, both levels of obstruction may coexist.

Unlike aortic valve stenosis, the valve area is not calculated from the Doppler or invasive hemodynamic data, and the gradient alone is used to determine the severity of the obstruction and guide therapy.

▶ Prognosis & Treatment

In severe untreated pulmonary valve stenosis, the average life expectancy is approximately 30 years. The natural history of medically treated mild (gradient < 50 mm Hg) or moderate (gradient 50–79 mm Hg) PS and surgically treated severe (gradient > 80 mm Hg) PS is excellent with a 25-year survival rate of 95%. Surgical valvotomy via a pulmonary artery incision has been extremely effective in long-term relief of pulmonary valve obstruction. Although approximately 50% of patients have mild-to-moderate regurgitation following surgery, it is seldom of hemodynamic significance, and reoperation is rarely necessary.

In children treated conservatively for PS, the likelihood of eventually requiring surgery is dependent on the initial gradient: less than 25 mm Hg, 5%; 25–49 mm Hg, 20%; and 50–79 mm Hg, 76%. In the adult, the indication for treatment of pulmonary valve stenosis is a peak systolic gradient in excess of 50 mm Hg. When the gradient is between 40 and 50 mm Hg, the decision to treat is based on the presence of symptoms, the age of the patient, and the degree of RVH (by echocardiography or ECG). Echocardiography, before and after exercise, may be an important technique to assess RV function in the presence of an increased gradient.

As mentioned earlier, most patients (including adults) with pulmonary valve stenosis are currently treated with percutaneous balloon valvuloplasty. The Registry of the Valvuloplasty and Angioplasty of Congenital Anomalies has listed 35 patients over the age of 20, among them a 76-year-old man. No significant complications occurred in adult patients, and the gradient was reduced from approximately 70 mm Hg to 30 mm Hg, with about 50% of the residual gradient caused by infundibular hypertrophy. Ongoing assessment of these patients indicate sustained long-term relief of the pulmonary valve gradient with progressive infundibular remodeling causing further reduction in the outflow tract gradient over time. Recent technical improvements leading to the development of low-profile balloon have decreased the risk of pulmonary regurgitation after dilatation. Based on these results, percutaneous balloon valvuloplasty appears to be the treatment of choice in adults with pulmonary valve stenosis. Severe pulmonary valve insufficiency after either balloon or surgical valvotomy is uncommon, but patients should be evaluated every 5–10 years for this complication. Even when PS is associated with severe infundibular stenosis and tricuspid regurgitation, the long-term results from balloon valvuloplasty are excellent.

Bashore TM. Adult congenital heart disease: right ventricular outflow tract lesions. *Circulation.* 2007;115(14):1933–47. [PMID: 17420363]

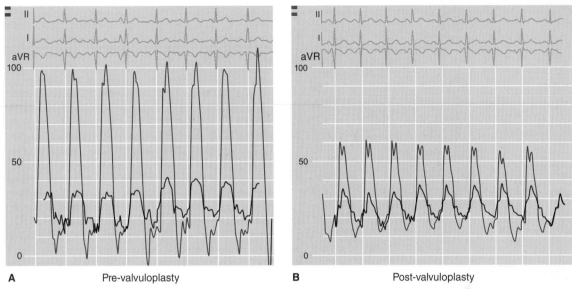

A Pre-valvuloplasty   **B** Post-valvuloplasty

▲ **Figure 31–5.** Hemodynamic tracings in pulmonic stenosis. **A:** Predilation: Peak gradient of 65 mm Hg between right ventricle (RV) and pulmonary artery (PA). **B:** Postdilation: Residual gradient of 20 mm Hg between RV infundibulum and pulmonary artery.

Baumgartner H, et al. Guidelines on the management of valvular heart disease (version 2012): the Joint Task Force on the Management of Valvular Heart Disease of the European Society of Cardiology (ESC) and the European Association for Cardio-Thoracic Surgery (EACTS). *Eur J Cardiothorac Surg.* 2012;42(4):S1–S44. [PMID: 22922698]

Fawzy ME, et al. Long-term results (up to 17 years) of pulmonary balloon valvuloplasty in adults and its effects on concomitant severe infundibular stenosis and tricuspid regurgitation. *Am Heart J.* 2007;153(3):433–8. [PMID: 17307424]

ATRIAL SEPTAL DEFECT

ESSENTIALS OF DIAGNOSIS

▶ A widely split S_2 without respiratory variation ("fixed split") and a midsystolic murmur are characteristic.

▶ RV conduction delay ("incomplete right bundle branch block") with vertical QRS axis (ostium secundum ASD) and superior axis (ostium primum ASD) on ECG.

▶ Prominent pulmonary arteries and RV enlargement (decreased retrosternal air space) on chest radiograph. Increased pulmonary vascular markings.

▶ RV dilatation, increased pulmonary artery flow velocity, and left-to-right atrial shunt by contrast and Doppler echocardiography.

▶ Oxygen step-up within the right atrium; right-sided catheter can pass into the left atrium across the defect.

▶ General Considerations

ASDs make up 10% of congenital heart disease cases in newborns and are regularly encountered as new diagnoses in adults. The defects vary in size from the smallest fenestrated ASD (a few millimeters) to the largest defect—the complete absence of the atrial septum, or common atrium. The most common interatrial communication is a patent foramen ovale that is anatomically and physiologically not classified as an ASD.

Classification of ASDs is according to location (Figure 31–6): ostium secundum in the region of the fossa ovalis, ostium primum in the lower portion of the atrial septum (actually part of an atrioventricular [AV] canal defect, discussed later), sinus venosus in the upper part of the septum near the entrance of the superior vena cava or at the entrance of the inferior vena cava, and unroofed coronary sinus (communication between the coronary sinus and left atrium). Important associated abnormalities include anomalous drainage of the right upper pulmonary vein into the superior vena cava associated with a superior sinus venosus ASD, a persistent left superior vena cava draining to the coronary sinus with secundum or primum ASDs, and a cleft anterior mitral leaflet and mitral regurgitation associated with an ostium primum ASD. Ostium primum ASD is a common cardiac anomaly in trisomy 21 (Down syndrome) and is part of the spectrum of AV septal "canal" defects (discussed later). There is an approximately 2:1 female predominance for ostium secundum ASDs, while the sex ratio for ostium primum and sinus venosus ASDs is approximately 1:1. An autosomal dominant inheritance pattern has been demonstrated in some patients with ostium secundum

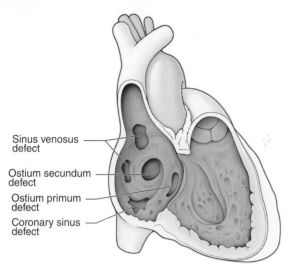

▲ **Figure 31–6.** Anatomic location of atrial septal defects.

Sinus venosus defect

Ostium secundum defect

Ostium primum defect

Coronary sinus defect

ASD with associated first-degree AV block, and cases of ASD in monozygotic twins have been reported. Recent studies have implicated mutations in the genes *gata4*, and *nkx2-5* in nonsyndromic ASDs, whereas point mutations in the gene *tbx5* are known to cause the Holt-Oram syndrome (ASD and limb defects).

The pathophysiologic consequences of an ASD depend on the quantity of blood shunted from the systemic to pulmonary circulation. The size of the shunt is in turn dependent on the size of the defect and the relative compliance of the RV and LV. Little or no shunting occurs immediately after birth because of the high pulmonary vascular resistance (PVR), but as resistance falls, the more compliant RV receives the shunted blood mainly in diastole, when all four chambers are in communication. In the compensated patient with ASD, pulmonary resistance is usually low. The older adult with the LV diastolic abnormalities of hypertension, coronary artery disease, and aging may experience increased left-to-right shunting and, consequently, right heart failure. While pulmonary resistance may increase, the development of Eisenmenger physiology is unusual after the age of 25. Atrial arrhythmias, especially atrial fibrillation, are common over the age of 50.

▶ **Clinical Findings**

A. Symptoms & Signs

The young adult with an uncorrected ASD and normal pulmonary artery pressures is usually asymptomatic, with normal or minimally diminished exercise tolerance. After the age of 30, however, exertional dyspnea and atypical chest pain increase in frequency. As mentioned earlier, the frequency of atrial arrhythmias increases with age and occurs in

a high percentage of patients over the age of 50 who have not been treated surgically. Signs and symptoms of RV failure may occur because of pulmonary hypertension or as a result of long-standing volume overload.

Important findings of the physical examination in an uncomplicated ASD include a prominent RV impulse along the lower left sternal border; a palpable pulmonary artery; a systolic ejection murmur, caused by increased flow across the pulmonic valve, which does not vary in intensity with respiration; and the almost pathognomonic fixed split second heart sound. When the Q_p:Q_s exceeds 1.5-2:1, there may be an associated right-sided diastolic flow rumble and S_3 gallop from increased flow across the tricuspid valve. The patient with ostium primum ASD usually has a holosystolic murmur of mitral regurgitation. If pulmonary hypertension is present, P_2 is increased and a high-pitched murmur of pulmonary regurgitation (Graham Steell murmur) may be audible. Signs of RV failure with elevated jugular venous pressure and venous congestion may be apparent in the later stages of this disease.

B. Diagnostic Studies

1. Electrocardiography and chest radiography—The ECG shows an RV conduction delay ("incomplete right bundle branch block" [IRBBB]) in 90% of cases (Figure 31–7). In ostium secundum and sinus venosus ASDs, the QRS axis is vertical or rightward. In the patient with ostium primum ASD, the axis is superior and leftward. Abnormal sinus node function in patients with sinus venosus ASD often results in an ectopic atrial rhythm with a superior P-wave axis.

The chest radiograph shows prominent main and branch pulmonary arteries with a small aortic knob and RV enlargement. The right atrium may appear enlarged. In the absence of pulmonary hypertension, the lung markings are increased as a result of increased pulmonary blood flow.

2. Echocardiography—The findings on TTE include right-heart enlargement and increased pulmonary artery flow. Color-flow Doppler often can identify the interatrial flow, especially in the subcostal four-chamber view. An intravenous saline contrast injection should be used in all patients with these findings to exclude an unsuspected ASD. In the presence of an ASD, a negative contrast effect can be seen in the right atrium as the unopacified left atrial blood is shunted from left to right. A small degree of bidirectional shunting nearly always is present, and microbubbles can be seen in the left atrium as a result of right-to-left shunting. The shunting across a patent foramen ovale is purely right to left and occurs only during transient (eg, Valsalva maneuver, coughing) or persistent elevations in right atrial pressure.

Pulmonary artery pressure can be estimated from the peak velocity of the tricuspid regurgitant jet. Echocardiographic measurements may be used to determine shunt flow, eliminating the need for an invasive assessment. In adults, however, the TTE is somewhat limited in quantifying the magnitude of shunts and the size of the defect and in

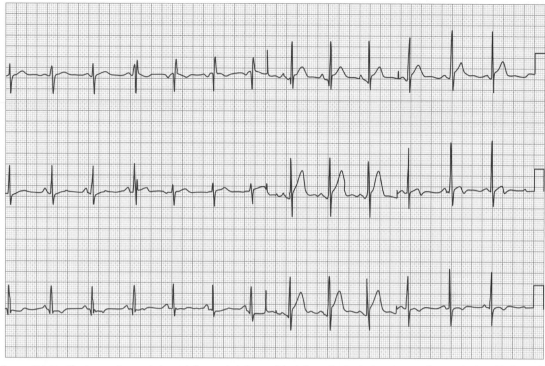

▲ **Figure 31–7.** Electrocardiograph in atrial septal defect with right-axis deviation, incomplete right bundle branch block, and right ventricular hypertrophy.

locating sinus venosus defects or anomalous pulmonary veins. As noted earlier, TEE has been found to be more accurate in determining the size and location of atrial communications (Figure 31–8). Biplanar and multiplanar transesophageal views are particularly useful in identifying sinus venosus type ASD (Figure 31–9).

3. Cardiac catheterization—In some younger individuals with unequivocally large defects on noninvasive imaging, diagnostic cardiac catheterization may be avoidable. In others, however, invasive studies may be necessary to accurately quantitate the shunt, measure PVR, and exclude coronary artery disease. Right-heart catheterization with repeated blood sampling for oxygen saturation demonstrates an oxygen step-up (ie, an increase in saturation) from the vena cava to the right atrium. In general, the higher the pulmonary arterial oxygen saturation, the greater is the shunt, with a value greater than 90% suggesting a large shunt. The ratio of pulmonary to systemic flow can be calculated by the following formula:

$$\frac{Q_P}{Q_S} = \frac{(S_{AO_2} - M_{VO_2})}{(P_{VO_2} - P_{AO_2})}$$

Where S_{AO_2}, M_{VO_2}, P_{VO_2}, and P_{AO_2} are systemic arterial, mixed venous, pulmonary venous, and pulmonary arterial blood oxygen saturations, respectively. M_{VO_2} is calculated using the Flamm equation, $[(3 \times SVC) + IVC]/4$, where SVC is the oxygen saturation of blood from the superior vena cava and IVC is the oxygen saturation of blood from the inferior vena cava.

A PVR that is more than 70% of the systemic vascular resistance suggests significant pulmonary vascular disease, and closure is best avoided. Pulmonary vasodilator therapy may be used, and occasionally, pulmonary resistance decreases enough to consider closure.

▶ **Prognosis & Treatment**

Although patients with an uncorrected ostium secundum ASD generally survive into adulthood, their life expectancy is not normal; older natural history studies showed a 50% survival beyond age 40. The mortality rate after the age of 40 is about 6% per year. Small ASDs (a Q_p:Q_s < 1.5–2:1) may cause problems only in the advanced years, when hypertension and coronary artery disease cause reduced LV compliance, resulting in increased left-to-right shunting, atrial arrhythmias, and potential biventricular failure. Severe pulmonary hypertension develops during young adulthood in only 5–10% of patients with large shunts (Q_p:Q_s > 2:1). Although most adults with ASDs have mild-to-moderate pulmonary hypertension, the late

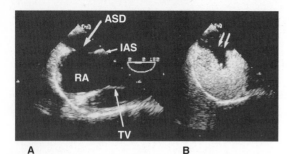

▲ Figure 31–8. Transesophageal echocardiogram in a patient with an ostium secundum atrial septal defect (ASD). **A:** The image clearly demonstrates the position of the ASD in the midportion of the interatrial septum (IAS). **B:** The image is obtained after intravenous injection of agitated saline, which opacifies the right atrium (RA). The negative contrast effect produced by the unopacified left atrial blood entering the RA is clearly demonstrated (*double arrow*). TV, tricuspid valve.

development of severe pulmonary hypertension in older adults appears to be quite rare. Pregnancy, in the absence of pulmonary hypertension, is usually uncomplicated. Another potential complication of ASD (including even the smallest patent foramen ovale) in the adult patient is paradoxical embolization. Endocarditis is rare in patients with ASD, and

prophylaxis is not routinely recommended unless associated lesions with higher risk exist.

The natural history of sinus venosus ASDs is similar to that of ostium secundum defects, although many of these patients have associated partial anomalous pulmonary venous connection. Adults with an ostium primum ASD are less commonly encountered and may have additional complications resulting from mitral regurgitation caused by the cleft leaflet (see the discussion on AV canal defects, later in this chapter).

Ostium secundum ASDs have been surgically repaired for more than 40 years. No late cardiac deaths occurred in those who had early surgical repair of ASDs (before the age of 18) among patients in a large registry. Patients with elevated pulmonary systolic pressure (> 40 mm Hg) at the time of surgery have the poorest survival rate, especially if they are older than 40 at the time of operation.

Despite the poorer surgical results in adults older than 40 years, closure is superior to medical therapy and is recommended in patients with predominant left-to-right shunts (Q_p:Q_s > 1.5–2:1) and PVR less than 10 units/m². Although mortality rates increase when the resistance exceeds this level, surgery can be performed safely in many patients with PVR between 10 and 15 units/m²; pulmonary vasodilator therapy should be considered in these patients before closure. Surgery will improve functional class and eliminate the risk of paradoxical embolization, but closure does not reduce the incidence of atrial arrhythmias.

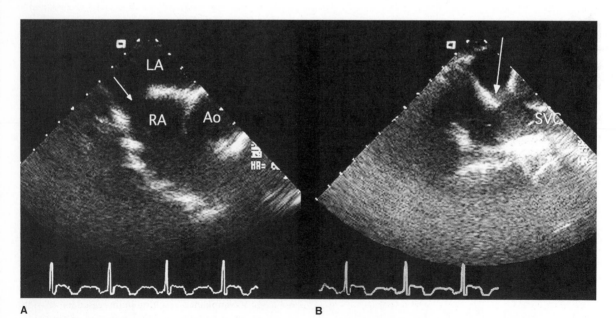

▲ Figure 31–9. Transesophageal echocardiography in a 50-year-old man with a sinus venosus atrial septal defect. **A:** Horizontal view showing the defect (*arrow*) in the superior portion of the interatrial septum. **B:** The defect (*arrow*) is clearly demonstrated in this longitudinal plane view. Ao, aorta; LA, left atrium; RA, right atrium; SVC, superior vena cava.

Percutaneous device closure is widely available, and retrospective studies have suggested comparable results with device closure and surgical closure. Therefore, device closure has become the standard of care for appropriately selected adolescents and adults with ostium secundum defects.

Adult patients with initially small shunts (Q_p:Q_s < 1.5) should undergo continued echocardiographic surveillance because the shunt may increase over time owing to a progressive decline in LV compliance.

In patients with patent foramen ovale who have suffered embolic phenomena, device closure has become a standard intervention, although evidence from a randomized controlled trial is lacking.

Attie F, et al. Surgical treatment for secundum atrial septal defects in patients > 40 years old. A randomized clinical trial. *J Am Coll Cardiol.* 2001;38(7):2035–42. [PMID: 11738312]

Garg V, et al. GATA4 mutations cause human congenital heart defects and reveal an interaction with TBX5. *Nature.* 2003;424(6947):443–7. [PMID: 12845333]

Patel A, et al. Transcatheter closure of atrial septal defects in adults > or = 40 years of age: immediate and follow-up results. *J Interv Cardiol.* 2007;20(1):82–8. [PMID: 17300410]

Webb G, et al. Atrial septal defects in the adult: recent progress and overview. *Circulation.* 2006;114(15):1645–53. [PMID: 17030704]

VENTRICULAR SEPTAL DEFECTS

 ESSENTIALS OF DIAGNOSIS

▶ History of murmur appearing shortly after birth.

▶ Holosystolic murmur at left sternal border radiating rightward.

▶ Left atrial and LV or biventricular enlargement.

▶ High-velocity color-flow Doppler jet across VSD.

▶ Increased pulmonary flow velocities.

▶ General Considerations

Because of the tendency for many VSDs to close spontaneously (see later discussion) and the tendency of larger defects to produce CHF in early childhood, it is relatively uncommon to encounter adults with previously undiagnosed VSDs of hemodynamic consequence. In adults, VSDs are usually either small and hemodynamically insignificant or large and associated with Eisenmenger syndrome. The importance of identifying the former is that they pose an ongoing risk of endocarditis and the potential complication of progressive aortic regurgitation. Eisenmenger syndrome is discussed later in this chapter.

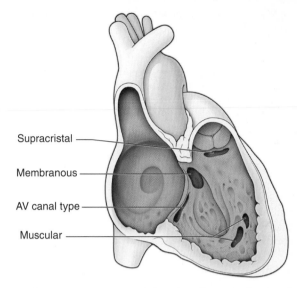

▲ **Figure 31–10.** Anatomic location of ventricular septal defects (VSDs).

Classifications of VSDs can be based on anatomic location or physiology. The anatomic classification includes defects of both the membranous and muscular portions of the ventricular septum (Figure 31–10). Membranous VSDs can be subdivided into supracristal (also known as doubly committed subarterial), perimembranous (the inlet portion of the membranous septum), and malalignment (found in TOF with an overriding aorta) defects. The muscular VSDs, often multiple, may be located in the inlet or outlet regions or within the trabecular portion of the septum. Classifying VSDs physiologically is based on the size of the defect as well as the relative vascular resistances within the systemic and pulmonary circulation. A high-pressure gradient exists across a small restrictive VSD, with normal or mildly elevated pulmonary artery pressure and predominant left-to-right shunting. A large nonrestrictive VSD permits equalization of RV and LV pressures with obligatory pulmonary hypertension (in the absence of RV outflow-tract obstruction) and bidirectional shunting. The smallest VSD (maladie de Roger) is characterized by a hemodynamically insignificant shunt, a loud murmur, and an intermediate to high risk of endocarditis.

In the infant, left-to-right shunting occurs only when PVR falls below systemic vascular resistance, and the murmur usually becomes audible in the first month of life. With a large nonrestrictive defect, PVR may not fall; if the defect is not surgically closed by age 2, irreversible pulmonary hypertension may ensue. The volume overload caused by a large restrictive VSD may cause CHF in the first 6 months of life. Approximately 40% of VSDs close spontaneously by age 3, and a smaller percentage close before age 10. Generally, the smaller defects are more likely to close, but even in infants with heart failure, 7% will experience spontaneous closure.

Three late complications of VSD are worth mentioning. Tricuspid regurgitation may rarely result when the septal leaflet of the tricuspid valve is deformed by the ventricular septal aneurysm that causes spontaneous closure of a perimembranous VSD. Aortic regurgitation is common in patients with doubly committed subarterial VSDs (supracristal, or outlet, VSDs), as a result of herniation of the right aortic sinus into the defect; it also occurs in those with perimembranous VSDs. Infundibular PS from hypertrophy of the RV outflow tract can develop, functionally dividing the RV into inflow and outflow segments, a condition termed "double-chambered right ventricle." If a sufficient pressure gradient develops, RV systolic pressure can exceed LV systolic pressure, and right-to-left shunting can occur across the VSD. The resultant hypoxia may only occur during exercise.

▶ Clinical Findings

A. Symptoms & Signs

The young adult with an uncorrected VSD and normal pulmonary artery pressures is usually asymptomatic, with normal or minimally diminished exercise tolerance. Like those with ASDs, exertional dyspnea often develops in patients with VSDs after the age of 30 when the Q_p:Q_s exceeds 2–3:1. Individuals with smaller shunts rarely report symptoms. The most disabled group with pulmonary hypertension and cyanosis (Eisenmenger physiology, or syndrome) will be discussed later.

Physical findings depend on the size of the VSD. The patient with uncomplicated VSD is acyanotic, and the LV apical impulse is displaced laterally, suggesting LV volume overload, and may be hyperdynamic. A holosystolic murmur occurs, often associated with a systolic thrill, heard best in the fourth or fifth intercostal space along the left sternal border, with radiation to the right parasternal region. Because of the increased flow across the mitral valve, an S_3 gallop and a diastolic rumble may be present. Additional signs of tricuspid insufficiency (prominent jugular venous *v* wave and systolic murmur) or aortic valve regurgitation (diastolic blowing murmur, increased arterial pulses) will be present in patients with these complications.

B. Diagnostic Studies

1. Electrocardiography and chest radiography—In the presence of a large shunt, the ECG is suggestive of LVH or biventricular hypertrophy, with biphasic QRS complexes in the transitional precordial leads. Evidence of left or right atrial enlargement is present in only about 25% of patients.

Cardiac enlargement with an increased cardiac silhouette is evident on chest radiograph only in the presence of a large left-to-right shunt. In the absence of pulmonary hypertension, there is evidence of pulmonary vascular engorgement with a plethora of the peripheral vasculature as well as enlargement of the proximal vessels. Left atrial enlargement may be evident on the lateral chest radiograph.

It is important to remember that in most adults with a small VSD (< 1.5–2:1 shunt), both the ECG and radiograph are normal, even in the presence of a loud murmur. On the other hand, the presence of pulmonary hypertension alters the ECG and radiograph findings.

2. Echocardiography—Two-dimensional and Doppler echocardiography can usually define the location and often the size of a VSD, although accurate Doppler shunt quantitation may not be possible in the adult. There is evidence of left atrial and LV dilatation. The right-heart chamber dimensions are usually normal, although the main pulmonary artery may appear dilated. The presence of RVH usually signifies pulmonary hypertension or associated PS (with right-to-left shunting and cyanosis). Usually only the largest defects, often located in the membranous septum, can actually be visualized echocardiographically (Figure 31–11). The aneurysmal pouch of a ventricular septal aneurysm may be seen in the parasternal short-axis view just below the aortic valve in the inlet portion of the septum near the septal leaflet of the tricuspid valve. Saline contrast administration shows a negative contrast effect within the RV, and a small degree of bidirectional shunting is sometimes present, with microbubbles appearing in the LV.

Color-flow Doppler imaging demonstrates a high-velocity (aliased) systolic jet across the ventricular septum into the RV. The location of the jet provides the best guide to the location of the defect. In the parasternal short-axis view, the jet from a membranous VSD may be seen in the region of

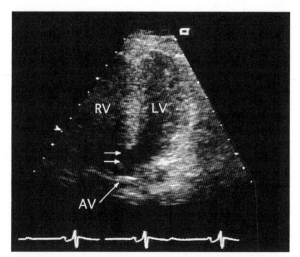

▲ **Figure 31–11.** Transthoracic echocardiogram in a 40-year-old woman with a large membranous ventricular septal defect (*double arrow*). The right ventricle (RV) was enlarged because of pulmonary hypertension. AV, aortic valve; LV, left ventricle.

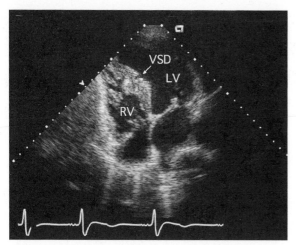

▲ **Figure 31–12.** Transthoracic echocardiogram in a 45-year-old woman with a small muscular ventricular septal defect (VSD). LV, left ventricle; RV, right ventricle.

the tricuspid valve (perimembranous) or toward the pulmonary artery (doubly committed subarterial, or supracristal). Muscular VSD jets are best seen in the apical or subcostal four-chamber views (Figure 31–12).

In continuous wave Doppler, the peak velocity of the jet across the ventricular septum provides the peak systolic LV-RV gradient (using the modified Bernoulli equation). Subtracting this gradient from the systolic blood pressure gives the peak RV systolic pressure. In the absence of a pressure gradient across the RV outflow tract—including the pulmonary valve (which should be carefully sought)—the RV systolic pressure is equivalent to the pulmonary artery systolic pressure. Additional Doppler evidence of the left-to-right shunt is found in the increased pulmonary artery flow velocity.

In the postrepair patient, the VSD patch may or may not be apparent, depending on the size of the original defect. Once endothelialized, the patch may not cause acoustic shadowing (or distal echo blockout). Color-flow Doppler may demonstrate patch leaks at the peripheral suture lines of the patch in a small percentage of patients. Spontaneous closure of a VSD involving juxtaposed tricuspid valve tissue may cause significant tricuspid regurgitation. Varying degrees of aortic regurgitation may be present and are most often associated with membranous or supracristal VSDs.

3. Cardiac catheterization—Although the diagnosis is often made noninvasively, the decision to close a VSD rests on accurate measurements of the shunt ratio and the level of PVR. Catheterization is therefore often necessary for therapeutic decision making.

Right-heart catheterization with sequential measurements of oxygen saturation reveals a step-up within the body

of the RV. As with an ASD, the higher the RV oxygen saturation, the greater is the degree of shunting. For the calculation of Q_p:Q_s, the same formula is used as for ASD, except that the mixed venous blood sample is drawn from the right atrium. Pulmonary artery pressures and vascular resistance should be measured, and a gradient across the RV outflow tract, including the infundibulum and the pulmonary valve, must be excluded. Left ventriculography in the cranial left anterior oblique projection will reveal the location of the defect as contrast enters the RV.

▶ Prognosis & Treatment

As previously mentioned, adults with large, uncorrected VSDs are uncommonly encountered. With an uncorrected VSD, the overall 10-year survival rate after initial presentation is 75%. Survival is adversely affected by functional class greater than New York Heart Association class I, cardiomegaly, and elevated pulmonary artery pressure (> 50 mm Hg). As in patients with ASD, surgery is generally recommended when the magnitude of the systemic-to-pulmonary-shunt ratio exceeds 2:1. Other indications for surgery may include recurrent endocarditis and progressive aortic regurgitation.

In patients with small VSDs treated either conservatively or with surgery, outcomes are identical for patients with a Q_p:Q_s < 2.0, normal PVR, no LV volume overload or VSD-related aortic regurgitation, and no symptoms of exercise intolerance.

Surgery for closure of VSDs has been available for more than 50 years, and long-term follow-up data are available. Surgery prior to age 2—even in infants with a large VSD, high pulmonary blood flow, and preoperative pulmonary hypertension—almost always prevents the development of pulmonary vascular obstructive disease. In patients who underwent surgery during the 1960s and 1970s, there is an approximately 20% incidence of residual left-to-right shunt and a persistent risk of endocarditis. Ventricular arrhythmias and right bundle branch block (RBBB) are more common with a repair performed via right ventriculotomy (eg, muscular or subarterial VSD); when possible, the right atrium is the preferred approach. The risk of sudden death and complete heart block is low. Most patients who have VSDs repaired in childhood survive to lead normal adult lives.

Devices have been developed for percutaneous closure of both muscular and perimembranous VSDs. Muscular VSD occluders have been approved by the U.S. Food and Drug Administration and are commercially available in the United States. Initial case series suggest high success rates and low complication rates. Reported complications (in nine patients) include conduction anomalies and aortic or tricuspid regurgitation. More extensive follow-up data are needed before device implantation becomes routine.

Aboulhosn J, et al. Common congenital heart disorders in adults: percutaneous therapeutic procedures. *Curr Probl Cardiol.* 2011;36(7):263–84. [PMID: 21704232]

Gabriel HM, et al. Long-term outcome of patients with ventricular septal defect considered not to require surgical closure during childhood. *J Am Coll Cardiol.* 2002;39(6):1066–71. [PMID: 11897452]

Penny DJ, et al. Ventricular septal defect. *Lancet.* 2011;377(9771): 1103–12. [PMID: 21349577]

PATENT DUCTUS ARTERIOSUS

 ### ESSENTIALS OF DIAGNOSIS

▶ Continuous machinery-like murmur, loudest below the left clavicle.

▶ Left ventricular hypertrophy.

▶ Pulmonary plethora, left atrial and ventricular enlargement; in older adults, calcification of the ductus on chest radiograph.

▶ Left atrial and ventricular dilatation with normal right-heart chambers on echocardiography.

▶ Continuous high-velocity color Doppler jet with retrograde flow along lateral wall of main pulmonary artery near left branch.

▶ General Considerations

The patent ductus arteriosus (PDA) is a remnant of the normal fetal circulation. In the fetal circulation, superior vena cava blood enters the right atrium and characteristically is directed across the tricuspid valve into the RV. It is then delivered into the systemic circulation via the ductus arteriosus, which connects the left pulmonary artery to the descending aorta just distal to the insertion of the left subclavian artery (Figure 31–13). In the normal full-term newborn, the ductus closes within the first 10–15 hours following birth. If the ductus fails to close after birth when PVR falls, the direction of blood flow within the ductus reverses, producing a left-to-right shunt. CHF usually develops within the first year of life in patients with nonrestrictive PDA (large left-to-right shunts). As with VSD, it is relatively unusual—but by no means rare—to encounter an adult with uncorrected PDA.

An anatomic variant of the PDA is the aortopulmonary window (see Figure 31–13), which is usually a relatively large communication between the ascending aorta and the main pulmonary artery. The pathophysiology is similar to that of the PDA and is dependent on the size of the shunt and the level of PVR. The degree of pulmonary hypertension depends on the directly transmitted aortic pressure, which in turn depends on the size of the channel and the amount of pulmonary blood flow. If LV failure occurs, pulmonary venous hypertension may contribute further to the pulmonary hypertension. In a small number of patients, PVR rises above systemic vascular resistance and the shunt reverses. Because the site of the PDA is distal to the left subclavian, the head and neck vessels continue to receive oxygenated blood—but the descending aorta receives the desaturated blood, with the development of differential cyanosis.

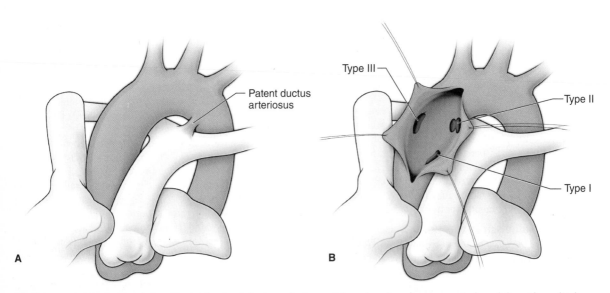

▲ **Figure 31–13.** Anatomic locations of patent ductus arteriosus (**A**) and aortopulmonary window (**B**), with multiple distinct anatomic locations possible.

When present in isolation, the PDA may lead to heart failure from pulmonary overcirculation. In conjunction with other defects, however, it may represent the sole pulmonary (eg, pulmonary atresia with intact ventricular septum) or systemic (eg, aortic atresia) blood supply, and survival may depend on persistent patency.

▶ **Clinical Findings**

A. Symptoms & Signs

The mothers of patients with PDA may have a history of maternal rubella, and the patient may have had a murmur since infancy. If CHF has not developed by age 10, most patients will be asymptomatic as adults. CHF develops in a few patients in their 20s and 30s, however, and presents as exertional dyspnea, chest pain, and palpitations.

The patient is almost always acyanotic; but when cyanosis and clubbing are present, the upper extremities are usually spared. Thus, the lower extremities and sometimes the left hand may show clubbing and cyanosis, but the right hand and head are always pink. The pulse pressure may be widened, and the pulses are collapsing. The LV impulse is hyperdynamic and often laterally displaced. The classic murmur of the uncomplicated PDA is best heard below the left clavicle and gradually builds to its peak in late systole; it is continuous through the second heart sound and wanes in diastole. There may be a pause in late diastole or early systole. With a significant LV volume overload caused by a large shunt, an S_3 gallop and a diastolic murmur of relative mitral stenosis (similar to that of the large VSD) may be present. The murmur varies as PVR increases and shunting reverses, first with a decrease in the diastolic component and then a decrease in the systolic component. Finally, the murmur is silent and the physical findings are consistent with pulmonary hypertension (see Eisenmenger Syndrome).

B. Diagnostic Studies

1. Electrocardiography and chest radiography—The ECG is normal when the shunt is small; it shows left atrial and ventricular hypertrophy in the presence of a large shunt. When pulmonary hypertension is present and the shunt is predominantly right to left, the ECG may show P-pulmonale, right-axis deviation, and evidence of RVH.

The chest radiograph is also normal in the presence of a small shunt. With a significant shunt, LV prominence is evident with an enlarged cardiac silhouette and pulmonary vascular plethora. In the presence of pulmonary hypertension, pruning of the peripheral pulmonary vessels is present, with prominence of the central pulmonary arteries. The ductus may be calcified in the older adult.

2. Echocardiography—The two-dimensional echocardiogram shows left atrial and ventricular enlargement, but imaging of the ductus itself is usually difficult in the adult.

Color-flow Doppler imaging is diagnostic and reveals continuous high-velocity flow within the main pulmonary artery near the left branch. Flow is predominantly retrograde within the pulmonary artery and can be detected by continuous wave Doppler. In an aortopulmonary window, continuous color flow is detected, but it is most often antegrade, which distinguishes it from the flow through a PDA. Pulmonary artery pressure can be estimated from the almost ubiquitous tricuspid regurgitant jet.

3. Cardiac catheterization—Right-heart catheterization is performed to measure the pulmonary artery pressure, PVR, and flow ratio ($Q_p:Q_s$). The oxygen step-up is at the level of the pulmonary artery, and when the ductus is large enough, the descending aorta can be entered from the pulmonary artery. The ductus can also be seen during aortography in the left lateral projection. Because echocardiography is noninvasive and diagnostic, cardiac catheterization may become exclusively therapeutic in the future. Techniques for coil and, more recently, device occlusion are well established and currently represent the treatment of choice for simple PDAs in many institutions. Thus, catheterization should be combined with a therapeutic intervention.

▶ **Prognosis & Treatment**

Patients who survive into adulthood with a large uncorrected PDA generally have CHF or pulmonary hypertension (with right-to-left shunting and differential cyanosis) by about age 30. Most adults with PDA and normal or only mildly elevated PVR (< 4 units) are either asymptomatic or mildly impaired and can undergo surgical ligation or percutaneous closure with good results. In the group with severely elevated PVR (> 10 units/m²), survival is poor. Approximately 15% of patients older than 40 years of age may have calcification or aneurysmal dilatation of the ductus, which can complicate surgery. Surgical ligation or percutaneous coil or device occlusion of a PDA can be performed with low morbidity and mortality and is recommended—independent of the size of the shunt—because of the high risk of endocarditis in uncorrected cases. Division of an isolated restrictive PDA in childhood can be curative of congenital heart disease. If repaired after childhood, the morbidity and mortality rates depend on the degree of pulmonary hypertension, LV volume overload, and calcification of the ductus. Unless persistent shunting is present following a surgical ligation, endocarditis prophylaxis is not recommended after the sixth postoperative month.

Masura J, et al. Long-term outcome of transcatheter patent ductus arteriosus closure using Amplatzer duct occluders. *Am Heart J.* 2006;151(3):755.e7–755.e10. [PMID: 16504649]

Schneider DJ, et al. The patent ductus arteriosus in term infants, children, and adults. *Semin Perinatol.* 2012;36(2):146–53. [PMID: 22414886]

COARCTATION OF THE AORTA

ESSENTIALS OF DIAGNOSIS

▶ Elevated systolic blood pressure in the upper extremities (always in right arm); normal or diminished systolic blood pressure in lower extremities (and often left arm); radial-femoral pulse delay.

▶ LVH, LV prominence, "3" sign, rib notching on chest radiograph.

▶ Visualization of the coarctation by imaging.

▶ Distal aortic pressure drop by Doppler echocardiography or catheterization.

▶ General Considerations

Coarctation of the thoracic aorta predominates in males, is often associated with a congenitally abnormal aortic valve, and is a congenital narrowing of the aorta, usually in the region of ductal insertion. The most common location is distal to the origin of the left subclavian artery (postductal; Figure 31–14), but the narrowing may also be proximal (preductal). Infrequently, a preductal coarctation is present in combination with an anomalous origin of the right subclavian artery, causing reduced pressures in the right upper extremity. There is considerable variability in the degree and extent of narrowing, ranging from a localized shelf to a long tubular narrowing. Multiple discrete sites are rarely encountered. Coarctation of the abdominal aorta is less common than that of the thoracic aorta; it is found equally in males and females and presents with symptoms of claudication. Additional coexisting problems may include congenital mitral valve disease and aneurysms of the circle of Willis (the latter are present in approximately 25% of patients with coarctation). Coarctation is frequently seen as part of a syndrome. Approximately 50% of patients have an associated bicuspid aortic valve. Long, tubular narrowing should alert the clinician to the possibility of Williams syndrome, whereas preductal coarctation is frequently seen in Turner syndrome. Collateral circulation to the distal aorta develops mainly via the subclavian and intercostal arteries, in addition to the vertebral and anterior spinal arteries.

Aortic coarctation is usually diagnosed during childhood in the asymptomatic phase by routine examination of blood pressure and femoral pulse palpation. Aortic coarctation is approximately two to five times more common in boys than in girls. In cases of severe obstruction, infants may have CHF. Symptoms may arise in the adult during the 20s and 30s, and evidence of coarctation should always be sought in patients of this age group presenting with hypertension. Early detection and repair are highly desirable because repair forestalls the associated accelerated development of coronary artery disease.

▶ Clinical Findings

A. Symptoms & Signs

The adult with uncorrected coarctation is usually asymptomatic. When symptoms occur, they are nonspecific: exertional dyspnea, headache, epistaxis, and leg fatigue. CHF can occur in the adult with long-standing hypertension secondary to coarctation. Additional significant complications, usually

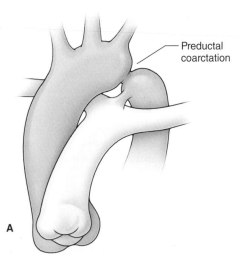

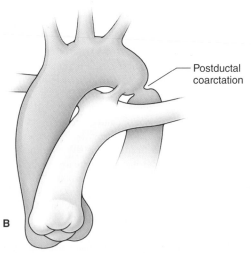

▲ **Figure 31–14.** Anatomic features of aortic coarctation. **A:** Preductal coarctation, in which differential cyanosis may occur. **B:** Postductal coarctation.

occurring between the ages of 15 and 40, include aortic rupture or dissection of the proximal thoracic aorta or an aneurysm distal to the coarctation, infective endocarditis on an associated bicuspid aortic valve or endarteritis at the site of coarctation, and cerebrovascular accidents, which are most often due to rupture of an aneurysm of the circle of Willis.

The systolic blood pressure is elevated in the right arm and often the left arm, with reduced systolic blood pressures in the lower extremities. Diastolic blood pressures are not usually affected. Simultaneous palpation of the radial and femoral pulses reveals delayed arrival of the femoral pulse. Adult patients with highly developed collateral circulation may no longer exhibit these signs, however, and a clinically recorded difference between upper and lower extremity blood pressure will underestimate the coarctation gradient. The jugular venous pulse is normal, the carotid upstroke is usually brisk, and the aorta may be palpable in the suprasternal notch. Cardiac examination reveals a nondisplaced, but forceful, LV impulse. The first heart sound is normal, and the aortic component of the second heart sound may be accentuated. A late systolic murmur is present (as a result of the coarctation) that is best heard between the scapulae to the left of the spine. The murmur caused by collateral flow through the intercostal and internal mammary arteries is longer, but it is not necessarily continuous. An ejection click and systolic murmur as well as a blowing diastolic murmur of aortic regurgitation may be associated with a bicuspid aortic valve.

B. Diagnostic Studies

1. Electrocardiography and chest radiography—The ECG is nonspecific, with LVH and, in the later stages, left atrial enlargement. As in other patients with long-standing hypertension, atrial fibrillation may occur.

On the other hand, the radiograph finding of rib notching is highly specific, although it is not 100% sensitive even in adults. Notching is present on the bottom of the rib where the intercostal arteries are located. In preductal coarctation (ie, proximal to the left subclavian artery), the rib notching is present only on the right side, and, in abdominal coarctation, it is limited to the lower ribs. Another classic radiograph finding is the "3" sign, with the aortic arch and dilated left subclavian artery forming the upper curvature and the dilated distal aorta forming the lower. There may be radiologic evidence of LV and atrial enlargement.

2. Echocardiography—It is extremely difficult to identify the actual site of the coarctation in the adult patient with precordial two-dimensional echocardiography. Doppler evidence of flow acceleration in the descending aorta from the suprasternal notch, however, can often identify obstruction even when images are suboptimal. The peak systolic velocity can be used to estimate the gradient, but the presence of persistent antegrade flow in diastole (Figure 31–15A) and decreased acceleration time beyond the coarctation provide additional confirmation of hemodynamic significance. Further localization of the coarctation is now possible with

imaging of the descending aorta in the longitudinal plane during multiplanar TEE. The anatomy of the aortic valve should be carefully defined, and careful Doppler interrogation for evidence of stenosis or insufficiency is essential.

3. Magnetic resonance angiography and computed tomography angiography—MRA can localize and define the extent of narrowing with a high degree of accuracy (Figure 31–15B) and provides estimates of the presence of collateral flow to the distal aorta. Aneurysmal dilatation is visible, and postoperative evaluation is possible. Computed tomography (CT) angiography provides excellent anatomic definition but cannot provide any physiologic information.

4. Cardiac catheterization—Aortography is necessary only when the diagnosis is not adequately confirmed clinically or the anatomy cannot be fully defined noninvasively. Premature coronary disease is common, and if it is clinically suspected, coronary arteriography should be performed. Balloon dilatation with or without stent placement across native and recurrent coarctation has been attempted in cases of discrete narrowing (see later discussion).

▶ Prognosis & Treatment

The importance of identifying coarctation in adults lies in the tendency toward LVH and CHF, premature coronary artery disease, and cerebral hemorrhage. In an autopsy series of uncorrected coarctation, 50% of patients had died by about age 30 and 90% by age 60. Proximal aortic rupture, aortic dissection, and cerebral hemorrhage often occur before the age of 30, and the incidence of CHF continues to increase after the age of 40.

Surgery for correcting coarctation presents a considerable challenge in patients over the age of 15 years because of large intercostal aneurysms and atheromatous changes in the aorta near the shelf. It should be noted that surgical repair even in childhood is often only palliative, and these patients require continued surveillance, particularly in the presence of associated cardiac lesions or preoperative systemic hypertension. Hypertension persists in approximately one-third of patients operated on after the age of 14. The major determinants of long-term survival following repair of aortic coarctation are the presence of associated lesions and the age at operation. The postsurgery cardiac mortality rate after age 20 is approximately 5% in patients with isolated coarctation. Causes of late cardiovascular deaths (in order of frequency) include coronary artery disease, sudden death, aortic regurgitation and heart failure, hypertension and heart failure, and cerebrovascular accidents. Approximately 10% of patients require subsequent cardiovascular surgery, the majority for aortic valve replacement. The incidence of recurrent coarctation requiring surgery or percutaneous intervention varies significantly depending on surgical technique and can be 16–60%, with the highest recoarctation rates generally associated with earlier operation.

The surgical methods of repair have undergone considerable evolution since their initial introduction in the late 1950s.

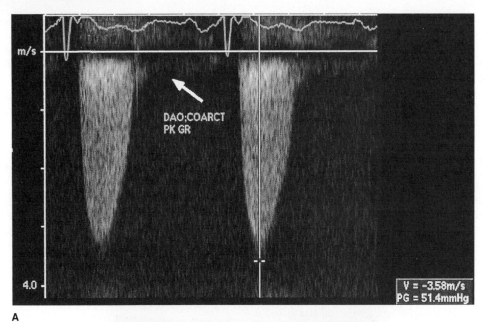

A

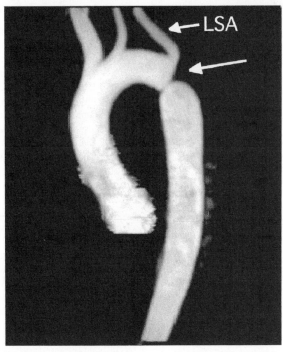

B

▲ **Figure 31–15. A:** Continuous wave Doppler from transthoracic echocardiogram in a patient with coarctation of the descending aorta (DAO). There was a peak gradient (PK GR) of 51.4 mm Hg with runoff in diastole (*arrow*). **B:** Three-dimensional reconstruction of a magnetic resonance angiogram of the thoracic aorta demonstrates a discrete coarctation (*lower arrow*) in the typical location after the take-off of the left subclavian artery (LSA).

In part this is due to the considerable morphologic variability that has precluded using a single method for correction. The removal of the abnormal coarctation tissue as occurs in an end-to-end anastomosis is most desirable, but depending on other factors, a subclavian flap repair or an interposition graft may be necessary. Less reliance is placed on the patch angioplasty because long-term studies have shown late aneurysm formation due to thinning of the posterior wall.

Over the last 10 years, endovascular repair of coarctation has become a popular treatment option. Furthermore, the advent of balloon-expandable stents has reduced the complication rate associated with balloon angioplasty alone. Complications of stent implantation can be classified into three categories: technical (stent migration or fracture, balloon rupture, and overlap of the brachiocephalic vessels), aortic (intimal tear, dissection, and aneurysm formation), and peripheral vascular (cerebral vascular accident, peripheral embolization, and injury to access vessels). Compared with surgical therapy, endovascular stenting of native coarctation has a similar morbidity and mortality but is associated with a significantly higher incidence of recoarctation, need for reintervention, and persistent hypertension. In light of these differences, there is ongoing controversy about the best treatment approach for adults and adult-sized adolescents with native coarctation of the aorta. There is general agreement, however, that recoarctation in adults can be managed by percutaneous transluminal balloon angioplasty, with or without stent implantation.

Because of the risk of recoarctation and of complications such as aortic aneurysm, periodic surveillance with MRI or with CT aortography is recommended in the adult after repair, irrespective of technique. It is essential to screen women of childbearing age for postrepair aortic dilatation because the risk of aortic dissection or rupture during pregnancy is high. The need to screen for intracranial aneurysms is controversial.

Connolly HM, et al. Intracranial aneurysms in patients with coarctation of the aorta: a prospective magnetic resonance angiographic study of 100 patients. *Mayo Clin Proc.* 2003;78 (12):1491–9. [PMID: 14661678]

Godart F, et al. Intravascular stenting for the treatment of coarctation of the aorta in adolescent and adult patients. *Arch Cardiovasc Dis.* 2011;104(12):627–35. [PMID:22152515]

Pádua LM, et al. Stent placement versus surgery for coarctation of the thoracic aorta. *Cochrane Database Syst Rev.* 2012;5:CD008204. [PMID: 22592728]

EBSTEIN ANOMALY

 ESSENTIALS OF DIAGNOSIS

▶ History of dyspnea, atypical chest pain, or intermittent cyanosis.

▶ Palpitations associated with supraventricular arrhythmias and preexcitation syndrome.

▶ Right parasternal lift, widely split S₁, systolic clicks, and systolic murmur of tricuspid regurgitation (without inspiratory accentuation).

▶ Right atrial enlargement, RV conduction defect of RBBB type, posteriorly directed delta waves with accessory pathway by ECG. Frequent first-degree AV block.

▶ Normal or reduced pulmonary vascularity without pulmonary artery enlargement, right atrial enlargement, normal left-sided cardiac silhouette on chest radiograph.

▶ Apical displacement of septal tricuspid valve leaflet; variable degrees of tricuspid regurgitation originating from apical portion of RV; and enlarged right atrium on echocardiography.

▶ General Considerations

Ebstein anomaly is characterized by deformity of the tricuspid valve with apical displacement of the septal and posterior leaflets (Figure 31–16) and their adhesion to the RV wall. The anterior leaflet is elongated and has been described as sail-like. Tricuspid regurgitation arises from the apically displaced site of leaflet coaptation with considerable variability

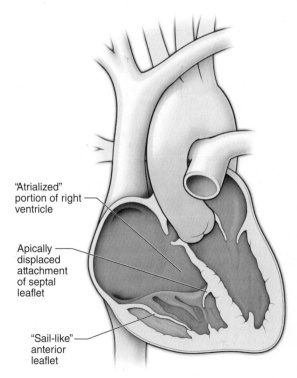

"Atrialized" portion of right ventricle

Apically displaced attachment of septal leaflet

"Sail-like" anterior leaflet

▲ **Figure 31–16.** Anatomy of Ebstein anomaly.

in the extent of tricuspid leaflet displacement and the degree of tricuspid regurgitation. The portion of the RV proximal to the leaflets is atrialized (thinned), and if the remaining RV is diminutive in size, pump function may be inadequate. Cyanosis may be present as a result of right-to-left shunting across an ASD or patent foramen ovale in the presence of significant tricuspid regurgitation or elevated right atrial pressures. Interatrial septal defects, including patent foramen ovales, are the most common associated anomaly, occurring in 80–90% of patients with Ebstein anomaly.

Tremendous variability exists in the morphologic abnormalities and clinical presentation of patients with Ebstein anomaly. In severe cases, CHF or cyanosis may be present during infancy. At the opposite end of the spectrum, a mildly affected adult may be asymptomatic or symptomatic only because of supraventricular tachyarrhythmias. The latter are an important feature of Ebstein anomaly, which is associated with preexcitation in 25–30% of patients. The accessory pathway is usually posteroseptal or posterolateral in location.

▶ Clinical Findings

A. Symptoms & Signs

Cyanosis may be the most important clinical feature in early life, but in older patients, long-standing RV volume overload and right atrial distention result in CHF. Dysrhythmias, including the Wolff-Parkinson-White syndrome, are frequent. Adult patients may have dyspnea, arrhythmias, decreased exercise tolerance, and intermittent or exercise-induced cyanosis (with associated right-to-left shunting across an ASD or patent foramen ovale).

Physical examination reveals right parasternal lift, widely split S_1, systolic clicks (from delayed tricuspid valve closure, the "sail" sounds), and the systolic murmur of tricuspid regurgitation. The latter does not usually increase in intensity during inspiration, because the noncompliant RV cannot accept an increase in venous return. On the other hand, the right atrium is compliant, and systemic venous congestion is uncommon; the jugular venous pulse is therefore usually normal. S_3 and S_4 gallops may be present, as may an early diastolic snap from the opening of the elongated anterior leaflet.

B. Diagnostic Studies

1. Electrocardiography and chest radiography—The ECG shows evidence of right atrial enlargement and an RV conduction defect of the RBBB type. The PR interval may be prolonged, except in the presence of an accessory pathway. In 25–30% of patients, ECG findings are consistent with Wolff-Parkinson-White syndrome; the PR interval is short, and delta waves from a posterolateral or posteroseptal bundle of Kent are evident (Figure 31–17). Atrial fibrillation may be present in older patients.

The chest radiograph shows normal or reduced pulmonary vascularity without pulmonary artery enlargement; it also shows cardiac enlargement to the right of the sternum caused by right atrial enlargement. The LV and left atrium are normal in size.

2. Echocardiography—The classic M-mode description of this anomaly included increased excursion of the anterior tricuspid valve leaflet and delayed tricuspid valve closure (> 40 ms) following mitral valve closure. Two-dimensional and Doppler echocardiography are diagnostic in most adults. The four-chamber apical and subcostal views provide most of the necessary information. The right atrium is enlarged and the RV is usually small, consisting of the atrialized portion and the remaining pumping chamber. The septal, and possibly the posterior, leaflet of the tricuspid valve is apically displaced, and color-flow Doppler imaging shows the regurgitant jet arising from the apical point of coaptation (Figure 31–18). The degree of tricuspid regurgitation can be estimated from the extent of right atrial filling by color flow and from the density of the continuous wave Doppler signal. The pulmonary artery systolic pressure estimated from the continuous wave tricuspid regurgitation jet is nearly always normal.

Although color-flow imaging may reveal a patent foramen ovale or an ASD, it is mandatory to perform a saline contrast examination to reliably exclude these sources of right-to-left shunting. When precordial echocardiography is inadequate, TEE can be used to exclude associated lesions of the atrial septum.

3. Cardiac catheterization—During right-heart catheterization, simultaneous recordings of an RV electrogram and a right atrial pressure tracing are obtained with a catheter in the atrialized portion of the RV. This finding is considered pathognomonic of Ebstein anomaly, but catheterization is rarely necessary for diagnosis.

▶ Prognosis & Treatment

The chance of surviving to age 50 is about 50%, with survival dependent on the degree of the anatomic and physiologic abnormalities. As mentioned, 25–30% of patients have supraventricular arrhythmias, many associated with accessory pathways that are now amenable to catheter ablation. Tricuspid annuloplasty and repair with RV plication have been challenging. The success of these approaches has traditionally been limited, with approximately 50% of patients requiring tricuspid valve replacement. Newer techniques, such as the Carpentier and "cone" techniques, promise to reduce further the need for valve replacement. Improvement in exercise tolerance following tricuspid valve replacement or repair has been observed, especially in patients with associated ASD. In patients with severe morphologic variants, a Fontan-like procedure (see Palliative Surgical Procedures) may be the only suitable choice. In patients who are symptomatic predominantly on the basis of exercise-induced cyanosis, device closure of the interarterial septal defect may be adequate treatment.

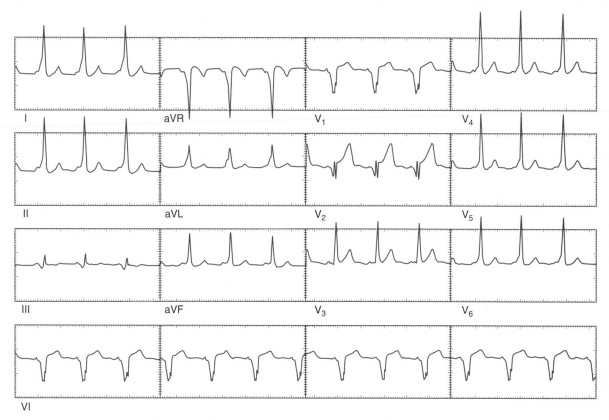

I aVR V₁ V₄
II aVL V₂ V₅
III aVF V₃ V₆
VI

▲ **Figure 31–17.** Electrocardiogram in Ebstein anomaly with associated Wolff-Parkinson-White syndrome.

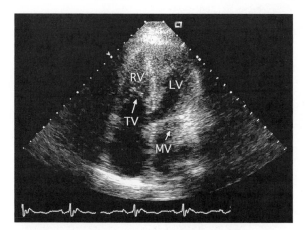

▲ **Figure 31–18.** Transesophageal echocardiogram in a 50-year-old woman with Ebstein anomaly. This four-chamber view shows the apically displaced tricuspid valve (TV) in relation to the normal mitral valve (MV). LV, left ventricle; RV, right ventricle.

Attenhofer Jost CH, et al. Ebstein's anomaly. *Circulation.* 2007;115(2):277–85. [PMID: 17228014]

da Silva JP, et al. The cone reconstruction of the tricuspid valve in Ebstein's anomaly: early and midterm results. *J Thorac Cardiovasc Surg.* 2007;133:215–23 [PMID: 17198815]

Paranon S, et al. Ebstein's anomaly of the tricuspid valve: from fetus to adult: congenital heart disease. *Heart.* 2008;94(2): 237–43. [PMID: 18195130]

CONGENITALLY CORRECTED TRANSPOSITION OF THE GREAT ARTERIES

 ESSENTIALS OF DIAGNOSIS

► Prominent left parasternal impulse, soft S₁, accentuated A₂, soft or inaudible P₂.

► PR prolongation, variable degrees of AV block, Q waves in right precordial leads with absence in left precordial leads on ECG.

► Absence of left-sided aortic knob on chest radiograph.

► Rightward and posterior pulmonary artery with leftward and anterior aorta, apical displacement of right-sided AV valve, coarsely trabeculated left-sided systemic ventricle with moderator band (the morphologic RV) on cardiac imaging.

► General Considerations

In congenitally corrected transposition of the great arteries (C-TGA, also abbreviated as l-TGA), the visceroatrial relationship is normal with the right atrium to the right of the left atrium (Figure 31–19). The systemic venous blood drains into the right atrium and through a bileaflet (mitral) valve into a morphologic LV pumping into a posterior and rightward pulmonary artery. The pulmonary venous blood drains into the left atrium and through a trileaflet tricuspid valve into a morphologic RV pumping into an anterior and leftward aorta. This occurs because of atrial-ventricular discordance (ventricular inversion), which causes the RV to be located to the left of the LV. The great arteries are transposed, with the aorta arising from the RV and the pulmonary artery rising from the LV. The result is physiologic correction of the circulation, in that oxygenated blood comes into the left atrium, goes to the anatomic right ventricle, and then flows out of the aorta. The patient is acyanotic, and early symptoms typically result from associated lesions such as PS, VSD, and heart block.

The most common complications are complete heart block (occurring with an incidence of approximately 2% per year) and other associated anomalies, most commonly VSD, subvalvular PS, and abnormalities of the systemic AV valve. Coronary anomalies are uncommon, and the coronary circulation is usually concordant; that is, a right coronary artery supplies the RV. Eventually, the systemic ventricle (a massively hypertrophied RV) is subject to pump failure, even in cases of isolated C-TGA. The relative degree of PS and the size of the VSD determine whether cyanosis is present. In the absence of PS, the patient with a large VSD may have CHF due to the volume overload of the systemic ventricle and is at risk for pulmonary vascular disease.

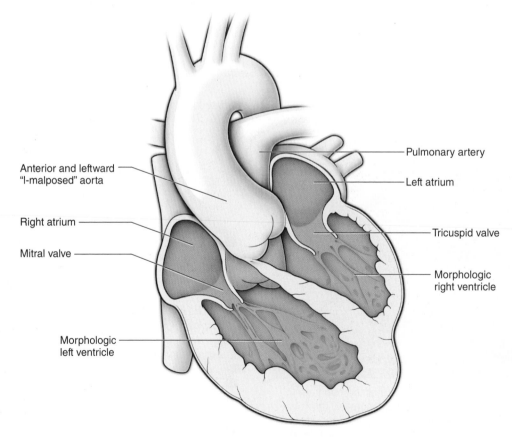

▲ **Figure 31–19.** Anatomy of congenitally corrected transposition of the great arteries. LV, left ventricle; RV, right ventricle.

The male:female ratio is approximately 1.5:1. While familial recurrence has been reported, no genetic linkage has been identified.

▶ Clinical Findings

A. Symptoms & Signs

Most patients with isolated C-TGA are asymptomatic in childhood and young adulthood, although formal cardiopulmonary exercise testing typically reveals lower VO_{2max} than in healthy controls. The highly prevalent complication of complete heart block may present with syncope, sudden death, or, less dramatically, exercise intolerance. More often, the clinical picture is dominated by associated lesions.

Exertional dyspnea and easy fatigability may develop with systemic AV valve regurgitation. Pulmonary venous congestion from pump failure of the anatomic RV may occur in middle age.

The physical examination depends largely on the associated anomalies. The left parasternal impulse is prominent as a result of the hypertrophied systemic ventricle. In the presence of a prolonged PR interval, S_1 is diminished in intensity. The proximity of the aorta to the chest wall causes an accentuated A_2; conversely, the posterior displacement of the pulmonary valve causes a soft or inaudible P_2. Systolic thrills occur in the presence of PS, with and without VSD. If PS is present, the murmur is best heard in the third left intercostal space, radiating to the right. The murmur of a VSD is usually typical, but the murmur of left-sided AV valve regurgitation radiates to the left sternal border in C-TGA.

B. Diagnostic Studies

1. Electrocardiography and chest radiography—The ECG and radiologic findings of C-TGA are dominated by its associated lesions. The ECG shows variable degrees of AV block, from simple PR prolongation to complete heart block. The absence of Q waves in leads I, V_5, and V_6 or the presence of Q waves in leads V_4R or V_1 is characteristic of the condition. This pattern results because the ventricular septal depolarization proceeds from the morphologic LV to RV (Figure 31–20). The typical chest radiograph finding in isolated C-TGA is a straight, left upper cardiac border, formed by the ascending aorta and loss of the pulmonary trunk contour.

2. Echocardiography—The anatomic features of isolated C-TGA are usually apparent by TTE, even in adults. TEE may be useful in defining the anatomy of associated lesions such as infundibular obstruction and the severity of left-sided AV valve regurgitation. In the basal parasternal short-axis view, the aortic valve is anterior and usually to the left of the pulmonic valve. Because the two great arteries arise in parallel, there is a "figure-eight" appearance, rather than the usual arrangement of the pulmonary artery in long axis

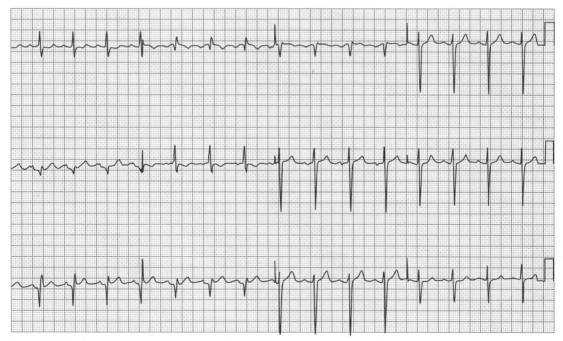

▲ **Figure 31–20.** Electrocardiograph in congenitally corrected transposition of the great arteries with associated pulmonic stenosis and ventricular septal defect.

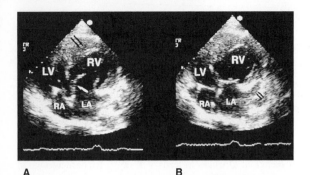

▲ **Figure 31–21.** Apical transthoracic echocardiographic views in a patient with congenitally corrected transposition of the great arteries. **A:** The moderator band is clearly visualized (*double arrow*) in the left-sided morphologic right ventricle (RV). **B:** The narrow-based atrial appendage (*double arrow*) clearly identifies this as a left atrium (LA). The RV is spherically dilated, reflecting the pressure overload of this chamber. The left ventricle (LV) is small and compressed. RA, right atrium. The left-sided atrioventricular (AV) valve is a morphologic tricuspid valve and the right-sided AV valve is a morphologic mitral valve.

surrounding the aortic valve. On careful inspection, the coronary arteries can be identified as they emerge from the aortic root. In the long-axis view (obtained from a more vertical and leftward scan), the aorta arises from the posterior ventricle, and its valve is not in fibrous continuity with the AV valve. The heavily trabeculated and hypertrophied RV with its moderator band is posterior and to the left, and the smoothly trabeculated LV is anterior and to the right (Figure 31–21). The systemic AV (anatomically a tricuspid) valve has three leaflets and septal attachments, is apically displaced, and may show variable degrees of regurgitation. In contrast, the subpulmonary AV (anatomically a mitral) valve has two leaflets and no septal attachments.

It is essential to identify associated lesions because these are the primary determinants of survival, specifically a VSD and infundibular pulmonary valve stenosis. Doppler echocardiography should be used to determine the pulmonary valve gradient and to identify any pulmonary hypertension. Autopsy studies of patients with C-TGA have documented abnormalities of the pulmonary venous AV valve in greater than 90% of cases. The most common of these is an Ebstein-like deformity. The leaflets of this systemic tricuspid valve are displaced apically, and the chordae tendineae are short and thickened. Clinically significant tricuspid systemic AV valve regurgitation has been reported in 20–50% of patients with C-TGA.

3. Cardiac catheterization—When noninvasive data are diagnostically conclusive, the role of cardiac catheterization is for preoperative evaluation in patients with surgically remediable lesions. The pulmonary artery may be difficult to enter; fluoroscopically, the venous catheter is noted to enter a posterior and rightward vessel. The PVR must be measured to rule out irreversible pulmonary vascular disease in patients with VSD. Although angiography can indicate the abnormally positioned great arteries, it is important only for identification of anomalous coronary arteries, which are infrequently encountered.

▶ **Prognosis & Treatment**

Survival in C-TGA is usually determined by other associated lesions, but even in its isolated form, survival may not be normal. The natural history and postoperative outcome of patients with C-TGA and the commonly associated lesions of VSD and PS are known to be less satisfactory than those of patients with normal AV connections and similar intracardiac lesions. The propensity for AV conduction abnormalities and for tricuspid valve dysfunction and the much-debated capability of the RV to function adequately in the systemic circulation may all affect survival.

A frequent feature of C-TGA is the development of complete heart block, estimated to occur at a rate of about 2% per year. AV conduction abnormalities of varying degrees are seen in nearly 75% of patients with this anomaly; many will require permanent pacemaker insertion. Periodic surveillance for the development of high-degree AV block is important: sudden death may be the first manifestation of this complication. However, it is the morphologic abnormalities of the tricuspid valve resulting in severe valvular dysfunction/regurgitation that have been shown to be the most critical determinant for survival. The systemic RV in C-TGA appears to be less tolerant than an anatomic LV of similar degrees of valvular incompetence, and there is an acceleration of the usual vicious cycle of ventricular remodeling, hypertrophy, and dysfunction in response to volume overload. The RV's inability to cope with significant tricuspid regurgitation leads to decreased contractility and annular dilation that in turn exacerbates the degree of regurgitation. Theoretically, the anatomic RV is subject to progressive pump failure from the obligatory pressure overload of the systemic circulation, potentially hastened by systemic hypertension, coronary artery disease, and volume overload from a regurgitant AV valve. Because the circulation is functionally corrected, the indications for surgery are those of the associated lesion requiring surgery (eg, VSD with a $Q_p:Q_s$ of 2:1, VSD with PS causing cyanosis). Repair or replacement of the tricuspid valve may be indicated; however, 10-year survival after surgical intervention is low. A "double switch" operation has been proposed for patients whose tricuspid valves are severely insufficient. An atrial switch combined with an arterial switch (see the section on Transposition of the Great Arteries) in the absence of LV outflow obstruction or with a **Rastelli** procedure (RV to pulmonary artery conduit) has been successfully performed. After surgery, the LV and mitral valve are restored to systemic circulation. Improvement in tricuspid valve function in a low-pressure RV has been documented after these operations. This procedure carries significant risk, and late complications relating to the atrial switch component (baffle obstruction, sick sinus syndrome) are of additional concern. Heart transplantation remains the final option for patients with C-TGA, intractable tricuspid regurgitation, and RV failure.

Graham TP Jr, et al. Long-term outcome in congenitally corrected transposition of the great arteries: a multi-institutional study. *J Am Coll Cardiol.* 2000;36(1):255–61. [PMID: 10898443]

Wallis GA, et al. Congenitally corrected transposition. *Orphanet J Rare Dis.* 2011;6:22. [PMID: 21569592]

Warnes CA. Transposition of the great arteries. *Circulation.* 2006;114(24):2699–709. [PMID: 17159076]

▼ OTHER ACYANOTIC CONGENITAL DEFECTS

Partial anomalous pulmonary venous return usually involves abnormal drainage of the right upper pulmonary vein into the superior vena cava and is often associated with sinus venosus ASD. Other sites of drainage include the coronary sinus and the inferior vena cava (scimitar syndrome). The need for surgical correction depends on the presence or degree of pulmonary venous obstruction and on the size of the shunt, which in turn is related to the number of pulmonary veins draining into the pulmonary circulation. As a rule, more than one anomalously draining pulmonary vein is required to produce a hemodynamically significant shunt.

AV septal defects (also known as **endocardial cushion defects** or **AV canal defects,** both terms referring to abnormalities of derivatives of the endocardial cushions of the embryonic AV canal) are particularly common in children born with trisomy 21. These defects include an ostium primum ASD, a membranous VSD, and a mitral valve malformation, consisting of a cleft in the anterior leaflet or anterior and posterior bridging leaflets (Figure 31–22). Irreversible pulmonary vascular disease with shunt reversal may lead to cyanosis (see section on Eisenmenger Syndrome) and is extremely common in the adult who has had no attempt at repair. Residual mitral regurgitation is often encountered following repair. Even when the valve is competent in the early postoperative period, late regurgitation occurs in a small percentage of patients.

Coronary artery anomalies are seen not uncommonly as an isolated defect in the adult patient. They are found in approximately 1% of patients undergoing coronary arteriography and in approximately 0.3% of autopsies. An anomaly of particular importance is the left main coronary artery arising from the pulmonary trunk. This may present in infancy as cardiomyopathy and CHF from myocardial ischemia and systolic dysfunction. Sufficient myocardial collaterals from the right coronary artery may develop in a small number of patients, which allows survival into adulthood. Physical examination may reveal a continuous murmur, and clinical assessment may be remarkable for angina pectoris,

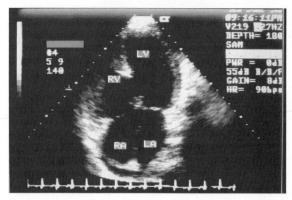

▲ **Figure 31–22.** Apical four-chamber view from a transthoracic echocardiogram in a patient with atrioventricular septal defect and Down syndrome. The crux of the heart is missing, and a large ostium primum atrial septal defect and large ventricular septal defect are evident. LA, left atrium; LV, left ventricle; RA, right atrium; RV, right ventricle.

myocardial infarction, dyspnea, syncope, and sudden death. Treatments include surgical closure of the left main artery with possible bypass to the left anterior descending artery or primary reanastomosis of the anomalous artery from the pulmonary artery to the aorta or the subclavian artery. There are many anatomic variations of the less severe coronary anomalies. When the left coronary artery arises from the right or noncoronary cusp and passes between the aorta and pulmonary artery, however, the patient is at increased risk for ischemia and sudden death. This diagnosis should be considered in young patients with exertional chest pain. TEE may identify anomalous coronary ostia. Although MRA or CT angiography may be diagnostic in skilled hands, coronary angiography is currently the diagnostic gold standard. The role for surgery in these patients is controversial and is usually reserved for patients with unequivocal evidence of ischemia and for young, athletic patients, who are at the highest risk for sudden cardiac death.

Coronary arteriovenous fistulas are more likely than serious coronary anomalies to permit survival to adulthood. Large fistulas draining into the right side of the circulation may be associated with a sizable shunt and can rarely present with CHF in infancy. Coronary steal may occur, leading to myocardial ischemia. In the adult, there may be a history of exertional dyspnea or chest pain and a continuous murmur on physical examination. TTE detects the dilated fistulous coronary artery in approximately 50% of patients. Abnormal continuous jets within the cardiac chambers (RV is most common) or in the pulmonary artery seen in color-flow Doppler should suggest this diagnosis. Cardiac catheterization showing the dilated coronary artery and fistulous communication confirms the diagnosis.

Congenital **sinus of Valsalva aneurysms** may coexist with supracristal VSDs and have the potential for catastrophic rupture with development of acute severe aortic regurgitation or pericardial tamponade. Although the perforation may be subacute with mild regurgitation, it nonetheless poses an ongoing risk for endocarditis. Echocardiography, with a transesophageal approach if necessary, is diagnostic. Surgical repair with a pericardial patch is indicated when rupture is present.

Angelini P. Coronary artery anomalies: an entity in search of an identity. *Circulation.* 2007;115(10):1296–305. [PMID: 17353457]

Misuraca L, et al. Coronary artery anomalies and their clinical relevance. *Monaldi Arch Chest Dis.* 2011;76(2):66–71. [PMID: 22128609]

Taylor AM, et al. Coronary artery imaging in grown up congenital heart disease: complementary role of magnetic resonance and x-ray coronary angiography. *Circulation.* 2000;101(14):1670–8. [PMID: 10758049]

▼ CYANOTIC CONGENITAL HEART DISEASE

Patients with cyanotic congenital heart disease have arterial oxygen desaturation resulting from the shunting of systemic venous blood to the arterial circulation, or from cardiac anatomy that mandates mixing of systemic and pulmonary venous blood. The shunting can occur at the level of the atrium (ASD), the ventricle (VSD), or the great vessels (PDA or aortopulmonary window), or in the lungs (pulmonary arteriovenous malformations or venovenous collaterals). If a right-to-left shunt is present, it implies a right-sided obstruction distal to that level or the presence of pulmonary vascular obstructive disease causing reversal of flow through a previously left-to-right shunting lesion.

There are many specific congenital cardiac lesions that cause cyanosis, and each of the specific diagnoses may have its own variations, making memorization of a comprehensive list of diagnoses difficult. However, the spectrum of basic cyanotic congenital lesions can be remembered as the "5 Ts": TOF, (complete) transposition of the great vessels, total anomalous pulmonary venous return, tricuspid atresia, and truncus arteriosus communis. The many remaining lesions can generally be thought of as variants of these basic diagnoses. The pathophysiology of each of these lesions is discussed in the respective section. Untreated cyanotic heart disease carries an extremely high mortality rate in the infant and child; therefore, most patients reaching adulthood have had reparative or palliative surgery. Those who reach adulthood without surgery are usually those with TOF or irreversible pulmonary vascular disease (eg, Eisenmenger syndrome) from underlying congenital cardiac lesions.

The importance of recognizing cyanotic heart disease in the adult lies not only in the potential for possible surgical or nonsurgical intervention but is also important for appropriate management of the extracardiac manifestations of long-standing cyanosis. The systemic complications of cyanotic heart disease include the development of hematologic and metabolic disorders. Neurologic abnormalities include infectious, hemorrhagic, and hypoxic disorders.

Hematologic disorders in adults with cyanotic congenital heart disease can significantly influence morbidity and mortality rates. Secondary erythrocytosis has been classified as either **compensated** or **decompensated.** Patients with compensated erythrocytosis are in equilibrium with stable hematocrits, no evidence of iron depletion, and few (if any) symptoms of hyperviscosity. Even with hematocrits above 70%, they do not appear to be at increased risk for cerebrovascular accidents and do not require phlebotomy. Patients with decompensated erythrocytosis have increased hematocrits (> 65%) with symptoms. Because iron deficiency and dehydration may also produce hyperviscosity, these conditions should be excluded and, if present, treated before phlebotomy is undertaken. Generally, phlebotomy is not recommended for patients with hematocrits of less than 65%. A bleeding diathesis is also associated with cyanotic heart disease; it is usually mild and requires no specific therapy except for the avoidance of heparin and aspirin. Because severe life-threatening bleeding can occur during surgical procedures, preoperative phlebotomy to attain a hematocrit just below 65% is recommended. Associated abnormalities include thrombocytopenia and hyperuricemia secondary to increased red cell turnover. Urolithiasis and urate nephropathy rarely occur, but gout is common. The last problem can be managed with conventional therapy, taking care to avoid the antiplatelet properties of anti-inflammatory agents. In managing CHF in cyanotic patients, diuretics must be used judiciously in order to avoid dehydration, which may exacerbate hyperviscosity, and thrombotic risk. These patients may also be more susceptible to digoxin toxicity.

Counseling of the young adult with reference to contraception, pregnancy, and exercise is especially important in this group of patients.

Palliative surgical procedures for complex cyanotic congenital heart disease performed during infancy or childhood in the early years of pediatric cardiothoracic surgery were associated with unique physical findings and specific complications. These procedures, such as aortopulmonary anastomoses (Waterston, Potts, Blalock-Taussig) and atrial switches (Senning and Mustard), are still commonly encountered in adult patients. These procedures may produce unique physical findings and specific complications, which are discussed later (see Palliative Surgical Procedures). Most of these procedures are no longer performed in children, since surgical techniques that optimize physiology and reduce complications have evolved over the years.

Foster E, et al. Task force 2: special health care needs of adults with congenital heart disease. *J Am Coll Cardiol.* 2001;37(5):1176–83. [PMID: 11300419]

TETRALOGY OF FALLOT & PULMONARY ATRESIA WITH VENTRICULAR SEPTAL DEFECT

 ESSENTIALS OF DIAGNOSIS

- ▶ History of exercise intolerance and squatting during childhood.
- ▶ Central cyanosis, mildly prominent RV impulse, murmur of PS (with sufficient pulmonary blood flow) and absent P_2.
- ▶ Mild RVH; occasionally, LVH.
- ▶ Chest radiograph shows classic boot-shaped heart (coeur en sabot) in severe cases without left-to-right shunt; LV enlargement and poststenotic pulmonary artery dilatation in milder cases; right-sided aortic arch in approximately 25% of patients.
- ▶ Echocardiogram shows RVH, overriding aorta, large perimembranous VSD, and obstruction of the RV outflow tract (subvalvular, valvular, supravalvular, or in the pulmonary arterial branches).
- ▶ Gradient across pulmonary outflow tract, normal pulmonary artery pressures, equalization of RV and LV pressures.
- ▶ Possibly anomalous branches of right coronary artery crossing RV outflow tract on coronary angiography.

▶ General Considerations

TOF is the most common form of cyanotic congenital heart disease. Without surgical intervention, most patients die in childhood; however, occasionally an acyanotic patient with only mild-to-moderate PS and minimal right-to-left shunting is encountered (pink TOF). Although it is called a tetralogy, only the membranous nonrestrictive VSD, PS, and dextroposition of the aorta contribute to the pathophysiology of this disorder (Figure 31–23). The severity of PS determines the RV systolic pressure and thus the degree of right-to-left shunting. The PS can be valvular or, more commonly, infundibular with an obstructing muscular band in the RV outflow tract. The other two components of the tetralogy include the aortic override and the secondary RVH. Both cyanotic and acyanotic patients are at high risk for endocarditis, much like patients with complicated VSD.

Common associated anomalies include ASD (15%; the pentalogy of Fallot or Cantrell), right-sided aortic arch (25%, most commonly seen in pulmonary atresia with VSD), and anomalous coronary distribution (about 10%). It is important to identify the origin of the left anterior descending artery from the right coronary cusp preoperatively because the artery courses over the RV infundibulum, a potential incision site for the repair. TOF is a form of conotruncal malformation that may occur in conjunction with DiGeorge syndrome. The chromosome 22q11.2 microdeletion is present in as many as 8–35% of patients with TOF, and routine screening for the deletion is now recommended for affected patients to guide appropriate management and identify those patients whose offspring will be at increased risk for congenital heart disease. In addition, mutations in the genes encoding the cardiac transcription factor NKX2-5 and the Notch-1 ligand Jagged have been reported in patients with TOF.

▶ Clinical Findings

A. Symptoms & Signs

The patient with TOF was typically a blue baby, cyanotic at birth. There is usually a history of exercise intolerance and squatting during childhood. Characteristic "tet spells," which are typified by episodic faintness and worsening cyanosis, are believed to be due to infundibular spasm and are generally diminished or absent by adulthood. Worsening cyanosis also occurs during exercise because of the associated systemic vasodilation and increased right-to-left shunt.

In severe cases of PS or atresia, the patient may have had life-saving surgical palliation with an aortopulmonary shunt. In the past, total repairs were not attempted until school age, but they are now being performed in infancy in most centers.

Physical examination reveals cyanosis and, less frequently, clubbing. The precordium is generally quiet, although a mild RV heave may be present. The intensity and duration of the pulmonic flow murmur vary with the degree of PS; P_2 is usually absent. In cases of pulmonary atresia with VSD (an extreme form of TOF), P_2 is absent by definition, and a continuous murmur may be audible over the back due to aortopulmonary collaterals. Patients who have had a "classic" Blalock-Taussig shunt, anastomosis of the subclavian to the side of the pulmonary artery, will have an absent pulse in the ipsilateral arm and a continuous murmur as long as the shunt is patent and functioning properly. A "modified" Blalock-Taussig shunt, interposing a small Gore-Tex tube between the subclavian artery and the pulmonary artery, preserves the brachial pulse and is easily occluded at the time of intracardiac repair. In patients who have had intracardiac repair, a low-pitched pulmonary regurgitation murmur is commonly audible. When the murmur occurs only in early diastole, it suggests clinically important residual regurgitation.

B. Diagnostic Studies

1. Electrocardiography and chest radiography—The ECG findings depend on the severity of the PS and the relative degree of shunting. If PS is severe, RVH is usually evident. If the PS is mild and the shunt is predominantly left to right, LVH may be evident. P waves are usually normal. Following intracardiac repair with infundibular resection, RBBB and varying forms of heart block are common.

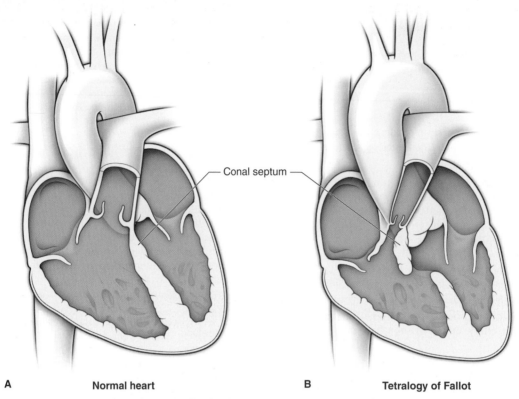

Conal septum — Conal septum

A   Normal heart   B   Tetralogy of Fallot

▲ **Figure 31–23.** Anatomy of tetralogy of Fallot (TOF). Note that in TOF, the conal septum is displaced anteriorly and to the right, resulting in a smaller pulmonary artery orifice and subpulmonic obstruction.

Postoperative atrial and ventricular arrhythmias are well-recognized complications. A QRS duration of > 180 ms has been shown to correlate with significant RV dilatation due to pulmonic regurgitation after surgical repair and to predict sudden cardiac death in patients with repaired TOF.

The radiographic findings also depend on the underlying individual pathophysiology. The typical boot-shaped coeur en sabot is seen when PS is severe and the LV is small. In these cases, pulmonary blood flow is reduced. Poststenotic pulmonary artery dilatation and a right-sided aortic arch may be visible on chest radiograph.

2. Echocardiography—Transthoracic two-dimensional and Doppler echocardiography demonstrates the features of this defect in its native and repaired state. The typical findings in patients with unrepaired TOF include severe RVH and a thickened, malformed pulmonary valve with poststenotic dilation. Alternatively, the level of stenosis may be primarily infundibular, with marked hypertrophic narrowing of the RV outflow tract (Figure 31–24). Systolic color-flow aliasing and a continuous wave Doppler gradient are detectable across the RV outflow tract or pulmonic valve. Two-dimensional imaging reveals a perimembranous

VSD with evidence of right-to-left shunting by color-flow imaging; the peak velocity of the VSD jet seen by spectral Doppler is usually low, reflecting the low interventricular gradient. The aortic root is variably enlarged and overrides the VSD. Aortic insufficiency, usually mild, may be present. Multiplanar TEE is particularly suited to define the anatomy of the RV outflow tract and the pulmonary valve when precordial imaging is difficult. In pulmonary atresia with VSD, aortopulmonary collaterals arising from the descending aorta can also be imaged by TEE.

Complications of TOF repair that can be detected noninvasively by echocardiography include residual outflow obstruction, pulmonary valve regurgitation, RV outflow-tract aneurysms, and VSD patch leak. In rare cases, an anomalous left anterior descending artery that was severed during surgery results in an LV apical aneurysm. Late LV systolic dysfunction has been increasingly recognized after TOF repair and is a risk factor for sudden cardiac death.

3. Magnetic resonance imaging—MRI has become an important noninvasive imaging modality in the assessment of patients with conotruncal anomalies, including TOF. Advantages include the ability to obtain accurate measurements

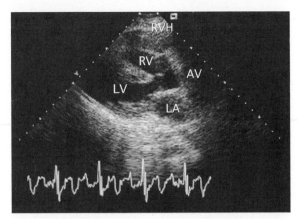

A

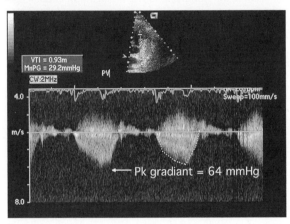

B

▲ **Figure 31–24.** Transthoracic echocardiogram in patient with tetralogy of Fallot. **A:** The parasternal long-axis view shows the ventricular septal defect, overriding aorta. **B:** Continuous wave Doppler signal across the right ventricular outflow tract shows a high-velocity, late-peaking jet. This demonstrates severe outflow tract obstruction. The late peak suggests a component of dynamic obstruction due to the hypertrophied infundibulum. AV, aortic valve; LA, left atrium; LV, left ventricle; Pk, peak; RV, right ventricle; RVH, right ventricular hypertrophy.

of RV size and ejection fraction, and pulmonic regurgitant fraction.

4. Cardiac catheterization—Cardiac catheterization reveals a gradient across the pulmonary outflow tract, usually normal pulmonary artery pressure, and equalization of RV and LV pressures. Angiography may better define the anatomy of the RV outflow tract and the size of the VSD (this information is usually available noninvasively). Coronary arteriography may demonstrate anomalous origins of the left coronary artery.

5. Other laboratory findings—Arterial saturation is variably reduced, and secondary erythrocytosis is present in the adult who has had no reparative surgery. In those with adequate surgical repair, arterial saturation should be normal.

▶ **Prognosis & Treatment**

Only 11% of individuals born with this lesion survive without palliative surgery beyond the age of 20, and only 3% survive beyond the age of 40. Because the PS protects TOF patients from the development of pulmonary hypertension, however, they are almost always surgical candidates as adults. Medically, it is important to avoid systemic vasodilator therapy in the patient whose TOF is uncorrected because a reduction in arterial blood pressure can increase right-to-left shunting. Endocarditis is relatively common in unrepaired TOF.

Total intracardiac repair with closure of the VSD and correction of the pulmonary or infundibular stenosis is indicated in the cyanotic patient to reduce symptoms and forestall complications attributable to cyanosis. The infundibulum is incised and resected to alleviate obstruction, with patching of the RV outflow tract or pulmonary annulus when necessary. The indications for surgery in the occasional acyanotic patient with TOF are similar to those of a patient with VSD. Important considerations prior to surgery include the presence of anomalies in the pulmonary and coronary arteries (approximately 15% and 35%, respectively). In pulmonary atresia with VSD, survival depends on the presence of well-developed bronchopulmonary or systemic-to-pulmonary collaterals. **In the rare adult with uncorrected pulmonary atresia with VSD,** surgical repair is either more complicated, requiring multiple procedures, or is not feasible.

In patients who undergo intracardiac repair for TOF, potentially significant postoperative anatomic sequelae are possible, including residual outflow obstruction, pulmonary valve regurgitation, RV aneurysms, and VSD patch leak. Pulmonary regurgitation may develop as a consequence of surgical repair of the RV outflow tract as well as with placement of a patch to enlarge the pulmonary artery annulus (transannular). Although even substantial regurgitation can be tolerated for long periods, enlargement of the RV eventually occurs, with resultant RV dysfunction, and repair or replacement of the pulmonary valve may be required.

A recent large retrospective study of risk stratification for arrhythmia and sudden death in these patients underscores the importance of vigilant assessment of ECG parameters (QRS duration) and hemodynamic characteristics (pulmonary regurgitation/obstruction) with timely intervention as a means of modifying the risk for sudden cardiac death in these patients. Appropriately timed surgical replacement of the regurgitant pulmonic valve has been shown to stabilize QRS prolongation and to reduce the incidence of ventricular arrhythmias when combined with cryoablation. It is hoped that two current trends in surgery will further reduce the incidence of arrhythmias. The first is avoidance of RV outflow-tract incisions by either a transatrial or transpulmonary approach. Second, earlier surgical intervention may allow less time for the development of ventricular fibrosis. Given the frequency of ventricular tachycardia and sudden cardiac death in these patients, clinicians should remain vigilant for symptoms of palpitations. Some experts advocate routine annual screening with a Holter monitor and referral for electrophysiologic study upon finding nonsustained ventricular tachycardia or complex ectopy, although no consensus exists at this point.

Ghai A, et al. Left ventricular dysfunction is a risk factor for sudden cardiac death in adults late after repair of tetralogy of Fallot. *J Am Coll Cardiol.* 2002;40(9):1675–80. [PMID: 12427422]

Knauth AL, et al. Ventricular size and function assessed by cardiac MRI predict major adverse clinical outcomes late after tetralogy of Fallot repair. *Heart.* 2008;94(2):211–6. [PMID: 17135219]

Pierpont ME, et al; American Heart Association Congenital Cardiac Defects Committee, Council on Cardiovascular Disease in the Young. Genetic basis for congenital heart defects: current knowledge: a scientific statement from the American Heart Association Congenital Cardiac Defects Committee, Council on Cardiovascular Disease in the Young: endorsed by the American Academy of Pediatrics. *Circulation.* 2007;115(23):3015–38. [PMID: 17519398]

Starr JP. Tetralogy of Fallot: yesterday and today. *World J Surg.* 2010;34(4):658–68. [PMID: 20091166]

Therrien J, et al. Impact of pulmonary valve replacement on arrhythmia propensity late after repair of tetralogy of Fallot. *Circulation.* 2001;103(2):2489–94. [PMID: 11369690]

EISENMENGER SYNDROME

ESSENTIALS OF DIAGNOSIS

▶ History of murmur or cyanosis in infancy, symptoms of dyspnea and exercise intolerance since childhood.

▶ Hemoptysis, chest pain, and syncope in the adult.

▶ Clubbing, cyanosis, and prominent P_2.

▶ Compensatory erythrocytosis, iron deficiency, and hyperuricemia.

▶ RVH; large central pulmonary arteries with peripheral pruning on chest radiograph.

▶ Severe RVH and right atrial enlargement, elevated pulmonary artery pressures, pulmonary regurgitation.

▶ Detection of bidirectional shunt.

▶ General Considerations

Three related, but not identical, clinical terms bear the name of Eisenmenger. The development of pulmonary hypertension in the presence of increased pulmonary blood flow is called the **Eisenmenger reaction. Eisenmenger syndrome** is a general term applied to pulmonary hypertension and shunt reversal in the presence of a congenital defect, including VSD, ostium primum ASD, AV canal defect, aortopulmonary window, or PDA. **Eisenmenger complex,** as originally described, is the association of a VSD with pulmonary hypertension and shunt reversal. The pulmonary hypertension usually develops before puberty; however, pulmonary vascular disease and the Eisenmenger reaction can occasionally develop after puberty in patients with ostium secundum ASDs.

In approximately 10% of patients with nonrestrictive VSDs, the pulmonary artery pressure does not fall normally in the neonatal period. Therefore, a large left-to-right shunt and CHF are not present. If the VSD goes undetected and the problem is not repaired before the infant reaches the age of 1 year, irreversible pulmonary vascular disease may result. The same is true for the other lesions associated with Eisenmenger syndrome. In patients with ostium secundum ASD, PVR almost always falls to normal levels in the neonatal period, and the development of irreversible pulmonary hypertension is far less common.

▶ Clinical Findings

A. Symptoms & Signs

Patients usually have a history of murmur during infancy, and cyanosis occurs later in childhood. Exertional dyspnea is the most commonly encountered symptom. Chest pain, hemoptysis, and presyncope are less common. Transient bacteremia can result in brain abscess as a result of right-to-left shunting and entry of bacteria into the cerebral circulation without the normal filtering through the pulmonary circulation.

Physical examination reveals cyanosis (involving the legs when the cause is PDA); cardiovascular examination is most remarkable for findings associated with pulmonary hypertension. The LV impulse is not displaced and an RV parasternal heave is present. The jugular venous pressure may be elevated in the presence of RV failure, and the *a* wave may be prominent. The first heart sound is normal, and P_2 is markedly accentuated. A systolic murmur of tricuspid regurgitation may be present, and a high-pitched diastolic murmur of pulmonary regurgitation (Graham Steell murmur) is common. In the presence of RV failure, hepatomegaly, ascites, and peripheral edema may be present.

B. Diagnostic Studies

1. Electrocardiography and chest radiography—The ECG shows evidence of right atrial enlargement and RVH with a rightward axis (Figure 31–25A). The presence of a leftward or superior axis suggests an ostium primum ASD or AV canal defect as the underlying cause (Figure 31–25B). Chest radiograph findings include RV enlargement with filling-in of the retrosternal air space, prominent proximal pulmonary arteries with pulmonary oligemia, and pruning of the peripheral pulmonary vessels.

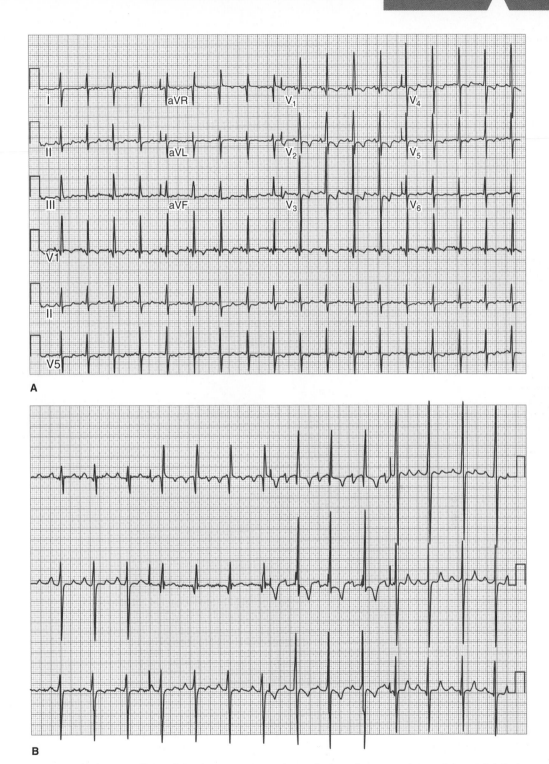

▲ **Figure 31–25. A:** Electrocardiograph in Eisenmenger syndrome from ostium secundum atrial septal defect with right ventricular hypertrophy and right-axis deviation. **B:** Electrocardiograph in Eisenmenger syndrome and atrioventricular canal defect with right ventricular hypertrophy and left anterior hemiblock.

2. Echocardiography—Severe RVH and right atrial enlargement is evident (Figure 31–26A). RV function may be normal until the late stages of the disease, at which time the right atrium enlarges. The LV appears small and underfilled; the septum deviates toward the LV. The level of shunt can be determined by two-dimensional imaging, aided by color-flow Doppler and saline contrast injection (Figure 31–26B). When a VSD is present, the flow velocity across the defect is low because of pressure equalization between the two ventricles. On the other hand, the tricuspid regurgitant velocity is increased and can be used to estimate the peak RV systolic pressure (Figure 31–26C). Pulmonary insufficiency with a high-velocity regurgitant jet is a frequent finding. Other valvular lesions are uncommon except in ostium primum ASD or AV canal defects, when mitral regurgitation is commonly present.

Eisenmenger syndrome can usually be differentiated from primary pulmonary hypertension noninvasively by TTE, although shunting across a patent foramen ovale may mimic an ASD with Eisenmenger syndrome and a PDA may be missed on color-flow Doppler in the presence of severe pulmonary hypertension. In these cases, further investigation with TEE or cardiac catheterization and sometimes cardiac MRI/MRA may be indicated.

3. Cardiac catheterization—The pathognomonic hemodynamic findings are elevated pulmonary artery pressure,

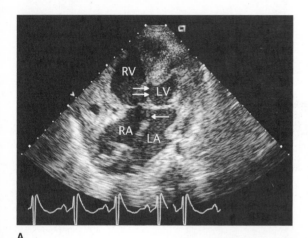

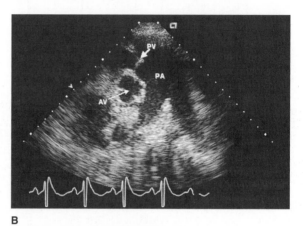

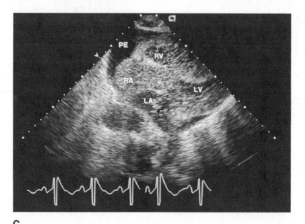

▲ **Figure 31–26. A:** Transthoracic echocardiogram in a 32-year-old woman with Down syndrome. She has Eisenmenger syndrome due to an atrioventricular septal defect. Four-chamber view shows hypertrophied right ventricular (RV) wall, ventricular septal defect (*double white arrow*), and ostium primum atrial septal defect (*single white arrow*). **B:** Parasternal short-axis view showing markedly dilated pulmonary artery (PA). **C:** Subcostal view after intravenous injection of agitated saline. The right atrium (RA) and right ventricle (RV) are opacified, and there is rapid appearance of contrast in the left atrium (LA) and ventricle (LV) (*double black arrow*). A moderate pericardial effusion (PE) is also noted. AV, aortic valve; PV, pulmonary valve.

increased PVR, and right-to-left shunting. The degree of residual left-to-right shunt should be measured. Oxygen should be administered during catheterization to determine whether pulmonary vascular reactivity persists. If PVR falls during oxygen or nitric oxide administration, increased left-to-right shunting can be measured. In this case, the patient may be a candidate for pulmonary vasodilator therapy and surgical repair.

4. Other laboratory findings—The arterial oxygen saturation by pulse oximetry or arterial blood gas measurements is markedly decreased. The hematocrit is elevated, with an overall increase in red cell mass. Iron deficiency is common, particularly after injudicious phlebotomies. Hyperuricemia caused by increased red cell turnover may be present.

▶ Prognosis & Treatment

Life expectancy is markedly shortened in patients with Eisenmenger syndrome; however, meticulous medical management can result in improved longevity in adults with this and other forms of cyanotic heart disease. The causes of death include uncontrollable hemoptysis (due to pulmonary infarction or pulmonary arteriolar rupture), arrhythmias with sudden death, progressive RV failure, and brain abscess.

The availability of a range of pulmonary vasodilators has revolutionized the management of Eisenmenger syndrome. Treatment with the oral agent bosentan has been shown in a large clinical trial to improve the functional status of these patients (see Chapter 30).

Surgical repair is contraindicated when the pulmonary vascular disease is fixed; that is, pulmonary resistance does not fall in response to oxygen or nitric oxide inhalation. In these patients, closure of the VSD (or other defects) increases the work of the RV, with a resultant excessively high mortality rate. Heart-lung transplantation offers hope for the adolescent and young adult with Eisenmenger syndrome, but the results support only guarded optimism. In addition, some centers are considering the feasibility of intracardiac repair in children after treatment with pulmonary vasodilator therapy to decrease the PVR.

Careful medical management of the complications of cyanotic congenital heart disease is crucial in these patients (see earlier section, Cyanotic Congenital Heart Disease). Counseling regarding contraception is crucial in these patients; pregnancy is accompanied by an unacceptably high rate of maternal and fetal mortality and is virtually contraindicated in patients with Eisenmenger syndrome (see later discussion).

Diller GP, et al. Pulmonary vascular disease in adults with congenital heart disease. *Circulation.* 2007;115(8):1039–50. [PMID: 17325254]

Galie N, et al; Bosentan Randomized Trial of Endothelin Antagonist Therapy-5 (BREATHE-5) Investigators. Bosentan therapy in patients with Eisenmenger syndrome: a multicenter, double-blind, randomized, placebo-controlled study. *Circulation.* 2006;114(1):48–54. [PMID: 16801459]

Gatzoulis MA, et al. Pulmonary arterial hypertension in paediatric and adult patients with congenital heart disease. *Eur Respir Rev.* 2009;18(113):154–61. [PMID: 20956136]

TRANSPOSITION OF THE GREAT ARTERIES

ESSENTIALS OF DIAGNOSIS

▶ History of cyanosis that worsens shortly after birth at the time of ductal closure.

▶ Prominent RV impulse, palpable and delayed A_2; murmurs from associated defects (eg, VSD, PS).

▶ Chest radiograph shows narrowing at base of heart in region of great vessels; prominent pulmonary vascularity unless PVR is increased.

▶ Right atrial enlargement, RVH; occasionally biventricular hypertrophy (with an associated VSD).

▶ Great arteries discordant with anterior and rightward aorta arising from the RV and leftward and posterior pulmonary artery arising from the LV. Atria and ventricles usually in normal position with severe RVH.

▶ General Considerations

The key to the pathophysiology of transposition of the great arteries (D-TGA) is that the pulmonary and systemic circulations exist in parallel rather than in the normal series relationship (Figure 31–27). Survival after birth therefore depends on mixing saturated and desaturated blood via a PDA or an ASD or VSD. If an ASD or VSD does not coexist with D-TGA, an atrial communication must be created (usually percutaneously via an atrial balloon septostomy [the Rashkind procedure]) to permit survival in the newborn once the ductus closes. Prostaglandin E_1 may be given to restore or maintain patency of the ductus arteriosus; however, this does not always provide adequate mixing. When a VSD is present, the physiologic consequences depend largely on whether associated PS is present. In the absence of PS, there is a risk of pulmonary vascular disease because of the increased pulmonary blood flow; in the presence of PS, an aortopulmonary shunt may be necessary to increase pulmonary blood flow.

▶ Clinical Findings

A. Symptoms & Signs

More males (3:1) are affected by this condition. There is a history of cyanosis at birth that worsens shortly thereafter when the ductus closes. In the infant with a large VSD, heart failure can occur with lesser degrees of cyanosis. In addition to profound central cyanosis, physical examination reveals a prominent RV impulse and murmurs caused by associated

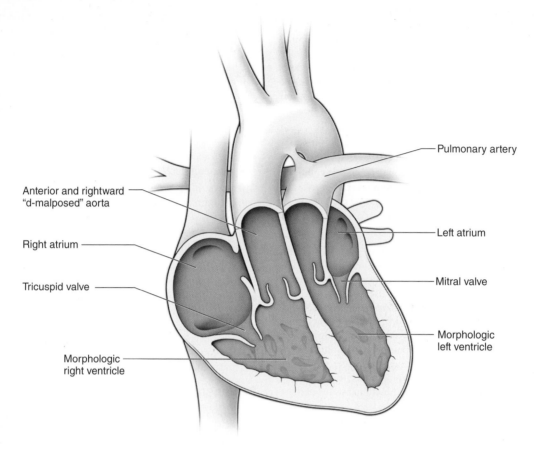

▲ **Figure 31–27.** Anatomy of transposition of the great arteries (D-TGA).

Labels:
- Pulmonary artery
- Anterior and rightward "d-malposed" aorta
- Left atrium
- Right atrium
- Tricuspid valve
- Mitral valve
- Morphologic left ventricle
- Morphologic right ventricle

defects (eg, VSD, PS). A$_2$ is typically loud and often palpable, as a consequence of the anterior malposition of the aortic valve. A$_2$ may also be delayed as a consequence of volume overload or RV dysfunction. The findings usually associated with a large PDA (see previous discussion of PDA) may be absent. The physical examination is often nondiagnostic and may actually provide more information about associated anomalies than about the presence of transposition.

B. Diagnostic Studies

1. Electrocardiography and chest radiography—The ECG usually demonstrates right atrial enlargement, a rightward QRS axis, and RVH. In the presence of a VSD, biventricular hypertrophy may be evident. The chest radiograph shows narrowing at the base of the heart in the region of the great vessels. In the newborn, prior to surgery, pulmonary vascularity is prominent unless pulmonary blood flow is limited by PS or, in older individuals, the PVR is increased by the associated pulmonary vascular disease. The RV and right atrium are prominent.

2. Echocardiography—The atria and ventricles are usually in the normal position with severe RVH. The great vessels are discordant with the anterior and rightward aorta arising from the RV, and leftward and posterior pulmonary artery arising from the LV. In the newborn, complete examination, using combined two-dimensional and color-flow Doppler imaging should confirm or exclude the presence of an associated ASD, VSD, or PS. In patients who have had an atrial switch operation, baffle obstruction and leaks can be detected by color-flow Doppler and contrast echocardiography. Late obstruction of the superior vena cava can be detected by contrast echocardiography with agitated saline injected into an arm vein, opacifying the inferior vena cava. After arterial switch procedures, echocardiography may show regurgitation of the neoaortic valve or stenosis of the neopulmonary valve or branches. MRI may also be helpful in determining the anatomy of the vena cava and pulmonary veins.

3. Cardiac catheterization—Invasive studies confirm the noninvasive diagnosis and the presence of associated defects. In the newborn, catheterization with a percutaneous atrial balloon septostomy is therapeutic and usually life-saving as well as diagnostic. The administration of intravenous prostaglandin E_1 to maintain ductal patency may preclude the need for an atrial septostomy if the oxygen saturations are adequate. In the adult with associated VSD, cardiac catheterization may be indicated to determine PVR or the severity of PS.

▶ Prognosis & Treatment

Without treatment, isolated D-TGA carries a mortality rate of greater than 90% in the first year of life. Infants with an ASD, a VSD, or a large PDA have higher oxygen saturations and better survival rates, but early surgery is indicated to prevent the development of irreversible pulmonary vascular disease.

Definitive repair of this defect was first undertaken in the early 1960s. The atrial switch operation (Mustard or Senning) redirects the pulmonary and systemic venous return at the atrial level. The atrial septum is excised, and using either a pericardial or prosthetic baffle, the systemic venous return is directed across the mitral valve into the left ventricle and the pulmonary venous return flows across the tricuspid valve into the RV. The postoperative physiology after an atrial switch procedure is similar to that of patients with C-TGA, in that the RV continues to supply the systemic circulation. Many of these patients have survived to lead productive lives; however, they are potentially faced with significant late postoperative complications, including sick sinus syndrome, atrial and ventricular tachyarrhythmias, baffle obstruction and leaks (approximately 15%), and systemic ventricular dysfunction (10–15%). The late (30-year) mortality rate is approximately 20%. Sudden (presumed arrhythmic) death and systemic ventricular failure are the most common causes of late death. Atrial arrhythmias are particularly common. In a large cohort study, sinus rhythm was present in 77% of patients at 5 years and only 40% of patients at 20 years. Atrial flutter, which may signal a higher risk for sudden death, was present in 14% of patients. Pacemaker implantation, which can pose technical challenges after atrial switch, was required in 11% of patients.

Repair since the early 1980s has favored the arterial switch procedure pioneered by Jatene. This repair reestablishes the LV as the systemic ventricle and has ameliorated many of such long-term complications of the atrial switch as arrhythmias, RV dysfunction, baffle stenosis, and tricuspid regurgitation.

Follow-up of patients after arterial switch procedures has recently become available. The late mortality rate is low, and good LV function and sinus rhythm have been maintained. Postoperative aortic regurgitation and the potential for development of coronary artery ostial stenosis and late supravalvular narrowing at the anastomotic sites are of concern but will require ongoing assessment.

Kammeraad JA, et al. Predictors of sudden cardiac death after Mustard or Senning repair for transposition of the great arteries. *J Am Coll Cardiol.* 2004;44(5):1095–102. [PMID: 15337224]

Legendre A, et al. Coronary events after arterial switch operation for transposition of the great arteries. *Circulation.* 2003; 108(Suppl 1):II186–90. [PMID: 12970230]

Losay J, et al. Late outcome after arterial switch operation for transposition of the great arteries. *Circulation.* 2001;104 (12 Suppl 1):I121–6. [PMID: 11568042]

Squarcia U, et al. Transposition of the great arteries. *Curr Opin Pediatr.* 2011;23(5):518–22. [PMID: 21849902]

Warnes CA. Transposition of the great arteries. *Circulation.* 2006; 114(24):2699–709. [PMID: 17159076]

TRICUSPID ATRESIA

 ESSENTIALS OF DIAGNOSIS

▶ History of either cyanosis (70%) or CHF (30%).

▶ Cyanotic patient with absent RV impulse and prominent LV impulse.

▶ Oligemic lung fields, right atrial and LV without RV enlargement in retrosternal airspace on chest radiograph.

▶ Evidence of LVH, absent or atretic tricuspid valve, ASD, small RV.

▶ General Considerations

Tricuspid atresia represents a spectrum of congenital defects characterized by the absence of connection between the right atrium and RV. In these patients, the tricuspid valve is absent or imperforate, the RV is hypoplastic, and the inflow portion of the RV is absent. Although an atrial communication is invariably present, the additional associated anomalies determine the ultimate pathophysiology and clinical presentation (Figure 31–28). Tricuspid atresia is usually classified according to the presence or absence of pulmonary stenosis and of malposition of the aorta and pulmonary artery. The great arteries are normally related in about 70% of the cases and are transposed in 30%. Pulmonary blood flow is supplied by either a PDA or aortopulmonary collaterals. Palliative surgery in this group is aimed at increasing pulmonary blood flow by a systemic venous or an arterial-to-pulmonary-artery shunt (see Palliative Surgical Procedures). A minority of patients will have a sufficiently large PDA to provide unrestricted pulmonary blood flow at the expense of ventricular volume overload, CHF, and the development of pulmonary vascular disease. In the 30% of patients born with tricuspid atresia and associated transposition of the great vessels, a VSD is usually present and no pulmonary obstruction is evident. These infants have CHF; pulmonary banding in the first year of life may prevent the development of irreversible pulmonary vascular disease and allow a later intracardiac repair to be performed.

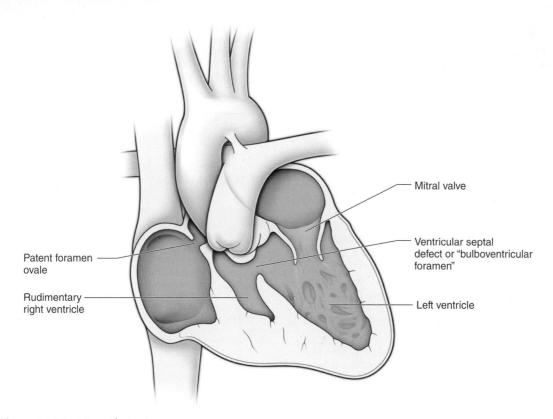

Mitral valve

Ventricular septal
defect or "bulboventricular
foramen"

Patent foramen
ovale

Rudimentary
right ventricle

Left ventricle

▲ **Figure 31–28.** Tricuspid atresia.

Adult survival without surgical intervention is rare. The clinical condition at presentation depends on the patient's underlying anatomy as well as the adequacy of the palliative procedure.

▶ Clinical Findings

A. Symptoms & Signs

A history of cyanosis predominates in patients with normally related great arteries, restrictive VSD, or PS or atresia. Patients with associated transposition of the great vessels and nonrestrictive VSD usually have a history of CHF from LV volume overload.

Physical examination is highly variable, but the absence of an RV impulse with a prominent LV impulse in a cyanotic patient suggests tricuspid atresia. The first heart sound is single, and the second heart sound often is as well. A continuous murmur may be present as a result of aortopulmonary collaterals or a Blalock-Taussig shunt.

B. Diagnostic Studies

1. Electrocardiography and chest radiography—The ECG reveals right atrial enlargement, LVH, and the absence

of right-sided precordial forces. This is the only cyanotic lesion associated with LVH at birth. In the adult, the chest radiograph usually shows oligemic lung fields and right atrial and LV prominence without RV enlargement in the retrosternal airspace.

2. Echocardiography and magnetic resonance imaging—Constant echocardiographic features include an absent or atretic, imperforate tricuspid valve, ASD, and a small RV. More variable features include the size of the RV, the presence and size of a VSD, the presence of pulmonary atresia or stenosis, and relationship of the great vessels (normal or transposed). Doppler examination can estimate the degree of PS and the gradient across the VSD. When PS is not present, the VSD gradient can be subtracted from the systolic arterial pressure to estimate the pulmonary artery systolic pressure. Color-flow Doppler imaging is helpful in confirming the pattern of flow and the site of the VSD (Figure 31–29). MRI can also be helpful in defining the anatomy.

3. Cardiac catheterization—Cardiac catheterization is used to determine operability by measuring PVR and the size of the pulmonary arteries. The RV cannot be entered through the right atrium, and the pulmonary artery (in the

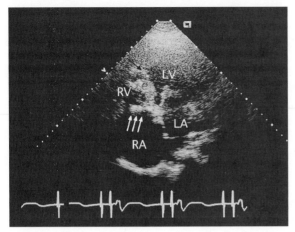

▲ **Figure 31–29.** Transthoracic echocardiogram in a 30-year-old woman with tricuspid atresia. This four-chamber view demonstrates the plate-like imperforate tricuspid annulus (*three white arrows*). The right atrium (RA) is markedly dilated, and the right ventricle (RV) is hypoplastic. A ventricular septal defect (*black arrow*) is noted. LA, left atrium; LV, left ventricle.

absence of atresia) must be entered from the LV through the VSD. Catheterization can also be used to assess the patency of palliative shunts.

▶ Prognosis & Treatment

Adults with tricuspid atresia will almost uniformly have undergone one or more operations to separate the pulmonary and systemic circulations. Patients with reduced pulmonary blood flow generally undergo a bidirectional Glenn procedure (superior vena cava to right pulmonary artery anastomosis) followed by a complete cavopulmonary anastomosis (Fontan procedure). Patients with increased pulmonary blood flow (typically those with associated d-malposition) may undergo pulmonary arterial banding as an initial procedure. The 1-year survival rate among patients who have not undergone palliative surgery is approximately 10%. Patients who have had successful modified Fontan procedures have widely variable outcomes, but routinely survive well into adulthood (see Palliative Surgical Procedures).

Lan YT, et al. Outcome of patients with double-inlet left ventricle or tricuspid atresia with transposed great arteries. *J Am Coll Cardiol.* 2004;43(1):113–9. [PMID: 14715192]

Mair DD, et al. The Fontan procedure for tricuspid atresia: early and late results of a 25-year experience with 216 patients. *J Am Coll Cardiol.* 2001;37(3):933–9. [PMID: 11693773]

Sittiwangkul R, et al. Outcomes of tricuspid atresia in the Fontan era. *Ann Thorac Surg.* 2004;77(3):889–94. [PMID: 14992893]

Wald RM, et al. Outcome after prenatal diagnosis of tricuspid atresia: a multicenter experience. *Am Heart J.* 2007;153(5):772–8. [PMID: 17452152]

PULMONARY ATRESIA WITH INTACT VENTRICULAR SEPTUM

 ESSENTIALS OF DIAGNOSIS

▶ History of cyanosis at birth, worsening at the time of ductal closure.

▶ Single S_2; continuous murmur is rare.

▶ Prominent LV forces.

▶ Oligemic lung fields, enlarged cardiac silhouette on chest radiograph.

▶ ASD, small RV, absent pulmonary valve. In adults, a palliative shunt or RV-to-pulmonary-artery conduit.

▶ General Considerations

Pulmonary atresia with intact ventricular septum is rarely encountered as an unpalliated defect in the adult population. The pulmonary valve is absent or imperforate, and blood flow is entirely through a PDA in the newborn. As in tricuspid atresia, an atrial communication exists through which the left atrium receives all of the systemic and pulmonary venous return. The volume-overloaded LV pumps the total blood flow into the aorta, and in most cases, all the pulmonary blood flow is received retrograde via the ductus. When the ductus closes, cyanosis may worsen acutely, and pulmonary blood flow must be restored by a palliative shunt. The RV may be diminutive, normal, or increased in size, and the tricuspid valve is, respectively, atretic, normal, or severely regurgitant. The high pressure in the RV is decompressed through dilated coronary circulation (ie, coronary sinusoids) into the left or right coronary artery. The presence of the sinusoids directly relates to RV pressure and inversely to the amount of tricuspid regurgitation. These factors largely determine the clinical and echocardiographic findings.

▶ Clinical Findings

Patients have a history of cyanosis at birth that worsens shortly afterward, at the time of ductal closure. The physical examination is variable, and the findings depend on the size of the RV and the presence of tricuspid regurgitation. The chest radiograph may reveal oligemic lung fields and an enlarged cardiac silhouette, caused by the enlargement of the LV. The main pulmonary artery segment is concave. The echocardiogram most commonly shows an ASD; a hypertrophied RV wall with a small cavity; a patent but small tricuspid valve; and a thickened, immobile, atretic pulmonary valve with no Doppler evidence of blood flow through it. The ductus arteriosus is seen running vertically from the aortic arch to the pulmonary artery (ie, vertical ductus). In adults, a palliative shunt (see section on Tricuspid Atresia) or an RV-to-pulmonary-artery conduit is almost always present.

Cardiac catheterization reveals systemic or suprasystemic RV pressures, and the catheter cannot be passed from the RV to the pulmonic artery. Angiography of the RV fails to opacify the pulmonary arteries, and contrast may fill the sinusoidal vessels that often communicate with the coronary arteries.

▶ Prognosis & Treatment

Three categories of surgical intervention exist for infants with pulmonary atresia with intact ventricular septum. The intervention selected depends on the size of the RV and the presence or absence of coronary sinusoids or coronary artery anomalies. When the RV is of adequate size for anticipated future growth, a connection is established between the RV and main pulmonary artery to prepare for a two-ventricle repair. A systemic-to-pulmonary-artery shunt is performed at the same time. Generally, an RV-to-pulmonary-artery conduit (with or without a valve) can be placed in the older child. Problems from valvular obstruction or degeneration and conduit obstruction caused by pseudo-intimal thickening can be detected by Doppler echocardiography. A two-ventricle repair is not possible in the subset of these patients with severely hypoplastic RVs. Therefore, a systemic-to-pulmonary-artery shunt without the connection to the RV is performed, with anticipation of a Fontan procedure at a later date. Patients who have a rudimentary RV and sinusoidal channels serving as the major source of coronary circulation, with perfusion by desaturated blood, represent a special problem. Decompression of the RV by connection with the pulmonary artery may result in a reversal of coronary flow into the RV, thereby producing myocardial ischemia. If coronary anomalies are identified by an aortogram, the sinusoids are left alone, and a systemic-to-pulmonary-artery shunt is performed in anticipation of a future Fontan-type operation. Overall, the prognosis in pulmonary atresia is limited, and although palliative surgery improves longevity, these patients require careful surveillance for complications of the surgery in addition to the underlying cyanotic heart disease. An exciting therapeutic innovation of recent years for patients with a well-formed but imperforate pulmonic valve is the development of radiofrequency-assisted valve perforation followed by balloon valvotomy. This has permitted completely percutaneous repair of the defect, provided that there is a patent infundibulum and a non–RV-dependent coronary circulation. The first patients to have undergone this procedure will be entering adulthood shortly.

Alwi M. Management algorithm in pulmonary atresia with intact ventricular septum. *Catheter Cardiovasc Interv.* 2006;67(5): 679–86. [PMID: 16572430]

▼ OTHER CYANOTIC CONGENITAL HEART DEFECTS

It is increasingly common to encounter adults with complex forms of cyanotic congenital heart disease who have had some sort of palliative surgery. In addition to the conditions already discussed, there are many variants of the single-ventricular and double-outlet-ventricular anomalies. Most common among these are the **double-inlet LV, double-outlet RV, and hypoplastic left heart.** The anatomic features of the dominant ventricle that identify it as a right or left ventricle on echocardiography include the trabeculae (coarse in an RV, smooth in an LV), the presence of the moderator band (RV), the presence of septal attachments of the AV valve (RV), and the presence of conus tissue between the annuli of the AV and subarterial valves (RV). Sometimes a rudimentary second ventricle is present. In the absence of pulmonary or infundibular stenosis, pulmonary vascular disease is prevalent; subaortic stenosis and AV valve regurgitation are also common. Cyanosis is invariably present as a consequence of mixing of systemic and pulmonary venous blood. Survival into adulthood is more likely in patients with PS.

The defect in **truncus arteriosus communis** arises from a failure of the single truncus in the embryo to divide into pulmonary and aortic vessels; and the pulmonary artery, aorta, and coronary arteries arise from a single main trunk. Although the anatomy of this lesion varies, a VSD is always present. The single semilunar valve, often with more than three cusps, is usually incompetent. The LV is faced with not only the volume overload of both pulmonary and systemic circulations but also that caused by truncal valve regurgitation. Cyanosis is present as a consequence of shunting of blood from the RV into the truncus. The mortality rate in the first year of life from CHF is high. Pulmonary branch stenosis and increased PVR may improve prognosis by decreasing the likelihood of CHF. Treatment consists of closure of the VSD, surgical separation of the pulmonary arteries from the truncus, and placement of a valved conduit to connect them to the RV. Late sequelae include progressive truncal valve regurgitation, progressive pulmonary vascular disease, and the need for conduit revision because of patient growth and valve degeneration.

In **total anomalous pulmonary veins,** the pulmonary venous flow enters the right atrium either directly or by one of many possible connections including the coronary sinus, superior vena cava, inferior vena cava, portal vein, hepatic vein, and ductus venosus. Because the venous blood mixes in the right atrium, cyanosis is present. There is an atrial communication, and the degree of cyanosis depends on the size of the ASD and the PVR. If left untreated, most (80%) die within the first year of life. The subdiaphragmatic anomalous veins are more likely to be associated with pulmonary venous obstruction. Surgical correction consists of connecting the common pulmonary venous channel to the left atrium. Obstruction may recur following surgery in those patients in whom obstruction was originally present; in others, the postoperative course is usually uncomplicated.

▼ PALLIATIVE SURGICAL PROCEDURES

In cyanotic congenital heart disease associated with diminished pulmonary blood flow, palliative procedures have been aimed at increasing pulmonary blood flow by directly or indirectly shunting blood from the systemic veins or systemic circulation. These procedures have continued to evolve.

The **Fontan procedure** (with its many modifications), the final common pathway for single ventricle repair, obviates the need for an RV by rerouting the venous return from the superior and inferior vena cava directly to the pulmonary circulation, thus separating the systemic and pulmonary venous return. This operation was originally used in patients with tricuspid atresia but currently is the palliative procedure of choice for a variety of congenital heart defects, including hypoplastic left heart syndrome and morphologic single ventricle when the pulmonary bed has been protected by congenital or palliative (ie, pulmonary band) stenosis. The Fontan procedure performed in adulthood carries a relatively low perioperative risk and leads to relief of cyanosis and improved functional class. However, arrhythmias, protein-losing enteropathy, and progressive systemic ventricular dysfunction remain ongoing concerns. The extracardiac Fontan procedure (direct cavopulmonary anastomosis) may decrease the incidence of arrhythmias. Thromboembolic disease is also a major cause of morbidity and mortality among patients after the Fontan procedure, and this recognition has led some cardiologists to advocate prophylactic anticoagulation in these patients. However, insufficient data exist to support a blanket recommendation on this issue. The modified, or bidirectional, **Glenn procedure** (superior vena cava to confluent pulmonary artery) can be used as a staging procedure for a future Fontan procedure or as a palliative shunt that can increase pulmonary blood flow when a Fontan is contraindicated because of poor ventricular function. Because right atrial distention does not occur, atrial arrhythmias may be less common.

In cyanotic patients with inadequate pulmonary blood flow (eg, TOF, pulmonary and tricuspid atresia), early surgical **systemic-to-pulmonary shunts** are life-saving procedures. The **Waterston** (ascending-aorta-to-pulmonary-artery) and **Potts** (descending-aorta-to-pulmonary-artery) shunts have been largely abandoned because of the high frequency of pulmonary hypertension, stenosis distal to the shunt sites, and considerable difficulty with surgical take down, but adult patients with these types of shunts are still infrequently encountered. Pulmonary artery pressure can be estimated noninvasively using the brachial artery systolic cuff pressure and continuous wave Doppler echocardiography to measure the gradient between aorta and pulmonary artery across the shunt. The classic **Blalock-Taussig shunt** (subclavian artery anastomosed to the pulmonary artery) has a much lower risk of pulmonary vascular disease, with preferential blood flow into one lung (usually the left). Even when pulmonary vascular disease develops in the ipsilateral lung, the other lung is usually protected and late intracardiac repair may be possible. Because the subclavian artery is diverted, the ipsilateral arm is pulseless. The modified Blalock-Taussig shunt (now more commonly performed)

uses a synthetic conduit and maintains perfusion to the arm. These shunts can become obstructed with recurrence of cyanosis, loss of the continuous murmur on physical examination, and decreased flow on Doppler echocardiography.

In the **Rastelli procedure,** extracardiac conduits from the right ventricle to the pulmonary artery may be used in pulmonary atresia and C-TGA with PS, truncus arteriosus, and double-outlet RV with PS. They can be synthetic (heterograft) or cadaveric (homograft) and may or may not contain valves. Problems are caused by valvular obstruction or degeneration and obstruction of shunts, baffles, and conduits. Continued clinical and noninvasive follow-up is essential in this group of patients.

▼ ARRHYTHMIAS IN CONGENITAL HEART DISEASE

Rhythm disturbances are a common source of morbidity among adult patients with congenital heart disease. Intra-atrial reentrant tachycardia (resembling atrial flutter) is particularly common in patients with prior atriotomies and atrial suture lines and is often poorly tolerated. Furthermore, the development of atrial flutter/intra-atrial reentrant tachycardia or atrial fibrillation may be a risk factor for sudden death. Modern interventional electrophysiologic techniques, using three-dimensional mapping and radiofrequency ablation, have expanded treatment options, and early electrophysiologic consultation should be considered for patients with complex congenital heart disease and recurrent atrial arrhythmias. Ventricular tachycardia is relatively common in patients with prior ventriculotomies (particularly for TOF repair) and with myopathic ventricles. Clinicians should have a low threshold to perform Holter monitoring in these patients, and some advocate routine annual testing in patients with TOF. Sinus node dysfunction occurs frequently in patients with atrial isomerism or with prior Fontan or atrial switch operations. The resultant bradycardia is associated with a higher rate of intra-atrial reentrant tachycardia or atrial fibrillation in these patients. AV node dysfunction is commonly seen in patients as a consequence of surgery and also in patients with AV septal defect and C-TGA. The indications for pacing are similar to those in the general population, although an awareness of the patient's anatomy is important because patients with atrial switch procedures or single ventricles often require placement of epicardial pacing leads.

▼ PREVENTION OF INFECTIVE ENDOCARDITIS

The risk of infective endocarditis remains an issue of ongoing concern in many patients with congenital cardiac defects. The absolute magnitude of risk varies considerably from one lesion to another and is also dependent on whether the patient has been surgically treated. In 2007, the American Heart Association revised its guidelines regarding infective endocarditis prophylaxis. The revised guidelines suggest a much more conservative approach to the use of prophylactic antibiotics. Broadly speaking, infective endocarditis prophylaxis is now recommended in only three groups of patients with congenital heart disease: (1) those with unrepaired cyanotic congenital heart disease, including patients with palliative shunts and conduits; (2) those with a defect completely repaired (either surgically or by catheter-based intervention), using prosthetic material or device, during the first 6 months after the procedure; and (3) those with repaired congenital heart disease who have residual shunts at the site of or adjacent to the site of a patch or device. The risk of endocarditis in individual lesions is summarized in Table 31–1.

▼ GENETIC COUNSELING & PREGNANCY

As many young adults with congenital heart disease have entered or are about to enter their reproductive years, genetic counseling and prepregnancy consultation are an important component of their care. The risk of congenital heart defects increases to 5–10% (higher in specific disorders) in the offspring of patients with congenital heart disease. Preconception genetic counseling and genetic testing are indicated for patients with syndromic congenital heart disease as well as for patients with nonsyndromic congenital heart disease and a family history of congenital heart disease. In addition, testing for the 22q11 deletion is indicated in patients with TOF, truncus arteriosus, aortic arch anomalies, or VSD who display at least one other feature of the 22q11 deletion syndrome (including dysmorphic facies, cleft palate, hypernasal speech, learning disabilities, behavioral or psychiatric disorders, thymic abnormalities, or hypocalcemia).

Most patients with acyanotic congenital heart disease can successfully carry a pregnancy to term. A small number of conditions place the patient and fetus at high risk during pregnancy. These include unrepaired cyanotic heart disease, Eisenmenger syndrome with severe pulmonary vascular disease/pulmonary hypertension, Marfan syndrome with a dilated aortic root, severe LV outflow obstruction, and moderate to severe systolic dysfunction of the systemic ventricle. Patients with these conditions should be advised against pregnancy. Other patients should be risk-stratified with respect to their tolerance of the anticipated hemodynamic changes of pregnancy and labor, namely expansion of intravascular volume, reduction of vascular resistance, and augmentation of cardiac output. It is therefore helpful to assess exercise tolerance prior to conception. Maternal and fetal mortality rates vary with functional class: in New York Heart Association (NYHA) class I, they are 0% and 0.4%, respectively; in NYHA class IV, the rates are 30% and 6.8%, respectively. Although pulmonary edema occurs less commonly than in patients with acquired heart disease, it may be useful to assess ventricular function noninvasively

prepartum and in the early months of pregnancy. Patients with significant congenital heart disease should receive close follow-up during pregnancy by a cardiologist and should receive care in a high-risk obstetric clinic. Fetal echocardiography should be offered when the parent or a previous child is affected. Prophylaxis during vaginal delivery is generally recommended for those at high risk for endocarditis (see Table 31–1). For a complete discussion of pregnancy in patients with heart disease, please see Chapter 33.

▼ RECOMMENDATIONS FOR EXERCISE & SPORTS PARTICIPATION

General recommendations regarding exercise should be individualized to the patient following a complete clinical and noninvasive evaluation. Exercise testing and Holter monitoring should be included in this evaluation to define exercise capacity and detect significant asymptomatic arrhythmias. No exercise restrictions are recommended for patients with small or repaired ASDs, VSDs, or PDAs, repaired AV septal defects, repaired total or partial anomalous pulmonary venous connection, mild PS, repaired coarctation, or repaired congenital coronary artery anomalies, or patients with D-TGA who have had an arterial switch procedure. Patients with moderate PS, mild aortic stenosis, completely repaired TOF, or AV septal defect with moderate mitral regurgitation should be restricted to moderate dynamic and isometric exercise. Patients with Ebstein anomaly, D-TGA after atrial switch procedure, C-TGA, or univentricular heart/Fontan circulation should be restricted to moderate dynamic exercise and mild isometric exercise. Patients with moderate aortic stenosis or TOF with residual disease should be restricted to mild dynamic and static exercise. Patients with Eisenmenger syndrome should be restricted to mild dynamic exercise.

▼ ACQUIRED HEART DISEASE IN ADULTS WITH CONGENITAL HEART DISEASE

It is important not to ignore the presence of acquired heart disease in adults with congenital heart disease. Acquired and congenital heart lesions may interact in unexpected ways, for example, the association of rheumatic mitral stenosis causing increased shunting across an ASD in Lutembacher syndrome. Impaired diastolic function from hypertension or coronary artery disease in a patient with an ASD may also increase the magnitude of the left-to-right shunt. Similarly, increased systemic vascular resistance from hypertension in a patient with a VSD may worsen the shunt. The clinician must exclude coronary artery disease as a cause of chest pain in adults with congenital aortic stenosis and pulmonary hypertension. In addition, the progression of atherosclerotic coronary disease may be accelerated in association with aortic coarctation.

Table 31–1. Endocarditis in Adults with Congenital Heart Disease

Defect	M:F	Associated Defects	Risk of Endocarditis
Acyanotic			
Bicuspid AV	4:1	Coarctation	High
Valvar PS	1:1	VSD (see TOF), Noonan syndrome	Low (mild PS), intermediate (severe PS)
ASD secundum	1:2	Mitral valve prolapse	Low
ASD primum	1:1	Bridging AV valve leaflets, trisomy 21	Intermediate (with MR)
AV septal defect			
VSD	1:1	PS (see TOF), AR	Intermediate-high (unoperated or with AR)
			Low (operated without AR)
PDA	1:2–3	Coexists with many complex syndromes	Low (ligated), intermediate (patent)
Coarctation	2:1	Bicuspid AV	Low (operated[1]), intermediate (without treatment)
C-TGA	M > F	VSD, infundibular PS	Low (isolated C-TGA)
Ebstein anomaly	1:1	ASD	Low-intermediate
		PFO	
Coronary AV fistulae	1:1		Intermediate
Cyanotic			
TOF	1.5:1	RAA, ASD	Intermediate
Eisenmenger syndrome	M < F	VSD, ASD, PDA	Low
Tricuspid atresia	1:1[2]	Pulmonary atresia, ASD, VSD	?
Pulmonary atresia with intact septum	1:1		?
D-TGA	2–4:1	ASD, PFO, PDA, VSD, PS, RAA	Intermediate
Postoperative			
Fontan			Variable
Glenn			Variable
Blalock-Taussig			High
RV-PA conduit			High

[1]Unless there is associated bicuspid AV.
[2]In tricuspid atresia with transposition, M > F.
AR, aortic regurgitation; ASD, atrial septal defect; AV, aortic valve; C-TGV, congenitally corrected transposition of the great vessels; F, female; M, male; MR, mitral regurgitation; PA, pulmonary artery; PDA, patent ductus arteriosus; PFO, patent foramen ovale; PS, pulmonic stenosis; RAA, right-sided aortic arch; RV, right ventricle; TOF, tetralogy of Fallot; VSD, ventricular septal defect.

Harris IS. Management of pregnancy in patients with congenital heart disease. *Prog Cardiovasc Dis.* 2011;53(4):305–11. [PMID: 21295672]

Hirth A, et al. Recommendations for participation in competitive and leisure sports in patients with congenital heart disease: a consensus document. *Eur J Cardiovasc Prev Rehabil.* 2006;13(3):293–9. [PMID: 16926656]

Pierpont ME, et al; American Heart Association Congenital Cardiac Defects Committee, Council on Cardiovascular Disease in the Young. Genetic basis for congenital heart defects: current knowledge: a scientific statement from the American Heart Association Congenital Cardiac Defects Committee, Council on Cardiovascular Disease in the Young: endorsed by the American Academy of Pediatrics. *Circulation.* 2007;115(23):3015–38. [PMID: 17519398]

Walsh EP, et al. Arrhythmias in adult patients with congenital heart disease. *Circulation.* 2007;115(4):534–45. [PMID: 17261672]

Cardiac Tumors

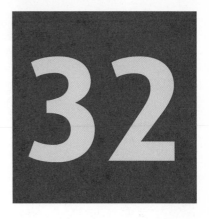

32

Bill P.C. Hsieh, MD
Rita F. Redberg, MD, MSc

ESSENTIALS OF DIAGNOSIS

▶ An uncommon but important differential diagnosis of cardiac masses.

▶ Diagnosis is suspected by history, physical examination, and imaging characteristics and confirmed by biopsy of mass.

▶ General Considerations

Cardiac tumors arise either as a primary tumor of the heart or more commonly from metastasis of a distant noncardiac primary tumor. Because of the low incidence and nonspecific clinical manifestations, cardiac tumors have often been diagnosed incidentally during evaluation of a seemingly unrelated problem or misdiagnosed as other cardiac conditions. A high index of suspicion in combination with characteristic cardiovascular imaging study is essential for rapid identification of cardiac tumors.

A. Metastatic Cardiac Tumors

Metastatic cardiac tumors are a 100-fold more common than primary tumors. Cardiac metastases often present as pericardial effusions; myocardial, coronary, and intracavitary involvement occur uncommonly, in order of decreasing frequency. The tumor that has the highest predilection for metastasis to the heart is disseminated malignant melanoma, which occurs in 50–65% of afflicted patients (Figure 32–1). The common noncardiac sources of metastatic cardiac neoplasms are neoplasm of the lungs, hematopoietic (lymphoma and leukemia) and gastrointestinal cancers (esophageal and liver), breast cancer, and renal cell carcinoma. Cancers from the respiratory system have been consistently shown to be the most common source of cardiac metastasis in different series; the relative proportion of other primary noncardiac

malignancy for cardiac metastasis varies according to the local cancer incidence.

Malignant cells from any single source can metastasize to the heart via multiple routes and can often seed in multiple cardiac structures. For example, adenocarcinoma of the colon can metastasize to the heart by lymphatic or hematogenous spread, usually affecting first the pericardium and then the myocardium. Cardiac metastases that occur in patients with colon cancer are usually preceded by involvement of other organs. Metastases to the endocardium have been reported in renal cell carcinoma, which can also extend into the inferior vena cava, and the tumor thrombus occasionally involves the right atrium (Figure 32–2).

Butany J, et al. A 30-year analysis of cardiac neoplasm at autopsy. *Can J Cardiol.* 2005;21(8):675–80. [PMID: 16003450]

B. Primary Tumors

Primary tumors of the heart are rare, with an incidence from 0.001–0.03% reported in unselected autopsy studies. Although myxoma has been traditionally reported to be the most frequent tumor type in adults, increasing utilization of imaging studies has revealed similar frequency of papillary fibroelastoma. In the pediatric population, rhabdomyomas represent the most common type (Table 32–1).

1. Benign—The majority (75–80%) of primary cardiac tumors are benign and therefore potentially curable.

A. MYXOMAS—These tumors account for approximately half of benign cardiac tumors and are usually found in patients between 30 and 60 years old, with a mean age of onset of 51 years. They occur predominantly in women; although most are isolated or sporadic, they can also be familial or complex. Less than 10% of myxomas are familial and are apparently transmitted in an autosomal dominant pattern. Familial myxoma presents earlier in life, with a mean age of onset of 25 years. Complex cardiac myxomas or the familial

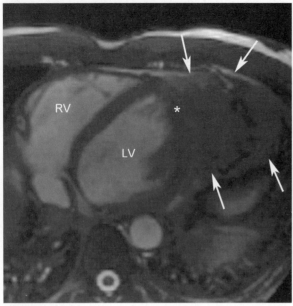

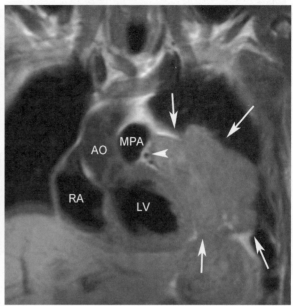

A   B

▲ **Figure 32–1.** Magnetic resonance imaging of the heart in a 50-year-old man who presented with dyspnea on exertion, 3 months after a diagnosis of melanoma on his back was made. A large pericardial mass was demonstrated on (**A**) bright blood-cine steady-state free precession image in axial plane. The *arrows* show the extension of the mass into the pleural space and possibly lung parenchyma. The *asterisk* indicates different texture of the myocardial signal, suggesting myocardial invasion of the mass. (**B**) Coronal black-blood T1-weighted image showing extension of the mass anteriorly and superiorly to impinge on the proximal left anterior descending artery (*arrow head*). Biopsy of the mass confirmed metastatic melanoma. AO, aorta; LV, left ventricle; MPA, main pulmonary artery; RA, right atrium; RV, right ventricle. (Courtesy of Karen Ordovas).

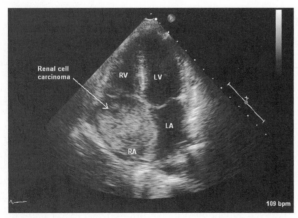

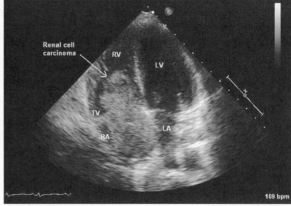

A   B

▲ **Figure 32–2.** Transthoracic echocardiogram in a 65-year-old man with a history of renal cell carcinoma in whom dyspnea and lower extremity edema developed. **A:** The apical four-chamber view shows a large mass most likely representing metastatic renal cell carcinoma in the right atrium. **B:** During diastole, the tumor prolapses through the tricuspid valve. LA, left atrium; LV, left ventricle; RA, right atrium; RV, right ventricle; TV, tricuspid valve.

Table 32–1. World Health Organization Classification of Tumors of the Heart

Benign tumors and tumor-like lesions
   Cardiac myxoma
   Rhabdomyoma
   Papillary fibroelastoma
   Lipoma
   Cardiac fibroma
   Hemangioma
   Histiocytoid cardiomyopathy
   Hamartoma of mature cardiac myocytes
   Adult cellular rhabdomyoma
   Inflammatory myofibroblastic tumor
   Cystic tumor of the atrioventricular node
Malignant tumors
   Metastatic tumors
   Angiosarcoma
   Rhabdomyosarcoma
   Fibrosarcoma and myxoid fibrosarcoma
   Leiomyosarcoma
   Liposarcoma
   Cardiac lymphomas
   Synovial sarcoma
   Undifferentiated pleomorphic sarcoma
   Epithelioid hemangioendothelioma
   Malignant pleomorphic fibrous histiocytoma
Pericardial tumors
   Metastatic pericardial tumors
   Solitary fibrous tumor
   Malignant mesothelioma
   Germ cell tumors

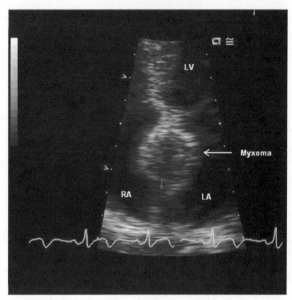

▲ **Figure 32–3.** Transthoracic echocardiogram in an apical four-chamber view showing a mass in the interatrial septum. The mass was resected and found to be an atrial myxoma. LA, left atrium; LV, left ventricle; RA, right atrium.

Carney complex may include such features as multiple pigmented skin lesions (lentigines), myxoid fibroadenomas of the breast, tumors of the pituitary and testes, and primary pigmented nodular adrenocortical disease. Carney complex appears to be genetically heterogenous with gene localization on chromosome 2p16 and chromosome 17q22-24. The majority of Carney complex appears to be caused by a mutation in the *PRKAR1α* gene that encodes the R1α regulatory subunit of the cyclic adenosine monophosphate–dependent protein kinase A (PKA). Patients with familial or complex myxomas are more likely than those with sporadic myxomas to have multiple (30–50%) and recurrent (12–22%) tumors. This occasional recurrence of myxomas and a few reported cases of invasion of surrounding tissue by the tumor suggest that myxomas have some low-grade malignant features.

Macroscopically, myxomas are pedunculated and gelatinous in consistency; the surface may be smooth, irregular, or friable. Friable or villous, myxomas are associated with a higher risk of embolization, whereas larger tumors with a smooth surface tend to present with obstructive cardiovascular symptoms. Microscopically, myxoma is characterized by islands of tumor cells with variable shapes (round,

elongated, or polyhedral) scattered throughout pale-staining extracellular matrix. The tumor cells are thought to be derived from mesenchymal cardiomyogenic precursor cells.

Most myxomas (74%) occur in the left atrium, although they can occur in any chamber (right atrium, 18%; right ventricle, 4%; left ventricle, 4%) or on any valve. They often arise from the endocardial surface of the left atrium with a stalk attached to the interatrial septum close to the fossa ovalis (Figure 32–3). When a myxoma occurs in the ventricles, it almost always originates from the free wall. Although asymptomatic myxomas have been recognized, most patients experience one or more effects from the classic triad of constitutional, embolic, and obstructive manifestations. (For details, refer to the section on Clinical Findings.)

Rothenbuhler A, et al. Clinical and molecular genetics of Carney complex. *Best Pract Res Clin Endocrinol Metab.* 2010;24(3): 389–99. [PMID: 20833331]

B. Papillary fibroelastomas—These tumors account for 7–8% of cardiac tumors. They are usually discovered postmortem, with an autopsy incidence of 0.002–0.33%, although their premorbid detection rate is rising with the increasing use of echocardiography (Figure 32–4). They are usually found in patients older than 60 years of age, although they have been reported in patients from 3 to 86 years old. A profusion of

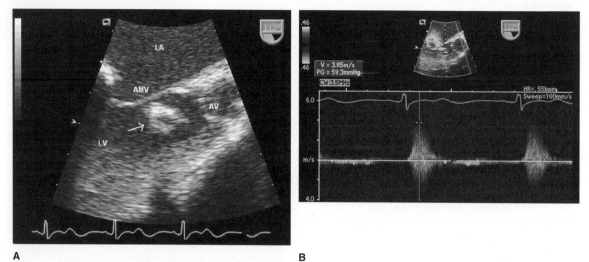

A   **B**

▲ **Figure 32–4.** Transesophageal echocardiogram to evaluate a mass found on a transthoracic echocardiogram in a 75-year-old man who suffered from dizziness. **A:** An irregular mass attached to the ventricular side of the anterior mitral leaflet is shown in this 113° long-axis view. The location on the downstream side of the valve and the frond-like surface are highly suggestive of a papillary fibroelastoma (*arrow*). **B:** Doppler signal demonstrating left ventricular outflow tract obstruction caused by the mass during systole. AMV, anterior mitral valve leaflet; AV, aortic valve; LA, left atrium; LV, left ventricle.

names—cardiac papilloma, papillary fibroma, giant Lambl excrescence, and papillary endocardial tumor—have been used to describe what is properly a papillary fibroelastoma. These tumors (first described as small filiform projections on the cusps of aortic valves) have multiple papillary fronds and look like a sea anemone, attached to the endocardial surface of the valves by a small pedicle.

Papillary fibroelastomas can form a nidus for platelet and fibrin aggregation and lead to systemic or cerebrovascular emboli. They are most commonly identified on the valves, arising on the left-sided valvular structures much more frequently than the right-sided ones. A literature review of 725 reported cases of papillary fibroelastoma found 44% of the tumors arising from the aortic valve, followed by mitral valve in 35%, tricuspid valve in 15%, and pulmonary valve in 8%. Other less common locations, such as the chordae, papillary apparatuses, left ventricular septum, left ventricular outflow tract, left ventricular free wall, and the left atrium, have also been reported. Clinical manifestations include such conditions as cerebral embolism, myocardial infarction, sudden death, pulmonary embolism, and syncope. Surgical excision is generally recommended in the symptomatic individual. Mobile tumors have been suggested to be independent predictors of the occurrence of death or nonfatal embolization.

Anastacio MM, et al. Surgical experience with cardiac papillary fibroelastoma over a 15-year period. *Ann Thorac Surg.* 2012; 94(2):537–41. [PMID: 22626753]

C. LIPOMAS—These tumors should not be confused with lipomatous hypertrophy of the interatrial septum, which is a nonneoplastic condition caused by adipose cell hyperplasia. Cardiac lipomas account for about 8% of primary cardiac tumors; they occur as solitary, circumscribed, encapsulated tumors with a wide range of size and weight. They can arise from epicardial surface and grow into the pericardial space, confined in the myocardium, or grow from subendocardium into the ventricular chamber.

D. FIBROMAS—Approximately three-quarters of all fibromas occur in the pediatric population. The second most common benign tumor of childhood, they have been reported in patients from age 2–57 years. Almost always solitary, fibromas can occur in any chamber but are most commonly found in the ventricular myocardium—usually in the anterior wall of the left ventricle and interventricular septum—and in the right ventricle (Figure 32–5). These tumors are often large, between 4 and 7 cm in diameter, and exert a mass effect. They are also associated with ventricular arrhythmias and heart failure; when arising from the ventricular septum, they can be associated with sudden death. Unlike lipoma, fibromas are not distinctly encapsulated, which makes complete resection more challenging.

Pozzi M, et al. Conservative management of left ventricle cardiac fibroma in an adult asymptomatic patient. *Int J Cardiol.* 2012;161(3):e61–2. [PMID: 22592025]

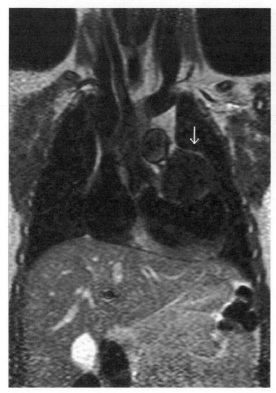

A

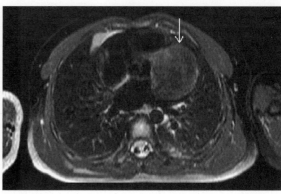

B

▲ **Figure 32–5. A:** Coronal T2-weighted spin-echo magnetic resonance image of the heart through the level of the left ventricular anterior wall and the aortic valve. A mass is visualized emanating from the anterior wall of the left ventricle (*arrow*). The mass is mildly heterogeneous with mild T2 hypointensity relative to the myocardium. **B:** Transaxial T2-weighted image demonstrates predominantly peripheral enhancement. These findings are suggestive of a cardiac fibroma. (Courtesy of C. Higgins.)

E. RHABDOMYOMAS—Rhabdomyomas are the most common benign cardiac tumor in children, usually occurring before the age of 1 year. In fact, an intracavitary mass discovered incidentally in a pediatric patient is suggestive of rhabdomyoma until proven otherwise. There are frequently multiple tumors, occurring equally in the right and left ventricles or the atria; the valves are spared (Figure 32–6). They range in size from a few millimeters to a few centimeters and are white to yellow. Rhabdomyomas are often associated with tuberous sclerosis, more frequently seen in those with mutations in the *TSC2* gene compared to the *TSC1* gene. Spontaneous regression is well established in the pediatric population, although tumor enlargement and de novo appearance have been observed during puberty. Unless the patient is symptomatic, surgical intervention is often unnecessary. When surgical resection is indicated, partial tumor resection has not been found to be inferior to complete resection.

Padalino MA, et al. Surgery for primary cardiac tumors in children: early and late results in a multicenter European Congenital Heart Surgeons Association study. *Circulation.* 2012; 126(1):22–30. [PMID: 22626745]

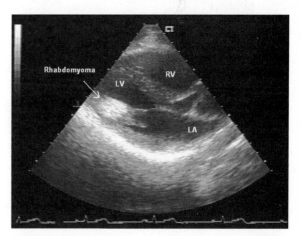

▲ **Figure 32–6.** Transthoracic echocardiogram in parasternal long-axis view showing a rhabdomyoma in the left ventricle of a patient with tuberous sclerosis. LA, left atrium; LV, left ventricle; RV, right ventricle.

F. CARDIAC HAMARTOMAS (ONCOCYTIC CARDIO-MYOPATHY)—Also known as histiocytoid cardiomyopathy or Purkinje cell hamartoma, these tumors are seen in children and infants. Hamartomas occur as flat sheets of cells on the endocardial or epicardial surfaces of the left ventricle and may present as ventricular arrhythmia. As many as 50% of cardiac hamartomas undergo involution with time, and recent data suggest that conservative management is appropriate. Controlling the arrhythmia medically, when possible, obviates the need for surgery.

G. HEMANGIOMAS—Accounting for 5–10% of all primary benign cardiac tumors, these benign vascular tumors occur in three histologic types: capillary, cavernous, or mixed. They occur in a wide age distribution from age 2 weeks to 65 years old and can be isolated or be in multiple locations. They are located in any of the cardiac chambers. They usually appear as a hyperechoic lesion on echocardiogram, but cystic appearance has been noted (Figure 32–7).

Fathala A. Left ventricular cardiac cyst: unusual echocardiographic appearance of a cardiac hemangioma. *Circulation*. 2012; 125(17):2171–2. [PMID: 22547757]

2. Malignant—Twenty five percent of all primary cardiac tumors have malignant characteristics.

A. SARCOMAS—Comprising 50–75% of all primary cardiac malignancies, cardiac sarcomas are the most common malignant cardiac tumors in adults, with a predilection for patients between the third and fifth decades. Angiosarcomas are the most common histologic subtype, followed by rhabdomyosarcomas, fibrosarcomas, and osteosarcomas. Because angiosarcomas usually occur in the right atrium or pericardium, right-sided failure, pericardial disease, or vena caval obstruction can be the presenting manifestations. The tumor is extensively infiltrative of cardiac structures, and metastatic spread at the time of diagnosis is common (Figure 32–8). The tumor can be diagnosed by lung biopsy if pulmonary metastases are present. Cardiac Kaposi sarcoma is a type of angiosarcoma found in immunocompromised individuals, such as those with acquired immunodeficiency syndrome (AIDS). Angiosarcomas are usually found on the epicardial or pericardial surface. Rhabdomyosarcomas have been reported in all age groups with a male predominance; in children, they constitute the most common malignant cardiac tumors. Fibrosarcomas have the characteristic "white fish flesh" appearance, composed of spindle cells. They occur equally in the left and right sides of the heart, are often multiple, extensively infiltrative, and protrude into a cardiac chamber or the pericardium. A valve is affected in half the cases. Osteosarcomas have been found in patients ranging in age from 24 to 67 years. They usually originate in the posterior wall of the left atrium, near the entrance of the pulmonary veins, and can be intramural or intracavitary. Osteosarcomas can metastasize to the thyroid, skin, and lungs. They exhibit the same gross

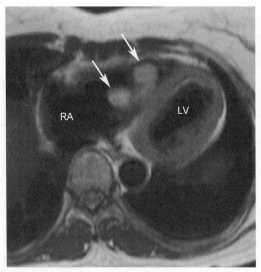

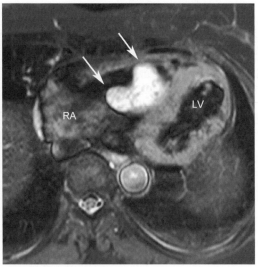

A **B**

▲ **Figure 32–7.** (**A**) Axial plane black-blood T2-weighted and (**B**) T2-weighted fast-spin echo with fat suppression images in a 60-year-old woman who had two right ventricular masses discovered incidentally on an echocardiogram. These masses are intermediate signal intensity between fat and myocardium, which increase in signal intensity with fat saturation pulse sequence. These characteristics are suggestive of hemangioma. LV, left ventricle; RA, right atrium. (Courtesy of Karen Ordovas.)

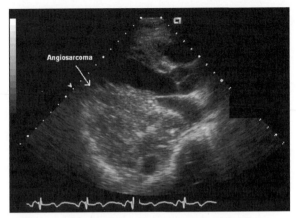
Angiosarcoma

▲ **Figure 32–8.** Transthoracic echocardiogram in a 60-year-old woman who had a 2-month history of dyspnea and palpitations. A parasternal long-axis view shows an infiltrating mass involving the left ventricular posterior wall and left atrium. A biopsy of the mass showed angiosarcoma.

and microscopic appearance as osteosarcoma of the bone. Leiomyosarcomas have rarely been reported in the heart. When they do occur, they are found in an older age group (> 55 years) and mainly in the posterior wall of the left atrium. Primary cardiac liposarcomas occur in younger patients (28–37 years) and are found in the right atrium or left ventricle and on the mitral valve.

Irrespective of histologic type, common features that predict more benign disease course are left atrium location, low-mitotic activity and scarce cellular pleomorphism, and absence of metastasis or necrosis. The overall prognosis of cardiac sarcomas is very poor, with mean survival ranging from 9.6 to 16.5 months.

Orlandi A, et al. Cardiac sarcomas: an update. *J Thorac Oncol.* 2010; 5(9):1483–9. [PMID: 20651614]

B. Lymphomas—Although cardiac involvement is seen (at autopsy) in 25% of patients with lymphoma, primary cardiac lymphoma is extremely rare, with a prevalence of 1–2% of all primary cardiac tumors, and found predominantly in immunocompromised individuals. Largely composed of diffuse large B-cell lymphoma, it can involve any area of the heart, with the highest frequency arising from the right side of the heart, particularly the right atrium. The infiltrative nature of this disorder can lead to conduction abnormalities, large pericardial effusion, and even congestive heart failure symptoms from restriction. Metastasis can occur to distant organs after seemingly successful eradication of the primary cardiac source. These factors may account for the dismal prognosis, with a median survival of 7 months after initial diagnosis.

Miguel CE, et al. Primary cardiac lymphoma. *Int J Cardiol.* 2011; 149(3):358–63. [PMID: 20227122]

C. Malignant fibrous histiocytomas—Also classified as undifferentiated pleomorphic sarcomas, this malignancy usually arises in the left atrium, with the potential to obstruct mitral orifice and cause heart failure symptoms. These malignant tumors have a high likelihood of recurrence and metastasis after surgical resection with a median survival of 1 year after treatment.

Okamoto K, et al. Malignant fibrous histiocytoma of the heart: case report and review of 46 cases in the literature. *Intern Med.* 2001;40(12):1222–6. [PMID: 11813848]

3. Tumors that may be benign or malignant

A. Mesotheliomas—These tumors are the most common primary pericardial tumors; they present with pericarditis, tamponade, or constriction. Benign mesotheliomas of the atrioventricular node may produce heart block. There is a 2:1 male predominance, and adults are most frequently afflicted. Pericardial mesotheliomas usually cover most of the parietal and visceral surfaces encasing the heart, with only superficial invasion of adjacent myocardium. Unlike pleural mesotheliomas, pericardial mesotheliomas are not consistently linked to asbestos exposure. Responses to radiation and chemotherapy are poor; surgical pericardiectomy offers a palliative measure

Sharma PS, et al. Primary malignant pericardial mesothelioma presenting as effusive-constrictive pericarditis. *J Invasive Cardiol.* 2011;23(8):E197–9. [PMID: 21828406]

B. Paraganglioma—These extra-adrenal tumors can produce catecholamines and cause symptoms of heightened sympathetic activity. The majority are not hormonally active and are located in the pericardium; the active tumors arise from the visceral autonomic paraganglia of the left atrial wall. Because they are supplied by multiple cardiac blood vessels, complete excision is difficult. Perioperative α- and β-adrenergic blockade should be performed. Partly because of hormonally active nature, early detection is possible, which may account for the high 10-year survival rate—84% in some series where complete resection was performed.

Huo JL, et al. Cardiac paraganglioma: diagnostic and surgical challenges. *J Card Surg.* 2012;27(2):178–82. [PMID: 22273468]

▶ Clinical Findings

Cardiac tumors are challenging to diagnose because there are no specifically identifiable symptoms. The anatomic location and size of the tumor rather than the histopathology

Table 32–2. Clinical Manifestations of Cardiac Neoplasms

Endocardial
  Thromboembolism: cerebral, coronary, pulmonary, systemic
  Cavitary obliteration or outflow tract obstruction
  Valve obstruction and valve damage
  Constitutional manifestations
Myocardial
  Arrhythmias, ventricular or atrial
  Conduction abnormalities
  Electrocardiographic changes
  Systolic or diastolic left ventricular dysfunction
  Coronary involvement: angina, infarction
Pericardial
  Pericarditis
  Pericardial effusion
  Arrhythmias
  Tamponade
  Constriction
Valvular
  Valvular damage, obstruction, or regurgitation
  Congestive heart failure
  Sudden death or syncope

determine the clinical findings (Table 32–2). For example, small intracavitary tumors that cause obstruction of flow may produce symptoms earlier than would large, infiltrative intramural tumors. In addition to producing obstruction, arrhythmias, and myocardial dysfunction, cardiac tumors (particularly myxomas, which produce interleukin-6) may also present with constitutional symptoms, such as weight loss, fatigue, fever, arthralgias, or symptoms and signs mimicking vasculitis.

As with other forms of cardiac mass, there are no specific physical findings for cardiac tumors. The one physical sign that may raise the suspicion for a cardiac tumor is the tumor plop, which is caused by the obstruction of the mitral valve orifice by the tumor. The sound occurs later than the opening snap of a stenotic mitral valve and earlier than an S_3, which can be difficult to distinguish with auscultation. The coexistence of other cardiac auscultatory signs of mitral stenosis without a history of rheumatic fever should raise the possibility of a left atrial tumor.

Overall, myxomas are associated with a mitral diastolic murmur in 75% of cases; mitral regurgitation murmur in 50%; pulmonary hypertension in 70%; right-sided heart failure in 70%; pulmonary emboli in 25%; anemia in 33%; elevated erythrocyte sedimentation rate in 33%; and a third heart sound (the tumor plop) in 33%.

▶ Diagnostic Studies

Advances in noninvasive imaging techniques have facilitated the early diagnosis of cardiac tumors and increased the accuracy and complexity of information available to both the cardiologist and the cardiac surgeon. Echocardiography, computed tomography (CT), magnetic resonance imaging (MRI), and positron emission tomography (PET) have replaced plain radiographs and angiography.

A. Echocardiography

Echocardiography is the initial diagnostic modality of choice. In general, the sensitivity of both the transthoracic and transesophageal echocardiography is highest for endocardial lesions because the mass is easily distinguished from the echolucent chamber; the sensitivity is slightly lower for intramyocardial lesions and lowest for pericardial tumors. Despite its inconsistency in image quality secondary to varying degree of chest structure interference between different individuals, transthoracic echocardiography offers a superior acoustic window for the left ventricle and, therefore, is more sensitive in detecting a left ventricular tumor. On the other hand, transesophageal echocardiography has the advantage of providing better resolution for valvular and posterior structures that are distant from the anterior chest wall, such as the left and right atria, superior vena cava, and the descending thoracic aorta. Because of its superior image resolution and transesophageal approach, intraoperative transesophageal echocardiography has proven extremely useful to the surgeon for the guidance of tumor resection, particularly in cardiac sarcoma. Increasingly, transesophageal echocardiography is also used to aid cardiac biopsy and guide surgical intervention, helping to ensure that there is no residual tumor and that the repaired structures are free of defects (Figure 32–9). Follow-up echocardiography is recommended after resection of a tumor, particularly a myxoma, where there is a significant recurrence rate of 5%.

Newer echocardiographic techniques are being increasingly used to determine tissue characterization of the tumor. Perfusion contrast enhancement of the tumor may be suggestive but not diagnostic of malignant or vascular tumors, because benign tumors and thrombi can exhibit contrast enhancement. Real-time three-dimensional echocardiography provides accurate estimation of the tumor size, compared with two-dimensional transthoracic or transesophageal echocardiography.

Zaragoza-Macias E, et al. Real time three-dimensional echocardiography evaluation of intracardiac masses. *Echocardiography.* 2012;29(2):207–19. [PMID: 22283202]

B. Computed Tomography

Conventional, nongated CT scanning is most useful in diagnosing paracardiac masses in the region of the pericardium. It can differentiate tissue types and help identify their extent within the lungs, mediastinum, pericardium, and cardiac chambers. The evaluation can be improved with contrast enhancement (Figure 32–10).

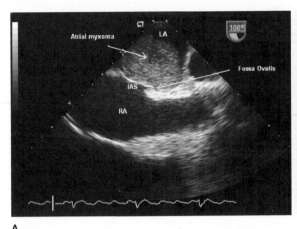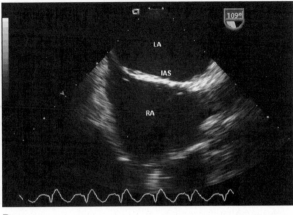

A   B

▲ **Figure 32–9.** (**A**) Intraoperative transesophageal echocardiogram in the bicaval view, showing a left atrial myxoma attaching to the fossa ovalis of the interatrial septum. (**B**) Postoperative transesophageal echocardiogram shows complete resection of the atrial myxoma with intact interatrial septum. IAS, interatrial septum; LA, left atrium; RA, right atrium.

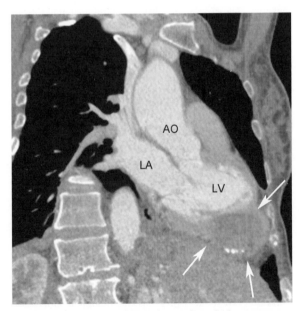

▲ **Figure 32–10.** Contrast-enhanced, multidetector computed tomography image of the heart in coronal section. This 40-year-old female with a history of ovarian cyst complained of chest pain. A cystic mass with calcification involving the myocardium and pericardium was noted incidentally. The mass was resected and found to be a teratoma. AO, aorta; LA, left atrium; LV, left ventricle. (Courtesy of Karen Ordovas.)

CT is also superior in identifying tumor involvement of the pericardium when there is no pericardial effusion and in identifying nodular pericardial thickening. CT may be useful when the mediastinum, pleura, and lungs must also be examined to provide therapeutic guidance and management of cardiac tumors. This modality can show a complete cross section of all cardiac, mediastinal, pulmonary, and thoracic structures (in contrast to angiocardiography), without the anatomic restrictions of echocardiography. Additional advantages of cardiac CT over MRI for cardiac mass imaging include identification of calcified mass and superior safety in patients with implanted device and dialysis patients.

Two techniques have been developed to reduce the poor temporal resolution and motion blurring seen in the conventional single-slice CT. Multidetector row CT with electrocardiogram (ECG) gating allows a complete chest survey with high-resolution images to be performed in 10–15 minutes. Ultrafast CT, known as the electron-beam computed tomography (EB-CT), using continuous high-speed scanning with 50–100 ms exposures, improves the detection of paracardiac and intracardiac masses and produces images with excellent spatial and density resolution. The technique also allows a movie mode, adding information to the static images; because it avoids superimposition of other tissues, it is useful in evaluating multiple masses.

C. Magnetic Resonance Imaging

MRI is a three-dimensional technique that can be used to supplement the information provided by echocardiography about cardiac masses. The high natural contrast between the blood pool and cardiovascular structures allows internal cardiac structures to be visualized by this technique. The direct

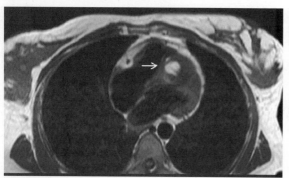 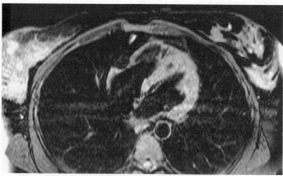

A　　　　　　　　　　　　　　　　　　　　　　**B**

▲ **Figure 32–11.** T1-weighted transaxial spin-echo magnetic resonance image of the heart through the level of the interventricular septum. **A:** A high-signal-intensity mass (*arrow*) is seen embedded in the distal anteroseptum. **B:** During fat saturation pulse application, the mass loses its bright signal, suggesting the diagnosis of a cardiac lipoma. (Courtesy of C. Higgins.)

multiplanar imaging capability of MRI is advantageous in demonstrating vessels and vessel/mass relationships.

The main strength of MRI for cardiac mass imaging is the potential for tissue characterization. Fibrous tissue remains at low signal intensity on T2-weighted images, whereas tumors have increased signal intensity. Fat-rich tissues, such as the lipomas, can be accurately characterized by using the fat suppression technique (Figure 32–11). Tumors and thrombi can be distinguished by using the inversion recovery scouting sequence or gadolinium injection, which enhances masses with rich vascular supply. Delayed enhancement with gadolinium injection is indicative of necrosis or nonviable tissues, which are often located in the center of a tumor where the cells have outgrown the blood supply.

Functional assessment should be included as part of a complete MRI study of a cardiac mass. Using long- and short-axis cine imaging, the mobility of the mass and its hemodynamic consequence can be evaluated. Furthermore, myocardial tagging allows examination of intramyocardial strain pattern, which helps differentiate contractile from noncontractile tissue. This is particularly useful in determining whether a segment of intramyocardial thickening represents a tumor, such as rhabdomyoma, or hypertrophied myocardium.

MRI correctly identifies the etiology of cardiac masses about 75% of the time, while echocardiography (both transthoracic and transesophageal) only correctly diagnoses about one-third of cases. Thus, in many cases, a cardiac MRI or chest CT can help in diagnosis after an echocardiographic finding of a cardiac tumor. Myxomas can be diagnosed accurately by echocardiogram alone.

Buckley O, et al. Cardiac masses, part 1: imaging strategies and technical considerations. *AJR Am J Roentgenol.* 2011;197(5): W837–41. [PMID: 22021530]

D. Positron Emission Tomography

Whole-body 18-fluorodeoxyglucose (18F-FDG) PET has increasingly been used to diagnose cardiac metastasis in patients with renal cell carcinoma or lung cancer. Hybrid imaging using 18F-FDG PET/CT has been shown to be both sensitive and specific for distinguishing malignant from benign cardiac masses and may be helpful for this indication.

Rahbar K, et al. Differentiation of malignant and benign cardiac tumors using 18F-FDG PET/CT. *J Nucl Med.* 2012;53(6): 856–63. [PMID: 22577239]

▶ Differential Diagnosis

The differential diagnosis of cardiac masses includes tumors, thrombus, nonbacterial thrombotic endocarditis, infective endocarditis, or normal variant intracardiac or extracardiac structures. Imaging features that favor a diagnosis of tumor are a mobile, pedunculated appearance and an associated pericardial effusion. Masses that cross anatomic planes, from myocardium to pericardium or endocardium, are likely to be tumors. Clinical features are crucial in guiding the diagnosis of a cardiac mass. For example, left atrial thrombi are associated with mitral valve stenosis, enlarged left atrium, and atrial fibrillation, while ventricular thrombi are associated with cardiomyopathies or regional wall-motion abnormalities. Right atrial thrombi are seen in the setting of indwelling catheters or pacemaker wires (Figure 32–12). Nonbacterial thrombotic endocarditis is found in patients with malignancy or systemic lupus erythematosus.

Pericardial cysts can be identified by their unilocular nature and their location in either the right or left costophrenic angle. Diaphragmatic hernia can mimic a left atrial mass on transthoracic echocardiography. Transesophageal

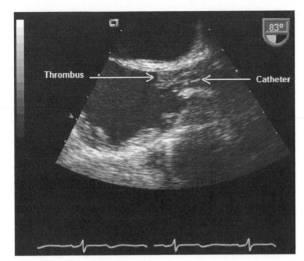

▲ **Figure 32–12.** Transesophageal echocardiogram in a 64-year-old hemodialysis patient for evaluation of fever. The bicaval view shows a thrombus forming around a catheter at the junction of the superior vena cava and the right atrium.

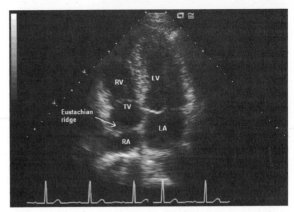

▲ **Figure 32–14.** Transthoracic echocardiogram in an apical four-chamber view showing a prominent eustachian ridge. LA, left atrium; LV, left ventricle; RA, right atrium; RV, right ventricle; TV, tricuspid valve.

echocardiography, on the other hand, can help diagnose the hernia by showing an extracardiac structure indenting the left atrium posteriorly and the swirling nonuniform echo densities within this structure caused by motion of the gastric contents.

Although lipomatous cardiac infiltration can mimic a tumor, it can be distinguished by its characteristic location (atrial septum) and dumbbell-shaped appearance (Figure 32–13). The shape is due to the thin fossa ovalis that separates the lipomatous atrial septum on either side.

The incidence of lipomatous septal hypertrophy increases with age and obesity. No intervention is required unless the hypertrophy causes arrhythmias or obstruction.

A number of normal variants of anatomic structures are occasionally confused with tumors. These include the Chiari network, a remnant of the sinus venosus seen in the right atrium; the eustachian valve, the valve of the inferior vena cava (Figure 32–14); the septum spurium, a superior fold of the coronary sinus opening; and the thebesian valve, the valve of the coronary sinus.

▶ Treatment

A. Pharmacologic Therapy

Surgery remains the mainstay of treatment for all cardiac tumors. Pharmacologic therapy has no role in the management of benign cardiac tumors. In cardiac sarcoma, adjuvant chemotherapy using doxorubicin-containing regimens has not been shown to prolong survival. In recent years, anecdotal success has been reported with paclitaxel, but no systematic studies are available to support survival benefit. The use of chemotherapy in tumor cytoreduction in preparation for surgical resection and palliation of unresectable disease might be of value in selected cases. Unlike sarcoma, primary cardiac lymphoma is thought to be more responsive to chemotherapy. However, because of the infiltrative nature of lymphoma and its potential brisk response to chemotherapy, the tumor melt phenomenon may increase mortality in the first cycle of chemotherapy. Using a CHOP (cyclophosphamide + doxorubicin + vincristine + prednisone)–based regimen, combined with radiation or surgery (or both) in certain cases, one-third of patients may experience complete remission, and a median survival of 1 year has been observed. More recently, promising results have been

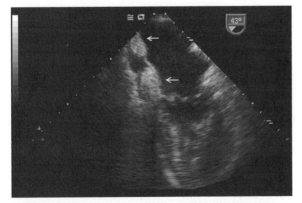

▲ **Figure 32–13.** Transesophageal echocardiogram in 43° long-axis plane showing lipomatous hypertrophy of the interatrial septum (*arrows*). Note the dumbbell-shaped appearance.

obtained with monoclonal CD20 antibody (rituximab) and autologous stem cell transplant.

Hamidi M, et al. Primary cardiac sarcoma. *Ann Thorac Surg.* 2010; 90(1):176–81. [PMID: 20609770]

B. Radiation

Adjuvant radiotherapy can be helpful for prolonging survival of patients with cardiac lymphoma if total surgical excision is not successful or curative for malignant tumors. Primary cardiac sarcomas, however, are relatively radio-insensitive. Radiotherapy may have a role in local disease management, but its effect in prolonging survival has not been demonstrated in a systematic manner despite some anecdotal reports of success.

C. Surgery

Because of embolic complications and the limited capacity of the heart to tolerate space-occupying lesions, most cardiac tumors—benign or malignant—require prompt surgical removal. The surgical techniques vary for tumors located in left heart, right heart, or pulmonary artery.

1. Benign tumors—Myxomas should be removed expeditiously because of their high embolic potential. Lipomas are often asymptomatic and do not require further treatment. Because large papillary fibroelastomas, particularly if they are more than 1 cm, mobile, and located on the left heart, are a nidus for platelet aggregation and embolization, resection is recommended. Small papillary fibroelastomas, such as Lambl excrescences, on an elderly patient's aortic leaflets need not be resected. Present data suggest a conservative approach to treatment of rhabdomyomas in asymptomatic patients. Although surgery is indicated for symptomatic patients (a large mass can cause inflow and outflow obstruction), it can be difficult because these tumors tend to be multiple, nonencapsulated, and embedded in the myocardium. Patients may need inotropic support in the postoperative period because of the extensive surgical dissection, which often involves the myocardium. Fibromas are often large (4–7 cm in diameter); prompt surgery is recommended. Excision may remove much ventricular myocardium. Complete excision is recommended, because any fibroma that remains may be a focus for ventricular arrhythmias. Reconstructive surgery with a synthetic patch may be necessary.

2. Malignant tumors—Although total surgical resection for sarcoma is often impossible, surgery is done to relieve compressive or obstructive symptoms in some cases. Surgery is rarely performed to remove metastatic tumor masses unless a cure of the primary tumor is highly likely. In addition to high in-hospital mortality rate, surgery for malignant tumors remains palliative without effective adjuvant therapy. Prognosis of malignant cardiac tumor is overall extremely poor.

Rice DC, et al. Left heart sarcomas. *Methodist Debakey Cardiovasc J.* 2010;6(3):49–56. [PMID: 20834212]

D. Cardiac Transplantation

Cardiac transplantation can be an alternative therapy for unresectable cardiac tumors when infiltration by fibroma is too extensive for excision. This approach remains experimental and is limited by the potential for posttransplant recurrence, which may be accelerated by immunosuppressive therapy. In rare cases where radical resection of the tumor and ex vivo repair of the heart are possible, autotransplantation instead of allogeneic transplantation should be attempted.

Coelho PN, et al. Long-term survival with heart transplantation for fibrosarcoma of the heart. *Ann Thorac Surg.* 2010;90(2):635–6. [PMID: 20667366]

▶ Prognosis

The prognosis of metastatic tumors to the heart from distant sources is generally poor and is not different from the prognosis of other metastatic disease. For primary cardiac tumors, surgical resection usually results in cure of benign cardiac tumors. Approximately 1.5% of myxomas (12–22% in patients with familial or syndrome-related myxomas) recur within 10–15 years. Because of this small risk of recurrence, patients should be monitored with periodic echocardiography every 1–2 years for 15 years following the resection.

Long-term results for primary malignant tumors are disappointing, usually because of early metastatic or local spread or recurrence. In general, survival time appears to be inversely correlated with the tumor size and degree of regional tumor extension at the time of surgery. Mean survival for pericardial mesotheliomas is 6 months to 1 year, and for sarcomas, it is 3 months to 1 year with or without treatment. Localized disease arising from the left atrium with no necrotic tissues is associated with better prognosis in sarcomas. The survival of patients with treated primary cardiac lymphoma can be as long as 5 years, but as short as 1 month if left untreated.

Truong PT, et al. Treatment and outcomes in adult patients with primary cardiac sarcoma: the British Columbia Cancer Agency experience. *Ann Surg Oncol.* 2009;16(12):3358–65. [PMID: 19830494]

▶ Cardiac Toxicities from Oncologic Treatments

Because survival of patients with various oncologic conditions has improved, early or, especially, late adverse cardiac effects related to treatment can develop. Fortunately, because of increasing recognition of some of these potential toxicities, modern treatment protocols have been modified to minimize side effects. Nevertheless, it is important to recognize some of the adverse outcomes related to earlier treatments. At the same time, clinicians need to be cognizant of potential late effects of contemporary therapy (Table 32–3).

Table 32–3. Cardiotoxicity Induced by Chemotherapeutic Agents

Chemotherapeutic Agent	Adverse Effect
Anthracyclines/anthraquinolones	
Doxorubicin, daunorubicin, epirubicin/mitoxantrone	QT prolongation, ST-T segment changes, arrhythmias, left ventricular (LV) dysfunction, myopericarditis
Alkylating agents	
Cisplatin	Myocardial ischemia, thrombotic events (deep vein thrombosis or pulmonary embolism)
Cyclophosphamide	Hemorrhagic myopericarditis, acute heart failure, arrhythmias
Antimetabolites	
5-Fluorouracil, cytarabine, capecitabine	Myocardial spasm, ischemia, arrhythmia
Antimicrotubules	
Paclitaxel, vinca alkaloids	Sinus bradycardia, atrioventricular block, myocardial ischemia, pericardial effusion
Biologic response modifiers	
Interferons, interleukin-2	Hypotension/transient LV dysfunction
Topoisomerase inhibitors	
Etoposide	Hypotension
Differentiation agents	
All-*trans*-retinoic acid	Pulmonary edema, transient LV dysfunction, pericardial effusion
Arsenic trioxide	Prolonged QT, torsades de pointes
Monoclonal antibodies	
Trastuzumab	Transient LV dysfunction
Rituximab	Orthostatic hypotension
Small-molecule tyrosine kinase inhibitors	
Sunitinib, dasatinib, imatinib mesylate, lapatinib, erlotinib, sorafenib	Hypertension, myocardial ischemia, transient or permanent LV dysfunction

A. Chemotherapy

1. General consideration

A. ANTHRACYCLINES—Because of the common cardiotoxic effect and its broad application in oncology, this drug class is the most well-studied cardiotoxic chemotherapeutic agent. The most commonly used offending anthracyclines are daunorubicin and doxorubicin. Anthracyclines produce cardiotoxicity by reactive oxygen species formation and activation of apoptotic pathways, which cause irreversible myocyte death and neurohormonal-mediated ventricular remodeling in advanced cardiotoxicity.

Acute cardiotoxicity immediately after anthracycline infusion is uncommon (< 1% of cases). It can manifest as a transient decrease in ejection fraction with rarely clinical heart failure. Other subclinical manifestations of acute cardiotoxicity include ECG abnormalities such as QT prolongation, nonspecific ST-T segment abnormalities, tachy- or bradyarrhythmia, pericarditis, and myocarditis. These are often reversible within weeks after cessation of infusion. However, chronic cardiomyopathic effects are irreversible. The incidence has a bimodal pattern with the first early peak at 3 month after the treatment, and second late occurrence peaks at about 1 year after the last dose of treatment.

The most important risk factor for anthracycline-induced cardiac toxicity is the cumulative dose; a threshold cumulative dose of 450–500 mg/m^2 has been suggested to reduce cardiac toxicities. Other factors predisposing to increased risk of cardiotoxicity include female sex, very young age and old age, preexisting cardiac disease, concurrent or prior chest irradiation, and administration of multiple chemotherapeutic agents, particularly paclitaxel and trastuzumab.

B. TRASTUZUMAB—A recombinant humanized IgG monoclonal antibody that selectively binds to human epidermal growth factor receptor-2 (HER-2) has been reported to cause predominantly asymptomatic ventricular systolic or diastolic dysfunction. According to a recent report from the Surveillance, Epidemiology, and End Results (SEER)-Medicare database, trastuzumab use in breast cancer has increased by more than eightfold from 2000 to 2007; after excluding patients with preexisting cardiac disease or risk factors for heart failure, the incidence of developing heart failure or cardiomyopathy among older women (67–94 years old) with breast cancer in association with trastuzumab use was noted to be substantially higher compared to previous reports in younger women. The adjusted 3-year incidence for heart failure or cardiomyopathy associated with trastuzumab use alone was 32.1%, whereas the incidence was 41.9% with combined anthracycline and trastuzumab therapy. This report highlights the important contribution of age and the additive effect of anthracycline to trastuzumab-induced cardiotoxicity.

The mechanism of cardiotoxicity is thought to be secondary to inhibition of cardiomyocyte protective pathways, mediated by the HER-2 signaling and its ligand neuregulin-1. Therefore, by losing the innate cardiac repair mechanism, the incidence is higher in those receiving concomitant cardiac toxic chemotherapy and those with older age and history of chest irradiation. Unlike anthracycline toxicity, trastuzumab-related cardiac dysfunction is not dose dependent; prompt resolution of ventricular dysfunction with drug withdrawal or standard heart failure therapy has been reported over a mean interval of 1.5 months.

C. CYCLOPHOSPHAMIDE—The cardiotoxicity of this alkylating agent is also dose dependent. However, unlike the anthracyclines, it is the total dose per infusion that determines the probability for cardiac injury, not the cumulative dosage. For example, cyclophosphamide in a high-dose protocol, 120–170 mg/kg, can cause cardiac injury over 1–7 days after the initiation of the first dose. The spectrum of cardiac toxicity can range from decreased QRS amplitude, repolarization abnormalities, tachyarrhythmias, and heart block to asymptomatic pericardial effusion and heart failure. Acute-onset heart failure can occur in as many as 28% of patients receiving high-dose cyclophosphamide. Hemorrhagic myopericarditis leading to pericardial effusion and tamponade is a unique complication from this chemotherapeutic agent, which usually occurs within the first week after the treatment. It is caused by endothelial capillary damage and red cell extravasation. Pericardiocentesis is usually not necessary for hemorrhagic pericardial effusion. Analgesics and corticosteroids with serial echocardiographic monitoring are effective treatment.

D. RETINOIC ACID—Retinoic acid produces a syndrome in up to 25% of cases, with manifestations of fever, dyspnea, pleural and pericardial effusion, pulmonary infiltrates, and peripheral edema. Transient myocardial dysfunction can occur in 17% of patients receiving this vitamin A derivative agent. This syndrome is usually responsive to corticosteroid therapy.

E. PACLITAXEL—Paclitaxel commonly leads to ECG changes and cardiac rhythm disturbances; atrioventricular conduction abnormalities, complete heart block, and even asystole have been reported. Fortunately, these conduction abnormalities are usually reversible with the termination of treatment. Thus, continuous ECG monitoring is advised during treatment.

F. 5-FLUOROURACIL—This antimetabolite agent is frequently associated with myocardial ischemia probably by provoking coronary spasm. The cardiotoxicity is not dose dependent and can occur with conventional doses of 1000 mg/m^2 daily for 4–5 days. The risk is fourfold higher in those with preexisting coronary artery disease. Stress testing and coronary angiography before commencing 5-fluorouracil (5-FU) therapy may be considered to risk stratify coronary events in high-risk patients, although acute coronary syndrome has been reported in those with normal coronary arteries. In general, ECG changes resolve following termination of treatment, and anginal symptoms are responsive to

conservative medical treatment. Prophylactic treatment with nitrates and calcium channel blockers has been used without consistent effects. Atrial or ventricular arrhythmias and ventricular dysfunction unrelated to myocardial ischemia are other potential complications of 5-FU therapy.

G. INTERLEUKIN-2—This immunomodulator produces a capillary leak syndrome and causes cardiovascular changes that mimic septic shock syndrome. In severe cases, ventricular arrhythmias and profound cardiac systolic function depression can occur. The syndrome usually subsides after treatment cessation and supportive treatment; however, it may take up to 6 days after the last dose for some patients to completely regain normal hemodynamics.

H. TYROSINE KINASE INHIBITORS—Only small-molecule tyrosine kinase inhibitors that target specific kinases expressed in the myocardium have been reported to be linked to adverse cardiac effects. Such kinase inhibitors include sunitinib, dasatinib, imatinib mesylate, lapatinib, and erlotinib. The cardiotoxic effects of tyrosine kinase inhibitors occur in 2–4% of patients, and the effects have ranged from hypertension, myocardial ischemia, and asymptomatic left ventricular dysfunction to clinical heart failure. While clinical experience is still accumulating, some anecdotal data have reported reversibility of left ventricular dysfunction with drug discontinuation. With the advent of newer tyrosine kinase inhibitors targeting a broader spectrum of cancer cells, clinicians should have an elevated level of vigilance for cardiac injury caused by these agents.

2. Prevention—Most preventive strategies have been adopted to reduce acute cardiotoxicity in patients receiving anthracyclines. Measures to prevent early- or late-onset chronic cardiotoxicity have been less well studied. Minimizing the total cumulative dose is the primary strategy; other modifications to the delivery of anthracyclines that can reduce the risk of anthracycline-induced cardiomyopathy include continuous infusion protocol, liposome encapsulation, and molecular modification (such as mitoxantrone and epirubicin). Several prophylactic agents have been studied; the most commonly used agent is dexrazoxane chelation. Despite its effectiveness in preventing left ventricular dysfunction, this agent may attenuate antitumor effects of chemotherapy and has not been shown to prolong overall survival. In small randomized trials, β-blockers and angiotensin receptor blockers have been shown to preserve left ventricular ejection fraction in the acute chemotherapy infusion phase. In general, because of inconsistent effectiveness, potential side effects, and cost issues, the adoption of these strategies is limited to those who are at high risk for developing cardiotoxicity.

Other than the known clinical risk factors that predispose to cardiac injury, persistently elevated troponin and natriuretic peptide levels during and after chemotherapy administration have been found to be predictive of future development of left ventricular dysfunction. However, the timing and frequency of testing and the clinical effectiveness of therapy guided by these biomarkers remain topics of ongoing investigation. In clinical practice, imaging modalities such as echocardiography and radionuclide angiography provide more direct means of left ventricular function surveillance; screening intervals of 3 to 4 months during the therapy, and 6 to 8 months after completion of therapy, are commonly adopted. Absolute declines in left ventricular ejection fraction by 20% or more or to less than 45% are considered criteria for discontinuation of anthracyclines. In patients with equivocal results on serial monitoring, endomyocardial biopsy may be necessary.

Chen J, et al. Incidence of heart failure or cardiomyopathy after adjuvant trastuzumab therapy for breast cancer. *J Am Coll Cardiol.* 2012;60(24):2504–12. [PMID: 23158536]

Shaikh AY, et al. Chemotherapy-induced cardiotoxicity. *Curr Heart Fail Rep.* 2012;9(2):117–27. [PMID: 22382639]

3. Treatment—In those who have developed chemotherapy-induced cardiomyopathy, standard heart failure therapy with β-blockers and angiotensin-converting enzyme inhibitors has been shown to improve left ventricular ejection fraction in nonrandomized, noncontrolled trials. In advanced cardiomyopathy, patients should be managed similarly as for cardiomyopathy of other etiologies, except that cardiac transplantation is usually not considered until 5 years after the cancer is cured to ensure no recurrence.

B. Radiation

Acute radiation cardiac injury is rare. The highest risk oncologic populations for chronic radiation-induced heart disease are those who received mediastinal radiation for Hodgkin lymphoma during childhood and those who received a total dose of 30–40 Gy or a dose per fraction of more than 2 Gy in any left-sided chest radiation. The incidence has declined significantly in recent years with contemporary radiotherapy delivery systems, using intensity-modulated radiotherapy, three-dimensional treatment planning with dose volume

Table 32–4. Clinical Manifestations of Radiation-Induced Heart Disease

Pericardial disease
Acute pericarditis
Delayed pericarditis
Pericardial effusion
Constrictive pericarditis
Myocardial disease
Ventricular dysfunction
Myocarditis
Restrictive cardiomyopathy
Valvular heart disease
Predominantly mitral and aortic valves
Electrical conduction disturbances
Coronary artery disease

histogram, and cardiac sparing lead block. Any structure of the heart can be involved (Table 32–4). Pericardial involvement is the most common cardiac complication, which usually appears 6–12 months following radiation therapy. Progressive fibrosis of the pericardium will result in late complications such as constrictive pericarditis. A history of past irradiation to the chest and unexplained signs or symptoms of right-sided venous congestion should raise the index of suspicion for constrictive pericarditis. Unlike pericardial complications, the development of accelerated coronary atherosclerotic disease, mainly in the left anterior descending and the right coronary arteries, will not be apparent until 10–15 years after the radiation therapy. Other than maintaining a high level vigilance for this disease entity and implementing life-long cardiac surveillance, the diagnostic and therapeutic strategies for radiation-induced heart disease are not different from those in general cardiology practice.

Filopei J, et al. Radiation-induced heart disease. *Cardiol Rev.* 2012; 20(4):184–8. [PMID: 22314140]

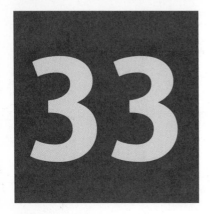

Cardiovascular Disease in Pregnancy

Kirsten Tolstrup, MD

ESSENTIALS OF DIAGNOSIS

► Pregnancy.

► History of heart disease.

► Symptoms and signs of heart disease.

► Echocardiographic or other objective evidence of heart disease.

▶ General Considerations

Cardiovascular disease occurs in up to 4% of pregnancies, but the incidence is increasing due to improved prognosis of women with congenital heart disease and a trend toward older maternal age. The unique hemodynamic changes associated with pregnancy make diagnosis and management of heart disease in pregnant patients a challenge to the physicians, who must consider not only the patient but also the risks to the fetus.

In general, the normal hemodynamic changes associated with pregnancy are well tolerated by those who have a normal cardiovascular system, valvular regurgitation, and left-to-right intracardiac shunts. On the other hand, the highest maternal and fetal morbidity and mortality is seen with severe obstructive valvular lesions, severe aortic disease (dilated thoracic aorta or uncorrected coarctation), New York Heart Association (NYHA) class III or IV heart failure, uncontrolled hypertension, and cyanotic congenital heart disease. As a rule, spontaneous vaginal delivery, often with use of vacuum extraction or forceps to facilitate stage 2 of labor to avoid the hemodynamic stress associated with pushing, is preferred. Cesarean section, with few exceptions, should be reserved for obstetric indications.

Roos-Hesselink JW, et al. Outcome of pregnancy in patients with structural or ischemic heart disease: results of a registry of the European Society of Cardiology. *Eur Heart J.* 2013;34(9):657–65. [PMID: 22968232]

Sahni G, et al. Cardiovascular disease in pregnancy. *Cardiol Clin.* 2012;30:11–12. [PMID: 22813373]

▶ Cardiovascular Physiology of Normal Pregnancy

Normal pregnancy is accompanied by significant physiologic changes, although the specific mechanisms remain virtually unknown (Table 33–1). This increased hemodynamic burden of pregnancy may unmask previously unrecognized heart disease. The normal signs and symptoms associated with pregnancy, such as shortness of breath, fatigue, and exercise intolerance, may obscure the diagnosis of heart disease. The clinician must, therefore, have a thorough knowledge of these normal changes and the aspects of the history and physical examination that suggest the presence of heart disease.

A. Blood Volume

The increase in maternal blood volume begins as early as the sixth week of pregnancy, peaks at approximately 32 weeks of gestation, and stays at that level (40–50% higher than pregestational levels) until delivery. A rapid rise in blood volume is typically noted until mid-pregnancy, after which the rise is slower. The plasma volume shows a more rapid and significant rise than the red blood cell mass, accounting for the appearance of *physiologic anemia during pregnancy*. The levels of hemoglobin and hematocrit may be as low as 11 g/dL and 33%, respectively. Iron supplementation may mitigate the drop in hemoglobin. The increased blood volume is maintained until after delivery, when a spontaneous diuresis occurs. At the same time, there is an increased venous return due to the relief of vena caval compression after delivery. These rapid postpartum changes in blood volume are critical for patients with underlying heart disease.

Table 33–1. Cardiovascular Changes in Normal Pregnancy

	First Trimester	Second Trimester	Third Trimester	At Term
Blood volume	+	+ +	+ + +	↑ 30–50%
Heart rate	+	+ +	+ + (+)	↑ 15–20 bpm
Stroke volume	+	+ + (+)	+	
Cardiac output	+	+ + (+)	+	↑ 30–50%
Systolic blood pressure	–	–	No change	↓ 5–10 mm Hg c/w midpregnancy
Diastolic blood pressure	–	– –	–	
Pulse pressure	+	+ +	+	
Systemic vascular resistance	–	– – –	– –	
Pulmonary vascular resistance	–	– –	–	
Left ventricular end-diastolic pressure	+	+ +	No change	
Venous compliance and volume	+	+ +	+	
Red blood cell mass	+	+	+	↑ 15–20%

Data from Fujitan S. *Crit Care Med.* 2005;33:S354.

B. Cardiac Output

One of the most significant changes during pregnancy is the increase in cardiac output, which begins to rise during the first trimester and peaks around the 25th week of gestation and then levels off. Total cardiac output increases up to 50% over pregestational levels. Cardiac output is the product of stroke volume and heart rate. During the early part of pregnancy, the increase in cardiac output is predominantly the result of an increase in stroke volume, augmented by increased intrinsic myocardial contractility. Numerous studies have shown a gradual increase in left ventricular systolic function attributed to left ventricular afterload reduction due to the low-resistance runoff of the placenta. The rise in left ventricular systolic function begins in early pregnancy, peaks in the 20th week, and then remains constant until delivery. As pregnancy advances, heart rate increases and stroke volume mildly decreases. The increased cardiac output in late pregnancy is maintained because of the increased heart rate. The heart rate increase typically peaks around 32 weeks gestation, reaching 15–20 bpm above the prepregnancy heart rate. There is a significantly greater increase in cardiac output in twin gestations compared with singletons.

A unique aspect of pregnancy is the hemodynamic changes induced by a change in a patient's position. When the patient is in the supine position, the gravid uterus induces profound mechanical compression of the inferior vena cava, decreasing venous return to the heart, and thus, cardiac output. A change from the supine to the left lateral position results in a 25–30% increase in cardiac output because of an increase in stroke volume.

C. Blood Pressure and Vascular Resistance

Systolic and diastolic pressures drop during pregnancy. A small decrease in systolic blood pressure begins in the first trimester, peaks at midgestation, and returns to or exceeds prepregnancy levels at term. The diastolic blood pressure decreases more than the systolic blood pressure, due to a significant fall in systemic vascular resistance, and results in a wider pulse pressure. The systemic blood pressure increases during pregnancy with the patient's age and parity. It also varies with the patient's position. The highest levels are recorded early in the pregnancy when the patient is upright, and the lowest levels occur when she is supine. During the latter part of pregnancy, the effect of position on systemic blood pressure depends on the relative degrees of inferior vena cava and aortic compression. It is recommended to use automated cuff measurements as there may be absence of the fifth Korotkoff sound in some pregnant women. Total vascular resistance, including both the systemic and the pulmonary, decrease during pregnancy. The mechanism for the fall in resistances is poorly understood but is attributed to the low-resistance circulation of the pregnant uterus and to hormonal changes (progesterone and prostaglandin among many) associated with pregnancy. The systemic vascular resistance (SVR) drops approximately 10% in the first trimester and reaches nadir around 20 weeks of gestation with SVR around 35% less than baseline. There is a small increase in SVR toward the end of pregnancy.

Fujitani S, et al. Hemodynamic assessment in a pregnant and peripartum patient. *Crit Care Med.* 2005;33(10 Suppl):S354–61. [PMID: 16215359]
Ouzounian JG, et al. Physiologic changes during normal pregnancy and delivery. *Cardiol. Clin.* 2012;30:317–29. [PMID: 22813360]

▶ Etiology & Symptomatology

A. Congenital Heart Disease

Because the medical and surgical treatment of uncorrected or surgically corrected congenital heart diseases (CHD) has improved, more women are surviving into adulthood and may become pregnant. It is recommended that patients with CHD consult with a cardiologist experienced in adult CHD and a maternal-fetal specialist before conception. The prevalence of cardiac complications greatly depends on the type of congenital lesion; regurgitant lesions are typically tolerated well, while stenotic lesions carry a higher risk. The risk for all-comers is estimated to be up to 13%, with the predominant symptoms being congestive heart failure/pulmonary edema and arrhythmias. Maternal *mortality* primarily occurs

in women with Eisenmenger syndrome. Obstetric complications are not increased, except in cases of hypertension and thromboembolic disease (2%). Premature delivery occurs in about 16%, and children small for gestational age are also common. Overall, offspring mortality is around 4%. The risk of recurrence of congenital malformations in the offspring depends on the type and ranges from 0.6% to 10%.

Only a few conditions place a patient at a high risk to advise against pregnancy (Table 33–2). High-risk patients with severe cyanotic CHD, marked decreased functional capacity, symptomatic severe obstructive lesions, or Eisenmenger syndrome should be advised against pregnancy.

1. Acyanotic heart disease

A. ATRIAL SEPTAL DEFECT—Secundum atrial septal defect is the most common congenital cardiac abnormality encountered during pregnancy. Patients with uncomplicated atrial septal defects usually tolerate pregnancy with little problem. Patients may not be able to tolerate the acute blood loss that can occur at the time of delivery because of increased shunting from left to right caused by systemic vasoconstriction associated with hypotension. Patients with symptomatic or hemodynamically significant lesions should have these closed percutaneously or surgically prior to pregnancy to decrease the incidence of thromboembolism and arrhythmias. Percutaneous closure can be performed during pregnancy but is reserved for decompensated patients. The incidence of supraventricular arrhythmias may increase in older pregnant patients, which may result in right ventricular failure and venous stasis leading to paradoxical emboli. Low-dose aspirin, once daily after the first trimester until

Table 33–2. High-Risk Conditions That Warrant Advice against Pregnancy

	Condition	Maternal Risk	Fetal Risk
1.	Cyanotic congenital heart disease	4–34% MI/stroke/death	12–40% miscarriage
2.	Eisenmenger syndrome	35% death	30% miscarriage, 15–20% fetal loss
3.	Severe pulmonary hypertension (> 75% of systemic blood pressure)	30–40% death	10% fetal loss
4.	NYHA class III/IV symptoms	10–56% death	30% fetal loss
5.	Severe symptomatic obstructive valvular lesions	56–78% CHF or pulmonary edema	11% death 33–66% preterm delivery
6.	Marfan syndrome with thoracic aorta > 4.0 cm	11–50% risk of dissection	50% risk of inheriting the syndrome 4–20% risk of fetal/neonatal death
7.	Loeys-Dietz syndrome	9% death in nonpregnant with aorta < 4.5 cm	50% risk of inheriting the syndrome

CHF, congestive heart failure; MI, myocardial infarction; NYHA, New York Heart Association.
Data from Crawford MH. *Cardiology.* 2001; Drenthen W. *J Am Coll Cardiol.* 2007;49:2303–2311; Hameed A. *J Am Coll Cardiol.* 2001;37:893–899; Silversides CK. *Am J Cardiol.* 2003;91:1382–1389; Elkayam U. *J Am Coll Cardiol.* 2005;46:223–230; Lind J. *Eur J Obstet Gynecol Reprod Biol.* 2001;98:28–35; Elkayam U. *Ann Intern Med.* 1995;123:117–122; Sliwa K. *Lancet.* 2006;368:687–693; Williams JA. *Ann Thorac Surg.* 2007;83:757–763.

delivery, may help prevent clot formation. Patients should use compressive stockings, and all intravenous lines should have air filters. Pulmonary hypertension from an atrial septal defect usually occurs late in life, past the childbearing years. However, if there is severe pulmonary hypertension (Eisenmenger syndrome), pregnancy should be avoided. Bacterial endocarditis prophylaxis is not recommended. Vaginal delivery is preferred over cesarean section. Risk of CHD in the offspring is estimated to be 8–10%.

B. Ventricular septal defect—Most isolated ventricular septal defects have closed by adulthood. Women with ventricular septal defects generally fare well in pregnancy if the defect is small and pulmonary artery pressure is normal. Congestive heart failure and arrhythmia are reported only in patients with decreased left ventricular systolic function prior to pregnancy. Endocarditis prophylaxis during delivery is not recommended. Air filters should be used on intravenous lines to avoid paradoxic embolism. Large ventricular septal defects with pulmonary hypertension are a contraindication to pregnancy.

C. Atrioventricular septal defect (endocardial cushion defect)—This defect includes a large central defect that may lie above the valve (atrial septal defect) or may extend to variable degrees above and below the atrioventricular valve. The defect can therefore be small or large. Many of these are repaired in childhood. While most complete atrioventricular canal defects are seen in Down syndrome, most partial defects are seen in non–Down syndrome patients. Adult patients without repair may be asymptomatic or may have symptoms of congestive heart failure, arrhythmias, and pulmonary hypertension with cyanosis. The key to good pregnancy outcome is exclusion of hemodynamically significant residual lesions, pulmonary hypertension, and cyanosis prior to conception. Trisomy 21 patients have a 50% risk of transmitting trisomy 21 and other genetic defects to their offspring.

D. Congenital aortic stenosis—This is most commonly caused by a congenital bicuspid aortic valve. The prevalence in the general population is 1–2% but may be as high as 9–21% in some families, where the condition appears to be autosomal dominant with reduced penetrance. The condition is usually more common in men (2:1 ratio). In patients with congenital aortic stenosis, the outcome during pregnancy depends on the severity of the obstruction. Pregnancy is usually well tolerated in mild-to-moderate aortic stenosis (aortic valve area [AVA] 1.0–2.0 cm^2). Patients with severe aortic stenosis with a valve area of < 1.0 cm^2 and mean transvalvular gradients greater than 40 mm Hg may experience an increased risk of complications (from 10–44%), although death is very rare, and fetal morbidity is increased. The increased cardiac output and decreased SVR of pregnancy creates an additional hemodynamic burden in these patients. Syncope, cerebral symptoms, dyspnea, angina pectoris, and even heart failure may occur for the first time during pregnancy. Ideally valve replacement should be performed before pregnancy in symptomatic patients with severe aortic stenosis or if the left ventricular ejection fraction is below 50%. Valvuloplasty, if needed, is preferred over surgery during pregnancy. As part of the bicuspid aortic valve syndrome, the aortic root often will be dilated, evidence that the condition is not only a disease of the valve but of the connective tissue as well. When the aortic root is dilated, there is an increased risk of aortic dissection during pregnancy, and such events have been reported when the aorta is greater than 40 mm, although the true incidence is unknown. The risk of aortic dissection is higher than in the general population but not as high as in Marfan syndrome. Current guidelines would advise counseling and consideration for prophylactic aortic root repair if the aorta exceeds 45 mm. Obtaining serial echocardiograms at least every 3 months to monitor progression of root dilatation appears prudent. Hemodynamic monitoring during labor and delivery should be performed in patients with moderate-to-severe aortic stenosis. Endocarditis prophylaxis is not recommended for vaginal delivery. Cesarean section is recommended in the presence of critical aortic stenosis, aortic aneurysm, or dissection. The risk for the condition in the offspring is variable but at least 4%.

E. Pulmonic stenosis—The natural history of pulmonic stenosis favors survival into adulthood even with severe obstruction to right ventricular outflow. Mild-to-moderate pulmonic stenosis (mean gradient < 40 mm Hg) usually presents no increased risk during pregnancy. Patients with severe pulmonic stenosis may occasionally tolerate pregnancy without the development of congestive heart failure. Vaginal delivery is tolerated well. Ideal treatment consisting of balloon valvuloplasty should be performed before conception but may be performed safely during pregnancy if necessary. The risk in the offspring is about 3.5%.

F. Coarctation of the aorta—In uncomplicated coarctation of the aorta, pregnancy is usually safe for the mother but may be associated with fetal underdevelopment because of the diminished uterine blood flow. The blood pressure may decrease slightly, as during normal pregnancy, but still remains elevated. Maternal deaths in these patients are usually the result of aortic rupture or cerebral hemorrhage from an associated berry aneurysm of the circle of Willis. Patients with the greatest risk during pregnancy are those with severe hypertension or associated cardiac abnormalities, such as bicuspid aortic valves. Treatment consists of limitation of physical activity and maintenance of systolic blood pressure around 140 mm Hg for fetal circulation; β-blockers are preferred and should be continued through delivery. Generally, vaginal deliveries are recommended unless there are obstetric indications for a cesarean delivery. Good pain management for labor and delivery is very important in order to minimize maternal cardiac stress and help to control blood pressure. In cases of severe gradient across the coarctation or associated bicuspid valve with dilated aorta, cesarean section should be considered. Surgical treatment should be reserved for patients in whom complications develop (eg, aortic dissection, uncontrollable hypertension, and refractory heart failure).

G. PATENT DUCTUS ARTERIOSUS—Most patients with a patent ductus arteriosus undergo repair in childhood. A normal pregnancy can be expected in patients with small-to-moderate shunts and no evidence of pulmonary hypertension. Patients with a large patent ductus arteriosus, elevated pulmonary vascular resistance, and a reversed shunt are at greatest risk for complications during pregnancy. The decreased SVR associated with pregnancy increases the right-to-left shunt and may cause intrauterine oxygen desaturation. Patients in whom heart failure develops are treated with digoxin and diuretics. Closure of the patent ductus arteriosus may be done safely during pregnancy using a percutaneous ductal occluder device. The preferred mode of delivery is vaginal in most patients, with hemodynamic monitoring considered at the time of delivery. The risk of patent ductus arteriosus occurring in an offspring is about 4%.

2. Cyanotic heart disease

A. TETRALOGY OF FALLOT—This is the most common cyanotic CHD found in pregnant patients. The syndrome consists of pulmonary stenosis, right ventricular hypertrophy, an overriding aorta, and a ventricular septal defect. The decrease in SVR, the increased cardiac output, and the increased venous return to the right heart augment the amount of right-to-left shunt and further decrease the systemic arterial saturation. Acute blood loss during postpartum hemorrhage is particularly dangerous because venous return to the right heart is impaired. The labile hemodynamics during labor and the peripartum period may precipitate cyanosis, syncope, and even death in surgically untreated women. Patients with uncorrected or partially corrected tetralogy of Fallot are advised against becoming pregnant because they have a high rate of miscarriages (12–40%) as well as a high risk of heart failure (15–25%), arrhythmias (5%) and stroke, myocardial infarction (MI), or death (4–34%). Patients who have had good surgical repair with no important hemodynamic residual lesions and good functional capacity may anticipate successful pregnancies, although the risk of arrhythmias may be increased. Pregnancy is usually well tolerated even in the setting of severe pulmonary regurgitation, as long as right ventricular function is no more than mildly depressed and sinus rhythm is maintained. Antibiotic prophylaxis is recommended for patients with uncorrected tetralogy of Fallot and those in whom prosthetic material has been placed within 6 months. Screening for 22q11.2 microdeletion should be considered in patients with conotruncal abnormalities before pregnancy to provide appropriate genetic counseling. In the absence of a 22q11 deletion, the risk of a fetus having CHD is approximately 4–6%. Fetal echocardiography should be offered to the mother in the second trimester.

B. TRANSPOSITION OF THE GREAT ARTERIES (TGA)—TGA implies that each great artery arises from the wrong ventricle. TGA is atrioventricular concordance with ventriculoarterial discordance, and the aorta arises from the systemic right ventricle while the pulmonary artery arises from the nonsystemic left ventricle. Most adults born with TGA will have had one or more operations in childhood. Comprehensive evaluation is recommended before pregnancy in all patients with TGA and prior repair. The risk of pregnancy depends on the type(s) of repair. For patients after atrial baffle, major prepregnancy concerns include ventricular function assessment, systemic atrioventricular regurgitation, and atrial arrhythmias. The physiologic stresses of pregnancy, although clinically well tolerated late after an atrial baffle procedure, carry an increased risk of right ventricular dysfunction that may be irreversible. Isolated reports are available on the outcome of pregnancy after the arterial switch procedure: In the absence of important cardiovascular residua, pregnancy is well tolerated. A comprehensive anatomic and functional assessment, including assessment of coronary artery anatomy, is recommended before a patient proceeds with pregnancy. Patients who had the atrial baffle should have antibiotic prophylaxis before vaginal delivery.

C. EISENMENGER SYNDROME—This syndrome may occur due to several types of CHD and is characterized by systemic-level pulmonary hypertension with right-to-left or bidirectional shunt with deoxygenation. The right-to-left shunt and deoxygenation will increase with the decrease in SVR occurring with pregnancy. The risk of maternal and fetal morbidity and mortality is so high that patients are advised against becoming pregnant. There is a 35% chance of death in the mother and 15–30% chance of offspring mortality.

3. Surgically corrected congenital heart disease—The obstetric care of patients who have had surgical correction of a CHD requires an understanding of the type of surgical procedure, the sequelae, and the hemodynamic consequences. Although atrial flutter may occasionally develop following surgical closure, the successful closure of an uncomplicated atrial septal defect results in no increased maternal risk during pregnancy. Surgical closure of a patent ductus arteriosus that is not associated with pulmonary hypertension is also not associated with maternal complications during pregnancy. In pulmonary hypertension that develops before surgical closure, the decrease in the pulmonary vascular resistance may not be complete, and complications during pregnancy will depend on its severity. Correction of congenital pulmonary stenosis with either surgery or balloon dilatation that leaves little or no transvalvular gradient presents no difficulty to pregnant patients. Surgical correction of coarctation of the aorta with complete relief of the obstruction decreases the development of associated hypertension and the risk of aortic rupture during pregnancy. Successful repair

of tetralogy of Fallot with little residual gradient across the pulmonary outflow tract and relief of the cyanosis should result, with careful management, in a normal pregnancy. Pregnancy after repair of complex CHD is increasingly encountered. In such patients, the outcome depends on the mother's functional status, the type of repair, the sequelae, and the cardiovascular response to an increase in stress.

Drenthen W, et al. Outcome of pregnancy in women with congenital heart disease: a literature review. *J Am Coll Cardiol*. 2007; 49(24):2303–11. [PMID: 17572244]

Franklin WY, et al. Congenital heart disease in pregnancy. *Cardiol Clin*. 2012;30:383–94. [PMID: 22813364]

Warnes CA, et al. ACC/AHA 2008 guidelines for the management of adults with congenital heart disease: a report of the ACC/AHA Task Force on Practice Guidelines: developed in collaboration with the American Society of Echocardiography, Heart Rhythm Society, International Society for Adult Congenital Heart Disease, Society for Cardiovascular Angiography and Interventions, and Society of Thoracic Surgeons. *Circulation*. 2008;118:714–833. [PMID: 19038677]

B. Valvular Heart Disease

No randomized controlled trial data are available to guide decision making for pregnant women with valvular heart disease. However, many patients with valvular heart disease can be treated successfully through their pregnancy with conservative medical treatment, focusing on optimization of intravascular volume and systemic load. Ideally, symptomatic patients should be treated before conception. Drugs, in general, should be avoided whenever possible. Antibiotics for infective endocarditis prophylaxis for uncomplicated vaginal delivery are not indicated, unless a prosthetic valve was placed within 6 months. Although there are few supportive data, antibiotic prophylaxis is often given for complicated vaginal deliveries.

1. Mitral valve disease

A. MITRAL STENOSIS—Mitral stenosis is the most commonly encountered acquired valvular lesion in pregnancy and is almost always caused by rheumatic heart disease. Mitral stenosis may be first diagnosed during pregnancy and is the valvular disorder most likely to develop serious complications during pregnancy. Increased left atrial pressure and even pulmonary edema due to a decrease in diastolic filling time during the tachycardia of pregnancy may develop in women who were previously asymptomatic. In critical mitral stenosis, due to a large diastolic gradient (even at rest), any demand of increased cardiac output results in a significant elevation in the left atrial pressure and pulmonary edema. The most common symptoms include dyspnea, fatigue, orthopnea, and dizziness or syncope, symptoms that may be difficult to distinguish from normal effects of pregnancy. Signs and symptoms of mitral stenosis may develop

for the first time during pregnancy. The greatest danger is in late pregnancy and labor due to increased heart rate and cardiac output, blood volume expansion, and intensified oxygen demand. Pulmonary edema may occur immediately after delivery even after uncomplicated labor when the blood returns from the decompressed inferior vena cava. Mild-to-moderate mitral stenosis (mean diastolic pressure gradient < 10 mm Hg) may be managed safely with the use of diuretics to relieve pulmonary and systemic congestion and β-blockers to prevent tachycardia to optimize diastolic filling. If diuretics are needed before the third trimester, then there is a high chance that additional measures such as balloon dilatation, commissurotomy, or early delivery may be needed, and close follow-up is needed. Diuretics, β-blockers, digoxin, or direct-current cardioversion for atrial fibrillation should be instituted in cases of hemodynamic compromise, taking into consideration maternal safety. Refractory cases and patients with severe mitral stenosis with heart failure and those with significant pulmonary hypertension prompt mechanical relief, either by percutaneous balloon valvuloplasty or surgery, preferably before conception. Patients with a history of acute rheumatic fever and carditis should continue receiving penicillin prophylaxis.

B. MITRAL REGURGITATION—Mitral regurgitation (most commonly due to mitral valve prolapse) in the absence of NYHA class III or IV heart failure symptoms is generally tolerated well during pregnancy, even if severe. The decrease in systemic blood pressure in pregnancy may reduce the amount of mitral regurgitation. Left ventricular dysfunction, if severe, may precipitate heart failure. Medical management includes use of diuretics; in rare instances, surgical management is necessary, preferably mitral valve repair, which is indicated for severe, acute regurgitation or ruptured chordae and uncontrollable heart failure symptoms. In the future, percutaneous mitral valve repair may be an option for severe, symptomatic mitral regurgitation during pregnancy.

C. MITRAL VALVE PROLAPSE—Mitral valve prolapse is the most common heart disease encountered in pregnancy. Patients without comorbidity, such as a connective tissue, skeletal, or other cardiovascular disorders, tolerate pregnancy. The click and murmur become less prominent during pregnancy. No special precautions for isolated mitral valve prolapse are required. Antibiotic prophylaxis is not recommended. The incidence of complications of the mitral valve prolapse (3%) is similar in pregnant and nonpregnant patients.

2. Aortic valve disease

A. AORTIC STENOSIS—Aortic stenosis in pregnancy is most commonly caused by a congenital bicuspid aortic valve (see previous section).

B. AORTIC REGURGITATION—Isolated chronic aortic regurgitation without left ventricular dysfunction is usually tolerated well. Even if patients are symptomatic, they can often be treated medically with salt restriction, diuretics, and vasodilators. The most common causes are rheumatic disease, bicuspid aortic valve, endocarditis, and a dilated aortic root. Surgery is only indicated for patients with refractory (NYHA class III or IV) symptoms. Acute aortic regurgitation, as in nonpregnancy, is not well tolerated and should be regarded as a surgical emergency.

3. Pulmonic and tricuspid valve disease

A. PULMONIC VALVE REGURGITATION—Pulmonic valve regurgitation may occur in isolation or in combination with other heart lesions. Isolated pulmonic regurgitation can be managed conservatively.

B. TRICUSPID VALVE DISEASE—Tricuspid valve disease may be congenital or acquired. Isolated tricuspid valve disease can be managed successfully with diuretics. Special care should be given to diuretic-induced hypoperfusion.

4. Prosthetic heart valves—Females with a prosthetic heart valve can usually tolerate the hemodynamic burden of pregnancy without difficulty. The function of the prosthesis can be evaluated and monitored throughout the pregnancy with noninvasive Doppler echocardiography. Two types of heart valves are available with their own distinct risks and advantages: tissue valves and mechanical prostheses. The main differences between the types are durability, risk of thromboembolism, valve hemodynamics, and effect on fetal outcome.

Tissue valves (bioprostheses) may be selected for a pregnant patient to avoid anticoagulation and risk of thromboembolism and should be considered in women of childbearing age who desire a pregnancy if there are no other indications for anticoagulation and if the patient accepts the eventual need for replacement of the prosthesis. Bioprostheses in young women in general are associated with an increased risk of structural valve deterioration. Recent data suggest that this risk is not further increased with pregnancy. The risk of failure is estimated to be at least 50% in 10 years and higher if in the mitral position. Therefore, most women of childbearing age will need reoperation, and the risk of a second open-heart surgery should be considered when discussing the risk with the patient. The newer pericardial bioprostheses may offer better durability, but not enough data are available at the moment to make an estimate of the risk. Homografts appear to have a very low risk of failure even in younger patients and also offer superior hemodynamic profiles over other valves and should therefore be considered when possible.

Mechanical valves are indicated in pregnant patients with other coexisting heart disorders requiring anticoagulation (eg, atrial fibrillation, apical thrombus, or history of thromboembolism). Maternal thromboembolism complicates 4–14% of pregnancies in women with mechanical valves despite a therapeutic international normalized ratio (INR), with a reported mortality of 1–4%. This complication is more likely in patients with the older generation valves (caged-ball, tilting disk) in the mitral position but is also reported in the newer bileaflet valves. The choice of prosthetic valve and the safe method of anticoagulation are, therefore, still of concern in pregnant patients and need further study.

Unfortunately, significant maternal and fetal risk of either hemorrhage or thrombosis with the accompanying use of warfarin or heparin remains a major problem. The decision on the choice of anticoagulation should therefore be made with both the patient and the physician after full discussion of potential risks and benefits, and the risk of pregnancy in patients with prosthetic heart valves should be discussed in detail with the patient and the family prior to conception.

The incidence of warfarin embryopathy (nasal hypoplasia, hypoplasia of extremities, and mental retardation) is estimated to be 5–30% when the fetus is exposed during the critical period of organogenesis between the fourth and eighth gestational weeks. The risk of miscarriage and still birth is estimated to be 15–56%, depending on the series. Some studies indicate that the risk may be very low if the woman can be controlled on 5 mg or less of warfarin, and the earlier studies reporting a very high incidence of adverse effects may have been with the use of higher doses. Unfractionated heparin, which does not cross the placenta, is believed to be safe for use during pregnancy; however, due to increase in plasma volume and increased renal excretion, the drug needs to be administered in higher doses and with increased frequency. There is a small risk of osteopenia resulting in fractures and in heparin-induced thrombocytopenia. Low-molecular-weight heparin (LMWH) may provide an advantage in terms of less bleeding and a more predictable response. There is increasing evidence that LMWH can be used for prevention of mechanical valve thrombosis during pregnancy. To adequately prevent thrombosis and prevent bleeding, both peak and trough anti-Xa levels should be measured (Table 33–3), and compliance with dosing is of utmost importance. In almost every instance of reported valve thrombosis with LMWH, subtherapeutic anti-Xa levels were found. Anti-Xa activity should be measured once weekly for the first 4 weeks and later at least once every 2 weeks. High-risk cases may benefit from addition of low-dose aspirin. Table 33–3 shows a recommended regimen for anticoagulation in mechanical prosthetic heart valves taking into account the risk of the patient as well as the risk of side effects from the drugs. Patients with prosthetic heart valves should be managed by cardiologists and obstetricians experienced with this high-risk group.

5. Infective endocarditis—Underlying structural abnormalities of the heart predispose patients to the development of infective endocarditis. The most common cause is rheumatic heart disease, with others being mitral valve prolapse, injecting drug abuse, and iatrogenic procedures. The estimated incidence of infective endocarditis during pregnancy is 0.005–1.0% of all pregnancies. Although it is rare, the development of infective endocarditis during pregnancy

Table 33–3. Recommended Approach for Anticoagulation Prophylaxis in Women with Prosthetic Heart Valves during Pregnancy

	Higher Risk	Lower Risk
Conditions	First-generation prosthetic heart valve (eg, Starr-Edwards, Bjork Shiley) in the mitral position Atrial fibrillation History of thromboembolism while receiving anticoagulation therapy	Second-generation prosthetic heart valve (eg, St. Jude Medical, Medtronic-Hall) in mitral position Any mechanical prosthetic heart valve in the aortic position
Treatment	Warfarin (INR 2.5–3.5) to 35–36th week, then UFH (aPTT ≥ 2.5) to parturition + aspirin 80–100 mg per day OR UFH (aPTT ≥ 2.5) or LMWH (predose anti-Xa ~0.7, peak 1.0–1.4) for 12 weeks, followed by warfarin (INR 2.5–3.5) to 35–36th week, then UFH (aPTT ≥ 2.5) + aspirin 80–100 mg/day	LMWH (trough anti-Xa ~0.6, peak 1.0–1.4) to 35–36 weeks, then UFH (aPTT ≥ 2.0) to parturition OR LMWH (trough anti-Xa ~0.6, peak 1.0–1.4) for 12 weeks, or UFH (aPTT ≥ 2.0), followed by warfarin (INR 2.5–3.0) until 35–36th week, then UFH (aPTT ≥ 2.0) to parturition.

aPTT, activated partial prothrombin time; INR, international normalized ratio; LMWH, low-molecular-weight heparin; UFH, unfractionated heparin.
Modified, with permission, from Goland S. *Cardiol Clin*. 2012;30:395–405.

can have devastating consequences, with maternal and fetal mortality rates estimated to be 22% and 15%, respectively. The clinical diagnosis and the management of infective endocarditis in pregnancy are the same as for nonpregnant patients (see Chapter 22); however, special consideration must be given to the diagnostic and therapeutic approaches during pregnancy to reduce the risk to the fetus.

6. Rheumatic heart disease—Despite an overall decline in the incidence of rheumatic heart disease in Europe and North America, rheumatic valvular disease remains common in women of childbearing age.

The cardiac involvement in acute rheumatic fever is a pancarditis involving the endocardium, myocardium, and pericardium. It is the involvement of the endocardium, including the valvular and the subvalvular apparatus, that gives rise to the acute manifestations as well as causes the development of chronic rheumatic valvular heart disease. The specific valvular conditions are described in previous sections. The mitral valve is most commonly affected, followed by the aortic valve, and less frequently the tricuspid and pulmonic valves.

Mild rheumatic fever may be difficult to diagnose in pregnancy due to tachycardia, functional murmur, and anemia. The management of acute rheumatic fever is similar in pregnant and nonpregnant patients and consists of bed rest, anemia correction, and penicillin. In severe cases, vasodilators, positive inotropes, or even surgery may be required. Echocardiography can be performed safely during pregnancy to delineate myocardial and heart valve function.

American College of Cardiology/American Heart Association Task Force on Practice Guidelines; Society of Cardiovascular Anesthesiologists; Society for Cardiovascular Angiography and Interventions; Society of Thoracic Surgeons, Bonow RO, et al.

ACC/AHA 2006 guidelines for the management of patients with valvular heart disease: a report of the American College of Cardiology/American Heart Association Task Force on Practice Guidelines (writing committee to revise the 1998 Guidelines for the Management of Patients With Valvular Heart Disease): developed in collaboration with the Society of Cardiovascular Anesthesiologists: endorsed by the Society for Cardiovascular Angiography and Interventions and the Society of Thoracic Surgeons. *Circulation*. 2006;114(5):e84–231. [PMID: 16880336]
Goland S, et al. Anticoagulation in pregnancy. *Cardiol Clin*. 2012; 30:395–405. [PMID: 22813365]
Pieper PG, et al. Pregnancy in women with prosthetic heart valves. *Neth Heart J*. 2008;16:406–11. [PMID: 19127317]
Traill TA. Valvular heart disease and pregnancy. *Cardiol Clin*. 2012; 30:369–81. [PMID: 22813363]

C. Myocarditis

This inflammatory process is either focal or diffuse and involves the heart musculature. Of all the infectious and noninfectious causes, viral infection with enterovirus, most commonly **coxsackie B virus**, accounts for most of the cases, but adenovirus, parvovirus B19, cytomegalovirus, Herpesviridae family, and more lately H1/N1 influenza virus have been implicated. Acute rheumatic fever is discussed in the previous section. Other important causes include **acquired immunodeficiency syndrome (AIDS)** and **Chagas disease** due to *Trypanosoma cruzi*, which is the most common cause in South and Central America. Only a few cases of myocarditis have been reported in pregnancy. Clinical manifestations range from incidental finding of silent myocarditis to overt heart failure with hemodynamic collapse. In the acute stage, the electrocardiogram (ECG) is almost always abnormal, showing Q waves with ST- and T-wave changes, which may mimic acute MI. The erythrocyte sedimentation rate (ESR) and cardiac enzymes are usually elevated. Viral cultures may or may not be helpful. Noninvasive imaging studies may reveal regional wall motion abnormalities. Although endomyocardial biopsy is the gold standard for the diagnosis of myocarditis, a negative result does not rule it out, and rarely does the biopsy aid in diagnosing the etiology or guide management. Therefore, endomyocardial biopsy is not routinely recommended. All pregnant women in whom myocarditis is suspected should be hospitalized. Therapy is supportive, with bed rest; avoidance of strenuous activity; and treatment of heart failure with digoxin, diuretics, and vasodilators. Angiotensin-converting enzyme (ACE) inhibitors should be avoided because of the risk of fetal anomalies. Administration of corticosteroids and immunosuppressive therapy has been controversial and has demonstrated no proven benefit. Potential complications of myocarditis include arrhythmia, heart blocks, and cardiogenic shock. Anticoagulation should be seriously considered, especially for patients with severe left ventricular dysfunction.

Chan K, et al. Unusual association of ST-T abnormalities, myocarditis and cardiomyopathy with H1N1 influenza in pregnancy: two case reports and review of the literature. *J Med Case Rep.* 2011;5:314. [PMID: 21756329]

D. Cardiomyopathy

1. Peripartum cardiomyopathy (PPCM)—This rare but distinct form of heart failure with left ventricular dysfunction occurs during pregnancy or postpartum. Classically, it is described as occurring between the last month of pregnancy and 5 months postpartum, but cases that do not appear different have been reported from week 17 of pregnancy to 6 months postpartum. PPCM remains a diagnosis of exclusion. The prevalence appears to be increasing, but this is most likely due to increased diagnosis with the common use of echocardiography. Its estimated incidence in the United States is 1 in 2000–4000 deliveries and is higher in other countries such as South Africa (1 in 1000) and Haiti (1 in 300). Its cause is unknown but is probably multifactorial. Risk factors include age greater than 30 years, patients with history of hypertension and preeclampsia, twin (or greater) pregnancies, and African American women in the United States. Histopathology reveals a dilated heart with pale myocardium, but myocardial biopsy is of little value. Because signs and symptoms of normal pregnancy resemble heart failure, PPCM is easily missed or diagnosed late in the course. PPCM usually presents with dyspnea, cough, orthopnea, paroxysmal nocturnal dyspnea, fatigue, palpitations, and chest pain. Echocardiography is central to diagnosis. The echocardiogram demonstrates dilated left ventricle with marked overall impairment of systolic function. Pulmonary artery catheter placement should be considered for optimized treatment of these patients. Medical therapy is essentially supportive and similar to that for other forms of heart failure and includes salt restriction, diuretics,

digoxin, and afterload reduction with hydralazine (the drug of choice). ACE inhibitors are contraindicated during pregnancy because of associated fetal central nervous system anomalies but can be used after delivery. There is no good evidence for the use of immunoglobulin, although it has been tried in some small trials. A possible promising specific treatment is the use of bromocriptine, a prolactin antagonist. It is believed that the increased oxidative stress as seen with PPCM transforms prolactin to an antiangiogenic and proapoptotic protein with harmful effect on the microvasculature. A small South African study demonstrated improved outcome, and it is expected this may be followed by larger trials in other geographic locations. Heparin should seriously be considered for treating possible thromboembolic phenomena in pregnant patients with very low left ventricular ejection fraction (< 35%). In cases refractory to medical therapy, use of an intra-aortic balloon pump for temporary stabilization and left ventricular assist device as a bridge to transplant is indicated.

Most patients recover partially or even completely, typically within 2–6 months after delivery. There is distinct geographical variation in the rate of recovery, which appears to be at least 50% in the United States but no more than 20–40% in other countries and in women of African American descent. Mortality rates also vary, and recent data from the United States estimate a mortality rate of 0–19%. Mortality in other regions appears higher (15–40%). There is an increased risk of death with increasing age, multiparity, and African American ethnicity and when diagnosis is delayed. Women with a history of PPCM have a significant risk of deleterious fetal and maternal outcome in subsequent pregnancies, even if their left ventricular function has returned to normal. The risk in subsequent pregnancies is around 20% if left ventricular systolic function is normal and around 45% if function has not recovered. Patients who have had fulminant courses and whose left ventricular function has remained depressed should be advised against becoming pregnant again. Women with severe symptoms refractory to medical therapy should terminate the pregnancy as this often results in improvement of symptoms and cardiac function. Recovery of left ventricular function may continue beyond 6 months, and repeat echocardiograms are recommended.

Elkayam U, et al. Peripartum cardiomyopathy. *Cardiol Clin.* 2012; 30:423–40. [PMID: 22813368]
Sliwa K, et al. Evaluation of bromocriptine in the treatment of acute severe peripartum cardiomyopathy: a proof-of-concept pilot study. *Circulation.* 2010;121:1465–73. [PMID: 20308616]

2. Hypertrophic cardiomyopathy—This primary myocardial disease shows a characteristic hypertrophy of the left or right ventricular myocardium. The hypertrophy is asymmetric and most commonly involves the intraventricular septum (asymmetric septal hypertrophy). Pathophysiologic mechanisms include presence of a hyperdynamic left ventricle, obstruction of left ventricular outflow tract, mitral regurgitation, and myocardial ischemia. Prevalence in the young population (age 23–35 years) is 2 per 1000. A large number of patients are asymptomatic. Severe illness is manifested by poor functional capacity, heart failure, and sudden death.

Dyspnea is the most common symptom, with others being chest pain (which may be postprandial), dizziness, syncope, and palpitations. In younger patients, sudden death may be the first manifestation, with an annual incidence in the population being 6%. Physical examination varies from normal to characteristic findings in patients with high gradients. The auscultatory hallmark is a diamond-shaped, grade 3–4/6 systolic murmur, heard best at apex radiating to the left sternal border. The murmur increases in intensity during the strain phase of the Valsalva maneuver. Electrocardiogram shows ventricular hypertrophy, ST and T changes, and Q waves in inferolateral leads. Ventricular arrhythmias are commonly seen on Holter monitoring. Echocardiography diagnostically demonstrates asymmetric septal hypertrophy (with a ratio of septum to posterior wall thickening exceeding 1.5) and decreased septal motion.

Most patients do well during pregnancy. High-risk pregnant patients with a higher likelihood of worsening symptoms during pregnancy include those who were symptomatic prior to pregnancy and asymptomatic patients with left ventricular dysfunction. Increased incidence of supraventricular as well as ventricular arrhythmia in pregnancy has been reported. Maternal hypertrophic cardiomyopathy does not influence fetal outcome, although in about half of the patients, it is familial with autosomal dominant inheritance and confers a 50% risk for affecting the child. Genetic counseling is therefore recommended, and a detailed discussion regarding risks and a thorough evaluation of the patient are required prior to conception.

In asymptomatic patients, outcome is usually good, but close monitoring is recommended. Therapy needs to be individualized in symptomatic patients. β-Blockers have been used most frequently and relatively safely in symptomatic patients but are not recommended for routine use. Of the calcium channel blockers, verapamil has been used sporadically in pregnant patients. Dual-chamber pacing for arrhythmia has been shown to be beneficial but is reserved for severely symptomatic cases refractory to medical therapy. Surgical myectomy has not yet been reported in pregnancy. Atrial fibrillation occurs in 10% of the patients, leading to an increased risk of systemic emboli and hemodynamic worsening. Sotalol, procainamide, and direct-current cardioversion have all been used to treat pregnant patients. Prophylactic placement of an implantable cardioverter-defibrillator should be considered in patients with high-risk features similar to nonpregnant patients. Alcohol septal ablation may reduce symptoms but does not alter prognosis. Hemodynamic monitoring with a pulmonary catheter is recommended for clinical deterioration encountered during labor and delivery and should be considered even in asymptomatic patients. Fortunately, the strain of vaginal delivery is well tolerated in women with hypertrophic cardiomyopathy. Cesarean section is reserved for obstetric indications. Epidural anesthesia should be avoided. Magnesium should be used for tocolysis if needed.

Autore C, et al. Risk associated with pregnancy in hypertrophic cardiomyopathy. *J Am Coll Cardiol.* 2002;40(10):1864–9. [PMID: 12446072]

E. Coronary Artery Disease

Coronary artery disease is a leading cause of death in women in the United States. Coronary artery disease kills more women than the next 16 leading causes of death combined. The incidence of MI during pregnancy and postpartum is estimated to be 3–7 in 100,000 and predominantly antepartum or intrapartum. Because of a trend toward older childbearing age, the incidence of coronary artery disease may be increasing. Earlier studies reported a mortality rate of 37–50% due to MI during pregnancy. However, recent data suggest the rate is much lower at 5–11%, possibly due to improved diagnosis and use of percutaneous coronary intervention in acute coronary syndromes during pregnancy. It is not clear if pregnancy itself increased the risk of MI. The known risk factors include age (30-fold increased if older than 40 years compared with younger than 20 years), hypertension, diabetes mellitus, smoking, and thrombophilia (Table 33–4). The causes of MI in pregnancy include atherosclerosis, congenital lesions (anomalous origin of coronary artery), inflammatory diseases of coronary arteries (Kawasaki disease), connective tissue (eg, Ehlers-Danlos) or vasospastic disorders, and spontaneous coronary artery dissection, which may account for up to 30% of cases. Only around 40% of the women who undergo coronary angiography will have atherosclerotic lesions as a cause of the MI. Coronary artery dissections may be seen at any time during the pregnancy but are much more common in the peripartum period (50%) or postpartum (34%). Most MIs that occur during pregnancy are anterior and transmural, involving the left anterior descending artery. Successful treatment of acute MI during pregnancy with thrombolytic therapy has been reported, but given the risk of placental and fetal bleeding, percutaneous coronary intervention is the preferred treatment for acute ST elevation MI in pregnancy. When percutaneous coronary intervention is indicated, bare-metal stents should be used. β-Blockers are the mainstay of medical therapy. Non-ST elevation acute coronary syndromes should be managed conservatively unless there are high-risk features where angiography may be considered. While coronary artery bypass grafting carries similar risk for the woman as in nonpregnancy, there is an increased risk of fetal mortality (10–19%). The most common presentation is angina pectoris. Patients with a high index of suspicion should undergo a stress test for risk stratification. Due to risk to the fetus, submaximal exercise at 70% of maximum

Table 33–4. Risk Factors for Pregnancy-Related Acute Myocardial Infarction

Risk Factor	Univariate Risk Odds Ratio	P Value	Multivariate Risk Odds Ratio	P Value
Age, years				
< 20 (Ref)	1		1	
20–24	2.4	NS	1.9	NS
25–29	4.3	0.02	3.3	NS
30–34	9.5	< 0.01	6.7	< 0.01
35–39	20.5	< 0.01	16.0	< 0.01
≥ 40	31.6	< 0.01	15.2	< 0.01
Race				
White (Ref)	1		1	
Black	1.4	NS	1.4	NS
Hispanic	0.5	0.02	0.8	NS
Condition				
Hypertension	11.7	< 0.01	21.7	< 0.01
Diabetes	3.2	< 0.01	3.6	< 0.01
Smoking	6.2	< 0.01	8.4	< 0.01
Anemia	2.0	< 0.01	1.6	NS
Thrombophilia	22.3	< 0.01	25.6	< 0.01
Preeclampsia	1.6	0.03	0.1	< 0.01
Postpartum bleeding	2.1	0.02	1.8	NS
Transfusion	7.4	< 0.01	5.1	< 0.01
Postpartum infection	2.5	0.04	3.2	0.02

NS, not significant.
Modified, with permission, from James AH. *Circulation*. 2006;113:1564–1571.

predicted heart rate is recommended, preferably with fetal monitoring. Left ventricular function needs to be assessed to determine the choice of therapy and predict likelihood of survival. The normal physiologic changes of pregnancy may precipitate myocardial ischemia and heart failure in women with left ventricular impairment caused by an infarct. Troponin I remains the most useful marker for monitoring pregnant women for a myocardial injury because it is undetectable during normal labor and delivery, although women with preeclampsia and gestational hypertension may have mildly elevated levels. Lipid-lowering drugs of the statin type are contraindicated during pregnancy due to reported teratogenicity, and the risk clearly outweighs the potential benefit. Efforts should be made to limit myocardial oxygen consumption, particularly during late pregnancy and delivery, in women with known coronary artery disease.

James AH, et al. Acute myocardial infarction in pregnancy: a United States population-based study. *Circulation*. 2006; 113(12):1564–71. [PMID: 16534011]
Roth A, et al. Acute myocardial infarction associated with pregnancy. *J Am Coll Cardiol*. 2008;52:171–80. [PMID: 18617065]
Sahni G. Chest pain syndromes in pregnancy. *Cardiol Clin*. 2012; 30:343–67. [PMID: 22813362]

F. Arrhythmias

Most arrhythmias occurring during pregnancy are benign. Sinus tachycardia, sinus arrhythmia, sinus bradycardia, atrial premature beats, and ventricular premature beats are very common during pregnancy. These are easily diagnosed using standard diagnostic tools such as 12-lead ECG and Holter monitoring. These arrhythmias are hemodynamically insignificant and require no treatment, and the patient can be reassured of their innocence. The occurrence of more complex arrhythmias should, however, raise the suspicion of underlying cardiac disease. Symptomatic arrhythmias, which are rare during pregnancy, may develop during an otherwise uncomplicated pregnancy or in association with underlying cardiac disease. In fact, cardiac arrhythmias may be the first manifestation of cardiac disease during pregnancy.

1. Supraventricular arrhythmias

A. PAROXYSMAL SUPRAVENTRICULAR TACHYCARDIA—The most common arrhythmia encountered during pregnancy is paroxysmal supraventricular tachycardia (PSVT), either atrioventricular nodal reentry tachycardia or resulting from an accessory pathway (see below); it has been estimated to occur in approximately 3% of pregnant patients. In patients with a previous history of PSVT, the frequency and severity of the episodes may increase during pregnancy. The symptoms of PSVT are dyspnea, lightheadedness, and anxiety in patients without underlying cardiac disease. In patients with underlying cardiac abnormalities, angina, heart failure, and syncope may occur as a result of myocardial ischemia and decreased cardiac output. Although there is concern about the effects of hypotension on the fetus during these episodes, women with PSVT do not have an increase in perinatal complications. Patients should have an echocardiogram to excluded structural heart disease. The Valsalva maneuver and carotid massage are less effective in pregnant women as compared with nonpregnant women. Intravenous adenosine, verapamil, or metoprolol are all effective in terminating the tachycardia. Maintenance therapy should only be considered if the arrhythmia is recurrent, and then verapamil or metoprolol may be a good choice. Ablation procedures should be avoided during pregnancy due to the radiation risk on the fetus.

B. ATRIAL FLUTTER AND ATRIAL FIBRILLATION—Atrial flutter, which is uncommon during pregnancy, and atrial fibrillation are usually found in patients with underlying cardiac disease. The hemodynamic consequences and the associated symptoms depend on the underlying cardiac status and the ventricular rate during the tachycardia. During pregnancy, atrial fibrillation is most commonly found in association with mitral stenosis. The development of this arrhythmia in these patients may precipitate congestive heart failure and embolic events. Consideration should be given to anticoagulation therapy if persistent. β-Blockers, verapamil, and digoxin are preferred for long-term rate control, whereas verapamil, metoprolol, or diltiazem usually will slow the heart rate acutely.

C. WOLFF-PARKINSON-WHITE SYNDROME—This preexcitation syndrome usually occurs in patients without underlying cardiac disease. Patients with Wolff-Parkinson-White (WPW) syndrome may have recurrent arrhythmias—most commonly, atrioventricular reentry tachycardia, atrial fibrillation, or atrial flutter. The hemodynamic effects of the associated arrhythmias are related to the type of arrhythmia and the ventricular rate. Many patients with WPW syndrome are asymptomatic, but pregnancy is associated with an increased incidence of arrhythmias in women with this syndrome. WPW may present with an irregular wide complex tachycardia, which is best treated with procainamide.

2. Ventricular arrhythmias

A. PREMATURE VENTRICULAR COMPLEXES—Premature ventricular complexes (PVCs) are relatively common in pregnant women and may be associated with complaints of palpitations. Pregnant women with PVCs and no underlying cardiac disease have an excellent prognosis and require no treatment. Reassurance to the patient is frequently all that is required, along with avoidance of such aggravating factors as smoking and stimulants.

B. VENTRICULAR TACHYCARDIA—Defined as the occurrence of three or more consecutive ventricular complexes, ventricular tachycardia is a serious cardiac arrhythmia that, if sustained, can lead to death. Ventricular tachycardia is rare during pregnancy, but when it occurs, it is usually associated with underlying cardiac disease. The most common cardiac abnormalities associated with ventricular tachycardia are mitral valve prolapse, valvular disease, and cardiomyopathy. The prognosis for patients with nonsustained ventricular tachycardia (< 30 seconds in duration) and no underlying cardiac disease is excellent. In such patients, the ventricular tachycardia is catecholamine-sensitive, and extreme exercise should be avoided. In some patients, therapy with β-adrenergic blocking drugs may be indicated. Sustained ventricular tachycardia (> 30 seconds in duration) or hemodynamically significant ventricular tachycardia is usually associated with underlying cardiac disease, and therapy with antiarrhythmics is usually indicated. Such patients should also undergo evaluation for such precipitating factors as myocardial ischemia, electrolyte imbalance, congestive heart failure, digitalis intoxication, stimulants, and hypoxia. Drugs that can be used are procainamide, lidocaine, or sotalol. Amiodarone should be avoided. In hemodynamically unstable patients, immediate direct-current cardioversion should be performed. Patients with aborted sudden death, syncopal ventricular tachycardia, or ventricular fibrillation or flutter should have an implantable cardioverter-defibrillator implanted, preferably under echocardiographic guidance.

3. Heart blocks—First-degree heart block is evident as PR prolongation on the ECG and results from an increased time of conduction through the atrioventricular junction. First-degree heart block is primarily associated with rheumatic heart disease or digitalis therapy and does not usually require therapy. Second-degree heart block can be divided into two types: Mobitz type I (Wenckebach) and Mobitz

type II. Mobitz type I is characterized by progressive lengthening of the PR interval until an impulse is blocked. It is a relatively benign disorder and occurs when vagal tone is increased. Treatment is seldom indicated. Mobitz type II is a sudden block of conduction without previous prolongation of the PR interval. It often precedes the development of complete heart block. It is rare during pregnancy but may occur in association with rheumatic heart disease or infections. If the ventricular rate is slow and the patient is symptomatic, treatment with permanent pacing is indicated.

Complete heart block can be congenital or acquired. Its onset is usually prior to the pregnancy, and it rarely progresses. Approximately half the cases of complete heart block occurring during pregnancy have an associated ventricular septal defect. Other causes include ischemic heart disease, myocarditis, and rheumatic heart disease. The need for pacemaker therapy depends on the ventricular escape rate. Symptoms are rare at a rate of 50–60 bpm; if the rate suddenly slows, however, syncope may develop. Permanent pacing is indicated in such patients.

McAnulty JH. Arrhythmias in pregnancy. *Cardiol Clin.* 2012;30: 425–34. [PMID: 22813367]

Trappe HJ. Acute therapy of maternal and fetal arrhythmias during pregnancy. *J Intensive Care Med.* 2006;21(5):305–15. [PMID: 16946446]

G. Pericardial Diseases

Pericarditis is usually a mild, self-limited disease. Its incidence, diagnosis, and treatment are similar in pregnant and nonpregnant patients. Most pregnancies, even the complicated ones, may safely reach full term. Idiopathic pericarditis is the most common cause of pericardial disease, others being trauma, infections (viral, bacterial, fungal, tuberculosis), radiation, and collagen vascular diseases.

Sharp, stabbing chest pain that is exacerbated in the supine position and relieved by leaning forward is the most common complaint. Pathognomonic finding of pericardial friction rub is best heard with the diaphragm of the stethoscope over the second and fourth intercostal spaces in midclavicular line or the left sternal border, with the patient leaning forward and inspiring deeply. Characteristic ST-segment elevations with upward concavity and upright T waves have been reported in 80% of patients with acute pericarditis. Echocardiography is an important diagnostic modality and may reveal thickened pericardium, pericardial effusion, and, most importantly, cardiac tamponade.

Pregnant patients in whom pericarditis is suspected who present with ECG changes, tachycardia, and ill appearance should be hospitalized for complete bed rest. Nonsteroidal anti-inflammatory drugs (NSAIDs), aspirin, and indomethacin are effective analgesics that may be used safely before 20 weeks gestation. After 20 weeks gestation, prednisone not to exceed 25 mg/day is the preferred drug. Colchicine should be avoided. Corticosteroids should be avoided in tuberculosis.

Pericardiectomy is reserved for severe, relapsing pericarditis, refractory to medical treatment. Symptoms of a complicating pericardial effusion with cardiac tamponade mimic the symptoms of pregnancy and include shortness of breath, dyspnea on exertion, and fatigue. Echocardiogram will quickly establish the diagnosis. Treatment for symptomatic cardiac tamponade is percutaneous drainage with surgical pericardial window reserved for refractory cases.

Asymptomatic pericardial effusion is frequently encountered in all trimesters, most commonly in the third (up to 40%), but resolves postpartum. Pericardial constriction has been rarely reported in pregnancy, although it could occur as a pericarditis sequel. Most patients have dyspnea, marked edema, and ascites in the latter half of pregnancy. Diuretics, corticosteroids, and pericardiectomy (reserved for refractory cases and associated with reasonable maternal and fetal risk) have all been used to treat pericardial constriction in pregnant patients. Preterm delivery and fetal death have been reported.

Imazio M, et al. Diagnosis and management of pericardial disease. *Nat Rev Cardiol.* 2009;6:743–51. [PMID: 23419899]

H. Pulmonary Hypertension

1. Pulmonary arterial hypertension (World Health Organization class I)

—This entity is defined as *mean* pulmonary artery pressure by right heart catheter of more than 25 mm Hg at rest, a pulmonary capillary wedge pressure or left ventricular end-diastolic pressure ≤ 15 mm Hg, and pulmonary vascular resistance > 3 Wood units. Within this class is primary pulmonary hypertension, which poses a significant risk to pregnant women, with mortality approaching 40%, warranting prevention of pregnancy or early therapeutic abortion (see Table 33–2). However, should these women become pregnant, several options are available. The most common presenting symptoms are dyspnea, fatigue, chest pain, palpitations, syncope or near-syncope, and Raynaud phenomenon. Characteristic physical findings are a result of markedly increased pulmonary pressures, leading to right ventricular hypertrophy and failure with decreased cardiac output. The echocardiogram reveals elevated pulmonary artery pressures, right atrial enlargement, right ventricular hypertrophy, and tricuspid regurgitation. A new onset or worsening of symptoms is commonly seen in the second and third trimesters.

Treatment options include inhaled nitric oxide, calcium channel blockers, sildenafil, epoprostenol (class B), and iloprost (class C). Incidents of premature labor and delivery are high. Patients should lie in the left lateral decubitus position to improve cardiac output. Planned vaginal delivery seems to be safe in stable patients. Epidural anesthesia has been used in most reported cases. Patients should be monitored for 7–10 days postpartum prior to discharge to ensure stability. Patients with primary pulmonary hypertension should be considered for anticoagulation treatment with low-molecular-weight heparin.

Huang S, et al. Treatment of arterial hypertension in pregnancy. *Am J Health Syst Pharm.* 2007;64:1922–6. [PMID: 17823103]

2. Thromboembolic disease—Venous thromboembolic disease is a leading cause of morbidity and mortality during pregnancy and postpartum and accounts for 20% of maternal deaths in the United States. Venous thromboembolism affects pregnant women five times more frequently than nonpregnant women. It is estimated to complicate 2 in 1000 pregnancies. The diagnosis is complicated by symptoms similar to usual pregnancy symptoms such as shortness of breath, tachycardia, and leg swelling. As many as up to 33% of deep venous thrombosis cases may occur in the first trimester, although the risk is highest postpartum (five times higher than during the pregnancy). The immediate postpartum period risk for pulmonary embolism is 15 times greater than during the pregnancy. Risk factors for venous thromboembolism include age > 35 years, body mass index > 30 kg/m^2, a family or personal history of deep venous thrombosis or pulmonary embolism, varicose veins, smoking, or any known hypercoagulable state, as well as multiple previous pregnancies. Pulmonary embolism will occur in 15–24% of patients with untreated deep venous thrombosis and may be fatal in 15%. Diagnosis of deep venous thrombosis should be made with compression ultrasound or impedance plethysmography. Magnetic resonance imaging (MRI) can be performed to diagnose iliac thrombosis. The diagnosis of pulmonary embolism is complicated by the similarities of deep venous thrombosis and pulmonary embolism symptoms with the normal pregnancy symptoms (leg swelling and dyspnea) and the need to avoid radiation in the pregnant patient. The American Thoracic Society recommends initial screening chest x-ray and, if normal, to proceed to a ventilation-perfusion scan, which is considered safe throughout pregnancy. To further decrease radiation, consideration should be given to performing perfusion scan alone, or one may use dose-reduction techniques and use xenon-133 over technetium-99m. If there is no defect, then pulmonary embolism would be very unlikely. If the chest x-ray is abnormal, the test of choice would be a pulmonary angiogram. Except in the first trimester, pulmonary angiogram exposes the fetus to less radiation than a helical computed tomography (CT) scan, and the theoretical risk of exposing the fetus to iodine has not manifested in current studies. An echocardiogram may support the diagnosis of acute embolus by demonstrating right heart enlargement without hypertrophy and elevated pulmonary artery pressure. Hypokinesis with relative sparing of the right ventricular apex may be seen.

The main treatment for deep venous thrombosis during pregnancy consists of heparin, although warfarin can be given after the first trimester until 35 weeks gestation. If unfractionated heparin is used, a target activated partial prothrombin time should be 2.0–2.5. If an LMWH is used, the patient should be monitored with anti-Xa levels. Pulmonary embolism, if stable, should be treated with intravenous heparin for at least 5 days. Oral anticoagulation should be continued for 6 months thereafter. In unstable pulmonary embolism, consideration to thrombolysis and embolectomy should be given. An inferior vena caval filter may also be needed.

McLaughlin VV, et al. ACCF/AHA 2009 expert consensus document on pulmonary hypertension. *J Am Coll Cardiol.* 2009; 53:1573–619. [PMID: 19389575]

I. Diseases of the Aorta

1. Marfan syndrome—Marfan syndrome is an inheritable autosomal dominant connective tissue disorder of the fibrillin gene on chromosome 15 with a prevalence of 1 in 3000–5000 individuals. It involves the ocular, skeletal, and cardiovascular systems. Patients are predisposed to aortic dissection or actual rupture of the aorta most commonly originating in the ascending portion during pregnancy, most likely in the third trimester. High-risk patients have significant associated cardiac abnormalities, such as mitral valve prolapse, mitral and aortic regurgitation, and an aortic root greater than 4.0 cm in diameter. All women with Marfan syndrome planning to become pregnant should undergo a screening transthoracic echocardiogram. High-risk patients (aortic root > 4.0 mm or rapidly progressive dilatation) should have elective surgery before conception, preferably with valve-sparing surgery if no significant aortic regurgitation is present. If the diagnosis is made during pregnancy, β-blockers are strongly recommended, with some authorities advocating prompt termination of pregnancy with aortic repair. Close follow-up with echocardiography should be performed. Women at increased risk for complications during pregnancy should be advised against attempting a pregnancy that may be associated with a 50% maternal mortality rate (see Table 33–2). Patients with no dissection or aortic root enlargement can deliver vaginally with epidural anesthesia and facilitated stage 2 of labor. However, if there is aortic root enlargement, aortic regurgitation, or rapid progression of the aorta size, cesarean delivery is recommended. The risk of the offspring inheriting the disorder is 50%.

2. Loeys-Dietz syndrome—This syndrome is caused by genetic mutation in transforming growth factor (TGF)-β with autosomal dominant inheritance with variable clinical expression. The most common manifestations are aortic aneurysms with a high risk of dissection, hypertelorism, bifid uvula or cleft palate, generalized arterial tortuosity, and aneurysms throughout the arterial tree. Loeys-Dietz syndrome may be misdiagnosed as Marfan syndrome, but patients with Loeys-Dietz syndrome will have normal fibrillin gene. Women with this syndrome should be advised against pregnancy due to the risk of aortic dissection with normal aortic diameter and a risk for uterine rupture during pregnancy.

Hiratzka LF, et al. 2010 ACCF/AHA/AATS/ACR/ASA/SCA/SCAI/SIR/STS/SVM guidelines for the diagnosis and management of patients with thoracic aortic disease: executive summary. *J Am Coll Cardiol.* 2012;55:1509–44. [PMID: 20359588]

Williams JA, et al. Early surgical experience with Loeys-Dietz: a new syndrome of aggressive thoracic aortic aneurysm disease. *Ann Thorac Surg.* 2007;83(2):S757–63. [PMID: 17257922]

J. Hypertension

Hypertension affects 12% of pregnancies and is responsible for 18% of maternal deaths in the United States, but may be on the rise. Risk factors include African American ethnicity, age greater than 45 years, and women with diabetes. Hypertension in pregnancy causes increased rates of intracerebral hemorrhage, placental abruption, intrauterine growth retardation, prematurity, and intrauterine death. Hypertensive disorders in pregnancy can be divided into four groups: (1) chronic, persistent hypertension (blood pressure ≥ 140/90 mm Hg before pregnancy or before the 20th gestational week, or persisting beyond the forty-second postpartum day); (2) gestational hypertension (hypertension developing beyond the 20th gestational week, not associated with preeclampsia or eclampsia and resolving within 42 days postpartum); (3) preeclampsia/eclampsia (hypertension beyond the 20th gestational week with > 300 mg protein/24 hours or > 30 mmol/L in spot urine sample; eclampsia includes presence of seizures); (4) preeclampsia superimposed on chronic hypertension (onset of preeclampsia symptoms in woman with chronic hypertension beyond 20 weeks gestation). Elevated measurements should be confirmed on two occasions, and the patient should be supine in the left lateral position and having rested for at least 10 minutes. The degree of blood pressure elevation does not correlate with risk for eclamptic seizures. Ambulatory blood pressure monitoring may be of value and improve risk prediction. The drug treatment of choice for mild hypertension is methyldopa. Treatment should be initiated if blood pressure is > 150/100 mm Hg. For severe hypertension, drugs such as hydralazine, labetalol, and nifedipine can be used. Target diastolic blood pressure is 80–105 mm Hg depending on the risk.

Vest AR, et al. Hypertension in pregnancy. *Cardiol Clin.* 2012; 30:407–23. [PMID: 22813366]

Vidaeff AC, et al. Acute hypertensive emergencies in pregnancy. *Crit Care Med.* 2005;33(10 Suppl):S307–12. [PMID: 16215352]

▶ Clinical Findings

A. History

The evaluation of heart disease in pregnancy is difficult due to the normal anatomic and physiologic changes of pregnancy. Therefore, taking a careful history is very important and should include a history of rheumatic fever, valvular disorder, arrhythmia, CHD, coronary risk factors or established coronary artery disease, and cardiac surgery.

B. Symptoms & Signs

Reduced exercise tolerance and fatigue are the most common symptoms reported in pregnant women, probably due to increased body weight and anemia. Dizziness, light-headedness, or even syncopal episodes may occur during the latter part of pregnancy because mechanical compression of the uterus on the inferior vena cava decreases venous return and thus the cardiac output. Palpitations are also a frequent complaint but usually are not associated with a significant arrhythmia. Dyspnea and orthopnea, probably due to hyperventilation, are also reported.

C. Physical Examination

The physical examination of pregnant patients with normal cardiovascular systems changes because of the increased hemodynamic burden. The evaluation of patients with suspected heart disease during pregnancy requires a thorough knowledge of the normal physiologic changes (see Table 33–1).

A normal pregnant patient has a slightly fast resting heart rate, large pulse, slightly widened pulse pressure, and warm extremities. Jugular venous distention is seen starting at the 20th week. Edema of the ankles and legs is commonly encountered in late pregnancy. A prominent but unsustained left ventricular impulse may be palpated in late pregnancy and may simulate the volume overload seen in aortic or mitral regurgitation. The auscultatory findings of normal pregnancy begin late in the first trimester and usually disappear 2–4 weeks after delivery. During cardiac auscultation, the first heart sound is loud and exhibits an exaggerated splitting. The second heart sound during late pregnancy is often increased and may exhibit persistent expiratory splitting, especially with the patient in the left lateral position. A third heart sound has been reported to be frequent in late pregnancy. However, because of its association with heart failure, the presence of a third heart sound should lead to further investigation of underlying heart disease, especially in women with symptoms and other signs suggestive of heart disease. A fourth heart sound is rarely heard during a normal pregnancy and may indicate hypertensive heart disease or presence of ischemia.

Systolic murmurs are common during pregnancy and result from the increased blood volume and hyperkinetic state. Most frequently, they are innocent early systolic murmurs, grade 1–2/6, that are best heard at the lower left sternal border and over the pulmonary area, radiating to the suprasternal notch or to the left of the neck. They usually represent vibrations created by ejection of blood into the pulmonary trunk. A cervical venous hum or mammary souffle heard best in the right supraclavicular area in a supine position is a benign systolic, or a continuous, murmur occurring in late pregnancy (Table 33–5). Diastolic heart murmurs are unusual and usually represent valvular abnormalities.

D. Diagnostic Difficulties

Although systolic murmurs are common, the finding of a diastolic murmur is rare during a normal pregnancy and

Table 33–5. Cardiovascular Signs and Symptoms in Normal Pregnancy

Symptoms
Fatigue
Orthopnea
Dyspnea
Decreased functional capacity
Dizziness
Syncope
Physical signs
Jugular venous distention
Displaced left ventricular apical impulse
Right ventricular heave
Palpable pulmonary impulse
Increased intensity of the first heart sound
Persistent splitting of the second heart sound
Systolic ejection murmur at the left lower sternal border or pulmonary
   area with radiation to the neck
Cervical venous hum, mammary souffle

should warrant further diagnostic evaluation. Both systolic and diastolic murmurs associated with cardiac disease can increase or decrease in intensity during pregnancy. Innocent flow murmurs and benign vascular murmurs usually decrease in the sitting position. The systolic murmurs of aortic or pulmonic stenosis usually increase in intensity because of the increased cardiac output and blood volume. The diastolic murmur of mitral stenosis is also increased and may even be first detected during pregnancy. The augmented blood volume and the increased heart rate of pregnancy shorten the diastolic filling period and increase the rate of blood flow across the mitral valve. In contrast, murmurs of mitral or aortic regurgitation may soften or even disappear during pregnancy as a result of the decrease in peripheral vascular resistance. The circulatory changes of pregnancy also affect the auscultatory findings in cardiac abnormalities, such as mitral valve prolapse and hypertrophic cardiomyopathy, which are dependent on volume. The increase in left ventricular volume during pregnancy may attenuate or abolish the click and late systolic murmur typical of mitral valve prolapse. The systolic murmur of hypertrophic obstructive cardiomyopathy may also decrease or disappear as the left ventricular volume increases during pregnancy.

E. Diagnostic Studies

1. Electrocardiography—The ECG is an important diagnostic technique that can indicate the presence of underlying cardiac abnormalities. Cardiac chamber hypertrophy, myocardial ischemia and infarction, pericarditis, myocarditis, conduction abnormalities, and the presence of atrial and ventricular arrhythmias may be detected by ECG. In patients with suspected cardiac arrhythmias, ambulatory Holter monitoring may be indicated. During normal pregnancy, sinus tachycardia, a shift of the axis to the left or

right, may be observed, and transient ST abnormalities are common.

2. Echocardiography—Transthoracic echocardiography is an important diagnostic noninvasive study that can be performed safely in pregnancy. The intracardiac structures can be evaluated for abnormalities of the great vessels, cardiac chambers, and heart valves. Chamber sizes and ventricular function can also be measured.

During the echocardiographic examination, the normal physiologic changes that occur with pregnancy should be kept in mind. When the patient is evaluated in the left lateral position, an increase in the diastolic dimensions of the right and left ventricles is common because of volume increases that occur with a normal pregnancy. Because of the increase in the left ventricular dimensions, mitral valve prolapse may improve or disappear during pregnancy. Right and left atrial dimensions may also increase slightly; these changes increase as the pregnancy progresses. Small pericardial effusions are common throughout pregnancy in healthy women, but with highest incidence in the last trimester.

Doppler echocardiography provides reliable quantitative and qualitative information regarding the presence and severity of valvular stenosis and regurgitation. Doppler echocardiography can measure the valve area and gradients across stenotic valves. Small degrees of pulmonary, tricuspid, and mitral regurgitation have frequently been found in normal individuals, whether pregnant or not. In patients with CHD (corrected or uncorrected), Doppler echocardiography can detect the presence of intracardiac shunts and estimate the shunt ratios by determining the right and left cardiac outputs. It can measure pulmonary artery systolic pressure to assess the effects of the valvular lesions and intracardiac shunts on the pulmonary circulation.

Transesophageal echocardiography (TEE) provides superior images of the intracardiac structures and great vessels, providing the same detailed analysis of cardiac structure, function, and hemodynamic assessment possible with transthoracic echocardiography. TEE can be used for patients in whom the transthoracic examination is technically suboptimal and for those with suspected prosthetic or native valve dysfunction, infective endocarditis, CHD, or aortic dissection. Although experience with TEE during pregnancy has been limited, the procedure should be considered in pregnant patients for whom the risks are less than the possible benefit. The procedure should be performed by an experienced echocardiographer, and fetal monitoring, in addition to the routine monitoring of the patient, should be available (Table 33–6).

3. Exercise tolerance test—Little is known about the safety of an exercise test to establish ischemic heart disease in pregnancy. Fetal bradycardia, marked hypoxia, acidosis, and severe hypothermia at peak exercise have been reported. In light of these facts, the use of a submaximal stress test (approximately 70% of the maximal predicted heart rate) with close fetal monitoring is recommended, until more information regarding its

Table 33–6. Normal Diagnostic Test Findings in Pregnancy

Electrocardiogram
Sinus tachycardia
Increased incidence of arrhythmias
QRS axis deviation
Increased amplitude of R wave in lead V_2
ST segment and T-wave changes
Small Q waves
Echocardiogram
Mildly increased biatrial size
Increased biventricular dimensions
Mildly increased left ventricular systolic function
Small pericardial effusion
Increased tricuspid valve diameter
Mild tricuspid, pulmonic, and mitral regurgitation
Chest roentgenogram
Increased lung markings
Horizontal positioning of the heart
Straightened left upper cardiac border

safety is available. Maximal oxygen consumption, unchanged in pregnancy, could be used for the assessment of the functional status in cardiac patients during pregnancy.

4. Chest radiography—The usefulness of chest films during pregnancy is limited because of the potential hazard to the fetus from radiation exposure. Whenever a chest film is believed necessary, the abdominopelvic area should be shielded with lead to minimize exposure. The normal cardiac changes of pregnancy, such as chamber enlargement and the horizontal position of the heart because of the elevation of the diaphragm, should not be misinterpreted as cardiac disease. Newer and more accurate techniques such as Doppler echocardiography have largely replaced chest films in the evaluation of cardiac structure and function. Chest x-rays are recommended as part of the evaluation of the pregnant patient suspected of having acute pulmonary embolism.

5. Radionuclide studies—Myocardial perfusion scans and radionuclide ventriculography should be avoided, if possible, especially in the first trimester of pregnancy because of the risk of rare but possible fetal malformations. Also, in women of childbearing age, the incidence of coronary heart disease is low, and other noninvasive techniques, such as exercise echocardiography, can be used to assess coronary artery disease. In cases of suspected pulmonary embolism, a limited ventilation-perfusion scan (only performing the perfusion phase) may be performed weighing out the risks and the benefits. The minimal dose of isotope possible should be used, and xenon-133 is preferred over technetium-99m.

6. Computed tomography—CT scanning imposes ionizing radiation to the mother and in part to the fetus and should only be used if no other imaging modalities can provide the diagnostic information. Using specific low-dose protocols, the amount of radiation with a CT scan may be less than that of a radionuclide scan. For certain studies, iodine contrast is used, which may carry a small risk for hypothyroidism in the fetus, although newer studies have not been able to detect this. At present, it appears the only time CT angiography benefit may outweigh the risk is in pregnant women suspected of pulmonary embolism. Aortic dissections should be evaluated by TEE or MRI.

7. Magnetic resonance imaging—MRI provides multiplanar images of the body with excellent soft-tissue contrast without the use of ionizing radiation. MRI is, in general, regarded as safe in pregnancy. However, safety data are limited. Therefore, MRI should be limited to cases where ultrasonography is inconclusive and where patient care depends on further imaging. Gadolinium contrast should be avoided.

8. Pulmonary artery catheterization—Bedside hemodynamic monitoring can be performed with a balloon-tipped pulmonary artery catheter. In most patients, inflating the balloon permits flotation of the catheter through the right heart without the need for fluoroscopy. With the catheter in the pulmonary artery, the balloon is inflated until it occludes a small vessel; the pulmonary artery wedge pressure obtained reflects the left ventricular end-diastolic pressure. Pulmonary artery pressures and cardiac output can also be measured. The placement of a balloon flotation catheter should be considered during the early stages of labor in any patient with cardiac disease who has been symptomatic during the pregnancy. Furthermore, because of postpartum hemodynamic changes, hemodynamic monitoring should be continued for up to 48 hours following delivery.

9. Cardiac catheterization—In some patients with cardiac disease who decompensate during pregnancy, complete diagnostic information cannot be obtained by noninvasive methods alone. This is particularly important when surgical intervention is contemplated. Cardiac catheterization in these patients may need to be performed during pregnancy. Because the radiation required for the performance of this technique has potentially adverse effects on the fetus, cardiac catheterization should be performed only if the needed information cannot be obtained by any other means. Whenever possible, cardiac catheterization should be performed after major organogenesis has occurred (> 12 weeks after the last menses). The radial approach is the preferred method to minimize the risk of radiation exposure to the abdomen, which should be lead shielded. The exposure to x-rays should be reduced to a minimum; catheter position can be guided in some cases by Doppler and contrast echocardiography.

▶ Treatment

A. Pharmacologic Treatment

Treatment of the pregnant patient with cardiac disease requires the collaborative consultation of the obstetrician and cardiologist at regular intervals during gestation and careful planning for delivery with the anesthesiologist. All cardiovascular drugs during pregnancy should be avoided, if possible, especially in the first trimester. Most cardiovascular drugs cross the placenta and are secreted into the breast milk, mandating a detailed evaluation of risk-to-benefit ratio (Table 33–7).

1. Heart failure—Treatment of heart failure is more challenging in pregnant patients than in nonpregnant women. Salt restriction and activity limitation are extremely important. In patients with pulmonary congestion, medical therapy should begin with digoxin. Although digoxin has been safely used during pregnancy for many years, blood levels should be monitored to avoid toxicity. Diuretics, although not teratogenic, may cause impaired uterine blood flow

and placental perfusion, and hence should only be used in severely symptomatic patients. Thiazide diuretics have been associated with neonatal thrombocytopenia, jaundice, hyponatremia, and bradycardia, and loop diuretic are preferred.

Afterload is already reduced during pregnancy; hence, further reduction in afterload may only be beneficial in selected cases. Hydralazine, the most frequently used afterload-reducing agent during pregnancy, is a direct arteriolar dilator and has not been associated with adverse fetal effects. ACE inhibitors are contraindicated in pregnancy due to their associated increased risk of premature delivery, low birth weight, fetal hypotension, renal failure, bony malformations, persistent patent ductus arteriosus, respiratory distress syndrome, and even death. Angiotensin II receptor blockers

Table 33–7. Alphabetical List of the Commonly Used Cardiovascular Medications, Their Potential Fetal Side Effects, and Overall Safety

Drugs	Potential Side Effects	Safety
ACE-I	IUGR, prematurity, low birth weight, neonatal renal failure, bony malformations, limb contractures, patent ductus arteriosus, death	Contraindicated
Adenosine	Limited data (in first trimester only)	Safe
Amiodarone	IUGR, prematurity, hypothyroidism, prolonged QT in the newborn	Unsafe
ARB	Same as ACE-I	Contraindicated
β-Blockers	Fetal bradycardia, hypoglycemia and apnea at birth, IUGR, uterine contraction initiation	Safe
Calcium channel blocker	Maternal hypotension leading to fetal distress, birth defects	Verapamil safe
Digoxin	Low birth weight	Safe
Disopyramide	Uterine contraction initiation	Safe
Diuretics	Hyponatremia, bradycardia, jaundice, low platelets, impaired uterine blood flow	Potentially unsafe
Heparin	None reported	Probably safe
Hydralazine	None reported	Safe
Lidocaine	CNS depression due to fetal acidosis with high blood levels	Safe
Mexiletine	IUGR, fetal bradycardia, neonatal hypoglycemia, and hypothyroidism	Safe
Nitrates	Fetal bradycardia	Probably safe
Nitroprusside	Thiocyanate toxicity	Potentially unsafe
Procainamide	None reported	Safe
Quinidine	Premature labor, fetal VIII cranial nerve damage with high blood levels	Safe
Sotalol	Limited data; bradycardia, reports of death	Probably safe
Warfarin	Embryopathy, in utero fetal hemorrhage, CNS abnormalities	Unsafe

ACE-I, angiotensin-converting enzyme inhibitor; ARB, angiotensin receptor blockers; CNS, central nervous system; IUGR, intrauterine growth retardation.

have similar adverse reactions and are thus rendered unsafe. Data on nitrates are limited and require further evaluation. β-Blockers may be used safely, although atenolol should be avoided.

2. Arrhythmias—During pregnancy, any precipitating factors of arrhythmia should be avoided or corrected. In general, conservative treatment of cardiac arrhythmias is indicated. Direct-current cardioversion is the treatment of choice in patients with hemodynamic compromise due to arrhythmia. Although no antiarrhythmic is completely safe during pregnancy, most are tolerated well and are relatively safe. Drugs with the longest record of safety should be used as first-line therapy. Digoxin, although one of the safest drugs for treating arrhythmia during gestation, may cause increased risk of prematurity and intrauterine growth retardation. Adenosine has been reported safe and successful in terminating supraventricular tachycardias during pregnancy.

Quinidine, with minimal fetal risk, has the longest record of being used safely and effectively in the treatment of both atrial and ventricular tachycardia during pregnancy. When quinidine is indicated during pregnancy, blood levels should be closely monitored because drug interactions with warfarin may develop excessively prolonged prothrombin time, with the potential for hemorrhage. Procainamide has also been used safely and is the drug of choice in the treatment of wide-complex tachycardias.

Amiodarone is associated with fetal hypothyroidism, smaller size at birth for date of gestation, and prematurity, and is also secreted in breast milk. Amiodarone is thus reserved only for treating life-threatening arrhythmias or those refractory to other medical therapy. Verapamil, although used during pregnancy, should be discontinued at the onset of labor to avoid dysfunctional labor and postpartum hemorrhage.

β-Adrenergic blocking agents are relatively safe and have frequently been used in pregnant patients to treat arrhythmia, hypertrophic cardiomyopathy, and hyperthyroidism. Propranolol is a nonselective β-blocker that has been used frequently during pregnancy. Fetal and newborn heart rate, blood glucose levels, and respiratory status should be monitored closely.

Lidocaine may be used for ventricular tachycardia, especially in the setting of an acute MI, but it requires close monitoring of blood levels.

3. Thrombosis and thromboembolism—Even though increased concentrations of clotting factors and platelet adhesiveness and decreased fibrinolysis in pregnancy result in an overall increased risk of thrombosis and embolism, the actual incidence of venous thromboembolism during pregnancy is lower than previously reported. The gestational age at presentation appears to be equally distributed. Pulmonary embolism cases are reported to occur most commonly in the postpartum period and are strongly associated with a cesarean section. About 40% of asymptomatic patients with deep venous thrombosis may indeed have a pulmonary embolism.

The major indications for anticoagulants during pregnancy include the presence of mechanical heart valves and prophylaxis for recurrent pulmonary thromboembolism. Some patients with rheumatic heart disease with atrial fibrillation and cardiomyopathies may also be candidates for anticoagulation during pregnancy. The best method of anticoagulation in a pregnant patient is still controversial. A recommended regimen is suggested in Table 33–3.

Warfarin has been associated with fetal wastage due to spontaneous abortion and stillbirths, optic nerve atrophy and blindness, microcephaly, mental retardation, and even death due to intracranial hemorrhage. Its use in the first trimester is associated with warfarin embryopathy in 5–30% of newborns, a syndrome comprising nasal bone hypoplasia and epiphyseal stippling. The risk may be less if the patient can be controlled on a daily dose of 5 mg or less. Warfarin poses significant risks to both the mother and the fetus during labor and delivery; however, breastfeeding women can be prescribed warfarin because it is not secreted in the breast milk. In the second trimester, warfarin is the treatment of choice, with INR monitoring. Therefore, warfarin should be given only after the 12th gestational week and should be stopped before delivery around 35th week.

Heparin is generally the drug of choice for anticoagulation in pregnant patients, unless there is a very high risk for thromboembolism (see section on prosthetic heart valves). As soon as pregnancy is diagnosed, oral anticoagulants should be discontinued, and subcutaneous heparin, with a goal partial thromboplastin time (PTT) of 2–2.5 times normal, should be initiated. If LMWH is used, anti-Xa levels (peak and trough) should be monitored. Complications of unfractionated heparin administration include thrombocytopenia, alopecia, and osteoporosis. At the 36th week of gestation, subcutaneous heparin should be switched to intravenous route. To avoid the risk of bleeding during labor and delivery, heparin should be discontinued 24 hours prior. Anticoagulation should then be resumed 4 hours after delivery if no bleeding complications.

Low-dose aspirin has been safely used in pregnancy. Dipyridamole should not be used in a pregnant patient. Thrombolytic therapy has been used safely and effectively but should be avoided whenever possible.

4. Endocarditis prophylaxis—The American Heart Association does not recommend prophylaxis for infective endocarditis in pregnant patients. However, many obstetrician do decide to administer antibiotics in high-risk patients at time of rupture of the membranes in patients undergoing vaginal delivery. The patients considered highest risk are those with mechanical prosthetic heart valves, those with a history of infective endocarditis, and those with uncorrected or recently corrected cyanotic CHDs or with residual defects. In addition, patients with a known infection should be treated.

Frishman WH, et al. Cardiovascular drugs in pregnancy. *Cardiol Clin.* 2012;30:463–91. [PMID: 22813371]

Nishimura RA, et al. ACC/AHA 2008 guideline update on valvular heart disease: focused update on infective endocarditis: a report of the American College of Cardiology/American Heart Association Task Force on Practice Guidelines. *J Am Coll Cardiol.* 2008;52:676–85. [PMID: 18702976]

B. Surgical Treatment

Ideally, most cardiac diseases requiring surgical correction are diagnosed and treated before the patient becomes pregnant, so the data are anecdotal. In general, cardiac surgery in pregnant patients is not associated with significant maternal risk but may cause fetal wastage. Fetal risk has been reported to be as high as 33%. Pregnant women requiring cardiac surgery need utmost care, adequate valve selection, and anticoagulation to ensure a good outcome.

Surgery should be reserved for severely symptomatic patients and those who are refractory to medical therapy, and it should be avoided in the first trimester, if possible. Procedures not involving cardiopulmonary bypass are preferred because of associated risks of fetal bradycardia and hypoperfusion.

C. Labor & Delivery

Labor and delivery are periods of maximal hemodynamic stress during pregnancy. Pain, anxiety, and uterine contractions all contribute to altered hemodynamics. Oxygen consumption is higher, and cardiac output is increased up to 50%. Both systolic and diastolic pressures are increased significantly during uterine contractions, especially in the second stage. Anesthesia and analgesia during labor and delivery may affect oxygen consumption, but they do not reduce increased cardiac output secondary to uterine contractions.

Acute decompensation may develop in patients with pre-existing cardiac disease. This increase in preload and cardiac output can be devastating in a patient with limited cardiac reserve or an obstructive valvular lesion. Patients at greatest risk for complications during labor and delivery include those with significant pulmonary hypertension and those in NYHA functional class III or IV.

The preferred method of delivery is vaginal, with careful attention paid to pain control by regional anesthesia to avoid tachycardia. Postpartum hemorrhage and excessive fluid intake should be prevented. Invasive hemodynamic monitoring may be needed in some cases to guide treatment rapidly during labor and delivery. In these patients, the monitoring should be continued for at least 24–48 hours after delivery or until hemodynamic stability is ensured. Cesarean section, with few exceptions, should be performed only for obstetric indications because it can also create blood loss and fluid shifts. Regardless of the delivery method, however, effective pain control is absolutely essential.

▶ Prognosis

Maternal mortality and morbidity rates during pregnancy depend on the underlying cardiac lesion and the functional status of the patient (see Table 33–2). The greatest risk of maternal mortality (25–50%) is for patients with pulmonary hypertension, Eisenmenger syndrome, NYHA class III and IV, and Marfan syndrome with a dilated aorta. Pulmonary vascular disease prevents the adaptive mechanisms of normal pregnancy and makes labor, delivery, and the early postpartum period particularly problematic. Moderate-to-severe mitral stenosis, aortic stenosis, the presence of mechanical prosthetic valves, uncomplicated coarctation of the aorta, uncorrected CHDs (without Eisenmenger syndrome), and Marfan syndrome with a normal aorta are associated with a 5–10% mortality rate. Left-to-right shunts, pulmonary valve disease, corrected CHD, bioprosthetic valves, and mild-to-moderate mitral stenosis have a mortality rate of less than 1%.

The functional status of a patient should be classified according to the NYHA classification system. Patients in class I or II can be expected to undergo pregnancy with a less than 0.5% risk of death.

Endocrinology & the Heart

Eveline Oestreicher Stock, MD

Endocrinology involves the study of glands that secrete hormones into the circulation for effects at distant target sites. Classic endocrine glands include organs like the pituitary gland, thyroid and parathyroid glands, pancreatic islets, adrenal glands, ovaries, and testes. It is now clear that hormones are also secreted from nontraditional endocrine organs and play critical roles in the regulation of physiologic processes. Examples of such organs include the heart (natriuretic peptides), kidney (renin and erythropoietin), adipose tissue (leptin, adiponectin, and irisin), and gut (cholecystokinin and incretins). Once in the circulation, hormones bind to receptors on target tissues to elicit biological effects. Target tissues for some hormones (eg, glucocorticoid, thyroid hormone) can be numerous, reflecting the wide distribution of receptors, while other tissues may have a more limited distribution (eg, androgens). Because hormone receptors can be so ubiquitous throughout the body, the presence or absence of a single hormone can have multiple effects on one or more organ systems, including the cardiovascular system. This chapter considers most of the common and some uncommon endocrinopathies that can affect the heart, addressing specifically how they can be recognized and treated to best restore cardiovascular health.

THYROID & THE HEART

The cardiovascular signs and symptoms of thyroid disease are some of the most characteristic and clinically relevant signs and symptoms seen. Both hyperthyroidism and hypothyroidism produce changes in cardiac contractility, myocardial oxygen consumption, cardiac output, blood pressure, and systemic vascular resistance. Although it is well known that hyperthyroidism can produce atrial fibrillation, it is less well recognized that hypothyroidism predisposes to ventricular dysrhythmias. The importance of the recognition of the effects of thyroid disease on the heart is highlighted by the recognition that restoration of normal thyroid function in almost all cases reverses the abnormal cardiovascular changes.

Thyroid disease is quite common, affecting approximately 9–15% of the adult female population and a smaller percentage of males. This gender-specific prevalence likely results from autoimmune causes for the most common forms of thyroid disease, such as Graves and Hashimoto disease. However, with advancing age, especially beyond the eighth decade of life, the incidence of disease in males increases to equal that of females.

Thyroid hormone regulates oxidative and metabolic processes throughout the body by directing cellular protein synthesis at the nuclear level. Nongenomic actions of thyroid hormones have also been recognized based on rapid tissue responses that take place before RNA transcription could occur and by recognition of triiodothyronine (T_3) and thyroxine (T_4) binding sites outside of the nucleus. Both overproduction and underproduction of thyroid hormone can disrupt normal metabolic function. Under the control of pituitary release of thyroid-stimulating hormone (TSH), the thyroid gland secretes T_4 and T_3, mostly bound to plasma proteins. The free, or unbound, fraction of hormone negatively feeds back at the level of the hypothalamus and pituitary to suppress further release of thyroid-releasing hormone (TRH) and TSH.

▶ Cardiovascular Effects of Thyroid Hormones

The mechanism of thyroid hormone–induced dysfunction is multifactorial. Thyroid hormones increase the number of β-adrenergic receptors in the heart and skeletal muscle, adipose tissue, and lymphocytes. They also amplify catecholamine action at a postreceptor site. The heart rate increases due to increased sinoatrial activity, a lower threshold for atrial activity, and shortened atrial repolarization. These last two factors also create a favorable substrate for the generation of atrial fibrillation (AF), and a similar effect on ventricular myocardium has been associated with ventricular arrhythmias. In addition, vascular volume increases due to activation of the renin–angiotensin system, and there is increased contractility due to increased metabolic demand and the direct effect of T_3 on cardiac muscle. Systemic vascular resistance decreases because of T_3-induced peripheral vasodilation. The sum of these effects is a dramatic increase in cardiac output, frequently to more than 7 L/min.

Many of the clinical manifestations of thyrotoxicosis appear to reflect increased sensitivity to catecholamines. Therapy with β-adrenergic blocking agents is often helpful in controlling these sympathomimetic manifestations of thyroid hormone excess.

In addition, thyroid hormone has numerous effects on coagulation, such as shortened activated partial thromboplastin time, increased fibrinogen levels, and increased factor VIII and factor X activity, and clinical sequelae such as stroke are seen in patients with thyrotoxicosis, even in sinus rhythm. Although undocumented paroxysmal AF may contribute to embolic phenomena, studies suggest that hyperthyroidism is associated with a prothrombotic state and ischemic stroke independent of atrial arrhythmias.

1. Hyperthyroidism

ESSENTIALS OF DIAGNOSIS

▶ Low (suppressed) thyroid-stimulating hormone levels (below the lower range).

▶ High free T_4, total T_4, and free thyroxine index, and/or high free T_3 or total T_3 radioimmunoassay.

▶ High 24-hour radioactive iodine uptake in Graves disease or toxic multinodular goiter; low uptake in thyroiditis or exogenous cause.

▶ Goiter (often with bruit) and exophthalmos in Graves disease.

▶ General Considerations

In general, thyrotoxicosis is the clinical syndrome that results when tissues are exposed to high levels of circulating thyroid hormones. Short-term hyperthyroidism is characterized by a high cardiac output state with an increase in heart rate and cardiac preload and a reduction in peripheral vascular resistance, resulting in a hyperdynamic circulation. Cardiac preload (left ventricular end-diastolic volume) is increased as a consequence of the increase in blood volume and the enhancement of diastolic function. The reduction in systemic vascular resistance is responsible for decreased renal perfusion pressure and subsequent activation of the renin–angiotensin–aldosterone system, resulting in increased sodium absorption and blood volume. In experimental studies, thyroid hormone induced physiologic cardiomyocyte hypertrophy by acting on intracellular signaling pathways. In humans, long-term exposure to thyroid

hormone excess may exert unfavorable effects on cardiac structure and function because it may increase left ventricular mass, arterial stiffness, and left atrial size and may induce diastolic dysfunction, thereby impairing left ventricle performance. However, because thyroid hormone excess does not induce cardiac fibrosis, these changes are reversed once euthyroidism is restored.

In most instances, thyrotoxicosis is due to hyperactivity of the thyroid gland, or hyperthyroidism. Occasionally, thyrotoxicosis may be due to other causes such as excessive ingestion of thyroid hormone. The various forms of hyperthyroidism are listed in Table 34–1.

▶ Clinical Findings

A. History

A family history of thyroid disease should be investigated, including a history of goiter, as well as immunologic disorders such as type 1 diabetes, rheumatoid disease, pernicious anemia, vitiligo, or myasthenia gravis, which may be associated with an increased incidence of autoimmune thyroid disease. Iodine ingestion in the form of amiodarone, an iodine-containing antiarrhythmic drug, or intravenous iodide-containing contrast media used in angiography and computed tomography (CT) scanning may induce hyper- or hypothyroidism. Lithium carbonate, used in the treatment of bipolar disorder, can also induce hypothyroidism, goiter, and more rarely, hyperthyroidism. Residence in an area of low dietary iodide is associated with iodine deficiency goiter (endemic goiter). Exposure to ionizing radiation in childhood has been associated with increased incidence of thyroid disease.

B. Symptoms & Signs

Patients with hyperthyroidism often complain of weight loss despite an increased appetite; this helps distinguish this condition from other wasting conditions such as cancer or acquired immunodeficiency syndrome (AIDS) where appetite is usually diminished. A fine resting tremor of the hands is noticed, along with nervousness, anxiety, insomnia, mood swings, and irritability. Heat intolerance and diaphoresis are seen. Proximal muscle weakness and muscle wasting may be prominent. An increased number of bowel movements or diarrhea may occur due to accelerated transit in the gut. Thyroid enlargement, thyrotoxic eye signs (eg, lid retraction, proptosis, periorbital edema, conjunctival redness, extraocular muscle involvement) and tachycardia are commonly seen. In patients over age 60, cardiovascular and myopathic manifestations predominate; the most common presenting complaints are palpitations, dyspnea on exertion, tremor, nervousness, and weight loss.

Patients with overt and subclinical hyperthyroidism are at increased risk of cardiac death, although the exact mechanism leading to this effect is not well established. The increased risk of cardiac mortality might be a consequence of the increased risk of atrial arrhythmias and of the risk of

Table 34–1. Causes of Hyperthyroidism

Etiology	Comments
Graves disease	Symmetric smooth goiter, ophthalmopathy, elevated ^{131}I uptake, homogeneous uptake on thyroid scan, TSH receptor antibodies
Toxic multinodular goiter	Nodular goiter, nonhomogeneous uptake on thyroid scan
Autonomous thyroid nodule	Single large "hot" nodule on thyroid scan, suppressing rest of thyroid tissue
Thyroiditis	
Subacute	Tender firm goiter, low ^{131}I uptake, transient high ESR
Radiation	Tender goiter, low ^{131}I uptake, high ESR; occurs after ^{131}I therapy
Painless (silent)	Nontender goiter, low ^{131}I uptake, normal ESR
Postpartum	Nontender goiter, low ^{131}I uptake, antithyroid antibodies, transient; tends to recur with each pregnancy
Exogenous	
Amiodarone	Low or normal ^{131}I uptake
Iatrogenic	Absent goiter, low serum thyroglobulin, low ^{131}I uptake
Factitious	Absent goiter, low serum thyroglobulin, low ^{131}I uptake
Iodine induced	Low ^{131}I uptake, high 24-hour urinary iodide excretion; history of iodine ingestion or exposure (contrast agents)
Rare causes	
Struma ovarii	Low ^{131}I uptake in thyroid; positive uptake in the ovary
Trophoblastic tumor	Very high hCG
Metastatic follicular carcinoma	Usually obvious metastases on ^{131}I scan
TSH-producing adenoma	TSH not suppressed, tumor on CT or MRI of pituitary; consider if gland regrows after thyroidectomy or ^{131}I treatment

CT, computed tomography; ESR, erythrocyte sedimentation rate; hCG, human chorionic gonadotropin; ^{131}I, radioactive iodine; MRI, magnetic resonance imaging; TSH, thyroid-stimulating hormone.

heart failure (HF) in these individuals, especially in elderly patients. In particular, thyrotoxic AF has been associated with an increased risk of cerebrovascular and pulmonary embolism. Furthermore, autoimmune hyperthyroidism has been associated with autoimmune cardiovascular involvement: pulmonary arterial hypertension, myxomatous cardiac valve disease, and autoimmune cardiomyopathy have been reported in patients with Graves disease with higher frequency than in the general population.

AF is the most common cardiac complication of hyperthyroidism, occurring in an estimated 10–25% of overtly hyperthyroid patients compared with 0.4% of the general population. High-normal thyroid levels or subclinical hyperthyroidism is also associated with an increased risk of developing AF. The prevalence of AF in both populations increases with age; other risk factors for AF in thyrotoxic patients include male sex, valvular heart disease, ischemic heart disease, and congestive HF. In the elderly, AF may be the only manifestation of thyrotoxicosis, a condition known as **apathetic hyperthyroidism.** Other atrial dysrhythmias, such as paroxysmal atrial tachycardia and atrial flutter, are unusual. Ventricular arrhythmias usually indicate underlying cardiac disease.

The overall incidence of arterial embolism or stroke in thyrotoxic AF appears to be increased, but the reported range varies widely in clinical trials (8–40%). The recommendations for thromboembolic prophylaxis are controversial.

The American College of Cardiology/American Heart Association (ACC/AHA) guidelines state that, although the topic is controversial and increased risk has not been definitively proven, anticoagulation treatment is recommended "in the absence of a specific contraindication, at least until a euthyroid state has been restored and heart failure has been cured." It should be noted that the effect of vitamin K antagonists is affected by the patient's thyroid status—elevated thyroid levels increase the anticoagulation effect, and antithyroid agents (such as propylthiouracil or methimazole) may diminish the effect. Careful monitoring of anticoagulation levels is required during the treatment of patients with AF and hyperthyroidism. Given the lack of clear evidence, the ACC/AHA classification of thyrotoxicosis as a moderate thromboembolic risk factor appears reasonable, and the recommendation to initiate anticoagulation when there are no contraindications appears to be warranted. More evidence-based trials are needed to clarify this issue.

Other cardiac manifestations of hyperthyroidism are symptomatic HF (which occurs in approximately 6% of patients) and pulmonary arterial hypertension. Less than 1% of patients with hyperthyroidism develop dilated cardiomyopathy with left ventricular systolic dysfunction. Hyperthyroid patients most commonly complain of exercise intolerance and exertional dyspnea, which are largely explained by inadequate increase in cardiac output during exercise. Impaired exercise tolerance in these patients is a sign that the hyperthyroid heart cannot further accommodate the increase in cardiovascular demand during physical exercise. Changes in loading conditions, loss of sinus rhythm, or a reduction in myocardial contractility may further impair the efficiency of the cardiovascular system in hyperthyroid patients, thereby inducing congestive HF. The development of orthopnea, paroxysmal nocturnal dyspnea, peripheral edema, and neck vein distension may indicate the progression to advanced HF. However, the clinical manifestations and degree of HF in hyperthyroid patients depend on a variety of factors, including the patient's age, the cause and severity of hyperthyroidism, and the underlying cardiac conditions. Often, thyrotoxicosis precipitates exacerbation of angina when the increased demands placed on the heart by the thyrotoxic state are accompanied by the underlying fixed atherosclerotic lesions of coronary artery disease. The angina improves once the thyrotoxicosis is treated, and frank myocardial infarction precipitated by thyrotoxicosis is rare.

In most conditions, a goiter is present. Absence of a goiter, especially in a young person, should raise the suspicion of factitious hyperthyroidism; elderly patients, however, may not have a palpable goiter in the presence of disease.

The precordium is hyperdynamic, and loud heart sounds and systolic ejection murmurs may be heard, reflecting increased cardiac flow across the valves. The pulse is rapid and bounding. The skin has an unusually soft and velvety texture and is often sweaty. There is proximal muscle weakness, with patients often having difficulty rising from a squatting position. Deep tendon reflexes are hyperreflexic, and a resting tremor is present. Dermopathy or localized edema may be present on the shins (pretibial myxedema, also known as *peau d'orange*).

In younger patients, especially young women, Graves disease is the most common cause of thyrotoxicosis. Graves disease is an autoimmune disease in which antibodies to the

TSH receptor stimulate both excessive thyroid growth and thyroid hormone production. The disease may occur at any age, with a peak incidence in the 20- to 40-year age group. These patients typically have a symmetric goiter (often with a bruit) with or without exophthalmos. Toxic multinodular goiter is a more common diagnosis in patients over the age of 40. Usually these goiters are large and nodular (as the name suggests). Iatrogenic or factitious thyrotoxicosis should always be considered; these patients typically have no goiter, and the thyroglobulin level is suppressed. Clinicians should suspect hyperthyroidism in patients with persistent sinus tachycardia and AF, unexplained congestive HF, or unstable angina.

C. Diagnostic Studies

1. Electrocardiography & echocardiography—Sinus tachycardia is usually present, although any supraventricular tachycardia can be seen. AF occurs in 10–20% of hyperthyroid patients; its prevalence in the population at large is 0.4%. On echocardiography, a hypercontractile state is seen with rapid filling of a highly compliant ventricle. Increased left ventricular mass and cardiac hypertrophy can also be seen.

2. Laboratory findings—Diagnosis is made by measurement of thyroid function tests (Table 34–2). TSH should be suppressed below the lower limit of detection, and the free T_4 or free thyroxine index (FTI) should be elevated, confirming the diagnosis. If the free T_4 or FTI is normal, measurement of total or free T_3 is recommended to rule out a condition known as **T_3 thyrotoxicosis**, in which the serum T_4 level is normal but the total or free T_3 is elevated. If the only abnormality is a suppressed TSH level, subclinical hyperthyroidism versus a systemic nonthyroidal illness must be considered. Thyroid function tests should be repeated after any period of illness to determine whether the abnormal

Table 34–2. Tests in Hyperthyroidism

Condition	T_4	T_3	TSH	^{131}I Uptake
Graves disease	↑, N	↑	↓	↑↑↑
Multinodular goiter	↑, N	↑	↓	↑↑
Solitary nodule	↑, N	↑	↓	↑ or N
Early subacute and silent thyroiditis	↑	↑	↓	↓
Exogenous T_4	↑	↑	↓	↓
Exogenous T_3	↓	↑	↓	↓
Iodine-induced	↑	↑	↓	↓
Ectopic	↑, N	↑	↓	↓
TSH-producing pituitary tumor	↑, N	↑	↑, N	↑

^{131}I, radioactive iodine; N, normal; T_3, triiodothyronine; T_4, thyroxine; TSH, thyroid-stimulating hormone.

thyroid function tests have resolved and were due to non-thyroidal illness.

Although only about one-third of patients have eye involvement clinically, enlarged muscles can be detected by imaging in over 90% of patients. If eye signs are present, the diagnosis of Graves disease can be made without further tests. If eye signs are absent and the patient is hyperthyroid (with or without goiter), a radioactive iodine uptake (RAIU) test should be done. Elevated RAIU is seen in Graves disease, toxic multinodular goiter, and occasionally, an autonomously functioning thyroid nodule. In contrast, a decreased RAIU is seen in thyroiditis and exogenous hyperthyroidism. A low RAIU is also found in patients who are iodine-loaded or who are taking T_4 therapy. Thyroid scans rarely add any useful information to a good physical examination in patients with diffusely enlarged thyroid glands. In Graves disease, the scan typically shows an enlarged symmetric gland with homogeneous uptake. Thyroid scans are occasionally helpful in identifying an adenoma or multinodular gland, in which one or more cold spots are seen. Other tests that may be helpful, include measurement of antithyroid antibodies (antimicrosomal or thyroid peroxidase antibodies) or TSH receptor antibody (TSAb), which are relatively specific for patients with Graves disease. Thyroglobulin levels will be suppressed in patients with factitious or iatrogenic thyrotoxicosis.

▶ Treatment

Treatment is directed at rapidly improving symptoms and reducing demands on the heart. The mainstay of treatment is accomplished by preventing thyroid hormone synthesis and release with **antithyroid drugs**, followed by radioactive iodine thyroid ablation (Table 34–3); surgery may also be indicated. β-Blockers are most commonly used to improve symptoms. If the tachycardia is considered to be significantly deleterious in patients with HF, esmolol, which has a rapid onset of action and short half-life, may be given intravenously; it should be stopped—with rapid reversal—if HF worsens. Tremor and tachycardia will improve almost immediately with β-blocker therapy, although systolic and diastolic contractile performance will not change due to direct effects of thyroid hormone on cardiac muscle. Of the oral β-blockers, propranolol is preferred because it also prevents the peripheral conversion of T_4 to T_3. The dose should be titrated to the patient's pulse and is usually 20–80 mg four times daily. Occasionally, high doses (100–320 mg four times daily) of propranolol are required in thyroid storm.

Thionamides are used to prevent thyroid hormone release and synthesis, by blocking iodine oxidation, organification, and iodotyrosine coupling. Propylthiouracil (PTU) and methimazole are the thionamides used in the United States. Because they deplete intrathyroidal stores of thyroid hormone, they circumvent the precipitation of thyroid storm that can result from radiation thyroiditis after radioactive iodine ablation. Doses typically begin at 50–100 mg three times daily of PTU and 10–30 mg daily of methimazole. Methimazole may be preferred because of its once-a-day dosing and lower incidence of side effects, such as the potential for severe hepatotoxicity with PTU. PTU is preferred in pregnant women, in the first trimester, because of rare

Table 34–3. Agents Used to Treat Hyperthyroidism

Agent	Dose	Mechanism of Action
Thionamides		
Propylthiouracil	50–300 mg, PO three times daily	Inhibits thyroid hormone synthesis Inhibits T_4 conversion to T_3
Methimazole	10–60 mg, PO once daily	Inhibits thyroid hormone synthesis
β-Blockers		
Propranolol	10–80 mg, PO q6–8h	Decreases β-adrenergic activity; decreases T_4 conversion to T_3
Atenolol	50–100 mg/day PO	Decreases β-adrenergic activity
Nadolol	80–160 mg/day PO	Decreases β-adrenergic activity
Metoprolol	100–200 mg/day PO	Decreases β-adrenergic activity
Iodides		
SSKI	5 drops PO q6–8h	Prevents thyroid hormone release
Lugol	5 drops PO q6–8h	Prevents thyroid hormone release
Ipodate	3 g PO q2–3 days or 0.5 g/day	Prevents thyroid hormone release
Radioactive iodine	Calculated dose	Destroys overfunctioning thyroid
Other agents		
Lithium	300 mg PO three times daily (monitor blood levels)	Prevents thyroid hormone release
Hydrocortisone	50–100 mg IV q6–8h	Decreases peripheral conversion of T_4 to T_3; prevents thyroid hormone release

IV, intravenous; PO, oral; SSKI, saturated solution of potassium iodide; T_3, triiodothyronine; T_4, thyroxine.

teratogenic effects of methimazole. These drugs are typically withdrawn 3–5 days prior to radioactive iodine ablation and restarted 3–5 days after ablation. Thionamides are known to cause nausea and rash (in about 5% of patients) and, of most concern, agranulocytosis (in about 0.5% of patients). Agranulocytosis is often heralded by severe sore throat and fever and requires immediate cessation of antithyroid drug therapy. Thus, all patients receiving antithyroid drugs are instructed to stop the drug and contact their physician to obtain a complete blood count if sore throat or fever develops during treatment.

Other drugs, including lithium, iodides, and corticosteroids, are usually reserved for the prevention of life-threatening conditions such as thyroid storm; occasionally, they are used for patients with severe congestive HF or unstable angina secondary to thyrotoxicosis. Lithium prevents thyroid hormone release, and the dosage is determined by monitoring therapeutic serum levels. Iodides abruptly prevent the release of thyroid hormone. They **must** be used in conjunction with thionamides because rebound or escape occurs commonly. Doses are usually 3–5 drops of a supersaturated potassium iodide solution or Lugol solution (50 mg of iodide per drop) every 6–8 hours.

Parenteral corticosteroids are usually given in stress doses for thyroid storm. Corticosteroids inhibit thyroid hormone secretion and prevent peripheral conversion of T_4 to T_3. Doses are usually 50–100 mg of hydrocortisone every 6–8 hours.

Radioactive iodine (^{131}I) is the preferred and definitive treatment for thyrotoxicosis in patients with a high RAIU. Because thyroid tissue is the only tissue that requires iodine (for thyroid hormone synthesis), ^{131}I is used for thyroid gland destruction. The advantages of radioactive iodine include the fact that usually only a single treatment is needed and that it is relatively safe and inexpensive. Because the treatment usually requires 3–6 months to resolve the hyperthyroidism, most patients will require interim therapy with thionamides during that time. The patient is usually rendered hypothyroid as a result of the treatment and is then treated with long-term thyroid hormone replacement.

Patients with multinodular goiters, who have lower RAIU (than do patients with Graves disease), often have an inadequate response to ^{131}I and may require re-treatment or surgery. Pregnant patients should not receive ^{131}I and should, therefore, be treated with PTU, with or without β-blockers, or with subtotal thyroidectomy in the second trimester.

Aspirin, nonsteroidal anti-inflammatory drugs, and—rarely—corticosteroids are used if painful thyroiditis is present. Thyroiditis is reversible and requires short-term therapy only. β-Blockers can be used temporarily to improve thyrotoxic symptoms.

Treatment of congestive HF and AF is essentially the same as for a euthyroid individual. Treatment should include use of a nonselective β-blocker (eg, propranolol) or a selective $β_1$-blocker (eg, metoprolol) to normalize the heart rate. The physician should be aware, however, that treatment of AF is limited to control of the ventricular rate because cardioversion will not be successful as long as the thyrotoxicosis is present. In addition, patients may be relatively resistant to digoxin. Usually, sinus rhythm returns within 6 weeks with resolution of the thyrotoxic state. Older patients with underlying cardiac disease may not spontaneously revert and may require cardioversion. Anticoagulation should be considered until the patient is euthyroid and in sinus rhythm.

Once the patient becomes euthyroid, the hyperdynamic cardiovascular manifestations disappear. AF should convert to normal sinus rhythm in more than 60% of patients, and angina should improve because of decreased demands on the heart.

▶ Prognosis

The prognosis is generally excellent for most hyperthyroid conditions. Graves disease and autonomously functioning thyroid nodules usually respond well to ^{131}I and do not recur. As noted previously, multinodular goiters may be relatively resistant to ^{131}I and may ultimately require subtotal thyroidectomy. Despite surgical treatment, multinodular goiters frequently recur.

Frost L, et al. Hyperthyroidism and risk of atrial fibrillation or flutter: a population-based study. *Arch Intern Med.* 2004; 164(15):1675–8. [PMID: 15302638]

Klein I, et al. Thyroid disease and the heart. *Circulation.* 2007; 116:1725–35. [PMID: 17923583]

Sheu JJ, et al. Hyperthyroidism and risk of ischemic stroke in young adults: a 5-year follow-up study. *Stroke.* 2010;41(5):961–6. [PMID: 20360542]

2. Hypothyroidism

ESSENTIALS OF DIAGNOSIS

▶ TSH levels above normal range (primary hypothyroidism).

▶ Low free T_4 or low FTI.

▶ General Considerations

Hypothyroidism is a clinical syndrome resulting from thyroid hormone deficiency, which results in a generalized slowing down of metabolic processes, with slowed heart rate, diminished oxygen consumption, and deposition of glycosaminoglycans in extracellular spaces, particularly in skin and muscle; in extreme cases, the clinical syndrome of **myxedema** occurs, which is associated with hypothermia, hypoventilation, hypotension, and central nervous system signs. Overt hypothyroidism affects ~3% of the adult female population; it is estimated that anywhere from 0.5% to 5.0% of the adult population of the United States has underlying hypothyroidism.

Hypothyroidism is associated with accelerated atherosclerosis, likely from the accompanying hyperlipidemia and diastolic hypertension seen in these patients. Hypothyroid patients have other atherosclerotic cardiovascular disease risk factors, such as increased C-reactive protein and homocysteine, and appear to have increased risk of stroke. The atherosclerosis is especially pronounced in the presence of hypertension; however, angina is uncommon, and the incidence of myocardial infarction is not increased. This is probably due to the decreased metabolic demands placed on the heart in the hypothyroid state. More commonly, angina is precipitated or worsened by rapid thyroid hormone replacement.

▶ Clinical Findings

A. Symptoms & Signs

1. Systemic symptoms & signs—Hypothyroidism is an insidious disease and may be subtle in its progression and presentation. Patients typically complain of weight gain (although morbid obesity does not occur), weakness, lethargy, fatigue, depression, muscle cramps, constipation, cold intolerance, dry skin, and coarse hair. Women often have menstrual disorders (most commonly, menorrhagia), and men may have impotence or decreased libido.

2. Cardiovascular symptoms & signs—Cardiovascular findings are the opposite of those found in hyperthyroidism. There is a decrease in cardiac output because of reduced ventricular contractility, bradycardia, increased peripheral resistance, and reduced blood volume. The hemodynamic alterations resemble those of congestive HF except that pulmonary congestion does not occur, and pulmonary artery and right ventricle pressures are often normal. In addition, cardiac output and systemic vascular resistance increase normally in response to exercise, unlike HF from other causes.

Cardiac enlargement may occur due to a combination of interstitial edema, left ventricular dilatation, and pericardial effusion. Myxedematous HF can be distinguished from other causes in that it responds to exercise with an increased heart rate; improves with thyroid hormone replacement, but not digitalis and diuretics; rarely results in pulmonary congestion; and exhibits high protein content effusions.

B. Physical Examination

Hypothermia, bradycardia with weak arterial pulses, and mild hypertension are characteristic vital signs. The hypertension may be due to increased peripheral resistance. Thyroid hormone replacement will normalize blood pressure in approximately one-third of these patients. The patient may appear pale, with periorbital edema and facial puffiness. Hair and skin are usually coarse and dry. Goiter is present in patients with Hashimoto thyroiditis, congenital enzyme deficiencies, iodine deficiency, and thyroid hormone resistance; it is also present in patients taking amiodarone and antithyroid drug therapy such as thionamides and lithium.

Percussion of the chest may reveal pleural effusions. Distant heart sounds are present, especially if a pericardial effusion is present. Reflexes are characteristically delayed in the return phase. Nonpitting edema may be present as a result of the deposition of mucopolysaccharides. Severe hypothyroidism can progress to myxedema coma, and anasarca may be present. In the presence of congestive HF, pitting edema may be superimposed on the nonpitting edema.

C. Diagnostic Studies

1. Electrocardiography & echocardiography—Electrocardiographic (ECG) changes include low-voltage QRS complexes and flattened or inverted T waves, sinus bradycardia, and prolonged PR and QT intervals. Prolonged QT may increase ventricular irritability and, rarely, induce torsade de pointes; this is reversible by treatment. Atrial, ventricular, and intraventricular conduction delays are three times as likely in patients with myxedema as in the general population. Pericardial effusion is probably partly responsible for these ECG changes.

Pericardial effusions occur in as many as 30% of all hypothyroid patients. Cardiac tamponade is unusual because of the slow accumulation of fluid, which does not increase pericardial pressure excessively.

2. Laboratory findings—Asymptomatic hypothyroid individuals, such as the elderly, frequently go unrecognized. By far, the most common cause of hypothyroidism in the United States is Hashimoto thyroiditis. Other causes of hypothyroidism are listed in Table 34-4.

The combination of elevated serum TSH and low serum free T_4 is diagnostic of primary hypothyroidism. Serum T_3 levels are variable and may be within normal range. The absence of an elevated TSH level indicates either nonthyroidal illness or hypothalamic–pituitary dysfunction. Occasionally, TSH level is mildly elevated (usually < 10 mU/L) in the face of a normal T_4 level. Subclinical hypothyroidism, as opposed to recovery from a nonthyroidal illness, must be considered. These patients are typically asymptomatic but are at intermediate risk for cardiovascular disease when compared with euthyroid or frankly hypothyroid individuals.

Antithyroid antibodies (antimicrosomal or thyroid peroxidase antibodies) are elevated in Hashimoto thyroiditis. Creatine kinase isoenzymes are increased in hypothyroidism; the isoenzyme pattern is usually MM and not MB. Hypothyroidism is a common cause of hyperlipidemia; 95% of hypothyroid individuals will have elevated low-density lipoprotein (LDL) cholesterol, and 70% will have elevation in both LDL cholesterol and triglycerides. Anemia of chronic disease may be seen, as well as hyponatremia from impaired free-water clearance.

▶ Treatment

T_4 therapy usually reverses the cardiovascular manifestations associated with hypothyroidism. Treatment with T_4, which is available in pure form and is stable and inexpensive,

Table 34–4. Causes of Hypothyroidism

Causes	Comments
Destructive	
Radioactive iodine ablation	No palpable thyroid tissue
Thyroid surgery	Scar evident
External radiation to neck	History of malignancy
Infiltrative diseases	Diagnose by fine-needle aspirate
Autoimmune	
Hashimoto thyroiditis	Goiter, antithyroid antibodies
Following Graves disease	History of Graves; may have ophthalmopathy
Hereditary or congenital	
Congenital dyshormonogenesis	Goiter, usually diagnosed in childhood
Thyroid hormone resistance	Rare, familial
Iodine deficiency	Rare in United States (iodine added to salt)
Drug-induced	
Lithium	Goiter, on lithium, usually with underlying predisposition to thyroid disease
Thionamides	History of hyperthyroidism
Iodines	Wolff-Chaikoff effect
Pituitary/hypothalamic failure	Other hormone deficiencies usually apparent

is recommended. Because T_4 is converted to T_3 in peripheral tissues, both hormones become available once T_4 is administered. Desiccated thyroid is now considered obsolete; it contains both T_4 and T_3 (as liothyronine). T_3 is unsatisfactory because of its rapid absorption, short half-life, and transient effects. The half-life of T_4 is 7 days, so it is given once daily. It is well absorbed, and blood levels are monitored following TSH levels. Replacement doses of T_4 vary according to the patient's age and body weight. Regarding cardiovascular effects of T_4 supplementation, one of the most important considerations with thyroid hormone replacement therapy is the speed of rendering the patient euthyroid. Young patients without evidence of cardiac disease can be replaced with full doses of T_4. Patients over the age of 55 or patients with evidence or suspicion of cardiac disease require slow and judicious use of thyroid hormone replacement to prevent exacerbation of angina or precipitation of myocardial infarction. The typical regimen would begin with 25 mcg (0.025 mg/day) or one-fourth of a normal replacement dose and increase the dose gradually after 6- to 8-week intervals based on serum TSH measurements; it may take several months to reach full replacement doses (100–150 mcg/day).

Patients with unstable angina and hypothyroidism may be specially challenging to treat because of the risk of exacerbating the angina. Very small doses of hormone should be used, and the dosage increments must be made slowly over a longer-than-usual time. If necessary, angioplasty or coronary artery bypass grafting (CABG) should be recommended, after which—if revascularization is complete—thyroid hormone replacement can occur at the usual dosage and rate. Such a strategy is likely to result in better surgical outcomes with improved morbidity and mortality. Adjustments in anesthesia and drug doses should be made because their decreased metabolic clearance makes hypothyroid patients very sensitive to these agents.

Treatment of myxedema coma is controversial. Many authors recommend high initial doses of intravenous T_4 (400 mcg) to saturate receptors and replenish diminished stores, followed by 100 mcg/day. Others prefer a more conservative approach of 50–100 mcg/day intravenously. Stress doses of hydrocortisone should also be administered (100 mg intravenously every 6–8 hours) because hypothyroidism and adrenal insufficiency frequently coexist, and thyroid hormone replacement may precipitate adrenal crisis.

▶ **Prognosis**

In the absence of coexisting heart disease, treatment with thyroid hormone and restoration of a euthyroid status correct the hemodynamic, ECG, and serum enzyme alterations and restore heart size to normal. Therapy is lifelong, and relapses occur if the patient is noncompliant or taken off therapy for any reason.

Flynn RW, et al. Mortality and vascular outcomes in patients treated for thyroid dysfunction. *J Clin Endocrinol Metab.* 2006;91(6):2159–64. [PMID: 16537678]
Hak AE, et al. Subclinical hypothyroidism is an independent risk factor for atherosclerosis and myocardial infarction in elderly women: The Rotterdam Study. *Ann Intern Med.* 2000;132(4):270–8. [PMID: 10681281]

Monzani F, et al. Effect of levothyroxine on cardiac function and structure in subclinical hypothyroidism: a double blind, placebo-controlled study. *J Clin Endocrinol Metab.* 2001;86(3):1110–5. [PMID: 11238494]

Tielens ET, et al. Changes in cardiac function at rest before and after treatment in primary hypothyroidism. *Am J Cardiol.* 2000;85(3):376–80. [PMID: 11078310]

Toft AD, et al. Thyroid disease and the heart. *Heart.* 2000;84(4):455–60. [PMID: 10995425]

3. Effect of Heart Disease on Thyroid Function

Acute or chronic illness, such as occurs with myocardial infarction, congestive HF, and during the postoperative period of cardiopulmonary bypass, can make the interpretation of thyroid function tests difficult. Levels of T_3 and T_4 can drop as much as 20–40%, the so-called euthyroid sick syndrome. TSH is inhibited centrally and can be suppressed further by use of drugs, such as dopamine or corticosteroids, to undetectable levels. As recovery from the underlying illness occurs, the TSH level may rise above normal into the hypothyroid range. Consequently, patients with significant cardiovascular disease in a coronary care unit are likely to have abnormal thyroid function tests. The interpretation of low serum thyroid hormones with acute or chronic illnesses should be done with great caution because of the importance of distinguishing between hypothyroidism and the euthyroid sick syndrome. There is no evidence to support thyroid hormone replacement in the latter patients, and it may be potentially harmful.

4. Cardiovascular Drugs & the Thyroid

Overall incidence of thyroid dysfunction in patients receiving amiodarone is estimated to be between 2% and 24%. Amiodarone-induced thyrotoxicosis (AIT) is more common in countries with low iodine uptake, and amiodarone-induced hypothyroidism is more common in areas that are iodine replete.

AIT may occur at any time during or even after amiodarone treatment, particularly in patients with an underlying predisposition to thyroid disease, such as those who have a goiter. Presenting symptoms and signs include weight loss, weakness, tremor, or new or recurrent atrial tachyarrhythmias. Classic symptoms may be masked by the antiadrenergic effects of amiodarone. Biochemical diagnosis is straightforward if the T_3 or free T_3 level is elevated and the TSH level is suppressed to undetectable levels.

Pathogenesis is complex and can involve excessive thyroid hormone synthesis from the iodine load (so called type I AIT) or destructive thyroiditis (type II AIT). Features of both types of AIT are listed in Table 34–5.

Therapy for AIT may be complex and requires knowledge of the underlying pathogenesis. In type I AIT, thionamides should be used to block further organification of iodine and synthesis of hormones. Larger than usual doses are often required (methimazole 40–60 mg/day or PTU 600–800 mg/day) because the iodine-rich gland is resistant to thionamide therapy. Potassium perchlorate (800–1000 mg/day for 15–45 days), a drug that inhibits iodine uptake into the gland, can also be used, although with caution because agranulocytosis, aplastic anemia, and nephrotic syndrome have occurred at doses > 1.5 g. Discontinuation of amiodarone may be recommended and necessary in some cases. Thyroidectomy can be undertaken in severe cases unresponsive to medical therapy.

Type II AIT can be treated with high-dose corticosteroids (prednisone 30–40 mg/day or equivalent) for 3 months with a gradual slow taper to minimize recurrence. Discontinuation of amiodarone is usually not necessary because the thyroiditis resolves within several weeks to months and rarely recurs.

Table 34–5. Features of Amiodarone-Induced Thyrotoxicosis

	Type I	Type II
Pathogenesis	Excess hormone synthesis due to excess iodine	Excess hormone release due to thyroid tissue destruction
Goiter	Often present; multinodular or diffuse	Occasionally present; small diffuse, firm, may be tender
Autoantibodies	May be present	Usually absent
Interleukin-6	Normal/elevated	Markedly elevated
Radioactive iodine uptake	Low or normal	Low or suppressed
Color-flow Doppler	Normal or increased flow	Decreased flow
Thyroid ultrasound	Nodular, hypoechoic, large	Normal size, homogeneous thyroid tissue
Therapy	Methimazole or PTU, perchlorate may be necessary, thyroidectomy may be an option	Steroids
Subsequent hypothyroidism	No, unless thyroidectomy performed	Possible

PTU, propylthiouracil.

If the two types of AIT cannot be distinguished, therapy with both corticosteroids and antithyroid drugs should be started.

Like amiodarone, radiologic contrast material containing iodine, such as that used in cardiac catheterizations, has the potential for causing transient thyrotoxicosis.

Daniels GH. Amiodarone induced thyrotoxicosis. *J Clin Endocrinol Metab*. 2001;86(1):3–8. [PMID: 11231968]

Martino E, et al. The effects of amiodarone on the thyroid. *Endocrinol Rev*. 2001;22(2):240–54. [PMID: 11294826]

PARATHYROID & THE HEART

Parathyroid hormone (PTH) is mainly responsible for the regulation of ionized calcium levels by concerted effects on three main target organs: bone, intestinal mucosa, and kidney. It participates in the regulation of calcium, phosphate, and magnesium homeostasis throughout the body. Although PTH itself has few effects on the heart, an excess or deficiency of this hormone can affect the cardiovascular system indirectly through its regulation of calcium.

1. Hyperparathyroidism

ESSENTIALS OF DIAGNOSIS

▶ Inappropriately normal or elevated PTH levels.

▶ Serum calcium level above upper limit of normal (> 10 mg/dL) corrected for serum albumin, or ionized calcium level higher than upper limit of normal range.

▶ Increased 24-hour urine calcium excretion (> 200 mg).

▶ Elevated alkaline phosphatase.

▶ Decreased serum phosphate level.

▶ General Considerations

Primary hyperparathyroidism is most commonly due to overproduction of PTH from a parathyroid adenoma in about 80% of cases, and typically causes hypercalcemia. Rare causes include parathyroid hyperplasia in familial cases, often in the setting of a multiple endocrine neoplasia (MEN) syndrome; parathyroid carcinoma is a rare, accounting for 1–2% of cases. Secondary hyperparathyroidism occurs in hypocalcemic states in which the lack of negative feedback of calcium to the parathyroid glands results in overproduction of PTH and is usually seen in the setting of chronic hypocalcemia, vitamin D deficiency, or renal failure. Tertiary hyperparathyroidism can occur when chronic overstimulation of the parathyroid gland (as in renal failure) causes the autonomous release of PTH.

When the disorder is detected in an outpatient setting, the most common diagnosis is primary hyperparathyroidism from a parathyroid adenoma. Although parathyroid hyperplasia is rare, it is usually found in the setting of a rare hereditary condition of MEN. MEN type I comprises hyperparathyroidism, pituitary adenoma, and pancreatic islet cell tumor; MEN II consists of hyperparathyroidism, medullary thyroid carcinoma, and pheochromocytoma. Granulomatous disease, such as tuberculosis or histoplasmosis, can cause hypercalcemia by increased $1\text{-}\alpha\text{-hydroxylase}$ activity, which converts the inactive 25-hydroxy vitamin D to the active 1,25-dihydroxy vitamin D. All patients with hypercalcemia should be queried regarding calcium (including over-the-counter calcium carbonate antacids) and vitamin intake to rule out milk-alkali syndrome and vitamin D and A toxicity. Thyrotoxicosis can cause hypercalcemia because of increased bone turnover. Adrenal insufficiency is another cause of hypercalcemia.

When detected in an inpatient setting, hypercalcemia is usually the harbinger of malignancy and portends a poor prognosis. Malignancies associated with hypercalcemia include bone metastases; multiple myeloma; lymphoma; leukemia; and squamous cell cancers, primarily of the head and neck, which secrete PTH-related peptide. This can bind to PTH receptors and cause PTH-like effects.

The hyperparathyroid state, by altering serum calcium and PTH, has the potential to adversely affect the cardiovascular system. Hypertension; left ventricular hypertrophy (LVH); hypercontractility; arrhythmias; and calcific deposits in the myocardium, aortic and mitral valves, and coronary arteries have all been described. Some but not all studies have demonstrated an increased incidence of cardiovascular death that seems to correlate with the degree and duration of disease.

▶ Clinical Findings

A. Symptoms & Signs

1. Systemic symptoms & signs—Most patients with chronic hyperparathyroidism are asymptomatic and are detected through finding of hypercalcemia in routine laboratory testing. Nonspecific symptoms include fatigue, depression, difficulty in concentrating, personality changes, and vague aches and pains. Muscle weakness with characteristic electromyographic changes is also seen. Dyspepsia, nausea, and constipation can occur, likely secondary to hypercalcemia, but there is probably no increase in the incidence of peptic ulcer disease. The articular manifestations include chondrocalcinosis in up to 5% of patients.

2. Cardiovascular symptoms & signs—Arrhythmias are uncommon, but acute hypercalcemia can cause bradycardia and first-degree heart block. Acute elevation of calcium may cause hypertension, although this may be due to renal damage from nephrocalcinosis and elevated peripheral vascular resistance—a direct effect of calcium on the vascular smooth muscle cells. LVH is noted in as many as 80% of patients referred for parathyroidectomy and can be reversible, particularly in normotensive individuals. Valvular sclerosis, on the other hand, does not appear to improve after parathyroidectomy but also does not appear to progress. Several studies in Europe have reported increased cardiovascular morbidity and mortality in patients with otherwise asymptomatic hyperparathyroidism. However, the survival benefit was not observed until 15 years after parathyroidectomy in the largest study published to date. A population-based study from the United States did not find an increase in mortality in patients with primary hyperparathyroidism. In this study of 435 patients, cardiovascular mortality was reduced in patients with primary hyperparathyroidism compared with age- and gender-matched residents of the same community (relative risk, 0.6; 95% confidence interval, 0.4–0.8). One explanation for the incongruent mortality data is that more patients in the U.S. studies had mild disease with lower serum calcium levels (mean calcium, 10.9 mg/dL [2.7 mmol/L]) and fewer symptoms than patients in the European studies, where average calcium levels were significantly higher.

B. Physical Examination

Calcium deposition in the cornea, or band keratopathy, may be noted. In hyperparathyroidism secondary to renal failure, calcium and phosphate may precipitate in the soft tissues and in and around joints. These precipitants are usually readily seen on radiograph and palpated on physical examination and, if severe, can limit mobility of the joints.

C. Diagnostic Studies

1. Electrocardiography & echocardiography—Hypercalcemia decreases the plateau phase of the cardiac action potential, reflected by a shortened ST segment and a reduced QT interval. The QT interval corrected for heart rate is probably the most reliable ECG index of hypercalcemia. With severe hypercalcemia (calcium level > 16 mg/dL, or 4 mmol/L), the T wave widens, tending to increase the QT interval.

Echocardiography reveals a high incidence of LVH and calcification of aortic and mitral valves as well as the coronary tree and myocardium. Several studies have shown improvement after successful parathyroidectomy in subjects with symptomatic hyperparathyroidism.

2. Laboratory findings—Typically, both serum calcium and ionized calcium are elevated, with an inappropriately normal or elevated PTH. Other causes of hypercalcemia are accompanied by a suppressed or low-normal PTH. The 24-hour urine calcium level is usually more than 200 mg. Phosphate levels are usually low or low-normal because PTH has a phosphaturic effect on the kidney, and a hyperchloremic metabolic acidosis is present because of the bicarbonaturic effect of PTH. Alkaline phosphatase levels may be elevated, especially in the setting of hyperparathyroid bone disease.

▶ Treatment & Prognosis

Parathyroidectomy is the definitive treatment for hyperparathyroidism and is indicated in all patients with symptoms as well as patients believed to be at high risk for progressive disease. In experienced hands, the cure rate for a single parathyroid adenoma is more than 95%; the success rate in parathyroid hyperplasia is lower due to missed glands and recurrent hyperparathyroidism. Parathyroidectomy is a difficult surgery; the parathyroid gland is small and may be located throughout the neck or upper mediastinum. Preoperative assessment to locate not only the adenoma, but also to find the other glands and determine whether or not they are normal in size is key; intraoperative PTH testing has also improved outcomes. Complications of surgery include damage to the recurrent laryngeal nerve and inadvertent removal of all parathyroid tissue, leading to permanent hypoparathyroidism, a condition difficult to treat.

Successful parathyroidectomy normalizes calcium, phosphate, PTH, and alkaline phosphatase levels while improving bone density, decreasing the risk of kidney stones, slowing the progression of renal insufficiency, diminishing LVH, and improving symptoms. Hypertension may persist or progress in a percentage of patients, most likely the result of nephrocalcinosis and irreversible renal impairment. Postoperative hypocalcemia is common and may be transient or permanent. If it is permanent, the patient will require lifelong calcium and vitamin D replacement.

There is no definitive medical treatment for primary hyperparathyroidism, so medical treatment is less preferable than surgery, unless the patient has a contraindication to the latter. Current medical treatment is limited and includes administration of the bisphosphonates, pamidronate or risedronate, and high-dose estrogen in postmenopausal women. The effects of estrogen are on the skeletal responses to PTH; the levels of PTH do not fall. Newer treatments, such as calcimimetic agents, activate the calcium-sensing receptor in the parathyroid gland, thereby inhibiting PTH secretion, and may offer an alternative to surgery. One calcimimetic drug, cinacalcet, is Food and Drug Administration (FDA) approved for the treatment of secondary hyperparathyroidism in patients on dialysis. It is also used in patients with parathyroid cancer and for the treatment of severe hypercalcemia in patients with primary hyperparathyroidism unable to undergo parathyroidectomy. Drugs on the horizon include calcitriol analogues that inhibit PTH secretion directly, but do not stimulate gastrointestinal calcium or phosphate absorption, and drugs that block the PTH receptor.

Andersson P, et al. Primary hyperparathyroidism and heart disease—a review. *Eur Heart J.* 2004;25(20):1176–87. [PMID: 15474692]

Bilezikian JP. Primary hyperparathyroidism when to operate and when to observe. *Endocrinol Metab Clin North Am.* 2000; 29(3):465–78. [PMID: 11033756]

Bilezikian JP, et al. Clinical practice. Asymptomatic primary hyperparathyroidism. *N Engl J Med.* 2004;350:1746–51. [PMID: 15103001]

Bilezikian JP, et al. Guidelines for the management of asymptomatic primary hyperparathyroidism: summary statement from the third international workshop. *J Clin Endocrinol Metab.* 2009;94:335–9. [PMID: 19193908]

Bollerslev J, et al. Effect of surgery on cardiovascular risk factors in mild primary hyperparathyroidism. *J Clin Endocrinol Metab.* 2009;94:2255–61. [PMID: 19351725]

Peacock M, et al. Cinacalcet HCl reduces hypercalcemia in primary hyperparathyroidism across a wide spectrum of disease severity. *J Clin Endocrinol Metab.* 2011;96:E9–18. [PMID: 20943783]

Rubin MR, et al. The natural history of primary hyperparathyroidism with or without parathyroid surgery after 15 years. *J Clin Endocrinol Metab.* 2008;93:3462–70. [PMID: 18544625]

2. Hypoparathyroidism

Hypoparathyroidism usually occurs in the postoperative setting after neck or thyroid surgery. Acquired hypoparathyroidism not related to surgery is most often an autoimmune disease. Other causes of hypoparathyroidism due to parathyroid gland destruction, all very rare, include radiation and storage or infiltrative diseases of the parathyroid glands (hemochromatosis, Wilson disease, granulomas, or metastatic cancer). Symptomatic hypoparathyroidism has also been described in association with human immunodeficiency virus (HIV) infection. Functional hypoparathyroidism can occur in patients with magnesium deficiency by inducing PTH resistance, which occurs when serum magnesium concentrations fall below 0.8 mEq/L (1 mg/dL or 0.4 mmol/L), or by decreasing PTH secretion, which occurs in patients with more severe hypomagnesemia. The hypocalcemia cannot be corrected with calcium; the patients must be given magnesium.

Symptoms include tingling around the mouth and in the hands and feet. Cardiovascular manifestations are rare. The physical examination reveals positive Chvostek and Trousseau signs. Laboratory evaluation reveals a low serum calcium or ionized calcium with a low or inappropriately low normal PTH level. Hypoparathyroidism is associated with a prolonged QT interval on the ECG because of ST segment lengthening; the T wave is usually normal. Impaired left ventricular function has been reported. Restoration of eucalcemia may improve cardiac function.

Goltzman D, et al. Hypoparathyroidism. In: *Primer on the Metabolic Bone Diseases and Disorders of Bone Metabolism.* New York: Wiley, 2006;6:216.

Lehmann G, et al. ECG changes in a 25-year-old woman with hypocalcemia due to hypoparathyroidism. *Chest.* 2000;118(1):260–2. [PMID: 10893393]

ADRENAL & THE HEART

1. Pheochromocytoma

ESSENTIALS OF DIAGNOSIS

- ▶ Biochemical evidence of excess catecholamines.
- ▶ Adrenal tumor or tumor along the sympathetic chain (paraganglioma).
- ▶ Headache, palpitations, and sweating in conjunction with either hypertension (may be paroxysmal) or orthostatic hypotension.
- ▶ Pressor response to anesthesia induction or to antihypertensive or sympathomimetic drugs.

▶ General Considerations

Catecholamine-secreting neoplasms, or pheochromocytomas, can be life-threatening and cause hypertension, arrhythmia, and hyperglycemia. One case per 2 million persons is diagnosed annually in this country, accounting for less than 0.1% of underlying primary causes of hypertension. Despite the rarity of this condition, its importance cannot be overstated because correct diagnosis and treatment lead to cure and a missed diagnosis can be fatal. Ninety percent of pheochromocytomas are located in the adrenals; 10% arise from extra-adrenal chromaffin tissue along the sympathetic chain and are known as paragangliomas. Cardiac pheochromocytomas arising from the visceral autonomic paraganglia (atrium or interatrial septum) or branchiomeric paraganglia (branchial arch) are extremely rare. Approximately 10% are malignant, and recurrences can be seen in 6–23% of cases.

Most pheochromocytomas secrete predominantly norepinephrine; about 15% secrete mainly epinephrine. The majority of pheochromocytomas occur sporadically; occasionally (about 10% of cases), they are seen as part of a familial syndrome such as MEN IIa (hyperparathyroidism, medullary thyroid cancer, pheochromocytoma), MEN IIb (pheochromocytoma, medullary thyroid carcinoma, mucosal neuromas, marfanoid habitus), or von Hippel-Lindau disease (cerebelloretinal hemangioblastomas, pheochromocytoma, pancreatic islet cell tumors, renal cell cysts, testicular cysts). Affected family members may have only one manifestation of these syndromes. All members of the family should be screened for pheochromocytomas up until the age of 40 because of the potentially life-threatening nature of these tumors.

▶ Clinical Findings

A. Symptoms & Signs

1. Systemic symptoms & signs—The release of catecholamines from the tumor is unpredictable and usually causes paroxysmal attacks of headache, palpitations, and sweating. Together with hypertension, these three symptoms, when present, have a diagnostic specificity of 94% and sensitivity of 91%. When this triad of symptoms is absent, pheochromocytoma can be excluded with 99.9% certainty. Patients may also complain of increased nervousness, irritability, and an impending sense of doom. Mild abdominal pain and constipation are relatively common. Pallor and hyperventilation may be noted on examination. The clinician should suspect a pheochromocytoma in any patient in whom a sudden elevation of blood pressure develops during anesthesia induction.

2. Cardiovascular symptoms & signs—The effects of catecholamines on the heart are mediated by β_1-receptors and include increased heart rate, enhanced contractility, and augmented conduction velocity—all of which contribute to an increase in cardiac output. Eighty-five percent of patients will have hypertension, which can be either sustained, labile (with hypotension and hypertension), or paroxysmal. Patients without hypertension most likely secrete dopa or dopamine, which can be vasodilating. Orthostatic hypotension is often noted, and the combination of severe hypertension and orthostasis should suggest the possibility of pheochromocytoma. Light-headedness and syncope occur rarely.

Both dilated and hypertrophic cardiomyopathies and myocarditis have been described with pheochromocytoma, and exposure to high levels of catecholamines can cause contraction-band necrosis and fibrosis. The cardiomyopathy is reversible if the excessive catecholamine stimulus is removed early, before extensive replacement fibrosis takes place. Chest pain, angina, and acute myocardial infarction may occur in the absence of coronary artery occlusive disease. Catecholamine-induced increases in myocardial oxygen consumption, myocarditis, and coronary artery spasm likely contribute to the infarction. Cardiac arrhythmias such as atrial and ventricular fibrillation occur, especially in the setting of surgical resection of the tumor. Sudden death is not an uncommon presentation for patients with pheochromocytoma. Pulmonary edema and shock may also be presentations of such patients; shock may be associated with myocarditis or infarction, or it may follow a hypertensive crisis.

B. Physical Examination

Sustained or paroxysmal hypertension is common. Orthostasis is also often seen, and noncardiogenic pulmonary edema of obscure origin has also been described. Retinal hemorrhage or papilledema is a rare occurrence.

C. Diagnostic Studies

1. Electrocardiography & imaging—ECG changes are common; nonspecific ST-T wave changes and prominent U waves may be seen. Sinus tachycardia, sinus bradycardia, and atrial and ventricular tachyarrhythmias have all been noted and may be associated with palpitations. Conduction disturbances, including right and left bundle branch block, and signs of LVH sometimes occur.

Clinically significant cardiomyopathy and increased left ventricular mass have been noted on echocardiography. CT and magnetic resonance imaging (MRI) are useful for localizing the tumors. Occasionally, radionuclide imaging with ^{123}I-metaiodobenzylguanidine is used to detect small tumors, but its sensitivity can be affected by drugs such as labetalol.

2. Laboratory findings—Elevations in plasma catecholamines or their metabolites are necessary for the diagnosis in addition to localization imaging studies. The most useful tests are 24-hour collections of urinary metanephrines and free catecholamines. Most clinicians favor urinary or plasma metanephrines as the initial screening test. In general, if the results are equivocal, plasma catecholamines should be measured. Plasma catecholamines must be collected after placement of an intravenous catheter for 30 minutes, with the patient resting supine, preferably in a quiet room to avoid release of catecholamines from pain or emotional arousal. False-positive results should be minimized by avoiding drugs, foods, and conditions that affect the tests (Table 34–6).

Table 34–6. Drugs, Foods, and Conditions That Artificially Increase or Decrease Tests for Pheochromocytoma

Test	Increase	Decrease
Metanephrines, VMA	Sympathomimetics: amphetamines, ephedrine, nasal decongestants, bronchodilators	Large doses of ganglionic blockers: guanethidine, reserpine
Catecholamines	Levodopa Rapid clonidine withdrawal Excess banana ingestion Nitroprusside, nitroglycerin Theophylline, aminophylline Severe stress Diseases: intracranial lesions, psychosis, Guillain-Barré, lead poisoning, eclampsia, hypoglycemia, carcinoid, acute porphyria, acrodynia, quadriplegia, amyotrophic lateral sclerosis Fluorescent substances: quinidine, chloral hydrate, tetracyclines, niacin, erythromycin, quinine, bretylium, methenamine, methocarbamine	Fenfluramine Renal insufficiency Malnutrition, dysautonomia, quadriplegia
Catecholamines	Ethanol, isoproterenol, methyldopa, MAO inhibitors, phenothiazines, α-methyl p-tyrosine, methenamine, bilirubin, labetalol	
Metanephrines	Ethanol, methyldopa, MAO inhibitors, benzodiazepines, phenothiazines	Radiopaque media: Renografin, Hypaque-M, Renovist, Cardiografin, Urografin, Conray
VMA	Lithium, nalidixic acid, methocarbamol, glycerol guaiacolate, p-aminosalicylic acid, salicylates, mephenesin, sulfonamides, chocolate, citrus, tea, vanilla, coffee	Ethanol, MAO inhibitors, disulfiram, clofibrate, mandelamine, salicylates

MAO, monoamine oxidase; VMA, vanillylmandelic acid.

Occasionally, suppressive pharmacologic testing may be needed, if all prior testing is equivocal and clinical suspicion is high. The clonidine suppression test is the most widely used. The test is performed by measuring plasma catecholamines at rest and 3 hours after oral administration of 0.3 mg of clonidine. In patients with pheochromocytoma, catecholamines remain unchanged because tumor secretion is unaffected by the centrally acting clonidine. Patients with essential hypertension, on the other hand, will decrease their catecholamine levels to less than 500 pg/mL.

3. Localization studies—Initial localization is usually done either with CT or MRI of the abdomen, and these studies are able to detect approximately 95% of pheochromocytomas or paragangliomas. However, since paragangliomas can arise in the chest, a chest scan may be required. Confirmation that a tumor or mass is a paraganglioma or a pheochromocytoma is usually done with either ^{123}I-metaiodobenzylguanidine (MIBG) or ^{18}F-flurodeoxyglucose positron emission tomography (PET) scanning. Unfortunately, these scans are only 78% sensitive for these tumors. They can also be helpful in detecting metastasis. MIBG is a guanidine derivative that resembles norepinephrine and is actively transported into the adrenal medullary cells. False-negative MIBG scans are seen in about 15% of cases; certain drugs such as tricyclic antidepressants, cyclobenzaprine, amphetamines, phenylpropanolamine, haloperidol, nasal decongestants, cocaine, diet pills, reserpine, and phenothiazines can increase the rate of false-negative scans. Labetalol reduces MIBG uptake; the scan can still be done, but with suboptimal sensitivity.

▶ **Treatment**

Treatment involves the prevention of cardiovascular complications such as myocardial infarction, HF, hypertensive crisis and stroke, arrhythmias, and sudden death; it also involves surgical removal of the tumor. Recent advances in localizing imaging studies and the emergence of laparoscopic adrenalectomy along with proper preoperative medical preparation have reduced morbidity and mortality significantly. Patients need to be treated with oral antihypertensives and stabilized hemodynamically prior to surgery. Preoperative α- and β-blockade is used to reverse the effects of excessive catecholamines and prevent crisis. Because most pheochromocytomas secrete norepinephrine, α-blockade should be given first to prevent aggravation of hypertension and precipitation of coronary spasm or pulmonary edema from unopposed α-receptor stimulation. The most frequently used combination of drugs is phenoxybenzamine, started at 10 mg/day (patients with more severe hypertension may receive a starting dose of 10 mg twice daily). The dose may be increased by 10 mg every 2 days until blood pressure falls to an average of 130/85 mm Hg while sitting or until symptomatic orthostatic hypotension occurs. Hypotension occurs more frequently in patients who are normotensive between hypertensive paroxysms. Most clinicians gradually increase antihypertensive medications over 2

or more weeks. Treatment with phenoxybenzamine increases heart rate but decreases the frequency of ventricular arrhythmias. Patients are in general volume depleted and should be encouraged to hydrate well. Ideally, patients should be admitted for administration of intravenous fluids at least 1 day prior to surgery. Phenoxybenzamine has a long half-life of about 24 hours, can cause orthostasis, and should be titrated according to the severity of the orthostasis before the β-blocker is added.

β-Adrenergic blockers are generally not prescribed until treatment has been started with either an α-adrenergic blocker or a calcium channel blocker. Blocking the vasodilating β_2 receptors without previously blocking the vasoconstricting α_1 receptors can lead to hypertensive crisis when serum norepinephrine levels are high. β-Blockade can be used to reduce β-adrenergic symptoms such as flushing, palpitations, or tachycardia. Nonselective β-blockers (β_1 and β_2 blockers), such as nadolol, propranolol, pindolol, and timolol, block the vasodilating arterial β_2 receptors and should not be administered to patients with pheochromocytoma or paragangliomas. Labetalol and carvedilol are nonselective β-blockers that additionally block the α_1 receptor. Labetalol is used to treat patients with pheochromocytomas, but it can initially aggravate hypertension. β-Blockers that selectively block β_1-adrenergic receptors such as atenolol, bisoprolol, esmolol, and metoprolol induce reduction in heart rate without unopposed α-receptor–mediated rise in blood pressure. However, at high doses, these β-blockers also block β_2-adrenergic receptors and can cause a paradoxical worsening of hypertension. Extended-release metoprolol is the preferred oral preparation; esmolol is the preferred intravenous agent.

Metyrosine is a drug that inhibits the enzyme tyrosine hydroxylase, which catalyzes the first reaction in catecholamine biosynthesis (rate-limiting step). Because of side effects, it is usually reserved for treatment of hypertension in patients with metastatic or inoperable pheochromocytoma. It can be used preoperatively if the hypertension is difficult to control. Doses are 250 mg three times daily, increased by increments of 250–500 mg to a maximum of 4 g/day.

Patients should be warned to avoid vigorous exercise, particularly bending or heavy lifting, which can aggravate hypertension. They should also avoid large amounts of foods containing tyramine, a precursor to catecholamines, such as red wine, tap beers, aged dairy products, fermented or picked fish, liver, soybeans, tofu, overripe fruit, brewer's yeast pills, marmite, and vegemite.

▶ **Prognosis**

Perioperative mortality overall has dropped to about 2.4% due to improved medical preparation and surgical technique, but reported morbidity rates can be as high as 25%. Surgical complication rates are higher in patients with severe hypertension and in patients undergoing reoperations. Surgical morbidity and mortality risks can be minimized by meticulous preoperative preparation, accurate tumor localization, and supportive intraoperative care.

Nonmalignant surgically resected pheochromocytoma has a 5-year survival rate of 95%. Risk factors for death include large tumors (> 5 cm), metastatic disease, and local tumor invasion. In malignant disease, the 5-year survival is less than 50%. If a surgical cure is achieved before the cardiovascular system has been irreparably damaged, cardiovascular health will be completely restored. In 25% of patients, hypertension persists due to underlying essential hypertension or irreversible vascular or renal damage but is usually well-controlled with standard antihypertensive agents. However, in this instance, a search for a second or residual tumor should be considered.

Patients with a history of pheochromocytoma require long-term postoperative surveillance and aggressive treatment for cardiovascular risk factors. They have increased long-term risk of death from cardiovascular causes.

Duh QY. Evolving surgical management for patients with pheochromocytoma. *J Clin Endocrinol Metab*. 2001;86(4):1477–9. [PMID: 11297570]

Eisenhofer G, et al. Biochemical diagnosis of pheochromocytoma: how to distinguish true- from false-positive test results. *J Clin Endocrinol Metab*. 2003;88:2656–66. [PMID: 12788870]

Havekes B, et al. Detection and treatment of pheochromocytomas and paragangliomas: current standing of MIGB scintigraphy and future role of PET imaging. *Q J Nucl Med Mol Imaging*. 2008;52:419–29. [PMID: 19088695]

Liao WB, et al. Cardiovascular manifestations of pheochromocytoma. *Am J Emerg Med*. 2000;18(5):622–5. [PMID: 10999582]

Pacak K, et al. Pheochromocytoma: recommendations for clinical practice from the First International Symposium. October 2005. *Nat Clin Pract Endocrinol Metab*. 2007;3(2):92–102. [PMID: 17237836]

Plouin PF, et al. Factors associated with perioperative morbidity and mortality in patients with pheochromocytoma: analysis of 165 operations at a single center. *J Clin Endocrinol Metab*. 2001;86(4):1480–6. [PMID: 11297571]

2. Adrenal Insufficiency

ESSENTIALS OF DIAGNOSIS

▶ Inability to increase cortisol levels above 20 mg/dL in response to synthetic adrenocorticotropic hormone (ACTH) during rapid ACTH stimulation testing.

▶ Orthostatic hypotension, salt wasting (urine), and hyperkalemia in primary adrenal insufficiency (Addison disease).

▶ Hyponatremia in both primary and secondary (pituitary) adrenal insufficiency.

▶ Elevated ACTH in Addison disease.

▶ Hypovolemic shock, hypoglycemia, and fever in adrenal crisis.

▶ General Considerations

Deficient production of glucocorticoids, mineralocorticoids, or both results in adrenal insufficiency. This is classified into two types: primary adrenal insufficiency, or Addison disease, in which the adrenal cortex is destroyed; and secondary adrenal insufficiency, in which adrenocorticotropic hormone (ACTH) hyposecretion leads to decreased production of adrenal glucocorticoids.

Today, the most common cause of Addison disease is autoimmune destruction of the adrenal cortex. Adrenal hemorrhage, metastasis, AIDS, and granulomatous diseases (such as tuberculosis and histoplasmosis) are other etiologic considerations. Adrenal hemorrhage usually occurs in the setting of anticoagulation. The most common cause of secondary adrenal insufficiency is withdrawal of corticosteroids, which suppresses the hypothalamic–pituitary–adrenal axis and therefore causes glucocorticoid deficiency. Adrenal insufficiency is rare in the general population, with an incidence of < 0.01%. However, the overall risk of adrenal insufficiency is increased in critically ill patients, especially those over the age of 55 who are hypotensive and require pressors. Estimates are that, in this setting, adrenal insufficiency is present in 30–40%.

▶ Clinical Findings

A. Symptoms & Signs

1. Systemic symptoms & signs—Glucocorticoid deficiency causes fatigue, anorexia, nausea, vomiting (and therefore weight loss), hypotension, and hypoglycemia. Mineralocorticoid or aldosterone deficiency causes renal sodium and bicarbonate wasting, resulting in hyponatremia, hyperkalemia, acidosis, and profound dehydration. Acute adrenal insufficiency or crisis occurs when the patient is exposed to stresses such as infection, trauma, and surgery, and cannot compensate adequately with augmented glucocorticoid release.

2. Cardiovascular symptoms & signs—Hypotension, often orthostatic, is present in 90% of patients and may cause syncope. Chronic adrenal insufficiency is characterized by decreased systemic vascular resistance and decreased myocardial contractility. On the other hand, acute adrenal insufficiency can have variable cardiac function with low, normal, or high systemic vascular resistance, cardiac output, and capillary wedge pressure. Thus, in acute adrenal insufficiency—which can be superimposed on a setting of chronic adrenal insufficiency—the patient may be in hypovolemic shock, accompanied by fever, volume depletion, depressed mentation, nausea, vomiting, abdominal pain, and hypoglycemia. Patients often seem as though they have an acute abdominal emergency and can mistakenly be taken for exploratory surgery—which can be lethal in this setting. Shock and coma can rapidly progress to death, if untreated. Adrenal crisis should be considered in any patient with unexplained hypovolemic shock.

B. Physical Examination

The classic physical examination finding for chronic primary adrenal insufficiency is hyperpigmentation of the skin and mucous membranes, especially over pressure points such as the knuckles, toes, elbows, and knees and also in scars, palmar creases, nail beds, areolae, and the perianal and perivaginal areas. The hyperpigmentation is caused by increased levels of ACTH, which is released along with melanocyte-stimulating hormone and stimulates the melanocyte receptor. Vitiligo is a clue that the adrenal insufficiency is autoimmune in nature. Calcification of the pinna and the loss of pubic and axillary hair from decreased production of adrenal androgens may also be seen. In secondary adrenal insufficiency, patients lack the hyperpigmentation; the presence of cushingoid features suggests glucocorticoid withdrawal.

C. Diagnostic Studies

1. Electrocardiography & echocardiography—ECG findings include sinus bradycardia, sinus tachycardia, nonspecific T-wave changes, peaked T waves if hyperkalemia is prominent, and low voltage and a shortened QT interval if hypercalcemia is present. Echocardiography reveals small cardiac chambers with normal function.

2. Laboratory findings—Hyponatremia, hyperkalemia, hypercalcemia, hypoglycemia, and acidosis are seen in Addison disease. Patients with secondary adrenal insufficiency will not have hyperkalemia because their renin and angiotensin system is able to stimulate aldosterone production. A normocytic, normochromic anemia with lymphocytosis and eosinophilia is seen on the blood smear.

The rapid ACTH stimulation test is used to diagnose adrenal insufficiency. Administration of synthetic ACTH (cosyntropin) causes an elevation of cortisol within 30–60 minutes. Failure to increase cortisol to 20 mg/dL confirms the insufficiency. An ACTH level can help distinguish primary from secondary causes; hypersecretion is characteristic of primary adrenal insufficiency only.

In the setting of critical illness, the diagnosis of adrenal insufficiency is more problematic. Although it is well known that stress such as that seen with hypotension, inflammation, sepsis, or surgery results in elevated cortisol levels, the definition of adrenal insufficiency in this setting is less clear. Most authors believe that a stress cortisol level in critically ill patients should be > 25 mcg/dL. When the level of stress is uncertain, the low-dose corticotropin stimulation test (1 mcg) can be used. Failure to increase stimulated cortisol to > 25 mcg/dL indicates the need for treatment with corticosteroids.

▶ Treatment

The treatment of adrenal crisis is lifesaving. If the patient is in serious shock, delay of treatment to make the diagnosis of adrenal crisis is both unwise and dangerous. Patients should receive stress doses of corticosteroids, such as 100 mg of hydrocortisone intravenously every 6–8 hours, starting immediately. Saline volume resuscitation along with glucose infusion is necessary to correct volume and electrolyte abnormalities. A search for the underlying precipitant, such as infection, should be undertaken and treated as necessary. Once the patient is safely over the crisis, corticosteroids can be slowly withdrawn, and the diagnosis of adrenal insufficiency confirmed. An alternative approach would be to use dexamethasone, 2–4 mg intravenously initially, which does not interfere with the cortisol assay; perform the rapid ACTH stimulation test; and then switch to hydrocortisone. The treatment of chronic Addison disease involves both glucocorticoid and mineralocorticoid replacement.

Rivers EP, et al. Adrenal insufficiency in high-risk surgical ICU patients. *Chest.* 2001;119(3):889–96. [PMID: 11243973]

Zaloga GP, et al. Hypothalamic-pituitary-adrenal insufficiency. *Crit Care Clin.* 2001;17(1):25–41. [PMID: 11219233]

3. Cushing Syndrome

▶ General Considerations

The term **Cushing syndrome** refers to excess cortisol in the circulation. **Cushing disease** is the state of hypercortisolemia caused by an ACTH-producing pituitary adenoma. Other causes of Cushing syndrome are ectopic ACTH production from tumors, such as small-cell carcinoma of the bronchus; primary adrenal disease, such as glucocorticoid-secreting adrenal tumors; or the exogenous use of corticosteroids. **Pseudo-Cushing syndrome** refers to patients who, on screening, appear to have hypercortisolemia but have relatively few physical signs. These patients typically are alcoholic or obese or have psychiatric conditions. Confirmatory testing for Cushing syndrome is normal in pseudo-Cushing.

Patients with Cushing syndrome typically have central obesity, hypertension, hyperlipidemia, and hyperglycemia; it is not surprising that they are at risk for coronary artery disease. The longer the duration of the hypercortisolemia, the greater is the risk of coronary disease and congestive HF.

▶ Diagnostic Considerations

Diagnosis requires three steps: screening, confirmation, and determination of the cause. Screening tests are a 24-hour urine collection for free cortisol or a 1-mg overnight dexamethasone suppression test. Patients with Cushing or pseudo-Cushing syndrome will have an elevated urinary free cortisol level, and 1 mg of dexamethasone will not suppress their cortisol to less than 5 mg/dL. Confirmation requires a low-dose (2 mg/day) dexamethasone suppression test, with or without corticotropin-releasing factor testing. True Cushing syndrome will not suppress with low-dose testing. To determine cause, an ACTH level should be performed. Elevated ACTH indicates a pituitary tumor or ectopic production of ACTH. Low ACTH levels indicate adrenal disease. High-dose (8 mg) dexamethasone suppression testing and the cortisol-releasing hormone stimulation test are the main tests used to differentiate pituitary from ectopic sources of ACTH. Inferior petrosal sinus sampling should be reserved for patients with confusing hormonal testing who have a pituitary adenoma on imaging studies or in patients in whom an ectopic source of ACTH is suspected. Imaging should be done after the biochemical workup is completed to localize the tumor.

▶ Treatment

Treatment involves surgical removal of the pituitary tumor, with or without radiation, in Cushing disease; removal of the adrenal tumor; or removal of the ectopic source of ACTH production. If these procedures are not feasible, medical treatment can be done, using adrenolytic therapy, such as mitotane, or adrenocortical-blocking drugs, such as aminoglutethimide, metyrapone, or ketoconazole.

Boscaro M, et al. The diagnosis of Cushing's syndrome: atypical presentations and laboratory shortcomings. *Arch Intern Med.* 2000;160(20):3045–53. [PMID: 11074733]
Newell-Price J, et al. Cushing's syndrome. *Lancet.* 2006;367(9522): 1605–17. [PMID: 16698415]

4. Primary Hyperaldosteronism

▶ General Considerations

The increased and autonomous production of aldosterone by the adrenal gland is known as primary hyperaldosteronism. Consequences of excessive aldosterone production include sodium retention, with plasma volume expansion and hypertension; renal loss of potassium and bicarbonate, causing hypokalemia and metabolic alkalosis; and suppression of renin and angiotensin synthesis. Hyperaldosteronism is the most common secondary cause of hypertension. As many as 9–20% of cases referred to hypertension clinics have primary hyperaldosteronism.

Patients usually come to medical attention because of hypertension, and the incidence of hypokalemia is low and depends on sodium intake. The hypertension may be moderately severe, requiring several antihypertensives; malignant hypertension, however, is rare. Despite the sodium retention, edema is not a feature of hyperaldosteronism; the kidney can presumably compensate for the excess sodium.

Patients with primary aldosteronism, when matched for age, blood pressure, and the duration of hypertension, have greater left ventricular mass compared to patients with other types of hypertension, including essential hypertension, pheochromocytoma, and Cushing syndrome. Overexpression of aldosterone is thought to contribute to myocardial fibrosis (especially following myocardial infarction) and vascular fibrosis. Mineralocorticoid receptors are located in the kidney, heart, blood vessels, and brain. High dietary salt intake has been shown to be an independent predictor for left ventricular wall thickness and mass in patients with primary aldosteronism, but not essential hypertension. Although data are limited, dietary salt restriction may help reduce cardiovascular risk in these patients.

Randomized controlled trials have demonstrated improved survival in patients with HF treated with the mineralocorticoid receptor antagonists spironolactone and in patients with left ventricular dysfunction after a myocardial infarction treated with eplerenone (a selective mineralocorticoid receptor antagonist), providing further evidence for the adverse cardiovascular effects of excess aldosterone.

▶ Diagnostic Considerations

Nonsuppressible (primary) hypersecretion of aldosterone is an underdiagnosed cause of hypertension. The diagnosis should be considered in any hypertensive patient with spontaneous hypokalemia, resistant hypertension, or adrenal incidentaloma, or in patients in whom secondary hypertension is suspected. However, it is increasingly recognized that a large number of patients with primary aldosteronism due to an adrenal adenoma and, more commonly, those with adrenal hyperplasia are **not hypokalemic** at presentation for reasons that are not well understood. With increasing use of the plasma aldosterone–to–plasma renin activity ratio as a screening test for primary aldosteronism in hypertensive patients, more normokalemic patients are being identified. In a multicenter review using this approach, approximately 60% of patients with primary aldosteronism were not hypokalemic. This issue has also been addressed in hereditary disorders such as glucocorticoid-remediable aldosteronism (GRA; in which the aldosterone promoter responds to ACTH, causing excess release of aldosterone) and Liddle syndrome (in which there is a gain-of-function mutation in the collecting tubule sodium channel gene). In both of these disorders, many affected family members have hypertension but a normal plasma potassium concentration.

With increasing use of the plasma aldosterone–to–plasma renin activity ratio to screen hypertensive patients for primary aldosteronism, more nonhypokalemic patients are being identified. The 2008 Endocrine Society guidelines recommend that the plasma aldosterone concentration–to–plasma renin activity (PAC/PRA) ratio be used for case detection of primary aldosteronism. The test is performed by measuring morning (preferably 8:00 AM due to circadian rhythm of aldosterone secretion), ambulatory, paired, random plasma aldosterone concentration (PAC) and plasma renin activity (PRA). The definition of an abnormal PAC/PRA ratio is laboratory dependent. Basal PRA should be suppressed in primary hyperaldosteronism, and PAC should be elevated (> 9 ng/dL) with an elevated aldosterone/renin ratio. The mean value for the PAC/PRA ratio in normal subjects and patients with essential hypertension is 4 to 10, compared with more than 30 to 50 in most patients with primary aldosteronism. The PAC/PRA ratio is denominator-dependent, and the lower limit of detection varies among the different PRA assays. Some labs may have a lower limit of detection for PRA of 0.6 ng/mL per hour compared with 0.1 ng/mL per hour; thus, the cutoff for a "high" PAC/PRA ratio is laboratory dependent and, more specifically, PRA assay dependent. It is for this reason that an increased PAC is part of the diagnostic requirement (usually > 15 ng/dL [416 pmol/L]).

If the patient has an elevated PAC/PRA ratio, the diagnosis can be further confirmed by demonstrating failure of the elevated aldosterone to suppress normally with fludrocortisone or saline loading. The patient must discontinue any antihypertensives that affect the renin–angiotensin–aldosterone axis for 3–6 weeks before salt suppression testing; α-adrenergic blockers can be used to control blood pressure. The patient is typically placed on a high-salt diet (> 120 mEq/day) with sodium chloride supplementation for 3–4 days to suppress aldosterone; on the last day of the high-salt diet, a 24-hour urine is collected to test for aldosterone, sodium, and creatinine. If urinary Na is > 200 mEq and aldosterone is > 12 mcg, unsuppressibility of aldosterone is documented. After confirmation of hyperaldosteronism, imaging of the adrenals should be performed with CT to look for hyperplasia versus adenoma. In equivocal cases, adrenal vein sampling for aldosterone can be performed.

▶ Treatment

Treatment for adenoma involves surgical resection. In as many as 70% of patients, this cures the hypertension and hypokalemia. The blood pressure, however, may require several months following surgery to return to normal. Medical therapy for patients who are not surgical candidates or those with hyperplasia includes the aldosterone antagonists spironolactone (100–200 mg/day) or eplerenone (25–100 mg/day), the diuretic amiloride (10–40 mg/day), and calcium channel blockers.

Funder JW, Carey RM, Fardella C, et al. Case detection, diagnosis, and treatment of patients with primary aldosteronism: an endocrine society clinical practice guideline. *J Clin Endocrinol Metab.* 2008;93:3266-81. [PMID 18552288]

Pimenta E, et al. Cardiac dimensions are largely determined by dietary salt in patients with primary aldosteronism: results of a case-control study. *J Clin Endocrinol Metab.* 2011;96:2813–20. [PMID: 21632817]

Pitt B, et al. Eplerenone, a selective aldosterone blocker, in patients with left ventricular dysfunction after myocardial infarction. *N Engl J Med.* 2003;348:1309–21. [PMID: 12668699]

ACROMEGALY & THE HEART

ESSENTIALS OF DIAGNOSIS

▶ Elevated somatomedin C.

▶ Inability to suppress growth hormone to less than 2 ng/mL during glucose tolerance test.

▶ Pituitary adenoma found on magnetic resonance imaging.

▶ General Considerations

Acromegaly is caused by the excessive secretion of growth hormone (GH) by a pituitary adenoma in an adult; gigantism occurs in children. Characteristic clinical manifestations are due to the chronic effects of GH, mediated through insulin-like growth factor 1 (IGF-1 or somatomedin C) in the liver and the periphery. Bony overgrowth is the classic feature, particularly of the skull and mandible; they also present with organomegaly and premature death, often due to cardiovascular, cerebrovascular, and respiratory dysfunction. In rare cases, ectopic GH-releasing hormone secretion due to carcinoid, small-cell, islet cell, and other tumors can cause acromegaly.

▶ Clinical Findings

A. Symptoms & Signs

1. Systemic symptoms & signs—Excessive GH causes bony, soft tissue, and visceral overgrowth. Patients may also complain of symptoms related to the local expansion of the tumor such as headache or bitemporal hemianopsia. Impotence, galactorrhea, and amenorrhea may result from cosecretion of prolactin or the destruction of normal gonadotrophs by the tumor. Other symptoms include excessive sweating, hoarseness, carpal tunnel syndrome, polyuria, and polydipsia.

2. Cardiovascular symptoms & signs—Cardiac dysfunction and HF are major causes of death in acromegalics. The older the patient and the longer the duration of disease, the more likely acromegalic cardiomyopathy will develop. The most striking clinical feature is concentric biventricular hypertrophy with inadequate filling leading to both systolic and diastolic dysfunction. Cardiomegaly occurs in about 15% of cases. Cardiac enlargement may be secondary to hypertension, atherosclerotic disease, or rarely due to acromegalic cardiomyopathy. Histologic findings include interstitial fibrosis, collagen deposition, myofibrillar derangement, lymphomononuclear infiltration, and myocyte apoptosis resembling myocarditis.

Other factors can potentially contribute to the cardiac dysfunction. The coexistence of hypertension, diabetes, or both in this condition can accelerate the progression to cardiac hypertrophy and HF. Hypertension, the most common cardiovascular finding in acromegalics, occurs in about 25% of patients, is usually mild in nature, and is easily treated with antihypertensives. The mechanism of the hypertension may be due to increased sodium and extracellular fluid retention with increased plasma volume.

Because of the role of GH as a counterregulatory hormone for hypoglycemia, most acromegalics have either glucose intolerance or frank diabetes, which may explain their increased incidence of premature coronary artery disease. Untreated acromegaly is associated with hypertriglyceridemia and elevated levels of apoprotein A-1, apoprotein E, fibrinogen, and plasminogen activator inhibitor-1 activity.

A rare disorder known as Carney syndrome involves any three of the following: GH-secreting pituitary tumors, cardiac or cutaneous myxoma, Sertoli cell tumors, cutaneous hyperpigmentation, and pigmented nodular adrenocortical disease. The myxomas seen in Carney syndrome are usually multiple and may involve more than one chamber. Family members should be screened with echocardiography.

B. Physical Examination

Because acromegaly is such an insidious disease, changes in the body occur gradually and usually go unnoticed until complications develop. Bitemporal hemianopsia may be detected on gross confrontation, indicating optic chiasm compression from the tumor. Thickened, oily skin, particularly of the face, and other facial changes, including thick lips, macroglossia, bulbous nose, frontal bossing, prominent cheek bones, hollow temporal fossa, and malocclusion with protrusion of the lower jaw, are usually seen. Synovial and periarticular swelling may be noted, and dorsal kyphosis, barrel chest, and spade-like hands with sausage-like digits are seen. The chest examination is most remarkable for galactorrhea. Abdominal examination may reveal generalized organomegaly.

C. Diagnostic Studies

1. Electrocardiography & echocardiography—Cardiomegaly may be present, even in the absence of hypertension, suggesting a direct effect of GH on the myocytes. Both symmetric and asymmetric cardiac hypertrophy have been reported on echocardiography. In early stages of the disease, both ventricular dimension and wall thickness are increased; therefore, relative wall thickness remains unchanged. In later stages, impaired diastolic filling and cardiac dilatation occur, leading to congestive HF.

ECG abnormalities include ST depression and nonspecific T-wave changes, LVH, and intraventricular conduction defects. Cardiac arrhythmias often occur, with ventricular ectopics and atrial fibrillation or flutter being the most frequent.

2. Laboratory findings—Diagnostic tests include random and glucose-suppressed GH levels, along with somatomedin C or IGF-1 levels. Because GH secretion is episodic, a random level alone is rarely helpful. Normally, GH is suppressed to less than 2 ng/mL in response to glucose infusion. Other findings often associated with acromegaly include hyperglycemia, hyperphosphatemia, and hypertriglyceridemia.

▶ Treatment

The goal in treating acromegaly is to normalize GH and IGF-1 concentrations in order to prevent early cardiovascular mortality. Treatment includes surgical removal of the pituitary adenoma with postoperative radiation therapy, or medical therapy with octreotide (200–500 mcg/day subcutaneously), a somatostatin analog, or bromocriptine (5–30 mg/day). More recently, sustained-release somatostatin analogs with activities lasting up to 1 month, such as octreotide LAR and lanreotide acetate, are becoming more popular and are the treatment of choice for patients with residual GH hypersecretion following surgery. The dopamine agonist, cabergoline, may be added to somatostatin analog therapy to improve control of GH levels. Many authors have suggested that once control of the disease occurs, defined as a GH level of < 2 ng/mL and a normal age-adjusted IGF-1 level, the progression of cardiac disease can be arrested and cardiovascular mortality reduced.

Colao A, et al. Growth hormone and the heart. *Clin Endocrinol (Oxf)*. 2001;54(2):137–54. [PMID: 11207626]
Fazio S, et al. Cardiovascular effects of short-term growth hormone hypersecretion. *J Clin Endocrinol Metab*. 2000;85(1):179–82. [PMID: 10634384]
Melmed S. Medical progress: acromegaly. *N Engl J Med*. 2006;335(24):2558–73. [PMID: 17167139]
Vitale G, et al. Cardiovascular complications in acromegaly. *Minverva Endocrinol*. 2004;29(3):77–88. [PMID: 15282442]

GROWTH HORMONE DEFICIENCY

Unlike acromegaly, in which cardiac involvement has been appreciated for many decades, the cardiac abnormalities associated with adult GH deficiency (GHD) have only recently been recognized. GHD is associated with abnormal body composition with increased fat mass, abnormal lipid metabolism, impaired capacity for exercise, decreased bone mineral density, decreased quality of life, and a risk of increased mortality from cardiovascular disease that is approximately twice that found in the normal population. Myocardial infarction, cardiac failure, and cerebrovascular accidents are the main causes of death.

The precise mechanisms responsible for the increase in cardiovascular disease are unknown, but a characteristic hypokinetic syndrome has been described. In this syndrome, a decrease in left ventricular and septal wall thickness is noted on echocardiography along with low heart rate and blood pressure. One study using radionuclide angiography has noted decreased left ventricular ejection fraction (LVEF) compared with that in controls.

Most commonly, adult GHD results from childhood onset of GHD that continues throughout life. Thus, the patient with a history of pituitary or hypothalamic disease, childhood-onset GHD, cranial irradiation, or trauma is a candidate for GHD testing. Testing consists of provocative stimulation with an insulin tolerance test. A biochemical diagnosis of adult GHD is determined by a subnormal response, for example, a peak level of GH < 5 ng/mL. Testing should not be performed in patients with ischemic heart disease or seizure disorder. Treatment is initiated with a daily subcutaneous injection of 2–5 mcg/kg/day of GH and can be titrated to 10–12 mcg/kg/day. Side effects are dose-dependent and consist of fluid retention and carpal tunnel syndrome.

GH therapy has been implicated in the health of the endothelium and increases nitric oxide production in in vitro studies. In humans with GHD, short-term treatment has been shown in various studies to increase cardiac mass, decrease carotid intimal medial thickness, reverse early atherosclerotic changes in major arteries, and possibly improve the vasodilatory function of the endothelium. However, the hypertrophic effect of long-term replacement with GH appears to subside over time. It remains to be seen if GH replacement therapy will reduce the prevalence of cardiovascular disease in this population.

Colao A, et al. Growth hormone and the heart. *Clin Endocrinol (Oxf)*. 2001;54(2):137–54. [PMID: 11207626]

CARCINOID TUMORS & THE HEART

▶ General Considerations

Carcinoid tumors are neuroendocrine tumors containing vasoactive secretagogues and are found in the gastrointestinal tract, urogenital tract, or the pulmonary bronchioles. Although these tumors can secrete a number of hormones, including ACTH and GH-releasing hormone, they most commonly secrete serotonin and serotonin metabolites. The presentation of the patient depends on the location of the carcinoid. Symptoms include flushing of the head and neck, with liver metastases, and bronchospasm with pulmonary carcinoid.

A unique endocrine effect of carcinoid tumors is fibrotic plaque-like thickenings on the endocardium of the tricuspid and pulmonic valves, atria, and ventricles. Deposition may also be seen on the superior and inferior venae cavae, pulmonary artery, and coronary sinus. The right side of the heart is affected predominantly, and although left-sided heart disease may occur, it is of lesser significance. Thickening of the valves results in tricuspid regurgitation and pulmonic stenosis. If the tricuspid regurgitation is severe, right-sided HF and cardiomegaly result. Nearly half of patients who die of carcinoid die of congestive HF.

Elaboration of serotonin by the tumor is believed to mediate the fibrosis; however, lowering serotonin levels does not cause regression of the plaques. Diagnosis is made by documenting more than 30 mg of 5-hydroxyindoleacetic acid (a serotonin metabolite) in a 24-hour urine collection. Normal individuals secrete less than 10 mg in 24 hours, and values between 10 and 30 mg are equivocal. Testing must be done while the patient has been on a diet free of serotonin-rich foods for several days. Localization should be attempted with bowel series, CT, somatostatin receptor scintigraphy, or PET. All patients with carcinoid should have echocardiography to look for heart involvement.

▶ Treatment

Treatment is surgical removal of the tumor if it has not metastasized. Synthetic somatostatin (octreotide) has been shown to shrink tumor metastases in addition to decreasing serotonin levels. Unfortunately, the heart disease does not improve with reduction of serotonin levels, and some patients will require valve replacement.

Ganim RB, et al. Recent advances in carcinoid pathogenesis, diagnosis and management. *Surg Oncol*. 2000;9(4):173–9. [PMID: 11476988]
Kulke MH. Clinical presentation and management of carcinoid tumors. *Hematol Oncol Clin North Am*. 2007;21(3):433–55. [PMID: 17548033]
Moller JE, et al. Prognosis of carcinoid heart disease: analysis of 200 cases over two decades. *Circulation*. 2005;112(21):3320–7. [PMID: 16286584]

DIABETES MELLITUS & THE HEART

▶ General Considerations

Myocardial infarction is the leading cause of death in patients with type 2 diabetes. The incidence of coronary artery disease and myocardial infarction in diabetic patients is two to five times more common than in age-matched controls. Cardiovascular risk is also increased in patients with type 1 diabetes, although the absolute risk is lower than for type 2 diabetes. Two types of vascular disease are seen: macrovascular disease, causing atherosclerosis and arteriosclerosis; and microvascular disease, producing retinopathy, nephropathy, neuropathy, and microangiopathy in the heart. Microangiopathy may explain the existence of congestive HF in diabetic patients without demonstrable coronary artery disease. Macrovascular disease develops prematurely in diabetic patients and is usually severe, with a striking predominance in diabetic women. Diabetics with no history of coronary heart disease (CHD) have risk for major cardiovascular events equal to that in established CHD. Consequently, the Adult Treatment Panel III has designated diabetes as a "CHD risk equivalent," with a 10-year risk for major cardiovascular events (risk of myocardial infarction and coronary death) of more than 20%.

A large body of evidence now links the increased risk of atherosclerosis to a combination of factors present in diabetes such as hyperlipidemia, abnormalities of platelet adhesiveness, coagulation factors, hypertension, and oxidative stress and inflammation leading to endothelial dysfunction. The evidence is particularly striking in persons with type 1 diabetes with microalbuminuria and proteinuria; however, endothelial dysfunction also occurs in patients with type 2 diabetes and normal urinary albumin excretion as well as in patients with insulin resistance who are normoglycemic. Once established, endothelial dysfunction induces changes in vascular tone, reactivity, and function that contribute to the progression of vascular disease. Insulin sensitizers, hypolipidemic therapy, and angiotensin-converting enzyme inhibitors have all been shown to improve endothelial function.

Hyperinsulinemia and insulin resistance have been postulated to relate directly to both hypertension and CHD in type 2 diabetes. The so-called "metabolic syndrome" is a constellation of metabolic risk factors that includes obesity, insulin resistance, elevated triglycerides, low high-density lipoprotein, hypertension, and fasting hyperglycemia. It enhances the risk for CHD at any given LDL level. To achieve maximum benefit from risk factor modification, the underlying insulin-resistant state must be a primary target of therapy.

▶ Clinical Findings

Angina and myocardial infarction in persons with diabetes are often manifested by atypical symptoms. Painless myocardial infarction may occur, and unusual pain patterns may delay diagnosis. Diabetic patients have a high mortality rate from myocardial infarction; recurrence is frequent, and the long-term prognosis is poor, with a higher incidence of congestive HF and ventricular rupture. Diabetic men have a 2.4-fold increase in HF, but diabetic women have a particularly high incidence: 5.1 times that of persons without diabetes. Diabetic cardiomyopathy occurs even in the absence of epicardial vessel disease, causing some investigators to hypothesize a preponderance of small-vessel disease. Autonomic neuropathy frequently occurs and results in sympathetic denervation manifested by a fixed tachycardia with subsequent parasympathetic damage that results in lowering of the heart rate. Complete autonomic cardiac denervation finally occurs, resulting in a heart rate that is no longer responsive to physiologic stimuli such as standing.

Echocardiographic studies may show abnormal systolic and diastolic function, with impaired diastolic filling as one of the earliest manifestations of diabetic cardiomyopathy. Various studies in diabetic patients have shown delayed opening of the mitral valve, a longer preejection period, and a shorter left ventricular ejection time, resulting in decreased left ventricular filling and contractility. Other studies have shown an increase in contractility in patients with diabetes of recent onset. Left ventricular dysfunction is likely multifactorial, reflecting the effects of hypertension, microvascular disease, and coronary atherosclerosis.

▶ Treatment

Large intervention studies of risk factor reduction in diabetes are lacking, but it is reasonable to assume that reducing risk factors would have a beneficial effect. Every 1 mmol/L (38.7 mg/dL) decline in LDL cholesterol results in a 21% decrease in cardiovascular events. A decrease in systolic blood pressure by 10 mm Hg can decrease cardiovascular mortality by 20–40%. Similarly, the risk of acute myocardial infarction increases by 5.6% for every additional cigarette smoked per day.

Lifestyle changes, including diet and exercise; oral hypoglycemics; insulin sensitizers; and insulin remain the mainstay of therapy for hyperglycemia. Tight glucose control decreases the progression and development of diabetic microvascular complications in patients with both type 1 and type 2 diabetes. For the prevention of microvascular

disease, a target hemoglobin A1c level of less than 7%, which corresponds with mean glucose levels of 150 mg/dL, is recommended. Intensive glycemic control aiming for near-normal levels has been shown to have a substantial beneficial effect (58% reduction in major cardiovascular disease events) on macrovascular outcomes in type 1 diabetes, when the intervention is done early in the disease course and after one to two decades of therapy. However, to date, few trials examining tight glucose control have shown any reduction in macrovascular disease, and it is still unclear whether tight glucose control influences CHD risk. In the acute setting, the evidence of benefit from strict glycemic control with insulin therapy in patients with acute myocardial infarction is limited. There is a positive association between the serum glucose at the time of myocardial infarction and mortality in patients with and without diabetes, but it is not fully understood as to whether strict glycemic control during hospitalizations for acute myocardial infarction improves outcomes.

Target lipid levels are similar to those for patients with established CHD and include a LDL of < 100 mg/dL, triglycerides < 150 mg/dL, and high-density lipoprotein > 45 mg/dL in women and > 55 mg/dL in men. Lowering LDL cholesterol reduces first events in patients without known coronary disease and secondary events in patients with known CHD. The Adult Treatment Panel III National Cholesterol Education Program (NCEP) guidelines, published in 2001, with an update in 2004, include initiation of lifestyle and drug management with the primary goal of reducing LDL cholesterol level to < 100 mg/dL in individuals with CHD, diabetes, or > 20% 10-year Framingham risk. In response to more recent trial results, the NCEP has recommended lowering the LDL target goals to < 70 mg/dL with at least 30–40% reduction for very high-risk individuals, such as those with acute coronary syndrome or diabetes and to < 100 mg/dL for those at moderately high risk. The value of intensive cholesterol reduction is best documented for patients with CHD in the recent IVUS, ASTEROID, and PROVE-IT trials, studying atherosclerosis progression and coronary events, respectively. Their statement acknowledges that the recent trials have failed to demonstrate an LDL cholesterol level below which coronary risk does not decrease.

When drug therapy is indicated for reducing LDL cholesterol, statins are generally initiated as first-line therapy. Exceptions include pregnancy, hepatic disease, or history of myopathy while on these agents. Resins, nicotinic acid, or ezetimibe can be added if LDL cholesterol levels are not reduced to goal. Pharmacologic therapy for hypertriglyceridemia includes fibrates, nicotinic acid, and omega-3 fatty acids. Fibrates and nicotinic acid are also effective in raising low high-density lipoprotein, particularly when high triglycerides are present.

The American Diabetes Association recommends lowering blood pressure to 130/80 mm Hg or less. Diabetic patients often require more intensive antihypertensive therapy to reach this goal; the majority need two to three drugs concomitantly. Early and vigorous antihypertensive therapy with angiotensin-converting enzyme inhibitors or angiotensin receptor blockers should be first-line therapy. The Antihypertensive and Lipid-Lowering Treatment to Prevent Heart Attack Trial (ALLHAT) randomized 33,357 subjects (age 55 or older) with hypertension and at least one other CHD risk factor (including 12,063 individuals with diabetes). In this trial, chlorthalidone appeared to be superior to amlodipine and lisinopril at lowering blood pressure, reducing the incidence of cardiovascular events, and with respect to tolerability and cost.

Aspirin (81–325 mg daily) inhibits thromboxane synthesis by platelets and is effective in reducing cardiovascular morbidity and mortality in patients who have a history of myocardial infarction or stroke. It is unclear if aspirin prevents primary cardiovascular events in people with diabetes. The current recommendation is to give aspirin to people with diabetes who are at increased risk for cardiovascular events, such as most men older than 50 years and women older than 60 years of age with one or more additional risk factor such as smoking, hypertension, dyslipidemia, family history of premature CHD, and albuminuria. Contraindications for aspirin therapy include aspirin allergy, bleeding tendency, recent gastrointestinal bleeding, or active liver disease. The Early Treatment Diabetic Retinopathy Study (ETDRS) showed that aspirin does not increase the incidence or severity of bleeding (vitreous/preretinal hemorrhages) in diabetic proliferative retinopathy or alter its course. Thus, it appears that there is no contraindication to aspirin use in patients with proliferative retinopathy.

Treatment of CHD for diabetic patients is similar to that for nondiabetic persons with some important caveats. Endothelial dysfunction and the platelet and coagulation disturbances characteristic of type 2 diabetes have been postulated to affect morbidity and mortality in the setting of unstable angina, non–ST segment elevation myocardial infarction, and after percutaneous transluminal coronary angioplasty (PTCA), stenting, and CABG. Diabetic patients have higher rates of adverse outcomes and restenosis in these settings. Early and midterm follow-up of diabetic patients after revascularization indicates that the incidences of myocardial infarction and repeat revascularization are reduced in patients undergoing CABG compared with those treated by balloon angioplasty alone. Percutaneous coronary intervention (PCI) with bare metal stents has reduced the need for reintervention after PCI in the early–mid-term; however, repeat revascularization in diabetic patients continues to be substantially higher after PCI. Advances in PCI include the use of drug-eluting stents and adjunctive drug therapies, such as abciximab. Glycemic control is an important determinant of outcome after revascularization in diabetic patients, and the impact of tight glycemic control after PCI was investigated in the Bypass Angioplasty Revascularization Investigation 2 in Diabetes (BARI-2D) study that tested whether increasing a patient's sensitivity to insulin produced by the pancreas would be superior to insulin injections in patients with *stable* coronary artery disease.

Overall, the study found there was little difference between insulin sensitization and insulin administration with respect to rates of death and cardiovascular events at 5 years. This trial also evaluated the effects of prompt revascularization by CABG or PCI versus medical therapy; patients who underwent CABG had better outcomes, especially those with diabetes and multivessel coronary artery disease. Results from the BARI-2D trial, combined with other randomized trials comparing PCI with CABG surgery, have so far shown that diabetics with multivessel coronary artery disease undergoing CABG have a survival advantage and reduced rates of subsequent cardiovascular events compared to PCI. Improvements in PCI and CABG surgery are leading to better results in diabetic patients, and future clinical trials are needed to answer many unanswered questions. Until future trial results become available and new technologies and medical therapies emerge, aggressive secondary prevention and ongoing management of CHD in the setting of diabetes will continue to pose a challenge.

BARI 2D Study Group. A randomized trial of therapies for type 2 diabetes and coronary artery disease. N Engl J Med. 2009; 360:2503–15. [PMID: 19502645]

Bhatt DL, et al. Abciximab reduces mortality in diabetics following percutaneous coronary intervention. J Am Coll Cardiol. 2000;35(4):922–8. [PMID: 10732889]

Booth GL, et al. Relation between age and cardiovascular disease in men and women with diabetes compared with non-diabetic people: a population-based retrospective cohort study. Lancet. 2006;368(9529):29–36. [PMID: 16815377]

Brooks RC, et al. Clinical trials of revascularization therapy in diabetics. Curr Opin Cardiol. 2000;15(4):287–92. [PMID: 11139093]

Calles-Escandon J, et al. Diabetes and endothelial dysfunction: a clinical perspective. Endocr Rev. 2001;22(1):36–52. [PMID: 11159815]

Colin B, et al. Coronary heart disease in patients with diabetes: part II: recent advances in coronary revascularization. J Am Coll Cardiol. 2007;49(6):643–56. [PMID: 17291929]

Expert Panel on Detection, Evaluation and Treatment of High Blood Cholesterol in Adults. Executive summary of the third report of the National Cholesterol Education Program (NCEP) Expert Panel on Detection, Evaluation and Treatment of High Blood Cholesterol in Adults (Adult Treatment Panel III). JAMA. 2001;285(19):2486–97. [PMID: 11368702]

Gæde P, et al. Multifactorial intervention and cardiovascular disease in patients with type 2 diabetes. N Engl J Med. 2003; 348(5):383–93. [PMID: 12556541]

Goldberg IJ. Clinical review 124: diabetic dyslipidemia: causes and consequences. J Clin Endocrinol Metab. 2001;86(3):965–71. [PMID: 11238470]

Hammoud T, et al. Management of coronary artery disease: therapeutic options in patients with diabetes. J Am Coll Cardiol. 2000;36(2):355–65. [PMID: 10933343]

Hu G, et al. The effect of diabetes and stroke at baseline and during follow-up on stroke mortality. Diabetologia. 2006;49(10):2309–16. [PMID: 16896934]

Huang ES, et al. The effect of interventions to prevent cardiovascular disease in patients with type 2 diabetes mellitus. Am J Med. 2001;111(8):633–42. [PMID: 11755507]

McFarlane SI, et al. Insulin resistance and cardiovascular disease. J Clin Endocrinol Metab. 2001;86(2):713–8. [PMID: 11158035]

Roffi M, et al. Platelet glycoprotein IIb/IIIa inhibitors reduce mortality in diabetic patients with non-ST-segment-elevation acute coronary syndromes. *Circulation*. 2001;104(23): 2767–71. [PMID: 11733392]

Stratton IM, et al. Association of glycaemia with macrovascular and microvascular complications of type 2 diabetes (UKPDS 35): prospective observational study. *BMJ*. 2000;321(7258):405–12. [PMID: 10938048]

Vega GL. Results of expert meetings: obesity and cardiovascular disease. Obesity, the metabolic syndrome, and cardiovascular disease. *Am Heart J*. 2001;142(6):1108–16. [PMID: 11717620]

Zhang F, et al. Percutaneous coronary intervention (PCI) versus coronary artery bypass grafting (CABG) in the treatment of diabetic patients with multi-vessel coronary disease: a meta-analysis. *Diabetes Res Clin Pract*. 2012;97(2):178–84. [PMID: 22513345]

▶ Effects of Diabetes on Peripheral Vascular Disease

Diabetes accelerates the rate of atherosclerosis in larger arteries; plaque formation is often diffuse, but tends to localize in areas of turbulent blood flow, such as at the bifurcation of the aorta or other large vessels. Clinical manifestations of peripheral vascular disease include ischemia of the lower extremities, impotence, and intestinal angina. Lower extremity arterial disease is clinically identified by intermittent claudication and/or the absence of peripheral pulses in the lower legs and feet. These clinical manifestations reflect decreased arterial perfusion of the extremity. However, there is evidence that a history of intermittent claudication and the palpation of peripheral pulses are unreliable techniques for the detection of peripheral arterial disease. The sensitivity of an abnormal posterior tibial pulse is better than an abnormal dorsalis pedis pulse (sensitivity and specificity of 70% and 90%, respectively, versus sensitivity of only 50% for dorsalis pedis); this artery is congenitally absent in 10–15% of the population. Greater accuracy has been achieved with noninvasive testing using Doppler ankle-brachial pressure ratios, measurement of reactive hyperemia after exercise, pulse reappearance time, ultrasound duplex scanning, and plethysmography. The American Diabetes Association and AHA recommend annual screening for peripheral arterial disease in patients with diabetes. Measurement of toe pressures has received a great deal of attention because of their predictability in defining individuals at high risk of gangrene, ulceration, and infection associated with occlusive arterial disease, even in patients with noncompressible vessels. Reduced toe pressures are highly associated with progression of lower extremity arterial disease to gangrene, ulceration, and the need for amputation.

The incidence and prevalence of peripheral arterial disease increase with age and with duration of diabetes. Many elderly diabetic persons have peripheral vascular disease (PVD) at the time of diabetes diagnosis. Concurrent peripheral neuropathy with impaired sensation makes the foot susceptible to trauma, ulceration, and infection. These factors contribute to progression to gangrene and osteomyelitis and, ultimately, to amputation. Critical limb ischemia and gangrene of the feet in patients with diabetes are 30 times more frequent than in age-matched controls. Diabetes accounts for approximately 50% of all nontraumatic amputations in the United States. A second amputation within a few years after the first is very common. PVD increases mortality, particularly if foot ulcerations, infection, or gangrene occur. Three-year survival after an amputation is < 50%.

Prevention is critically important; by the time PVD becomes clinically evident, it may be too late to salvage an extremity or requires costly resources. The Diabetes Control and Complications Trial (DCCT) showed a beneficial trend of glycemic control on vascular disease in insulin-dependent diabetes mellitus, but this trend was not statistically significant. Perhaps with longer follow-up the beneficial effect on vascular disease could be demonstrated.

ESTROGENS & THE HEART

1. Hormone Replacement Therapy

The net benefit of estrogen or combined estrogen-progestin replacement therapy in postmenopausal women is still uncertain. Based on extensive observational data, estrogen was thought to be cardioprotective, and estrogen replacement therapy was routinely prescribed for both primary and secondary prevention of CHD. However, prospective data from the Women's Health Initiative (WHI) combined estrogen-progestin trial reported an increase in CHD risk. Furthermore, the Heart and Estrogen/Progestin Replacement Study (HERS-I and -II), other controlled trials, and two meta-analyses were unable to demonstrate a protective effect of estrogen replacement therapy on the heart. HERS demonstrated a 52% increased risk of major coronary events within the first year of the trial. During the second year, risk was equal in the two groups, and by years 4–5, risk was higher in the placebo group. The early increase in risk suggests that hormone replacement therapy (HRT) may predispose to thrombosis, arrhythmia, or ischemia. The WHI unopposed estrogen trial did not report an increase in CHD events, although stroke and venous thromboembolism were increased, as was seen in the combined estrogen-progestin trial. Further follow-up analysis has suggested that younger postmenopausal women taking postmenopausal hormone therapy (unopposed or combined) are *not* at increased risk for CHD.

The Effects of Estrogen Replacement on the Progression of Coronary Artery Atherosclerosis (ERA) trial demonstrated that postmenopausal HRT is not beneficial in the short term (3 years) in preventing progression or inducing regression of coronary atherosclerosis in women with established CHD who undergo angiography.

It should be noted that both HERS and ERA were designed to examine the role of HRT in secondary prevention. The WHI is the first trial examining the effect of HRT in primary prevention and was terminated in early 2002 due to increased risk of invasive breast cancer. Rates of CHD, stroke, deep venous thrombosis, and pulmonary embolism were higher in women receiving HRT. Therefore, postmenopausal HRT cannot be recommended solely for prevention of CHD.

Most now agree that estrogen is a reasonable therapy when used short-term for menopausal symptoms, but it should not be prescribed for either primary or secondary prevention of CHD.

Canonico M, et al. Hormone therapy and venous thromboembolism among postmenopausal women: impact of the route of estrogen administration and progestogens: the ESTHER study. *Circulation.* 2007;115:840–5. [PMID: 17309934]

Hulley S, et al. Randomized trial of estrogen plus progestin for secondary prevention of coronary heart disease in postmenopausal women. Heart and Estrogen/progestin Replacement Study (HERS) Research Group. *JAMA.* 1998;280(7):605–13. [PMID: 9718051]

Rossouw JE, et al. Postmenopausal hormone therapy and risk of cardiovascular disease by age and years since menopause. *JAMA.* 2007;297:1465–77. [PMID: 17405972]

Rossouw JE, et al; Writing Group for the Women's Health Initiative Investigators. Risks and benefits of estrogen plus progestin in healthy postmenopausal women: principal results from the Women's Health Initiative randomized controlled trial. *JAMA.* 2002;288(3):321–33. [PMID: 12117397]

Shufelt CL, et al. Timing of hormone therapy, type of menopause, and coronary disease in women: data from the National Heart, Lung, and Blood Institute-sponsored Women's Ischemia Syndrome Evaluation. *Menopause.* 2011;18:943–50. [PMID: 21532511]

2. Oral Contraceptives

Oral estrogen-progestin contraceptives have long been touted as risks for deep venous thrombosis, myocardial infarction, and stroke that occurred with the early high-dose pills. However, the reduction in estrogen content has increased safety substantially. Because myocardial infarction is an extremely rare event in otherwise healthy women of reproductive age, even a doubling of the risk would result in an extremely low attributable risk, but the risk in older women who smoke outweighs the risk of an unwanted pregnancy. The increased risk in myocardial infarction and cardiovascular mortality reported in epidemiologic studies was seen among women over the age of 35 who were cigarette smokers. These studies included women who used both high- (≥ 50 mcg ethinyl estradiol) and low-dose (≤ 35 mcg ethinyl estradiol) oral contraceptives. However, the absolute risk of a myocardial infarction in a nonsmoker using a pill containing 20–40 mcg of ethinyl estradiol is very low. For women using contraceptive patch and vaginal ring, the numbers of myocardial infarctions have been too low to estimate risk; no excess risk has been noted with progestin-only formulations. General consensus is that that the risk of oral contraceptive use is unacceptable for women over 35 who smoke. On the other hand, for younger women, the benefits of oral contraceptives appear to outweigh the risks, even among heavy smokers, as long as there is no personal or family history of thromboembolic disease. Women who have taken an oral contraceptive appear not to be at increased risk for CHD later in life.

Lidegaard Ø, et al. Thrombotic stroke and myocardial infarction with hormonal contraception. *N Engl J Med.* 2012;366:2257–66. [PMID: 22693997]

Merz CN, et al. Past oral contraceptive use and angiographic coronary artery disease in postmenopausal women: data from the National Heart, Lung, and Blood Institute-sponsored Women's Ischemia Syndrome Evaluation. *Fertil Steril.* 2006;85:1425–31. [PMID: 16600235]

Rosondaal FR, et al. Female hormones and thrombosis. *Arterioscler Thromb Vasc Biol.* 2002;22(2):201–10. [PMID: 11834517]

Schiff I, et al. Oral contraceptives and smoking, current considerations: recommendations of a consensus panel. *Am J Obstet Gynecol.* 1999;180:S383–4. [PMID: 10368525]

Connective Tissue Diseases & the Heart

Carlos A. Roldan, MD

The connective tissue diseases are immune-mediated inflammatory diseases, primarily of the musculoskeletal system; however, they frequently also involve the cardiovascular system. The most important of these diseases are systemic lupus erythematosus, rheumatoid arthritis, scleroderma, ankylosing spondylitis, polymyositis/dermatomyositis, and mixed connective tissue disease. They affect the valve leaflets, coronary arteries, pericardium, myocardium, conduction system, and great vessels with different rates of prevalence and degrees of severity. Although heart involvement in patients with connective tissue diseases contributes significantly to their morbidity and mortality rates, there is a large discrepancy between clinically recognized heart disease, echocardiography studies, and postmortem series. Furthermore, the pathogenesis, natural history, and effects of therapy are incompletely understood. Increased awareness and better understanding of the cardiovascular diseases associated with connective tissue diseases may lead to earlier recognition and treatment with consequent decreased morbidity and mortality. Finally and of importance, patients with connective tissue diseases and associated heart disease should be managed by both cardiologists and rheumatologists given the potential morbidity and mortality of their heart disease and the complexity and potential harm of their pharmacotherapy.

SYSTEMIC LUPUS ERYTHEMATOSUS

ESSENTIALS OF DIAGNOSIS

▶ Musculoskeletal and mucocutaneous manifestations of systemic lupus erythematosus (SLE).

▶ Libman-Sacks vegetations, atrioventricular (AV) valve regurgitation, myocarditis, vascular thrombotic disease, and SLE.

▶ Cardioembolism and SLE.

▶ Acute pericarditis with antinuclear antibodies detected in the pericardial fluid.

▶ General Considerations

Systemic lupus erythematosus (SLE) is a multisystem chronically recurrent inflammatory disease that affects the musculoskeletal, mucocutaneous, visceral, and central nervous systems. Symptoms include fatigue, myalgias, arthralgias or arthritis, photosensitivity, and serositis. The prevalence of SLE varies widely, from 4 to 250 cases per 100,000 persons. It is more frequent in a patient's relatives than in the general population. SLE is predominantly seen in females, with a female-to-male ratio of 10:1. The pathophysiology of the disease is related to the multiorgan deposition of circulating antigen–antibody complexes and activation of the complement system, leading to humoral- and cellular-mediated inflammation.

Although SLE affects the cardiovascular system with varied frequency and degrees of severity, cardiovascular disease is the fourth most important cause of death in SLE patients (after infectious, renal, and central nervous system diseases) during the earlier course of disease, but later on, cardiovascular disease is a predominant cause of their death. The most significant SLE-associated heart diseases are valvular heart disease, arterial or venous thrombosis and systemic thromboembolism, coronary artery disease (CAD), and pericarditis. Myocarditis or cardiomyopathy and cardiac arrhythmias or conduction disturbances are less common.

Regarding the pathogenesis of SLE-associated cardiovascular disease, it is believed, as it is for the primary disease, that the immune complex deposition and complement activation lead to an acute, chronic, or recurrent inflammation of the valve leaflets, endocardium, vascular endothelium, pericardium, myocardium, or conduction system. The presence in these tissues of immune complexes, complement, antinuclear antibodies, lupus erythematosus cells, mononuclear inflammatory cells, necrosis, hematoxylin bodies, and deposits of fibrin and platelet thrombi support this theory. Many studies suggest that antiphospholipid antibodies (aPL) (immunoglobulin [Ig] A, IgG, or IgM anticardiolipin antibodies [aCL], lupus-anticoagulant [LA], or antibodies to plasma phospholipid-binding protein β_2-glycoprotein I) cause cardiovascular injury. These antibodies, present in as many as half of SLE patients, are directed against negatively charged phospholipids present in the membrane of endothelial cells causing endothelial dysfunction, endocardial and/or vascular injury, and increased endocardial, arterial, and/or venous thrombogenesis.

1. Valvular Heart Disease

▶ General Considerations

Valvular heart disease is the clinically most important and frequent of the SLE-associated cardiovascular manifestations. Valvular heart disease is associated with an increased morbidity and mortality of SLE patients. It has been categorized as vegetations (Libman-Sacks endocarditis), leaflet thickening, valve regurgitation, and infrequently, valve stenosis. Although the true prevalence of clinically recognized valve disease is unknown, recent transesophageal echocardiography (TEE) series showed rates of at least 40%. Although not consistently demonstrated, rates of valve disease are probably higher in patients who have had SLE for more than 5 years, in those treated with corticosteroids, in those with higher disease damage scores, in those with moderate to high levels of aPL, and in those older than 50 years of age.

The pathogenesis of SLE valve disease includes (1) an immune complex–mediated inflammation with subendothelial deposition of immunoglobulins and complement leading to an increased expression of $\alpha_3\beta_1$-integrin on the endothelial cells; (2) increased amount of collagen IV, laminin, and fibronectin; (3) proliferation of blood vessels; (4) inflammation and fibrosis; and finally, (5) commonly associated increased local or systemic thrombogenesis.

The proposed mechanisms of valve damage by aPL include (1) binding of aPL, which induces activation of endothelial cells and upregulation of the expression of adhesion molecules, secretion of cytokines, and abnormal metabolism of prostacyclins; (2) increased oxidized low-density lipoprotein (LDL) (LDL taken up by macrophages leads to macrophage activation and further damage to endothelial cells); (3) aPL interference with the regulatory functions of prothrombin and with the production of prostacyclin and endothelial relaxing factor, protein C, protein S, and tissue factor; and (4) a heparin-like–induced thrombocytopenia. All of these factors lead to increased vasoconstriction, platelet aggregation, and thrombus formation.

A. Valve Vegetations, or Libman-Sacks Endocarditis

Considered pathognomonic of SLE-associated valve disease, noninfective valve vegetations are almost exclusively seen on the mitral and aortic valves. Most vegetations are located on the coaptation portions of the leaflets, the atrial side for the mitral valve, and the aortic vessel or ventricular side for the aortic valve. The valve vegetations are usually sessile, are less than 1 cm² in size, have irregular borders and heterogeneous echodensity, and have no independent motion (Figures 35–1 and 35–2). Most valves with vegetations have associated thickening or regurgitation. Although valve vegetations have been seen more commonly in younger persons (< 40 years), their temporal association with SLE activity, severity, duration, and therapy has been variable.

Pathologic examination reveals that active Libman-Sacks vegetations have central fibrinoid necrosis with fibroblastic proliferation and fibrosis, surrounded by mononuclear and polymorphonuclear cellular infiltration, small hemorrhages, and platelet or fibrin thrombus. Healed vegetations have central fibrosis, minimal or no inflammatory cell deposition, and no or hyalinized and endothelialized thrombus. Active, healed, and mixed vegetations can be seen in the same valve.

B. Valve Thickening

Leaflet thickening with or without abnormal mobility results from replacement of the normal spongiosum and endothelial

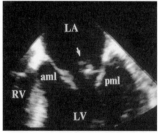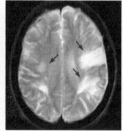

A   B

▲ **Figure 35–1.** Recurrent strokes and mitral valve thickening with a large Libman-Sacks vegetation in a 47-year-old woman with systemic lupus erythematosus. **A:** This transesophageal echocardiographic (TEE) four-chamber view shows diffuse thickening predominantly of the mid and tip portions of the anterior (aml) and posterior (pml) mitral leaflets. A large vegetation with heterogeneous echoreflectance and irregular borders is noted on the atrial side of the posterior mitral leaflet (*arrow*). Moderate mitral regurgitation was present. LA, left atrium; LV, left ventricle; RV, right ventricle. **B:** This T_2-weighted magnetic resonance imaging of the brain demonstrates generalized cortical atrophy, multiple areas of old cerebral infarcts characterized by loss of both gray and white matter (*arrows*) in a cortical and subcortical pattern. Also, multiple areas of deep white matter abnormality consistent with widespread ischemic cerebrovascular disease are noted.

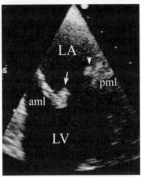
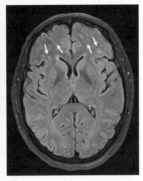

A   **B**

▲ **Figure 35–2.** Mitral valve Libman-Sacks vegetations in a 37-year-old woman with systemic lupus erythematosus and a stroke. **A:** This close-up transesophageal echocardiographic view demonstrates a Libman-Sacks vegetation on the atrial side and tip of the anterior mitral leaflet (aml) (*arrow*) and a second vegetation on the midportion of the posterior leaflet (pml) (*arrowhead*). Associated diffuse thickening of both mitral leaflets is also noted. Moderate mitral regurgitation was demonstrated by color Doppler. LA, left atrium; LV, left ventricle. **B:** This fluid-attenuated inversion recovery magnetic resonance imaging of the brain demonstrates multiple and bilateral frontal subcortical white matter abnormalities (*arrows*) consistent with small cerebral infarcts.

layers by postinflammatory fibrous tissue and infrequently by calcification. Valve thickening may be seen in up to half of patients; it is generally diffuse, with greater involvement of the middle and tip portions (see Figures 35–1 and 35–2). When leaflet thickening is localized, the basal, middle, and tip portions are equally affected. Valve thickening predominantly affects the mitral and aortic valves and is commonly associated with valve regurgitation, valve vegetations, or both. In young patients with no atherogenic risk factors, associated valve calcification is uncommon (< 5%). However, in middle-age patients with traditional atherogenic risk factors, mitral annular and aortic valve calcifications are common (20%).

C. Valve Regurgitation

This abnormality is predominantly mild in severity and therefore usually clinically silent. Although the prevalence of regurgitation is similar for the mitral, tricuspid, and pulmonic valves (about 50–75%) and the lowest for the aortic valve (25%), the mitral and aortic valves are those most commonly associated with complications. Mitral or aortic valve stenosis associated with respective valve regurgitation is uncommon.

▶ Clinical Findings

A. Symptoms & Signs

Unless it is severe, valve disease is generally asymptomatic or overshadowed by the musculoskeletal and systemic inflammatory symptoms. However, subclinical valve disease is commonly first manifested with cardioembolism. Recent studies report that valve disease detected by TEE, especially mitral valve vegetations, are two to four times more common in patients with focal ischemic brain injury on magnetic resonance imaging (MRI), in those with stroke or transient ischemic attack (TIA), and in those with nonfocal neuropsychiatric manifestations of cognitive dysfunction, acute confusional state, seizures, or psychosis (see Figures 35–1 and 35–2). In these series, valve vegetations were strong independent predictors of brain injury and focal or nonfocal neuropsychiatric manifestations. These data suggest that valve disease in lupus patients is a source of fibrin or platelet macro- or microembolism to the brain. Also, severe valve regurgitation resulting from recurrent or acute native and bioprosthetic valvulitis, noninfective mitral valve chordal rupture, or infective endocarditis may occur in ≤ 4% of patients per year. Infective endocarditis can mimic, accompany, or trigger a flare of SLE and lead to severe valvular dysfunction, heart failure, and death from septicemia. Similarly, a flare of SLE can clinically and echocardiographically mimic infective endocarditis (pseudo-infective endocarditis). A low white count, elevated aPL and anti-DNA antibodies, depressed complements, and negative or low C-reactive protein support the diagnosis of active SLE with pseudo-infective endocarditis.

B. Physical Examination

The physical findings of musculoskeletal and mucocutaneous disease generally predominate in SLE patients, even in those with cardiovascular disease. If moderate-to-severe mitral or aortic regurgitation or stenosis is present, the auscultatory findings found on physical examination will be typical. Less significant degrees of regurgitation (these are the majority) may not be clinically detected or may be mistaken for functional murmurs related to fever, anemia, hypertension, or volume overload. In patients with focal (stroke and TIAs) and nonfocal neuropsychiatric syndromes of seizures, confusional state, and cognitive dysfunction, cardioembolism from Libman-Sacks vegetations should be considered.

C. Diagnostic Studies

1. Electrocardiography—Results of electrocardiographic (ECG) studies are nonspecific. Left atrial abnormality and left ventricular (LV) hypertrophy can be seen in patients with chronic and severe aortic or mitral regurgitation.

2. Chest radiography—Cardiomegaly with LV and left atrial enlargement may be seen in the presence of significant mitral or aortic regurgitation.

3. Echocardiography—Transthoracic color-flow Doppler echocardiography (TTE) is the most commonly applied technique for the diagnosis of SLE-associated valve disease. This technique accurately determines the presence and severity of valve regurgitation or stenosis and abnormal leaflet thickening, but not of vegetations. The prevalence of Libman-Sacks vegetations by TTE is less than 10%. This technique will also detect associated increased wall thickness, chamber enlargement, ventricular diastolic or systolic dysfunction, and associated left atrial and pulmonary hypertension. TEE is superior to TTE in detecting and characterizing SLE-associated valve masses and leaflet thickening. TEE detects valve vegetations in up to 35% of patients. Considering TEE as the standard, TTE has a low sensitivity (63% overall, 11% for valve vegetations), low specificity (58%), low negative predictive value (40%), and a moderate positive predictive value (78%) for detection of Libman-Sacks endocarditis. By serial TEE, Libman-Sacks vegetations resolve, appear de novo, or change their morphology over time and may not be temporally related to SLE activity, severity, duration, or therapy. Therefore, TEE is indicated to exclude sources of cardioembolism in patients with a focal neurologic defect or in patients with a nonfocal neurologic deficit (moderate or worse cognitive dysfunction, seizures, acute confusional state, or psychosis) and cerebral infarcts on MRI, and in patients with suspected complicating infective endocarditis. Although there are limited data, three-dimensional TEE may further improve the diagnosis and characterization of Libman-Sacks endocarditis.

▶ Treatment

A. Specific Anti-inflammatory Therapy

Currently, prospective data are limited regarding whether corticosteroids, disease-modifying antirheumatic drugs (DMARDs) such as antimalarials (hydroxychloroquine and chloroquine), immunosuppressive therapy (eg, methotrexate, azathioprine, cyclophosphamide, mycophenolate), biologic response modifiers (eg, rituximab, belimumab, intravenous immunoglobulin), and plasmapheresis are beneficial in treating acute SLE-associated valve disease. In general, acute valvulitis complicated with valve vegetations and/ or moderate or worse valve regurgitation may be associated with active SLE disease, and therefore, treatment focuses on managing both active SLE disease and endocardial inflammation with anti-inflammatory (pulse corticosteroids) and immunosuppressive agents.

B. Long-Term Anticoagulation

Long-term anticoagulation is beneficial in patients with Libman-Sacks vegetations and previous systemic embolism independently of aPL. The role of antiplatelets or anticoagulants in patients with vegetations but no clinical evidence of embolism has not been defined, but probably should be considered.

C. Other Therapy

Diuretics, vasodilators, valve repair, or prosthetic valve replacement is indicated in severe symptomatic valve disease, including those cases complicated by infective endocarditis. The mortality rate associated with valve repair may be similar to the rate in those without SLE, but for valve replacement in SLE patients, it is twice that for patients without SLE.

2. Pericarditis

▶ General Considerations

Pericarditis, with or without effusion or pericardial thickening, is common in postmortem series. Also, about half of lupus patients suffer at least one episode of symptomatic pericarditis. Most episodes are acute and are frequently associated with active SLE and valvulitis, myocarditis, pleuritis, or nephritis. Cardiac tamponade or constrictive pericarditis rarely occurs (< 2%).

▶ Clinical Findings

A. Symptoms & Signs

The diagnosis of pericarditis is based on clinical manifestations rather than on the echocardiogram, because an effusion or pericardial thickening is frequently absent. Symptomatic pericarditis is generally acute and uncomplicated and is most commonly seen during flare-ups of the disease. Asymptomatic pericardial disease may be present in some patients. It is manifested by incidentally detected small effusions in most cases and far less frequently by pericardial thickening found on echocardiography. Asymptomatic pericardial disease is generally seen in patients with stable disease that is either mildly active or in remission. Occasionally, acute pericarditis, cardiac tamponade, or both may be the initial manifestation of SLE. Chronic constrictive pericarditis is rare. Infectious pericarditis is rare but catastrophic and most commonly caused by *Staphylococcus aureus*. Finally, a pericardial effusion in SLE patients may also be secondary to severe uremia or nephrotic syndrome.

Because it is frequently symptomatic, acute pericarditis is the SLE-related cardiovascular disease most often detected clinically. It may present with fever, tachycardia, pleuritic chest pain, and, on auscultation, the presence of a pericardial rub. If a large effusion is present, decreased heart sounds, jugular venous distention, and pulsus paradoxus may be noted.

B. Laboratory Findings

Pericarditis typically yields serofibrinous, fibrinous, or, rarely, serosanguineous exudative fluid containing low complement level and antinuclear antibodies. By immunofluorescence, the pericardium shows granular deposition of immunoglobulins and C3.

C. Diagnostic Studies

1. Electrocardiography—The ECG most frequently shows no abnormalities or nonspecific ST segment and T-wave changes. The characteristic diffuse ST segment elevation with upward concavity and PR segment depression of acute pericarditis are common. Low voltage or electrical alternans may also be seen if a large pericardial effusion is present.

2. Chest radiography—The chest radiography is generally of little diagnostic value because most patients with acute pericarditis have no—or only small—pericardial effusions. If a large pericardial effusion is present, cardiomegaly with a characteristic water-bottle shape may be seen.

3. Echocardiography—Since pericardial chest pain can be masked by musculoskeletal or pleural pain, echocardiography has complementary diagnostic value. Echocardiography may demonstrate small pericardial effusions or none. Small, asymptomatic pericardial effusions have also been found in up to 20% of SLE patients hospitalized with active disease. However, the absence of an effusion on echocardiography does not exclude a clinically suspected pericarditis. In cases of pericarditis with large pericardial effusion and clinically suspected cardiac tamponade, echocardiography may demonstrate right atrial or ventricular diastolic collapse and significant respiratory variability of the mitral or tricuspid Doppler inflows, indicating the need for therapeutic pericardiocentesis. Also, echocardiographically guided pericardiocentesis has been successfully performed in lupus patients with hemodynamically significant pericardial effusions. In addition, serial follow-up echocardiography after pericardiocentesis or after anti-inflammatory therapy is helpful to guide the need of future interventions. Echocardiography is less useful in detecting pericardial thickening or calcification in cases of suspected chronic pericardial constriction.

4. Computed tomography and magnetic resonance imaging—These techniques are preferred methods for assessing pericardial thickening when the echocardiogram suggests constriction.

▶ Treatment

A. Medical Therapy

Pericarditis is an indicator of serositis and of severely active SLE disease. Therefore, for severe pericarditis, immunosuppressive therapy with intravenous methylprednisolone or high-dose oral corticosteroids, followed by intravenous cyclophosphamide, plasmapheresis, rituximab, or oral mycophenolate, can be considered. For more indolent, recurrent, or chronic pericarditis, antimalarials (hydroxychloroquine or chloroquine), colchicine, methotrexate, mycophenolate, or intravenous belimumab can be used. The use of nonsteroidal anti-inflammatory drugs (NSAIDs) is frequently limited by associated renal disease, thrombocytopenia, or anticoagulation.

B. Surgical Therapy

Pericardiocentesis should be performed when large effusions are unresponsive to medical therapy and when cardiac tamponade or complicating infectious pericarditis with effusion is suspected.

Pericardiectomy has been performed in isolated cases of SLE-associated chronic pericardial constriction.

3. Myocarditis or Cardiomyopathy

▶ General Considerations

Myocarditis can be seen in autopsy series in up to 80% of patients with SLE; by contrast, only 20% of cases can be clinically detected. Myocardial disease in SLE patients has four principal causes. First, a primary acute, chronic, or recurrent myocarditis is the most common. Primary myocarditis may be associated with acute pericarditis (myopericarditis). Primary myocarditis with LV diastolic and, rarely, global or regional systolic dysfunction occurs in at least 10% of patients. Rarely, acute myocarditis complicated with heart failure may be the initial manifestation of active SLE. An association of cellular antigen Ro (SS-A) and La (SS-B) antibodies and this type of myocarditis has been established, but their primary pathogenic role is still undefined. The second most common cause of myocardial diastolic and uncommonly systolic dysfunction results from endothelial dysfunction–mediated microvascular CAD. Small-vessel vasculitis or epicardial coronary arteritis is rare. The third cause is myocardial dysfunction resulting from severe mitral or aortic regurgitation. Finally, a rare and potentially reversible chloroquine sulfate–induced dilated or restrictive cardiomyopathy has been reported.

▶ Clinical Findings

A. Symptoms & Signs

Acute myocarditis typically manifests with fever, tachycardia, chest pain, and, rarely, symptoms of heart failure, arrhythmias, or conduction disturbances. Acute myocarditis may clinically, electrocardiographically, and by laboratory mimic acute myocardial infarction. The myocarditis is generally mild and usually does not cause LV systolic dysfunction. However, up to one-third of young patients with active SLE have asymptomatic diastolic dysfunction. Occasionally, severe dilated cardiomyopathy is seen. Characteristic manifestations of an acute coronary syndrome will be present in those patients with myocardial dysfunction secondary to coronary arteritis, coronary atherosclerosis, small-vessel vasculitis, acute coronary thrombosis without underlying atherosclerosis, or coronary embolism from aortic or mitral valve noninfective vegetations.

If diastolic or systolic dysfunction is present, tachycardia, fourth and third heart sounds, pulmonary rales, and edema may be found.

B. Diagnostic Studies

1. Electrocardiography—Nonspecific ST segment and T-wave abnormalities and atrial or ventricular ectopic complexes are common. Rarely, atrial or ventricular tachyarrhythmias can be detected.

2. Chest radiography—Cardiomegaly may be present if dilated cardiomyopathy has developed.

3. Echocardiography—Generally, no abnormalities are detected in acute myocarditis. When the myocarditis is severe, diffuse or regional wall motion abnormalities may be observed. Doppler echocardiography series, including tissue Doppler, strain, and strain rate in asymptomatic young patients without systemic or pulmonary hypertension and normal LV systolic function, have demonstrated up to one-third of LV and right ventricular (RV) diastolic dysfunction, predominantly of impaired relaxation. Diastolic dysfunction occurs three to four times more frequently in patients with active SLE. In unselected patients, the prevalence of asymptomatic LV systolic dysfunction is low ($\leq 3\%$). These abnormalities may be related to subclinical acute or recurrent myocarditis, microvascular CAD, or hypertension.

4. Radionuclide studies—Either first-transit or gated-acquisition radionuclide angiography also can be used to assess ventricular systolic and diastolic dysfunction, wall motion abnormalities, and chamber enlargement. In up to one-third of SLE patients, this technique has shown an abnormal ventricular function response to exercise, as evidenced by a fall or subnormal rise in ejection fraction and the appearance of new or worsened wall motion abnormalities indicative of myocarditis or CAD. Reversible, fixed, or mixed myocardial perfusion defects can be seen in patients with normal epicardial coronary arteries indicative of active or past myocarditis or abnormal coronary flow reserve or microvascular disease.

5. Magnetic resonance imaging—This technique improves the detection of subclinical and clinical myocarditis. Patchy epicardial and intramyocardial delayed gadolinium enhancement is characteristic of postinflammatory myocardial fibrosis.

6. Endomyocardial biopsy—Tissue samples may demonstrate SLE-associated myocarditis or cardiomyopathy when a clinical or serologic diagnosis cannot be made.

7. Cardiac biomarkers—Mild elevation of troponin I will be more common than elevation of creatine phosphokinase (CPK) and may occur in the absence of ECG or echocardiographic abnormalities.

▶ Treatment
A. Specific Anti-inflammatory Therapy

As for pericarditis, myocarditis usually indicates severely active SLE disease, and therefore, in-patient intravenous pulse cyclophosphamide or oral mycophenolate in addition to intravenous methylprednisolone (1–2 mg/kg/day) can be considered. Once patients are considered stable, outpatient therapy with oral mycophenolate, antimalarials (hydroxychloroquine or chloroquine), methotrexate, azathioprine, or intravenous belimumab or rituximab is used and the corticosteroids are gradually tapered. This therapy is usually continued for 6–12 months, and corticosteroids are titrated down based on overall SLE and cardiac clinical response.

B. Other Therapy

Symptomatic therapy with NSAIDs or other analgesics, bed rest, and ECG monitoring for detection of arrhythmias are indicated. If symptomatic dilated cardiomyopathy is present, standard therapy of diuretics, vasodilators, and digoxin therapy are used.

4. Thrombotic Diseases
▶ General Considerations

Deep venous thrombosis, pulmonary embolism, and peripheral or cerebral arterial thrombosis are common in SLE patients. Acute coronary thrombosis or thromboembolism in the absence of angiographic CAD has also been reported. Both arterial and venous thrombotic events have been associated with aPL. Patients with SLE are subject to intracardiac thrombosis and cerebral or systemic thromboembolism independently of or exacerbated by aPL. Current data support that SLE cerebrovascular disease is commonly associated and likely causally related to cardioembolism from Libman-Sacks endocarditis. In recent series, mitral or aortic valve vegetations were two to four times more common and strong independent predictors of focal ischemic brain injury on MRI; stroke or TIA; and nonfocal neurologic dysfunction, such as cognitive dysfunction, acute confusional state, or seizures (see Figures 35–1 and 35–2). In fact, microembolic events during transcranial Doppler echocardiography are common in patients with cerebral ischemic events.

▶ Clinical Findings
A. Symptoms & Signs

Although acute pleuritic chest pain and tachycardia could be related to the presence of pericarditis, pleuritis, or pneumonitis, they should prompt the suspicion of pulmonary embolism and deep vein thrombosis (DVT). Focal and nonfocal transient or permanent neurologic deficits are commonly due to cardioembolism from valvular disease and rarely due to vasculitis or cerebritis or atherosclerosis.

B. Laboratory Findings

Antiphospholipid antibodies are highly associated with venous or arterial thrombotic events. However, these antibodies can be present in SLE patients without thrombosis and infrequently in patients who do not have SLE. Therefore, routine measurement of aPL to identify patients at high thrombotic risk and as a basis for prophylactic antiplatelet or anticoagulant therapy is still undefined.

C. Diagnostic Studies

1. Transesophageal echocardiography—TEE should be considered in SLE patients with focal neurologic deficits, in those with nonfocal neurologic deficits and focal brain injury on brain MRI, and in those with peripheral arterial thrombosis to exclude cardioembolism from Libman-Sacks vegetations.

2. Doppler echocardiography, plethysmography, scintigraphy, or venogram—These imaging methods of the lower extremities should be performed if DVT is suspected.

3. High-resolution computed tomography of the chest or pulmonary ventilation-perfusion scan—These methods should be considered if pulmonary embolism is clinically suspected.

▶ Treatment

A. Specific Anti-inflammatory Therapy

Corticosteroids or immunosuppressive agents may be beneficial in patients with active SLE and noninfective vegetations with or without thrombosis or thromboembolism.

B. Other Therapy

Anticoagulation with warfarin is the therapy of choice in patients with DVT, pulmonary embolism, and noninfective valve vegetations and stroke or TIA or suspected embolic cerebral infarcts on MRI.

5. Coronary Artery Disease

▶ General Considerations

Postmortem studies in SLE patients have demonstrated at least a 25% prevalence of CAD, but clinically evident disease or arteritis is probably less common. Clinical and subclinical functional or small-vessel CAD is more frequent than epicardial coronary disease in clinical series.

After controlling for traditional risk factors for CAD, the risk of functional (abnormal coronary vasodilation or microvascular disease) or subclinical atherosclerotic epicardial CAD in the form of coronary artery calcifications in lupus patients is three to eight times higher than matched controls. This form of subclinical CAD is predictive of a higher risk for future cardiovascular events (myocardial infarction [MI], stroke, death). Risk factors for CAD in SLE patients are a longer mean duration of the disease, a longer mean duration and dose of prednisone therapy, a high disease activity and damage score, lupus nephritis, and SLE-induced dyslipidemia (high levels of LDL phenotype B [the atherogenic phenotype], low levels of high-density lipoprotein [HDL], high levels of proinflammatory HDL, and high levels of triglycerides). Although, a high Framingham risk score is also an important predictor, this score by itself underestimates these patients' cardiovascular risk.

The proposed pathogenetic mechanisms for CAD include activation of cellular and humoral immunity (including aPL) with activation of macrophages, CD4$^+$CD28$^-$ T cells, and dendritic cells. The cytotoxicity of these cells to the endothelium and vascular wall results in decreased production of prostacyclin and prostaglandin I and consequently in increased vasoconstriction. Also, vascular wall cytotoxicity results in an increased thrombosis via release of platelet-derived growth factor and thromboxane A$_2$. Cytotoxic cells also produce interferon-γ, which destabilizes atherosclerotic plaques by suppressing synthesis of collagen, increased proliferation of smooth muscle cells, and activation of macrophages to release free radicals and matrix metalloproteinases. Other proposed pathogenetic mechanisms for CAD include increased oxidation of LDL and increased production of inflammatory cytokines and chemokines such as heat shock proteins, C-reactive protein, rheumatoid factor, tumor necrosis factor-α, and interleukins. These cytokines are expressed on the endothelium of coronary arteries, recruit inflammatory cells, promote abnormal vascular smooth cell proliferation, and induce oxidative stress, endothelial apoptosis, and further upregulation of adhesion molecules and chemokines. A final proposed pathogenetic mechanisms for CAD is exacerbation of dyslipidemia (high levels of very-low-density lipoproteins and triglycerides and low levels of HDL), homocysteinemia, and insulin resistance. Uncommon pathogenetic factors include coronary arteritis, in situ coronary thrombosis, or embolization from a Libman-Sacks vegetation.

▶ Clinical Findings

A. Symptoms & Signs

The presentation of CAD in SLE patients is not unique and involves stable or exertional angina, unstable angina, acute ST or non-ST elevation MI, or, rarely, heart failure from ischemic LV dysfunction. In addition, fatal MI can occur in SLE patients, and some data suggest an increased risk of myocardial rupture after MI in SLE patients treated with corticosteroids. Coronary arteritis should be suspected in a young patient with an acute ischemic syndrome, active SLE, and evidence of vasculitis affecting other organs. Also, coronary embolism or in situ thrombosis warrants consideration when MI occurs in the presence of a cardioembolic substrate (valve vegetations) or moderate to high levels of aPL.

B. Diagnostic Studies

Electrocardiography, exercise testing with or without perfusion scanning, and echocardiography can be used in SLE patients in whom CAD is suspected. However, the diagnostic value of these techniques is inferior to that in the general population due to their young age, female predominance, and lower prevalence of obstructive epicardial CAD. Electron-beam computed tomography (CT) has demonstrated a high prevalence (30–45%) of coronary calcification in asymptomatic patients. Cardiac MRI can detect subendocardial ischemia and small patchy areas of delayed contrast enhancement at rest and during exercise in up to 40% of patients with proven microvascular, but no epicardial, CAD on coronary angiography. A similarly high prevalence of perfusion abnormalities with normal coronary arteries has been reported using radioisotope myocardial perfusion imaging. Recent series in young SLE patients have also shown the development of premature carotid and aortic stiffness associated with intima media thickening and plaques, which may be markers of underlying premature epicardial or microvascular CAD. None of these techniques, including angiography, can reliably differentiate coronary arteritis from common coronary atherosclerosis. Suspected epicardial CAD may warrant coronary angiography because of the confounding clinical, echocardiographic, and myocardial perfusion features of functional or small-vessel CAD or lupus myocarditis.

► Treatment

A. Specific Anti-inflammatory Therapy

If coronary arteritis is suspected, in-patient intravenous cyclophosphamide or oral mycophenolate and high-dose corticosteroids (1–2 mg/kg/day) may be considered initially and continued on out-patient basis after patient clinical stabilization. The duration of high-dose therapy is usually for several weeks and tailored based on overall SLE and cardiac clinical response, but in these cases, long-term immunosuppression and antimalarial therapy are necessary to prevent recurrent disease. Corticosteroids may have some additional danger for myocardial rupture in patients with recent transmural MI.

B. Other Therapy

Except for the use of immunosuppressive agents in suspected arteritis, the medical therapy of acute and chronic epicardial CAD is not different from that in the general population. Both percutaneous coronary intervention (PCI) and bypass surgery have been successfully performed in SLE patients.

6. Cardiac Arrhythmias & Conduction Disturbances

► General Considerations

The prevalence of these abnormalities, including prolongation of the QT interval, is unknown. Although they are common with myocarditis and highly associated with the presence of anti-Ro/SS-A antibodies, no primary pathogenetic role of these antibodies has been demonstrated. Atrial fibrillation or flutter may be seen during episodes of acute pericarditis, myocarditis, pulmonary embolism, or pulmonary hypertension. Chronic conduction disturbances may be due to the inflammation and fibrosis of the conduction system frequently found at autopsy. ECG is the most valuable technique for detecting arrhythmias and conduction disturbances.

► Treatment

A. Specific Anti-inflammatory Therapy

Although experience is limited, acute high-degree atrioventricular (AV) blocks more commonly seen in association with acute myocarditis or myopericarditis may resolve with the use of intravenous immunosuppressives and high-dose corticosteroids, and these drugs should be used before considering permanent pacing.

B. Other Therapy

Temporary pacing is an alternative treatment for acute AV blocks. Permanent pacemakers should be used in cases of symptomatic high-grade AV blocks that are unresponsive to immunosuppressives and corticosteroids.

► Prognosis

The overall survival rate of SLE patients is about 75% over 10 years. If the heart, lung, kidney, or central nervous system is clinically involved, the prognosis is worse. Cardiovascular disease is the third major cause of mortality in SLE patients, after infectious and renal diseases early in the course of disease, but it becomes a predominant cause, especially CAD, at the later stage. Valvular disease, myocardial disease, and CAD are all known to decrease the survival of SLE patients.

Appenzeller S, et al. Acute lupus myocarditis: clinical features and outcome. *Lupus.* 2011;20(9):981–8. [PMID: 21478290]

Bengtsson C, et al. Cardiovascular event in systemic lupus erythematosus in northern Sweden: incidence and predictors in a 7-year follow-up study. *Lupus.* 2012;21(4):452–9. [PMID: 22065097]

Buss SJ, et al. Myocardial left ventricular dysfunction in patients with systemic lupus erythematosus: new insights from tissue Doppler and strain imaging. *J Rheumatol.* 2010;37(1):79–86. [PMID: 19955054]

Goykhman P, et al. Subendocardial ischemia and myocarditis in systemic lupus erythematosus detected by cardiac magnetic resonance imaging. *J Rheumatol.* 2012;39(2):448–50. [PMID: 22298279]

Nikpour M, et al. Relationship between cardiac symptoms, myocardial perfusion defects and coronary angiography findings in systemic lupus erythematosus. *Lupus.* 2011;20(3):299–304. [PMID: 21078763]

Roldan CA, et al. Premature aortic atherosclerosis in systemic lupus erythematosus: a controlled transesophageal echocardiographic study. *J Rheumatol.* 2010;37(1):71–8. [PMID: 19955049]

Roldan CA, et al. Transthoracic echocardiography versus transesophageal echocardiography for the detection of Libman-Sacks endocarditis: a randomized controlled study. *J Rheumatol.* 2008;35(2):224–9. [PMID: 18085739]

Shroff H, et al. Mitral valve Libman-Sacks endocarditis visualized by real time three-dimensional transesophageal echocardiography. *Echocardiography.* 2012;29(4):E100–1. [PMID: 22176492]

Zuily S, et al. Increased risk for heart valve disease associated with antiphospholipid antibodies in patients with systemic lupus erythematosus: meta-analysis of echocardiographic studies. *Circulation.* 2011;124(2):215–24. [PMID: 21690492]

RHEUMATOID ARTHRITIS

ESSENTIALS OF DIAGNOSIS

▶ Clinical evidence of rheumatoid arthritis.

▶ Granulomatous valve disease, predominantly of the mitral and aortic valves.

▶ Pericarditis and myocarditis with granuloma on biopsy.

▶ General Considerations

Rheumatoid arthritis is an immune-mediated chronic inflammatory disease characterized by morning stiffness, arthralgias, or arthritis, predominantly of the metacarpophalangeal or proximal interphalangeal joints; rheumatoid nodules; serum IgM or IgG rheumatoid factor and anticyclic citrullinated peptide (anti-CCP) antibody; and articular erosions seen on a radiograph. The disease prevalence is about 1%, and it affects females more than males with a ratio of 2–4:1. The natural history of the disease is such that the median life expectancy is reduced by 7 years in men and 3 years in women. The most common causes of death are articular and extra-articular complications such as atlantoaxial subluxation, cricoarytenoid synovitis, sepsis, heart disease, cardiopulmonary complications, and diffuse vasculitis. Rheumatoid arthritis patients with the worst prognosis are those with positive rheumatoid factor, nodular disease, and male gender.

Rheumatoid cardiovascular disease is produced by a nonspecific immune complex–mediated inflammation, vasculitis, or granulomatous deposition on the pericardium, myocardium, heart valves, coronary arteries, aorta, or the conduction system. Clinically apparent rheumatoid heart disease occurs in one-third of patients, compared with up to 80% in autopsy series. Rheumatoid heart disease may appear as pericarditis, myocarditis, valvular heart disease, atherosclerotic CAD, conduction disturbances, coronary arteritis, aortitis, or cor pulmonale. The sole presence of rheumatoid arthritis is now considered a primary pathogenic factor for premature development of CAD with also a threefold increase in cardiovascular events.

Predictors for clinically apparent cardiovascular disease vary among reported series and include male sex; disease duration; advanced age at the onset of the disease; hypertension; corticosteroid therapy early in the disease; long-standing disease; active extra-articular, erosive polyarticular, and nodular disease; systemic vasculitis; and high serum titers of rheumatoid factor, higher erythrocyte sedimentation rates (ESR), and higher levels of haptoglobin, von Willebrand factor, and plasminogen activator inhibitor. These findings suggest inflammatory and prothrombotic processes leading to cardiovascular disease. Heart disease is the third leading cause of death in patients with rheumatoid arthritis and accounts for nearly 40% of their mortality.

1. Rheumatoid Pericarditis

The prevalence of pericarditis is higher in hospitalized patients with active disease. Pericarditis generally follows the diagnosis of rheumatoid arthritis. There is a high association between pericarditis and IgG or IgM rheumatoid factor positivity, rheumatoid nodular disease, and ESR of > 55 mm/h. Rheumatoid pericarditis occurs by three mechanisms: a nonspecific immune complex inflammatory process, vasculitis, and, less frequently, granulomatous or nodular disease.

▶ Clinical Findings

A. Symptoms & Signs

Rheumatoid pericarditis is generally uncomplicated and most commonly is evidenced by typical pleuritic pain. About one-third of patients are asymptomatic. On physical examination, most will have a pericardial rub. Rarely, complicating cardiac tamponade or constrictive pericarditis may occur, generally in adult patients with active and severe disease of a longer duration and in those with extra-articular involvement. Dyspnea and orthopnea, edema, jugular venous distention, rales, pulsus paradoxus, Kussmaul sign, and hepatojugular venous distention are common when cardiac compression is present.

B. Laboratory Findings

Findings commonly associated with rheumatoid pericarditis include an ESR > 55 mm/h and high titers of rheumatoid factor. Pericardial fluid is exudative and serosanguineous, with a high protein content and high lactate dehydrogenase (LDH) but a characteristically low glucose level, and may contain rheumatoid factor. The cellular content is usually more than 2000 cells/mL, predominantly neutrophils. On pericardial biopsy (by immunofluorescence), granular deposits of IgG, IgM, C3, and C1q are seen in the interstitium and blood vessel walls of the pericardium.

C. Diagnostic Studies

1. Electrocardiography—An ECG commonly shows nonspecific ST segment and T-wave changes; a classic diffuse ST segment elevation and PR depression can be seen. Low voltage or electrical alternans may be seen with large pericardial effusions.

2. Chest radiography—The chest radiography is generally normal. Cardiomegaly is seen in patients with large pericardial effusions. Pericardial calcifications are rarely seen.

3. Echocardiography—This is the most important diagnostic technique for rheumatoid pericardial disease. The most common findings are pericardial effusion and pericardial thickening. Right atrial or ventricular diastolic compression may be seen with large pericardial effusions and may indicate tamponade hemodynamics. The presence of pericardial thickening and calcification without significant effusion and the presence of symptoms or signs of cardiac compression suggest constrictive pericarditis, which can be confirmed by cardiac catheterization. However, absence of pericardial abnormalities on echocardiography does not exclude the presence of pericarditis in a patient with typical symptoms or a pericardial rub. Finally, echocardiography is commonly used to guide pericardiocentesis.

4. Computed tomography or magnetic resonance imaging—These imaging methods are superior to echocardiography in detecting pericardial thickening and calcification in patients with suspected constrictive pericarditis.

▶ Treatment

Since hemodynamically significant pericarditis indicates active disease in the setting of rheumatoid arthritis, high-dose oral or intravenous pulse corticosteroids are used acutely to control pericardial inflammation, followed by long-term rheumatoid-specific chronic therapy, including methotrexate, sulfasalazine, antimalarials, leflunomide, tumor necrosis factor-α receptor blockers (infliximab, adalimumab, etanercept, golimumab, certolizumab), anti–B-cell (CD20) therapy (rituximab), T-cell stimulation inhibitors (abatacept), interleukin (IL)-6 receptor blocker (tocilizumab), or soluble IL-1 receptor antagonist (anakinra). If large pericardial effusions or tamponade are present, pericardiocentesis is also indicated. For chronic constrictive pericarditis, high-risk pericardiectomy has been performed. The use of intrapericardial corticosteroids at the time of pericardiocentesis is controversial but may be effective.

▶ Prognosis

The prognosis of rheumatoid arthritis in the presence of pericardial disease is unaltered when the pericardial involvement is mild. Large pericardial effusions with tamponade or chronic constrictive pericarditis, however, increase the morbidity and mortality rates among rheumatoid patients.

2. Rheumatoid Valvular Heart Disease

▶ General Considerations

Rheumatoid valvular heart disease is produced by a nonspecific acute, chronic, or recurrent immune complex inflammatory process, vasculitis, or deposition of granulomata on the valve leaflets. The inflammatory process consists of infiltration with plasma cells, histiocytes, lymphocytes, and eosinophils that lead to leaflet fibrosis, thickening, and retraction. The valve granulomata, which resemble rheumatoid nodules, are present inside any portion of the four valves, valve rings, papillary muscle tips, and atrial or ventricular endocardium. The aortic and mitral valves are most often affected. The granulomata are most commonly located at the basal or mid portion of the valves, are usually focal, and generally produce none or mild valve dysfunction.

Rheumatoid valvular heart disease is more commonly subclinical and can manifest in four forms: (1) healed valvulitis with residual leaflet fibrosis and regurgitation and rarely stenosis; (2) rheumatoid valve nodules (Figure 35–3A); (3) acute or recurrent valvulitis with variable degrees of regurgitation and with Libman-Sacks–like vegetations (Figure 35–3, B–D); and rarely, (4) aortitis with aortic root dilatation and aortic regurgitation. Acute and chronic valvulitis with resulting leaflet thickening and fibrosis is indistinguishable from that seen in SLE. In contrast, valve nodules appear to be unique to rheumatoid arthritis.

In previous series using TTE, rheumatoid valve disease has been reported in patients with long-standing rheumatoid disease and severe cases with erosive polyarticular and nodular disease, systemic vasculitis, and high levels of rheumatoid factor. In a recent TEE series, no correlation was found between valve disease and the duration, activity, severity, pattern of onset and course, extra-articular disease, serology, or therapy of rheumatoid arthritis. Therefore, a clinical or laboratory predictor or marker of rheumatoid valve disease is still undefined.

▶ Clinical Findings

A. Physical Examination

The physical examination in rheumatoid valve disease may not be revealing because in most cases the degree of valve dysfunction is mild. In the rare cases of acute mitral or aortic valvulitis resulting in severe valve regurgitation or acute severe valve regurgitation from "rupture" of a nodule or a large nodule affecting leaflets coaptation, classic auscultatory findings and associated signs of left or biventricular failure may be present. Uncommonly, a clinical syndrome of systemic embolism can result from a thrombus or a valve strand over imposed on a valve nodule or valve thickening or from Libman-Sacks–like vegetations complicating acute valvulitis.

B. Diagnostic Studies

1. Electrocardiography and chest radiography—The ECG and chest radiography have limited diagnostic value. Both techniques may show chamber enlargement in cases of severe valve disease.

2. Color-flow Doppler echocardiography—TTE is the most used test for detecting and assessing the severity of

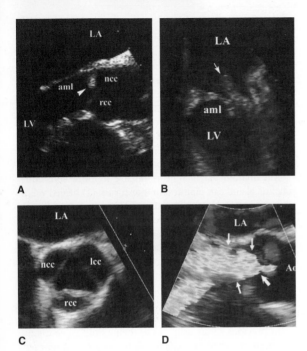

▲ Figure 35–3. A: Rheumatoid aortic valve nodule in a 48-year-old woman with rheumatoid arthritis. This transesophageal echocardiographic (TEE) longitudinal view of the left ventricular outflow tract demonstrates a well-defined nodule with oval shape and homogeneous soft tissue echoreflectance within the midportion of the aortic noncoronary cusp (ncc) (*arrowhead*). In contrast, the right coronary cusp (rcc) is normal. Aortic valve regurgitation was not demonstrated. aml, anterior mitral leaflet; LA, left atrium; LV, left ventricle. **B:** Severe mitral valvulitis with Libman-Sacks–like vegetations in a 52-year-old female with severe rheumatoid arthritis and recurrent transient ischemic attacks. This close-up four-chamber TEE view demonstrates marked thickening with soft tissue echoreflectance of the anterior and posterior mitral leaflets and a large and elongated soft tissue echoreflectant vegetation on the atrial side of the distal portion of the posterior mitral leaflet. After exclusion of infection, she was treated with warfarin, steroids, and tumor necrosis factor-α receptor inhibitors, and follow-up echocardiogram demonstrated remarkable improvement. **C and D:** Severe aortic valvulitis complicated by severe aortic regurgitation and subacute heart failure in a 47-year-old female with severely active rheumatoid arthritis. **C:** This basal short axis TEE view of the aortic valve shows diffuse thickening with soft tissue echoreflectance and decreased mobility of the non (ncc), left (lcc), and right (rcc) coronary cusps. **D:** Color Doppler longitudinal TEE view of the aortic valve (Ao) shows severe aortic regurgitation (*arrows*).

rheumatoid valve disease. In a recent series using TEE in 34 patients with rheumatoid arthritis, 20 patients (59%) had mainly left-sided valve disease (valve nodules in 11 [32%], valve thickening in 18 [53%], at least moderate mitral or mild aortic regurgitation in 7 [21%], and valve stenosis in 1 [3%]). *Valve nodules* were generally single and small (4–12 mm), of homogenous echoreflectance, and of oval shape with regular borders, typically located at the leaflets' basal or mid portions, and equally affected the aortic and mitral valves (see Figure 35–3A). In one patient, mitral and aortic valve thickening was associated with mitral valve Libman-Sacks–like vegetations (see Figure 35–3B). *Valve thickening* was equally diffuse or localized. When the thickening was localized, it affected any leaflet portion, was usually mild, involved the mitral and aortic valves similarly, and rarely involved the annulus and subvalvular apparatus (see Figure 35–3).

▶ **Treatment**

No specific anti-inflammatory therapy for rheumatoid valve disease has been established. The use of immunosuppressive agents or tumor necrosis factor-α receptor inhibitors in combination with corticosteroids, as noted earlier for pericarditis, in cases of acute severe valvulitis may result in significant improvement (see Figure 35–3, B–D). Also, in patients with Libman-Sacks–like vegetations, anticoagulation and anti-inflammatory therapy has resulted in improvement of valve masses and prevention of recurrent embolic events. Although no prospective trial data are available, prophylactic antiplatelet therapy may prevent cardioembolism in patients with valve nodules or thickening. Although the morbidity and mortality rates associated with valve surgery may be higher in patients with rheumatoid arthritis than in those without rheumatoid arthritis, mitral valve repair and mitral or aortic valve replacement or homograft root-and-valve replacement have been successfully performed in acute or chronic severe valve regurgitation.

3. Rheumatoid Myocarditis

▶ **General Considerations**

Rheumatoid myocarditis is observed in as much as 30% of patients in postmortem series but is rare in clinical and echocardiographic reports. Rheumatoid myocarditis is more common in patients with active and extra-articular disease, highly positive rheumatoid factor, and systemic vasculitis. Rheumatoid myocarditis may result from autoimmunity, vasculitis, or granulomata deposition; rarely, it is due to amyloid infiltration. Recently, a dilated or restrictive cardiomyopathy due to chloroquine therapy and characterized by myocyte enlargement due to perinuclear vacuolization and abundant myelinoid figures within myocytes has been reported. Unless granulomata are present, rheumatoid myocarditis is difficult to differentiate on histopathology from other types of myocarditis.

▶ Clinical Findings

The clinical presentation of rheumatoid myocarditis is similar to that for myocarditis from other causes. Most commonly, it is mild, asymptomatic, or overshadowed by other musculoskeletal disease manifestations and, therefore, often clinically unrecognized. When it is symptomatic, nonspecific symptoms of fatigue, dyspnea, palpitations, and chest pain may be present. The chest pain is usually pleuritic and probably reflects the presence of myopericarditis. Rarely, severe acute myocarditis with LV dysfunction may present as congestive heart failure or symptomatic atrial or ventricular arrhythmias.

A. Physical Examination

The cardiovascular exam is usually normal. In severe cases, fever and sinus tachycardia are common. First and second heart sounds are normal; a third or fourth heart sound may rarely be present. Functional systolic murmurs may be present. If myopericarditis is present, a pericardial rub may be detected.

B. Laboratory Findings

Myocarditis with LV diastolic or systolic dysfunction has been associated with the presence of anti-SS-A/anti-SS-B and anti-CCP autoantibodies. In the majority of cases, mild elevation of myocardial isoenzymes, such as troponin I, and less often of CPK-MB may be seen.

C. Diagnostic Studies

1. Electrocardiography—The ECG is often normal. When abnormal, the ECG shows nonspecific ST segment and T-wave abnormalities. AV conduction disturbances and atrial or ventricular ectopy can be detected. As a result of residual interstitial myocardial fibrosis, patients have higher dispersion of repolarization as manifested by prolongation of the uncorrected and corrected QT intervals.

2. Echocardiography—Recent series using pulse and tissue Doppler, transmitral color-flow propagation velocity, and myocardial performance index in young asymptomatic and nonhypertensive patients have demonstrated a high prevalence of diastolic dysfunction, predominantly of impaired relaxation. Also, longitudinal series have demonstrated a high incidence (40%) of clinical diastolic heart failure independent of traditional cardiovascular risk factors for diastolic dysfunction. Less commonly, echocardiography may show segmental wall motion abnormalities or diffuse LV contractile dysfunction and chamber dilatation in cases of severe myocarditis. The echocardiographic features of amyloidosis due to rheumatoid arthritis are nonspecific but may coexist or mimic rheumatoid constrictive pericarditis.

3. Radionuclide scanning—Scanning with indium-111, gallium-67, or technetium-99 may show focal patchy or diffuse myocardial uptake indicative of myocardial inflammation, necrosis, or both.

▶ Treatment & Prognosis

Limited data are available about the treatment of rheumatoid myocarditis. In-patient treatment with intravenous immunosuppressive therapy or tumor necrosis factor-α receptor blockers in combination with high-dose or pulse corticosteroids may be considered. This therapy may be continued orally on outpatient basis for several weeks and adjusted according to clinical course. Also, the incidence of new-onset heart failure in the setting of rheumatoid arthritis may decrease with tumor necrosis factor-α blocker therapy, although the use of these drugs in established heart failure may cause worsening or death, which is thus a contraindication to their use. Nonspecific therapy includes bed rest, analgesics, and cardiac monitoring for at least 48–72 hours. The natural history and prognosis of rheumatoid myocarditis are unknown.

4. Rheumatoid Coronary Artery Disease

▶ General Considerations

After controlling for traditional atherogenic risk factors, patients with rheumatoid arthritis have two to three times more epicardial and small-vessel CAD than matched controls. Except for aPL, the pathogenetic factors for these two types of CAD in rheumatoid patients are similar to those described for patients with SLE. Obstructive epicardial CAD is probably as common as abnormal coronary artery vasodilation or microvascular disease. Traditional atherogenic risk factors and Framingham and Reynolds scores underestimate the risk of CAD. Disease duration > 10 years, positive rheumatoid factor or anti-CCP antibody, and severe extra-articular manifestations are associated with arterial stiffness, are probably better predictors of carotid atherosclerosis and CAD, and predict a higher incidence of acute coronary syndromes. Patients older than 50 years are more prone to epicardial atherosclerotic CAD. About 66% of asymptomatic patients with established rheumatoid arthritis have coronary artery calcification on electron-beam CT, compared with 40% in those with recent onset or diagnosis of the disease. Mitral valve calcification on echocardiography is predictive of coronary artery calcification on CT, and a coronary calcification score > 100 on CT is predictive of future cardiovascular events (MI, congestive heart failure, stroke, and death). Patients with parameters of active and chronic inflammation have reduced small- and large-artery elasticity or associated plaques and have a twofold independent risk of MI, heart failure, stroke, and cardiovascular mortality compared with matched controls. Also, rheumatoid patients with acute coronary syndromes have a twofold higher recurrence rate of events and mortality than matched controls. Coronary

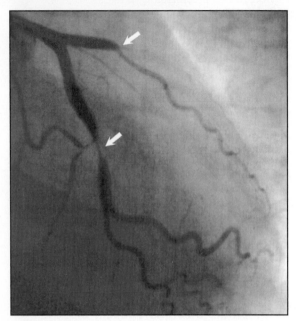

▲ **Figure 35–4.** Coronary arteritis complicated by a non–ST elevation myocardial infarction in a 47-year-old female with severely active rheumatoid arthritis. This left coronary artery angiogram demonstrates an occluded left anterior descending coronary artery (*upper arrow*) and a 90% stenosis of the circumflex artery (*lower arrow*). Successful stent placements on the anterior descending and circumflex arteries were performed. Since the patient also had associated severe aortic valvulitis (described in Figure 35–3, C and D) and clinical and serology data consistent with severely active rheumatoid arthritis, in addition to standard care for an acute coronary syndrome, the patient was also successfully treated with intravenous pulse corticosteroids and cyclophosphamide.

arteritis is rare and occurs in patients with rheumatoid nodules, overt vasculitis, rapidly progressive rheumatoid disease, and high titers of rheumatoid factor (Figure 35–4).

▶ Clinical Findings

A. Symptoms & Signs

Most patients with rheumatoid arthritis who have CAD are asymptomatic. Atherosclerotic CAD will manifest as chronic stable angina, unstable angina, or acute MI, whereas coronary arteritis is more commonly seen as unstable angina or acute MI.

Tachycardia, third or fourth heart sounds, and pulmonary rales, if LV failure is present, are seen during acute ischemic syndromes.

B. Diagnostic Studies

1. Electrocardiography—An ECG will show diagnostic Q waves indicative of previous MI, ST elevation or depression suggestive of epicardial or subendocardial ischemic injury, or T-wave inversion suggestive of ischemia.

2. Echocardiography—Resting and stress echocardiography are useful in the detection of wall motion abnormalities in those with obstructive CAD, but have decreased sensitivity for microvascular disease. Doppler TTE has also been used to assess coronary flow reserve in those with microvascular disease. During severe ischemia, echocardiography may show segmental wall motion abnormalities or myocardial scars if previous infarction has occurred. This technique will also determine the presence (or absence) of LV dysfunction and its severity.

3. Other tests—Patients with high ESR ($\geq$ 60 mm/h), C-reactive protein, serum amyloid, soluble vascular adhesion molecule-1, and interferon-γ have abnormal small- and large-artery vasodilatory response and are at increased risk for cardiovascular events and mortality. Electron-beam CT detects subclinical coronary artery calcification in patients with established disease.

Myocardial isoenzymes, such as troponin I (the most sensitive), CPK-MB, or LDH_1, may be elevated if myocardial necrosis has occurred. Exercise treadmill testing, with or without radionuclide scanning or echocardiography, can be used to detect suspected CAD. Coronary angiography should be considered when there is a high suspicion of CAD, an abnormal exercise treadmill test, or incapacitating symptoms. The diagnosis of coronary arteritis can be suspected if multiple stenotic lesions and aneurysmal lesions are found in the epicardial coronary arteries in a patient with severely active disease (see Figure 35–4).

▶ Treatment

In general, control of inflammation with tumor necrosis factor-α blockers, methotrexate therapy, and statins may reduce the development or progression of endothelial dysfunction, arterial stiffness, and premature atherosclerosis. Although experience in this area is limited, suspected severe and symptomatic coronary rheumatoid arteritis can initially be treated acutely with high doses of corticosteroids and, if refractory, with rituximab, plasmapheresis, or intravenous cyclophosphamide in conjunction with heparin, aspirin, nitrates, and calcium channel or β-blockers (see Figure 35–4). Limited data are available about PCIs in coronary arteritis, but if clinical circumstances allow it, it is reasonable to treat patients medically, and then reassess the need for PCI as the blood vessel may spontaneous heal and remodel. Symptomatic atherosclerotic CAD should be treated medically or with coronary revascularization as appropriate. Amelioration of inflammation with low-dose corticosteroids, tumor necrosis factor-α blockers, or statins may decrease the effects of vascular inflammation and dysfunction and consequently of coronary events. Furthermore, cyclooxygenase-2 selective inhibitors, which inhibit prostaglandin I-2 (a vasodilator and inhibitor of platelet aggregation), and NSAIDs increase the risk of acute coronary syndromes in rheumatoid patients. Finally, discontinuation of statin therapy may increase the risk of acute coronary syndromes.

5. Conduction Disturbances & Arrhythmias

▶ General Considerations

The prevalence and incidence of atrial arrhythmias, especially of atrial fibrillation, and consequently of stroke are 30% higher in rheumatoid arthritis patients than in matched controls. The prevalence of sinus or AV nodal or intraventricular conduction disturbances in patients with rheumatoid arthritis may not be different from that in age-matched controls in the general population. Possible mechanisms include premature CAD, acute inflammation of the sinus or AV node or His bundle (related to pancarditis), vasculitis of the arterioles supplying the conduction pathway, granulomata deposition in the conduction system, and amyloid infiltration.

▶ Clinical Findings

The mean age of patients with conduction disturbances is generally more than 60 years, and most of these patients have severe forms of rheumatoid arthritis with nodular disease, requiring chronic corticosteroid therapy. The conduction disturbances are generally mild, asymptomatic, and incidentally diagnosed by ECG.

A. Symptoms & Signs

In extremely rare cases, high-degree AV block may be evidenced with tiredness, dizziness, presyncope, or syncope. Although it is uncommon, complete AV block may be asymptomatic because the joint disease severely limits the patient's activity. Rarely, AV block is transient and can be reversed with anti-inflammatory therapy.

B. Diagnostic Studies

The best diagnostic methods are routine ECG, 24-hour or longer ECG monitoring, or both.

▶ Treatment

The treatment of severe and symptomatic high-degree AV or intraventricular blocks associated with acute myocarditis or valvulitis consists of temporary pacing and intravenous immunosuppressive therapy in combination with high-dose corticosteroids followed by chronic antirheumatoid therapy. Patients who are unresponsive to this therapy within 7–10 days should be considered for permanent pacemakers.

6. Rheumatoid Pulmonary Hypertension

▶ General Considerations

The causes of pulmonary hypertension with normal pulmonary venous pressure include serum hyperviscosity, interstitial fibrosis, obliterative bronchiolitis, and pulmonary vasculitis. Since patients with pulmonary arterial hypertension (defined as mean pulmonary artery pressure $\geq$ 25 mm Hg, pulmonary capillary wedge pressure or LV end-diastolic pressure $\leq$ 15 mm Hg, and a pulmonary vascular resistance of $\geq$ 240 dyn/cm^{-5} or $\geq$ 3 Wood units) have poor prognosis unless recognized and treated early with vasodilator therapy, it is essential to establish this diagnosis as accurately and as early as possible. The prevalence of these diseases is uncertain, but low. Since the mortality rate is high within 1 year of diagnosis, prompt diagnosis is vital. Lung biopsy or bronchoalveolar lavage may confirm pulmonary vasculitis and bronchiolitis obliterans, both of which are responsive to immunosuppressive therapy.

Severe pulmonary hypertension may lead to RV hypertrophy, enlargement, and diastolic followed by systolic dysfunction (cor pulmonale) and produce the symptoms and signs of right-sided heart failure.

▶ Clinical Findings

A. Symptoms & Signs

Dyspnea is a common manifestation of pulmonary hypertension and cor pulmonale. However, moderate pulmonary hypertension with or without mild cor pulmonale can be asymptomatic.

Findings on physical examination include a parasternal heave, split second heart sound with loud pulmonic component, tricuspid regurgitation, right-sided S_3 gallop, and rarely, hepatomegaly and edema.

B. Diagnostic Studies

1. Electrocardiography—An ECG may show right atrial and ventricular enlargement, right axis deviation, and/or right bundle branch block.

2. Color-flow Doppler echocardiography—This technique may show right atrial and ventricular enlargement, hypertrophy or dysfunction, tricuspid regurgitation, and evidence of high pulmonary artery systolic pressure. Pulmonary hypertension may not be accompanied by echocardiographic evidence of cor pulmonale, especially if the pulmonary artery pressure is less than 50 mm Hg. In controlled series of asymptomatic patients, the prevalence of pulmonary hypertension on echocardiography is five times higher in rheumatoid patients than in controls (21% versus 4%). Echocardiography can rule out left-sided heart disease as a cause of pulmonary hypertension. Echocardiography can also assess response to therapy.

3. Open-lung biopsy and bronchoalveolar lavage—These methods should be done if severe pulmonary vasculitis or bronchiolitis obliterans is suspected as the cause of pulmonary hypertension.

▶ Treatment & Prognosis

The treatment of pulmonary hypertension from pulmonary vasculitis or active inflammatory interstitial disease is intravenous immunosuppressive agents as noted previously in combination with high-dose corticosteroids, but the prognosis is poor, and most patients die within 1 year of diagnosis. However, the newer antirheumatoid therapies should be considered and may improve survival if the rheumatoid arthritis process can be controlled. The treatment of pulmonary arterial hypertension includes endothelin receptor antagonists, prostacyclins, and/or phosphodiesterase inhibitors.

Crowson CS, et al. Usefulness of risk scores to estimate the risk of cardiovascular disease in patients with rheumatoid arthritis. *Am J Cardiol.* 2012;110(3):420–4. [PMID: 22521305]

De Vera MA, et al. Statin discontinuation and risk of acute myocardial infarction in patients with rheumatoid arthritis: a population-based cohort study. *Ann Rheum Dis.* 2011;70(6):1020–4. [PMID: 21378405]

Evans MR, et al. Carotid atherosclerosis predicts incident acute coronary syndromes in rheumatoid arthritis. *Arthritis Rheum.* 2011;63(5):1211–20. [PMID: 21305526]

Kume K, et al. Tocilizumab monotherapy reduces arterial stiffness as effectively as etanercept or adalimumab monotherapy in rheumatoid arthritis: an open-label randomized controlled trial. *J Rheumatol.* 2011;38(10):2169–71. [PMID: 21807781]

Liang KP, et al. Increased prevalence of diastolic dysfunction in rheumatoid arthritis. *Ann Rheum Dis.* 2010;69(9):1665–70. [PMID: 20498217]

Lindhardsen J, et al. Risk of atrial fibrillation and stroke in rheumatoid arthritis: Danish nationwide cohort study. *BMJ.* 2012;344:e1257. [PMID: 22403267]

Roldan CA, et al. Characterization of valvular heart disease in rheumatoid arthritis by transesophageal echocardiography and clinical correlates. *Am J Cardiol.* 2007;100(3):496–502. [PMID: 17659935]

Targońska-Stepniak B, et al. The relationship between carotid intima-media thickness and the activity of rheumatoid arthritis. *J Clin Rheumatol.* 2011;17(5):249–55. [PMID: 21778898]

Westlake SL, et al. Tumour necrosis factor antagonists and the risk of cardiovascular disease in patients with rheumatoid arthritis: a systematic literature review. *Rheumatology (Oxford).* 2011;50(3):518–31. [PMID: 21071477]

SCLERODERMA

ESSENTIALS OF DIAGNOSIS

▶ Sclerotic skin, esophageal dysfunction, Raynaud phenomenon.

▶ Functional or structural small-vessel CAD.

▶ Multisegmental myocardial perfusion abnormalities.

▶ Diastolic heart failure.

▶ Pulmonary hypertension and cor pulmonale.

▶ General Considerations

Scleroderma, or systemic sclerosis, is a generalized disorder characterized by excessive accumulation of connective tissue; fibrosis; and degenerative changes of the skin, skeletal muscles, synovium, blood vessels, gastrointestinal tract, kidney, lung, and heart. Raynaud phenomenon, esophageal dysfunction, and sclerotic skin characterize the disease and are present in more than 90% of patients. The two major clinical variants are diffuse cutaneous (20% of cases) and limited cutaneous disease (80%). The less common diffuse type is characterized by skin thickening of the distal and proximal extremities and the trunk, with frequent involvement of the kidney, lung, or heart. In the more common limited type, which includes the CREST syndrome (calcinosis, Raynaud phenomenon, esophageal dysfunction, sclerodactyly, and telangiectasia), the skin changes are limited to the face, fingers, and distal portions of the extremities. A third, uncommon variant is the overlap syndrome, which includes scleroderma in association with other connective tissue disease.

The incidence of scleroderma is 10–20 per million population per year. The disease affects all races, is three times more common in women than in men, and usually occurs between the ages of 30 and 50 years. The diffuse cutaneous type has a poorer prognosis than does the limited type. The overall cumulative survival rates after 3, 6, and 9 years are 86%, 76%, and 61%, respectively. The prognosis is worst for males who are older than 50 years with lung, heart, or kidney disease. Pulmonary disease, including pulmonary hypertension and interstitial lung disease, and heart diseases are the major causes of death; these are followed by kidney disease, with a cumulative survival of only 20% at 7 years. The major causes of cardiac death are structural and functional microvascular ischemic heart disease, followed by refractory heart failure, sudden death, pulmonary hypertension, and pericarditis. Scleroderma cardiac disease manifests predominantly as microvascular CAD, myocarditis, and pulmonary hypertension with or without cor pulmonale. Pericarditis, conduction disturbances, and arrhythmias are less common. Clinically overt scleroderma heart disease is reported in less than one-fourth of patients; the rate rises to as high as 80% in autopsy series. Scleroderma heart disease is generally less common and less severe in the limited type than in the diffuse type.

1. Coronary Artery Disease

▶ Pathophysiology

Patients with scleroderma alone, independently of traditional atherogenic risk factors, have three times higher risk of developing CAD. In scleroderma, the intramyocardial coronary arteries and arterioles are affected by abnormally increased small-vessel vasoconstriction due to an immune-mediated endothelial cell injury and increased production of platelet-derived growth factor impairing the endothelial response to vasodilation. The intramyocardial coronary arteries and arterioles are also affected by mast cell degranulation of histamine, prostaglandin D_2, and leukotrienes C_4 and D_4, leading to coronary vasoconstriction. Also, obstructive microvascular disease occurs due to immune complex–mediated intimal inflammation, fibrinoid necrosis, stimulation of fibroblasts, collagen deposition, and ultimately vessel thrombosis. In contrast, the prevalence of epicardial atherosclerotic disease in patients with scleroderma is probably similar to that of a general population. The common finding on autopsy of myocardial contraction-band necrosis (necrotic myocardial cells with dense eosinophilic bands) is likely related to intermittent intramyocardial coronary spasm or intramyocardial Raynaud phenomenon. Furthermore, almost all patients with evidence of intramyocardial CAD have peripheral Raynaud phenomenon.

▶ Clinical Findings

A. Symptoms & Signs

Chest pain is uncommon; when present, it is related more commonly to pericarditis or esophageal reflux than to myocardial ischemia. Most patients, even with resting or stress-induced myocardial perfusion imaging defects or wall motion abnormalities, are asymptomatic. Although intramyocardial coronary vasospasm is the rule, severe vasospasm of the epicardial coronary arteries leading to transmural MI has rarely been reported.

B. Diagnostic Studies

1. Electrocardiographic exercise testing—This method has limited sensitivity because the prevalence of epicardial CAD in patients with scleroderma is low.

2. Radionuclide studies—Resting or exercise-induced multisegmental perfusion abnormalities are common; they are frequently reversed or improved with nifedipine or dipyridamole, which suggests recurrent vasospastic episodes leading to myocardial ischemia or fibrosis. Cold-induced reversible or partially reversible myocardial perfusion defects further support coronary vasospasm. On myocardial perfusion, most patients show fixed defects and some show reversible defects or both fixed and reversible defects (Figure 35–5). Most patients have normal LV function at rest despite the high frequency of perfusion defects, but almost half have an abnormal LV response (a failure to increase the ejection fraction > 5% from baseline) during exercise radionuclide ventriculography.

3. Echocardiography—Due to the predominant involvement of the intramyocardial coronary arteries, echocardiographic findings typical of transmural MI are uncommon. Using contrast-enhanced pulsed wave Doppler TTE in a series of 27 patients without clinical evidence of ischemic heart disease, reduction in coronary flow reserve (≤ 2.5) in the left anterior descending coronary artery during adenosine infusion was detected in 52% of patients, compared with 4% of matched controls. Reduction in coronary flow reserve is more common in the diffuse form of scleroderma and is related to the duration and severity of the disease. As a result of functional and, later on, of obliterative microvascular disease, LV and RV diastolic and uncommonly systolic dysfunction can occur. Occasionally, a transmural MI due to epicardial coronary vasospasm can occur, and its echocardiographic diagnosis relies on the same findings as those of atherosclerotic disease. The cold pressor test with simultaneous echocardiography demonstrates transient wall motion abnormalities in patients with angiographically normal or mild epicardial CAD.

4. Coronary angiography—This diagnostic study usually shows normal epicardial coronary arteries, a slow dye flow indicative of increased intramyocardial coronary resistance, and impaired coronary sinus blood flow indicative of abnormal coronary flow reserve.

▶ Treatment

Nifedipine and nicardipine have demonstrated short- and long-term improvement in the frequency and severity of angina and perfusion defects. Nitrates and captopril have shown similar beneficial effects. If coronary vasculitis is suspected, intravenous cyclophosphamide is used. Rituximab may be a salvage therapy that can be considered.

2. Myocarditis

▶ General Considerations

Two types of scleroderma myocardial disease are described. The most common is due to recurrent intramyocardial ischemia leading to fibrosis; the second and less common is an acute inflammatory myocarditis. Patients with scleroderma who have skeletal myopathy have twice the prevalence of myocardial disease, compared with patients without peripheral myopathy. Myocardial disease is also more common and severe in patients with diffuse cutaneous disease, anti-Scl70 antibodies, CAD, and who are older than 60 years.

Clinically apparent myocarditis is rare, but postmortem series report a high prevalence. Focal or diffuse myocardial fibrosis and contraction-band necrosis are common. Contraction-band necrosis typical of transient coronary occlusion and reperfusion is common but not pathognomonic. These pathologic findings differ from atherosclerotic myocardial disease by their lack of relation to coronary arteries and frequent involvement of the RV and subendocardium.

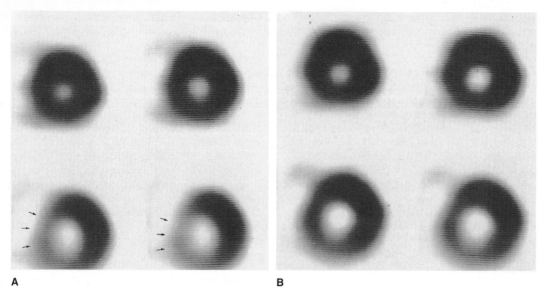

A　　　　　　　　　　　　　　　　　　　**B**

▲ **Figure 35–5.** Intramural coronary artery disease in a patient with scleroderma. **A:** This short axis postexercise perfusion scan of the left ventricle shows septal and inferoseptal wall ischemia (*small arrows*) that resolves on the resting images. **B:** This patient had normal epicardial coronary arteries.

▶ Clinical Findings

A. Symptoms & Signs

Focal or diffuse myocardial fibrotic disease may result in significant LV diastolic or systolic dysfunction, arrhythmias, and conduction disturbances. Patients with skeletal myopathy and those with myocarditis more commonly have clinical heart failure. Insidious symptoms are most common, and the physical findings of heart failure are similar to those of other conditions. Acute symptoms of heart failure and sudden death rarely occur.

B. Diagnostic Studies

If clinical or laboratory evidence of myositis is present, diagnostic screening for asymptomatic cardiac involvement with myocardial isoenzymes is warranted.

1. Electrocardiography—A septal infarction pattern is seen in some patients, correlating with septal or anteroseptal thallium perfusion abnormalities, despite the presence of normal epicardial coronary arteries. This may represent septal fibrosis.

2. Echocardiography—LV systolic dysfunction is uncommon in asymptomatic patients, but when associated with heart failure, it portends an 80% mortality rate at 1 year. In contrast, a high prevalence (30–50%) of LV diastolic dysfunction is seen in patients with either diffuse or limited cutaneous disease, compared with < 10% in controls.

Similarly, a high prevalence (40%) of RV diastolic dysfunction independently of pulmonary hypertension has been reported. LV diastolic dysfunction correlates with high levels of soluble vascular cell adhesion molecule-1 and ESR as well as the duration and severity of Raynaud phenomenon. Also, RV dysfunction in patients with normal pulmonary artery pressure improves with nicardipine therapy. These data support functional microvascular CAD as the cause of diastolic dysfunction. However, a decreased and heterogeneous integrated backscatter in the subendocardium by ultrasonic video densitometry in young, nonhypertensive patients supports interstitial collagen deposition and fibrosis as another cause of myocardial dysfunction.

3. Radionuclide studies—Radionuclide angiography demonstrates abnormal resting ejection fraction in 15% of patients. Myocardial perfusion scanning is a sensitive method for diagnosis and follow-up of the myocardial disease and for assessing therapeutic responses.

4. Magnetic resonance imaging—This technique can accurately detect myocardial inflammation, perfusion defects or ischemia, infarction or fibrosis, and aneurysms of the coronary arteries.

5. Endomyocardial biopsy—This technique has been used occasionally to diagnose scleroderma myocardial disease; however, the heterogenous and nonspecific pattern of involvement limits the sensitivity and specificity of this technique.

► Treatment

Calcium channel blockers may abolish or decrease the frequency and severity of episodes of ischemia and thereby of myocardial fibrosis, but this hypothesis has not been longitudinally tested. Although the use of intravenous immunosuppressive therapy (especially cyclophosphamide) and/or methylprednisolone in acute inflammatory myocarditis may be beneficial, supportive data are limited. Prednisone 30 mg and above has been associated with acute scleroderma renal crisis; thus, generally, if prednisone or methylprednisolone is used, the dose should be restricted to ≤ 25 mg. Recently, rituximab has been used for chronic scleroderma conditions, including myocarditis, with some success in case reports. Otherwise, symptomatic LV systolic or diastolic dysfunction is treated with current standard therapy.

► Prognosis

The presence of an S_3 gallop is indicative of LV systolic dysfunction and increases the risk of death by more than 500%. Patients with heart failure have a 100% mortality rate at 7 years, with the highest number (80%) occurring during the first year after diagnosis.

3. Conduction Disturbances & Arrhythmias

► General Considerations

Conduction defects occur in up to 20% of patients with scleroderma; the highest prevalence is seen in those patients with demonstrated myocarditis or myocardial perfusion defects. Fibrous replacement of the sinoatrial and AV nodes, bundle branches, and surrounding myocardium is seen on postmortem series of patients with conduction disturbances.

► Clinical Findings

A. Symptoms & Signs

Arrhythmias are common and frequently associated with active myocarditis. Atrial or ventricular premature contractions, supraventricular tachycardias, and nonsustained ventricular tachycardia are also common. Ventricular and supraventricular arrhythmias are more common in patients with diffuse cutaneous disease than in those with the limited type. Palpitations occur in 50% of patients. Syncope (Stokes-Adams attacks) can occur and is related to either high-degree AV block or ventricular arrhythmias; it may occasionally be the primary manifestation of scleroderma. Syncope can also occur in patients with severe pulmonary hypertension. Forty percent to 60% of cardiac deaths in patients with scleroderma who have active myocarditis may be sudden and related to ventricular arrhythmias.

B. Diagnostic Studies

1. Electrocardiography—Most patients have a normal ECG, which is highly predictive of normal LV function. The presence of left or right bundle branch block or bifascicular block generally correlates with resting or exercise-induced LV systolic dysfunction. Also, LV potentials on signal-averaged ECG, complex atrial and ventricular arrhythmias, or conduction abnormalities on ECG are common and correlate with LV dysfunction or myocardial perfusion defects.

2. Electrophysiologic studies—These studies show a high prevalence of abnormal sinoatrial and AV nodes and His-Purkinje function and conduction. However, electrophysiologic studies are recommended only for patients with syncope of undefined origin, for those with sustained ventricular tachycardia, or for survivors of sudden cardiac death.

► Treatment

A pacemaker is indicated for symptomatic high-grade conduction disturbances, and antiarrhythmic or implantable cardioverter-defibrillator therapy is appropriate for symptomatic ventricular arrhythmias.

► Prognosis

The presence on ambulatory ECG of frequent ventricular and supraventricular arrhythmias predicts a mortality risk two to six times higher than that of patients without arrhythmias. Because these arrhythmias are strong independent predictors of sudden cardiac death, 24-hour ambulatory ECG monitoring should be considered in patients with scleroderma to identify patients at high risk for sudden cardiac death. Cardiac conduction defects on the resting ECG also indicate a poor prognosis with a mortality rate of 50% by 6 years following diagnosis.

4. Pericarditis

► General Considerations

The pathogenesis of scleroderma pericardial disease is unknown and is usually clinically silent. A low clinical prevalence of pericardial disease contrasts with that of postmortem and echocardiographic series (~50%). Fibrinous pericarditis, chronic fibrous pericarditis, pericardial adhesions, and pericardial effusion are the pathologic types described.

► Clinical Findings

A. Symptoms & Signs

Pericardial disease is rarely the initial manifestation of scleroderma. Symptomatic pericardial disease occurs in less than 20% of patients. The most common clinical presentation is a chronic pericardial effusion with dyspnea, orthopnea, and edema; it is less frequently seen as an acute pericarditis with fever, pleuritic chest pain, dyspnea, and pericardial rub. Cardiac tamponade or pericardial constriction is rare. Symptomatic pericardial disease is two to four times more common in patients with the diffuse form of scleroderma than in those with the limited cutaneous form of the disease.

B. Diagnostic Studies

1. Echocardiography—Echocardiography commonly shows asymptomatic small pericardial effusions and uncommonly pericardial thickening. It can also confirm clinically suspected cardiac tamponade.

2. Computed tomography and magnetic resonance imaging—These imaging studies are important diagnostic adjuncts to echocardiography. They aid in the assessment of pericardial thickening or calcification in patients with suspected chronic constriction.

3. Other tests—Pericardial fluid aspirates are usually exudative without autoantibodies, immune complexes, or complement depletion. Antiphospholipid antibodies may be associated with pericardial disease.

▶ Treatment

Symptomatic pericarditis or significant pericardial effusions can be treated with NSAIDs. The role of immunosuppressive therapy and/or pulse corticosteroid therapy is less defined in these patients, and as noted earlier, if prednisone ≥ 30 mg is used, the risk of scleroderma renal crisis markedly increases. If tamponade is suspected, pericardiocentesis is usually successful. Corticosteroids alone are not effective in patients with large, chronic pericardial effusions.

▶ Prognosis

Patients with pericarditis and moderate pericardial effusion have a cumulative survival of only 25% after 6–7 years, with the highest mortality rates the first year after diagnosis. This high mortality rate is believed to be related to complicating or accompanying progressive renal failure in patients with chronic pericardial effusions and to sudden death in those with associated acute myopericarditis or myocarditis.

5. Valvular Heart Disease

The true prevalence of valvular heart disease in patients with scleroderma is unknown, but it is rarely recognized clinically. Postmortem series report a prevalence of up to 18%. Rarely, systemic embolism in association with echocardiographically defined noninfective mitral valve vegetations, similar to those of SLE, has been described. One echocardiographic series reported a 67% frequency of mitral regurgitation in scleroderma patients, compared with only 15% in controls. Nonspecific thickening of the mitral or aortic valves without significant regurgitation also can be seen. In addition, a disproportionately high clinical and echocardiographic prevalence of mitral valve prolapse has been described in patients with either diffuse or limited scleroderma.

6. Secondary Scleroderma Heart Disease

Secondary causes of scleroderma heart disease are related to pulmonary and systemic hypertension. Pulmonary fibrosis can occur in up to 80% and pulmonary hypertension with cor pulmonale in up to 40–50% of patients. Pulmonary arterial hypertension secondary to inflammatory vasculopathy or pulmonary vasospasm is less common, is more commonly associated with the limited cutaneous type and overlap syndrome, and portends good prognosis when responsive to vasodilator therapy. Abnormal pulmonary function tests, abnormal lung uptake of gallium and technetium-99m sestamibi, and radiographic abnormalities often precede cor pulmonale on echocardiography (Figure 35–6). In patients with pulmonary hypertension, a higher prevalence and severity of RV diastolic dysfunction independently of age and LV mass has been reported. An RV tissue Doppler E velocity of < 0.11 m/s selects patients with pulmonary artery pressure > 35 mm Hg. Patients with pulmonary hypertension of ≥ 36 mm Hg have decreased survival rates of 81%, 63%, and 56% at 1, 2, and 3 years, respectively, from the diagnosis.

In patients with pulmonary arterial hypertension, endothelin receptor antagonists, prostacyclins, and/or phosphodiesterase inhibitors should be considered. Oxygen, calcium channel blockers, and angiotensin-converting enzyme inhibitors may provide additional long-term benefits in these patients, but randomized controlled data are limited. Selected patients with severe scleroderma-related lung disease can undergo lung transplantation with similar morbidity and mortality to that of patients without scleroderma. Recently, in patients with active inflammatory interstitial lung disease, rituximab has been used in individual cases with some success.

Hypertension and hypertensive heart disease are generally related to renovascular disease. The prognosis is related to the severity of the heart disease.

Bernardo P, et al. Implantable cardioverter defibrillator prevents sudden cardiac death in systemic sclerosis. *J Rheumatol.* 2011; 38(8):1617–21. [PMID: 21632680]

Desai CS, et al. Systemic sclerosis and the heart: current diagnosis and management. *Curr Opin Rheumatol.* 2011;23(6):545–54. [PMID: 21897256]

Hinchcliff M, et al. Prevalence, prognosis, and factors associated with left ventricular diastolic dysfunction in systemic sclerosis. *Clin Exp Rheumatol.* 2012;30(2 Suppl 71):S30–7. [PMID: 22338601]

Kahan A, et al. Cardiac complications of systemic sclerosis. *Rheumatology (Oxford).* 2009;48(Suppl 3):iii45–8. [PMID: 19487224]

Kiatchoosakun S, et al. Right ventricular systolic pressure assessed by echocardiography: a predictive factor of mortality in patients with scleroderma. *Clin Cardiol.* 2011;34(8):488–93. [PMID: 21717471]

Mok MY, et al. Systemic sclerosis is an independent risk factor for increased coronary artery calcium deposition. *Arthritis Rheum.* 2011;63(5):1387–95. [PMID: 21538320]

Tyndall AJ, et al. Causes and risk factors for death in systemic sclerosis: a study from the EULAR Scleroderma Trials and Research

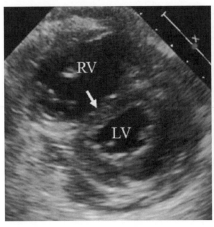
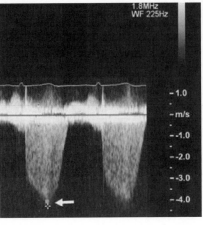
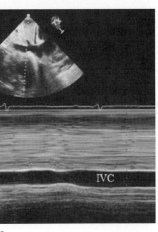

A   B   C

▲ **Figure 35–6.** A 48-year-old female with scleroderma and CREST syndrome and severe pulmonary hypertension, cor pulmonale, and right-sided heart failure due to severe interstitial lung disease. **A:** This parasternal transthoracic echocardiographic (TTE) short axis view demonstrates severe right ventricular (RV) dilatation and systolic dysfunction with associated abnormal interventricular septal motion of pressure and volume overload (flattening or inversion of the septum during late systole and early diastole and during mid to late diastole, respectively) (*arrow*). LV, left ventricle. **B:** Continuous wave Doppler shows a tricuspid regurgitation peak velocity of 4.1 m/s, equivalent to an RV systolic pressure of 67 mm Hg. **C:** Dilated inferior vena cava (IVC) with minimal diameter change with a sniff indicating a right atrial pressure of ≥ 15 mm Hg. Therefore, this patient's estimated pulmonary artery systolic pressure is 67 + 15 mm Hg = 82 mm Hg, which is consistent with severe pulmonary hypertension.

(EUSTAR) database. *Ann Rheum Dis.* 2010;69(10):1809–15. [PMID:20551155]

Yiu KH, et al. Left ventricular dysfunction assessed by speckle-tracking strain analysis in patients with systemic sclerosis: relationship to functional capacity and ventricular arrhythmias. *Arthritis Rheum.* 2011;63(12):3969–78. [PMID: 22127711]

Zöller B, et al. Risk of subsequent coronary heart disease in patients hospitalized for immune-mediated diseases: a nationwide follow-up study from Sweden. *PLoS One.* 2012;7(3):e33442. [PMID: 22438933]

ANKYLOSING SPONDYLITIS

ESSENTIALS OF DIAGNOSIS

▶ Characteristic lumbar spine and sacroiliac arthritis.

▶ Positive HLA-B27 assay.

▶ Aortic root sclerosis and dilation, leaflet thickening, and subaortic bump on echocardiography.

▶ Aortic regurgitation.

▶ General Considerations

Ankylosing spondylitis, also known as Marie-Strümpell or Bekhterev disease, is an inflammatory disorder that affects predominantly the vertebral and sacroiliac joints. It manifests itself as chronic low back pain and limitation of back motion and chest expansion. Less frequently, it affects the peripheral joints and extra-articular organs such as the heart. The disease is estimated to affect 1 in 2000 of the general population, predominantly white men less than 40 years old; the male-to-female ratio is 3–12:1. More than 90% of patients are positive for the histocompatibility antigen HLA-B27. Although the manifestations of the cardiovascular disease generally follow the arthritic syndrome by 10–20 years, they sometimes precede it. The most important cardiovascular manifestations of the disease are aortitis, with or without aortic regurgitation; conduction disturbances; mitral regurgitation; myocardial dysfunction; and pericardial disease. The clinical prevalence of cardiovascular disease in ankylosing spondylitis varies widely. The rates are higher in patients with more than 20 years of disease duration, in those who are older than age 50, and in those with peripheral articular involvement.

1. Aortitis & Aortic Regurgitation

▶ General Considerations

The pathogenesis of aortitis is still undefined. Increased platelet-aggregating activity and platelet-derived growth factor are believed to be pathogenetic factors in the characteristic proliferative endarteritis of aortic root disease. The inflammatory process also is mediated by plasma cells and lymphocytes. It occurs in the intima, media, and adventitia of the proximal aortic wall and sinus of Valsalva and results in a marked fibroblastic reparative response, fibrous thickening, and calcification, especially of the adventitia and intima. This process extends proximally to the aortic annulus, valve cusps, and adjacent commissures. The consequent dilatation and thickening of the aortic root and annulus and the thickening or retraction of the aortic valve cusps cause aortic regurgitation generally of mild to moderate degree. Severe aortic regurgitation is rare. The mitral valve is frequently involved by downward extension of the aortic root fibrosis into the intervalvular fibrosa and base of the anterior mitral leaflet. This often results in localized fibrotic thickening at the base of the anterior mitral leaflet forming the characteristic "subaortic bump."

▶ Clinical Findings

The most common and characteristic manifestation of ankylosing spondylitis–associated heart disease is proximal aortitis, with or without aortic regurgitation. Associated mitral valve disease is also common. Aortitis and aortic regurgitation are generally mild to moderate, clinically silent, and chronic. In rare cases, severe aortic regurgitation from severe acute or chronic aortitis or valvulitis or complicating infective endocarditis occurs. Clinically silent aortic root or valve disease, with or without aortic regurgitation, can be present in one-third of patients before the joint disease manifests itself. Although it happens rarely, severe aortic regurgitation may present with mild or no articular disease.

A. Physical Examination

The most common and salient clinical findings in patients with ankylosing spondylitis will be those of the articular disease because cardiac disease, when present, is generally mild to moderate and asymptomatic.

B. Diagnostic Studies

1. Chest radiography—The appearance of the cardiac silhouette and great vessels is usually normal. If severe aortic root disease or aortic regurgitation is present, the ascending aorta may appear dilatated or elongated, and LV and atrial enlargement may be noted.

2. Color-flow Doppler echocardiography—By TEE, aortic root thickening, increased stiffness, and dilatation are seen in 60%, 60%, and 25% of patients, respectively. Aortic valve thickening detected in 40% of patients is manifested mainly as nodularities of the aortic cusps. Mitral valve thickening seen in 30% of patients manifests predominantly as basal thickening of the anterior mitral leaflet, forming the characteristic "subaortic bump" (Figure 35–7).

Valve regurgitation seen in almost 50% of patients is moderate in one-third of them. Aortic root disease and valve

disease are related to the duration of ankylosing spondylitis but not to its activity, severity, or therapy. Associated LV enlargement, hypertrophy, and systolic or diastolic function can also be assessed.

3. Radionuclide ventriculography—This method can assess LV systolic or diastolic function and LV enlargement.

▶ Treatment

A. Medical Therapy

1. Specific anti-inflammatory therapy—Although limited data are available, immunosuppressives and corticosteroids should be considered in acute aortitis and valvulitis associated with ankylosing spondylitis. Corticosteroids, methotrexate, sulfasalazine, and especially tumor necrosis factor-α blockers have been used with some success.

2. Other therapy—Vasodilators can be used in patients with significant aortic regurgitation.

B. Surgical Therapy

Aortic valve replacement has been successfully performed in patients with severe and symptomatic aortic regurgitation.

2. Conduction Disturbances

Conduction disturbances occur in 30–35% of patients and are the second most common associated heart disease, although their pathogenesis is unknown. Although the prevalence of HLA-B27 is increased in patients with ankylosing spondylitis who have implanted pacemakers for heart block, it may be absent in these patients. Furthermore, because HLA-B27 may be present in 6% of normal patients, it cannot be implicated as a primary pathogenetic factor in ankylosing spondylitis–associated conduction disturbances. Conduction disturbances can be the result of the subaortic fibrotic process extending to the basilar septum, leading to destruction or dysfunction of the AV node, the proximal portion of the bundle of His, bundle branches, and fascicles. In fact, echocardiographic studies have demonstrated an association of conduction disturbances with aortic root thickening and subaortic bump.

▶ Clinical Findings

The prevalence of conduction disturbances varies greatly, but is at least 20%. AV blocks (first, second, and, rarely, third degree) are most frequent, followed by sinus node dysfunction (sinus arrhythmias, sinoatrial block, sinus arrest, and sick sinus syndrome) and bundle branch or fascicular block.

Patients with conduction disturbances are generally asymptomatic, and disturbances can be detected before clinically manifested in less than one-fifth of patients. The conduction disturbances can occasionally be transient, and symptomatic patients can be treated with temporary pacing.

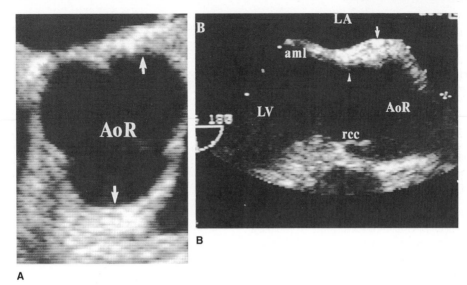

▲ **Figure 35–7.** Aortic root and valve disease in a patient with ankylosing spondylitis. **A:** This transesophageal basilar short axis view shows marked aortic root thickening, predominantly of the posterolateral and anteromedial walls (*arrows*). Mild aortic root dilation is present. **B:** Transesophageal basilar longitudinal close-up view of the aortic root also shows the marked thickening of the posterior wall (*arrow*) extending to the basilar portion of the anterior mitral leaflet (subaortic bump; *arrowhead*). Mild localized thickening of the right coronary cusp tip is noted. Moderately severe aortic regurgitation was detected on color-flow mapping. The distance between the dots at the edge of the image is 1 cm. aml, anterior mitral leaflet; AoR, aortic root; LA, left atrium; LV, left ventricle; rcc, right coronary cusp.

The prevalence of aortic root disease and valve regurgitation is high in the presence of conduction disturbances, in contrast to the small number of cases of aortic regurgitation in patients without conduction disturbances. Occasionally, severe conduction disturbances associated with symptoms requiring cardiac pacing may precede the diagnosis of ankylosing spondylitis. Therefore, unrecognized ankylosing spondylitis should be considered in patients with unexplained conduction disturbances or aortic regurgitation.

A. Physical Examination

Severe bradyarrhythmias will be clinically detected if patients are symptomatic; otherwise, conduction disturbances are generally incidentally detected with ECG.

B. Diagnostic Studies

ECG, including 24-hour ambulatory and event monitoring, can detect the described conduction disturbances.

▶ Treatment

A. Specific Anti-inflammatory Therapy

The role of anti-inflammatory therapy in patients with conduction disturbances is undefined, but a trial of high-dose prednisone to determine reversibility is indicated before permanent pacing is considered.

B. Other Therapy

Permanent pacing has been successfully performed. The most common indications for pacing are complete heart block and sick sinus syndrome.

3. Mitral Valve Disease

The prevalence of mitral valve disease is about 30%, but it is generally not significant and therefore frequently unrecognized. Mitral valve disease is generally asymptomatic and frequently incidentally detected by echocardiography. The pathogenesis of mitral valve disease is related to the extension of the aortic root fibrosis into the subaortic basilar portion of the anterior mitral leaflet, producing the characteristic subaortic bump. Mitral regurgitation results from either the decreased anterior leaflet mobility caused by the basilar subaortic bump or, less frequently, from LV dilatation caused by aortic regurgitation. Only a few cases of mitral regurgitation severe enough to require valve replacement have been reported.

4. Myocardial Disease, Coronary Artery Disease, Pericardial Disease, & Bacterial Endocarditis

Primary myocardial disease is rare. Although its pathogenesis is unknown, it is caused by a diffuse increase in the myocardial interstitial connective tissue and reticulum fibers.

It may manifest as LV systolic dysfunction and dilatation in up to one-fifth of patients. Doppler echocardiography series in patients younger than 50 years old with no clinical heart disease have uncommonly reported LV systolic dysfunction. In contrast, about one-third of patients have diastolic dysfunction, predominantly impaired relaxation. Diastolic dysfunction is unrelated to age, disease duration, or disease activity. Rarely, cardiac amyloidosis with diastolic heart failure has been reported. Rarely, secondary myocardial dysfunction relates to chronic volume overload of aortic or mitral regurgitation. If significant LV systolic or diastolic dysfunction is present, third or fourth heart sounds and pulmonary rales may be present. Echocardiography is the best diagnostic method to show primary or secondary LV dysfunction. Patients with ankylosing spondylitis have at least a twofold increase in CAD and systemic hypertension than matched controls. Although in general no specific therapy for primary myocardial disease has been defined, immunosuppressive and/or high-dose corticosteroid therapy may be considered in those with primary myocarditis if acute, and methotrexate or sulfasalazine chronically. Since tumor necrosis factor-α blockers can exacerbate congestive heart failure, only patients with normal LV systolic function should be treated with these agents.

Although the true prevalence of **pericardial disease** is unknown, it is rare in ankylosing spondylitis, and its pathogenesis is also undefined. It is generally asymptomatic and usually incidentally detected by echocardiography as pericardial thickening or small pericardial effusions. No specific therapy is available.

▶ Prognosis

The overall prognosis of patients with ankylosing spondylitis is good and almost comparable to that of a general population. In the past, the presence of severe cardiovascular disease significantly decreased the survival of these patients. Currently, improved diagnostic and therapeutic technologies have allowed early diagnosis, appropriate follow-up, and proper timing of valve replacement or pacemaker implantation in patients with cardiovascular disease. These factors have made the prognosis of ankylosing spondylitis with cardiovascular disease more benign.

Bremander A, et al. Population-based estimates of common comorbidities and cardiovascular disease in ankylosing spondylitis. *Arthritis Care Res (Hoboken)*. 2011;63(4):550–6. [PMID: 21452267]

Caliskan M, et al. Impaired coronary microvascular and left ventricular diastolic functions in patients with ankylosing spondylitis. *Atherosclerosis*. 2008;196(1):306–12. [PMID: 17169363]

Dik VK, et al. The relationship between disease-related characteristics and conduction disturbances in ankylosing spondylitis. *Scand J Rheumatol*. 2010;39(1):38–41. [PMID: 20132069]

El Maghraoui A. Extra-articular manifestations of ankylosing spondylitis: prevalence, characteristics and therapeutic implications. *Eur J Intern Med*. 2011;22(6):554–60. [PMID: 22075279]

Looi JL, et al. Valvulitis and aortitis associated with ankylosing spondylitis: early detection and monitoring response to therapy

using cardiac magnetic resonance imaging. *Int J Rheum Dis*. 2011;14(4):e56–8. [PMID: 22004242]

Luckie M, et al. Severe mitral and aortic regurgitation in association with ankylosing spondylitis. *Echocardiography*. 2009; 26(6):705–10. [PMID: 19594817131]

Okan T, et al. Ventricular diastolic function of ankylosing spondylitis patients by using conventional pulsed wave Doppler, myocardial performance index and tissue Doppler imaging. *Echocardiography*. 2008;25(1):47–56. [PMID: 18271873]

Palazzi C, et al. Aortitis and periaortitis in ankylosing spondylitis. *Joint Bone Spine*. 2011;78(5):451–5. [PMID: 21185758]

Peters MJ, et al. Ankylosing spondylitis: a risk factor for myocardial infarction? *Ann Rheum Dis*. 2010;69(3):579–81. [PMID: 19403516]

POLYMYOSITIS/DERMATOMYOSITIS

ESSENTIALS OF DIAGNOSIS

- ▶ Muscle weakness, characteristic skin lesions.
- ▶ Myocarditis and arrhythmias or conduction disturbances.
- ▶ Pericarditis, coronary arteritis, and valve disease.

▶ General Considerations

Polymyositis or dermatomyositis is an acquired, chronic, inflammatory myopathy that presents clinically as symmetric proximal muscle weakness of the extremities, trunk, and neck. Dermatomyositis differs from polymyositis by the presence of a rash on the face, neck, chest, and extremities, most commonly over the extensor surfaces, especially the dorsum of the hands and fingers. The incidence of polymyositis and dermatomyositis is estimated to be one to five new cases per million population per year in the United States. Overlap syndrome is the association of polymyositis/dermatomyositis with other connective tissue diseases, such as scleroderma, SLE, and rheumatoid arthritis. Rarely, polymyositis or dermatomyositis can be associated with the aPL syndrome. Adults in the fourth to sixth decades are most commonly affected. Both childhood polymyositis/dermatomyositis and that with malignancy are less common. Females, especially black females, are predominantly affected. A cumulative survival rate of 50–75% after 6–8 years has been reported. The major causes of death (in descending order) are malignancy, sepsis, and cardiovascular disease. Poor prognostic indicators of the disease include an age older than 45 years, cardiopulmonary disease, and cutaneous necrotic lesions.

▶ Clinical Findings

Polymyositis/dermatomyositis–associated heart disease is not uncommon and is manifested predominantly as myocarditis, leading more commonly (25–40%) to subclinical or clinical LV diastolic dysfunction and less often to LV systolic dysfunction and arrhythmias or conduction disturbances (25–30%). Dilated cardiomyopathy, pericarditis, coronary vasculitis, pulmonary hypertension with cor pulmonale, mitral valve prolapse, and hyperkinetic heart syndrome have also been reported. Clinically overt heart disease is less common than that found in postmortem series. Clinical heart disease is more common in polymyositis and overlap syndrome than in dermatomyositis or in malignant and childhood polymyositis/dermatomyositis. The presence of heart disease does not correlate with age or disease activity, severity, or duration and does not differ between men and women.

1. Myocarditis

Myocarditis is characterized at postmortem by diffuse interstitial and perivascular lymphocytic infiltration, contraction-band necrosis, and fibrosis. In one postmortem series, myocarditis was seen in half the patients, manifested equally as active myocarditis or focal myocardial fibrosis. Approximately 10% of them have dilated cardiomyopathy. Acute myocarditis as the principal manifestation of polymyositis has been reported in several cases presenting as a mimicker of acute MI, fatal cardiac arrhythmias, or heart failure. A high correlation has been demonstrated between myocarditis and active myositis. About half of patients with peripheral myositis, as indicated by uptake of technetium-99m pyrophosphate, also have myocardial uptake. Increased myocardial uptake is also frequently associated with depressed ejection fraction and abnormal wall motion (shown by radionuclide ventriculography or echocardiography), which is further supportive of myocardial inflammation. Myocarditis may manifest itself clinically as congestive heart failure or as dilated cardiomyopathy. However, recent small series using cardiac MRI in asymptomatic patients have shown late gadolinium-enhanced patchy epicardial and intramyocardial areas (predominantly in the septum and lateral walls) typical of postinflammatory myocardial fibrosis in almost half of patients. These findings suggest a high prevalence of subclinical myocarditis.

2. Arrhythmias & Conduction Disturbances

Right bundle branch block, left anterior fascicular block, bifascicular block, nonspecific intraventricular conduction block, left bundle branch block, and AV block can occur. Occasionally, conduction disturbances can progress to more severe forms, despite remission of the disease, and permanent pacing has been required in a few cases.

The prevalence of arrhythmias varies. The most common arrhythmias are premature ventricular and atrial beats. Supraventricular tachyarrhythmias and ventricular tachycardia are rare. Sudden cardiac death may occur in a small number of patients. Active myocarditis or residual myocardial

degeneration and fibrosis extending to the sinoatrial, AV nodal, and bundle branches explain the arrhythmias and conduction abnormalities.

3. Coronary Arteritis

The clinical prevalence is unknown. One postmortem series demonstrated the presence of coronary arteritis in 30% of patients, manifested as active vasculitis with intimal proliferation or as medial necrosis with calcification.

4. Valvular Heart Disease

Except for a higher prevalence of mitral valve prolapse, no other specific valve disease has been reported. The cause of mitral prolapse has not been determined.

5. Pericarditis

Acute uncomplicated pericarditis with small-to-moderate pericardial effusions has been described; acute pericarditis with cardiac tamponade and chronic constrictive pericarditis are rare. Pericarditis affects less than 20% of adults and a slightly higher percentage of children. Echocardiography, however, shows a prevalence of pericardial effusion, usually small, in up to 25% of adults and up to 50% of children. One large series reported a higher prevalence of pericarditis in overlap syndrome than in isolated polymyositis or dermatomyositis. Only rarely does pericarditis form part of the initial clinical presentation of polymyositis/dermatomyositis.

6. Pulmonary Hypertension, Cor Pulmonale, & Hyperkinetic Heart Syndrome

Both pulmonary hypertension secondary to interstitial lung disease and primary pulmonary vasculopathy leading to cor pulmonale have been found. In hyperkinetic heart syndrome, abnormally increased LV performance has been demonstrated in up to one-third of patients with polymyositis. The cause of this asymptomatic abnormality is unknown.

▶ Treatment & Prognosis

The consideration of immunosuppressive and corticosteroid therapy in patients with severely active disease complicated by myocarditis, pericarditis, or conduction disturbances is similar to that previously described for other connective tissue diseases. Usually high-dose corticosteroids are used acutely, and if the patient does not improve, intravenous immunoglobulin, cyclophosphamide, plasmapheresis, or rituximab can be considered. For chronic therapy, oral methotrexate, azathioprine, mycophenolate, or leflunomide can be used. In patients with pulmonary arterial hypertension, endothelin receptor antagonists, prostacyclins, and/or phosphodiesterase inhibitors should be considered.

Bazzani C, et al. Cardiological features in idiopathic inflammatory myopathies. *J Cardiovasc Med (Hagerstown)*. 2010;11(12):906–11. [PMID: 20625308]

Bhatia P, et al. Pericardial tamponade as the initial presentation in a patient with polymyositis. *J Clin Rheumatol*. 2010;16(6):298–9. [PMID: 20808173]

Dilaveris P, et al. Inducible ventricular tachycardia due to dermatomyositis-related cardiomyopathy in the era of implantable cardioverter-defibrillator therapy. *Circulation*. 2012;125(7):967–9. [PMID: 22354978]

Kato M, et al. The short-term role of corticosteroid therapy for pulmonary arterial hypertension associated with connective tissue diseases: report of five cases and a literature review. *Lupus*. 2011;20(10):1047–56. [PMID: 21676917]

Lu Z, et al. Cardiac involvement in adult polymyositis or dermatomyositis: a systematic review. *Clin Cardiol*. 2012;35(11):686–91. [PMID: 22847365]

Mavrogeni S, et al. Contrast-enhanced CMR imaging reveals myocardial involvement in idiopathic inflammatory myopathy without cardiac manifestations. *JACC Cardiovasc Imaging*. 2011;4(12):1324–5. [PMID: 22172790]

Odabasi Z, et al. Polymyositis presenting with cardiac manifestations: report of two cases and review of the literature. *Clin Neurol Neurosurg*. 2010;112(2):160–3. [PMID: 19910105]

Ong P, et al. Coronary artery spasm as a cause for myocardial infarction in patients with systemic inflammatory disease. *Int J Cardiol*. 2011;151(1):e32–4. [PMID: 21511348]

Schwartz T, et al. Cardiac dysfunction in juvenile dermatomyositis: a case-control study. *Ann Rheum Dis*. 2011;70(5):766–71. [PMID: 21216816]

MIXED CONNECTIVE TISSUE DISEASE

ESSENTIALS OF DIAGNOSIS

▸ Raynaud phenomenon, sclerodactyly.

▸ Myopathy.

▸ Pericarditis, pulmonary hypertension.

▸ High ribonucleoprotein antibody titers.

▶ General Considerations

Patients with mixed connective tissue disease are those with clinical findings of SLE, rheumatoid arthritis, scleroderma, and polymyositis. Characteristically, these patients have high titers of antibodies to nuclear ribonucleoprotein (RNP) and speckled antinuclear antibodies. Rheumatoid agglutinins also occur in more than half of patients. The disease occurs at all ages, affecting predominantly females (80%). Its prevalence is similar to that of scleroderma; it is more common than polymyositis, but less common than SLE. This disease has no particular racial or ethnic predominance. Primary cardiac involvement in mixed connective tissue disease is infrequent and less common than in other connective tissue diseases.

▶ Clinical Findings

A. Symptoms & Signs

Pericardial disease manifested as pericarditis, small pericardial effusions, or pericardial thickening is the most common. Pericarditis is more common in children, affecting almost half of patients. In rare cases, pericarditis complicated with cardiac tamponade can be the initial presentation of the disease (Figure 35–8). Mitral valve prolapse has also been reported in this disease, with an unusually high prevalence (30%). Verrucous thickening of the mitral valve and regurgitation have been rarely detected and are indistinguishable from those of SLE. Infrequently, supraventricular or ventricular arrhythmias and conduction disturbances have been reported. Functional or microvascular disease is the most common type of associated CAD. Acute coronary syndromes may also result from coronary vasospasm, in situ thrombosis, coronary embolism from a valve vegetation, and rarely arteritis. Myocarditis is characterized on histology by interstitial lymphocytic infiltrates and variable degrees of myocardial fibers necrosis and, when acute, can be reversible with corticosteroids and intravenous pulse cyclophosphamide. On echocardiography, the spectrum of the disease ranges from diastolic dysfunction to global or regional LV systolic dysfunction and heart failure. Acute myocarditis may mimic an MI and can be complicated by congestive heart failure and death. Because of the high frequency of pulmonary disease (80%) in patients with mixed connective tissue disease, pulmonary hypertension associated with pulmonary fibrosis or proliferative pulmonary vasculopathy of the small and medium-sized pulmonary arteries can occur, especially in patients with features of scleroderma. Pulmonary thromboembolism is rare.

The clinical manifestations of primary cardiac disease, pulmonary hypertension, and cor pulmonale associated with mixed connective tissue disease do not differ from the other connective tissue diseases.

B. Diagnostic Studies

The methods used to diagnose cardiac disease associated with mixed connective tissue disease are the same used for other connective tissue diseases.

▶ Treatment

Although limited data are available, the treatment of heart disease associated with active mixed connective tissue disease is similar to that described for other connective tissue diseases, and in particular, the immunosuppression closely parallels the therapy of heart and systemic disease in SLE, although therapy for vasospasm (Prinzmetal-type angina) is used more frequently. Endothelin receptor antagonists, prostacyclins, and/or phosphodiesterase inhibitors, and less often calcium channel blockers, have demonstrated both

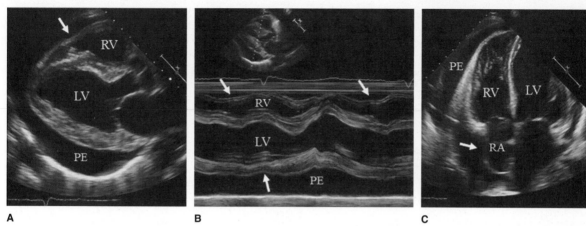

▲ Figure 35–8. A 70-year-old male with active mixed connective tissue disease with predominant features of diffuse scleroderma with a large pericardial effusion complicated with clinical and echocardiographic evidence of cardiac tamponade. **A:** This parasternal long axis transthoracic echocardiographic view demonstrates a large pericardial effusion (PE) predominantly posteriorly located and associated with right ventricular (RV) diastolic compression (*arrow*). **B:** This two-dimensional guided M-mode image from the parasternal long axis view demonstrates significant RV diastolic compression (*upper arrows*) and some degree of posterior left ventricular (LV) diastolic compression (*lower arrow*). **C:** This apical four-chamber transthoracic echocardiographic view demonstrates right atrial (RA) diastolic collapse (*arrow*). Therefore, the patient underwent urgent pericardiocentesis, and after all cultures returned negative, the patient was successfully treated with pulse corticosteroids and cyclophosphamide.

acute and sustained reduction in pulmonary vascular resistance in patients with pulmonary arterial hypertension.

▶ Prognosis

The overall mortality rate of patients with mixed connective tissue disease is 13% at 6–12 years. The prognostic implications of cardiac disease associated with mixed connective tissue disease are unknown.

Baldi S, et al. Efficacy of bosentan in the treatment of a patient with mixed connective tissue disease complicated by pulmonary arterial hypertension. *Clin Rheumatol.* 2010;29(6):687–90. [PMID: 19653056]

van der Net J, et al. Aerobic capacity and muscle strength in juvenile-onset mixed connective tissue disease (MCTD). *Scand J Rheumatol.* 2010;39(5):387–92. [PMID: 20604672]

Végh J, et al. Diastolic function of the heart in mixed connective tissue disease. *Clin Rheumatol.* 2007;26:176–81. [PMID: 16865311]

The Athlete & the Heart

Antonio B. Fernandez, MD
Paul D. Thompson, MD

▶ The patient has an extensive history of exercise training

▶ There may be profound sinus bradycardia, sinus arrhythmias, or atrioventricular conduction delays at rest that disappear with exertion.

▶ The athlete's heart may demonstrate four-chamber enlargement and mild left ventricular hypertrophy, but normal diastolic function and B-natriuretic peptide levels. The diastolic wall-to-volume ratio should be < 0.15 mm/m²/mL by magnetic resonance imaging.

▶ Morphologic changes reverse with detraining.

▶ General Considerations

The salutary physiologic effects of exercise training on the cardiovascular system have been studied extensively, but intense exercise training can produce cardiac adaptations that mimic pathological conditions. Consequently, clinicians should be aware of the normal cardiac structural and functional responses to exercise training in order to distinguish these changes from clinical disease that could also affect athletes.

A. Physiology of Exercise Training

The "athlete's heart" refers to the normal structural and physiologic cardiac adaptations to exercise training. Clinical characteristics of the athlete's heart include resting sinus bradycardia (occasionally profound), sinus arrhythmia, atrioventricular (AV) conduction delays, systolic flow murmurs, four-chamber enlargement, and an increase in cardiac mass, but usually normal or augmented ventricular systolic function.

The magnitude of these cardiac changes depends on a variety of factors including the duration and intensity of the exercise training, the body size of the athlete, the sport, and the physiologic demands of the exercise used to train for that sport. Sports can be roughly classified according to the type and intensity of the exercise performed and the degree of static and dynamic exercise required, but such classifications are innately flawed because they do not consider exercises used in training. Dynamic (isotonic) exercise and sports primarily involve changes in muscle length and joint movement with rhythmic contractions and small intramuscular force. Static (isometric) exercise and sports mainly involve large intramuscular force with little or no change in muscle length or joint movement. Most sports require elements of both.

The acute cardiovascular response to dynamic (aerobic) exercise includes a decrease in peripheral vascular resistance and increases in heart rate, stroke volume, cardiac output, systolic blood pressure, the arteriovenous oxygen difference, and oxygen consumption. Endurance exercise training increases maximal exercise capacity as measured by maximal oxygen uptake. This increase in exercise capacity is produced by increases in the arteriovenous oxygen difference and cardiac output due to increased stroke volume.

Endurance (aerobic) sports, such as long-distance running, and their required training produce the greatest reductions in heart rate and the largest increases in maximum oxygen consumption, cardiac output, stroke volume, and cardiac chamber dimensions. Endurance exercise predominantly produces a volume load on the left and right ventricles. Static or strength sports, such as weight lifting, in contrast, produce only small increases in oxygen consumption and minimal changes in cavity size, but may be associated with mild to modest increases in wall thickness, some of which may be due to increased body mass in such athletes. These changes in wall thickness with little change in chamber dimensions mimic the changes produced by pressure load.

B. Chamber Morphologic Adaptations to Endurance Training

The morphologic adaptations to endurance training have been characterized by echocardiography and magnetic resonance imaging. Cardiac remodeling occurs in approximately one-half of trained athletes. It consists of increases in left and right ventricular and left atrial cavity dimensions and volumes almost always associated with normal systolic and diastolic function (Figure 36–1). Few studies have examined right atrial size, but this may also be increased.

There can be overlap between the athlete's heart and mild forms of cardiac disease such as hypertrophic cardiomyopathy (Figure 36–2). The morphologic features of the athlete's heart are reversible with cessation of training so that cessation of exercise can help distinguish these two conditions. Many athletes resist the idea of detraining, however, so other approaches are often required.

C. Sudden Cardiac Death in Athletes

Clinicians require knowledge of the athlete's heart primarily because vigorous exertion increases the risk of sudden cardiac death during exercise in individuals with known or occult heart disease. Consequently, clinicians need to know what cardiac findings in athletes are normal and how to advise individuals with diagnosed cardiac disease concerning exercise.

The frequency of sudden cardiac death (SCD) in young athletes is not clearly defined, although the largest registry of such events estimates a rate in the United States of only 66 deaths per year. Other estimates have ranged from 1 in 23,000 to 1 in 300, 000 deaths in athletes per year. This variance is likely attributable to collection bias, incomplete identification of cases, and an imprecise denominator. A study of SCD in a defined population of American collegiate athletes suggested an incidence of SCD as high as 1 in 43,000 athletes.

The most common cause of SCD in athletes younger than 35 years of age in the United States is hypertrophic cardiomyopathy (HCM), accounting for up to one-third of sport-related deaths. Other frequent causes include congenital coronary artery anomalies, myocarditis, and aortic rupture, and less commonly, arrhythmogenic right ventricular cardiomyopathy, coronary artery disease, and conduction system abnormalities. In contrast, the most common cause of exertion-related SCD in the Veneto region of Italy is arrhythmogenic right ventricular cardiomyopathy, either because mandatory Italian screening has detected and eliminated athletes with HCM or because of population differences in the prevalence of disease. In contrast to young athletes, SCD in athletes over the age of 35 years is most frequently due to occult coronary artery disease (CAD), and multiple studies have documented an increase in acute myocardial infarction (MI) and SCD among older adults during vigorous exertion.

Endurance athlete

Untrained control subject

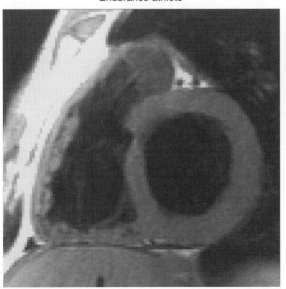 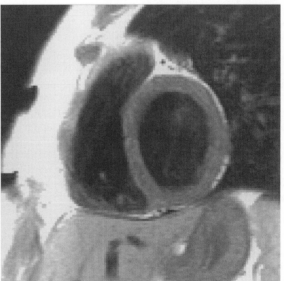

A **B**

▲ **Figure 36–1.** End-diastolic, T1-weighted, short axis slice from an endurance athlete (**A**) and an untrained control subject (**B**). Compared with the heart of the control subject, the endurance athlete's heart is characterized by an enlarged volume and a greater myocardial mass of both ventricles, while the proportions of the left and right heart are the same as in the untrained control subject. (Reproduced with permission from Jürgen Scharhag et al. *J Am Coll Cardiol* 2002;40:1856).

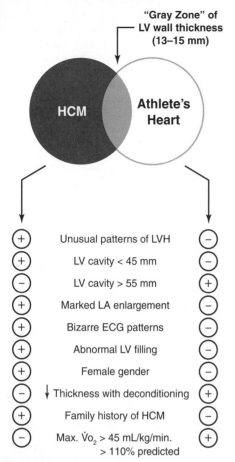

"Gray Zone" of
LV wall thickness
(13–15 mm)

HCM

Athlete's
Heart

(+)	Unusual patterns of LVH	(−)
(+)	LV cavity < 45 mm	(−)
(−)	LV cavity > 55 mm	(+)
(+)	Marked LA enlargement	(−)
(+)	Bizarre ECG patterns	(−)
(+)	Abnormal LV filling	(−)
(+)	Female gender	(−)
(−)	↓ Thickness with deconditioning	(+)
(+)	Family history of HCM	(−)
(−)	Max. $\dot{V}O_2$ > 45 mL/kg/min. > 110% predicted	(+)

▲ **Figure 36–2.** Clinical criteria used to distinguish non-obstructive hypertrophic cardiomyopathy (HCM) from athlete's heart when maximal left ventricular (LV) wall thickness is within shaded gray area of overlap, consistent with both diagnoses. ECG, electrocardiogram; LA, left atrium; LVH, left ventricular hypertrophy. (Adapted with permission from Maron BJ, et al. *Circulation.* 2006;114:1633.)

▶ Clinical Findings

A. Medical History & Physical Examination

As with all of medicine, the most important element of evaluating athletes and their clinical findings is the medical history, and in the medical history, the most important element is what prompted the athlete to obtain medical evaluation. Abnormalities found on screening examinations in an asymptomatic athlete have far less import than abnormalities found during the evaluation of a symptomatic individual. In our clinical experience, most clinical abnormalities found during screening ultimately turn out to be normal variants of the athlete's heart syndrome. Consequently,

dividing athletes into those with and without symptoms is an important initial approach to their evaluation.

The other key elements of the history are the athlete's exercise training history and his or her exercise performance. Marked changes in cardiac dimensions require considerable amounts of exercise training so that cardiac findings in an athlete with a short or low-level training history are of more concern than similar findings in an athlete with high volumes of training. It is also extremely useful to be able to assess the athlete's level of performance. Excellent endurance exercise performance requires a large cardiac stoke volume, so that excellent exercise capacity is reassuring but does not absolutely exclude important disease. Family history of cardiac disease or unexpected or unexplained sudden death (including drowning, unexplained car accidents, or sudden infant death syndrome) is also useful in evaluating young athletes since most conditions causing SCD during exercise in this group are congenital or inherited.

The evaluation of both symptomatic and asymptomatic athletes should include a thorough physical examination. Vital signs are usually notable for training bradycardia with a resting heart rate as low as 30 bpm in highly trained aerobic athletes. Asymptomatic adolescent athletes with heart rates in this range can participate without further evaluation. Athletes may also have an S_3 and S_4 gallop. Athletes frequently have classical flow murmurs related to their slower heart rates and concomitant increased stroke volume. These functional murmurs typically are systolic and less than IV/VI in intensity. They are typically present supine because of enhanced venous return in this position and absent with the athlete upright; they have no diastolic component and are associated with a normal physiologic split of the second heart sound. Because HCM is the most frequent cause of SCD in young athletes, auscultation during the Valsalva maneuver or after arising from the squatting position, either of which should decrease cardiac dimensions and increase the murmur of HCM, is useful.

Syncope is a common problem among athletes and a frequent reason for referral to a cardiologist. Syncopal events are significant if judged to be not neurocardiogenic (vasovagal) and if they occur during exercise. Postexertional syncope is a common phenomenon in athletes. It is usually benign and does not require further workup. Under normal circumstances, exercise increases cardiac output and decreases peripheral vascular resistance due to vasodilation. Syncope after exercise can occur because the increases in cardiac output and heart rate decrease more rapidly than does the peripheral vasodilation. The net effect when the individual stops exercising is an increase in vasodilation without the compensatory increase in heart rate and cardiac output, thus explaining postexertional syncope. In contrast, syncope during exercise usually suggests a cardiac origin, such as anomalous coronary artery anatomy or cardiac arrhythmias.

The American Heart Association (AHA) position on screening athletes before competition recommends a 12-point evaluation (Table 36–1). The historical elements are important,

Table 36–1. The 12-Element American Heart Association Recommendations for Preparticipation Cardiovascular Screening of Competitive Athletes

Medical history*
  Personal history
    1. Exertional chest pain/discomfort
    2. Unexplained syncope/near-syncope†
    3. Excessive exertional and unexplained dyspnea/fatigue, associated with exercise
    4. Prior recognition of a heart murmur
    5. Elevated systemic blood pressure
  Family history
    6. Premature death (sudden and unexpected, or otherwise) before age 50 years due to heart disease, in ≥1 relative
    7. Disability from heart disease in a close relative < 50 years of age
    8. Specific knowledge of certain cardiac conditions in family members: hypertrophic or dilated cardiomyopathy, long-OT syndrome or other ion channelopathies, Marfan syndrome, or clinically important arrhythmias
  Physical examination
    9. Heart murmur‡
    10. Femoral pulses to exclude aortic coarctation
    11. Physical stigmata of Marfan syndrome
    12. Brachial artery blood pressure (sitting position)§

*Parental verification is recommended for high school and middle school athletes.
†Judged not to be neurocardiogenic (vasovagal); of particular concern when related to exertion.
‡Auscultation should be performed in both supine and standing positions (or with Valsalva maneuver), specifically to identify murmurs of dynamic left ventricular outflow tract obstruction.
§Preferably taken in both arms.
Reproduced with permission from Maron BJ, et al. *Circulation* 2007;115:1643.

but young athletes often respond positively to many of these queries, again highlighting the importance of separating the evaluation of athletes with abnormalities found on screening from those presenting with symptoms.

B. Diagnostic Studies

1. Electrocardiogram—Many clinical and electrocardiographic (ECG) findings of concern in the general population are normal for athletes. The accuracy of the ECG interpretation is particularly difficult in young athletes due to ECG evolutionary changes that are related to age. Furthermore, there are inconsistencies in the definitions of ECG abnormalities and definite criteria for the diagnosis of several diseases. While the routine use of ECG for preparticipation screening remains controversial in young adults, its use remains a cornerstone of any cardiac evaluation in athletes with cardiac complaints. It is recommended as part of a routine evaluation for all masters athletes > 40 years of age since it occasionally identifies a prior MI.

Sinus bradycardia as low as 30 bpm, sinus arrhythmia, prolonged PR interval up to 300 ms, sinoatrial block, junction rhythms, and Wenckebach phenomenon are common in athletes due to a high resting parasympathetic tone and should not prompt further workup if the athlete is asymptomatic and has good exercise capacity and the abnormalities disappear during exercise.

QRS axis varies with age, but in athletes, mild right or left axis deviations should not trigger further evaluation unless there is history of pulmonary disease or systemic hypertension. An acceptable rage is between –30 and +115 degrees.

Incomplete right bundle branch block is extremely common in athletes. In contrast, complete block of either bundle, even in asymptomatic athletes, should prompt further investigation. Increased QRS amplitude is present in up to 80% of the athletes, but if the increased voltage is not accompanied by axis changes, repolarization changes, atrial abnormalities, or increased QRS width, it does not warrant further evaluation.

Small q waves may be present in athletes. The ECG in patients with HCM may also show q waves, but these "septal q's" are often seen in the inferior and/or lateral leads and suggest HCM if they are > 3 mm in depth and/or > 40 ms duration in at least two leads. Athletes with pathologic Q waves should be referred for further evaluation to exclude HCM (Table 36–2).

Early repolarization in V_3–V_6 with an elevated J point and peaked upright T waves is common in athletes and especially in those of African descent. The repolarization pattern may also include a domed ST segment followed by a biphasic or inverted T wave. These benign repolarization changes must be distinguished from the Brugada ECG pattern commonly present in leads V_1–V_2.

2. Other noninvasive cardiovascular evaluations—ECG and echocardiography are indicated when clinical, historical, or physical findings suggest the possibility of structural heart disease (valvular disease, HCM, arrhythmogenic right ventricular cardiomyopathy, or prior MI). Tilt table testing is often positive in athletes because of their resting bradycardia and large venous capacitance and thus should not be used or should be used cautiously in athletes to evaluate lightheadedness, syncope, or presyncope.

Echocardiography in highly trained endurance athletes may show evidence of four-chamber cardiac enlargement. Left ventricular end-diastolic dimensions can exceed 60 mm in 15% of athletes. Left ventricular wall thickness can occasionally exceed the upper normal limit of 12 mm. Values of 13–15 mm may be seen in normal athletes, although marked enlargement of > 16 mm is unusual, and the ratio of the septal to posterior wall thickness does not exceed 1.2. The left ventricular cavity in HCM typically has asymmetric wall thickening, although symmetric wall enlargement may occur and the cavity dimensions are usually small and < 45 mm. In contrast, the athlete's heart typically has symmetric mild increases in left ventricular wall thickness and an increase in left ventricular chamber size of 55 mm or greater.

Left atrial enlargement in athletes is also common, and anterior-posterior diameters > 40 mm, the upper limit of

Table 36-2. Electrocardiogram Abnormalities That Require Further Evaluation

LBBB RBBB IVCD	Any QRS >120 ms	
QRS axis deviation	More leftward than −30° More rightward than 115°	
QTc interval	>470 ms in males >480 ms in females <340 ms in any athlete	
Brugada pattern	Presence of Type 1 pattern: coved ST segment in V1 and V2 gradually descending into inverted T wave	
Pre-Excitation	Delta wave and PR interval <120 ms	
Ventricular extrasystoles, heart block, and supra-ventricular arrhythmia	Atrial fibrillation/flutter, supra-ventricular tachycardia, complete heart block or ≥2 PVCs in one 12 lead ECG	

ECG, electrocardiogram; IVCD, intraventricular conduction delay; LBBB, left bundle branch block; PVCs, premature ventricular contractions; RBBB, right bundle branch block.
Reproduced with permission from Uberoi A, et al. *Circulation.* 2011;124:746.

normal, exist in 20% of high-performance athletes. This increased atrial size may contribute to the observation that atrial fibrillation is more common in older athletes than in age-matched nonathletes.

Left ventricular diastolic function measured by tissue Doppler is normal in athletes despite the hypertrophy, and normal diastolic function can help distinguish the athlete's heart from pathologic hypertrophy. The systolic anterior motion (SAM) of the mitral valve and mitral leaflet elongation can help with the diagnosis of HCM. These changes could happen in HCM even when the walls are not severely thickened. Stress echocardiography could provoke SAM and can provide more information than at rest.

Cardiac MRI can also help distinguish athlete's heart from HCM. A left ventricular diastolic wall thickness–to–cavity volume ratio of < 0.15 mm/m^2/mL is useful in diagnosing athlete's heart. In HCM, intravenous gadolinium used in contrast-enhanced MRI is taken up by areas of myocardium with extra expanded cellular space indicating areas of fibrosis and scarring, also referred to as "late gadolinium enhancement" (LGE). LGE is not typical of the athlete's heart, especially in young athletes, but has been observed in older athletes with a history of life-long, intense exercise training.

Finally, detraining is another approach that could help to distinguish the athlete's heart from HCM. Three months of detraining should be sufficient to reverse the left ventricular hypertrophy of the athlete's heart and to distinguish this condition from HCM, although some studies suggest 6 months may be required. A decrease of > 2 mm in left ventricular wall thickness with detraining relative to peak training is more consistent with athlete's heart since patients with HCM should not demonstrate a change with deconditioning.

Corrado D, et al. Recommendations for interpretation of 12-lead electrocardiogram in the athlete. *Eur Heart J.* 2010;31:243–59. [PMID: 19933514]

Petersen SE, et al. Differentiation of athlete's heart from pathological forms of cardiac hypertrophy by means of geometric indices derived from cardiovascular magnetic resonance. *J Cardiovasc Magnetic Res.* 2005;7:551–8. [PMID: 15959967]

Scharhag J, et al. Right and left ventricular mass and function in male endurance athletes and untrained individuals determined by magnetic resonance imaging. *J Am Coll Cardiol.* 2002;40(10):1856–63. [PMID: 12446071]

Uberoi A, et al. Interpretation of the electrocardiogram of young athletes. *Circulation.* 2011;124;746–57. [PMID: 21824936]

▶ Integrating the Clinical Findings in Evaluating Athletes

Evaluating athletes, just like evaluating any patient, requires a careful integration of all aspects of the history, physical examination, and imaging findings. Clinicians should be careful of overreacting to borderline abnormalities found in asymptomatic athletes during screening. These often lead to "diagnostic creep" in which one borderline abnormality, such as a flow murmur, leads to other borderline abnormalities, with no clinician willing to diagnose normalcy. Such cases often are best handled by clinicians who have extensive experience dealing with athletes.

A. Preparticipation Screening

To prevent SCD in athletes, Italy has mandated by law the screening of all athletes ages 12 through 35 prior to participation in organized competitive sport. This is a state-subsidized national program that includes a history and physical, an ECG, and a 3-minute step test. The evaluation is performed by accredited sports medicine doctors specifically trained for this task. Further testing is done for abnormal findings or if there is a family history of sudden death or MI or a personal history of syncope or palpitations. The incidence of SCDs in 12- to 35-year-old athletes in one region of Italy, Veneto, has decreased since the implementation of this law due to decreases in deaths from arrhythmogenic right ventricular hypertrophy. No changes in the nonathlete population mortality rate occurred over the same period of time.

Based on this single-center data, the European Society of Cardiology (ESC) and the International Olympic Committee (IOC) recommended the addition of an ECG to preparticipation screening. In contrast to the Italian experience, mandated preparticipation ECG and exercise testing in Israel has had no effect on the incidence of SCD in athletes. The AHA has also proposed guidelines for screening athletes prior to participation, but the AHA guidelines do not recommend routine ECG screening. Consequently, whether or not athletes require a routine ECG prior to athletic participation is controversial, and preparticipation ECG is not presently recommended in the United States. Clinicians should perform such ECG screening in individual athletes when the clinical situation warrants such testing or to reassure anxious parents. In such screening, however, the clinician should be wary of the diagnostic creep noted earlier.

In 2001, the AHA also published recommendations for preparticipation medical evaluations for master athletes. These are individuals over the age of 35 who are involved in masters sports training programs and participate in organized competitions designed for older athletes. Exercise testing is recommended for masters athletes who have a moderate-to-high cardiovascular risk profile for coronary heart disease; this risk profile includes men > 40 years old and women > 50 years old (or postmenopausal) with one or more independent coronary risk factors (hypercholesterolemia or dyslipidemia, hypertension, current or recent cigarette smoking, diabetes mellitus, or a history of MI or sudden death in a first-degree relative < 60 years old). An exercise test is also recommended for masters athletes of any age with symptoms suggestive of coronary heart disease or those ≥ 65 years of age even in the absence of risk factors or symptoms. A positive test requires further evaluation to determine the coronary anatomy. Although these are the current AHA guidelines, we also regard the recommendation for routine exercise testing in asymptomatic individuals as controversial

since athletes frequently have false-positive ECG responses to exercise testing and there is limited clinical evidence to justify the routine revascularization of asymptomatic individuals, especially those with excellent exercise tolerance.

B. Recommendations for Sport Participation

Based on the routine history and physical examination prior to sport participation, the athlete should be either given clearance for participation, clearance to participate with activity limitations, or exclusion from participation pending further evaluation. If a cardiac diagnosis is made, limitations or exclusion might be warranted. The American College of Cardiology convened a consensus panel in 2005 to evaluate eligibility recommendations that are helpful once a diagnosis is made. This document summarizes experts' opinion regarding the type of sports the athlete is allowed to perform based on the cardiac pathology. Guidelines for sports participation for children with medical conditions have also been published and can assist in determining the level of sport recommended. Decisions should be individualized for each athlete since there are no definite data to determine the exercise risk for every cardiac condition, and guidelines are necessarily restrictive since they will be used by clinicians of varying ability. The decision to restrict sports participation should involve the athlete, the parents, and the coach.

Corrado D, et al. Cardiovascular pre-participation screening of young competitive athletes for prevention of sudden death: proposal for a common European protocol. Consensus Statement of the Study Group of Sport Cardiology of the Working Group of Cardiac Rehabilitation and Exercise Physiology and the Working Group of Myocardial and Pericardial Diseases of the European Society of Cardiology. *Eur Heart J.* 2005;26(5):516. [PMID: 15689345]

Maron BJ, et al. The heart of trained athletes: cardiac remodeling and the risks of sports, including sudden death. *Circulation.* 2006;114:1633–44. [PMID: 17030703]

Maron BJ, et al. Introduction: eligibility recommendations for competitive athletes with cardiovascular abnormalities-general considerations. *J Am Coll Cardiol.* 2005;45;1318–21. [PMID: 15837280]

Maron BJ, et al. Recommendations and considerations related to preparticipation screening for cardiovascular abnormalities in competitive athletes: 2007 update: a scientific statement from the American Heart Association Council on Nutrition, Physical Activity, and Metabolism: endorsed by the American College of Cardiology Foundation. *Circulation.* 2007;115:1643–55. [PMID: 17353433]

Maron BJ, et al. Recommendations for preparticipation screening and the assessment of cardiovascular disease in masters athletes: an advisory for healthcare professionals from the working groups of the World Heart Federation, the International Federation of Sports Medicine, and the American Heart Association Committee on Exercise, Cardiac Rehabilitation, and Prevention. *Circulation.* 2001;103(2):327–34. [PMID: 11208698]

Rice SG. Medical conditions affecting sport participation. American Academy of Pediatrics Council on Sports Medicine and Fitness. *Pediatrics.* 2008;121:841–8. [PMID: 18381550]

Wheeler MT, et al. Cost effectiveness of pre-participation screening for prevention of sudden cardiac death in young athletes. *Ann Intern Med.* 2010;152(5):276–86. [PMID: 20194233]

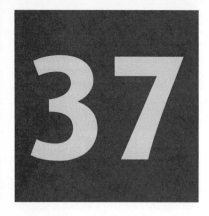

Thoracic Aortic Aneurysms & Dissections

John A. Elefteriades, MD

ANEURYSMS

ESSENTIALS OF DIAGNOSIS

▶ Ascending aortic diameter > 4 cm on imaging study.
▶ Descending aortic diameter > 3.5 cm on imaging study.

▶ General Considerations

In the ascending aorta, aneurysms tend to take on three common patterns, as indicated in Figure 37–1. These include the supracoronary aortic aneurysm, annuloaortic ectasia (marfanoid), and tubular diffuse enlargement.

The most common pattern is that of supracoronary dilatation of the ascending aorta. In this pattern of disease, the short segment of aorta between the aortic annulus and the coronary arteries remains normal in size. Sinuses are "preserved," meaning that the aorta indents normally, forming a "waist," near the level of the coronary arteries. For this type of aneurysm, a supracoronary tube graft suffices.

In the second type, annuloaortic ectasia, the aortic annulus itself becomes dilated, giving a shape to the aorta like an Erlenmeyer chemistry flask. In this type of disease, the segment of aorta between the annulus and the coronary arteries is diseased, dilated, and thinned. Sinuses are "effaced," meaning that the normal indentation, or waist, is lost. When surgery is required, the entire aortic root must be replaced.

In the third type of ascending aortic disease, the configuration is midway between the previous two patterns, that is, there is some dilatation of the annulus and root and some effacement of the sinuses, but these elements are not dramatic. The overall appearance is that of a large tube, rather than a flask. For such aortas, either supracoronary tube grafting or aortic root replacement may be appropriate.

The Crawford classification (Figure 37–2) is used to categorize the appearance of an aneurysm in the descending aorta and thoracoabdominal aorta. This classification is based on the longitudinal location and extent of aortic involvement, has implications for surgical strategy, and affects the risk of perioperative complications.

Type I aneurysms involve most of the thoracic aorta and the upper abdominal aorta. Type II aneurysms, the most extensive and most dangerous to repair, involve the entire descending and abdominal aortas. Type III aneurysms involve the lower thoracic and abdominal aortas. Type IV aneurysms are predominantly abdominal but involve thoracoabdominal exposure because of the proximity of the upper border to the diaphragm.

▶ Etiology

The genetics of Marfan disease, a well-known cause of aneurysms of the thoracic aorta, have been well delineated, with over 600 mutations identified at one locus on the fibrillin gene.

Increasingly, it is being appreciated that patients who do not have Marfan disease also manifest familial clustering of thoracic aortic aneurysms and dissections. Patients with aneurysms often answer one or both of the following questions affirmatively: "Do you have any family members with aneurysms anywhere in their bodies? Did any of your relatives die suddenly or unexpectedly of apparent cardiac causes?" Detailed construction of family trees on over 500 patients with thoracic aneurysm has indicated that 21% of aneurysm probands have a first-degree relative with a known or likely aortic aneurysm. The true number is certainly much higher, as these estimates are based only on family interview and not on head-to-toe imaging of relatives. Figure 37–3 shows the 21 positive family trees of the first 100 families analyzed. The most likely pattern of inheritance appears to be autosomal dominant with incomplete penetrance. A more recent analysis has shown that the location of the

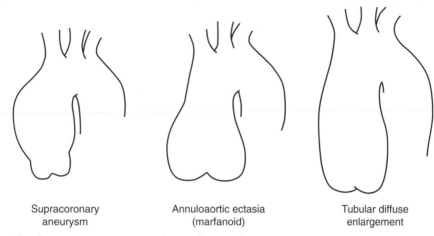

▲ Figure 37–1. The three common patterns of ascending aortic aneurysm.

Supracoronary
aneurysm

Annuloaortic ectasia
(marfanoid)

Tubular diffuse
enlargement

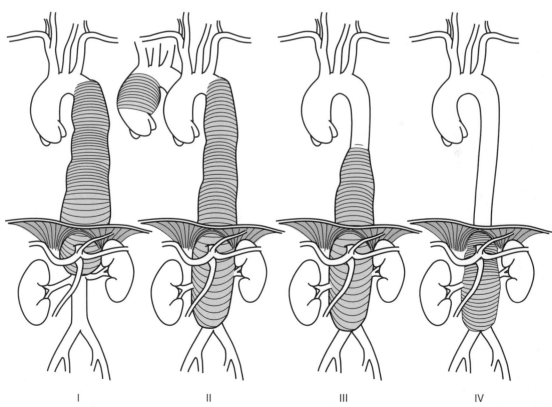

I II III IV

▲ Figure 37–2. The Crawford classification of descending and thoracoabdominal aneurysms. See text for description of each type. (Reprinted, with permission, from Edmunds LH Jr, ed. *Cardiac Surgery in the Adult.* New York: McGraw-Hill; 1997.)

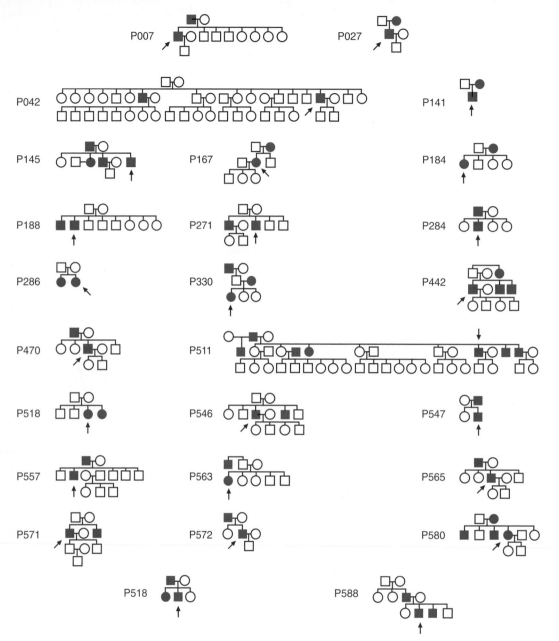

▲ **Figure 37–3.** The 21 positive family trees among the first 100 families assessed for genetic patterns of thoracic aortic disease.

proband's aneurysm largely influences the location of the aneurysms in the family members. If the proband has an ascending aneurysm, the likelihood is that the family members have ascending aneurysms. If, however, the proband has a descending aneurysm, it is likely that the family members have abdominal aortic aneurysms. These proband–family member observations are in keeping with the general concept that aneurysm disease divides at the ligamentum arteriosum:

Ascending and arch aneurysms represent one disease, largely nonarteriosclerotic, while descending and abdominal aneurysms represent another disease, largely arteriosclerotic.

Application of modern molecular genetic techniques is successfully making progress toward determining the specific genetic aberrations responsible for these family clusterings and for thoracic aneurysms in general. Original progress was made largely by linkage analysis of large families with multiple

Table 37–1. Current tabulation of genetic patterns of inheritance of thoracic aortic aneurysm and their underlying mutations.

Classification	Chromosome	Gene	Protein	Location	Frequency	Inheritance
Syndrome						
Marfan	15q21.1	FBN1	Fibrillin 1	ECM	1:5000-10,000	Dominant
Loeys-Dietz	3p24-25 9q33-34	TGFBR2, TGFBR1	TGFβ-R2 TGFβ-R1	Cell surface	Rare	Dominant
Ehlers-Danlos	2q24.3-31	COL3A1	Type III collagen	ECM	1:10,000-25,000	Dominant
ATS	20q13.1	SLC2A10	GLUT10	Intracellular	Rare	Recessive
AOS	15q22.2-24.3	Smad3	SMAD3	Intracellular	Rare	Dominant
TGFB2	1q41	TGFB2	TGFβ2	Intracellular	Rare	Dominant
Non-Syndromic						
TAAD2	3p24-25	TGFBR2	TGFβ-R2	Cell surface	~3 % of TAA	Dominant
TAAD4	10q23-24	ACTA2	Actin	Intracellular	10-15% of TAA	Dominant
TAAD5	9q33-34	TGFBR1	TGFβ-R1	Cell surface	~2 % of TAA	Dominant
TAAD-PDA	16p12-13 3q21.1	MYH11 MYLK	β-MHC MLCK	Intracellular Intracellular	1-2% of TAA ~1% of TAA	Dominant

Syndromic means associated with other, non-cardiac stigmata. Reproduced with permission from Pomianowski P, Elefteriades J. Genetics and genomics of thoracic aortic disease. Chiesa R, Melissano G, Zangrillo A. Aortic Surgery and Anesthesia "How To Do It". Arti Grafiche Colombo, Italy. 2012.

members affected. Now, as automated genomic analysis has become feasible and affordable, much scientific discovery has been made by direct exome sequencing. Milewicz, Dietz, Loeys, and others have succeeded in identifying specific familial aneurysm patterns and their underlying mutations (Table 37–1). Note that all of these disorders, except one, are transmitted in an autosomal dominant fashion (with decreased penetrance). Also note that the *ACTA2* disorder presents with aortic dissection at small diameters. These mutation-specific categorizations will soon allow personalized medicine based on the specific underlying mutation and its accompanying rupture and dissection patterns.

Examination of single nucleotide polymorphisms (SNPs) in the blood of hundreds of patients with thoracic aortic aneurysms via genome-wide surveys using large (> 30,000) SNP libraries has been accomplished. An "RNA signature" in the blood of patients with thoracic aortic aneurysm was found, which can predict with about 85% accuracy from a blood test alone whether the patient harbors a thoracic aortic aneurysm. This "signature" is composed of specific RNAs that are either markedly upregulated or markedly downregulated in aneurysm patients, compared with healthy controls.

Patients who have a genetic predisposition for aneurysm development, specifically those patients with annuloaortic ectasia or ascending dissection, are significantly protected from arteriosclerosis (Figure 37–4). Remarkably, they have less arterial medial thickness and less calcification than normal

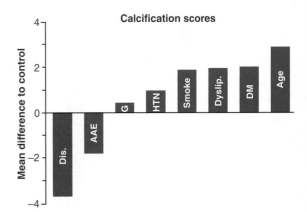

▲ **Figure 37–4.** Difference in overall calcification scores relative to the control group for all risk factors analyzed. Note that patients with ascending aortic dissection or annuloaortic ectasia are significantly "protected" from arteriosclerosis, manifesting lower calcification scores. AAE, annuloaortic ectasia; Age, age (in 10-year intervals); Dis, ascending aortic dissection; DM, diabetes mellitus; Dyslip, dyslipidemia; G, male gender; HTN, hypertension; Smoke, smoking history.

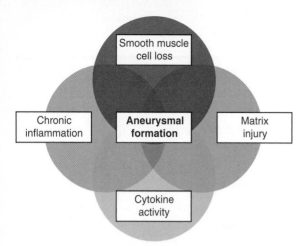

▲ **Figure 37–5.** Diagram illustrating the overlapping cellular and molecular processes that contribute to aortic aneurysm formation.

controls. It appears likely that the same mutations that promote lysis of the aortic wall also prevent plaque build-up.

Accepting that most patients with aneurysms have an underlying genetic predisposition to the condition, how does this genetic programming lead to the development of an aneurysm? Rapid progress is being made in elucidating these mechanisms. Aneurysm formation is currently thought to involve the following processes (Figure 37–5): extracellular matrix proteolysis, chronic inflammation, cytokine activity, and smooth muscle cell loss. The identification of these mechanisms raises the intriguing possibility of interfering pharmacologically with this pathophysiology, so aneurysm formation or progression can be stopped. The importance of the transforming growth factor-β (TGF-β) pathway in aneurysm formation has been demonstrated; the ability of angiotensin receptor–blocking medications (eg, losartan) to interfere with this pathophysiologic mechanism is being tested, and results of randomized, controlled studies will soon be available. At this time, however, it may be said that no specific pharmacologic strategy exists for delaying aneurysm progression. Results of trials of proteolytic antagonists and β-blockers have been underwhelming. The potential roles of statin medications, anti-inflammatory agents (cyclooxygenase [COX]-2 inhibitors), immunosuppressants (sirolimus), and antibiotics (doxycycline) are being investigated.

The proteolytic enzymes called matrix metalloproteinases (MMPs) are receiving extensive attention in aneurysm pathophysiology. These powerful enzymes are found in excess in thoracic aortic aneurysms (Figure 37–6) and are thought to play a major role in destroying the substance of the aortic wall, leading to decreased wall strength and, ultimately, dilatation and rupture.

The biologic changes in the aortic wall discussed earlier are vitally important, but hemodynamic forces need to be considered as well. As the ascending aorta reaches a diameter of 6 cm, the distensibility vanishes, so that the aorta

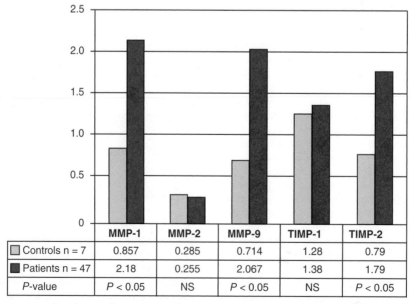

	MMP-1	MMP-2	MMP-9	TIMP-1	TIMP-2
Controls n = 7	0.857	0.285	0.714	1.28	0.79
Patients n = 47	2.18	0.255	2.067	1.38	1.79
P-value	P < 0.05	NS	P < 0.05	NS	P < 0.05

▲ **Figure 37–6.** Note overabundance of matrix metalloproteinase (MMP)-1 and MMP-9 in aortas of patients with thoracic aortic aneurysm, compared with controls. This information suggests an important role for MMP enzymes in the pathophysiology of aneurysm disease.

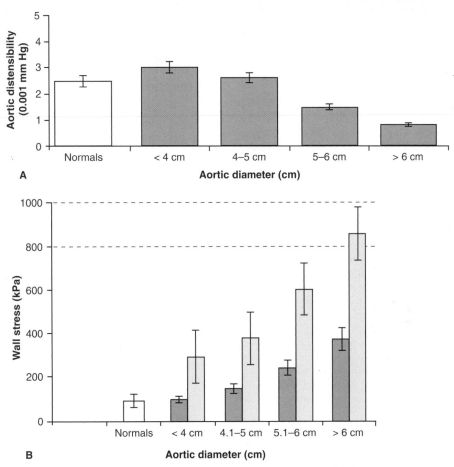

▲ **Figure 37–7. A:** Distensibility values in normal aortas and aortic aneurysms of different diameters. Distensibility of ascending aortic aneurysms decreases rapidly as diameter increases, to very low values at dimensions > 6 cm. At 6 cm, the aorta is essentially a rigid tube, unable to dissipate the force of systole by expanding phasically during the cardiac cycle. **B:** Exponential relationship between wall stress and aneurysm size in ascending aortic aneurysms. The dark columns represent a blood pressure of 100 mm Hg, and the light columns represent a blood pressure of 200 mm Hg. The lines at 800–1000 kPa represent the range of maximum tensile strength of the human aorta. Note that a patient with a 6-cm aneurysm and a blood pressure of 200 mm Hg (as during stress or extreme exertion) "flirts" with the limits of the ultimate strength of his or her aorta wall.

becomes essentially a rigid tube (Figure 37–7). Because of this rigidity, the force of systole can no longer be beneficially dissipated by elastic expansion of the aorta, and this translates into increased wall stress. Especially at high blood pressures, this wall stress becomes excessive, setting the stage for disruption of the aortic wall via rupture or dissection. It is instructive to note how closely this mechanical data dove-tail with the clinical behavior of the aorta: The mechanical properties deteriorate at 6 cm diameter, and that is precisely the hinge point for clinically manifest rupture and dissection.

▶ **Clinical Findings**

A. Natural History

The Yale computerized database now contains information on nearly 3000 patients with thoracic aortic aneurysm, including some 9000 tabulated serial imaging studies and 9000 patient-years of follow-up. This database and these methods of analysis have permitted assessment of multiple fundamental topics and questions regarding the natural behavior of the thoracic aorta and have shed light on appropriate criteria for surgical intervention.

1. How fast does the thoracic aorta grow?—Via specifically developed statistical methods designed to account for important potential sources of error, the annual growth rate of an aneurysmal thoracic aorta has been determined to be 0.12 cm on average. The descending aorta grows faster than the ascending aorta, at 0.19 cm/year compared with 0.07 cm/year. Also, the larger the aorta becomes, the faster it grows.

2. At what size does the aorta dissect or rupture?—Critical to decision making in aortic surgery is an understanding of when complications occur in the natural history of unrepaired thoracic aortic aneurysms. In the case of the thoracic aorta, the two complications that are vitally important are rupture and dissection. Knowing when these complications are likely to occur would permit rational decision making regarding elective, preemptive surgical intervention to prevent their occurrence.

Size criteria apply *only* to asymptomatic aneurysms. We are learning increasingly that the aorta can indeed "communicate" with us—via pain. Symptomatic (painful) aneurysms should be resected regardless of size. For ascending aneurysms, this pain is usually felt anteriorly, under the breastbone. For descending thoracic aneurysms, the pain is usually felt in the interscapular region of the upper back. For thoracoabdominal aneurysms, the pain is usually felt lower in the back and in the left flank. Other symptoms may occasionally be produced by thoracic aortic aneurysms, including bronchial obstruction, esophageal obstruction, and phrenic nerve dysfunction; these symptoms also constitute indications for surgical intervention.

Initial statistical analysis revealed sharp "hinge points" (Figure 37–8) in aortic size at which rupture or dissection occurred. For the ascending thoracic aorta, the hinge point occurs at 6.0 cm. By the time aortas reach this size, 31% have ruptured or dissected. For the descending aorta, the hinge point is located at 7.0 cm. By the time descending aortas reach this size, 43% have ruptured or dissected.

If a surgeon were to wait for the aorta to achieve the median size at time of complications in order to intervene, by definition rupture or dissection would have occurred in half of the patients (Figure 37–9). Accordingly, it is important to intervene before the median value is attained. The following recommendations take this factor into account, permitting preemptive surgical extirpation before rupture or dissection in most patients.

Current recommendations are listed in Table 37–2 and are based on the hinge points noted in Figure 37–8. Specifically, prophylactic extirpation of the aneurysmal ascending aorta is recommended when the aneurysm measures 5.5 cm; for the descending aorta, which does not rupture until a larger size, surgical intervention is recommended when the aneurysm measures 6.5 cm. Application of these criteria will prevent most ruptures and dissections, without prematurely exposing the patient to the risks and inconveniences of surgery. The efficacy of this management

algorithm has recently been documented in a large cohort of prospectively followed patients.

It is well-known that patients with Marfan disease are prone to unpredictable dissection at an early size. For this reason, earlier intervention is recommended for patients with Marfan disease as indicated in Table 37–2.

For patients with a positive family history, but without Marfan disease, the same criteria are applied as for Marfan disease, because malignant early behavior of the aneurysm in these patients may be seen as well.

If the patient has a positive family history, or if an afflicted family member has suffered rupture, dissection, or death, preemptive surgical extirpation is carried out earlier than otherwise.

Studies of aortic anatomy increasingly recognize that patients with a bicuspid aortic valve also have inherently deficient aortas. Therefore, lower intervention dimensions are used for patients with bicuspid aortic valve as well. Table 37–3 indicates that a bicuspid aortic valve is actually a more common cause of aortic dissection than Marfan disease. Table 37–3 compares the general incidence of Marfan disease with that of bicuspid aortic valve. Although the incidence of dissection is 5% for bicuspid valve disease, compared with 40% for patients with Marfan disease, bicuspid valve disease is so much more common that it causes more total cases of dissection than Marfan disease. This factor must be taken into account in planning surgical repair of the ascending aorta of the patient with a bicuspid aortic valve when the aorta is still in the aneurysmal stage and not yet a dissection.

3. What is the yearly rate of rupture or dissection for thoracic aortic aneurysms?—The preceding data indicate the cumulative *lifetime* rates of dissection or rupture by the time the aorta reaches a certain size. Determining the *yearly* risk of complications from the natural history of thoracic aortic aneurysm is more challenging because it requires extremely robust data. Such data must produce enough hard end points to permit analysis within a year's time for different size strata. Calculations of yearly rates of rupture or other complications based on size of the aorta have been produced. These yearly rates are expressed based simply on the size of the aorta (Figure 37–10).

These data all point to a diameter of 6 cm as a very dangerous size threshold. At or above this size, the yearly risk for rupture is about 4%, the yearly risk of dissection is about 4%, and the risk of death is about 11%. (Death is often directly related to catastrophic complications from the aneurysm.) The chance of any one of these phenomena occurring—rupture, dissection, or death—is 14%/year. As a mnemonic point of reference, a 6-cm aneurysm can be equated to about the diameter of a soft-drink can. When a thoracic aortic aneurysm reaches the diameter of a soda can, it has certainly attained the point where it poses a major risk to the patient.

These analyses should permit accurate decision making when seeing a patient during an office visit and considering

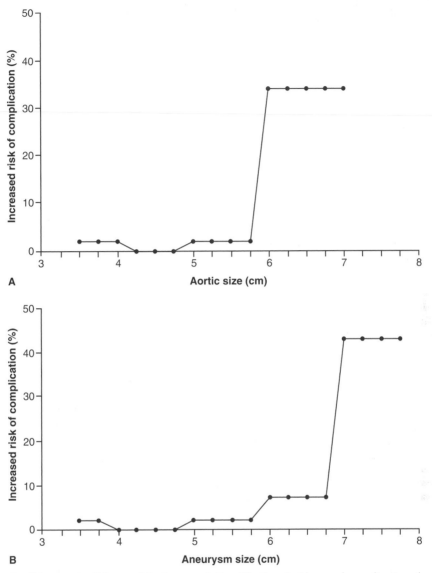

▲ **Figure 37-8.** The "hinge points" (*arrows*) in the cumulative, life-time incidence of complications (rupture or dissection) of thoracic aortic aneurysms, based on size. By the time the aorta reaches the dimensions on the *x*-axis, the percentage of patients shown on the *y*-axis has already incurred rupture or dissection. **A:** Curve for the ascending aorta. **B:** Curve for the descending aorta.

preemptive surgical extirpation of thoracic aneurysms. These data allow the physician to form a reasonable estimate of the individual patient's risk of dissection, rupture, or death for each future year of life, if the aorta is not resected. The risk of rupture, dissection, or death based on aortic size is presented graphically in Figure 37–10.

The question arises whether the same surgical intervention criteria should apply for a small woman as for a large man. It is true that a larger individual can be "allowed" a larger aorta, generally speaking. Conversely, even a moderate-sized aneurysm can be quite threatening in an individual of small stature. For this reason, adverse event rates (rupture or dissection) based on aortic size corrected for body surface area (BSA) have been analyzed. By plotting the aneurysm size along the horizontal scale and the BSA along the vertical scale, each particular patient can be classified into low-, medium-, or high-risk categories—thus taking account of the aneurysm size in relation to the patient's physical size.

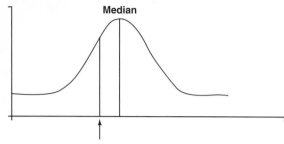

▲ **Figure 37–9.** A schematic representation of the importance of selecting a criterion for intervention before complications (rupture or dissection) commonly occur. Utilization of the median as the criterion level would allow half the population to realize a devastating complication before preemptive intervention. Accordingly, a criterion below the median is selected (*arrow*) to allow preemptive intervention before a large proportion of patients have suffered a complication.

B. Symptoms & Signs

Most thoracic aortic aneurysms are asymptomatic and are detected fortuitously during imaging of other thoracic structures. When they are symptomatic, deep visceral pain in the upper anterior chest or interscapular back can occur. This pain differs from angina pectoris because it is not necessarily precipitated by exertion nor relieved by rest or nitroglycerin. Often, it is rather constant and not influenced by body motion or position. All patients with chest pain should have a screening chest radiograph. Rupture of a thoracic aneurysm usually causes excruciating pain, accompanied by profound dyspnea as the chest fills with blood, and quickly results in shock. A large ascending aortic aneurysm occasionally may result in dysphagia or stridor due to esophageal or large airway obstruction. Rarely, a large aneurysm may cause bone pain due to pressure against thoracic skeletal structures.

C. Physical Examination

Physical examination is usually unremarkable. The presence of a murmur of aortic regurgitation should raise the suspicion of ascending aortic aneurysm, as should features suggestive of Marfan syndrome or related conditions. Rarely,

Table 37–2. Size Criteria for Surgical Intervention for Asymptomatic Thoracic Aortic Aneurysm

	Marfan	Non-Marfan
Ascending	5.0 cm	5.5 cm
Descending	6.0 cm	6.5 cm

an abnormal pulsation will be felt due to a large aneurysm contacting the chest wall.

D. Diagnostic Studies

The remarkable strides made in recent decades in three-dimensional body imaging have dramatically advanced the diagnosis and treatment of thoracic aortic aneurysm. Echocardiography (especially transesophageal) and computed tomography (CT) and magnetic resonance imaging (MRI) scans all yield images that clarify the presence, location, size, and extent of aneurysmal disease. An example of the precise imaging afforded by MRI is indicated for a specific, very extensive aneurysm in Figure 37–11.

In this era of specialized three-dimensional imaging, it is important not to forget the chest radiograph, which can often yield significant information about the thoracic aorta. An example is provided in Figure 37–12. Ascending aortic aneurysm presents as a bulge beyond the right hilar border. Arch aneurysm produces enlargement of the aortic knob. Descending thoracic aneurysm is often easily seen as a deviation of the stripe of the descending aorta, which normally runs parallel to and just left of the vertebral column.

▶ Treatment
A. Risks of Aortic Surgery

It is certainly helpful to know numerically and statistically the cumulative and yearly rates of rupture, dissection, and death imposed by an aortic aneurysm of a specific size. On the other hand, the equation is incomplete without consideration of the risks inherent in elective, prophylactic surgical extirpation of the thoracic aorta. Certainly these are major operations, and the surgical risks most feared include death, stroke, and paraplegia. However, these operations have become safer, reflecting increased surgical experience, improved perfusion techniques, improved (nonporous) grafts, effective antifibrinolytic agents for perioperative use, improved methods of spinal cord preservation, and the advent of centers specializing in aortic care and surgery. A recently published report emphasizes the "safety of thoracic aortic surgery in the present era." Mortality rates and rates of other complications after aortic surgery are quite low, especially for operations performed electively on stable patients, in whom the safety of ascending aortic and aortic arch surgery is as high as 98%. Table 37–4 shows the pertinent rates of morbidity and mortality.

B. Indications & Contraindications

By considering the rates of natural rupture, dissection, and death from the thoracic aneurysm itself versus the risks of operation, the physician can make an informed recommendation about elective, preemptive surgery. Once patients and their families are provided the natural history and surgical risk data, they often have strong opinions of their own. Some

Table 37–3. Aortic Manifestation of Connective Tissue Disease

	Incidence in General Population	Rate of Dissection (per affected individual)	Number of Dissections Caused (per 10,000 population)
Marfan syndrome	0.01% (1 in 10,000)	40%	0.4 persons
Bicuspid aortic disease	1–2% (100–200 in 10,000)	5%	5–10 persons

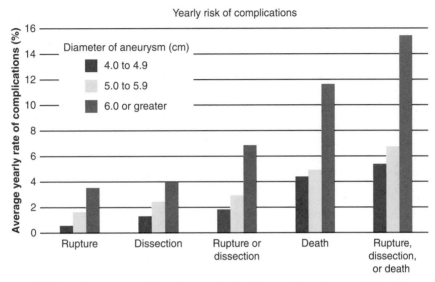

▲ **Figure 37–10.** Probabilities that rupture, dissection, or death will occur have been calculated for aortic aneurysms in the chest. The likelihood of these events jumps sharply for aneurysms that reach 6 cm or higher.

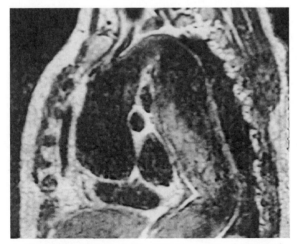

▲ **Figure 37–11.** Magnetic resonance scan of massively dilated aorta, which extends from the aortic valve to the iliac bifurcation. Note that the heart is compressed to a small shadow crushed between the elongated aorta and the diaphragm. This aneurysm was successfully resected in two stages.

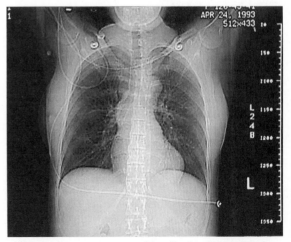

▲ **Figure 37–12.** An exemplary chest radiograph indicating that significant information about the aorta can be gleaned from this simple test. Note the bulge of the ascending aorta to the right of the upper mediastinal border. This young patient with Marfan disease suffered dissection at an ascending aortic dimension of 4.8 cm.

Table 37–4. Current Risks of Thoracic Aortic Surgery

	Mortality (%)	Stroke (%)	Paraplegia (%)
Ascending/arch	2.9	3.0	0.5
Descending/ thoracoabdominal	2.9	4.2	5.3

Data are for elective procedures, which is the category to whom surgical decision criteria are applied. Data from Achneck H, et al. Safety of thoracic aortic surgery in the present era. *Ann Thorac Surg.* 2007;84(4):1180–5.

patients are reluctant to undergo major surgery, with its significant attendant risks, for an asymptomatic problem. Most patients, however, seem to feel they will never be comfortable until the threatening aneurysm is resected.

One more very important general point needs to be considered. Once the aorta has dissected, the prognosis is thereafter adversely affected (Figure 37–13). Patients who required emergency surgery not only had a higher rate of early mortality, but their survival curve was dramatically poorer. Patients who elected for planned, nonemergent procedures showed a survival rate very similar to that of a normal population. The poor long-term outlook for patients

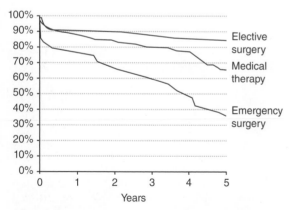

▲ **Figure 37–13.** Long-term survival rates based on treatment. Medically treated patients had, of course, smaller and less symptomatic aneurysms. Note particularly that patients having emergent surgery not only manifested a higher likelihood of perioperative mortality, but also had a poorer long-term outlook. On the other hand, patients who received elective surgery showed excellent survival rates, comparable to an age and sex-matched normal population. These data argue for elective, prophylactic extirpation of the aneurysmal aorta, before rupture or dissection can occur.

who required emergency surgery is due largely to the fact that, even after surgical replacement of portions of the aorta, the remainder of this vital organ will forever remain dissected. Because the aortic wall was deficient to start with, at half-thickness, after dissection, it is rendered even more vulnerable to subsequent enlargement and rupture.

C. Surgical Techniques

As discussed earlier, the type of operation for the ascending aorta is based on the pattern of aneurysmal pathology. For many patients, a supracoronary tube graft suffices (Figure 37–14A). For others, a composite graft, including both a valve and a graft, with obligate coronary artery reimplantation, is appropriate (Figure 37–14B). New valve-sparing aortic replacement procedures have been developed and are becoming increasingly popular (eg, David procedure).

The main debate regarding the procedure for ascending aortic operations and those on the aortic arch concerns the optimal means of protecting brain function during the time that anastomoses in the vicinity of the aortic arch are performed. Deep hypothermic circulatory arrest—a state of suspended animation, which is generally safe for 30–45 minutes or longer—is preferred by many surgeons, for its simplicity and effectiveness. In a study on 400 patients, the effectiveness of this remarkable technique as a sole means of brain preservation was confirmed. Retrograde cerebral perfusion—via the superior vena cava—has its advocates, although the actual amount of effective brain perfusion achieved by this means has been questioned. Direct perfusion of the head vessels—usually via a cannula in the innominate artery or cannulas in both the innominate and the left carotid artery—also has its supporters, despite its added complexity. Direct perfusion is gaining in popularity, and it does provide a margin of protection, especially for very complex arch reconstructions or for surgical teams relatively inexperienced with arch replacement. No technique has been demonstrated conclusively superior over the others.

For descending and thoracoabdominal operations, the technique of left atrial to femoral artery bypass has become extremely popular. This method takes strain off the heart by diverting blood away from the left ventricle. This approach mitigates the effect of high aortic cross-clamping on cardiac afterload. It also perfuses the lower body, especially the extremely vulnerable spinal cord. Despite decades of concerted attention, paraplegia from descending and thoracoabdominal aortic replacement continues to be a major clinical problem. The cause is multifactorial, with clamp time, air and particulate embolism, and disconnection of critical intercostal branches all playing a role. Besides the benefits of left atrial to femoral artery perfusion, most authorities feel that routine spinal fluid drainage and deliberate maintenance of a strong postoperative blood pressure (to encourage collateral blood flow) are also effective adjuncts against the complication of postoperative paraplegia.

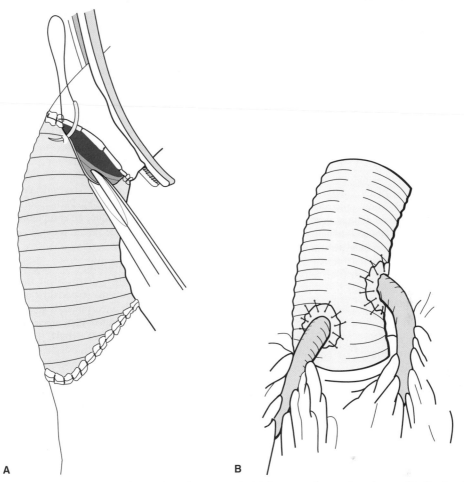

▲ **Figure 37–14. (A)** Supracoronary tube graft replacement and **(B)** composite graft replacement. (**A:** Reprinted, with permission, from Cooley DA, Wukasch DC. *Techniques in Vascular Surgery.* Philadelphia: WB Saunders; 1979.)

D. Specific Clinical Scenarios & Issues

1. Patient with pain, but aneurysm smaller than criteria—The answer to whether such an aorta should be replaced is a resounding yes. The dimensional criteria are specifically intended for asymptomatic patients. Any and all symptomatic aneurysms need to be resected because symptoms are a precursor to rupture. Aneurysm pain represents stretching or irritation of the aortic adventitia, the adjacent chest wall, the mediastinal pleura, or some other structure impinged on by the expanding aneurysm. Even an aorta smaller than the criterion can rupture or dissect. Such a patient is of extreme concern, and preemptive resection is needed. In one case, a patient complained of typical pain of an ascending aortic aneurysm. The aorta was 5.0 cm. Because the medical team thought this was too small for resection, they underestimated the symptoms at presentation. The aorta subsequently ruptured, and the

patient died within 48 hours. This point cannot be overemphasized: The size criteria are explicitly intended only for asymptomatic patients; *all symptomatic aneurysms need to be resected.*

2. Differentiating aneurysm pain from musculoskeletal pain—This very important point is not always easy to determine, even in the most experienced hands. The patient usually has a good sense of whether the pain is originating from muscles and joints. The clinician usually gets an additional understanding by asking the following questions:

a. Is the pain influenced by motion or position? (If so, it is probably musculoskeletal.)

b. Do you have a history of lumbosacral spine disease or chronic low back pain? (If so, the symptoms may not be aortic in origin.)

c. Do you feel the pain in the interscapular back? (An affirmative answer indicates an almost certain relationship to thoracic aortic aneurysm.)

Presume that the pain is aortic in origin if no other cause can be conclusively established. This is the only approach that can prevent rupture.

3. Appropriate interval for serial aortic imaging—

Patients with a thoracic aortic aneurysm should be monitored indefinitely. Stable, asymptomatic patients can undergo imaging about once every 2 years, remembering that the aneurysmal aorta grows at a relatively slow 1 mm/year. In case of new onset of symptoms, imaging should be done promptly, regardless of the interval from the prior scan. For new patients, for whom only one size data point is available, imaging should be done at short intervals until the behavior of aorta is understood. Imaging may be done every 3–6 months for new patients with moderately large aortas. Remember to compare the present scan with the patient's *first* scan, not with the last prior scan. That is the way to detect growth. Many patients have suffered because scans were only compared with the last prior scan, and major growth went undetected.

4. Choice of imaging modality for serial follow-up—

Three quality imaging techniques are currently available: echocardiography (ECHO), CT scan, and MRI. If echocardiography is chosen, it is important to remember that a standard transthoracic echocardiogram cannot see the distal ascending aorta, the aortic arch, or the descending aorta with conclusive accuracy because of intervening air-containing lung tissue. Supplement such studies with a periodic CT scan or MRI, which can visualize the entire aorta. The choice between CT and MRI may depend on ease of availability and radiologic expertise in a particular environment. Both modalities can image the entire aorta extremely well. Elevated creatinine or contrast allergy may contraindicate CT and instead favor MRI. The need to evaluate complex aortic lesions in multiple imaging planes would also favor MRI (although very recently, concerns have been raised about the risk to the kidneys of gadolinium contrast agents used for MRI scanning). Of course, indwelling metallic foreign objects, such as pacemakers or metal artifacts from previous surgery, may make CT the necessary choice instead of MRI. The advantages and limitations of echocardiography and CT are shown in Figure 37–15. Both echocardiography and CT are required for complete evaluation of the entire aorta.

5. Evaluation of family members—

The data on familial inheritance has become strong enough that the treating physician is obligated to recommend that family members be evaluated. Physicians of family members should be made aware that aneurysm disease has been diagnosed in the family. A CT scan is recommended for adult males and for females beyond childbearing age. For children and for females of childbearing age, echocardiography of the ascending aorta and abdominal aorta is recommended.

Investigators hope to identify humoral markers or genetic aberrations that can be used for familial screening of the aneurysm trait in the very near future. Routine genetic testing is controversial. We now offer and encourage screening of patients and family members by "whole exome sequencing," which is generally covered by most large insurers.

6. Activity restrictions—

Continuation of any and all aerobic activities, including running, swimming, and bicycling, is recommended. Serious weight lifters, at peaks of exertion, can elevate systolic arterial pressure to 300 mm Hg. This type of instantaneous hypertension is, of course, not prudent for aneurysm patients. Weight lifters should limit themselves to one-half their body weight. The evidence for effort-induced aortic dissection is mounting. Participation in contact sports or those that might produce an abrupt physical impact, such as tackle football, snow skiing, water skiing, and horseback riding, is proscribed.

7. Role of stent grafting—

A word of caution is appropriate concerning stent grafts. Stent therapy has become routine for many patients (especially those with abdominal or descending aortic aneurysms). It is certainly less invasive and more easily tolerated than open surgical techniques. Specialists, however, must avoid "irrational exuberance." Owing to the high need for subsequent conventional surgery after abdominal aneurysm stent placement, the recent large, multicenter Eurostar study questioned the very efficacy and advisability of stent grafting. Endoleak, stent dislodgement, and aneurysm expansion or rupture were disturbingly widespread in medium-term follow-up. It should be remembered that stents were designed to keep tissue from encroaching on the vessel lumen, not to keep the vessel from expanding. One noted authority believes that the aneurysmal aorta essentially "ignores" the stent graft, dilating regardless of the stent, at its own pace (personal communication, Dr. L. Svennson). Also remember that the natural history of the thoracic aorta is that aneurysms grow slowly, and that hard end points (rupture, dissection, and death) take years to be realized. For this reason, short-term stent studies are nearly meaningless. Long-term studies are needed. This newer modality should be approached with enthusiasm tempered by caution. Its advent should not at this point influence the decision about whether or not to intervene for a specific aneurysm; criteria (see earlier in chapter) should be met before any intervention, including stent therapy, is undertaken. Stent therapy appears especially well suited for patients with rupture of the descending aorta, in which setting a stent can be acutely life-saving.

Achneck HE, et al. Safety of thoracic aortic surgery in the present era. *Ann Thorac Surg.* 2007;84(4):1180–5. [PMID: 17888967]

Davies RR, et al. Novel measurement of relative aortic size predicts rupture of thoracic aortic aneurysms. *Ann Thorac Surg.* 2006;81(1):169–77. [PMID: 16368358]

Eleferiades JA, et al. Endovascular stenting for descending aneurysms: wave of the future or the emperor's new clothes? *J Thorac Cardiovasc Surg.* 2007;133(2):285–8. [PMID: 17258546]

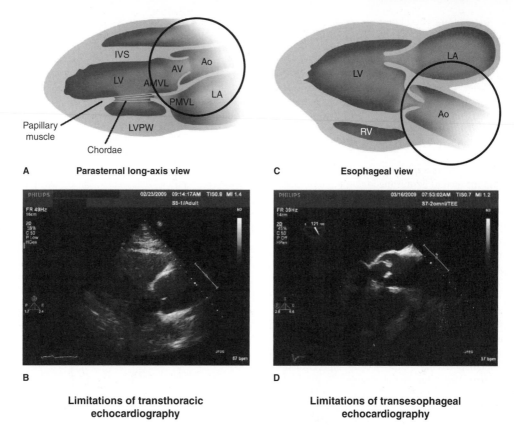

▲ **Figure 37–15. A and B:** Limited distance above the aortic valve (AV) for which the ascending aorta (Ao) can be seen on transthoracic echocardiography. Schematic **(A)** and actual echocardiographic **(B)** image. AMVL, anterior mitral valve leaflet; IVS, interventricular septum; LA, left atrium; LV, left ventricle; LVPW, left ventricular posterior wall. **C and D:** Limited distance above the aortic valve for which the ascending aorta can be seen on transesophageal echocardiography. The tracheal air column interferes with visualization of the upper ascending aorta. Schematic **(C)** and actual echocardiographic image **(D)**. RV, right ventricle. (**A and C:** Illustrations by Rob Flewell, used with permission. **B and D:** Elefteriades JA and Farkas EA. *J Am Coll Cardiol* 2010;55:841.)

Elefteriades JA, et al. Litigation in nontraumatic aortic diseases—a tempest in the malpractice maelstrom. *Cardiology.* 2008;109(4):263–72. [PMID: 17873491]

Elefteriades JA, et al. Thoracic aortic aneurysm: clinically pertinent controversies and uncertainties. *J Am Coll Cardiol.* 2010;55:841–57. [PMID: 20185035]

Danyi P, et al. Medical therapy of thoracic aortic aneurysms. *Trends Cardiovasc Med.* 2012;22:180–4. [PMID: 22906366]

Kroner BL, et al. The National Registry of Genetically Triggered Thoracic Aortic Aneurysms and Cardiovascular Conditions (GenTAC): results from phase I and scientific opportunities in phase II. *Am Heart J.* 2011;162(4):627–632.e1. [PMID: 21982653]

Kuzmik GA, et al. Natural history of thoracic aortic aneurysms. *J Vasc Surg.* 2012;56:565–71. [PMID: 22840907]

Pomianowski P, et al. Genetics and genomics of thoracic aortic disease. In: Chiesa R, et al., eds. *Aortic Surgery and Anesthesia "How to Do It."* Gessate, Italy: Arti Grafiche Colombo; 2012.

AORTIC DISSECTION

 ESSENTIALS OF DIAGNOSIS

► Usually middle-aged or elderly hypertensive men; occasionally, young patients with history of Marfan syndrome or other connective tissue disorder. Rarely, young women in late pregnancy or labor.

► Acute chest pain, frequently with hemodynamic instability.

► Possible appearance of shock but normal or elevated blood pressure.

► Various neurologic symptoms, such as Horner syndrome, paraplegia, and stroke.

► Absent or unequal peripheral pulses.
► Aortic regurgitation.
► Widened mediastinum on chest radiograph.
► Confirmatory aortic imaging study.

► General Considerations

A. Terminology

Aortic dissection refers to a splitting of the layers of the aortic wall (within the media) permitting longitudinal propagation of a blood-filled space within the aortic wall. Aortic dissection is thought to be the most common cause of death related to the human aorta (Figure 37–16).

Three related but distinct entities—acute aortic transection, rupture of aortic aneurysm, and aortic dissection—are commonly confused, both in substance and in terminology (Figure 37–17). **Acute aortic transection** is a traumatic phenomenon, with disruption of the wall of the aorta, without a propagating dissection. The aortic wall is intrinsically normal and resistant to the dissection process. **Rupture** of aortic aneurysm is self-explanatory; however, confusion in terminology may arise if an acute aortic transection or an acute aortic dissection happens to rupture—a common eventuality. **Acute aortic dissection** refers to the very specific process of separation of layers of the aortic wall discussed fully in this chapter. For dissection to occur, the aortic wall must nearly always be affected by structural disease of the media.

Recent years have brought recognition of two important variants of aortic dissection: intramural hematoma (IMH) and penetrating aortic ulcer (PAU) (Figure 37–18).

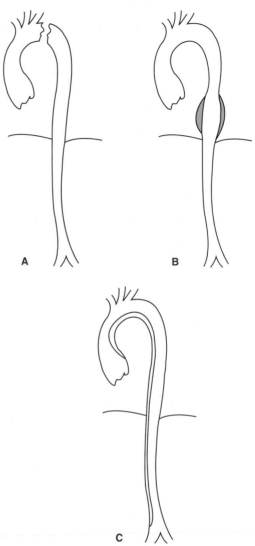

▲ **Figure 37–17.** Frequently confused terminology. See text for a description of the very different disorders of acute aortic transection **(A)**, ruptured aortic aneurysm **(B)**, and acute aortic dissection **(C)**.

IMH of the aorta differs from typical dissection in that there is no flap defining a true and a false lumen, and the hematoma (on axial imaging) is located circumferentially around the aortic lumen, rather than obliquely oriented across the aortic lumen. Whether the IMH arises from a small intimal tear (not detected radiographically) or from a rupture of a vasa vasorum within the aortic wall remains controversial. The clinical course is variable; the hematoma may persist, reabsorb (returning the aorta to a normal appearance), lead to aneurysm with the possibility of rupture, or

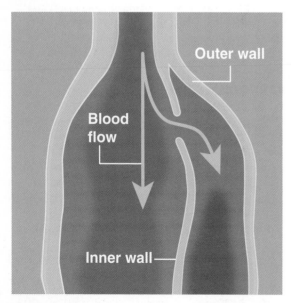

▲ **Figure 37–16.** Schematic depiction of aortic dissection.

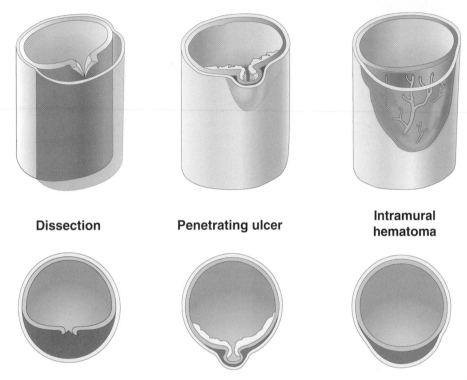

Dissection   **Penetrating ulcer**   **Intramural hematoma**

▲ **Figure 37–18.** Schematic of variant forms of aortic dissection: typical dissection, penetrating ulcer, and intramural hematoma. A true dissection has to have a flap.

convert to dissection. PAU involves a local penetration deep into the wall of the aorta, resembling a penetrating ulcer of the stomach. This lesion disrupts the internal elastic lamina and erodes into the media, which in some cases may mimic or initiate aortic dissection, pseudoaneurysm formation, IMH, or rupture. Extensive arteriosclerosis is a common accompaniment of PAU (see Figure 37–18).

It is important to recognize that IMH and PAU are diseases of advanced age. In addition, it is important point to mention that although branch vessel occlusion is part and parcel of typical aortic dissection, the variants of aortic dissection PAU and IMH never occlude branch vessels.

The general management of these lesions is still a matter of debate. Most authorities believe that descending aortic IMH and PAU can be managed medically, with "anti-impulse" therapy (see Treatment section). However, early (but not immediate) surgical intervention is preferred in suitable operative candidates to preempt rupture due to a high incidence of death from rupture. Some of the discrepancy in recommendations also has to do with regional differences: In Japan, IMH behaves in a more benign fashion than in the Western world, perhaps reflecting fundamental genetic differences in the aortic wall or differences in body size and aortic dimension. Stent therapies are often applied for IMH or PAU.

For ascending variant dissections IMH and PAU, most authorities agree on aggressive immediate surgical intervention, although one recent paper from Japan challenges the need for routine surgery, even in this anatomic location.

B. Anatomic Classification

Aortic dissections may be ascending (type A) or descending (type B). The two patterns are determined by the location of the inciting intimal tear. Tears occur in two very specific locations: (1) in the ascending aorta, 2–3 cm above the coronary arteries, and (2) in the descending aorta, 1–2 cm beyond the left subclavian artery. The first type of tear produces ascending dissection and the second, descending dissection. Please note that ascending dissections usually go around the aortic arch to involve the descending and abdominal portions of the aorta (Figure 37–19).

▶ Clinical Findings
A. Symptoms & Signs

Aortic dissection produces intense, severe pain, often described as tearing or shearing in quality. This pain is sudden in onset (a differentiating feature from the pain of

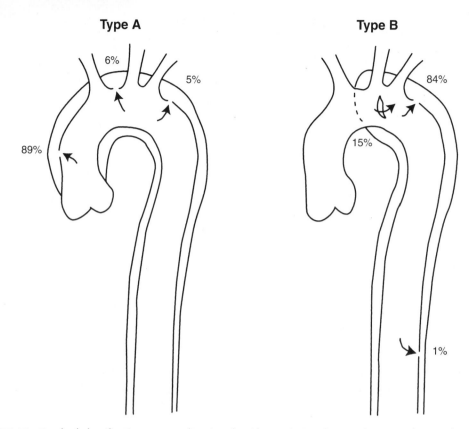

Type A

6%

5%

89%

Type B

84%

15%

1%

▲ **Figure 37–19.** Stanford classification system. (Reprinted, with permission, from Daily PO, et al. *Ann Thorac Surg.* 1970;10:244.)

myocardial infarction) and very severe in intensity. Most patients describe this as the most intense pain of their lives, more intense even than childbirth or kidney stone. The pain of ascending dissection is felt in the anterior chest, substernally, and that of a descending dissection is felt posteriorly, between the scapulae. The "tearing," "shearing," "knife-like" quality of the pain is quite consistent with the pathophysiology. The pain can migrate downward, into the flank or pelvis, as the dissection process propagates distally. Impending aortic rupture should be considered when pain subsides and later recurs. On occasion, painless dissection does occur, perhaps as often as in 15% of patients; this is usually picked up later, on a routine imaging study done for another reason.

B. Diagnostic Studies

1. Chest radiography—Chest radiography is a useful screening test. Many, if not most, aortic dissections occur in the setting of a chronic aortic aneurysm. To the astute observer, chronic thoracic aneurysms can be visualized on a chest radiograph. The enlarged ascending aorta will protrude to the right of the upper mediastinal border, an arch aneurysm will show as an exaggerated aortic knob, and a descending aortic

aneurysm will be visible as a left-deviated stripe of the descending aorta. In case of aortic dissection, chest radiography will usually provide additional clues: most commonly, widening of the mediastinal shadow, pleural effusion, or inward displacement of aortic medial calcification.

2. Three-dimensional imaging methods—Multiple types of three-dimensional imaging modalities are pertinent in aneurysm disease and aortic dissection, and all have excellent sensitivity and specificity: transesophageal echocardiography (TEE), CT scanning, and MRI. Many patients undergo a TEE and either a CT or an MRI. The CT or MRI shows the three-dimensional structure of the entire aorta. The TEE, while partially blinded to the aortic arch and abdominal aorta, provides information about pericardial effusion and tamponade, valve function, and left ventricular function. TEE images both ascending and descending aortas well.

The primary diagnostic criterion for aortic dissection by CT or MRI is demonstration of two contrast-filled lumens separated by an intimal flap. Sensitivity and specificity of CT and MRI for diagnosis of aortic dissection are approaching 100%. TEE does not lag far behind in accuracy. Contrast aortography, once the gold standard, has fallen by the wayside for diagnosis of aortic dissection, being more invasive and not offering nearly the amount of three-dimensional anatomic information afforded by CT, MRI, and TEE.

▶ Differential Diagnosis

The imaging studies discussed earlier provide specific information that rules in or out the presence of aneurysm or dissection. The main diagnostic issue involves (1) maintaining a high index of suspicion for aneurysm disease and (2) being aware of the protean presentations of aneurysm disease. In particular, aortic dissection has been called "the great masquerader" because it can produce symptoms related to virtually any organ. A high index of suspicion is required to establish the diagnosis promptly, since the presentations of aortic dissection are so myriad and mimic a wide array of other diseases. Specifically, all patients admitted with chest pain without obvious cause should have their thoracic aorta imaged. Patients with a ruptured or dissected thoracic aorta often "masquerade" as heart attacks. It is especially important to rule out aortic dissection in patients about to be treated for myocardial infarction, as administration of thrombolytic drugs in patients with acute aortic dissection is associated with a high mortality rate.

Among conditions for which aortic dissection can be confused are myocardial infarction, musculoskeletal chest pain, pericarditis, pleuritis, pneumothorax, pulmonary embolism, cholecystitis, ureteral colic, appendicitis, mesenteric ischemia, pyelonephritis, stroke, transient ischemic attack, and primary limb ischemia. Especially troublesome to clinicians in emergency departments are patients with abdominal symptoms and signs without apparent abdominal cause; aortic dissection must be considered in such patients.

Given the extensive differential diagnosis, aggressive, objective diagnostic testing is necessary when the possibility of aortic dissection is considered. The diagnosis is most strongly suggested when migratory chest and back pain of less than 24 hours in duration arises in a patient with a history of hypertension. The following recommendations are made for the physicians who are the first to evaluate such patients: (1) Keep aortic dissection (and ruptured thoracic or abdominal aneurysm) in the differential diagnosis. (2) Image freely and liberally to rule out aortic pathology. A CT scan can exclude all three major chest diagnoses likely to result in death: coronary artery disease, pulmonary embolism, and aortic aneurysm or dissection. The modern 64-slice scanners are ideal for this purpose. (3) Remember the D-dimer test. A negative D-dimer, which is most commonly applied to rule out pulmonary embolism, also rules out aortic dissection. The clot that forms in the false lumen of an aortic dissection liberates D-dimer quite strikingly. This simple blood test is nearly 100% sensitive in picking up aortic dissection. (4) Remember to look at the aorta, even if the CT scan is ordered for other, especially abdominal, examination.

Attention to these recommendations will also serve to discourage litigation for failure to diagnose aortic dissection.

▶ Treatment

A. Pharmacotherapy

Most patients will require intensive medical therapy for acute aortic dissection, either as sole treatment or as a stabilizing measure until appropriate surgical therapy is undertaken.

It has been recognized that aortic dissection propagates more vigorously when either blood pressure or force of cardiac contraction are excessive. Accordingly, blood pressure needs to be controlled in patients with acute aortic dissection or other acute aortic syndromes, including aortic rupture or impending rupture. Nitroglycerin and nitroprusside are usually used for this purpose, because of their effectiveness, their rapid onset of action, and their quick cessation of action upon discontinuation. Blood pressure should be reduced as low as possible without producing neurologic dysfunction or oliguria. Usually, the severity of general occlusive vascular disease determines how low the blood pressure can safely be taken. The blood pressure may be lowered to 90–100 mm Hg initially, until the patient's response can be evaluated. For older patients with extensive end-organ vascular disease, lowering the blood pressure pharmacologically to 120–130 mm Hg may need to be satisfactory.

However, to lower blood pressure by afterload reduction alone would actually increase the sheer stress on the aortic wall. It is crucial to decrease the force of cardiac contraction (Figure 37–20). The morphology of the arterial pulse

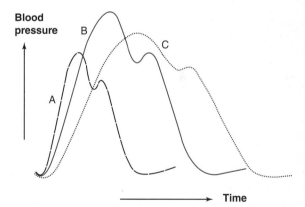

▲ **Figure 37–20.** Diagram of aortic pressure curves under various conditions. The continuous line **(B)** represents the baseline state. Administration of a vasodilator agent such as nitroprusside is represented by the dashed curve **(A)**. There is significant decrease in pressure levels and acceleration in heart rate, but this is accompanied by a steepest slope of the ascending portion of the curve (increased dp/dt_{max}). β-Blockade administration is represented by the dotted line **(C)**. Although the degree of pressure lowering is usually smaller, the drug negative inotropic and chronotropic effects result in decreased impulse and dp/dt_{max}.

wave must be blunted by decreasing the force of cardiac contraction. The *dp/dt*, reflected in the upslope of the initial portion of the aortic pulse wave, must be decreased, usually by administering a short-acting β-blocker, such as esmolol. Another approach is administration of the α- and β-adrenergic antagonist labetalol by intravenous infusion. When β-blocking drugs are contraindicated, calcium channel blockers are a reasonable substitute.

Together, the afterload reduction and the β-blockade are referred to as "anti-impulse" therapy for acute aortic dissection. Regardless of whether the dissection is ascending or descending, or whether or not the patient will be taken emergently to the operating room, such therapy must be instituted—to discourage rupture or extension of the dissection.

Anti-impulse therapy is the appropriate initial response once the diagnosis of any type of acute aortic dissection or related process is made. Often, such therapy is undertaken while imaging studies are being performed to confirm the diagnosis of aortic dissection and define the anatomic type, location, and extent of the process. Definitive therapeutic decisions and treatments will follow.

B. Surgical Treatment

For acute aortic dissection, the following guidelines regarding definitive therapy apply.

Ascending aortic aneurysms require urgent surgery because death from intrapericardial rupture, aortic regurgitation, or myocardial infarction from coronary artery involvement usually occurs in patients who do not undergo surgery. The dissection layers are reapproximated as a "sandwich" between layers of Teflon felt (Figure 37–21). Overall survival at experienced centers is about 85% for patients with acute type A aortic dissection. The exact surgical procedure performed, vis-à-vis the proximal aortic root and the coronary arteries, varies depending on the circumstances. For patients in whom dissection occurs in the setting of Marfan disease or other cause of annuloaortic ectasia (proximal root enlargement), the aortic valve, aortic root, and ascending aorta are replaced with a prefabricated "composite graft" including both a valve and a graft (see Figure 37–14B).

Descending dissections, in the absence of specific vascular complications, do well with medical management (short- and long-term "anti-impulse" therapy with β-blockers and afterload-reducing medication). If a specific complication occurs, this is addressed directly by surgery ("complication-specific" approach to descending aortic dissection). Ninety-one percent of patients survived the initial hospitalization (type B aortic dissection is "milder" than type A dissection), and about 66% had a completely uncomplicated course while receiving anti-impulse medical therapy alone. The majority of complications were related to vascular malperfusion of specific organs. Stent therapy for acute or chronic type B dissection is controversial.

The subacute and chronic stages of aortic dissection are managed differently. Once the patient with type A dissection has been brought safely through surgery, or the type B patient has been stabilized with anti-impulse therapy, the patient is observed closely for the first month, with repeat aortic imaging. After that point, it is uncommon for the dissection to extend, cause symptoms, or rupture in the short-term to mid-term. The patients are then monitored the same as those with chronic aneurysm. Over years, enlargement of the dissected aorta will develop in some patients and require resection. The same dimensional criteria for surgical intervention can be applied as for nondissected aneurysms. It is usually the most proximal portion of the descending aorta, just beyond the subclavian artery, that dilates first and requires surgical replacement.

▶ Prognosis

Aortic dissection is often fatal without early diagnosis and aggressive treatment. The presenting symptoms and signs are so myriad and nonspecific (see earlier in chapter) that dissection may be overlooked initially in up to 40% of cases; in fact, the diagnosis is not made until postmortem examination in a disturbingly large fraction of patients. This can be a frequent cause of litigation, and guidelines have recently been outlined so litigation can be avoided. Few other conditions demand such prompt diagnosis and treatment, since the mortality rate of untreated dissection approaches 1–2% per hour during the first 48 hours, 89% at 14 days, and 90% at 3 months.

Aortic dissection can result in death in four ways: (1) intrapericardial rupture (of an ascending dissection), (2) acute aortic regurgitation (from an ascending aortic dissection), (3) free rupture into the pleural space (of a descending dissection), and (4) occlusion of any branch of the aorta (with consequent organ ischemia).

Branch vessel occlusion comes about via impingement on the true lumen of any branch vessel (coronaries to iliacs) by the distended false lumen (Figure 37–22). The acute aortic regurgitation of an ascending dissection may be very poorly tolerated, compared with chronic aortic regurgitation, because the sudden nature allows no time for cardiac adaptation. Cardiogenic shock may result.

Several general advances promise to mitigate the scourge of aortic diseases on society: Aortic aneurysms are diagnosed more frequently (incidentally) due to widespread application of imaging techniques for other reasons (echocardiography, CT, MRI). Aortic aneurysms are diagnosed more frequently (deliberately) due to increasing recognition that these are inherited diseases, and family members are screened. Advances in genetics are increasingly facilitating the recognition of specific mutations underlying aortic diseases in specific patients and their families. Personalized therapy will soon be possible. Advances in genetics hold promise for effective screening tests for the general population. Surgical therapies have become extremely safe.

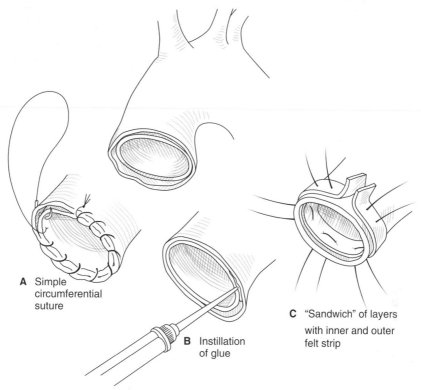

▲ **Figure 37–21.** Alternate methods of dealing with the dissection prior to anastomosis.

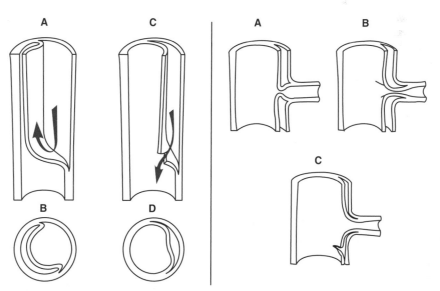

▲ **Figure 37–22.** Depiction of means by which the dissected lumen can compromise the true lumen, seen in various planes. The figures on the left look at the aorta itself. Note the relief of impingement when the flap fenestrates (images left, C and D, and right, C).

Appropriate intervention criteria have been developed that permit evidence-based preemptive surgical intervention to prevent rupture and dissection. Near-normal prognosis is maintained, provided that surgery is carried out before onset of aortic dissection. Public awareness of aneurysm disease has increased.

Elefteriades JA. What operation for acute Type A dissection? *J Thorac Cardiovasc Surg.* 2002;123(2):201–3. [PMID: 11828276]

Hatzaras IS, et al. Role of exertion or emotion as inciting events for acute aortic dissection. *Am J Cardiol.* 2007;100(9):1470–2. [PMID: 17950810]

Hatzaras I, et al. Weight lifting and aortic dissection: more evidence for a connection. *Cardiology.* 2007;107(2):103–6. [PMID: 12821554]

Jonker FH, et al. Open surgery versus endovascular repair of ruptured thoracic aortic aneurysms. *J Vasc Surg.* 2011 May; 53:1210–6. [PMID: 21296537]

Nienaber CA, et al. Strategies for subacute/chronic type B aortic dissection: the Investigation of Stent Grafts in Patients with Type B Aortic Dissection (INSTEAD) trial 1-year outcome. *J Thorac Cardiovasc Surg.* 2010;140(6 Suppl):S101–8. [PMID: 21092774]

Tittle SL, et al. Midterm follow-up penetrating ulcer and intramural hematoma of the aorta. *J Thorac Cardiovasc Surg.* 2002; 123(6):1051–9. [PMID: 12063450]

Index

Note: Page numbers followed by *t* indicate tables; those followed by *f* indicate figures.